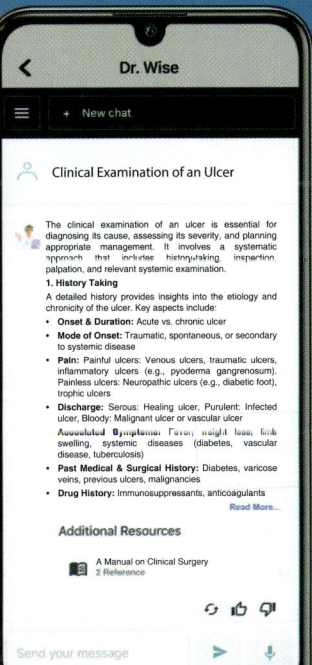

A Manual on
Clinical Surgery

With New Diagnostic Algorithms, Special Investigations and Differential Diagnosis

EIGHTEENTH EDITION

Somen Das
MBBS (Cal.) FRCS (Eng. and Edin.)
Senior Consultant Surgeon

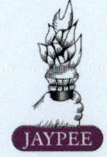

JAYPEE BROTHERS MEDICAL PUBLISHERS
The Health Sciences Publisher
New Delhi | London

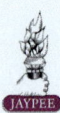
Jaypee Brothers Medical Publishers (P) Ltd.

Headquarters
Jaypee Brothers Medical Publishers (P) Ltd.
EMCA House
23/23-B, Ansari Road, Daryaganj
New Delhi - 110 002, India
Landline: +91-11-23272143, +91-11-23272703
+91-11-23282021, +91-11-23245672
Email: jaypee@jaypeebrothers.com

Corporate Office
Jaypee Brothers Medical Publishers (P) Ltd.
4838/24, Ansari Road, Daryaganj
New Delhi 110 002, India
Phone: +91-11-43574357
Fax: +91-11-43574314
Email: jaypee@jaypeebrothers.com

Overseas Office
J.P. Medical Ltd.
83 Victoria Street, London
SW1H 0HW (UK)
Phone: +44 20 3170 8910
Fax: +44 (0)20 3008 6180
Email: info@jpmedpub.com

Website: www.jaypeebrothers.com
Website: www.jaypeedigital.com

© 2025, Jaypee Brothers Medical Publishers

The views and opinions expressed in this book are solely those of the original contributor(s)/author(s) and do not necessarily represent those of editor(s) and publisher of the book.

All rights reserved. No part of this publication may be reproduced, stored or transmitted in any form or by any means, electronic, mechanical, photocopying, recording or otherwise, without the prior permission in writing of the publishers.

All brand names and product names used in this book are trade names, service marks, trademarks or registered trademarks of their respective owners. The publisher is not associated with any product or vendor mentioned in this book.

Medical knowledge and practice change constantly. This book is designed to provide accurate, authoritative information about the subject matter in question. However, readers are advised to check the most current information available on procedures included and check information from the manufacturer of each product to be administered, to verify the recommended dose, formula, method and duration of administration, adverse effects and contraindications. It is the responsibility of the practitioner to take all appropriate safety precautions. Neither the publisher nor the author(s)/editor(s) assume any liability for any injury and/or damage to persons or property arising from or related to use of material in this book.

This book is sold on the understanding that the publisher is not engaged in providing professional medical services. If such advice or services are required, the services of a competent medical professional should be sought.

Every effort has been made where necessary to contact holders of copyright to obtain permission to reproduce copyright material. If any have been inadvertently overlooked, the publisher will be pleased to make the necessary arrangements at the first opportunity.

Inquiries for bulk sales may be solicited at: jaypee@jaypeebrothers.com

A Manual on Clinical Surgery

First Edition : March, 1986
Second Edition : March, 1987
Third Edition : May, 1988
Fourth Edition : February, 1996
Fifth Edition : March, 2000
Sixth Edition : June, 2004
Seventh Edition : August, 2008
Eighth Edition : April, 2010
Ninth Edition : August, 2011
Reprint : December, 2011, June, 2011
Tenth Edition : January, 2013
Reprint : June, 2013, March, 2014, Novmber, 2014

Eleventh Edition : August, 2015
Reprint : May, 2016
Twelfth Edition : November, 2016
Reprint : June, 2017
Thirteenth Edition : February, 2018
Reprint : August, 2018
Fourteenth Edition : February, 2019
Reprint : August, 2019, December, 2019
Fifteenth Edition : May 2021
Reprint : October, 2021
Sixteenth Edition : August, 2022
Reprint : December, 2022

Seventeenth Edition 2024
Eighteenth Edition **2025**

ISBN: 978-93-6616-236-2

Printed in India

DEDICATED

To the Memory of My Father
Late Dr K Das FRCS (Eng. and Edin.)
and
To the Memory of My Mother

PREFACE TO THE EIGHTEENTH EDITION

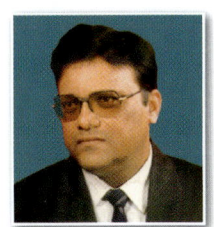

The enduring popularity of this book has inspired me to release this new edition. In the planning process, we made a firm commitment to ensure a comprehensive and up-to-date text. The field of surgery has evolved significantly in recent times, and every effort has been exerted to keep abreast of advancements in Clinical Surgery. While we describe the special investigation techniques in this edition, the underlying principle remains that effective surgical practice relies primarily on the skill and knowledge of the surgeon, with special investigations playing a secondary role.

We as surgeons emphasize the importance of clinical observations and the need to elicit accurate physical signs for a precise diagnosis. Despite the inclusion of newer, noninvasive methods, we caution against over-reliance on these techniques, as they may lead to delays and unnecessary costs. Therefore, we advocate a judicious use of investigations, with a focus on clinical diagnosis whenever feasible. Each chapter has undergone thorough revision and updating with incorporation of algorithms to approach to diagnosis in important chapters.

Launching of subsequent editions of a warmly received text is in some respects more of a challenge and I am fully aware of it. To what extent this goal has been met, only readers and time will tell. But at least I can assure that an ardent attempt was made.

This book was originally brought out to guide the new entrants to the surgical ward to answer the vexed question 'How to examine this case and come to a diagnosis?'. This original theme of the book has been maintained and adequate emphasis has been laid not only on 'what to do' but also on 'how to do' the various examinations to arrive at the provisional clinical diagnosis. More methods of examinations have been included in this edition with more illustrations to make the subject more understandable.

This manual has enjoyed great popularity in the Indian subcontinent and beyond. I express gratitude to the teachers who recommended this book to their students and believed it to be helpful in learning 'Clinical Surgery.' Thanks are also due to colleagues and patients who willingly participated in the photographic process. I owe a deep debt of gratitude to the multitude of students from this country and abroad who have shared their difficulties in understanding this subject. Their input has greatly aided in presenting this treatise in a more comprehensible manner, and I hope this edition proves even more helpful to them in learning 'Clinical Surgery.'

I would like to thank **Dr Shikhar Tripathi** for having assisted me with the editing and revision of this edition of the book. His contributions have been earnest and well rounded. He has proven to be an asset to the legacy that this book has built over the years.

13, Old Mayors' Court,
Kolkata — 700 005
March 2025

S Das

PREFACE TO THE FIRST EDITION

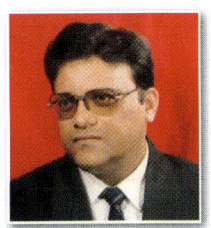

This manual is an attempt to provide an answer to the vexed question 'How shall I examine this case and come to a diagnosis?'. This is a question which confronts each and every clinician. Without doubt methods of history-taking and examination are different in various types of surgical diseases, e.g. a swelling in the neck, pain in a particular region of the abdomen, an ulcer in the leg, etc. Yet in the first chapter I have tried to formulate a general scheme of case-taking, so that the students can chalk out a common system of history-taking and physical examinations in all surgical cases. I think, this will be of great help to the students to build up a routine, which should be followed all throughout their careers. In subsequent chapters emphasis has been laid on the particular points of history-taking and special methods of physical examinations which are relevant to those diseases.

Each chapter begins with history-taking—the interrogations to be made to the patient, followed by the methods of physical examinations and special investigations which will be necessary for that particular case. While describing the methods of examinations I have not only mentioned 'what to do' but also have indicated 'how to do' aided by suitable illustrations. Emphasis has been laid on special investigations. The introduction of ever increasing sophisticated investigations over and above the basic techniques of history-taking and physical examination has helped the clinician to diagnose the cases more accurately. Ultimate aim of such a book is to teach how to arrive at a correct diagnosis and scope of special investigations in this regard cannot be underestimated. A number of illustrations have been used in this section to help the students in understanding particular investigations.

A reasoned explanation based on Anatomy, Physiology and Pathology has been included whenever necessary to explain most of the symptoms and signs. Diagnostic and prognostic significances have been discussed along with history-taking, various physical examinations and special investigations.

A list of differential diagnosis has been incorporated at the end of each chapter. This I think is very imporant and very helpful to the students. This I hope will make this book a complete one in its own field. Yet I have always tried to make this book handy. For this I have taken the advantage of photosetting which has accommodated much more matter in a single page. This book is in fact double the volume of its predecessor yet it looks so slim and handy. Coloured illustrations have been introduced to demonstrate in more details and more distinctly the figures of a few surgical conditions. I received request for this from various corners in the last few years.

I am grateful to my colleagues and many patients who voluntarily submitted themselves to the trouble of being photographed. I owe a deep debt of gratitude to the great mass of students from this country and abroad who have written to me and made me feel their difficulties in understanding this subject. If this book helps them in learning the ways of approach to Clinical Surgery, it will achieve its purpose.

13, Old Mayors' Court,
Kolkata — 700 005
March, 1986

S Das

CONTENTS

Chapter 1: General Scheme of Case Taking — 1
Chapter 2: A Few Special Symptoms and Signs — 14
Chapter 3: Examination of a Lump or a Swelling — 26
Chapter 4: Examination of an Ulcer — 68
Chapter 5: Examination of a Sinus or a Fistula — 85
Chapter 6: Examination of Peripheral Vascular Disease and Gangrene — 92
Chapter 7: Examination of Varicose Veins — 114
Chapter 8: Examination of the Lymphatic System — 126
Chapter 9: Examination of Peripheral Nerve Lesions — 142
Chapter 10: Diseases of Muscles, Tendons and Fasciae — 164
Chapter 11: Examination of Diseases of Bone — 171
Chapter 12: Examination of Bone and Joint Injuries — 195
Chapter 13: Examination of Injuries about Individual Joints — 207
Chapter 14: Examination of Pathological Joints — 246
Chapter 15: Examination of Individual Joint Pathologies — 259
Chapter 16: Examination of Head Injuries — 299
Chapter 17: Investigation of Intracranial Space-occupying Lesions — 314
Chapter 18: Examination of Spinal Injuries — 327
Chapter 19: Examination of Spinal Abnormalities — 335
Chapter 20: Examination of the Hand — 360
Chapter 21: Examination of the Foot — 374
Chapter 22: Examination of the Head and Face — 383
Chapter 23: Examination of the Jaws and Temporomandibular Joint — 390
Chapter 24: Examination of the Palate, Cheek, Tongue and Floor of the Mouth — 400
Chapter 25: Examination of the Salivary Glands — 415
Chapter 26: Examination of the Neck (Excluding the Thyroid Gland) — 427
Chapter 27: Examination of the Thyroid Gland — 438
Chapter 28: Examination of Injuries of the Chest — 462
Chapter 29: Examination of Diseases of the Chest — 469
Chapter 30: Examination of the Breast — 479

Chapter 31: Examination of a Case of Dysphagia — 504
Chapter 32: Examination of Abdominal Injuries — 516
Chapter 33: Examination of an Acute Abdomen — 527
Chapter 34: Examination of Chronic Abdominal Conditions — 559
Chapter 35: Examination of an Abdominal Lump — 596
Chapter 36: Examination of a Rectal Case — 617
Chapter 37: Examination of a Urinary Case — 635
Chapter 38: Examination of a Case of Hernia — 673
Chapter 39: Examination of a Swelling in the Inguinoscrotal Region or Groin — 692
Chapter 40: Examination of Male External Genitalia — 701
Index — 727

Online Examination Videos

1.	Examination of pain
2.	Examination of a swelling
3.	Examination of an ulcer
4.	Examination of a sinus or a fistula
5.	Examination of edema
6.	Examination of varicose veins
7.	Examination of peripheral nerve lesions
8.	Examination of muscles and tendons
9.	Examination of the shoulder joint
10.	Examination of the knee joint
11.	Examination of the wrist joint
12.	Examination of the elbow joint
13.	Examination of the hip joint
14.	Examination of the ankle and foot
15.	Examination of the spine
16.	Examination of head injuries
17.	Examination of the face

18.	Examination of the oral cavity
19.	Examination of the jaws and temporomandibular joint
20.	Examination of the salivary glands
21.	Examination of the neck
22.	Examination of the thyroid gland
23.	Examination of lymph nodes
24.	Examination of the chest
25.	Examination of the breast
26.	Examination of the abdomen
27.	Examination of the scrotum
28.	Examination of a ventral hernia
29.	Examination of an inguinal hernia
30.	Examination of the anorectal region
31.	Examination in a case of appendicitis
32.	Examination in a case of pancreatitis
33.	Examination in a case of cholelithiasis
34.	Examination in a case of peripheral vascular disease
35.	Examination in a case of acute abdomen
36.	Examination in a case of pneumothorax
37.	Examination in a case of ascites
38.	Examination in a case of thyroglossal cyst
39.	Examination in a case of nephrolithiasis
40.	Examination in a case of chest discomfort

Online Audio Case Files

1.	Right iliac fossa pain
2.	Right iliac fossa lump
3.	Right hypochondriac pain
4.	Epigastric pain

5.	Left hypochondriac pain
6.	Obstructive jaundice
7.	A case of painless hematuria
8.	A case of painless progressive jaundice
9.	Acute urinary retention
10.	Dysphagia
11.	A neck swelling
12.	A thyroid swelling
13.	A case of cervical lymphadenopathy
14.	A midline neck swelling
15.	A case of scrotal swelling
16.	Inguinal swelling
17.	A case of breast lump
18.	A case of nipple discharge
19.	A case of upper gi bleed
20.	A case of lowe gi bleed
21.	A case of acute abdomen
22.	A case of chronic abdominal pain
23.	A case of a nonhealing ulcer
24.	A case of a nonhealing wound
25.	A case of sudden-onset unilateral leg swelling
26.	A case of sudden-onset scrotal pain
27.	A case of back pain
28.	A case of chronic hip pain
29.	A case of shoulder pain
30.	A case of knee pain in a young athlete
31.	A case of hand deformity
32.	A case of foot ulcer
33.	A case of unilateral facial swelling
34.	A case of blunt abdominal trauma
35.	A case of chest trauma

36.	A case of burn injury
37.	A case of atraumatic limb swelling
38.	A case of postoperative fever
39.	A case of sudden onset chest pain
40.	A case of acute limb ischemia

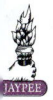
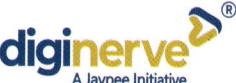

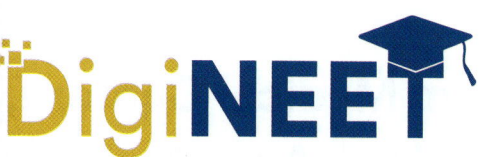

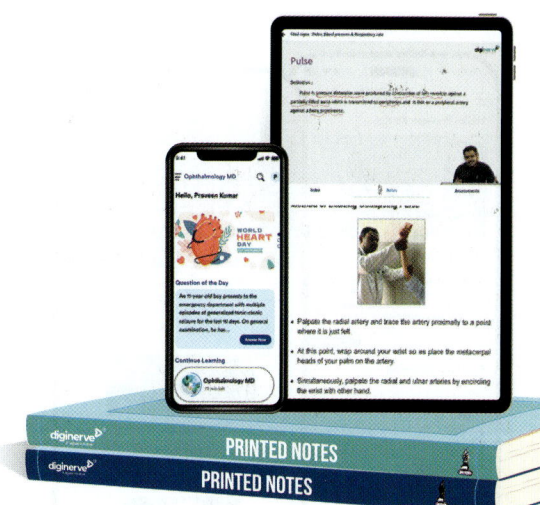

Simplify your undergraduate studies and NEET PG preparation with this comprehensive program covering all 19 subjects. Crafted by India's top faculty, it includes video lectures, printed notes, OSCEs, a QBank, test series, and the innovative Dr. Wise AI Chatbot.

Course Features

1400+ hrs Video Lectures

1500+ Topics in Notes

15000+ Questions in QBank

1800+ GEMS

450+ OSCEs

Test Series

Dr. Wise AI Chatbot

Drug Chart

Regular Webinars by Esteemed Faculty

Access Anytime, Anywhere

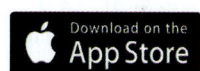
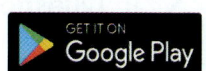

📞 +91-8800-418-418   ✉ marketing@diginerve.com

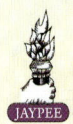
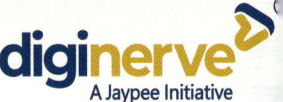

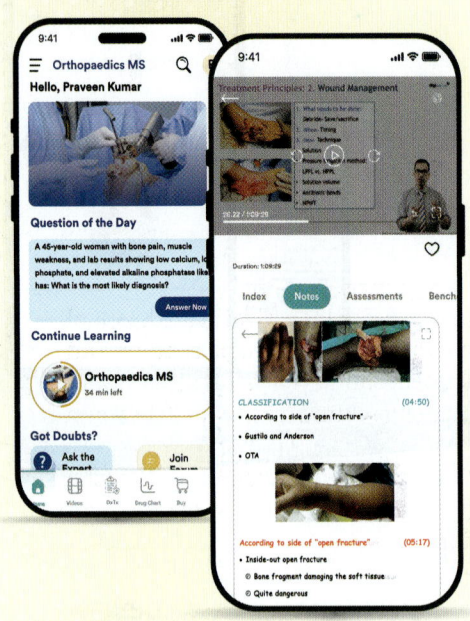

Premium Medical Content, Anytime, Anywhere

Trusted by 150K+ Users

20+ Courses   **3600+** Hrs of Video Content   **790+** Mentors

A host of features for UnderGrads, PostGrads and Professionals

Available on

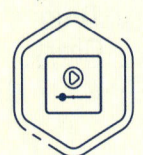 **Video Lectures**
 **Notes**
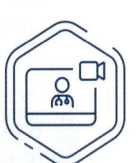 **OSCEs**

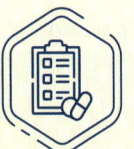 **Drug Chart**
 **Question Bank**
 **Dr. Wise AI Chatbot**

 +91-8800-418-418   marketing@diginerve.com

General Scheme of Case Taking

CHAPTER 1

In this chapter it will be narrated in brief, how to follow a patient from his arrival at the hospital or clinic up to his normal condition, i.e., after he has come round. It is a general scheme and applied to all patients whoever come to the surgeon. The student should learn this scheme and make it a reflex, so that he can apply this scheme to all his patients. Ultimately, this will become a habit in his professional career.

This general scheme includes—(1) History taking; (2) Physical examination; (3) Special investigation; (4) Clinical diagnosis; (5) Treatment—both medical and surgical; (6) Progress during postoperative period; (7) Follow-up; (8) Termination.

Case history taking

Step	Relevance in surgery	Clinical scenario (Appendicitis example)
History taking	Gather key details on symptoms, medical history, and risk factors.	A 25-year-old male presents with right lower abdominal pain, fever, and nausea. History reveals pain migrating from the umbilicus to the right iliac fossa.
Physical examination	Identify clinical signs supporting the suspected diagnosis.	Physical exam reveals tenderness at McBurney's point with rebound tenderness and guarding.
Special investigations	Confirm diagnosis and rule out differentials.	Blood tests show elevated WBCs; ultrasound confirms an inflamed appendix.
Clinical diagnosis	Correlate history, examination, and investigations to reach a final diagnosis.	Acute appendicitis is diagnosed, requiring urgent surgical intervention.
Treatment (Medical and surgical)	Decide on medical or surgical management based on diagnosis.	Laparoscopic appendectomy is performed under general anesthesia.
Postoperative progress	Monitor recovery, detect complications, and ensure healing.	Patient monitored for fever, wound infection, and bowel function recovery.
Follow-up	Assess long-term outcomes and detect recurrence early.	Postoperative review in 2 weeks confirms complete recovery with no complications.
Termination	Determine final outcome: recovery, chronic illness, or mortality.	Patient returns to normal activity; no recurrence after 6 months, case closed.

In the clinic, it is a good practice to start examining the patient when he walks into the room rather than to meet him undressed on a coach in a cubicle. It is helpful if the person, who accompanied the patient, remains by the side of the patient in the early part of the history-taking. He can provide valuable information about the type of injury the patient might have sustained, some details of the complaints or about changes in health or behavior of the patient in the recent past.

HISTORY-TAKING

1. **Particulars of the patient:** Before interrogating about the complaints of the patient, it is a good practice to know the patient first. That means the following headings should be noted in the history sheet:

Name: It is very important to know the patient by name. The patients like to be asked by name, as for example, 'Mr. Sirkar, how long are you having this problem?' This will not only help to elicit the history properly, but also it will be of psychological benefit to the patient just before the operation and in postoperative period. The patient is assured that you know him by name.

Age: Congenital anomalies mostly present since birth, e.g., cystic hygroma, cleft lip, cleft palate, sacrococcygeal teratoma, phimosis, etc. But a few congenital anomalies present later in life, such as persistent urachus, branchial cyst, branchial fistula, etc. Certain diseases are peculiar to a particular age. Acute arthritis, acute osteomyelitis, Wilms' tumor of the kidney are found mostly in infants. Sarcomas affect teenagers. Appendicitis is commonly seen in girls between 14 and 25 years of age. Though carcinomas affect mostly those who have passed 40 years of age, yet it must be remembered that *they should not be excluded by age alone.* Osteoarthritis and benign hypertrophy of the prostate are diseases of old age.

Sex: It goes without saying that the diseases, which affect the sexual organs, will be peculiar to the sex concerned. Besides these, certain other diseases are predominantly seen in a particular sex, such as diseases of the thyroid, visceroptosis, movable kidney, cystitis are *common in females,* whereas carcinomas of the stomach, lungs, kidneys are *common in males.* Hemophilia affects males only, although the disease is transmitted through the females.

Religion: Carcinoma of penis is hardly seen in Jews and Muslims owing to their religious custom of compulsory circumcision in infancy. For the same reason, phimosis, subprepucial infection, etc., are not at all seen in them. On the other hand, intussusception is sometimes seen after the month-long fast (Ramjan) in Muslims.

Social status: Certain diseases are more often seen in individuals of high social status, e.g., acute appendicitis; whereas a few diseases are more often seen in individuals of low social status, e.g., tuberculosis due to malnourishment and poor living conditions.

Occupation: Some diseases have shown their peculiar predilection towards certain occupations. As for example, varicose veins are commonly seen among bus conductors. Workers in aniline dye factories are more prone to urinary bladder neoplasms than others. Carcinoma of the scrotum is more commonly seen among chimney sweepers and in those, who work in tar and shale oil. Injury to the medial semilunar cartilage of the knee is common among footballers and miners. Enlargement of certain bursae may occur from repeated friction of the skin over the bursae, e.g., student's elbow, housemaid's knee, etc. Strain to the extensor origin from the lateral epicondyle of the humerus is commonly seen among tennis players and is known as 'tennis elbow'.

Residence: A few surgical diseases have got geographical distribution. Filariasis is common in Odisha, whereas leprosy in Bankura district of West Bengal. Gallbladder diseases are common in West Bengal and Bangladesh. Peptic ulcer is more commonly seen in northwestern part and southern parts of India as they are habituated to take more spicy foods. Bilharziasis is common in Egypt, sleeping sickness in Africa and hydatid disease in sheep-rearing districts of Australia, Greece, Turkey, Iran, Iraq, UK, etc. Tropical diseases, such as amoebiasis, are obviously common in tropical countries. 'Kangri' cancer **(Fig. 1.1)** is peculiar among the Kashmiri on their abdomen due to their habit of carrying the 'Kangri' (an earthenware filled with burning charcoal to keep themselves warm).

In this column, the students must not forget to write the full postal address of the patient for future correspondence.

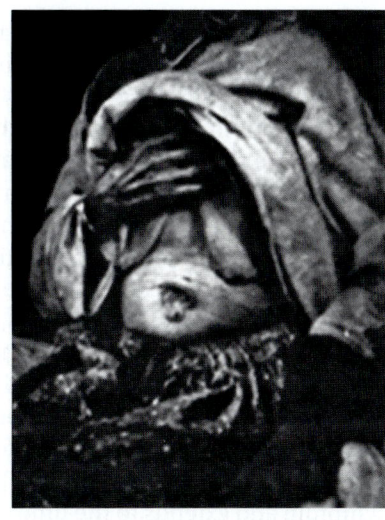

Fig.1.1: A kangri cancer on the abdomen of a Kashmiri.

Demographic details

Parameter	Relevance in surgery
Name	Builds rapport; useful for documentation.
Age	Some diseases are age-specific (e.g., Wilms' tumor in children, prostate hypertrophy in elderly).
Sex	Gender-specific conditions (e.g., ovarian cysts in females, prostate cancer in males).
Religion	Religious customs may influence surgical conditions (e.g., circumcision in Muslim/Jewish males reduces risk of penile carcinoma).
Social status	Higher socioeconomic groups → appendicitis; lower socioeconomic groups → tuberculosis.
Occupation	Certain jobs predispose to diseases (e.g., varicose veins in bus conductors, lung disease in coal miners).
Residence	Geographic prevalence of diseases (e.g., filariasis in Odisha, leprosy in West Bengal).

2. **Chief complaints:** The complaints of the patient are recorded under this heading in a chronological order of their appearance. The questions should be open ended, easily comprehensible by the patient, in a language that the patient understands. If the patient is asked, 'What are your complaints?' A few patients do not really understand what do you want to know and may start talking irrelevantly. In that case, he should be asked, 'What brings you here?'. You must also confirm the absence of key distinguishing symptoms to avoid missing important history, for example, in a case of swelling or lump, you must ask for any associated unwanted weight loss or night sweats to rule out malignancies. You should also know the duration of these complaints. For this, ask the patient, "How long have you been suffering from each of these complaints?" These should be recorded in a chronological order. As for example, in case of a sinus in the neck, the complaints may be put down in the following way:

(a) Swelling in the neck—1 year.
(b) Fever (mostly in the evening)—10 months.
(c) Slight pain in the swelling—6 months.
(d) Sinus in the neck—1 month.

If a few complaints start simultaneously, list them in order of severity.

The students should make it very clear that the patient was free from any complaint before the period mentioned by the patient, this is what we call negative history. For this, the student should ask the patient with sinus in the neck, "Were you perfectly well before the appearance of swelling in the neck?" This is very important, as very often the patients may not mention some of his previous complaints as he considers them insignificant or unrelated to his present trouble. But, on the contrary, this may give a very important clue to arrive at a diagnosis. As for example, a patient with rigidity and tenderness in right hypochondriac region of the abdomen may not have told you of his 'hunger pains' a few months back. But this simple hint at once tells you that this is a case of peptic perforation.

3. **History of present illness:** This history commences from the beginning of the first symptom and extends to the time of examination. This includes: (i) **the mode of onset** of the symptoms—whether sudden or gradual, as well as the cause of onset, if at all present; (ii) **the progress** of the disease with evolution of symptoms in the exact order of their occurrence; and lastly (iii) **the treatment** which the patient might have received—the mode of treatment and the doctor, who has treated. To know the mode of onset, the patient is asked, "How did the trouble start?" To know the progress of the disease, the patient is asked, "What is the next thing that happened?" or any such relevant question as the type of case may necessitate. *This should be recorded in the patient's own language* and not in scientific terms. The patient should be allowed to describe his own story of symptoms. They know more about their complaints than the doctors. But if they wander too far from the point, they should be put such questions as to bring them back into the matter. Never ask the question—"What are you suffering from?" The patient will obviously tell you his or another doctor's diagnosis, which you do not want to know. 'Leading questions' should not be put to the patients. By this, it is meant that questions, which yield only one answer, should not be asked. As for example, if the patient is asked like this—"Doesn't the pain move to the inferior angle of the right scapula?" Obviously a well-behaved patient will answer "Yes" to please you. So the question should be such that it leaves the patient with a free choice of answer. As for example, the question should be, "Does the pain ever move?" If the patient says, "Yes", you should ask, "Where does it go?" So the questions should not necessarily be 'leading', but to help the patient to narrate the different aspects of his symptoms to arrive at a definite diagnosis.

Sometimes *negative answers* are more valuable in arriving at a diagnosis and should never be disregarded. As for example, in case of a sinus on the cheek, absence of the history of watery discharge at the time of meals at once excludes the possibility of a parotid fistula.

History of present illness

Aspect	Description	Example questions
Mode of onset	Identify whether symptoms started suddenly or gradually.	"Did the symptoms begin suddenly or develop gradually?"
Cause of onset	Determine if an external factor (trauma, infection, stress) triggered the condition.	"Do you recall anything that may have triggered these symptoms?"

Contd...

Contd...

Aspect	Description	Example questions
Progress of disease	Track how the condition evolved from the first symptom to the present state.	"What were the first symptoms you noticed, and how did they change over time?"
Order of symptoms	List symptoms in the exact sequence they appeared for diagnostic clarity.	"Can you describe the symptoms in the order they appeared?"
Previous treatment	Document past medical interventions, medications, and treating doctors.	"What treatments have you tried before coming here? Did they help?"
Patient's own words	Encourage the patient to describe symptoms in their own words, avoiding medical jargon.	"How would you describe your pain/discomfort in your own words?"
Avoiding assumptions	Ensure the doctor does not infer symptoms but lets the patient provide details.	"Before these symptoms, were you feeling completely normal?"
Avoiding leading questions	Avoid yes/no questions that may force the patient into a biased response.	"Does the pain move? If so, where does it go?"
Clarifying unclear responses	Guide the patient back to relevant details if they stray from the topic.	"Earlier you mentioned nausea—can you explain when it started and how severe it was?"

4. **Associated diseases:** Patients may be suffering from associated medical diseases apart from the one which he/she is complaining of: diabetes, high blood pressure, asthma, tropical diseases, bleeding disorders, rheumatic fever or even rarely syphilis or gonorrhea. This history is highly important as these may require additional treatment.

5. **Past history:** *All the diseases* suffered by the patient, previous to the present one, should be noted and recorded in a chronological order. There should be mention of dates of their occurrence and the duration. This may have influence on the present condition. Peptic ulcer, acute pancreatitis, tuberculosis, gallbladder disease, appendicitis, etc., are important. Students should not forget to mention any of the *previous operations or accidents* which the patient might have undergone or sustained. The dates and the types of the operations should be mentioned in a chronological order.

6. **Drug history:** The patient should be asked about all the drugs he was on. Besides the fact that this will help to give a clue to the present illness or in the subsequent treatment, it has tremendous importance from anesthetic point of view. Special enquiry should be made about steroids, insulin, antihypertensives, diuretics, ergot derivatives, monoamine oxidase inhibitors, hormone replacement therapy, contraceptive pills, etc.

7. **History of allergy:** This is very important and should not be missed under any circumstances, while taking history of a patient. The patient should be asked whether he or she is allergic to any medicine or diet. It should be noted with red type on the cover of the history sheet. The

students should make it a practice and they will definitely find that this valuable practice will save many catastrophies.

8. **Personal history**: Under this heading, the patient's habit *of smoking* (cigarettes, cigar or pipe and the frequency), *drinking of alcohol* (quality and quantity), *diet* (regular or irregular, vegetarian or nonvegetarian, takes spicy food or not, etc.) are noted. It is also enquired about the *marital status* of the individual—whether married or single, a widow or a widower.

In women, *the menstrual history* must be recorded perfectly—whether the patient is having regular menstruation or not, the days of menstruation, whether any pain is associated with menstruation or not and last date of menstruation. The number of pregnancies and miscarriages are noted with their dates—whether the deliveries were normal or not, whether the patient had cesarean section or not and if so, for what reason. The patient is also asked whether there is any discharge per vaginum or not.

9. **Family history:** This is also important. Many diseases do recur in families. Hemophilia, tuberculosis, diabetes, essential hypertension, peptic ulcer, majority of the cancers particularly the breast cancer and certain other diseases like fissure-in-ano, piles, etc., run in families. So, the students must not forget to enquire about other members of the family, such as about the parents if they are still alive. How are they maintaining their health? Did they suffer from any major ailments? If they are dead, what were the causes of their deaths? You should also enquire about the brothers, sisters and children of the patient.

10. **History of immunization:** Children should be asked whether they have been immunized against diphtheria, tetanus, whooping cough, poliomyelitis, smallpox, tuberculosis, etc.

PHYSICAL EXAMINATION

This includes **General survey, Local examination** and **General examination**.

A. **GENERAL SURVEY:** Under this heading comes general assessment of illness, mental state, intelligence, build, state of nutrition, the attitude, the decubitus (position in bed), color of the skin, skin eruptions if present and pulse, respiration and temperature.

Physical examination starts when the patient enters the clinic. It requires daylight and of course a cooperative patient. In artificial light, one may miss the faint yellow tinge of slight jaundice. For complete examination, the patient should be asked to take off all his clothes and covered by only a dressing gown. For examining a female patient there must be an attendant nurse.

General assessment of illness: This is very important and should be assessed in the first opportunity. In case of severely ill patients, one should cut down the wastage of time to know other less important findings. The doctor should hasten into the treatment after rapidly going through the local examination to come to a probable diagnosis and to find out those signs which may help him to institute proper treatment.

Levels of consciousness

Level of consciousness	Description
Fully conscious	Alert, responds normally.
Confused	Disoriented in time/place/person.
Drowsy	Can be awakened but falls asleep quickly.
Stuporous	Responds to pain only.
Comatose	No response to pain.

Mental state and intelligence: In case of chronically ill patients, the doctor should always assess the mental state and intelligence of the individual. An intelligent patient will give a very good history on which the doctor can rely. On the other hand the doctor should not rely wholly on the history from the patient with very low intelligence.

Mental state (level of consciousness) is of particular importance in a head injury patient. There are five stages of level of consciousness—(1) Fully conscious with perfect orientation of time, space and person. (2) Fully conscious with lack of orientation of time and space. (3) Semiconsciousness (drowsy) but can be awakened. (4) Unconscious (stupor), but responding to painful stimuli. (5) Unconscious (coma) and not responding to painful stimuli. In all cases clinician must be well aware of the mental state of his patient.

Build and state of nutrition: Besides the fact that a few endocrine abnormalities become obvious from the build of the patient, a hint to clinical diagnosis may be achieved from a look on the build of the patient. As for example, a cachectic patient suffering from an abdominal discomfort with a lump, is probably suffering from carcinoma of some part of the gastrointestinal (GI) tract.

Attitude: This is very important and gives valuable information to arrive at a diagnosis. Patients with pain due to peritonitis lie still, whereas patients with colicky pain become restless and toss on the bed. Meningitis of the neck will show neck retraction and rigidity. An old patient after a fall, when lies helplessly with an everted leg, possibility of fracture of the neck of the femur becomes obvious.

Gait: This means the way the patient walks. Abnormal gait occurs due to various reasons—(a) Pain; (b) Bone and joint abnormalities; (c) Muscle and neurological diseases; (d) Structural abnormalities and (e) Psychiatric diseases. 'Waddling gait' is typical in bilateral congenital dislocation of hip and bilateral coxa vara. 'Trendelenburg gait' is typically seen in muscle dystrophies, poliomyelitis, unilateral coxa vara, Perthes' disease and different arthritis of the hip.

Facies: The face is the 'mirror of the mind' and the eyes are the 'windows of the mind.' Just looking at the face good clinician can assess the depth of the disease and effect of his treatment. The general diagnostic importance of the facies is enormous. Typical 'Facies hippocratica' in generalized peritonitis, 'Risus Sardonicus' in tetanus, 'Mask face' in Parkinsonism, 'Moon Face' in Cushing's syndrome and 'Adenoid facies' in hypertrophied adenoids are very characteristic and once seen is difficult to forget.

Decubitus: This means the position of the patient in bed. This is sometime informatory, e.g., in cerebral irritation the patient lies curled upon his side away from light.

Color of the skin: So far as the color of the skin is concerned, broadly the students should try to find out the presence of pallor, cyanosis or jaundice.

Pallor of the skin is seen in massive hemorrhage, shock and intense emotion. Anemic patients are also pale. One should look at the lower palpebral conjunctiva, mucous membrane of the lips and cheeks, nail beds and palmar creases for pallor.

Cyanosis, i.e., bluish or purplish tinge of the skin or mucous membrane which results from the presence of excessive amount of reduced hemoglobin in the underlying blood vessels. It may be either due to poor perfusion of these vessels (peripheral cyanosis) or due to reduction in the oxygen saturation of arterial blood (central cyanosis). For cyanosis to be observed, there must be a minimum of 5 g/dL of reduced hemoglobin in the blood perfusing the skin. So, cyanosis is not detectable in presence with severe anemia. **Peripheral cyanosis** is due to excessive reduction of oxyhemoglobin in the capillaries when the blood flow is slowed down. This may happen on exposure to cold (cold-induced vasoconstriction). It is also seen in patients with reduced cardiac output when differential vasoconstriction diverts blood flow from the skin to other more important organs, e.g., the brain, the kidney, etc. Peripheral cyanosis is looked for in the nail bed, tip of the nose, skin of the palm and toes.

Central cyanosis occurs from inadequate oxygenation of blood in the lungs. This may be due to diseases in the lungs or due to some congenital abnormalities of the heart where venous blood by-passes the lung and is shunted into the systemic circulation. For central cyanosis one should look at the tongue and other places as mentioned above. The tongue remains unaffected in peripheral cyanosis. Very occasionally cyanosis may be due to the presence of abnormal pigments, e.g., methemoglobin or sulfhemoglobin in the bloodstream. In these cases arterial oxygen tension is normal. This may occur due to taking of drugs such as phenacetin. Carbon monoxide poisoning produces a generalized cherry-red discoloration.

Jaundice is due to icteric tint of the skin, which varies from faint yellow of viral hepatitis to dark olive greenish yellow of obstructive jaundice. This is due to the presence of excess of lipid-soluble yellow pigments (mostly the bile pigments) in the plasma. The places where one should look for jaundice are—(i) sclera of the eyeball—for this the patient is asked to look at his feet when the surgeon keeps the palpebral fissure wide open by pulling up the eyelid, (ii) nail bed, (iii) lobule of the ear, (iv) tip of the nose, (v) undersurface of the tongue, etc. When the jaundice is deep and long standing, a distinct greenish color becomes evident in the sclerae and in the skin due to the development of appreciable quantities of biliverdin. Scratch marks may be prominent in the skin in obstructive jaundice as a result of pruritus which is believed to be due to retention of bile acids.

Jaundice may be confused with hypercarotenemia in which yellow pigment of carotene is inequally distributed and is particularly seen in the face, palms and soles but *not in the sclerae*. Such hypercarotenemia may occur occasionally in vegetarians and in those who eat excessive quantities of raw carrot.

Skin eruption: Under this heading comes macules, papules, vesicles, pustules, wheals, etc.

Macules—are alterations in the color of the skin, which are seen but not felt. They may be due to capillary naevi or erythemas which disappear on pressure, whereas purpuric macules do not blanch when pressed. **Papules**—are solid projections from the surface of the skin. It may be epidermal papule, e.g., a wart or a dermal papule, which will become less prominent if the skin is stretched, e.g., a granuloma of tuberculosis, reticulosis or sarcoidosis. **Vesicles**—are elevations of horny layer of the epidermis by collection of transparent or milky fluid within them. **Pustules**—are similar elevations of the skin as vesicles, but these contain pus instead of fluid within them. **Wheal**—is a flat edematous elevation of the skin frequently accompanied by itching. It is the typical lesion of urticaria and may be seen in sensitive persons provoked by irritation of the skin.

Pulse: This is an important index of severity of illness. Pulse gives a good indication as to the severity of acute appendicitis and thyrotoxicosis. Generally, it gives a good indication of the cardiovascular condition of the patient. Abnormalities of the heart and the vascular system, e.g., hypertension and hypotension are also revealed in pulse. Shock, fever and thyrotoxicosis are a few conditions, which are well reflected in pulse. Following points are particularly noted in pulse: (a) *Rate*—fast or slow, (b) *Rhythm*—regular or irregular, (c) *Tension* and *force* which indicate diastolic and systolic blood pressure respectively, (d) *Volume* which indicates pulse pressure, (e) *Character*, e.g., Water-hammer pulse of aortic regurgitation or thyrotoxicosis, pulsus paradoxus of pericardial effusion, etc., and (f) *condition of arterial wall,* e.g., atherosclerotic thickening, etc.

Respiration: The students will gradually learn the importance of respiration as a finding not only for diagnosis, but also to assess the condition of the patient under anesthesia and in early postoperative days. Tachypnea (fast breathing) is seen in fever, shock, hypoxia, cerebral disturbances, metabolic acidosis, tetany, hysteria, etc. Slow and deep respiration is an ominous sign in cerebral compression. Also note if there is any irregular breathing, e.g., Cheyne-Stokes respiration. In Cheyne-Stokes respiration there is gradual deepening of respiration or overventilation alternating with short periods of apnea.

Temperature: This is normally taken in the mouth or in the axilla of the patient. The temperature of the mouth is about 1°F higher than that of the axilla. Fever or high temperature is come across in various conditions, which the students will be more conversant in medical ward. But broadly, the students should know that there are three types of fever—the continued, the remittent and the intermittent. When the fever does not fluctuate for more than 1°C during 24 hours, but at no time touches the normal, it is described as *continued.* When the daily fluctuations exceed 2°C it is *remittent* and when the fever is present only for a few hours during the day, it is called *intermittent.* When a paroxysm of intermittent fever occurs daily, it is called *quotidian,* when on alternate days it is called *tertian* and when two days intervene between the consecutive attacks, it is called *quartan.*

B. **LOCAL EXAMINATION:** This is the most important part in the physical examination, as a careful local examination will give a definite clue to arrive at a diagnosis. By 'Local examination' we mean examination of the affected region. This should be done by *inspection* (looking at the affected part of the body), *palpation* (feeling of the affected part by the hands of the surgeon), percussion (listening to the tapping note with a finger on a finger placed on the affected part), *auscultation* (listening to the sounds produced within the body with the help of a stethoscope), *movements* (of the joints concerned), *measurement* (of the part of the body concerned) and *examination of the lymph nodes* draining the affected area. Detailed description of these examinations are discussed in subsequent chapters.

Inspection of the part should be carried out after complete exposure. *It should be compared with the corresponding normal side,* whenever possible. The importance of proper inspection cannot be overemphasized, as many of the surgical conditions can be diagnosed by looking at it with well-trained eyes. It is said that eyes do not see what mind does not know. So, a thorough knowledge of the whole subject is essential before one can train one's eyes for such good inspection.

Palpation will not only corroborate the findings seen in inspection, but also added informations with trained hands may not require any further examination to come to a diagnosis.

Percussion and **auscultation** are not so important as in the medical side for clinical diagnosis of surgical diseases. These are only important in a few surgical conditions, which will be discussed later in appropriate chapters.

Movements and **measurements** are important particularly in orthopedic cases, in fractures and in injuries of different nerves.

Local examination is never complete without the **examination of the draining lymph nodes.** More often than not the students forget to do this valuable examination and fail to diagnose many important cases.

C. **GENERAL EXAMINATION:** In chronic cases, one should always examine the patient as a whole, after completing the local examination. In acute cases, this examination may be omitted to save the valuable time. But even in acute cases, certain general examinations should be carried out either for anesthetic sake or for treatment point of view. General examination is required mainly for the following purposes:

1. *For the diagnosis and differential diagnosis:* For example, in case of retention of urine, one should examine the knee and ankle jerks and pupillary reflexes (Argyll Robertson pupil) to come to a diagnosis of Tabes dorsalis. Similarly, examination of the chest or spine should be carried out in an otherwise obscure abdominal pain to find out basal pleurisy or caries spine as the cause of pain. Sometimes the patient complains of pain in the knee when the pathology lies in the hip joint. Cases are on record when teenaged boy with the complain of pain in the right iliac fossa was referred to the hospital by the general physician as a case of acute appendicitis. Only after examination of the scrotum, the surgeon found torsion of the testis as the cause of pain and not appendicitis.

2. *For selecting the type of anesthetic:* The anesthetist should always examine the patient generally, particularly the heart and lungs to select the proper anesthetic. Sometimes the operation should be performed under local anesthesia in old and cardiac patients.

3. *To determine the nature of the operation:* In case of an inguinal hernia, one should examine the chest to exclude a cause of chronic cough, for enlarged prostate or for stricture of urethra as an organic cause of an obstruction to the outflow of urine and to exclude constipation as cause for increased abdominal pressure to initiate hernia. So, patients with these conditions, if operated on, will definitely come back with recurrence of hernia. At the same time, the surgeon should look for the tone of the abdominal muscles to determine whether herniorrhaphy or hernioplasty will give the best result.

4. *To determine the prognosis:* In a case of gastric cancer, if general examination reveals involvement of the supraclavicular glands, the prognosis is obviously grave. Similarly, cancer of the breast, if shows secondary metastases in bones and lungs, is considered to be in the last stage.

A list is given below to remember the points to be examined under the heading of 'general examination':

Head and neck
1. Cranial nerves—particularly the 3rd, 4th, 5th, 6th, 7th, 9th, 11th and 12th cranial nerves should be examined.
2. Eyes: Tests are done to know the visual field, condition of the conjunctiva and pupils (equality, reaction to light and accommodation reflex), movements of the eye and ophthalmic examination of the fundi.
3. Mouth and pharynx: Teeth and gum, movement of soft palate, the tongue and its undersurface, tonsils and lips for color, pigmentation (seen in Peutz-Jeghers syndrome) and eruptions.
4. Movements of the neck, neck veins and lymph nodes of the neck, carotid pulses and the thyroid gland.

Upper limbs
(1) General examination of the arms and hand with particular reference to their vascular supply and nerve supply (power, tone, reflexes and sensations). (2) Axillae and lymph nodes. (3) Joints. (4) Finger nails—clubbing or koilonychia.

Thorax
(1) Type of chest. (2) Breasts. (3) Presence of any dilated vessels and pulsations. (4) Position of the trachea. (5) Apex beat. (6) Lungs—as a whole, i.e., inspection, palpation, percussion

and auscultation. (7) The heart should be examined as a whole, i.e., palpation, percussion and auscultation.

Abdomen
(1) Abdominal wall—position of the umbilicus, presence of scars, dilated vessels, etc. (2) Abdominal reflexes. (3) Visible peristalsis or pulsation. (4) Generalized palpation, percussion and auscultation. (5) Hernial orifices. (6) Genitalia. (7) Inguinal glands. (8) Rectal examination. (9) Gynecological examination, if required.

Lower limbs
(1) General examination of legs and feet—with particular reference to the vascular supply and nerve supply (power, tone, reflexes and sensation). (2) Varicose vein. (3) Edema. (4) Joints.

Examination of the external genitalia
Sputum, vomit, urine, stool should be examined by naked eye and under microscope, if required.

PROVISIONAL DIAGNOSIS

At this stage the clinician should be able to make a provisional diagnosis. He should also keep in mind the differential diagnosis. He will now require a few investigations to come to the proper clinical diagnosis. The students should know how to diagnose common diseases first and then he should think for possibility of rare diseases. A word of the caution will not be irrelevant here that '*if you diagnose a rare disease, you will be rarely correct.*'

SPECIAL INVESTIGATIONS

Besides the routine examination of the blood, urine and stool, a few special investigations depending upon the provisional diagnosis will be required to arrive at a proper diagnosis. These are discussed in details in appropriate chapters.

CLINICAL DIAGNOSIS

After getting the reports of special investigations, the clinician should be able to give proper clinical diagnosis. By this we mean that not only the ailing organ is identified, but the type of pathological process at work and its extent in different directions is also understood. As for example, in carcinoma of the breast, one should mention under this heading the clinical stage of the disease and the various structures involved in metastasis. Similarly in case of inguinal hernia, the clinician should not only mention that whether it is direct or indirect, reducible or irreducible, but also should mention its content—either the intestine or omentum or a portion of urinary bladder.

TREATMENT

The students should record under this heading the details of medical treatment and the surgical treatment which the patient has received. While writing medical treatment the students should clearly mention the drugs given to the patient, their doses and duration of the treatment. In surgical treatment they should clearly mention the type of anesthesia given and type of operation performed.

In the operation note, the students should describe the operation under following headings:
(i) Type of anesthesia and anesthetics used;
(ii) Name of the anesthetist;
(iii) Name of the surgeons;
(iv) Position of the patient on the operation table;
(v) The type of incision made;
(vi) Technique of operation;
(vii) Closure;
(viii) Drainage—given or not.

PROGRESS

Daily progress of the patient starting from the time the patient came out of the operation theater should be clearly noted. Students should also mention if any investigation performed during the postoperative period, the dressings done during the period, condition of the wound, etc. The following postoperative monitoring parameters must be recorded:
(i) Vitals must be recorded every 4 hours in hemodynamically stable patients and continuously in vulnerable patients, using monitors.
(ii) Drain output monitoring
(iii) Signs of infection at surgical site
(iv) Pain assessment.

FOLLOW-UP

This resumes when the patient is discharged from the hospital and extends till he starts his normal active life. The students should learn how to make a discharge certificate mentioning in nutshell the diagnosis, special investigations performed, the treatment received and the postoperative advice. He should also mention the date when the patient should report to the outpatient clinic to let the surgeon know his progress and his complaints. Now the students should make a record of the days the patient came for follow-up and the advice given by the surgeon.

TERMINATION

To terminate the history sheet of the patient, the students should mention whether the patient was completely cured when his follow-up period ended or the patient was relieved of his symptoms but not cured or whether the patient died during his stay in hospital or in follow-up period. In case of death, the student should mention the cause of death and also make a note of the result of the postmortem examination, if carried out.

Chapter 1: General Scheme of Case Taking

Algorithm for General Scheme of Case Taking

Patient arrival and initial observation
- Observe general appearance, distress level, consciousness
- Note any immediate concerns (e.g., trauma, shock)

↓

History taking
- Record patient particulars (name, age, occupation, residence)
- Document chief complaints in chronological order

↓

Physical examination
- General survey: Check vital signs, mental status, nutrition
- Local examination: Inspect, plapate, percuss, ausculatate the affected area
- Systemic examination

↓

Special investigations
- Perform relevant lab tests (blood, urine, imaging)
- Order specific tests based on clinical suspicion (biopsy, CT, MRI, X-ray, endoscopy

↓

Clinical diagnosis
- Correlate history, physical exam, and investigations
- Differentiate between possible diagnoses
- Establish a working diagnosis

↓

Treatment plan
- Medical treatment: Medications, lifestyle changes, supportive care
- Surgical treatment: Decide on surgery type, preoperative preparation
- Discuss risks, prognosis, and expected recovery timeline

↓

Postoperative monitoring
- Monitor vitals, wound healing, pain, infections
- Adjust medications, ensure hydration/nutrition
- Address complications early

↓

Follow-up
- Schedule reviews at appropriate intervals
- Monitor for recurrence, complications, or residual symptoms
- Continue necessary medial therapy or rehabilitation

↓

Termination
- Recovery: Patient resumes normal activity, case closed
- Chronic illness: Requires long-term monitoring and intervention
- Death: Document cause, perform postmortem if needed

CHAPTER 2

A Few Special Symptoms and Signs

A few symptoms and signs are described in this chapter which I feel deserve special mention and are not thoroughly dealt with elsewhere.

PAIN

This is a very common symptom and all of us must have experienced pain sometime or the other. The word 'pain' is derived from Latin word 'poena' which means penalty or punishment. Pain should not be confused with 'tenderness'. The patient feels 'pain', while the doctor elicits 'tenderness'. Tenderness means pain which occurs in response to a stimulus given by somebody (usually from the doctor). So, pain is a symptom and tenderness is a sign.

Types of pain: Basically, four types of pain are noticed—(1) Superficial, (2) Segmental, (3) Deep or visceral and (4) Psychogenic or central.

1. *Superficial pain:* This occurs due to direct irritation of the peripheral nerve endings in the superficial tissue. Such irritation may be by chemical or mechanical or thermal or electrical. The superficial pain is sharp and can be pointed with a fingertip.
2. *Segmental pain:* This occurs due to irritation of a sensory nerve trunk or root. This is located in a particular dermatome of the body supplied by the affected sensory nerve trunk or root.
3. *Deep pain:* This pain occurs due to irritation of deep structures of the body, e.g., the deep fascia, the muscles, the tendons, the bones, the joints and the viscera. The pain sensation from the affected structure is conveyed to the brain either by somatic nerve or by the autonomic nervous system. The deep pain is vague compared to the superficial pain and may be one of the various types which are described below. The deep pain is vaguely localized in comparison to the superficial pain. The deep pain may be referred to some other area of the body due to common area of representation in the spinal cord (supplied by the same segment). The deep pain may cause involuntary spasm of the skeletal muscles supplied by the same spinal cord segment.
4. *Psychogenic pain:* In this condition pain arises from the brain, which may be a functional pain either emotional or hysterical or due to lesions in the thalamus or spinothalamic tract or due to causalgia.

Types of pain

Type of pain	Description	Example
Superficial pain	Sharp, well-localized pain due to irritation of peripheral nerve endings.	Skin burns, cuts
Segmental pain	Follows a dermatome due to sensory nerve root irritation.	Herpes zoster

Contd...

Contd...

Type of pain	Description	Example
Deep pain	Vague, poorly localized pain from deep structures like fascia, joints, and bones.	Bone fractures, arthritis
Psychogenic pain	Pain originating from emotional or neurological dysfunction.	Thalamic pain syndrome

Majority of the surgical patients come to the surgeon with the complaint of pain. A careful history must be taken about pain so that it may help to reach the diagnosis. If careful history is not taken about pain, it may frequently confuse the clinician to make wrong diagnosis. The followings are the various points which must be asked to know the cause of pain.

Original site of pain: The patient should be asked to locate the site of pain with his fingertip. It must be remembered that when the patient comes to the surgeon the site of pain may have changed. But it is highly important to know the original site of pain—'where did the pain start?' In many cases, particularly in abdominal pain, the patient may not be able to point with a fingertip, instead he uses his whole hand. So exact localization may not be possible particularly in case of deep pain originating in thoracic or abdominal viscus. A patient with acute appendicitis when brought to the surgeon may locate pain at the right iliac fossa. But when he is asked 'where did the pain start?' His answer is often 'in the umbilical region' and now it is in the right iliac fossa. This simple history is highly important to come to the diagnosis of acute appendicitis and this history only differentiates this condition from many others.

Origin and mode of onset: It may be possible to know from the patient the time of onset of pain and mode of onset. A long-continued pain with insidious onset indicates chronic nature of the disease, e.g., chronic pancreatitis, chronic peptic ulcer, subacute appendicitis, etc. Whereas recent onset of pain with sudden arrival indicates acute nature of the disease, e.g., acute pancreatitis, acute appendicitis, rupture of aneurysm, etc.

Enquire into 'how did the pain start?' When the pain starts after a trauma the cause of the pain must be traumatic, e.g., a sprain, or a fracture or dislocation or rupture of kidney or rupture of liver, etc.

Severity: This of course is not so important to come to a diagnosis. Individuals often react differently to pain. A severe pain to one person may be simple dull ache to another. However, a few diseases are known to produce severe pain, e.g., acute pancreatitis, biliary colic, perforated peptic ulcer, dissecting aneurysm of aorta, etc.

Nature of the pain: It is of great importance to know the character or nature of the pain. It often helps to come to a diagnosis. On the other hand patients may find it very difficult to describe the nature of their pain. The various types of pain are described below:

i. *Vague aching pain:* This is a mild continuous pain which has no other specific features.
ii. *Burning pain:* It is almost like a burning sensation caused by contact with a hot object. Burning pain is typically experienced in case of peptic ulcer or reflux esophagitis.
iii. *Throbbing pain:* It is a type of throbbing sensation which is typically felt in case of pyogenic abscesses.
iv. *Scalding pain:* It is also a type of burning sensation which is particularly felt during micturition in the presence of cystitis, acute pyelonephritis or urethritis.

v. Pins and needles sensation: It is typically felt in case of injury to the peripheral sensory nerve. As if pins and needles are being pricked in that area of the skin supplied by the affected sensory nerve.

vi. Shooting pain: It is typically felt in case of sciatica when pain shoots along the course of the sciatic nerve.

vii. Stabbing pain: It is a sudden, severe, sharp and short-lived pain. This is typically felt in acute perforation of peptic ulcer.

viii. Constricting pain: It means as if something is encircling and compressing from all directions the relevant part. The pain is often expressed as an iron band tightening around the chest. It is typical of angina pectoris.

ix. Distension: This type of pain is experienced in diseases of any structure encircled or restricted by a wall, e.g., a hollow viscus. When tension increases inside such hollow viscus it causes a pain which is typically described by the patient as a feeling of distension or 'tightness'.

x. Colic: A colicky pain occurs when the muscular wall of a hollow tube is attempting to force certain content of the tube out of it. A colicky pain has two features. Firstly, the pain appears suddenly, and it goes off as suddenly as it came. Secondly, the pain is of griping nature, may not be very excruciating and it is often associated with vomiting and sweating. Usually, four types of colics are seen in surgical practice—ureteric colic, biliary colic, intestinal colic and appendicular colic.

xi. Twisting pain—is a type of sensation as if something is twisting inside the body. Such sensation is often felt in case of volvulus of intestine, torsion of testis or ovarian cyst.

xii. 'Just a pain': Often a patient may not describe his pain. He often says that 'it is just a pain' and cannot describe the nature of the pain.

Progression of the pain: Now the patient should be asked 'how is the pain progressing?' (a) The pain may begin in a weak note and gradually reaches a peak or a plateau and then gradually declines. (b) It may begin at its maximum intensity and remains at this level till it disappears. (c) The severity of pain may fluctuate—its intensity may increase and decrease at intervals. This should be depicted in a graph.

Duration of the pain: Duration of pain means the period from the time of onset to the time of disappearance. Characteristically, the griping pain of intestinal colic is felt for less than a minute. The pain of angina of effort ceases within 5 minutes of resting, whereas that of a myocardial infarct may continue for hours.

Movements of pain: Pain may move from one place to the other and three types of such movements are noticed—(i) radiation, (ii) referred and (iii) shifting or migration of pain.

i. Radiation of pain: This means extension of the pain to another site whilst the original pain persists at its original site. The radiation of pain has almost the same character. The typical example is when a duodenal ulcer penetrates posteriorly. The pain in the epigastrium remains but at the same time the pain spreads or radiates to the back.

ii. Referred pain: When pain is felt at a distance from its source and there is no pain at the site of disease, it is called a referred pain. Irritation or inflammation of the diaphragm causes pain at the tip of the shoulder. Referred pain occurs when the central nervous system fails to differentiate between visceral and somatic sensory impulses from the same segment. In this case diaphragm is supplied by phrenic nerve (C3, 4 and 5) and the cutaneous supply of the shoulder is also C4 and C5. Diseases of the hip joint may be referred to the knee joint as both these joints are supplied by the articulate branches of the femoral nerve, obturator nerve and sciatic nerve.

iii. ***Shifting or migration of pain:*** In this condition pain is felt at one site in the beginning and then the pain is shifted to another site and the original pain disappears. This occurs when an abdominal viscus becomes diseased, the original pain is experienced at the site of distribution of the same somatic segment. But when the parietal peritoneum overlying the viscus is involved with the disease, the pain is experienced at the local site of the viscus. In case of acute appendicitis pain is first felt at the umbilical region which is also supplied by the T9 and 10 as the appendix, but later on pain is felt in the right iliac fossa when the parietal peritoneum above the appendix becomes inflamed.

Types of pain spread

Type	Definition	Example
Radiation	Pain spreads but remains at the original site.	Duodenal ulcer radiating to the back.
Referred pain	Pain is felt at a distant location, not at the source.	Diaphragmatic irritation causing shoulder pain.
Shifting pain	Pain starts at one site and later moves permanently.	Appendicitis: starts at umbilicus → moves to right iliac fossa.

Special times of occurrence: The patient should be asked if there is any special time of appearance of pain. Often patients with acute appendicitis give history that they feel pain on waking up in the morning, in fact pain awakens the patient. In case of duodenal ulcer pain is often complained at 4 PM in the afternoon and in the early morning at about 2-3 AM. This is 'hunger pain' and felt when food has passed out of the stomach and the stomach is empty. Migraine may occur especially in the morning, either every weekend or during menstruation. Headache of frontal sinusitis is often at its peak a few hours after rising.

Periodicity of pain: This is often characteristic in certain diseases. Sometimes an interval of days, weeks, months or even years may elapse between two painful attacks. Particularly in peptic ulcer, a periodicity is noticed and pain recurs in episodes lasting for 1 to several weeks, interspersed with pain free intervals of weeks or months. Trigeminal neuralgia often shows such periodicity and pain free intervals often last for months.

Precipitating or aggravating factors: This history is of great importance to come to a diagnosis. Alimentary tract pains may be made worse by eating particular types of foods. Musculoskeletal pains are often aggravated by joint movements. But certain typical factors should be given high consideration. Pain of appendicitis often gets worse on jolting, running and moving up the stairs. These movements also aggravate the pain of ureteric or vesical calculus. Pain of reflux esophagitis often becomes aggravated when the patient stoops. Pain of acute pancreatitis becomes worse when the patient lies down. Pain of peptic ulcer gets worse by ingestion of hot spicy food and drink. Pain of disc prolapse often gets aggravated on lifting weight from stooping position.

Relieving factors: Many pains subside spontaneously and the patient's statement must be carefully considered. Pain of peptic ulcer is often relieved by alkalies and antacids in 5-15 minutes but such relief neither appears immediately nor after 1 hour. Pain of acute pancreatitis is sometimes relieved to certain extent by sitting up in the bed in leaning forward position and the patient prefers to sit up throughout the night. Pain of reflux esophagitis due to sliding hiatus hernia is often relieved in propped up position. Colicky pain of intestinal obstruction often gets relieved on passing flatus. In perforative peritonitis any movement of the abdomen causes aggravation of pain and the patient gets some relief if he lies still.

Associated symptoms: Severe pain may be associated with pallor, sweating, vomiting and increase in pulse rate. Colicky pain is often associated with sweating, vomiting and clammy extremities. Migraine is often preceded by visual disturbances and accompanied by vomiting. Pain of acute pyelonephritis may be associated with rigor and high fever. Ureteric colic may be accompanied by hematuria. Biliary colic is often associated with presence of jaundice and pale stool. Excessive sweating and cold extremities are very common associated symptoms of leaking abdominal aneurysm, dissecting aneurysm, hemorrhagic pancreatitis, etc.

Conclusion: So, it is clear now that pain is a very important symptom in surgical cases and a careful history of the details of the pain may give very valuable clue to come to a diagnosis. Refer to flowchart for understanding how to approach a patient presenting with pain.

VOMITING

History of vomiting itself is not diagnostic of any condition. Vomiting may occur due to a wide variety of local and systemic disorders. Vomiting may occur from simple gastric irritation. Vomiting may occur in functional and organic disorders of the nervous system, e.g., fear, motion sickness, migraine, labyrinthine disorders, meningitis and intracranial tumor. Vomiting may occur from severe pain as in any colic. Amongst systemic conditions pregnancy, renal failure and metabolic disorders, e.g., diabetic ketoacidosis or hyperparathyroidism are important. A few drugs may cause vomiting, e.g., digoxin, morphine, etc.

In surgical practice vomiting may occur in peptic ulceration, pyloric stenosis (gastric outlet obstruction), acute cholecystitis, acute pancreatitis and intestinal obstruction. In some cases of intracranial tumor the vomiting is an important symptom.

Enquiry should be made about the frequency of vomiting, the time of day at which it occurs and also about the taste, color, quantity and smell of the vomitus.

The vomitus may be of the following types:
1. The vomitus may contain recent ingested material. Such vomitus may be acid in reaction when it is probably due to gastric outlet obstruction. If such vomitus is not acid in reaction the cause may be achalasia of the esophagus, benign or malignant stricture of the esophagus.
2. Vomit may contain bile to give yellow coloration of the vomitus.
3. Vomit containing upper small bowel contents may be green in color.
4. Feculent vomitus contains lower small bowel contents, brown and of fecal odor. This is characteristic of advanced low small bowel obstruction.
5. Vomit may contain feces. This may be due to abnormal communication between the stomach and transverse colon (gastrocolic fistula as a complication of gastric ulcer).
6. Vomit containing blood may be of various types. The bleeding may be copious. The vomit may present pure blood or clots. Such bleeding may come from gastric ulcer or esophageal varices. The blood in the vomit may be altered to blackish or dark brown in color in contact with gastric juice. This is due to conversion of hemoglobin to hematin. This altered blood gives the vomitus a *'coffee-ground'* appearance. Medicine containing iron or red wine may give rise to this type of vomitus. It must be remembered that blood in the vomit may have come from the nose or lungs which have been swallowed.

Types of vomitus

Type of vomitus	Possible cause	Example condition
Fresh blood	Upper GI bleeding	Esophageal varices
Coffee-ground	Altered gastric bleeding	Peptic ulcer disease
Fecal matter	Abnormal gastrocolic communication	Gastrocolic fistula
Bile-stained	Postpyloric obstruction	Duodenal obstruction

ITCHING

Itching or pruritus is not a very significant symptom so far as surgical conditions are concerned. The various causes of pruritus are mentioned below:

1. *Skin diseases:* Certain skin diseases cause pruritus and the patients should be advised to take physician's advise to cure these. Before any operation is performed such skin conditions must be cured first until and unless the surgical condition deserves immediate operative interference. These skin conditions are urticaria, scabies and eczema.

2. *Generalized diseases:* Persistent pruritus in the absence of obvious skin disease may be due to certain generalized diseases, e.g., thyrotoxicosis, obstructive jaundice, renal failure (uremia), hepatic failure, lymphoma and other malignancies. However, in old people with dry skin pruritus is common and is of no systemic significance. Diabetes mellitus is known to produce pruritus vulvae and pruritus ani.

3. *Local irritation:* Certain conditions of the anal canal may cause pruritus of the perianal region. These are discussed in Chapter 36. Local irritation by dirty under-clothes may also cause pruritus from local irritation. Fleas and mosquitoes also cause local irritation for itching. Threadworm is particularly known to cause pruritus ani.

4. *Drug induced:* Certain drugs may cause pruritus. Majority of these cases are due to allergic hypersensitivity and vary from person to person.

HICCUP

Hiccup is caused by spasmodic contractions of the diaphragm. Majority of these hiccups are of no significance and have been experienced by almost all of us without the presence of any organic disease. Three groups of hiccups are of some surgical importance and deserve mention. *The first group* occurs in *early postoperative period* and signifies upward pressure on the undersurface of the diaphragm due to increased abdominal pressure. This is often caused by dilated stomach or dilated coils of small intestine due to paralytic ileus or due to some intestinal obstruction. Obviously such hiccup requires introduction of a nasogastric tube and aspiration through such tube will cause diminution of intra-abdominal pressure and hiccup is relieved. Sometimes injection of pethidine or siquil may be required.

The *second group* is often due to peritonitis involving the diaphragmatic peritoneum. This sometimes causes repeated hiccup.

The *third group* is a common accompaniment of advanced renal failure. So in any case of hiccup the patient should be asked to protrude his tongue and brown dry tongue should indicate renal failure and immediate investigations should be performed in this line.

ABNORMAL SUPERFICIAL VEINS (VISIBLE VEINS)

When venous pressure is within normal limits with the head resting on a pillow, the external jugular vein is either invisible or visible only for a short distance above the clavicle. Only when there is raised venous pressure, *engorgement* of the external jugular vein occurs. Bilateral engorgement of neck veins indicates too much intravenous fluid infusion or myocardial failure. Unilateral engorgement may be due to pressure on the vein by enlarged lymph nodes, a tumor or a subclavian aneurysm. Bilateral or unilateral engorgement may also be due to presence of retrosternal goiter or due to something obstructing the superior vena cava.

Radiating veins from the umbilicus in the abdominal wall indicates obstruction to the portal venous system and this is known as the **caput medusae.**

Sometimes engorged superficial veins may be seen in the flank extending from the axilla to the groin. These are called inguinoaxillary veins and engorgement of such vein indicates obstruction of the inferior vena cava. In this case veins of both sides will be prominent. When vein of one side is affected, it indicates blockage of the common iliac or external iliac vein of that side.

For *varicose veins* of the lower limbs, *see* Chapter 7.

TONGUE

Examination of the tongue is quite important. Importance is probably much more in case of medical diseases, yet there is quite a big list of surgical cases in which examination of tongue is quite important.

The patient is always asked in 'general survey' to protrude the tongue for examination. **Inability to protrude the tongue** is due to ankyloglossia, tongue-tie (in case of children) or advance carcinoma of the tongue involving the floor of the mouth (in old age). While protruding the tongue may **deviate to one side**. Such deviation is due to hemiplegia of the tongue due to involvement its motor nerve supply the hypoglossal nerve mostly by carcinomatous lesion.

The tongue may be quite large (**macroglossia**). Such large tongue may be due to acromegaly, cretinism (in children), myxedema, lymphangioma, cavernous hemangioma and amyloidosis.

Tremor of the tongue after its protrusion is a very characteristic feature of primary thyrotoxicosis though delirium tremens and parkinsonism are other rare causes.

Color of the tongue is highly important. Its particularly reach blood supply with a capillary network close to the surface has made the color of the tongue dark red. Pale tongue (pallor) is seen in severe anemia. Discoloration of the tongue may be due to ingestion of color foods, e.g., lozenge, chocolates and certain fruits (black cherries or black berries). For other causes of pathological change of color, *see* Chapter 24.

Moistness is an indication of the state of hydration of the body. Dry tongue means the water content of the body is below standard and the patient is dehydrated. A dry, brown tongue may be found in later stages of severe illness, in acute intestinal obstruction and in advanced uremia.

Furring on the dorsum of the tongue is of little value as an indication of disease. It is often found in heavy smokers. A brown fur, the 'black hairy tongue' is due to a fungus infection. Furring may also result from local infection of the mouth (stomatitis), local infection of nose or throat (tonsillitis) or from the infection of the lungs (bronchitis or pneumonia).

Examination of papillae of the tongue is quite important. Generalized atrophy of papillae which produces a smooth and bald tongue is characteristic of vitamin B_{12} deficiency, iron-deficiency anemia or certain gastrointestinal disorders. In chronic superficial glossitis, whitish opaque areas of thickened epithelium (known as leukoplakia) are seen separated by intervening smooth and scarred areas, with no normal papillae seen on the dorsum of the tongue. In congenital fissuring the papillae are normal but the surface is interrupted by numerous irregular folds which run horizontally. In median rhomboid glossitis a lozenge-shaped area of loss of papillae and fissuring is seen in the midline anterior to the foramen cecum. It feels nodular and must be distinguished from lingual thyroid or carcinoma.

The sides and undersurface of the tongue should always be examined with a spatula to retract the cheeks and lips. Look for ulcers, which are often seen at the margins of the tongues. For details of findings of these examinations *see* Chapter 24.

Different appearances of tongue

Finding	Possible condition
Pale tongue	Anemia
Strawberry tongue	Scarlet fever, Kawasaki disease
Black hairy tongue	Fungal infection
Deviated tongue	Hypoglossal nerve palsy

■ NAILS (FIGS. 2.1A TO C)

Examination of the nails is important, though more so in medical cases. Well manicured nails are things of beauty and social asset. Injury is the most common cause of changes in the nails and may permanently impair their growths. A transverse groove at a similar level of each of the nails indicates a systemic disturbance and previous illness. Splinter hemorrhages under the nails are manifestations of systemic vasculitis caused by immune complexes which may cause hemorrhages in the skin and retina also. Multiple splinter hemorrhages suggest infective endocarditis. Long standing iron deficiency may make the nails brittle, then flat and ultimately spoon-shaped *(koilonychia)*, so this type of nail is seen in advanced cases of anemia and in Plummer-Vinson syndrome. Nails may be pitted in psoriasis which may also discolor and deform the nails which is often confused with fungal infection. Small isolated white patches are often seen in the nails of normal persons. Whitening of the nail bed *(Terry's nail)* is a manifestation of hypoalbuminemia. Bitten nails suggest anxiety neurosis. In *clubbing of the fingers,* the tissues at the base of the nail are thickened and the angle between the nail base and the adjacent skin of the finger is obliterated. There is swelling of the terminal phalanges which is due to interstitial edema and dilatations of the arterioles and capillaries. One can elicit fluctuation of the nail bed. The nail itself loses its longitudinal ridges and becomes convex from above downwards as well as from side-to-side. In advanced degree of clubbing there is swelling of the subcutaneous tissue over the base of the nail which causes the overlying skin to become tense, shiny and red. Gross degree of clubbing is found in association with severe chronic cyanosis, in congenital heart disease and in association with chronic suppuration within the chest, e.g., bronchiectasis and empyema. Lesser degree of clubbing may be found in

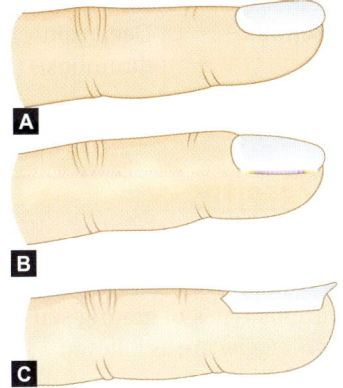

Figs. 2.1A to C: (A) Normal nail; (B) Clubbing; (C) Koilonychia.

carcinoma of the lung, pulmonary tuberculosis and in certain chronic abdominal conditions, e.g., polyposis of the colon, Crohn's disease and ulcerative colitis. Clubbing is also an important sign of subacute bacterial endocarditis when it may be associated with Osler's nodes, which are transient tender swellings in the pulp of the fingers and toes. *Nail bed infarcts* may occur in vasculitis especially in systemic lupus erythematosus and in polyarteritis.

PITTING ON PRESSURE

To confirm a suspicion of a subcutaneous edema, the cardinal sign is the indentation or *pitting* made on the skin by firm pressure maintained for a few seconds by the examiner's fingers or thumb. The pitting may persist for several minutes until it is obliterated by slow reaccumulation of the displaced fluid. So 'pitting on pressure' is a sign to detect subcutaneous oedema. Oedema may be generalized or local. *Generalized oedema* is often due to disorder of the heart, kidneys, liver, gut or diet. *Local edema* is more of surgical importance and may be due to venous or lymphatic obstruction, allergy or inflammation. Edema due to endocrine disorders particularly myxedema is also local oedema. Pretibial myxedema may be occasionally seen in thyrotoxicosis patients who are overzealously treated so that the patient is now symptom-free but presents with pretibial myxedema (myxedema in the subcutaneous tissue in front of the tibia) and probably persistent exophthalmos. The venous causes of edema have been well discussed in the chapter of 'Examination of varicose veins'. Localized edema from lymphatic causes has been described in the chapter of 'Examination of the lymphatic system'. Inflammatory causes are of main concern in surgical practice and in fact any inflammation starting from the bone to the skin causes edema of variable extent.

Causes of edema

Cause	Example condition	History taking questions
Cardiac	Congestive heart failure	"Do you experience shortness of breath or fatigue? Does swelling worsen at the end of the day?"
Renal	Nephrotic syndrome	"Have you noticed frothy urine or decreased urine output? Any history of kidney disease?"
Hepatic	Cirrhosis	"Do you have jaundice, abdominal swelling, or a history of alcohol use?"
Venous	Deep vein thrombosis (DVT)	"Do you feel pain or warmth in the swollen limb? Have you had prolonged immobility or recent surgery?"

CREPITUS

Two types of crepitus are seen in surgical cases—(1) **'Grating sensation'** in case of bone and joint pathologies and (2) **'Crackling sensation'** due to presence of air in the subcutaneous tissue. Various types of grating sensation *(crepitus)* which come across *in different bone and joint pathologies* are as follows:

Bone crepitus—can be heard when two fragments of a fracture are moved against each other. This examination has almost become obsolete as it induces pain and as facilities of X-ray examination are available almost in all rural health centers.

Joint crepitus—can be obtained when the affected joint is passively moved with one hand, while with the other hand placed on the joint is used to feel the crepitus. Joint crepitus are of three varieties—(i) *Fine crepitations* which are present in many subacute and chronic joint pathologies. (ii) *Irregular coarse crepitations* are detected in osteoarthritis. (iii) *'A click'* is a sign of loose body or displaced cartilage in the joint.

Crepitus of bursitis: This is occasionally heard when the lining of the bursa is rough or the fluid in the bursa contains small loose fibrinous particles.

Crepitus of tenosynovitis—is detected in a case of tenosynovitis, the typical example of which is De Quervain's disease at the lateral aspect of the wrist joint. The wrist joint is held tight and the patient is asked to open and close his fist, a crepitus is felt at the lateral aspect of the wrist joint just above radial styloid process at a point where the extensor pollicis brevis and abductor pollicis longus cross the extensor carpi radialis longus and brevis (*see* **Fig. 15.18**).

Crepitus of subcutaneous emphysema: In certain conditions a 'crackling sensation' is felt by the examining fingers due to presence of air in the subcutaneous tissue. If a stethoscope is placed over the area this crackling can be heard better. There are various causes which may give rise to subcutaneous emphysema (air bubbles in the subcutaneous tissue). These are as follows:

i. *Traumatic:* Fracture of ribs may injure the lung and air from the lung may extravasate into the subcutaneous tissue to cause subcutaneous emphysema. Fracture of nasal air sinus may cause subcutaneous emphysema of the face. Compressed air may perforate the thin bone at the apex of a tooth root in case of dental treatment allowing air to escape into the soft tissues. Similarly following tracheostomy such subcutaneous emphysema may be noticed.

ii. *Infective:* In gas gangrene subcutaneous crepitus is always detected.

iii. *Operative:* Air may become imprisoned during closure of an operative wound or traumatic wound. Subcutaneous crepitus from such condition may elude the surgeon to wrongly consider it to be due to gas gangrene.

iv. *Mediastinal emphysema* and later on subcutaneous emphysema of the neck, face and chest wall may complicate rupture of esophagus, *see* Chapter 31.

FECES

Examination of the feces is an important investigation, which is often ignored nowadays.

In all bowel disturbance cases, the stool should be examined.

Naked eye inspection: The following points should be noted—

1. ***The amount:*** Note whether the stool is copious or scanty and whether it is liquid or semiformed or formed or hard.

2. ***Color:*** Black stools are due to presence of hemorrhage in the intestine or due to ingestion of iron or bismuth. In case of hemorrhage high up in the intestine, the stools become dark, tarry-looking and offensive. *Pale-coloured stools* are due to failure of entrance of bile into the intestine, e.g., obstructive jaundice or due to rapid passage of stool through the intestine as in diarrhoea or due to abnormally high content of fat as in malabsorption syndrome or chronic pancreatitis.

3. ***Odor:*** Stools of jaundice are very offensive. The stools of acute bacillary dysentery are almost odorless, while those of amebic dysentery have a characteristic odor like that of semen.

4. *Abnormal stools*

i. **Slimy stools** are due to presence of excess of mucus and are often due to disorder of large bowel.

ii. **Purulent stools** are found in severe dysentery or ulcerative colitis.

iii. **Blood in stools** may be of different types—(a) *Bleeding from stomach and upper GI tract:* When blood comes from high in the intestinal tract, e.g., gastric ulcer or duodenal ulcer, the stools are black and tarry (sticky). This is known as **melaena**. The patients taking iron or bismuth also pass this type of stool but not sticky and are usually well formed. (b) Stools with dark red fragmented clots are seen *when there is bleeding in the small intestine,* e.g., from Meckel's diverticulum. But in case of massive gastroduodenal hemorrhage this type of stool may be found. (c) *When bleeding is from large intestine* the stools look dark red and jelly-like. (d) *Blood arising from rectum and anal canal:* In this case feces contain bright red blood either mixed or coating it

iv. **Steatorrhea:** The stools of steatorrhea are very large, pale, porridge-like and sometime frothy. These are apt to stick to the sides of lavatory pan and are difficult to flush away. This is also malodorous. Pancreatic insufficiency is the main cause, but there are also other causes which are described in the appropriate chapters.

v. **Pipestem stool:** This is seen in carcinomatous stricture of the rectum particularly in the annulus variety at the rectosigmoid junction.

vi. **Toothpaste stool:** This is occasionally seen in Hirschsprung's disease. The feces are expressed as toothpaste from a tube.

vii. **Meconium:** This is scanty, semiliquid, greenish black, odorless, sticky feces passed by newborn babies during first 3 days of life. After 7 days the stool becomes pale and putty-like in case of bottle-fed baby and thin yellow paste-type in case of breast-fed baby.

Types of stool

Type of stool	Clinical condition
black, Tarry (Melena)	Upper GI bleed (Peptic ulcer, varices)
Pale, Clay-colored	Biliary obstruction
Steatorrhea (Fatty stool)	Malabsorption syndromes (Pancreatic insufficiency)
Blood-streaked	Hemorrhoids, colorectal cancer

Algorithmic Approach to a Patient with Pain

Patient presents with pain

↓

Assess onset: Sudden or gradual?
- **Sudden:** Think **acute conditions** (e.g., appendicitis, myocardial infarction, perforated ulcer)
- **Gradual:** Consider **chronic conditions** (e.g., malignancies, chronic pancreatitis)

↓

Determine location: Localized or diffuse?
- **Localized pain:** Suggests a **specific organ involvement** (e.g., appendicitis → Right Iliac Fossa)
- **Diffuse pain:** Indicates **peritoneal irritation** (e.g., peritonitis, bowel obstruction)

↓

Assess nature of pain
- **Burning:** Peptic ulcer, GERD
- **Throbbing:** Abscess formation
- **Stabbing:** Perforated ulcer, pleurisy
- **Colicky:** Biliary colic, ureteric colic

↓

Check radiation: Is pain moving or referred?
- **Radiates to back:** Pancreatitis, AAA
- **Shoulder tip pain:** Diaphragmatic irritation (phrenic nerve)
- **Groin pain:** Ureteric colic

↓

Evaluate associated symptoms
- **Fever:** Infectious etiology (abscess, cholangitis)
- **Vomiting:** Obstruction, peritonitis
- **Jaundice:** Hepatobiliary pathology

↓

Consider exacerbating and relieving factors
- **Worsened by movement:** Peritonitis
- **Relieved by sitting up:** Pancreatitis
- **Relieved by antacids:** Peptic ulcer

↓

Narrow down likely diagnosis
Correlate history, examination, and pain pattern

↓

Order relevant investigations
- **Labs:** CBC, LFT, Amylase/Lipase, CRP
- **Imaging:** X-ray, Ultrasound, CT abdomen

↓

Confirm diagnosis and initiate treatment
- **Medical:** Pain relief, antibiotics, supportive care
- **Surgical:** Appendectomy, cholecystectomy, exploratory laparotomy

CHAPTER 3

Examination of a Lump or a Swelling

A '**Lump**' is a vague mass of body tissue.

A '**Swelling**' is a vague term which denotes any enlargement or protuberance in the body due to any cause. According to cause, a swelling may be *congenital, traumatic, inflammatory, neoplastic* or *miscellaneous*.

A '**Tumor**' or '**Neoplasm**' is a growth of new cells which proliferate independent of the need of the body. While *benign tumor* proliferates slowly with little evidence of mitosis and invasiveness to the surrounding tissues, *malignant tumor* proliferates fast with invasiveness and mitosis.

HISTORY: It is recorded as described in Chapter 1 with particular reference to the following points:

1. **Duration**: 'How long is the lump present there?' That means, you should ask the patient, 'When was the lump first noticed?' In case of congenital swellings, e.g., cystic hygroma, meningocele, sacrococcygeal teratoma **(Fig. 3.1)** they are likely to

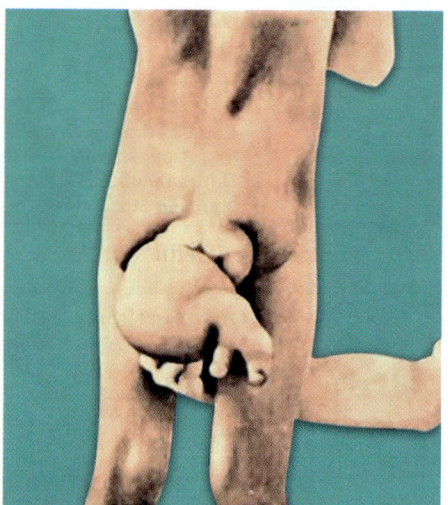

Fig. 3.1: Sacrococcygeal teratoma usually presents since birth. Rudimentary hand is seen in the tumor which develops from the totipotent cells.

be present since birth. One thing must be remembered that there is heaven and hell difference between 'The lump was first noticed two months ago' and 'The lump first appeared two months ago'. The former is the patient's finding and very often they feel its existence later than it actually appeared. A painless lump may be present for a long time without the patient's knowledge.

Lumps with shorter duration and pain are mostly inflammatory (acute), whereas those with longer duration and without pain are possibly neoplastic (benign). But the swellings with longer duration and with slight pain may be chronic inflammatory swellings whereas swellings with shorter duration may be neoplastic, mostly malignant.

2. **Mode of onset:** 'How did the swelling start'? It may have appeared just after a trauma (e.g., fractured displacement of the bone, dislocation of the joint or hematoma) or may have developed spontaneously and grown rapidly with severe pain (inflammation) or was noticed casually and the swelling was gradually increasing in size (neoplasm). Sometimes swelling may occur from pre-existing conditions, e.g., keloid may start from a scar of burn or otherwise **(Figs. 3.2A and 3.3)** or even from a pinprick in the ear **(Fig. 3.2B)**. Malignant melanoma generally develops from a benign naevus or a birthmark.

The neoplasms are mostly noticed casually and the patient says, 'I felt it during washing'. Or 'Someone else noticed it first and drew my attention.' These swellings are more dangerous and

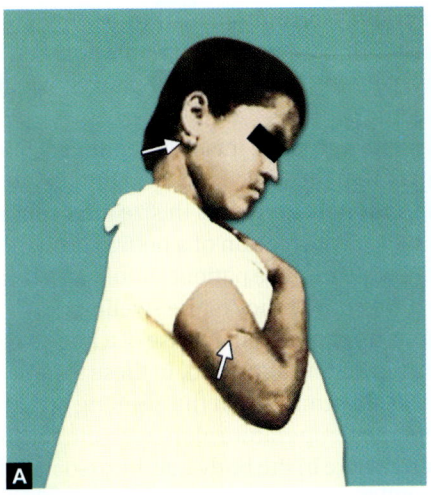 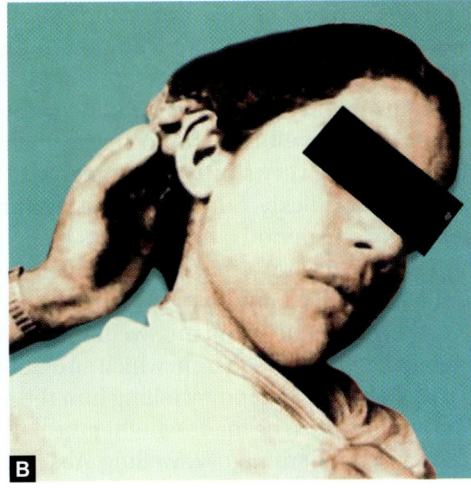

Figs. 3.2A and B: Keloids have developed in the scars of vaccination and ear pricks.

should invite more careful examination than those which are painful and mostly inflammatory or traumatic.

3. **Other symptoms associated with the lump:** PAIN is by far the most important symptom, which brings the patient to the doctor. Sometimes there may be other symptoms associated with the lump, such as difficulty in respiration, difficulty in swallowing, interfering with any movement, disfiguring, etc. The patient will definitely give the history of pain, but he may not give the history of other symptoms. So he must be asked relevant questions to find out if any symptom is associated with the lump.

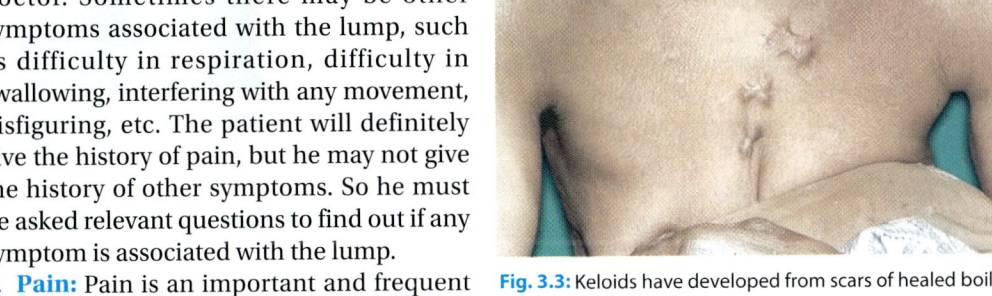

Fig. 3.3: Keloids have developed from scars of healed boils.

4. **Pain:** Pain is an important and frequent complaint of traumatic and inflammatory swellings, whereas pain is conspicuously absent in neoplastic swellings particularly in early stage. If the patient complains of pain associated with the lump, the surgeon should know precisely its nature, site and time of onset—whether appeared before the swelling or after it.

Nature of the pain: Whether the pain is throbbing which suggests inflammation leading to suppuration; or burning; or stabbing, i.e., the pain is sudden, sharp, severe and of short duration; or distending; or aching type.

Site: Sometimes the pain is referred to some other site than the affected one. As for example, in case of affection of the hip joint, the pain may be referred to the corresponding knee joint. But most often the pain is localized to the site of the swelling.

Time of onset: It is very important to know whether the pain preceded the swelling or the swelling preceded the pain. In the case of inflammation pain always appears before the swelling, but in case of tumors (both benign and malignant) swelling appears long before the patient will complain of pain. It cannot be impressed too strongly that *most malignant tumors be it in the* *stomach, kidney, rectum or breast, are painless to start with.* Pain only appears due to involvement of the nerves, deep infiltration, ulceration, fungation or associated inflammation and often indicates inoperability. The only exception is osteosarcoma in which mild pain is usually the first symptom and precedes the appearance of swelling.

5. **Progress of the swelling:** 'Has the lump changed its size since it was first noticed'? Benign growths grow in size very slowly and sometimes may remain static for a long time. Malignant tumors grow very quickly. Sometimes the swelling suddenly increases in size after remaining stationery for a long period—this suggests malignant transformation of a benign growth. If the swelling decreases in size—this suggests inflammatory lesion. The patient should also be asked whether he has noticed any change in the surface or in consistency of the swelling.

6. **Exact site:** Mostly the site of the swelling is obvious on inspection. In case of a huge swelling, the surgeon may be confused from which structure the swelling appeared. In these instances the patient may help the surgeon by telling him the exact site from which the swelling originated.

7. **Fever:** Enquiry must be made whether the patient ran temperature alongwith the swelling or not. This suggests inflammatory swelling. Abscess anywhere in the body may be associated with rise of body temperature—typical examples being axillary abscess, gluteal abscess, ischiorectal abscess, etc. Pyogenic lymphadenitis is often associated with fever. Sometimes Hodgkin's disease, renal carcinoma, etc., are also associated with peculiar fever.

8. **Presence of other lumps:** 'Whether the patient ever had or has any other lump'? Neurofibromatosis, diaphyseal aclasis, etc., will always have multiple swellings. Similarly, Hodgkin's disease generally shows multiple lymphoglandular enlargements **(Fig. 3.4)**. Abscesses may occur one after the other.

9. **Secondary changes:** Some swellings present secondary changes such as softening, ulceration, fungation, inflammatory changes, etc. The patients should be asked for the secondary changes specifically.

10. **Impairment of function**—particularly of the limb or spine may be associated with a swelling near about. Enquire about the nature of loss of movement and intensity of it and how much of it is due to the swelling. An osteosarcoma near knee joint may cause partial or total loss of knee movement. Similarly, a cold abscess from caries spine will cause limitation of movement of the spine.

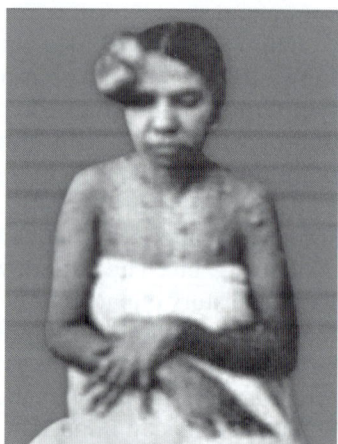

Fig. 3.4: Multiple swellings of neurofibromatosis (Von Recklinghausen's disease).

11. **Recurrence of the swelling:** If the swelling recurs after removal, this often indicates malignant change in a benign growth or the primary tumor was a malignant one. Certain other swellings are notoriously known to recur, e.g., Paget's recurrent fibroid. Cystic swelling may recur if the cyst wall is *not completely* removed.

12. **Loss of body weight:** Appearance of swelling may be associated with loss of body weight. This indicates that the swelling may be either a malignant growth or a cold abscess with generalized tuberculosis.

13. **Past history:** This may reveal presence of similar swelling or recurrence of swelling. Past history of syphilis or tuberculosis may offer clue to the present swelling.

14. **Personal history:** Habit of eating betel leaf, betel nut, slaked lime or tobacco, may be the etiological factor for growth in the mouth, tongue, cheek or lip. 'Chutta Cancer' of hard palate

is seen in women who smoke cigars with the burning ends in their mouths. 'Khaini Cancer' occurs due to mixture of lime and tobacco kept in the gingivolabial sulcus.

15. **Family history:** This is quite important, as many diseases have familial incidence. Tuberculosis, Von Recklinghausen's disease, many malignant tumors often recur among family members.

History in cases of lump or swelling

Aspect	Clinical significance	Key history taking questions
Duration	Short-duration lumps are often **inflammatory**, while long-duration lumps are **neoplastic**.	"When did you first notice the lump?" "Has it changed in size over time?"
Mode of onset	Sudden-onset lumps suggest **trauma or inflammation**; gradual-onset lumps suggest **neoplasia**.	"Did the lump appear suddenly or gradually?" "Was there any injury before it appeared?"
Pain	Painful lumps are **often inflammatory**; painless lumps may be benign or **malignant**.	"Is the lump painful?" "If yes, what is the nature of the pain?"
Growth pattern	Rapid growth suggests **malignancy or inflammatory processes**.	"Has the lump grown in size recently?"
Secondary changes	Ulceration, fungation, and discharge indicate **possible malignancy**.	"Have you noticed any changes in the lump, such as redness, ulceration, or pus?"
Family history	Some conditions, like **neurofibromatosis or malignancies, run in families**.	"Has anyone in your family had similar lumps or cancers?"

PHYSICAL EXAMINATION

GENERAL SURVEY: When a patient presents with a swelling, the patient should be looked at as a whole. Cachexia or malnutrition may be obvious in first look. The attitude of the patient is also very important. Abnormal attitude may be either due to a swelling like osteosarcoma pressing on the nerve leading to paresis or paralysis of the distal limb or the swelling may be a displaced fracture or dislocation and the limb assumes abnormal attitude due to that. Raised temperature and pulse rate are always associated with inflammatory swelling.

Examination of lump or swelling

Exam step	Findings and interpretation	Clinical example
Inspection	Look for **size, shape, color, pulsation, movement**.	Black color → **melanoma**; pulsatile → **aneurysm**.
Palpation	Assess **temperature, tenderness, consistency, mobility, fluctuation, transillumination**.	Hard, irregular, fixed lump → **malignancy**; fluctuant lump → **abscess/cyst**.
Percussion	Identify resonance or dullness over the swelling.	Resonant swelling → **hernia**; dull swelling → **solid tumor**.
Auscultation	Listen for bruits over vascular swellings.	Bruit heard → **arteriovenous malformation or aneurysm**.

LOCAL EXAMINATION

A. **INSPECTION:** It must be remembered that a good clinician always spends some time in observation. The students should make it a practice and should not hasten to touch the swelling as soon as he sees it.

In *inspection* the following points should be precisely noticed:

1. **Situation:** A few swellings are peculiar in their positions such as dermoid cysts are mostly seen in the midline of the body or on the line of fusion of embryonic processes, e.g., at the outer canthus of the eye—that means on the line of fusion between the frontonasal process and the maxillary process **(Fig. 3.5)** or behind the ear **(Fig. 3.6)** (post-auricular dermoid)— on the line of fusion of the mesodermal hillocks which form the pinna. Extragonal germ cell tumors like sacrococcygeal teratoma **(Fig. 3.7)** are also typically seen in midline (tail bone). It can also be anywhere on body like keloid formation due to abscess **(Fig. 3.8)**.

One must always note the extent of the swelling in vertical and horizontal directions on the case note.

2. **Color:** Color of the swelling sometimes gives a definite hint to the diagnosis. Black color of benign nevus and melanoma, red or purple color of hemangioma **(Fig. 3.47)** (according to whether it is an arterial or venous hemangioma), bluish color of ranula are obvious and diagnostic.

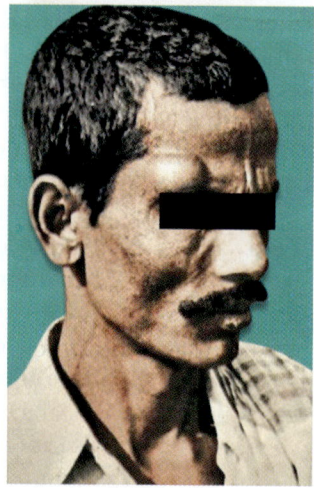

Fig. 3.5: Shows the typical site of the dermoid cyst at the outer canthus of the eye.

3. **Shape:** The shape of the swelling must be noted—whether it is ovoid, pear-shaped, kidney-shaped, spherical or irregular. Sometimes the students, by mistake, utter the term 'circular' to describe the shape of the swelling. A swelling cannot be circular as we do not know about the deeper dimension of the swelling. So, it is wiser to say 'spherical' to describe this swelling.

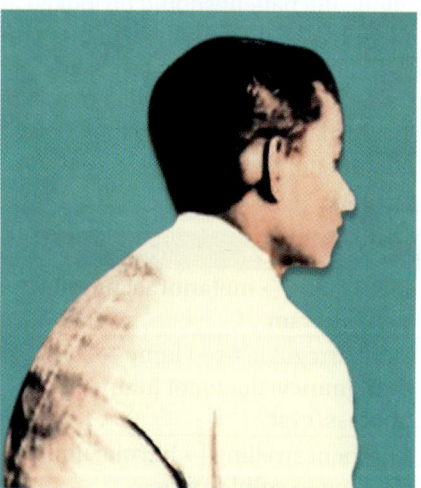

Fig. 3.6: Postauricular dermoid.

4. **Size:** To have firsthand knowledge about the swelling, one must know the size of the swelling. On inspection, we shall miss the deeper dimension, but shall have the other two dimensions. These must be mentioned clearly in your history sheet the vertical and horizontal dimensions.

5. **Surface:** On inspection, it may be difficult to have a clear idea about the surface of the swelling. But in certain swellings, the surface may be very much obvious and diagnostic, e.g., irregular numerous branched surface of a papilloma **(Fig. 3.9)**, cauliflower surface of squamous cell carcinoma **(Fig. 3.10)**, etc.

6. **Edge:** The edge of the swelling may be clearly defined or indistinct. The swelling may be pedunculated or sessile.

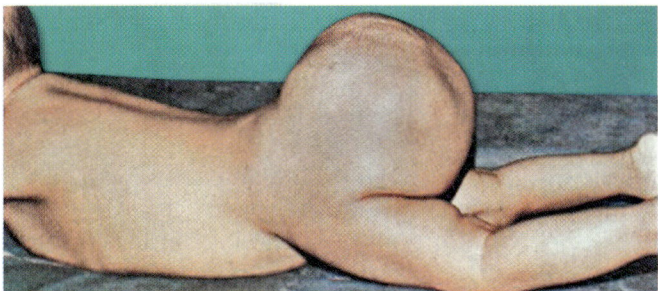

Fig. 3.7: A case of sacrococcygeal teratoma.

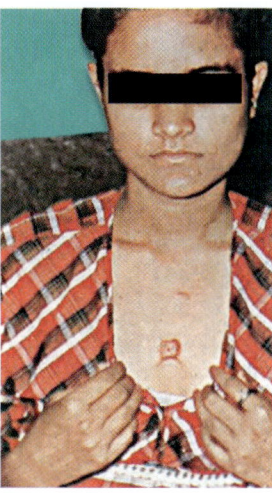

7. **Number:** This is important as this may give a clue to the diagnosis. Some swellings are always multiple, such as diaphyseal aclasis, neurofibromatosis, multiple glandular swellings, etc. Some swellings are more known to be solitary, e.g., lipoma, dermoid cyst, etc.

Fig. 3.8: A case of keloid in its typical position over the chest wall following a small abscess.

8. **Pulsation:** The swellings, arising from the arteries, are pulsatile, e.g., aneurysms and vascular growths, such as carotid body tumor. The swellings, which lie just superficial to the artery in close relation with it, will be pulsatile. This pulsation is called *transmitted pulsation*, whereas those which originate from the arterial walls give rise to *expansile pulsation*.

9. **Peristalsis:** Certain swellings are associated with visible peristalsis, e.g., congenital hypertrophic pyloric stenosis. A few swellings cause intestinal obstruction and thus show visible peristalsis.

10. **Movement with respiration:** Certain swellings arising from the upper abdominal viscera move with respiration, e.g., those arising from liver, spleen, stomach, gallbladder, hepatic and splenic flexures of the transverse colon.

11. **Impulse on coughing:** The swellings, which are in continuity with the abdominal cavity, the pleural cavity, the spinal canal or the cranial cavity, will give rise to impulse on coughing.

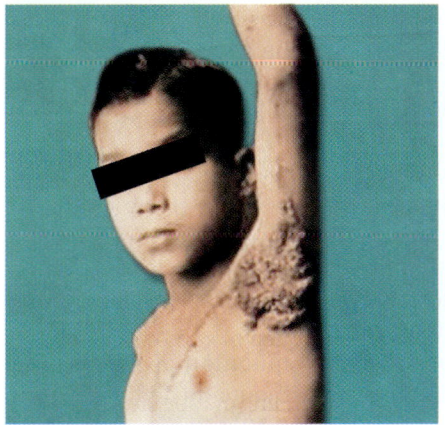

Fig. 3.9: Papilloma.

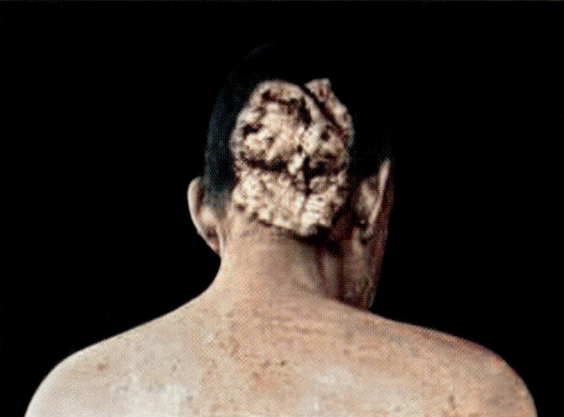

Fig. 3.10: Cauliflower surface of squamous cell carcinoma.

The patient is asked to cough and the swelling will be seen giving rise to an impulse while the patient is coughing. In case of children, crying will work as coughing.

12. **Movement on deglutition:** A few swellings which are fixed to the larynx or trachea move during deglutition, e.g., thyroid swellings, thyroglossal cysts, subhyoid bursitis and pre-or paratracheal lymph node enlargement.

13. **Movement with protrusion of the tongue:** A thyroglossal cyst moves up along with protrusion of the tongue showing its intimate relation with the thyroglossal tract.

14. **Skin over the swelling:** This will be *red and edematous*, where the swelling is an inflammatory one. The skin becomes *tense, glossy with venous prominence*, where the swelling is a sarcoma with rapid growth. Presence of a *black punctum* over a cutaneous swelling indicates sebaceous cyst. *Pigmentation* of the skin is seen in moles, nevi or after repeated exposures to deep X-rays. *Presence of scar* indicates either previous operation (when the scar is a linear one with suture marks), injury (a regular scar) or previous suppuration (when the scar is puckered, broad and irregular). Sometimes the skin over a growth looks like the peel of an orange—*Peau d' orange* **(Fig. 30.9)** which is due to edematous swelling from blockage of small lymphatics draining the skin. This is most peculiarly seen in breast carcinoma. Presence of *ulcer* on the skin over the swelling is examined as discussed in the next Chapter.

15. **Any pressure effect:** It is always essential to conclude the inspection by examining the limb distal to the swelling. In many cases this will give suggestion as to what may be the diagnosis. An axillary swelling with edema of the upper limb means the swelling is probably arising from the lymph nodes. Wasting of the distal limb indicates the swelling to be a traumatic one and the wasting is due to either nonuse of the limb or due to injury to the nerves **(Fig. 3.11)**. Sometimes a swelling may be seen in the neck with venous engorgement. This should immediately give rise to suspicion of possibility of retrosternal prolongation of the swelling, giving rise to venous obstruction.

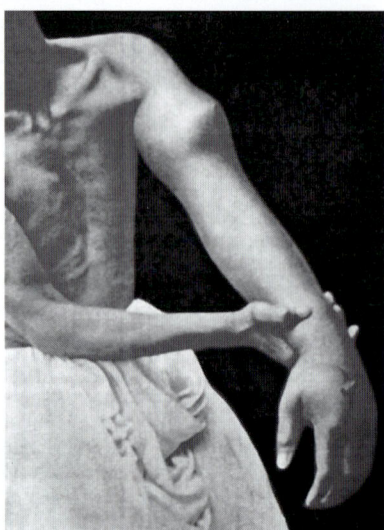

Fig. 3.11: Sarcoma of the left humerus interfering with venous return of the upper limb leading to excessive edema and wrist drop from nerve involvement.

B. PALPATION: This is the most important part of local examination which will not only corroborate the findings of inspection, but also will explore some other findings, which will give a definite clue to the diagnosis. The students must be very methodical in this examination and follow a definite order, which is given below, so that they would not miss any important examination. The students should also be very gentle in palpation not to hurt the patients and a few swellings may be malignant and may well spread into the system due to reckless handling.

1. **Temperature:** Local temperature is raised due to excessive vascularity of the swelling. It may be due to infection or due to well-vascularized tumor (e.g., sarcoma).

This examination should be done first in palpation, as manipulation of the swelling during subsequent examinations may increase the temperature without any definite reason. *Temperature of the swelling is best felt by the back of the fingers* **(Fig. 3.12)**.

2. **Tenderness:** It must be remembered that this is a sign, which is elicited by the clinician. When the patient complains of pain due to the pressure exerted by the clinician, the swelling

is said to be 'tender'. To elicit tenderness, one should be very gentle and should not give too much pain to the patient. It is a good practice to keep an eye on the patient's facial expression while palpating the swelling to note whether this is giving rise to pain or not. Inflammatory swellings are mostly tender, whereas neoplastic swellings are not tender.

3. **Size, shape and extent:** By palpation, one can have an idea about the deeper dimension of the swelling, which remains unknown in inspection. The vertical and horizontal dimensions of the swelling are also better clarified by palpation. It is a good practice to mention in cm the vertical and horizontal diameters and should be sketched on the history sheet clearly indicating the *position* of the swelling as well.

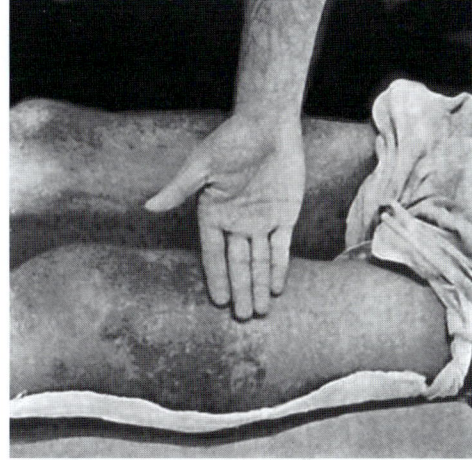

Fig. 3.12: Showing how to feel for local temperature with the back of the fingers which is more sensitive than the palmar surface.

The clinician should always try to find out the whole extent of the swelling. If a portion of the swelling disappears behind a bone, it should be clearly mentioned and its importance cannot be too impressed to the students.

4. **Surface:** With the palmar surfaces of the fingers, the clinician should palpate the surface of the swelling to its entirety. The surface of a swelling may be smooth (cyst), lobular with smooth bumps (lipoma), nodular (a mass of matted lymph nodes) or irregular and rough (carcinoma). Sometimes the surface of the lump may be varied according to variable consistency.

5. **Edge:** Very carefully, the edge or margin of the swelling is palpated **(Fig. 3.13)**. It may be well-defined or indistinct—merging imperceptibly into the surrounding structures. Broadly speaking, neoplastic swellings and chronic inflammatory swellings have well-defined margins. Benign growths generally have smooth margins whereas malignant growths have irregular margins. Acute inflammatory swellings have ill-defined or indistinct margins.

The margins are palpated by the tips of the fingers. Swellings with well-defined margins tend to slip away from the finger. Benign tumor such as lipoma is often confusing with a cyst. The benign tumor has a smooth margin, so has a cyst. The most important finding, which differentiates benign tumor like lipoma from the cyst is that the margin of the former slips

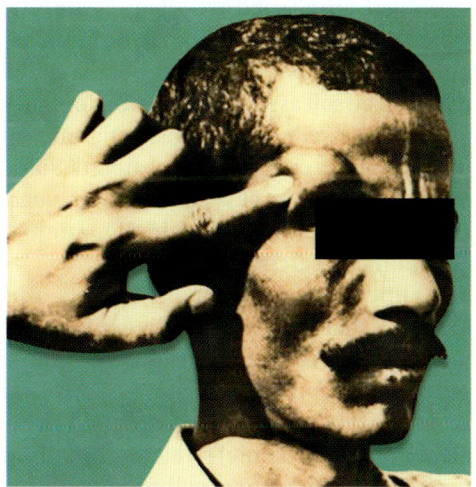

Fig. 3.13: Shows how to feel the margin of a swelling. The margin of a cyst yields to the palpating finger and does not slip away (cf. lipoma).

away from the palpating finger, but does not yield to it, whereas the margin of the latter yields to the palpating fingers and cannot slip away from the examining finger (Slip sign in **Figs. 3.14A and B**).

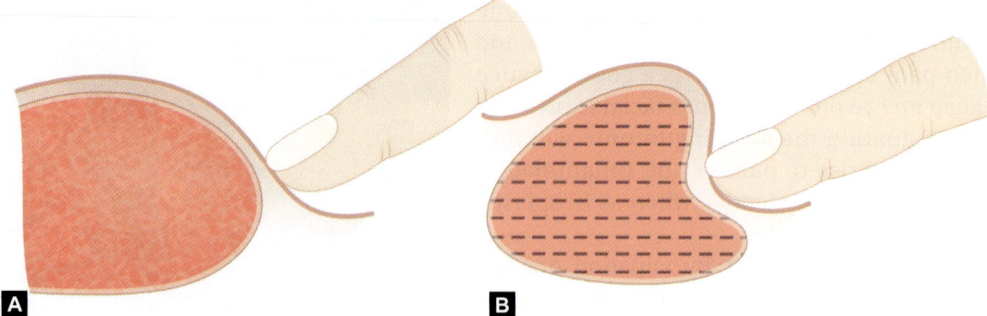

Figs. 3.14A and B: Slip sign: When the edge of a swelling is palpated, the margin of the solid swelling does not yield to the palpating finger but slips away from it; but in case of a cystic swelling the edge yields to the pressure of the palpating finger and does not slip away.

6. **Consistency:** The consistency of a lump may vary from very soft to very hard. It depends on what it is made up of (**Fig. 3.15**). When the swelling is of *UNIFORM consistency*, it gives a clue as to which anatomical structure it is derived from. It may be *soft*, e.g., lipoma; *cystic*, e.g., cysts and chronic abscesses; *firm*, e.g., fibroma; *hard* but yielding, e.g., chondroma, *bony hard*, e.g., osteoma or *stony hard*, e.g., carcinoma. The consistencies, just described, are all solid except the cystic one, which contains liquid within it. It should be borne in mind that consistency of a solid swelling may also be soft as seen in case of a lipoma. In case of gaseous swellings, e.g., gas gangrene, surgical emphysema, a *crepitus* may be heard. Sometimes the swelling may be of *VARIABLE consistency*. This variability often indicates malignancy—either carcinoma or sarcoma.

While palpating for consistency, one must look for whether the swelling is getting molded or not to pressure. It indicates that the content is a pultaceous or putty-like material. So, the swelling must be a sebaceous cyst or a dermoid cyst or even an abdominal (colonic) swelling containing fecal mass. Sometimes the swelling *pits on pressure*. This means that there is edematous tissue and most often the swelling is an inflammatory one.

7. **Fluctuation:** A swelling fluctuates, when it contains liquid or gas. This test should be carried out by one finger of each hand (**Fig. 3.16**). Sudden pressure is applied on one pole of the swelling.

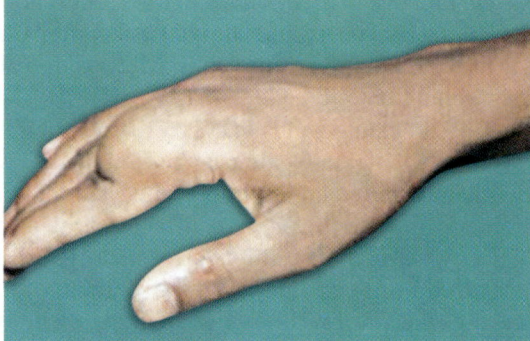

Fig. 3.15: Implantation dermoid at the dorsum of the left hand near the web between the index and the middle fingers.

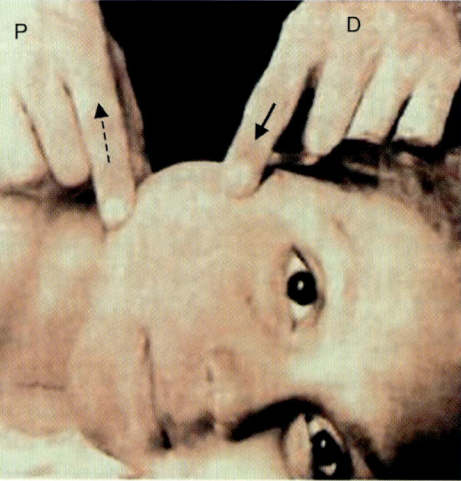

Fig. 3.16: Correct method of eliciting fluctuation. The fingers of the hand 'P' will remain passive and perceive the movement of the fluid displaced by the finger of the hand 'D'.

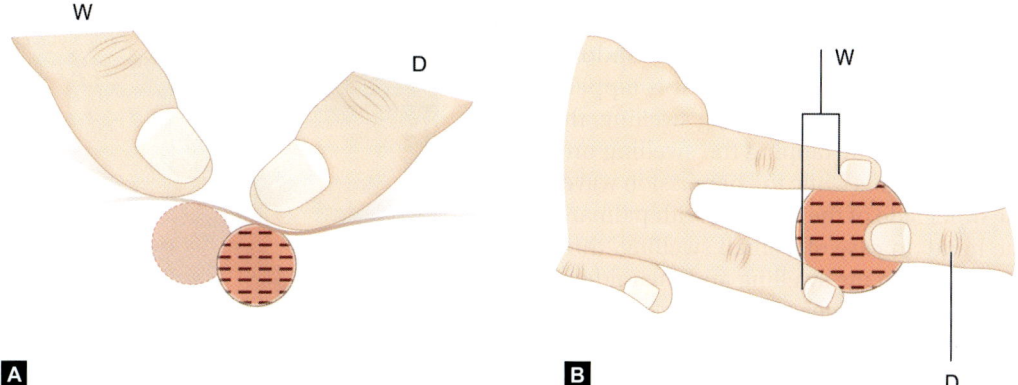

Figs. 3.17A and B: Shows the method of eliciting fluctuation in case of a small swelling. (A) shows how a small swelling may be displaced as a whole by the displacing finger (D) and it shifts towards the watching finger (W) to elicit a false sense of fluctuation even when the swelling is a solid one. (B) the correct method of eliciting fluctuation in case of a small swelling. Two fingers of the left hand (watching fingers 'W') are placed on two sides of the swelling and the index finger of the right hand (displacing finger 'D') is pressed on the swelling to displace the fluid within the swelling.

This will increase pressure within the cavity of the swelling and will be transmitted equally at right angles to all parts of its wall. If another finger of the other hand is placed on the opposite pole of the swelling, the finger will be raised passively due to increased pressure within the swelling. This means that the swelling is fluctuating **(Fig. 3.17A)**.

(i) *This test should always be performed in two planes at right angles to each other*. A fleshy muscle (e.g., quadriceps femoris) sometimes shows fluctuation at right angle to its fibers, but not along the line of its fibers. (ii) *The two fingers should be kept as far apart as the size of the swelling will allow*. (iii) In case of the *swelling, which is freely movable*, it should be held fixed with the thumb and forefinger of one hand, while the swelling is compressed on the other pole by the thumb and fingers of the other hand. The thumb and fore-finger, which have been used to fix the swelling, will feel increase of pressure within the swelling passively. Very often fluctuation is elicited in this manner in case of hydrocele. (iv) In case of *very small swelling*, which cannot accommodate two fingers, this test can be performed by simply pressing the swelling at its center. The swelling containing fluid, will be softer at the center than its periphery, while a solid swelling will be firmer at the center than its periphery. This test is known as **Paget's test** **(Fig. 3.17B)**. Another method is to keep two fingers of the left hand on the swelling so as to fix it and are called 'watching fingers'. Right index finger is used ('displacing finger') to press on the swelling to displace fluid inside the swelling which is felt by the 'watching fingers'. This test should be done in two planes at right angles to one another as the conventional method. The students should not try to perform traditional fluctuation test on a small swelling, as pressure exerted by one finger, will simply displace the swelling and fluctuation test cannot be performed. (v) *For very large swelling* more than one finger of each hand are used. Two or even three fingers may be used for providing pressure (displacing fingers) and palmar aspect of four fingers of the other hand may be used to perceive the movement of displaced fluid (watching fingers). (vi) *Very soft swellings sometimes yield false positive sense in fluctuation test.* The swellings which can be included in this list are: lipoma, myxoma, soft fibroma, vascular sarcoma, etc. But if the students become careful while performing the fluctuation test, they will easily realize that these swellings yield to pressure, but fail to expand in other parts of the swelling like a true fluctuant swelling.

8. **Fluid thrill:** In case of a swelling containing fluid, a percussion wave is seen to be conducted to its other poles when one pole of it is tapped as done in percussion. In case of a big swelling, this can be demonstrated by tapping the swelling on one side with two fingers while the percussion wave is felt on the other side of the swelling with palmar aspect of the hand. In case of a small swelling, three fingers are placed on the swelling and the middle finger is tapped with a finger of the other hand (as done in percussion), the percussion wave is felt by other two fingers on each side.

9. **Translucency:** This means that the swelling can transmit light through it **(Fig. 3.18)**. For this, it must contain clear fluid, e.g., water, serum, lymph, plasma or highly refractile fat. A swelling may be fluctuant as it contains fluid, but may not be translucent when it contains opaque fluid, such as blood or pultaceous

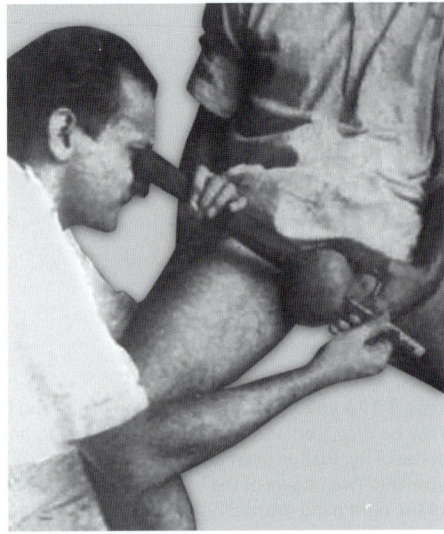

Fig. 3.18: Testing for translucency.

material (dermoid or sebaceous cyst). To carry out this test, darkness is essential. In day time, this can be achieved by a roll of paper, which is held on one side of the swelling, while a torch light is held on the other side of the swelling. The swelling will be seen to transmit the light, if it is a translucent swelling. The torch light should not be kept on the surface of the swelling, but on one side of the swelling, while the roll of paper on the other side so that the whole swelling intervenes between the light and the roll of paper. This will eliminate the possibility of false positive results.

10. **Impulse on coughing:** In palpation, this test corroborates the finding detected in inspection. The swellings, which are likely to give rise to impulse on coughing, are: (i) those, which are in continuity with the abdominal cavity (e.g., herniae, iliopsoas and lumbar abscesses), (ii) those, which are in continuity with the pleural cavity (e.g., empyema necessitatis) and (iii) those, which are in continuity with the spinal canal or cranial cavity (spinal or cranial meningocele).

The swelling is grasped and the patient is asked to cough. An impulse is felt by the grasping hand. Due to coughing, pressure is increased within the abdominal, pleural, spinal and cranial cavities. This increase in pressure is transmitted to the swelling, where the impulse is felt. *In case of children, this examination is performed when they cry* **(Figs. 3.19A and B)**.

11. **Reducibility:** This means that the swelling reduces and ultimately disappears when it is pressed upon. This is a feature of hernia. Lymph, varix, varicocele, saphena varix, meningocele, etc., are also reducible partly or completely.

12. **Compressibility:** In contradistinction to reducibility, compressibility means the swelling can be compressed, *but would not be disappeared completely*. The compressible swellings may not have connections with the abdominal, pleural, spinal or cranial cavity. These swellings are liquid-filled and are mostly vascular malformations, e.g., arterial, capillary or venous hemangiomas **(Fig. 3.20)**. Lymphangiomas are also compressible. The most important differentiating feature between a compressible swelling and a reducible swelling is that in case of the latter, the swelling completely disappears as the contents are displaced into the cavities from where they have come out and may not come back until and unless an opposite force, such as coughing or gravity

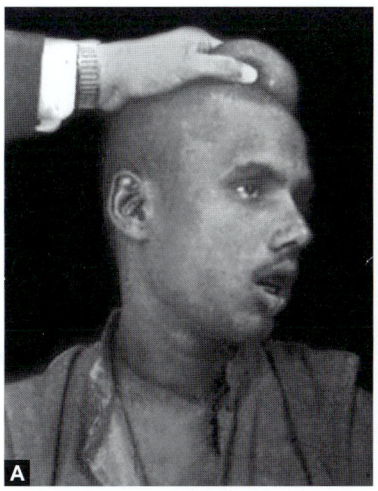
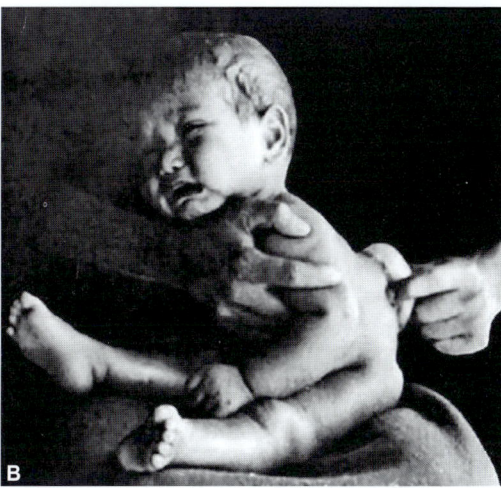

Figs. 3.19A and B: Note how to examine for impulse on coughing in case of an adult and a child.

is applied. But in case of the former, the contents are not actually displaced, *so the swelling immediately reappears* as soon as the pressure is taken off.

13. **Pulsatility:** A swelling may be pulsatile (i) if it arises from an artery (expansile pulsation), (ii) if it lies very close to an artery (transmitted pulsation) or (iii) if the swelling is a very vascular one (telangiectatic sarcoma). It is very easy to detect whether a swelling is pulsatile or not, yet the students miss this test and land up with great disaster (an aneurysm is sometimes incised by mistake considering it to be an abscess).

Two fingers, one from each hand, are placed on the swelling as far apart as possible **(Fig. 3.21)**. If the two fingers are raised with each throb of the artery, the swelling is a pulsatile one. When the two fingers are *not only raised, but also separated* with each beat of the artery, the pulsation is said to be an '**expansile**' one. When the two fingers are only raised, but *not separated*, the pulsation is said to be '**transmitted**'. In case of pulsatile swelling of the abdomen, the patient is placed in the knee-elbow position to determine whether it is an aneurysm of the abdominal aorta or a tumor lying in front of the abdominal aorta (transmitted pulsation). In case of the latter in this position pulsation ceases **(Figs. 3.22A and B)**.

14. **Fixity to the overlying skin:** The swellings, which originate from the skin (e.g., papilloma, epithelioma, sebaceous cyst, etc.) will be obviously fixed to the skin.

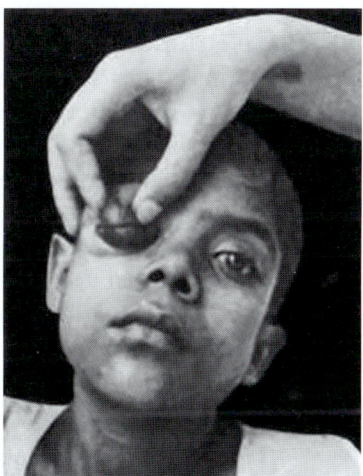

Fig. 3.20: Testing for compressibility in case of hemangioma of the upper eyelid.

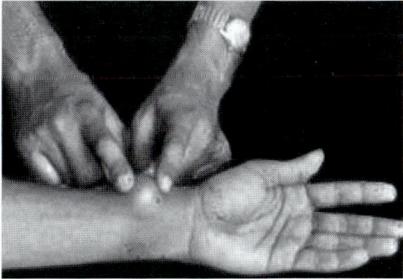

Fig. 3.21: Demonstration whether the pulsation is expansile or transmitted in nature.

They will invariably move along with the skin unless they are fixed to underlying structures by malignant infiltration (e.g., epithelioma).

In case of the subjacent swellings, the students should learn how to know whether the swelling is attached to the skin or not. For this, one can do one of the following tests: (i) The skin is made to move over the swelling. If it is fixed to the skin, the skin will not move. (ii) The skin over the swelling is pinched up in different parts. When the skin is not fixed, it can be easily pinched up, which may not be possible when the swelling is fixed to the skin.

15. Relations to surrounding structures: Clinically, the students should try to make out firstly the structure from which the swelling is originating and secondly whether the swelling is confined to its original structure or has invaded the other structures.

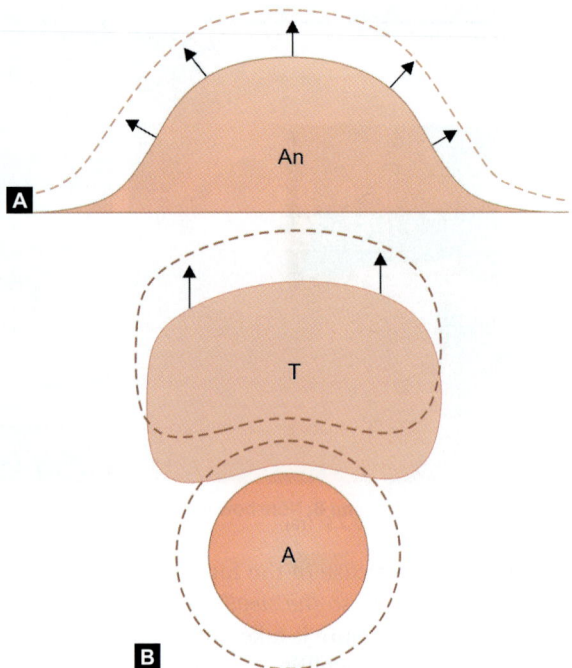

Figs. 3.22A and B: Diagnostic representation of expansile and transmitted pulsation. 'An' is aneurysm & 'A' is an artery. 'T' is the tumor. See the text.

The tumors, arising from the **subcutaneous tissue**, are free from the overlying skin and from the underlying *contracted* muscle. If a lipoma is pushed sideways, the skin will be seen puckering in some places over the tumor. This is due to the presence of some fibrous strands, extending from the capsule of the tumor to the overlying skin. The students often mistake in finding out whether the tumor is fixed to the underlying structure or not. Even if the tumor is fixed to the underlying deep fascia and muscle, the tumor can be moved sideways. But *if the underlying muscle is made taut*, the tumor cannot be moved if it is fixed to the muscle.

The tumors, arising from **the deep fascia**, will not be as mobile as those arising from the subcutaneous tissue. But it is very difficult to find out whether the tumor is fixed to the deep fascia or not as this fascia cannot be made taut apart from the muscle.

In case of the tumors arising from the **muscle**, the swelling can be moved with the muscle relaxed. To know that the tumor is fixed to the muscle, the patient should be asked to carry out such movement *against resistance* to throw the particular muscle into contraction. When the tumor is arising from overlying subcutaneous tissue, but is fixed to the muscle, the tumor will be *more prominent* and *cannot be moved along the line of the muscle fibers*. If the tumor is incorporated in the muscle, it will be fixed and *its size will be diminished* as soon as the muscle becomes taut. If the tumor lies deep to the muscle, it will *virtually disappear*, as soon as the muscle becomes taut.

Sometimes a swelling becomes evident only when the muscle contracts. This is due to *tear in the muscle or in the tendon* concerned.

Chapter 3: Examination of a Lump or a Swelling   39

HOW TO MAKE A MUSCLE TAUT BY PUTTING IT INTO CONTRACTION AGAINST RESISTANCE (FIGS. 3.23 TO 3.29)

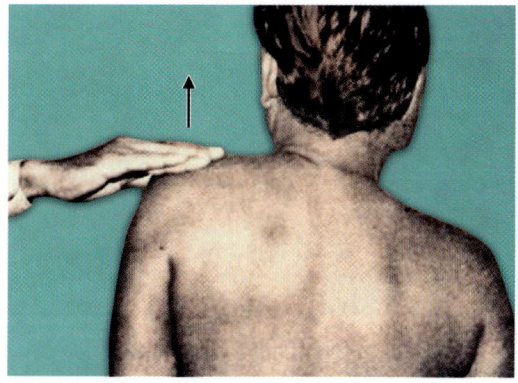

Fig. 3.23: Trapezius.

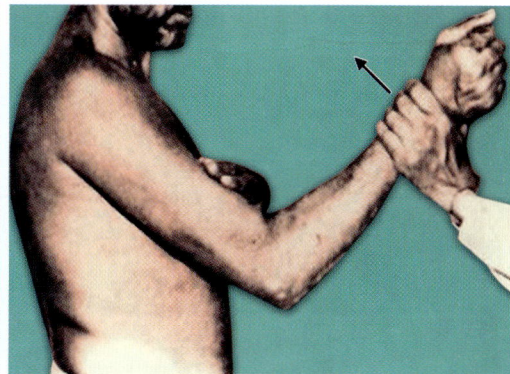

Fig. 3.26: Biceps brachii.

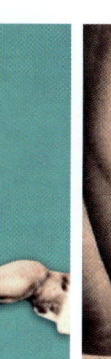

Fig. 3.24: Latissimus dorsi.

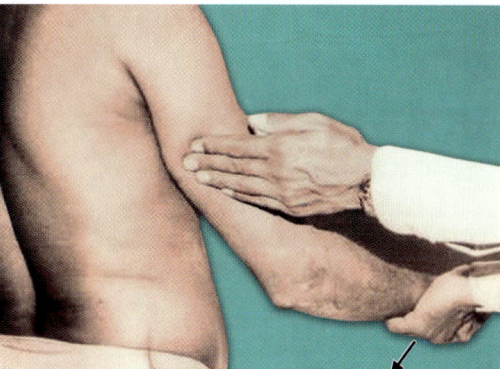

Fig. 3.27: Triceps.

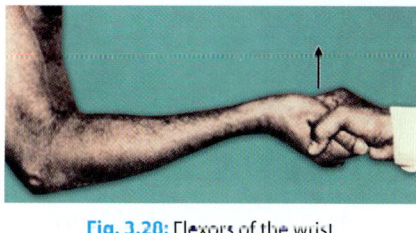

Fig. 3.28: Flexors of the wrist.

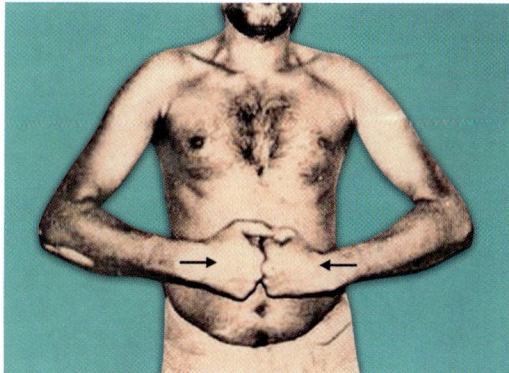

Fig. 3.25: Pectoralis major.

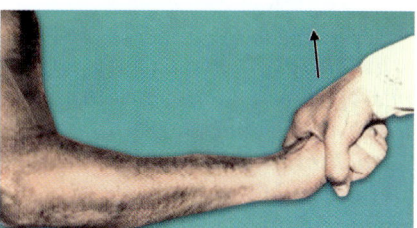

Fig. 3.29: Extensors of the wrist.

HOW TO MAKE A MUSCLE TAUT BY PUTTING IT INTO CONTRACTION AGAINST RESISTANCE (FIGS. 3.30 TO 3.36)

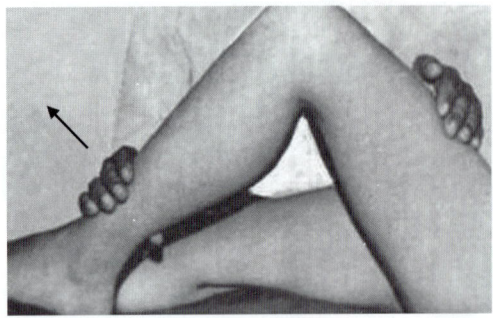

Fig. 3.30: Quadriceps femoris.

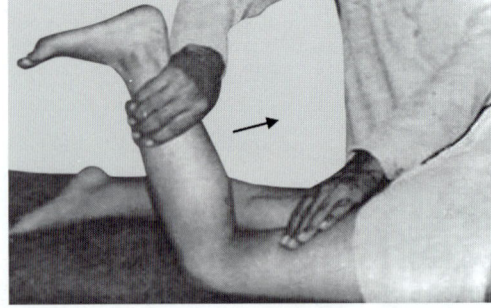

Fig. 3.33: The Hamstrings.

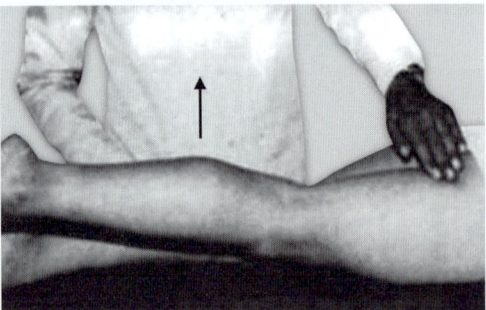

Fig. 3.31: Gluteus maximus.

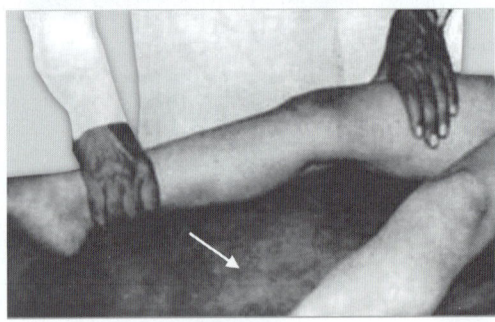

Fig. 3.34: Adductors of the thigh.

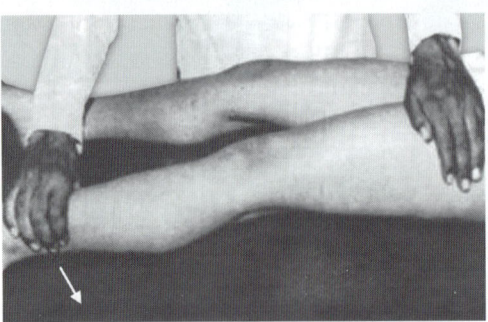

Fig. 3.32: Gluteus medius.

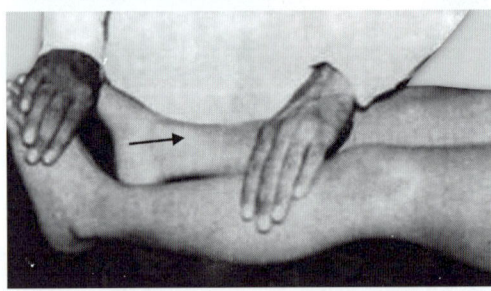

Fig. 3.35: Extensors of the ankle.

See the chapter of "Examination of Peripheral Nerve Lesions" for the actions of Trapezius, the Deltoid, the Serratus anterior and Brachioradialis and the chapter of "Examination of the Neck" for that of the Sternomastoid muscle. Any other muscle can be tested in the same way.

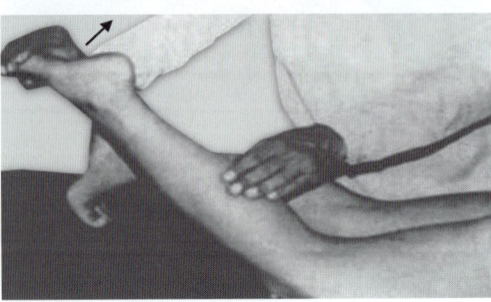

Fig. 3.36: Flexors of the ankle.

Swelling in connection with the tendon of a muscle moves along with **the tendon** and becomes fixed when the muscle is made taut against resistance **(Figs. 3.37 and 3.38)**.

Swellings, in connection with **the vessels** and **the nerves**, do not move along the line of the said vessel or the nerve but moves to a little extent at right angles to their axes.

Swelling in connection with a **bone**, is absolutely fixed even when the overlying muscle is absolutely relaxed and cannot be moved apart from the bone.

C. STATE OF THE REGIONAL LYMPH NODES: It cannot be impressed too strongly that no examination of a swelling is complete without the examination of the draining lymph nodes. The students should have knowledge of anatomy to find out which group of lymph nodes drain the particular area from which the tumor is originating. When the regional lymph nodes are enlarged, it is a good practice to examine the other groups of lymph nodes to exclude generalized lymphadenopathy.

D. PERCUSSION: The importance of this examination is not much in case of a swelling. Its sole place is to find out the presence of a gaseous content within the swelling, e.g., resonant note over a hernia; or to elicit slight tenderness, e.g., Brodie's abscess.

Hydatid thrill is a special sign in case of a hydatid cyst. The index, middle and ring fingers of the left hand are placed on the surface of the swelling so that the middle finger rests on the dome of the swelling and the other two fingers as placed as far apart as the size of the swelling will permit. The right middle finger is used to percussion the left middle finger and a sensation of thrill is felt by the other two fingers. This is due to displacement of the daughter cysts in the fluid of the mother cyst and then strike back the wall of the mother cyst to produce the typical 'hydatid thrill'.

E. AUSCULTATION: All pulsatile swellings should be auscultated to exclude presence of any bruits **(Fig. 3.39)** or murmurs. 'Machinery murmur' is heard in an aneurysmal varix.

F. MEASUREMENTS: This is important not only to find out increase in swelling at definite intervals, but also to find out if there is any wasting distal to the swelling.

G. MOVEMENTS: In case of a swelling, the students must not forget to examine the movements of the nearby

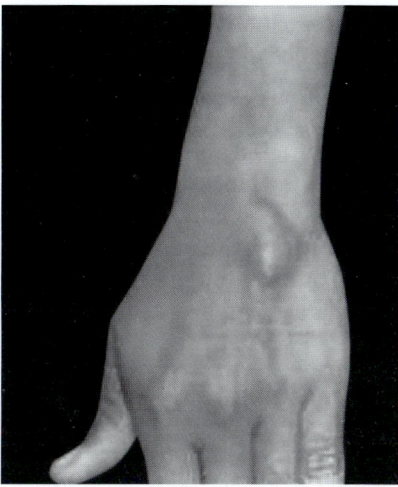

Fig. 3.37: Shows how the swelling in connection with the tendon moves along with the tendon.

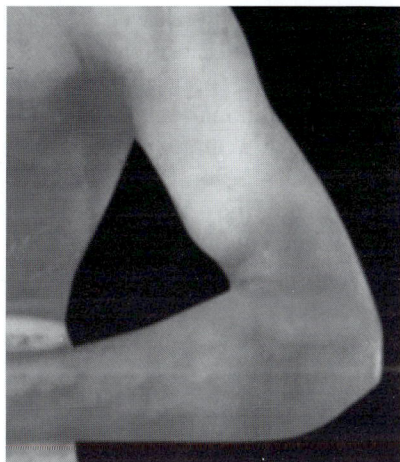

Fig. 3.38: Rupture of the long tendon of the biceps.

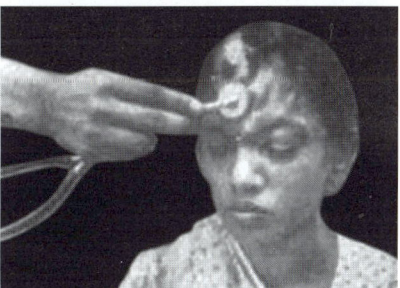

Fig. 3.39: Auscultating for a machinery murmur in an extensive cirsoid aneurysm.

joint to exclude any impairment. This should be noted in the history sheet and is of particular importance to find out if the swelling has involved the joint or not.

H. EXAMINATION FOR PRESSURE EFFECT: Swellings will inevitably exert pressure on the surrounding structures. Its effect must be noted by the following examinations:

(i) The arterial pulse distal to the swelling is felt. Sometimes the swelling may *press on the main artery* of the limb and causes weak pulse distally.

(ii) The *nerves may be affected* by the pressure of the swelling. This will cause wasting, paresis or paralysis of the muscles supplied by the nerve with or without sensory disturbances.

(iii) The swelling may even exert its pressure on the subjacent bone by eroding it. This is sometimes seen in aneurysm and dermoid cyst on the skull.

GENERAL EXAMINATION

It is very much tempting while examining a swelling to do all with the swelling and forget about the rest of the body. This will lead to innumerable misdiagnoses. So one must examine the patient as a whole.

In case of malignant swelling, the importance of general examination is well established. This will give an idea about the site of metastasis, if any. An enquiry should be made about cough, hemoptysis or pain in the chest for pulmonary metastasis. The *chest* should be examined very carefully for presence of consolidation and pleural effusion. *Liver* should always be examined as this may be the organ affected by metastasis. General examination of the *abdomen* should be carried out to exclude the possibility of peritoneal metastasis. The *spine*, the *pelvis*, the *trochanters of the femurs*, the *skull* should be examined to exclude bony metastasis **(Fig. 3.40)**.

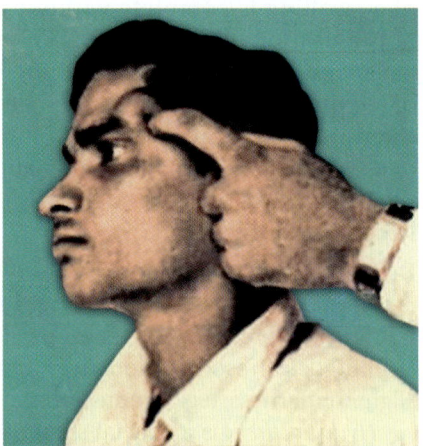

Fig. 3.40: Feeling for erosion of the skull in case of a dermoid cyst.

If the swelling is suspected to be a gumma or a condyloma, the patient should be examined generally to find out *other syphilitic stigmas* (*see* **Fig. 4.15**).

In case of lymph node enlargement, one should always examine the *other groups of lymph nodes* to find out the cause of lymphoglandular enlargement.

SPECIAL INVESTIGATIONS

1. Examination of the blood for total count (TC), differential count (DC), hemoglobin (Hb%), erythrocyte sedimentation rate (ESR) and sugar are very much informatory so far as the diagnosis of a swelling is concerned. Inflammatory swellings will obviously show leukocytosis (increased total count) and increased number of polymorphs in differential count. Chronic inflammatory swellings and malignant swellings will show increased ESR and low hemoglobin percentage (anemia). In case of recurrent abscesses and carbuncles, one should not forget to do the sugar estimation of the blood. Many a case of diabetes mellitus will be revealed through this test.

In case of syphilis, WC or Kahn test or complement fixation test of the serum is very important.

2. **In urine,** estimation of sugar is very important in case of recurrent abscesses and carbuncles to find out if the patient is suffering from diabetes.
3. **Aspiration** and examination of the aspirated material physically, chemically, microscopically and bacteriologically are very important in case of chronic cystic swellings.
4. **Fine needle aspiration biopsy (FNAB) or fine needle aspiration cytology (FNAC):** These investigations are often used nowadays to avoid extensive operation of open biopsy. A fine needle (of 22 or 23 gauge) fitted with a tight fitting syringe is used for this technique. The tissue aspirated is examined microscopically, chemically and bacteriologically. For cytology the cellular suspension obtained by aspiration is smeared on a slide. It is dried, fixed with absolute alcohol and stained with Papanicolaou technique.

    Exfoliative cytology—has little scope in case of a swelling. In this technique the cells shed from the tumor located in a hollow viscus is taken out and examined under microscope, stained (Papanicolaou) and unstained. This technique is particularly applied in case of GI tumors, respiratory tract tumors (sputum or through endoscope), urinary bladder (through endoscope) and female genital tract.
5. **X-ray** examination is indispensable in case of bony swellings and to find out if the subjacent bone has been eroded by an aneurysm or a dermoid cyst.

    Chest X-ray should be taken when pulmonary metastasis is to be excluded in case of a malignant growth.
6. **Skin test:** (a) **Tuberculin test**—if positive in infants and young children suggests tuberculous lesion. If this test is negative in adult, it can straightway exclude possibility of tuberculous origin of the swelling. (b) **Casoni's test** becomes positive in case of a hydatid cyst; but a negative result cannot exclude hydatid cyst.
7. **Ultrasonography:** This is a simple, inexpensive, non-invasive and safe technique. It produces mechanical vibrations at a high frequency which is imperceptible to human ear. These are detected by transducer and can measure depth and dimensions of various structures within the body. This technique is based on principle of reflection of sound waves of high frequency at the junction of different tissue levels in the body. The reflected echoes are converted in the transducer into small electrical changes. Images commonly are displayed on a television monitor as an electronic representation of the returning echoes. One dimensional or A-mode scan provides histogram of echo intensity along the line of tissue examined. In two dimensional or B-mode scan the morphologic structures are portrayed in two dimensions as the transducer can be moved in transverse, longitudinal or oblique directions. In 1974 Gray-scale imaging was introduced which renders varying echo intensities, as differing shades of gray with increased amount of information. Real-time imaging is a further step ahead in technology and provides more information. As ionizing radiation is not used, it is particularly safe and can be used in children and pregnant women.

    It is particularly used to determine whether a mass is solid or cystic.
8. **Computed tomography (CT scan):** This technique provides unique two-dimensional representation of differing radiographic densities throughout a cross-sectional volume of tissue. It avoids the confusing superimposition of organs and accurately records small variation in tissue density. Its limitations are its complexity and great expense. Radiation burden may become significant necessitating careful application. As the part of the body is evaluated in thin tomographic section many images may be required to completely evaluate large anatomic regions like abdomen. The whole body scan can be obtained through a series of transverse sections by gradually moving the body through a ring of tubes and detectors.

It provides more accuracy than that of ultrasonography in assessment of any growth, e.g., its size, shape, local spread and general dissemination. It helps in exact anatomical localization of deep seated masses even in obese individuals.

Three-Dimensional CT scan (3D CT scan)—is now available which provides three-dimensional picture of the structure or organ of the body. It is also possible with the help of the computer to resect or deduct a portion of the structure to get better view of the interior of the particular structure. In **Figure 3.41** a complete 3D CT scan of the cervical vertebrae with fracture-dislocation is shown and in **Figures 3.42A and B** a sagittal section of the same vertebrae are shown to see the inside of the spinal canal and to know how much it has been reduced by the fracture-dislocation which might have caused damage to the spinal cord.

9. **Magnetic resonance imaging (MRI) or nuclear magnetic resonance (NMR):** This is the latest and most potentially dramatic efficient diagnostic armamentarium. These images are derived from radiowaves emitted by protons, which when exposed to a magnetic field, can be excited by absorption of energy from radiofrequency pulses. Most protons in the body, are within water molecules and their properties differ from tissue to tissue, thus potentially making it possible to image a variety of structures in the body. For more details students are referred to page no. 564 of the same author's 'A Concise Textbook of Surgery'.

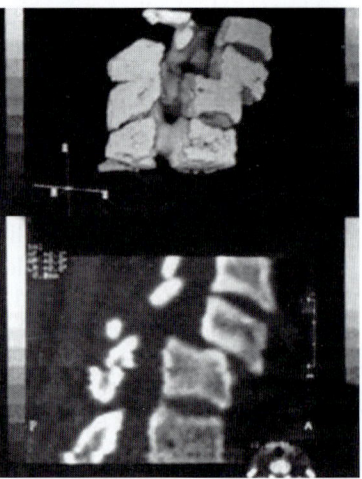

Fig. 3.41: The upper picture is a three dimensional CT Scan which shows fracture dislocation of cervical vertebra. Whereas the lower figure shows simple CT scan of the same case.

It provides a fine demonstration of soft tissues and bones for greater clarity of any swelling thereabout **(Fig. 3.43)**.

It is now *possible to use a contrast medium* for magnetic resonance tomography. The contrast medium used is known as Magnevist which is especially made for magnetic resonance tomography (MRT) and it is well tolerated by the body. It is eliminated from the body almost completely within 24 hours. Such contrast medium is mostly used in cranial and spinal MRT. After injection of Magnevist, the resulting opacification of areas with dysfunction of the blood-

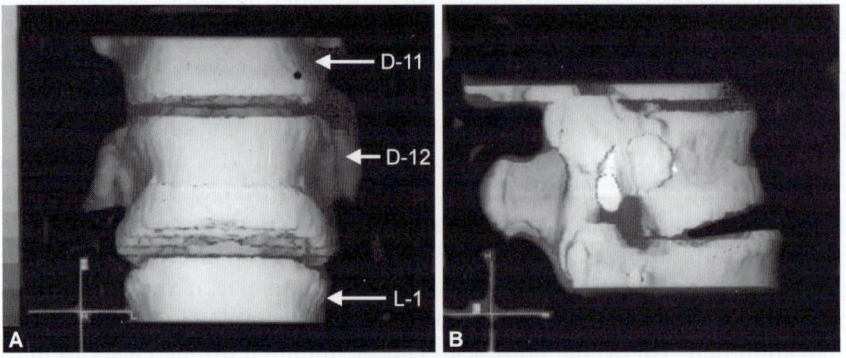

Figs. 3.42A and B: Shows AP and lateral views of three dimensional CT scan of a case of collapsed fracture of vertebra (D12).

brain barrier (e.g., glioblastoma) and of other intracranial and intraspinal lesions of noncerebral origin provides diagnostic information additional to that obtainable with a plain scan. The patient is to fast for 2 hours before the examination. The safety rules customary for MRI must be observed, e.g., exclusion of cardiac pacemakers and ferromagnetic implants. The dose required is administered intravenously as a bolus injection. The *contrast-enhanced* MRT (**Fig. 3.44**) is commenced immediately afterwards though optimal opacification is generally achieved within a period of about 45 minutes after the injection of Magnevist. In general, administration of 0.2 mL. Magnevist per kg body weight is sufficient for good opacification.

10. **Angiography:** For a few swellings this investigation is of value. For all aneurysmal swellings this investigation is a must. This investigation is also of value in differentiating a cyst from a tumor. In case of malignant tumor this investigation may show abnormal disposition of small arteries in and around the tumor as also the 'contrast pool' inside the tumor which is significant.

11. **Biopsy** is by far the most important investigation of a swelling. This is particularly done in case of suspected malignant tumors. The biopsy is generally taken from the margin of the tumor. The risk of spread of malignancy from biopsy is more theoretical than practical. There are various methods of biopsy:

a. **Needle biopsy:** In this method a hollow needle is introduced into the swelling and a core of tissue is taken out for histological examination. Various types of needles have been used for various organ swellings, e.g., Vim Silvermann needle for liver, Travenol Tru-cut needle for prostate through the perineum.

b. **Drill biopsy:** It is performed by an apparatus consisting of a small sharp cannula within which is attached a high speed compressor air drill. This is claimed to be better than needle biopsy and has been mostly used in case of breast lumps. The core of tissue obtained by this method is now examined for histopathological report. Accuracy has been claimed to the tune of more than 90% in case of breast lumps.

c. **Punch biopsy:** This method is more often used in case of tumor for hollow viscera or solid viscera. With punch biopsy forceps pieces of tissue are taken from the *margin* of the tumor along with surrounding normal tissue or from the *base* of the tumor. Typical four quadrant biopsy is taken from a big ulcer of the stomach.

d. **Open biopsy:** This is performed by operation. After getting access to the tumor a slice of tissue (incisional biopsy) or the whole of the tumor (excisional biopsy) is excised and then histopathological examination of the tumor is performed.

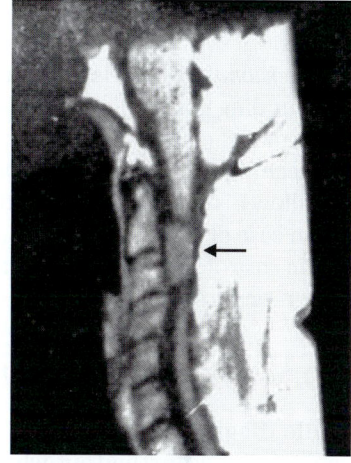

Fig. 3.43: MRI shows tumor of the spinal cord shown by arrow.

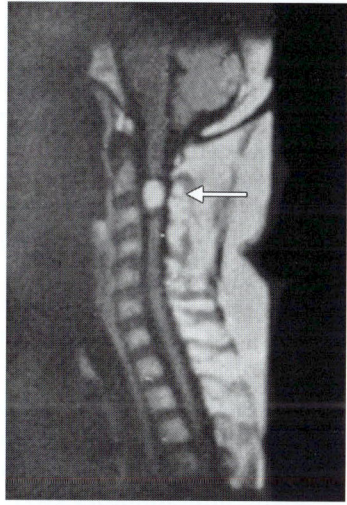

Fig. 3.44: MRI with contrast medium shows how clearly the spinal cord tumor can be delineated (shown by arrow).

Incisional biopsy—has the theoretical disadvantage of spreading the tumor to the adjoining tissues.

Excisional biopsy—is safe and better. It is done by excising the tumor with a margin of healthy surrounding tissue in case of malignant growth. But in case of confirmed benign tumors only the tumor is excised. It is better, as malignant change in a benign growth may be detected by this technique. The whole tumor can be examined histopathologically. It is also safe as it does not allow dissemination of the tumor. Whenever possible excisional biopsy should be carried out in case of suspected tumors.

12. In case of suspected malignant tumors, the patient should be **followed up** to find out if the tumor recurs or not.

DIAGNOSIS OF A SWELLING

While diagnosing a swelling, the clinician should first find out, whether the particular swelling is originating from—the *skin*, the *subcutaneous tissue*, the *muscles*, the *vessel*, the *nerve* or *bone* and secondly, the cause of the swelling—whether it is a *congenital, traumatic, inflammatory, neoplastic or otherwise*.

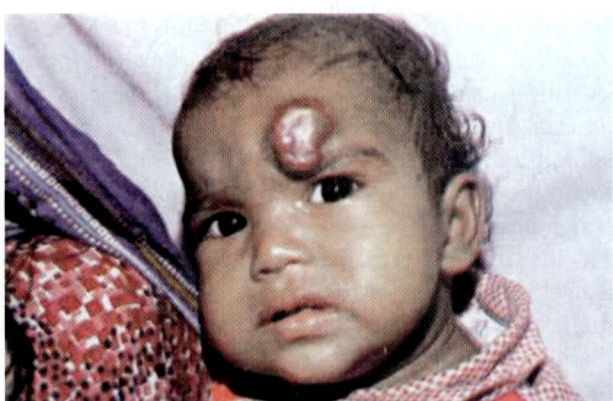

Fig. 3.45: Cavernous hemangioma on the face.

1. **Congenital** swellings are generally present since birth, e.g., hemangioma **(Fig. 3.45)**, cystic hygroma, meningocele, etc. A few swellings in this group may not appear since birth, but will make their appearance later in life, e.g., branchial cyst, dermoid cyst, thyroglossal cyst, etc.

2. **Traumatic** swellings develop immediately after a trauma, e.g., hematoma, fracture with displacement, dislocation, rupture of a muscle, etc.

3. **Inflammatory** swellings may be either of *acute* variety or *chronic* variety.

Acute inflammatory swellings present with redness (rubor), pain (dolor), heat (calor), swelling (tumor) and impairment of function (Functio laesa). Of these five signs and symptoms stress must be given to pain, redness and heat. Not infrequently a few rapidly growing sarcomas, e.g., osteosarcoma may mimic an acute inflammatory swelling with pain (which appears even before the swelling), redness, swelling, heat, etc. Probably *the differentiating features* in favor of acute inflammatory swelling which one should look for are tenderness, brawny induration and edema. Presence of fluctuation means presence of pus, which indicates that the swelling is an inflammatory one. Moreover, the related lymph nodes will be affected and will show signs of acute lymphadenitis. Though slight rise of body temperature is not unusual in sarcoma yet it is never of the hectic type, which may be noted in acute inflammation. Leukocytosis is a constant feature of acute inflammation, which may or may not be present in sarcoma.

Chronic inflammatory swellings will show the same signs and symptoms as the acute inflammatory swellings but in very much subdued form. In this case, swelling is more than the other features like pain, redness, heat, etc. Brawny induration and edema are conspicuous by their absence. So, at times it becomes rather difficult to differentiate chronic inflammatory swellings from malignancy. There may be slight rise of temperature, which may be associated with slight tenderness and fixity in a rapidly growing malignant growth. *The most important differentiating feature* is the history of occasional diminution in the size of the swelling, which goes in favor of an inflammatory swelling. A tumor always increases in size either rapidly or very slowly. It may even remain stationary for a long time but *never recedes*.

4. **Neoplastic** swellings may be either benign or malignant.

Benign tumors grow slowly, are encapsulated, move freely (fibroadenoma of the breast—better known as 'Breast Mouse'), hardly infiltrate the surrounding tissues and never metastasize either to the regional lymph nodes or to the distant organs. These tumors may undergo secondary changes of which malignant transformation seems to be the most common. **Malignant tumors** may be either carcinomas which arise from epithelial cells or sarcomas which originate from the connective tissues. As a rule, malignant tumors are notoriously known for their rapid growth and metastasis—either to the regional lymph nodes or to distant organs. Secondary changes such as ulceration and degeneration may be noticed in malignant growths. The students should always keep in mind that *pain is conspicuous by its absence* in malignant growths, barring osteosarcomas where pain precedes the swelling. Though too much importance cannot be given to the age of the patient, yet the students should know that the carcinoma affects the old and the sarcomas affect the young commonly.

Characteristics of benign and malignant growths:

Benign	Malignant
occurs at younger age.	Seen usually above 40 years of age, but may occur at younger age.
Symptoms	
1. Duration: Slow growth	1. Rapid growth
2. Pain: Usually absent	2. May be painful at late stage, barring osteosarcoma which is painful from the beginning
3. Loss of weight: Never seen	3. A feature of malignant growth
4. Loss of function: Usually not seen	4. Seen quite early

Benign	Malignant
signs	
1. Cachexia, anemia and loss of weight: Usually absent	1. Usually present
2. Mobility: Freely mobile	2. Fixed early due to infiltration
3. Surface: Usually smooth	3. Usually irregular
4. Margin: Definite and smooth	4. Not definite and irregular
5. Consistency: Usually firm	5. Either hard or of varying consistency.
6. Pressure effects: Usually absent	6. Often present
7. Regional lymph nodes: Not enlarged	7. Early involved and enlarged
8. Distant metastasis: Almost never seen	8. A feature of malignant growth—a late feature

Contd...

Contd...

Benign	Malignant
9. Secondary changes: Not seen	9. Often come across
10. Recurrence: Never recurs after excision	10. Often recurs after excision
Histology	
1. Cell differentiation: A feature of benign growth	1. Cells are usually undifferentiated
2. Polarity: Cells are arranged as parent tissue	2. Polarity is lost
3. Capsule: Always encapsulated	3. No capsule formation as local infiltration is the rule
4. Anaplasia: Not seen	4. A feature of malignant growth.
5. Nuclear structure: Same as the parent tissue without mitosis	5. Nucleus becomes larger, hyperchromatic with mitosis

It may so happen that a tumor may be benign to start with, but may undergo malignant transformation at some stage. The **malignant transformation** is recognized by—(i) Sudden increase in the size of the swelling; (ii) Increase in vascularity of the tumor with rise of local temperature; (iii) Fixity of the tumor and infiltration of the surrounding tissues, e.g., involvement of the facial nerve in case of a parotid tumor, or malignant change in a thyroid lobule is suspected when a patient complains of hoarseness of voice (due to involvement of recurrent laryngeal nerve) or dyspnea (due to involvement of the trachea) or dysphagia (due to involvement of esophagus); (iv) Secondary changes in the tumor either in the form of increase in pigmentation (e.g., malignant melanoma), ulceration and bleeding; (v) Appearance of pain, which is a late feature of malignant disease; (vi) Involvement of regional nodes; (vii) Appearance of distant metastasis.

In the differential diagnosis I shall only discuss the swellings arising from the *skin* and the *subcutaneous tissues*. The swellings originating from the muscle, tendon sheath, the vessel, the nerve or the bone are discussed in the appropriate chapters.

DIFFERENTIAL DIAGNOSIS

■ CONGENITAL

1. **DERMOID CYST (Sequestration dermoid):** This cyst generally develops in the line of embryonic fusion. So this cyst may appear anywhere in the midline of the body as also in places where the two embryonic processes meet each other, e.g., at the outer angle of the orbit **(Fig. 3.5)** (where the frontonasal process and the maxillary process fuse with each other), behind the pinna **(Fig. 3.6)** (postauricular dermoid), just below the tongue in the midline (sublingual dermoid), etc.

The characteristic features of the swelling will be similar to those of a cyst. There will be presence of fluctuation but translucency will be absent due to the presence of pultaceous material inside the cyst. The swelling is round and smooth and the margin will yield to the pressure of the finger and will not slip away (cf. lipoma). The swelling will be free from the skin and from the deeper structures. When the underlying structure is a bone an indentation in the bone may be felt at the margin of the swelling **(Fig. 3.40)**. Dermoid cyst in the scalp may be: (a) fully outside the skull bones or (b) outside the skull but attached to the duramater through defect in the skull or (c) partly extracranial and partly intracranial connected with a stalk or (d) fully intracranial lying between the skull and the dura (rarest). Sequestration dermoid never elicits impulse on coughing except the rare (e) type which occasionally may elicit impulse on coughing.

TUBULO DERMOID and **TERATOMATOUS DERMOID** are described in the same author's 'A Concise Textbook of Surgery' page 80 and are out of scope here.

Implantation or acquired dermoid (Figs. 3.46 and 3.15): It is *not a congenital swelling* in the true sense, but it is described here as it is included in the category of the dermoid cyst. It is actually a traumatic swelling and results from the surface ectoderm being driven into the subjacent tissue. So, the origin is more or less like a dermoid cyst but it is always a sequel of trauma. This is commonly seen in a finger or a hand from a needle prick or a prick with a thorn.

2. **HEMANGIOMAS:** These are vascular malformations or hamartomas and may arise from the capillary or the vein or the artery and accordingly called a capillary hemangioma or cavernous hemangioma or a plexiform (cirsoid) hemangioma respectively.

a. **Capillary hemangiomas (Figs. 3.47 and 3.48A)**—are bright red or purple colored patches of varying sizes. These are generally flat and not much raised above the skin surface. Pressure may cause complete disappearance or diminution of the color which returns immediately when the pressure is released. There are six varieties of capillary hemangioma which are well-known in surgical practice:

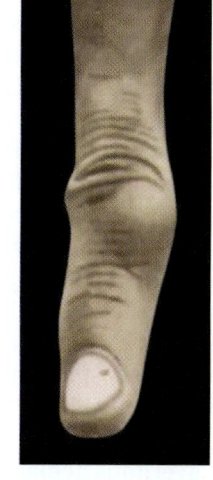

Fig. 3.46: Implantation dermoid in the middle finger.

(i) *Port-wine stain* is a diffuse telangiectasia with practically no swelling **(Fig. 3.48B)**.

(ii) *Salmon patch* is usually present since birth and often seen in the forehead or on the occiput. It usually disappears before first birthday.

(iii) *Spider nevus* has a central red spot with numerous radiating fine blood vessels like the legs of a spider. It is often seen over manubrium sterni. Spider nevus is often multiple and tend to increase in number over the years. It is mostly seen on the upper half of the trunk, face and arms. Spider nevi do not cause any change of skin temperature and are not tender. These fade completely when compressed with the finger and refill as soon as the pressure is released. Sometimes it may be acquired from a generalized disease like liver cirrhosis, tumors destroying the liver and tumors producing estrogen **(Fig. 3.48C)**.

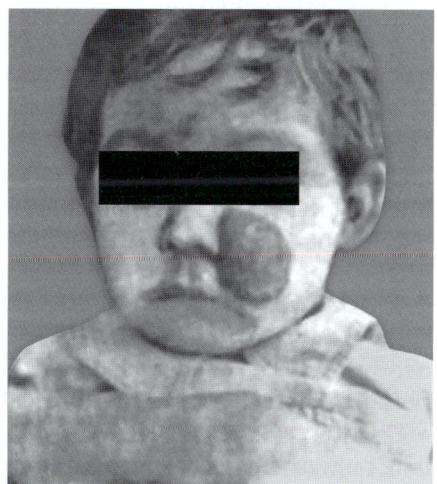

Fig. 3.47: Strawberry hemangioma (capillary hemangioma) of the cheek.

(iv) *Vin rose patch:* It is a congenital condition causing mild dilatation of intradermal subpapillary plexus giving rise to pale pink color to the skin. This can occur anywhere without any symptom. It is often associated with other vascular abnormalities, e.g., extensive hemangiomata, giant limb due to arteriovenous fistula and/or lymphoedema.

(v) **Campbell de Morgan spot:** This is caused by dilated capillaries fed by a single or cluster of arterioles giving rise to a bright red spot. It is about 1-3 mm in diameter. The cause is unknown. This condition is rarely seen in people less than 45 years of age. These appear suddenly one at a time, but gradually may become multiple often affecting one area of skin. These are symptomless. These are seen on both aspects of trunk, more on the upper half than the lower. Occasionally, may be seen on the limbs and almost unseen on the face. These are usually circular and have a sharp edge which may be raised. Important feature is that though these are collection of dilated capillaries, these are not totally compressible, but always fade.

(vi) **Strawberry angioma** is a sessile lobulated circumscribed swelling. Its surface looks like a strawberry. These generally appear at birth and often regress spontaneously a few months or years after birth. Incidence of multiple strawberry nevi is not unknown.

b. **Cavernous hemangioma (Fig. 3.49)**—is a bigger hemangioma than the preceding one. It consists of dilated spaces containing blood and gives rise to soft spongy bluish swelling, which is compressible and can be emptied by pressure but reappears on release of pressure. Common occurrence is seen in the lips, cheeks, face **(Fig. 3.45)**, brain, etc. It is interesting to know that surface hemangiomas are often associated with similar affection in the internal organs, e.g., hemangiomas of the face may be associated with hemangiomas of the brain on the same side. So, once hemangioma is discovered, all possible sites should be searched.

c. **Plexiform hemangioma**—is nothing but a network of dilated interwoven arteries like a bag of pulsating earth worms (**CIRSOID ANEURYSM—Fig. 3.50**).

d. **Congenital arteriovenous fistula**—is the result of persistence of congenital communication between the arteries and veins affecting the extremities usually. The diagnosis is made by warm limb, enlargement of the limb, localized bruit over the fistula, presence of varicose veins and insufficiency of the distal circulation. Acquired arteriovenous fistula may appear following trauma or may be created surgically for hemodialysis.

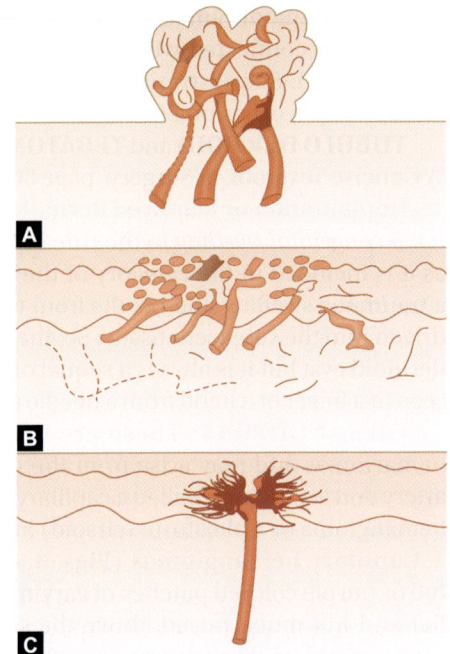

Figs. 3.48A to C: A schematic diagram to show: (A) Strawberry nevus; (B) Port-wine stain, which is a collection of dilated intradermal capillaries; (C) Spider nevus, in which there are visible radiating branches from a single arteriole.

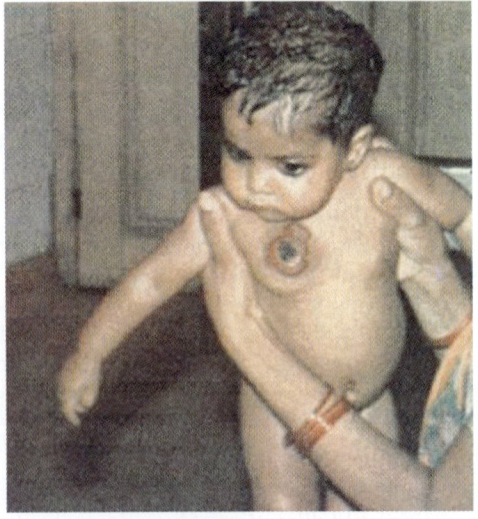

Fig. 3.49: Typical red color cavernous hemangioma on the chest of the baby (congenital).

e. **Glomangioma (glomus tumor):** It is not a congenital tumor in the true sense. It is a specialized arteriovenous communication surrounded by smooth muscle cells and large epithelioid or cuboidal cells called glomus cells. The sensory nerves (both medullated and nonmedullated) end at these epithelioid cells and make this tumor very much painful. Even the slightest pressure will give rise to an excruciating pain. The most common site of this tumor is just beneath the nail near the finger tip. It looks like a small reddish-blue spot. It does not blanch on pressure as a hemangioma. The tumors are subcutaneous and they can occur anywhere in the body, but are usually seen at the extremities of the limbs and often at subungual position. The lesion has a bluish tinge due to the blood content and the subungual lesions are usually 1–2 mL in size. It is a benign tumor which never turns malignant.

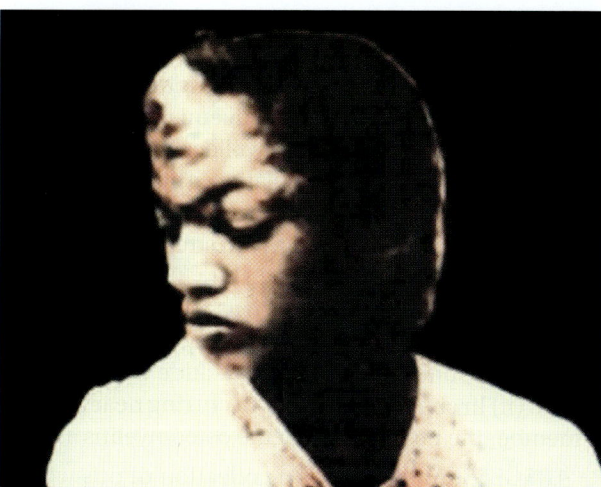

Fig. 3.50: Cirsoid aneurysm in the forehead.

■ TRAUMATIC

Traumatic swellings arising from the skin and subcutaneous tissues are rare. *Hematoma* following a trauma may give rise to swelling. The other important swelling in this connection is the *implantation dermoid* which has already been discussed under the heading of 'Dermoid Cyst.'

■ INFLAMMATORY

1. **ERYSIPELAS:** It is a spreading cuticular lymphangitis which may follow even a scratch. The causative organism is mostly *Streptococcus pyogenes*. The conditions which predispose this disease are debilitating state and poor health of the patient. The condition commences as a rose-pink rash which extends to the adjacent skin. The vesicles appear sooner or later over the rash and rupture. Serous discharge comes out from these vesicles. When it affects loose areolar tissues such as orbit, scrotum, etc., there is considerable swelling of the part due to edema of the subcutaneous tissue and thus very much resembles cellulitis.

   To distinguish between a true erysipelas and cellulitis the following points in favor of erysipelas should be borne in mind: (i) The typical rosy-red rash disappears on pressure and fills stiff; (ii) The raised rash of erysipelas has a sharply defined margin—which is better felt than inspected (this is the most important point); (iii) The vesicles of erysipelas contain serum in contradistinction to the cellulitis where they contain pus; (iv) In case of the face, Milian's ear sign, i.e., erysipelas can spread into the pinna (being cuticular affection) whereas cellulitis cannot, owing to close adhesion of the skin to cartilage of the ear.

2. **CELLULITIS:** It is a spreading inflammation of the subcutaneous and fascial tissues leading to suppuration, sloughing or even gangrene (especially in cases of diabetes) of the affected

part. The most common organism is again *Streptococcus pyogenes*. The organisms gain access through an accidental wound, however trivial it may be. The victims are generally diabetic or debilitated individuals with poor nutrition. It is a condition which requires intense attention of the surgeon as it may lead to septicemia and may turn fatal.

The affected part becomes swollen, hot and tender. The condition starts with redness, itching and stiffness at the site of inoculation. The part gradually looks brawny and becomes edematous which is demonstrated by pitting on pressure. There is no definite edge (cf. erysipelas). The lymph vessels may stand out as red streaks (lymphangitis), the regional lymph nodes draining the area become enlarged and show the picture of acute lymphadenitis. Varying degree of constitutional disturbances such as fever and toxemia are common.

The students should remember two things in connection with cellulitis. (i) In cellulitis of the scrotum, one should always exclude the possibility of presence of extravasation of urine with it. (ii) In children, cellulitis occurring near a joint (particularly the knee joint), one should remember the possibility of acute osteomyelitis as the most common cause of this condition.

3. **ABSCESS:** An abscess is a collection of pus within the body. There are three varieties of abscesses seen in surgical practice:

(i) **Pyogenic abscess:** This is the most common variety of abscess and may result from cellulitis or acute lymphadenitis. The organisms gain entry either directly through the penetrating wound or local extension from adjacent focus of infection or hematogenous or lymphatic spread from a distance. At first the infected part becomes red hot and quite tender. When pus develops, the pain takes a typical character of throbbing in nature. There will be brawny induration and edema (demonstrable by pitting on pressure). Fluctuation may or may not be present (as in parotid abscess).

(ii) **Pyemic abscess:** These are generally multiple in number, either develop simultaneously or a number of them crop up in succession only after one has been incised. This condition results when infective emboli circulating in the blood lodge in different parts of the body and give rise to multiple abscesses. The peculiarity of these abscesses are that they commonly occur in the subfascial plane and do not present the features of a common abscess. These are nonreacting in nature, i.e., acute features are absent. But constitutional disturbances are tremendous with high fever, rigor and toxemia.

(iii) **Cold abscess:** As the name suggests, this abscess is cold and nonreacting in nature. It does not produce hot and painful abscess as seen in pyogenic abscess. Brawny induration, edema and tenderness are conspicuous by their absence. Cold abscess is almost always a sequel of tubercular infection anywhere in the body commonly in the lymph nodes and bone. Caseation of the lymph nodes forms the cold abscess. The most common sites are at the neck and axilla. Sometimes cold abscesses are seen at the loin, at the back or at the side of the chest wall. These are sequel of tuberculous affection of the spine, ribs and posterior mediastinal group of lymph nodes. Cold abscesses may also originate from the ends of the bones and joints and gradually come to the surface through the fascial planes.

4. **BOIL** (Furuncle): Infection of a hair follicle with *Staphylococcus aureus* leads to this condition. It may be associated with perifolliculitis, which may proceed to suppuration. It starts with a painful and indurated swelling which gradually extends. There will be tremendous tenderness with surrounding edema. After a couple of days, there will be softening at the center on the summit of which a small pustule appears. It may burst spontaneously discharging greenish slough. After this, a deep cavity develops lined by granulation tissue, which heals by itself. Boils are common on the back and neck. Furuncle of the external auditory meatus is very painful as

the skin is more or less attached to the underlying cartilage and there hardly remains any space for the swelling to develop, so a great tension develops which leads to pain. Perianal boils when rupture form sinuses. Boils may lead to cellulitis particularly in those persons whose immunity is less. Boils may also lead to infection of the neighboring hair follicles where number of hair follicles are too many (e.g., axilla) leading to hydradenitis. Boils may lead to infection of the regional lymph nodes.

5. **CARBUNCLE:** It is a bigger form of boil and the causative organism is again *Staphylococcus aureus*. This is due to infective gangrene of the subcutaneous tissue where the infection has already spread. Generally men above 40 years of age are sufferers and they are mostly *diabetic*.

Carbuncles are commonly seen on the back, in the nape of the neck where the skin is coarse and the vitality of the tissue is less.

It commences as painful and stiff swelling which spreads very rapidly with marked induration. The overlying skin becomes red, dusky and edematous. Subsequently the central part softens, vesicles and later on pustules appear on the surface. These burst allowing the discharge to come out through several openings in the skin. The sieve like or cribriform appearance of the carbuncle is pathognomonic. These openings enlarge and ultimately coalesce to produce an ulcer at the floor of which lies the ashy-gray slough. Finally the slough separates leaving an excavated granulating surface, which heals by itself. The resistance of the individual is poor as in a diabetic subject. The sloughing process may extend deeply into the muscle or even bone. Constitutional symptoms and toxemia may vary according to the degree of the resistance of the individual.

NEOPLASTIC

1. BENIGN NEOPLASMS

PAPILLOMA: This is a simple overgrowth of all layers of the skin. Mostly it is a pedunculated growth having branched villous processes. It consists of a central axis of connective tissue, blood vessels and lymphatics. The surface is covered with epithelium in the form of squamous, transitional or columnar according to the site of the tumor.

Papilloma may appear at any age. Most common complaint is the swelling and nothing else. Sometimes, it may be injured to become red, swollen, ulcerated and even inflamed to present with the symptoms accordingly.

It may occur anywhere in the body. But here only the clinical features of the papilloma arising from the skin will be discussed. It may be papilliferous and pedunculated, which may vary in length starting from a long peduncle to a very short peduncle or even sessile. Cutaneous papilloma is soft and solid. It moves with the skin and its base is not indurated like an epidermoid carcinoma. Sometimes the surface of the growth may be hard, when it is called 'Horny papilloma'. *Complications* are ulceration, bleeding and malignancy.

Other common sites besides the skin are the lip, the tongue, the vocal cord, the colon, the rectum, the kidney, urinary bladder and the breast.

FIBROMA: This is a tumor of the fibrous tissue. Considering the wide spread distribution of the fibrous tissue in the body, true fibroma is of rare occurrence. Most fibromas are combined with other mesodermal tissues, such as fat (fibrolipoma), the muscles (fibromyoma), nerve sheath (neurofibroma), etc. The last named tumor may be seen in multiple numbers, which is called neurofibromatosis (Von Recklinghausen's disease).

Fibroma gives rise to a painless, firm, circumscribed swelling **(Fig. 3.51)**, which moves freely on the underlying structures. According to consistency, fibroma may be hard or soft (according to the amount of fibrous tissue it contains). Soft fibromas are often indistinguishable from sarcoma. *Paget's recurrent fibroid (desmoid tumor)*—an unusual type of fibroma arising from the rectus sheath is notorious for recurrence and stands in the borderline of malignancy.

LIPOMA: A lipoma is a cluster of fat cells which become overactive and so distended with fat that it produces a palpable swelling. This is the most common tumor of the subcutaneous tissue. It may occur anywhere in the body, hence it is known as *'universal tumor'*, but mostly seen in the back of the neck, shoulder and the back. Though subcutaneous lipoma is the most common and will be discussed in details, yet the students should keep in mind

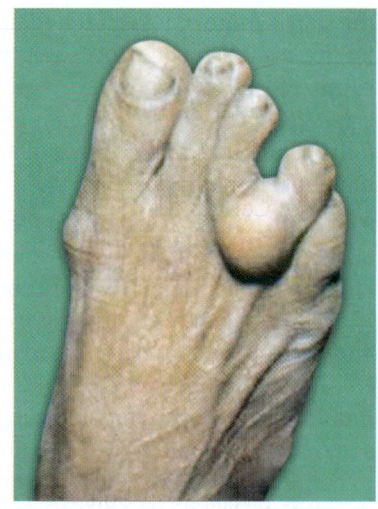

Fig. 3.51: Fibroma of the foot.

that lipoma may develop in other places, e.g., *intermuscular, subfascial, parosteal, subserous, submucous (GI tract), intraarticular, subsynovial, subdural or extradural* (spine).

There are mainly three varieties of lipoma—(1) Encapsulated variety; (2) Diffuse variety and (3) Multiple lipomas.

1. ***ENCAPSULATED SUBCUTANEOUS LIPOMA*:** This is the most common variety. Pathologically, it consists of normal fat which contains overactive fat cells and is arranged in lobules separated by fibrous septa and enclosed in a delicate capsule. A lipoma is usually small but it may attain very big size. Lipoma may occur at any age, but it is rarely seen in children. It is a painless, slowly growing, lobulated and soft swelling. It can occur anywhere in the body, though more commonly seen in the neck, in the back, around shoulder and in the upper limbs. The overlying skin is usually of normal color. Only in case of very large lipoma the skin may be stretched with dilated veins over the tumor. But such feature is more common in case of naevolipoma. The surface is smooth and lobulated. The edge is definite and slips under the palpating finger, which is known as *'slip sign'*. This sign is helpful to differentiate this condition from a cyst in which case the edge does not slip away from the palpating finger, but yields to it. Consistency is soft but does not fluctuate. In normal body temperature the fat remains almost in semiliquid condition and consequently slight fluctuation may be elicited and thus lipoma is often called a *'semifluctuant'* swelling. Though lipoma does not contain fluid, yet a large lipoma may transilluminate with the light from ordinary torch. A lipoma is a freely mobile swelling over the deeper structures such as muscles and fasciae. So a lipoma can be easily moved over a taut underlying muscle either along its long axis or at right angles to it. It is not attached to the skin, so that the skin over the swelling can be pinched up apart from the swelling. But there are fibrous strands which connect the capsule of the lipoma to the skin and that is why when the skin overlying the tumor is moved, there is dimpling on the skin **(Figs. 3.52 and 3.53)**.

Sometimes lipoma contains dilated blood vessels when it is called 'Naevolipoma'. If a lipoma contains excessive amounts of fibrous tissue, it is called 'Fibrolipoma'. When a lipoma contains nerve tissue, it becomes painful and is called 'Neurolipoma'.

Complications: A lipoma when present for a long time may undergo certain changes. This is particularly true in cases of lipoma in the subcutaneous tissue of the thigh, buttock or retroperitoneal lipoma. Such changes are: (i) myxomatous degeneration, (ii) saponification, (iii) calcification, (iv) infection, (v) ulceration due to repeated trauma and (vi) malignant change (liposarcoma), which the students should always keep in mind. Certain authorities believe that lipoma never turns into malignancy. If liposarcoma does occur (more often seen in the retroperitoneal tissue), it arises de novo and not in a benign lipoma.

2. **DIFFUSE VARIETY:** This is quite rare and does not possess the typical features of lipoma, hence it is often called '*Pseudolipoma*'. It is seen in the subcutaneous and intermuscular tissue of the neck and gradually may extend to the cheek. There is no capsule of this tumor. It hardly gives any trouble barring being unsightly. It is often found in persons taking excessive alcohol.

3. **MULTIPLE LIPOMAS:** It is often called 'Lipomatosis'. The tumors remain small or moderate in size and are sometimes painful as these contain nerve tissue and are called *neurolipomatosis*. These are mostly seen in the limbs and in the trunk. Lipomata of the different sizes and shapes may be seen. Macroscopically and microscopically these are not different from solitary lipoma. *Dercum's disease* (adiposis dolorosa) is a variety of this condition in which there are tender lipomatous swellings particularly affecting the trunk. This is more common in women.

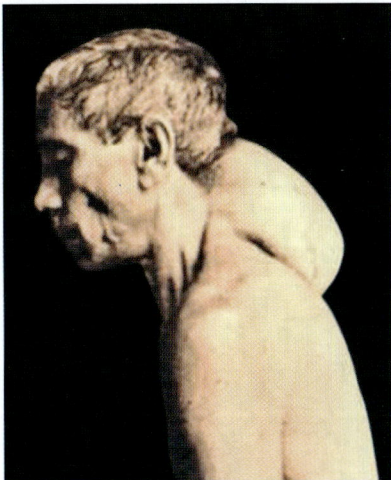

Fig. 3.52: A pedunculated lipoma at the nape of the neck.

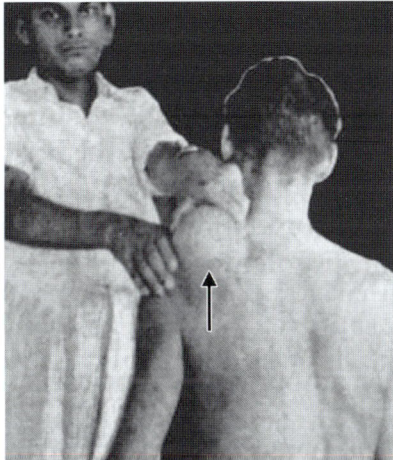

Fig. 3.53: Showing how a lipoma is freely mobile over a contracted muscle. The trapezius muscle has been made taut by shrugging the shoulder up against resistance with one hand and the lipoma is moved with the other hand.

NEUROFIBROMA: This tumor contains both neural (ectodermal) and fibrous (mesodermal) elements. Controversies still exist about its origin. This tumor should not be confused with *neurilemmoma (Schwannoma)*. Generally neurofibroma occurs in multiple number. But local or single neurofibroma is not unseen.

a. *Local neurofibroma (Fig. 3.54):* Neurofibroma may appear at any age but commonly seen in adults. It occurs in the subcutaneous tissue and presents as a slightly painful nodule, which is a firm, smooth swelling and can be moved in lateral direction but not along the direction of the nerve from which it arises. Paresthesia and tingle sensation along the distribution of the nerve are quite common. This is due to pressure effect of the tumor on the nerve fibers. **Complication** though rare yet occasionally seen and these are cystic degeneration and sarcomatous changes. 'Acoustic tumor' is an example of this variety when it arises from the 8th cranial nerve.

b. *Generalized neurofibromatosis (Von Recklinghausen's disease) (Figs. 3.55A and B):* These are multiple neurofibromas spread all over the body involving the cranial, the spinal and the peripheral nerves. The tumors are said to originate from the perineurium and epineurium.

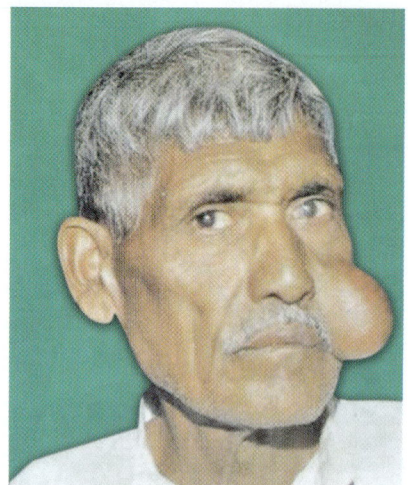

Fig. 3.54: A local neurofibroma affecting face.

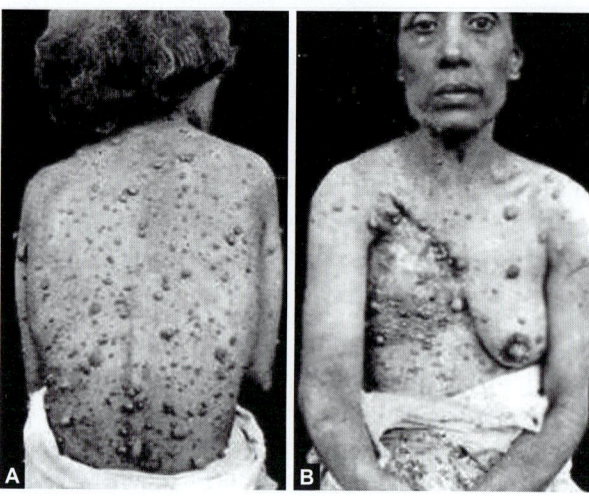

Figs. 3.55A and B: Von Recklinghausen's disease. See the text.

It is a *congenital (autosomal dominant)* disease. This condition may be associated with light brown pigmentation ('Cafe au Lait' patch), acoustic neuroma, pheochromocytoma, etc. Malignant change (neurofibrosarcoma) is seen in 5% of cases. Multiple nodules may present even at birth, but they may increase in size and number in subsequent years. The patient is almost covered with nodules of different sizes all throughout the body. Mostly they are in the subcutaneous tissue and some may even become pedunculated. The nodules vary in consistency from very firm (even hard) to soft nodules. Neurological disturbances are uncommon. **Complications** are: (a) Pigmentation of skin; (b) Neurological pressure symptoms, e.g., deafness in acoustic neuroma, spinal cord compression by 'Dumbbell tumor', mediastinal syndrome in case of mediastinal tumor; (c) Cystic degeneration; (d) Important sarcomatous change (neurofibrosarcoma); (e) It may be a part of multiple endocrine adenopathy type II B in which neurofibromas affecting lips, eyelids and face are associated with medullary carcinoma of thyroid, pheochromocytoma (hypertension) and hyperparathyroidism.

c. **Plexiform neurofibromatosis:** This tumor usually occurs in connection with the branches of fifth cranial nerve. The swelling is enormous with myxofibromatous degeneration and unsightly. It hangs down in folds. This tumor occasionally affects the upper limb and may be associated with generalized neurofibromatosis. Sarcomatous change is very rare in this condition **(Fig. 3.56)**.

d. **Elephantiasis neurofibromatosis:** In this condition the skin of the affected region becomes coarse dry and thickened resembling an elephant's skin. The subcutaneous tissue is replaced by fibrous tissue, which is enormously thickened and edematous. As differential diagnosis one

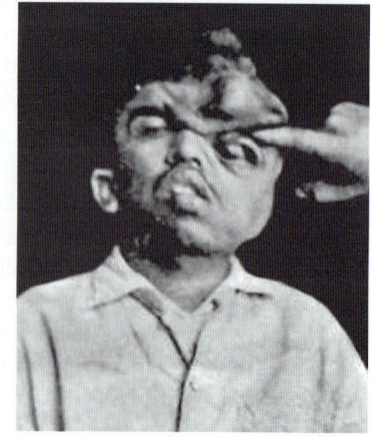

Fig. 3.56: Plexiform neurofibromatosis occurring in connection with the ophthalmic division of the trigeminal nerve.

must remember the *other causes of elephantiasis*. These are *filarial elephantiasis, following* en bloc excision of the lymph nodes for carcinoma of the breast or penis and *elephantiasis graecorum* of nodular leprosy affecting the face and forearm.

e. **Pachydermatocele (Fig. 3.57):** It can be described as a variant of plexiform neurofibromatosis, in which the neck is affected from where coils of soft tissue hang down resulting in an unsightly deformity.

SCHWANNOMA (NEURILEMMOMA): While neurofibroma is a benign tumor which contains a mixture of neural (ectodermal) and fibrous (mesodermal) elements, neurilemmoma arises from Schwann cell of neurilemma which is ectodermal in origin and is so rare as to be often forgotten. It is a benign, well encapsulated tumor, which forms a single, round or fusiform firm mass on the course of a large nerve. Schwannoma is white to gray, firm and well capsulated lesion. The most common site is the acoustic nerve, though this tumor has also been seen in the posterior mediastinum and in the retroperitoneal space. Multiple lesions are extremely rare. Neurilemmoma is a definite benign lesion and does not show any tendency to malignant transformation. Clinically, a mass of usually 1–2 cm may be detected along the course of a nerve. Radiating pain may be complained of along the distribution of the nerve. It gradually displaces the nerve fibers and the nerve fibers are never seen to be entangled into the tumor. It may often be asymptomatic, not tender, no nodal involvement and no tendency to malignant transformation.

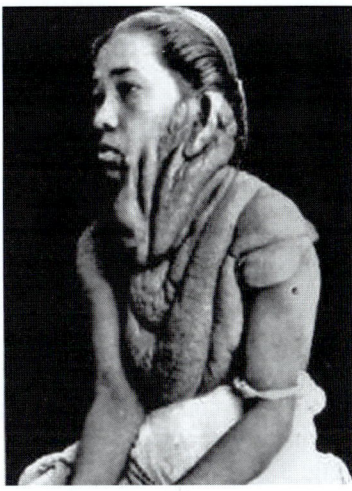

Fig. 3.57: Pachydermatocele—a rare variety of plexiform neurofibromatosis.

LYMPHANGIOMA: Lymphangioma is congenital in origin. Localized cluster of dilated lymph sacs in the skin and subcutaneous tissues which cannot connect into the normal lymph system grows into lymphangioma. Three types are usually seen—(a) Simple or capillary lymphangioma; (b) Cavernous lymphangioma and (c) Cystic hygroma.

a. **SIMPLE or CAPILLARY LYMPHANGIOMA:** This type presents as circumscribed lesion which appears as small vesicle or small blister or slightly elevated skin patch. These lesions are also called *lymphangioma circumscriptum*. The size varies from 0.5 to 4 mm in diameter. A large area of skin may be involved on the inner side of the thigh, buttock, on the shoulder or in the axilla. The whole lesion is soft and spongy. There may be multiple cysts or one or two large cysts. Fluctuation, fluid thrill and translucency test are always positive. The swelling is not compressible. The margins of the swelling are indistinct. The skin vesicles contain clear fluid which looks watery and yellow but blood in the vesicles turns them brown or dark red. The regional lymph nodes are usually not enlarged unless the cysts become infected. It must be remembered that the tissues between the cysts have normal lymph drainage and they are not edematous. The blood and nerve supply of the area of lymphangioma circumscriptum are also normal.

b. **CAVERNOUS LYMPHANGIOMA:** These present as bigger lymphatic swellings and are situated rather deep as compared to the capillary variety. It occurs commonly on the face, mouth, lips (causing enormous enlargement of the lip which is called macrocheilia), the neck, the tongue (a common cause of macroglossia), the pectoral region and axilla. The lesion is a soft and lobulated swelling containing single or multiple communicating lymphatic cysts. The swelling is obviously fluctuant and brilliantly translucent. The cyst is often interspersed among muscle fibers causing difficulty in dissection for excision of the cyst.

c. **CYSTIC HYGROMA:** This is the most common form of lymphangioma. This exhibits large cyst-like cavities containing clear watery fluid. It is in fact a collection of lymphatic sacs and probably represents a cluster of lymph channels that failed to connect into the normal lymphatic pathways **(Fig. 3.58)**. Majority (75%) of the cystic hygromata are seen in the neck **(Fig. 3.59)**. 20% are seen in the axilla and remaining 5% are found scattered in different parts of the body—in the mediastinum, groin, pelvis and even retroperitoneum.

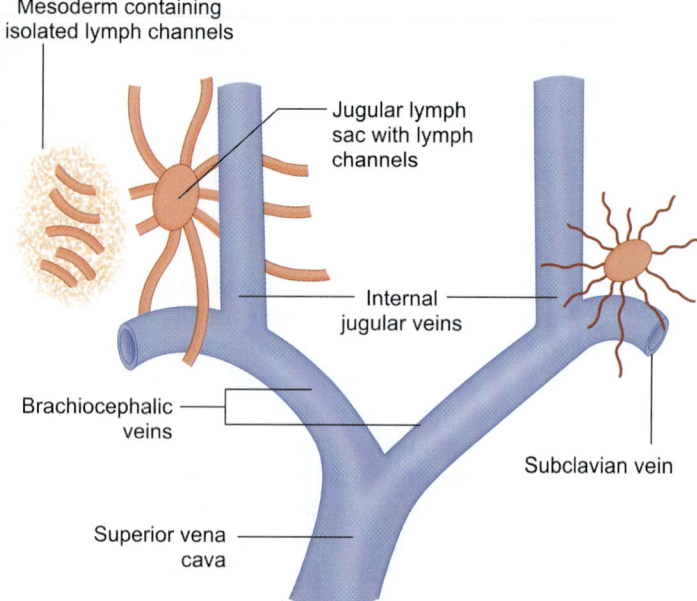

Fig. 3.58: Development of a cystic hygroma. The isolated lymph channels, which become segregated from the jugular lymph sac, form multilocular cystic hygroma at the root of the neck in the posterior triangle.

Macroscopically, cystic hygroma consists of multiple locules filled with lymph. In the depth the locules are bigger and towards the surface the locules become smaller and smaller in size. The content of the cyst is clear watery lymph or straw-colored fluid-containing cholesterol crystals and lymphocytes. The fluid does not coagulate.

It is mostly seen in children and is usually reported to be present since birth. Disfigurement is the main symptom. The swelling is painless, though occasionally may be painful when it becomes infected. This is a soft swelling which shows positive fluctuation and translucency test. In fact this

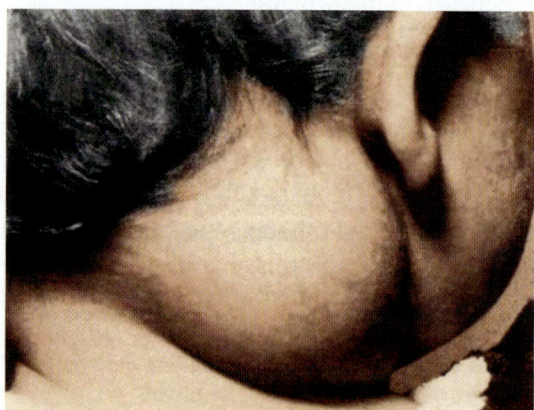

Fig. 3.59: Cystic hygroma at the right side of the neck of a baby.

is a brilliant translucent swelling unless it is infected or when bleeding occurs inside the cyst. It is partially compressible as fluid in one loculus can be compressed into the other. It is often called '*hydrocele of the neck*' particularly when it is unilocular. The regional lymph nodes should not be enlarged unless the lesion gets infected.

Complications rarely occur in such a lesion-like: (i) infection, (ii) rupture of the cyst leading to lymphorrhea; (iii) respiratory obstruction and rarely (iv) obstructed labor due to massive swelling before birth.

MOLES (pigmented naevus, freckles, benign melanoma) (Figs. 3.60A to C): 'Naevus' means a lesion which is present since birth. Although many of these may be present since birth, yet others appear later in life. This lesion contains an excess quantity of melanin, derived from melanocytes. The word 'benign melanoma' signifies that this growth is a benign neoplasm which means that its cells grow uncontrolled by the usual growth-limiting factors. But the histological feature of the mole is one of controlled overgrowth caused by excess stimulation, rather than excessive growth with normal stimulation. That is why a mole should better be called a 'Hamartoma' of melanocytes.

Every individual has a few moles at birth, and this number increases during life. Moles are more common in Caucasians living in hot countries, such as Australia, where the skin is exposed to more ultraviolet light. Though moles do occur in Negroes, but malignant change is very rare.

Disfiguring and black spot are the main symptoms. Moles can occur on any part of the body, though these are mostly seen on the limbs, the face and around the mucocutaneous junctions (the mouth and the anus). The color varies from light brown to black. Though amelanotic moles do exist, yet without pigment these moles cannot be recognized. Majority of the moles are 1–3 mm in diameter. Followings

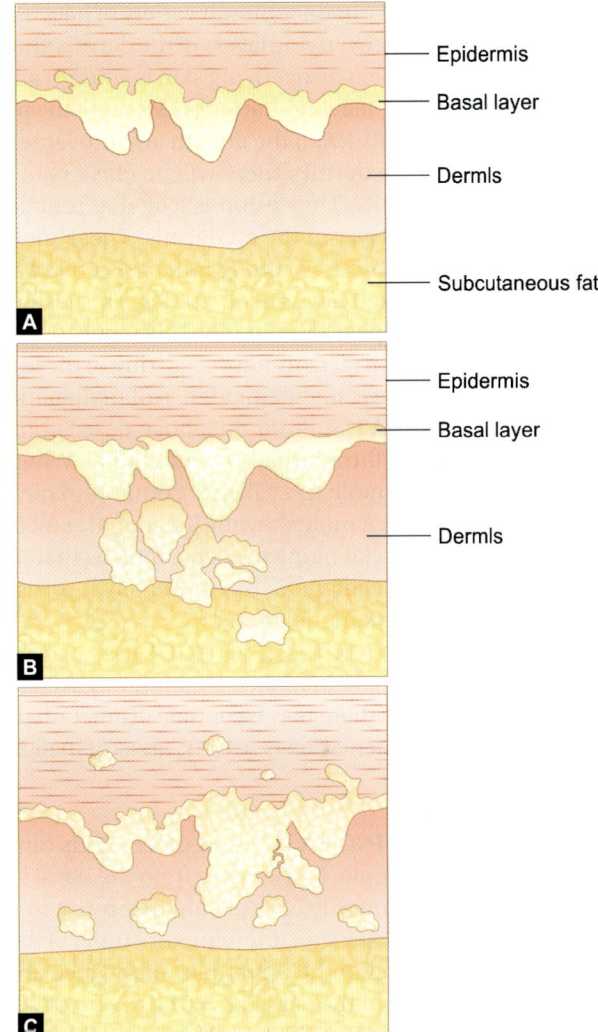

Figs. 3.60A to C: (A) **Normal skin**; (B) **Intradermal mole**, here the melanocytes conglomerate in the dermis and clinically this mole looks flat or raised, smooth or warty, hairy or non-hairy and it is always benign; (C) **Junctional mole**, here the melanocytes conglomerate in the epidermis and dermis, clinically it looks flat or raised, smooth or warty, is always non-hairy and may turn malignant.

are the various **types** of moles depending on the further proliferation and growth:

a. **HAIRY MOLE:** This is a common variety. It is flat and slightly raised above the level of the skin. It has a smooth or slightly warty epidermal covering. It has hairs growing from its surface. There are also sebaceous glands which may become infected. This causes increase in swelling and tenderness.

b. **NON-HAIRY OR SMOOTH MOLES:** This is also quite common. The surface is not elevated. The epithelium is smooth and there is no hair growing from its surface. The pigment is deeper than the hairy mole.

c. **BLUE NEVUS:** It is an uncommon variety of naevus. It is a type of mole which occurs deep in the dermis. The thick overlying layers of the dermis and epidermis mask the color of the melanin and make it look blue. The overlying skin is smooth and shiny. It is commonly seen on the face, dorsum of the hand, feet and buttocks (Mongolian spot) of babies or children.

d. **JUNCTIONAL NEVUS:** If the growth and movements of melanocytes stop before they have all migrated into the dermis, there will be clusters of cells of various stages of maturity in the epidermis and dermis. This lesion is called a 'Junctional nevus' as it is centered around the junctional or basal layer of the epidermis. These moles are immature, unstable and can turn malignant. *In fact majority of malignant melanoma begin in junctional nevi.* Junctional naevus is a smooth or elevated nevus of all shades. This lesion may occur anywhere in the body either from the birth or appear later in life. This nevus occurs more commonly on the palms, soles, digits and genitalia. In fact any nevi occurring in these areas should be considered as junctional nevi and hence there is higher incidence of malignant melanoma in these sites.

e. **COMPOUND NEVUS:** From the above description it is clear that two distinct varieties of mole are available—intradermal and junctional. When intradermal and junctional features are both present in one mole it is called a 'compound nevus'.

f. **JUVENILE MOLE:** A mole showing junctional activity before puberty is called a 'juvenile mole'. The reason for a special name of such a mole is that microscopically it looks so active that it is often thought to be malignant, but ultimately it turns into a mature benign intradermal mole and not into a malignant melanoma.

g. **HUTCHINSON'S FRECKLE (LENTIGO):** It is worthy of special note. This term is used to describe a large area of dark pigmentation. It is commonly seen on the face and neck in elderly people. The surface is smooth but there may be nodule of junctional activity and may turn malignant. Because the background pigmentation is so dark, areas of malignant change may pass unnoticed.

2. MALIGNANT

BASAL CELL CARCINOMA (Rodent ulcer): This tumor of low-grade malignancy is common in white-skinned people. It originates from the basal layer of the rete Malpighii of the skin. The exposed skin is commonly affected and exposure to sunlight or ultraviolet irradiation seems to be the predisposing factor, therefore Australia is the most commonly affected country. 90% of this tumor is found in the upper part of the face above the line drawn from the angle of the mouth to the lobule of the ear **(Fig. 3.61)**, the most common site being inner or outer canthus of the eye. Middle-aged or old people are usually the victims **(Figs. 3.62A and B)**.

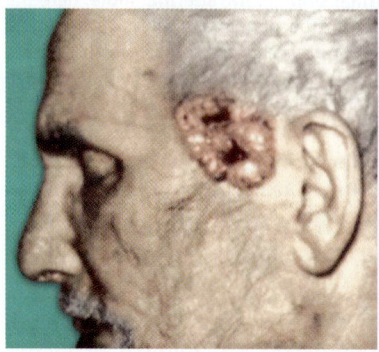
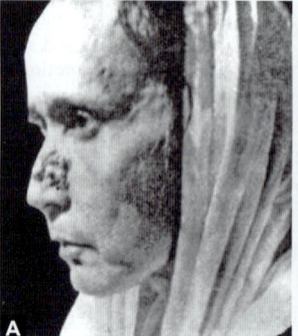
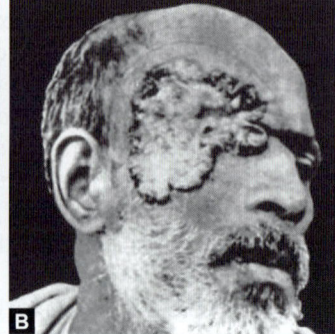

Fig. 3.61: Shows a typical case of basal cell carcinoma.

Figs. 3.62A and B: Basal cell carcinoma, mostly seen in the upper half of the face: (A) shows an early case whereas; (B) shows a late case of rodent ulcer.

It starts as a small brownish-red nodule with translucent color and shiny surface showing a network of capillaries. At this stage it is diagnosed due to its hardness, painlessness and presence of capillaries. Later on the tumor becomes ulcerated with a well-defined hard and raised edge (but not everted as seen in epithelioma) with a beaded appearance. There is a central scab but the margin gradually spreads and infiltrates into the surrounding tissues as well as deeper tissues even up to the bone. This characteristic feature of eroding the tissues, which come in contact with it, has given it the name '**rodent**'. At first it may itch, but at a later stage it may be painful if it has eroded any nerve.

Dissemination by lymphatic or blood vessels does not occur. So the *regional lymph nodes are not enlarged* and there will be no metastasis to the distant organs. There may be squamous celled carcinomatous change, though very rare.

SQUAMOUS CELL CARCINOMA (syn. epidermoid carcinoma or epithelioma): This is a more malignant tumor than the preceding one. The elderly people are the usual victims. It may affect the normal skin but there are a few predisposing factors which the students should keep in mind. These are previously irradiated skin, a long standing ulcer, e.g., varicose ulcer, scar from a burn (Marjolin's ulcer), repeated irritation of the skin by various chemicals such as dyes, tar, etc., and a few premalignant conditions such as Bowen's disease, Leukoplakia, Paget's disease, etc.

This tumor originates from prickle cell layer of the skin. It may give rise to sessile cauliflower mass or fungating ulcer *with raised and everted margin*. The base is always indurated and hard as also the edge. There may be blood-stained or purulent discharge if the tumor is secondarily infected. The regional lymph nodes are often involved as lymphatic spread is quite common and takes place early. But they may be involved by secondary infection and not due to metastasis only. Metastatic lymph nodes are hard in consistency and may invade the deeper structure to be fixed and inoperable.

MALIGNANT MELANOMA (Figs. 3.63A and B): It is a malignant tumor of melanocytes, which originate from the neural crest and so ectodermal in origin. It may occur de novo or in a benign mole. Malignant melanoma is rare before puberty, though it may even occur in children. Majority of patients range between 20 and 40 years of age. Girls are affected more than the boys in the ratio of 2 to 3 : 1. It is very common in Caucasians and extremely rare in Negroes. Melanocytes are stimulated by ultraviolet light. It is more commonly seen in the face, neck, soles, palms, digits, toes and external genitalia, which are common sites of junctional nevus. It may even occur in the choroid of the eye, in the meninges, in the rectum and anal canal and beneath the nail (which is called subungual melanoma), particularly in the thumb and great toe. The main symptom is cosmetic disfigurement caused by the enlarging lesion which brings the patient to the surgeon. Malignant melanoma is not painful, but it often itches. Sometimes lymph node enlargement or distant metastasis may be the first symptom. Color of the tumor may

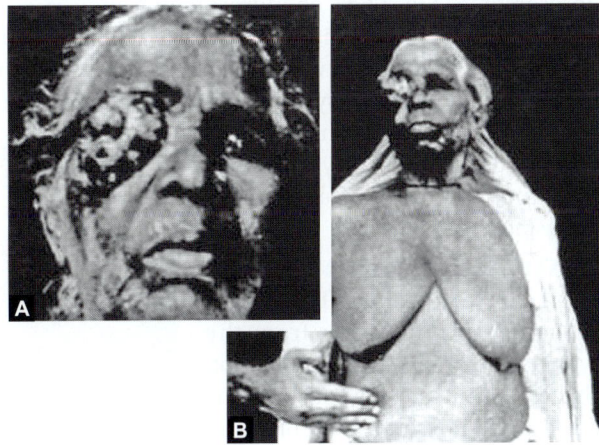

Figs. 3.63A and B: Malignant melanoma of the eye, the liver is being palpated for secondary deposits.

vary from pale pinkish-brown to black. Usually, there is a purple hue around the tumor due to rich blood supply. There is no increase of temperature and the tumor is not tender. The size varies considerably and clinically the tumor can be staged either according to Clark's level of invasion or according to Breslow, which is beyond the domain of this book and the students are referred to author's '**A CONCISE TEXTBOOK OF SURGERY**'. When the tumor is small it is covered with smooth epithelium. When the tumor is bigger the overlying epithelium may die from ischemic necrosis resulting in ulcer formation which is often covered with a crust. Bleeding and subacute infection are quite common in this tumor which make the surface often soft and boggy. The consistency of the tumor is usually firm. The regional lymph nodes are involved quite early and these are almost always enlarged when the patient presents to the surgeon. A halo of brown pigment may be seen in the skin around the tumor which indicates local infiltration of the tumor. Satellite nodules may be seen in the skin and subcutaneous tissue between the primary tumor and the nearest regional lymph nodes. This is due to lymphatic spread of the tumor by embolism which stops in the wall of the lymphatic and starts growing. These nodules are often hard in consistency. Malignant melanoma also metastasizes through bloodstream to the liver, lungs, bones and brain.

As mentioned earlier malignant melanoma may occur (90%) in a pre-existing benign mole. So one must remember the cardinal symptoms and signs of malignant change in a mole. These are: (i) Sudden increase in size. (ii) Change in color (the moles become darker which may be patchy; very occasionally malignant melanocytes do not produce melanin and the growth does not show dark color—**amelanotic melanoma**. (iii) Ulceration and bleeding with minor injury is quite characteristic. It may even bleed when the mole is rubbed off. (iv) There may be a pigmented halo around the tumor which indicates local spread and malignancy. Satellite nodules may also develop in the intradermal lymphatic. (v) Involvement of regional lymph nodes and distant organs, e.g., the liver, the lungs, the brain, etc., are indicative of malignancy.

SARCOMA: This is a malignant tumor of connective tissue. It may occur from any structure derived from mesoblastic origin. In contradistinction to the carcinomas, the sarcomas usually affect younger age group. These are rapid growing tumors and disseminate mainly by the blood stream (cf. carcinoma). Lymphatic spread does not occur early and is not important in these tumors. Sarcomatous cells produce similar tissue from which they originate, e.g., osteosarcoma, fibrosarcoma **(Fig. 3.64)**, chondrosarcoma, etc.

The tumors very rapidly infiltrate neighboring structures. The patients usually present with a big swelling with varying consistency, diffuse margin and the skin over the swelling becomes stretched, glossy with engorged veins. As the growth is very vascular, pulsation may be felt (telangiectatic sarcoma). As the blood-spread is very common, the lungs are often affected with metastasis.

SYNOVIAL SARCOMA (Syn. malignant synovioma): This highly malignant tumor arises from the synovial membrane of a joint, tendon sheath or a bursa. It may occur at any age but the boys of the second and third decades are usually affected.

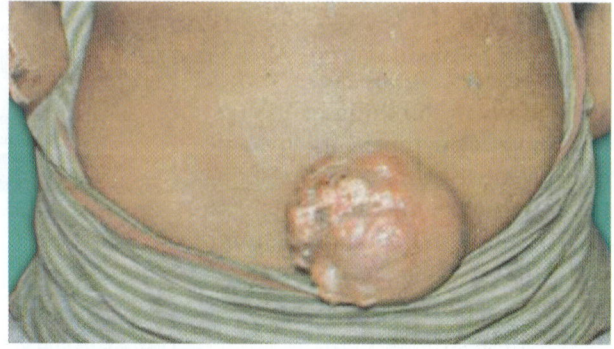

Fig. 3.64: Fibrosarcoma (a rare tumor) at the lower part of the back.

The patients usually present with a swelling at or near a joint, pain in the affected joint and limitation of movements of the said joint. X-ray shows a soft tissue shadow with flecks of calcification, but there is seldom any alteration of the joint line. Skiagraphy of the chest may reveal pulmonary metastasis. The diagnosis is confirmed by biopsy which will reveal mass of fusiform cells.

3. OTHER SWELLINGS

SEBACEOUS CYST (Fig. 3.65): This is a cyst of the sebaceous gland due to blockage of the duct of this gland which opens mostly into the hair follicle. The gland becomes distended by its own secretion. Obviously, it contains sebum, which is yellowish-white cheesy pultaceous material. Almost always there is a black spot on the swelling, which is the obstructed opening and is called *punctum*. This swelling is fixed to the skin but is quite movable over the deeper structures. Sebum can be squeezed out from this cyst through the punctum. Sometimes punctum is not visible, so other theories have come up to indicate its origin. These are—(i) it arises from a fragment of epidermal cell nest following blunt or penetrating injury; (ii) it arises from hair follicle. It is commonly seen in young adults, though no age is exempt. It may occur anywhere in the body except palm and sole, though it is commonly seen in the scalp, face and scrotum. It may be single or multiple. It is smooth and of round shape whose margin yields to the palpating finger. Fluctuation test is always present though transillumination test is always negative.

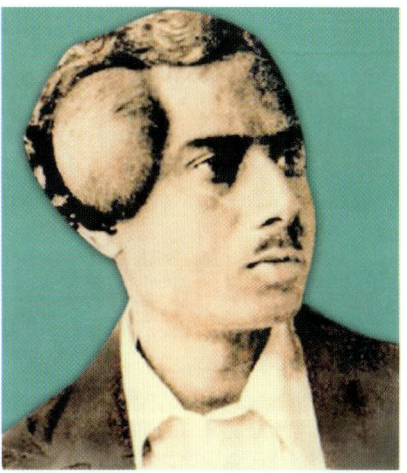

Fig. 3.65: Shows a big sebaceous cyst on the outer side of the forehead. Note the baldness over the cyst—a characteristic feature.

Complications are—(a) Infection when the cyst becomes enlarged and painful; (b) Ulceration; (c) Rupture and sinus formation; (d) Calcification; (e) Carcinomatous change; (f) Cock's peculiar tumor and (g) Sebaceous horn.

After the sebaceous cyst has been ruptured and chronic infection spreads to the surrounding tissues from the sebaceous cyst it may lead to a painful, boggy, fungating and discharging mass, quite often known as **Cock's peculiar tumor (Fig. 3.66)**.

Sometimes slow discharge of sebum from a wide punctum may harden as soon as it comes out to form a **Sebaceous horn (Figs. 3.67 and 3.68)**, which is nothing but inspissated sebaceous material.

CONDYLOMA: This is a manifestation of the secondary stage of syphilis. It is nothing but hypertrophy of the epidermis occurring at the mucocutaneous junction, e.g., angle of the mouth, anus **(Fig. 3.69)**, vulva, etc. It looks like a fungating, sessile, raised but flat growth with moist and sodden surface.

WARTS: These are patches of overgrown skin with hyperkeratosis. This may occur at any age but commonly found in children, adolescents and young adults. In the first few weeks these swellings grow up to their full sizes. The growth seems to be stimulated by a virus.

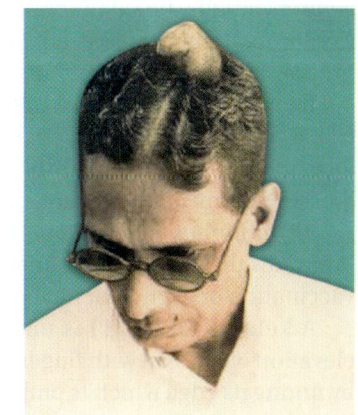

Fig. 3.66: Cock's peculiar tumor of the scalp.

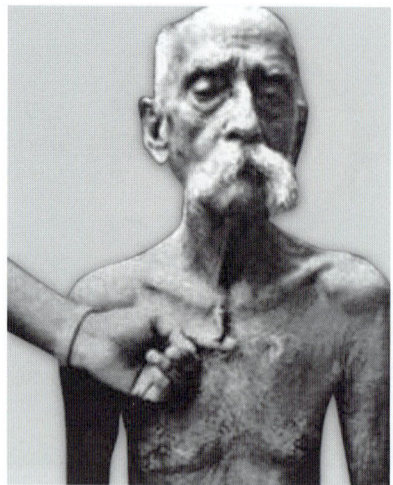

Fig. 3.67: Sebaceous horn.

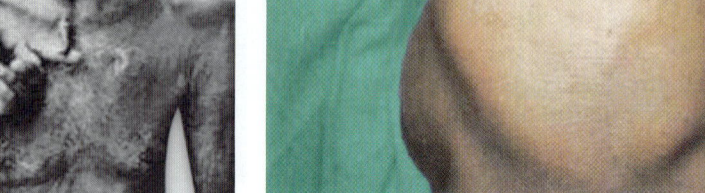

Fig. 3.68: Sebaceous horn over the knee.

The main complaint of the patient is disfiguring. Sometimes the warts become painful when they are repeatedly rubbed or become infected. These usually persist for quite a long time and even they disappear. Kiss lesions may appear in the skin where they frequently come into contact with warts. This condition frequently affects the hands, the face, the knees, the sole of the feet (plantar warts) and axilla. Warts are usually firm and covered with rough surface and filiform excrescences. This disease seems to be a familial one.

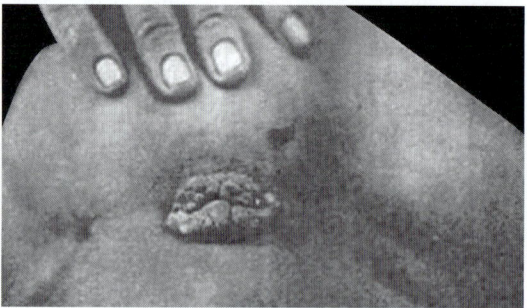

Fig. 3.69: Condyloma at the anus.

KELOID and **HYPERTROPHIC SCAR (Figs. 3.70A to C):** This is not a tumor but an overgrowth of the fibrous tissue which is concerned in wound healing and strengthening of the wound. A wound contains blood and fibrin, which is replaced by collagen and fibrous tissue and finally the fibrous tissue is organized to give the wound maximum strength. Nature controls this healing process in such a manner that normally the scars are thin with minimum fibrous tissue.

In abnormal cases there may be an excessive amount of fibrous tissue in the scar, which is called **hypertrophic scar.** Predisposing factors seem to be extra stimulus to the fibrous tissue formation during healing process. These are infection, excessive tension, the incision which crosses natural creases (Langer's lines), etc. In contradistinction to the hypertrophic scar, *in a keloid the fibrous tissue extends beyond the original wound* into the normal tissue and gradually infiltrates the surrounding healthy tissue. These often occur after burns, healing of an ulcer, vaccination or even after healing of small boils **(Figs. 3.2 and 3.3)**.

A **keloid (Fig. 3.71)** is unsightly, sometimes tender and itching. It is an irregular firm elevation of the skin with finger-like extensions. That the keloid is spreading can be determined by noting its edge which is pink and more tender. The following points should be remembered to differentiate a keloid from a hypertrophic scar: (i) it is itching, (ii) it is spreading, (iii) it is tender and (iv) it is vascular. The last but not the least point, which the students should always keep in mind, is its tendency to affect the Negroes and tuberculous patients.

CALLOSITY and **CORN:** These conditions are quite common and are not unknown to anybody. A callosity is a raised thickened patch of hyperkeratosis commonly seen in areas of the body which undergo excessive wear and tear and repeated minor traumas, e.g., gardener's hand. Histologically, there is increased thickening of the epidermis, particularly the stratum corneum and the granular layer.

A **corn** on the other hand is a circumscribed horny thickening, cone-like in shape with its apex pointing inwards and the base at the surface. Being circumscribed it is palpable as a nodule. It is thicker than a callosity and causes more concern to the patient. This occurs at the site of friction and often spontaneously disappears when the causing factor is removed. Histologically, it is composed of keratin masses with intact basal layers. It is often caused by ill-fitting and tight shoes chiefly affecting feet and toes.

KERATOACANTHOMA (Molluscum Sebaceum): It is a rapidly developing tumor composed of keratinizing squamous cells and is usually situated on the exposed areas of skin and resolves spontaneously even untreated. It is commonly seen in middle life or older age and males are affected more commonly than females (3:1). Predisposing factors are: (i) Exposure to Sun as this lesion is more often seen in the face, head and upper limbs, (ii) Contact with tar and mineral oil and (iii) Infection may play a role.

Pathologically, the tumor is situated in the dermis and globular in form. The epidermis is thin over the lesion from which it is separated by narrow connective tissue except at the mouth where the lesion and the epidermis are connected. The lesion is proliferating squamous cells arising from the sebaceous gland and progresses along the duct of the gland. This lesion is more often seen in places where there are plenty of sebaceous glands.

Clinically, this lesion presents as a firm, rounded reddish papule or nodule which gradually increases in size for first 6–8 weeks and may reach a size of about 2 cm in diameter. The bulk of the lesion is firm and rubbery, but the central core is hard. The epidermis over it is smooth and shiny. There may be telangiectases with reddish surface. The center contains horny plug

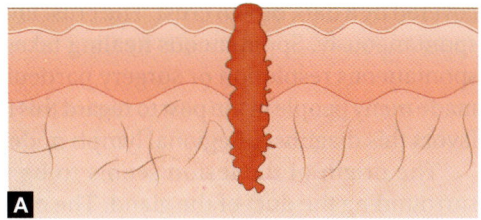
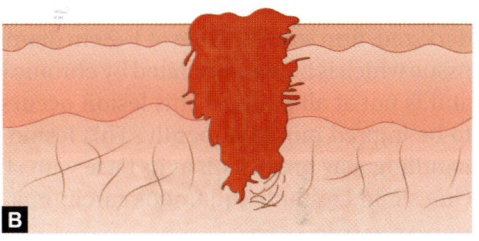
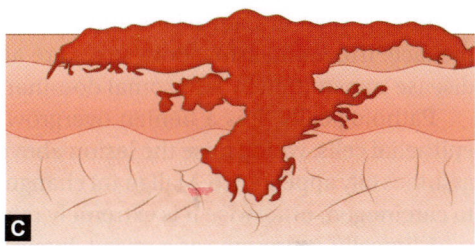

Figs. 3.70A to C: (A) Normal scar; (B) Hypertrophic scar; (C) Keloid.

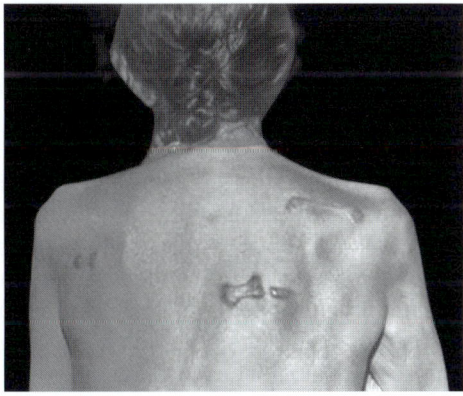

Fig. 3.71: Keloids at the back.

covered by a dark brown crust. The crust falls off, ulcer develops and the lesion starts regression spontaneously. Spontaneous healing takes about 6 months. Recurrence is noticed following spontaneous resolution or surgery particularly in lips and fingers. The progress of the growth made many people in the past to regard this lesion as an epithelioma, but spontaneous regression favors this diagnosis. Regional lymph nodes are not enlarged.

The origin of the lesion seems to be the sebaceous gland from which keratosis starts surrounding the duct of the gland. The cause is unknown. This lesion commonly affects older people and occurs mostly in the face or in places where there are plenty of sebaceous glands.

GRANULOMA PYOGENICUM (Pyogenic granuloma): This lesion looks like a hemangioma—dark, red, firm small nodule of 1–2 cm diameter. This lesion is an over-growth of the granulation tissue which is being stimulated by chronic infection. This *rapidly growing swelling* bleeds easily and is not at all painful. This lesion occurs mostly in the face and the hands which are likely to be injured more frequently. This lesion may become infected. It bleeds easily. Very rough handling may break it off at its base with slight bleeding, but only to reform within a few days. One should exclude squamous carcinoma.

SEBORRHEIC WART (senile wart or seborrheic keratosis or basal cell papilloma): This is a benign tumor which is mostly seen in the elderly and women at the time of menopause. It is commonly seen in Caucasians and rare among Indians and Negroes. It occurs commonly in the face, trunk and arms. Both sexes are almost equally involved. This seems to be a familial disease transmitted by autosomal dominant gene.

Pathologically, it is a benign overgrowth of the epidermis containing swollen abnormal epithelial cells, which raise the lesion above the level of normal skin. It is semitransparent and assumes oily appearance. Malignant change has been recorded particularly when skin is exposed to carcinogen, otherwise it is extremely rare.

Clinically, it presents as a raised, hypertrophic slightly greasy skin with rough papilliferous surface with distinct margin. Size varies from a few mL to 2–3 cm in diameter. It is a slow-growing lesion. It seldom bleeds by trauma which makes the lesion swell and turn brown, which may confuse this lesion with melanoma. This lesion may become infected and painful. It is a little firmer than normal skin and can be picked up. Regional lymph nodes are not enlarged.

SOLAR KERATOSIS (senile keratosis): As the name suggests it is a hyperkeratotic lesion of the skin and the predisposing factor is prolonged exposure of the skin to the sun. Obviously the common sites are the face, the ears, the dorsal aspects of the hands and fingers. The usual victims are old people who have engaged themselves very much in outdoor activities. At first the lesion occurs as thickened patch having yellowish-grey or brown color. It may turn into an ulcer with slight central cavity and raised plaque of skin at the periphery. This lesion is very much localized to the skin and its involvement to the underlying structure simply indicates malignant transformation. *It is a potentially malignant condition.* It takes about 10 years for malignant transformation and the result is squamous cell carcinoma which is slow-growing with little tendency to metastasize. Regional lymph nodes are not involved but if they are involved it indicates malignant transformation.

BOWEN'S DISEASE: *This is a precancerous condition.* The lesion looks-like brown indurated thickened mass covered with crust with well-defined edge. When crusts are removed the papules can be seen to have oozy, slightly bloody, papilliferous surface. The lesion may ooze serosanguineous discharge. The condition must be suspected and biopsy should be advised, which will reveal large clear cells as found in Paget's disease. It occurs equally in the exposed and covered areas, particularly at sites of repeated trauma. Its usual victims are the old people. 50% of patients will develop malignant cancer of the skin in about 6–8 years time.

Chapter 3: Examination of a Lump or a Swelling

Algorithmic Approach to a Patient with Swelling or Lump

Patient presents with a lump

↓

History taking
- **Duration:** Long-standing lumps → neoplastic; short-term lumps → inflammatory
- **Onset:** Sudden → trauma/infection; gradual → tumor
- **Pain:** Painful lumps → inflammatory/trauma; painless → neoplasm
- **Growth pattern:** Rapid growth → malignancy; slow growth → benign
- **Secondary changes:** Ulceration, discharge → malignancy

↓

Inspection
- **Size, shape, and color:** Helps in tumor identification
- **Pulsation:** Present in vascular swellings like aneurysms
- **Mobility:** Fixed lumps → malignancy; mobile lumps → benign

↓

Palpation
- **Temperature:** Increased → infection or highly vascular tumors
- **Tenderness:** Present in inflammatory swellings
- **Consistency:** soft → lipoma; hard → carcinoma; cystic → abscess/cyst
- **Fluctuation test:** Confirms the presence of fluid

↓

Percussion
- **Resonance:** Suggests a gaseous swelling (hernia, pneumothorax)
- **Dullness:** Indicates solid tumors or inflammatory swellings

↓

Auscultation
- **Bruit over swelling** → vascular lesions (arteriovenous malformation, aneurysm)

↓

Determine likely etiology
- Inflammatory (abscess, cellulitis, lymphadenitis)
- Neoplastic (benign vs malignant tumor)
- Congenital (dermoid cyst, meningocele, hemangioma)

↓

Order special investigations
- **FNAC** (fine-needle aspiration cytology)
- **Ultrasound** (cystic vs solid mass)
- **CT Scan/MRI** (extent and depth of tumor)
- **Biopsy** (definitive diagnosis)

↓

Confirm diagnosis and initiate treatment
- **Medical management:** Antibiotics, pain relief
- **Surgical management:** Excision, biopsy, tumor resection

CHAPTER 4

Examination of an Ulcer

An ulcer is a break in the continuity of the covering epithelium—skin or mucous membrane. It may either follow molecular death of the surface epithelium or its traumatic removal.

HISTORY: The following points are particularly noted in the history of a case of an ulcer:

1. **Mode of onset:** How has the ulcer developed—following a trauma or spontaneously? Traumatic ulcers generally heal by themselves if the traumatic agent is removed. But the ulcer may take a turn towards chronicity if the trauma continues that means traumatic agent persists, e.g., dental ulcer of the tongue. Again healing of an ulcer is delayed if it lies over a joint for want of rest.

Ulcers which originate spontaneously may follow swelling, which may be matted tuberculous lymph nodes or gumma or a rapidly growing malignant tumor [epithelioma **(Fig. 4.1)** or malignant melanoma]. Ulcers may be present in the leg with varicose veins or vascular insufficiency. Sometimes a malignant ulcer (Marjolin's) **(Fig. 4.2)** may develop on the scar of a burn **(Fig. 4.3**, *see* also **Fig. 4.12)**.

2. **Duration:** How long is the ulcer present there? An acute ulcer will be present for a shorter duration, whereas a chronic ulcer will remain for a long period **(Fig. 4.4)**. In this context, one must also

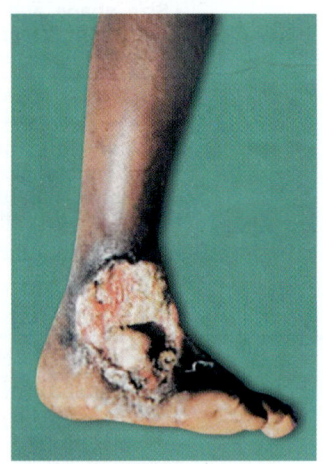

Fig. 4.1: Epitheliomatous ulcer.

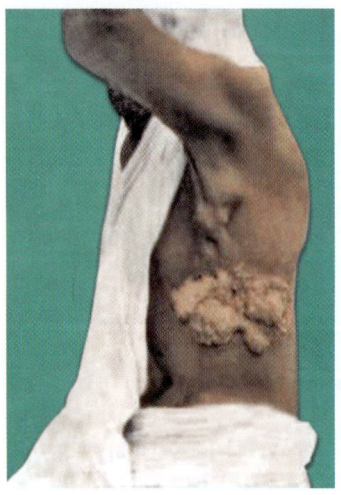

Fig. 4.2: Marjolin's ulcer developed at the loin from the scar of a burn.

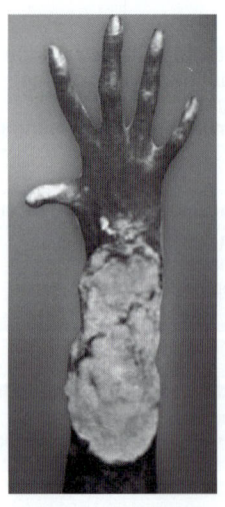

Fig. 4.3: Marjolin's ulcer developed in the scar of a burn.

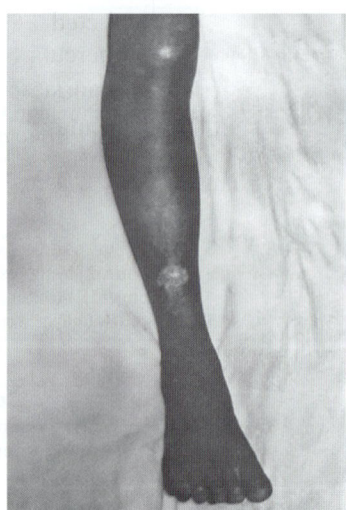

Fig. 4.4: Chronic ulcer in the leg, which refuses to heal.

know *the incubation period*, i.e., the time interval between the exposure and the onset of the ulcer. In Hunterian chancre (syphilis) this incubation period is 3–4 weeks, whereas in chancroid (soft sore) this period is about 3–4 days.

3. **Pain:** Is the ulcer painful? Only those ulcers associated with inflammation will be painful. Syphilitic ulcers and trophic ulcers resulting from nerve diseases (tabes dorsalis, transverse myelitis, peripheral neuritis) are painless. Tuberculous ulcers are slightly painful. Ulcers from malignant diseases such as epithelioma or basal-cell carcinoma are absolutely painless to start with and never become painful unless they infiltrate structures supplied by pain nerve endings.

4. **Discharge:** Does the ulcer discharge or not? If it discharges enquiry must be made about its nature—serum, pus or blood.

5. **Associated disease,** if present: Nervous diseases such as tabes dorsalis, syringomyelia, transverse myelitis and peripheral neuritis may result an ulcer (trophic or perforating ulcer). Generalized tuberculosis, nephritis or diabetes may lead to ulcer formation. Syphilis at the primary stage gives rise to chancre and in the tertiary stage gives rise to a gummatous ulcer.

History in ulcer patient

Aspect	Clinical significance	Key history taking questions
Mode of onset	Sudden-onset ulcers are **traumatic or infective**, gradual-onset ulcers may be **neoplastic or vascular**	"Did the ulcer appear suddenly or gradually?" "Was there an injury before it developed?"
Duration	Acute ulcers heal quickly, chronic ulcers indicate **persistent pathology (e.g., malignancy, ischemia, tuberculosis)**	"How long has the ulcer been present?"
Pain	Painful ulcers suggest **infection or vascular insufficiency**, painless ulcers suggest **neuropathic, syphilitic, or malignant** origin	"Is the ulcer painful?" "If yes, describe the nature of pain."
Discharge	Serous → Healing, Purulent → Infected, Blood-stained → Malignant/Tuberculous	"Does the ulcer discharge? If yes, what is its color and consistency?"
Systemic associations	**Diabetes, syphilis, tuberculosis, vascular diseases** may cause ulcers	"Do you have a history of diabetes, vascular disease, or tuberculosis?"

PHYSICAL EXAMINATION

GENERAL SURVEY: In case of ulcer, one should not give all attention to the ulcer only. Due consideration must be given to the general examination of the patient. Ulcer may well be a sequel of malnutrition, general atherosclerosis, syphilis, tuberculosis, etc.

LOCAL EXAMINATION

A. **INSPECTION:** The following points are particularly noted:

1. **Size and shape:** *Tuberculous ulcers* are generally oval in shape but their coalescence may give an irregular crescentic border. *Syphilitic ulcers* are similarly circular or semilunar to start

with but may unite to form a serpiginous ulcer. *Varicose ulcers* are generally vertically oval in shape. *Carcinomatous ulcers* are irregular in size and shape. The size of an ulcer is important to know the time which will be required for healing. A bigger ulcer will definitely take a longer time to heal. To record exactly the size and shape of an ulcer, a sterile gauge may be pressed on to the ulcer to get its measurements.

2. **Number:** Tuberculous, gummatous, varicose ulcers and soft chancres may be more than one in number.

3. **Position:** This is very important and often by itself gives a clue to the diagnosis. An ulcer on the medial malleolus of a lower limb which shows varicose veins, is obviously a *varicose ulcer* **(Fig. 4.5)**. *Rodent ulcers* are usually confined to the upper part of the face above a line joining the angle of the mouth to the lobule of the ear **(Fig. 4.6)**, occurring frequently near the inner canthus of the eye (*see* **Fig. 3.62B**). *Tuberculous ulcers* are commonly seen where tuberculous adenopathy is commoner, that means in the neck, axilla **(Figs. 4.7 and 4.8)** or groin. *Lupus*—a form of cutaneous tuberculosis occurs more frequently on the face **(Fig. 4.9)**, fingers and the hand. *Hunterian chancre* and soft sores will

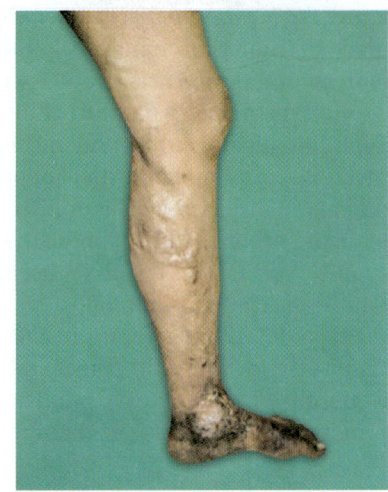

Fig. 4.5: Venous ulcer in its typical site. Note the varicose veins in the upper part of the leg and thigh.

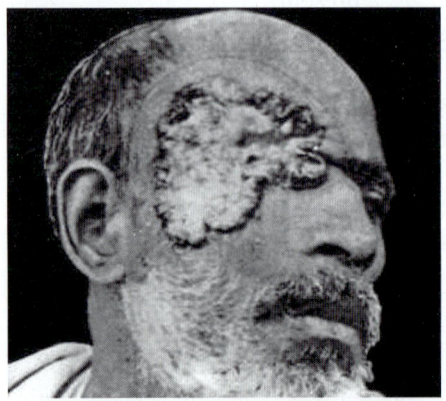

Fig. 4.6: Rodent ulcer in its late stage.

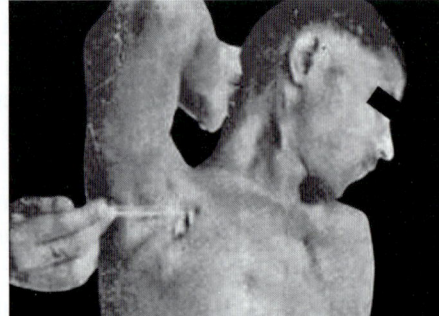

Fig. 4.7: Typical undermined edge of a tuberculous ulcer in the axilla. The probe can be easily insinuated between the edge and the floor of the ulcer. Also note the scars of healed tuberculous ulcer in the neck.

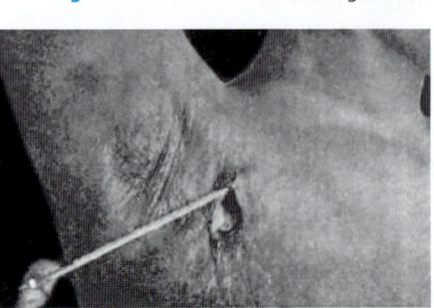

Fig. 4.8: Closer view of tuberculous ulcer in the axilla of patient in Figure 4.7.

obviously be found over the external genitalia. *Gummatous ulcers* are more commonly seen over the subcutaneous bones such as tibia, sternum, skull, etc. *Perforating* or *trophic ulcers* are commoner on the heel **(Fig. 4.10)** of the foot or on the ball of the foot, which carries maximum weight of the body. *Malignant ulcers* may occur anywhere in the body but more commonly seen on the lips, tongue, breast, penis and anus.

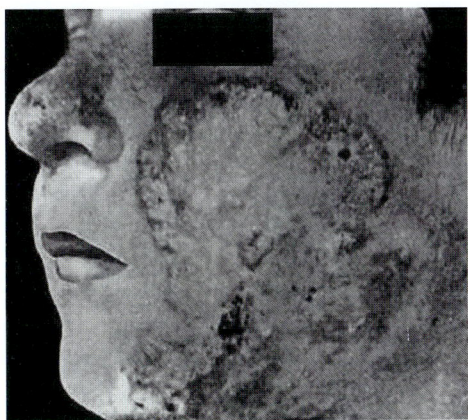

Fig. 4.9: Lupus vulgaris—a form of cutaneous tuberculosis occurring on the face.

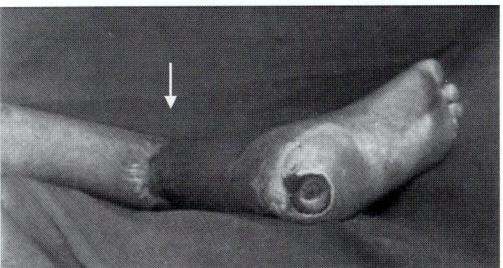

Fig. 4.10: Trophic ulcer at the heel resulting from nerve injury, the scar of which is shown by arrow.

4. **Edge:** This is another important finding of an ulcer which by itself not only gives a clue to the diagnosis of the ulcer but also to the condition of the ulcer. The term '*edge*' should not be confused with the term '*margin*' (*see* palpation in page 72). In a *spreading ulcer*, the edge is inflamed and edematous whereas in a *healing ulcer* the edge, if traced from the red granulation tissue in the center towards periphery, will show a blue zone (due to thin growing epithelium) and a white zone (due to fibrosis of the scar).

Five common types of ulcer edge are seen in surgical practice **(Figs. 4.11A to E)**:
(i) **Undermined edge**—is mostly seen in tuberculosis. The disease causing the ulcer spreads in and destroys the subcutaneous tissue faster than it destroys the skin. The overhanging skin is thin, friable, reddish blue and unhealthy. (ii) **Punched out edge**—is mostly seen in a gummatous ulcer or in a deep trophic ulcer. The edge drops down at right angle to the skin surface as if it has been cut out with a punch. The diseases which cause the ulcers are limited to the ulcer itself and do not tend to spread to the surrounding tissue. (iii) **Sloping edge** is seen mostly in healing traumatic or venous ulcers. Every healing ulcer has a sloping edge, which is reddish-purple in color and consists of new healthy epithelium. (iv) **Raised and pearly-white beaded edge**—is a feature of rodent ulcer. This type of edge develops in invasive cellular disease and becomes necrotic at the center **(Fig. 4.12)**. (v) **Rolled out (everted) edge**—is a characteristic feature of squamous-celled carcinoma or an ulcerated adenocarcinoma. This ulcer is caused by fast growing cellular disease, the growing portion at the edge of the ulcer heaps up and spills over the normal skin to produce an everted edge.

5. **Floor:** This is the exposed surface of the ulcer (cf. base). When floor is covered with red granulation tissue, the ulcer seems to be healthy and healing. Pale and smooth granulation tissue indicates a slowly healing ulcer. Wash-leather slough (like wet chamois leather) on the floor of an ulcer is pathognomonic of gummatous ulcer. One must be very careful to note what is there at the floor of an ulcer. A trophic ulcer penetrates down even to the bone, which forms the floor in this case. A black mass at the floor suggests malignant melanoma.

6. **Discharge:** The character of the discharge should be noted, its amount and smell. A healing ulcer will show scanty serous discharge, but a spreading and inflamed ulcer will show purulent discharge. Serosanguineous discharge is often seen in a tuberculous ulcer or a malignant ulcer. If the ulcer is infected with *B. pyocyanea*, the discharge will be greenish. It is always advisable to take a bacteriological swab of the ulcer.

7. **Surrounding area:** If the surrounding area of an ulcer is glossy, red and edematous, the ulcer is acutely inflamed. Very often the surrounding skin of a varicose ulcer is eczematous

and pigmented. A scar or a wrinkling in the surrounding skin of an ulcer may well indicate an old case of tuberculosis.

8. Even the **whole limb** should be examined in case of an ulcer. Presence of varicose vein and deep vein thrombosis will indicate the ulcer to be a varicose ulcer. Neurological insufficiency will indicate the ulcer to be a trophic one.

B. PALPATION

1. **Tenderness:** An acutely inflamed ulcer is always exquisitely tender. Chronic ulcers such as tuberculous and syphilitic ulcers are slightly tender. Varicose ulcers may or may not be tender. Neoplastic ulcers are never tender.

2. **Edge and margin:** These two terms should not be confused and both these terms demand separate entity. '*Margin*' is the junction between normal epithelium and the ulcer, so it is the boundary of the ulcer **(Fig. 4.13)**. '*Edge*' is the area between the margin and the floor of the ulcer. Activity is maximum at the margin and edge of the ulcer, though the degree of activity will vary according to the type of the ulcer.

In palpation the different types of the edge of the ulcers are corroborated with the findings of inspection. Besides this, a careful palpation of the edge and the surrounding tissue will give a clue to the diagnosis. Marked induration (hardness) of the edge is characteristic feature of a carcinoma, be it a squamous-celled carcinoma or adenocarcinoma. A certain degree of induration or thickness is expected in any chronic ulcer, whether it is a gummatous ulcer or a syphilitic chancre or a trophic ulcer.

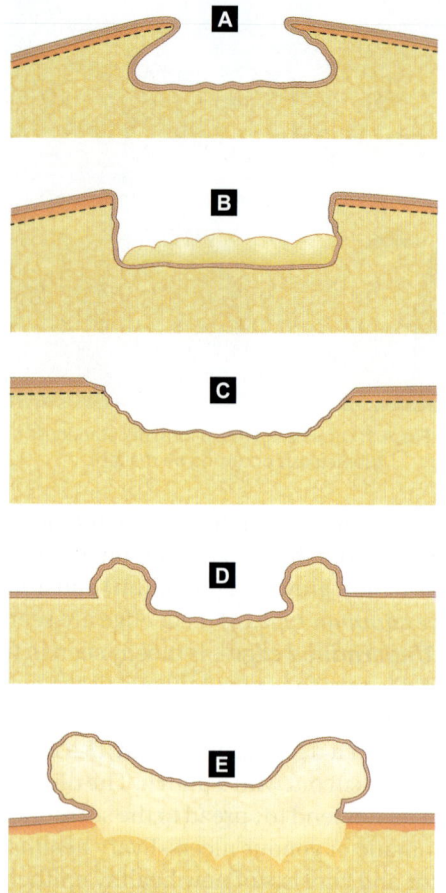

Figs. 4.11A to E: Diagrammatic representation of different types of edge of ulcers. (A) Undermined edge. (B) Punched out edge. (C) Sloping edge. (D) Raised and a pearly-white beaded edge of rodent ulcer. (E) Rolled out (everted) edge of an epithelioma.

3. **Base** (on which the ulcer rests): The students must understand the difference between the floor (i.e., exposed surface within the ulcer) and the base (on which the ulcer rests and it is better felt than seen) of an ulcer. If an attempt is made to pick up the ulcer between the thumb and the index finger, the base will be felt **(Fig. 4.14)**. Slight induration of the base is expected in any chronic ulcer but marked induration (hardness) of the base is an important feature of squamous-celled carcinoma and Hunterian chancre.

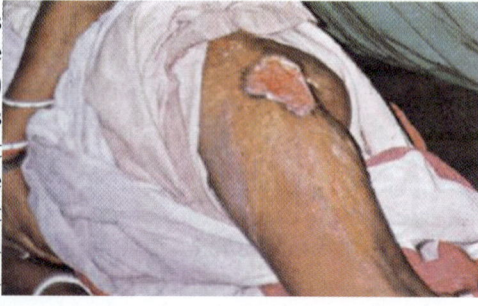

Fig. 4.12: A chronic ulcer in the gluteal region which has followed burn and is taking a turn towards Marjolin's ulcer.

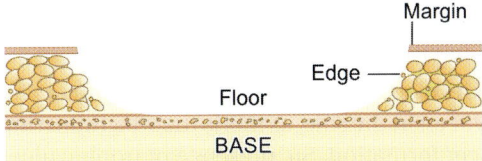

Fig. 4.13: Diagrammatic representation of various parts of an ulcer. See the text.

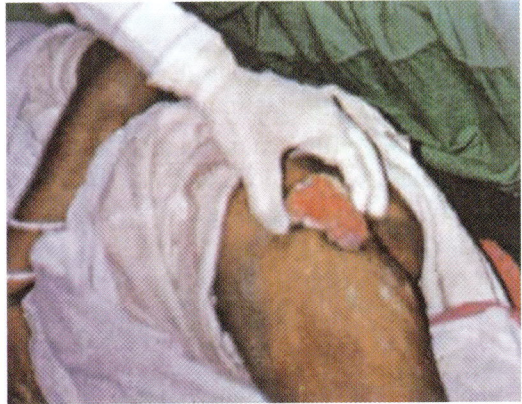

Fig. 4.14: Shows how to palpate for the base of the ulcer.

4. **Depth:** The students must make an assessment regarding depth of the ulcer. It can be recorded in the examination sheet in millimeters. Trophic ulcers may be as deep as to reach even the bone.

5. **Bleeding:** Whether the ulcer bleeds to touch or not? It is a common feature of a malignant ulcer.

6. **Relations with the deeper structures:** The ulcer is made to move over the deeper structures to know whether it is fixed to any of these structures. A gummatous ulcer over a subcutaneous bone (tibia or sternum) is often fixed to it. Malignant ulcer will obviously be fixed to the deeper structure by infiltration.

7. **Surrounding skin:** Skin around the ulcer must be palpated and examined. Increased temperature and tenderness of the surrounding skin indicates the ulcer to be of acute inflammatory origin. The mobility of the surrounding skin is examined. Fixity to deeper structures indicates the malignant nature of the lesion. Surrounding skin is tested for nerve lesion (loss of sensation or motor deficit). Try to feel the peripheral nerves around for abnormal thickening or tenderness. Feel the main arteries supplying the part. The artery may be blocked (atherosclerotic, Buerger's disease, Raynaud's disease) in case of arterial or ischemic ulcer. It is imperative to know the state of vein around the ulcer particularly when venous ulcer is suspected. Venous ulcer may or may not be associated with varicose veins of the limb.

C. **EXAMINATION OF LYMPH NODES:** This part of the examination is very important, but unfortunately the students often forget to do this. In *acutely inflamed ulcers*, the regional lymph nodes become enlarged, tender and show the signs of acute lymphadenitis. Later on, the nodes become soften to form an abscess. In *tuberculous ulcer* the lymph nodes become enlarged, matted and slightly tender. In *Hunterian chancre*, the regional lymph nodes remain discrete, firm and shotty. This type of lymph nodes is pathognomonic of hard (Hunterian) chancre. In *gummatous ulcers*, the lymph nodes are not usually involved. In *rodent ulcer* also the lymph nodes are not affected possibly because of the early obliteration of the lymphatics by the neoplastic cells. In *malignant ulcer* the nodes are stony hard and may be fixed to the neighboring structures in late stages. Simple enlargement of lymph nodes in malignant disease does not suggest lymphatic metastasis. The lymph nodes may be enlarged because of secondary infection rather than anything else. So palpation of the lymph nodes in case of malignant ulcer is very important. Stony hard consistency will suggest secondary involvement.

D. **Examination for vascular insufficiency**: When the ulcer is situated on the lower part of the leg, one should always search for *varicose veins* in the upper part of the leg or thigh. If there is no varicose vein and the cause of ulcer is not determined, the clinician must examine the condition of the arteries proximal to the ulcer. Atherosclerosis, Buerger's disease, Raynaud's disease, etc., may be the cause of the ulcer from poor circulation.

E. **Examination for nerve lesion:** Trophic ulcers develop as a result of repeated trauma to an insensitive part of the patient's body. This is mostly seen in the sole, as this is the weightbearing zone if there is sensory loss. It may well lead to ulcer formation. So, presence of trophic ulcer indicates some neurological (particularly sensory) disturbance, either in the form of tabes dorsalis or transverse myelitis or peripheral neuritis.

Examination of ulcer

Feature	Findings and interpretation	Clinical example
Size and shape	**Round/Punched-out:** Syphilis, trophic ulcer. **Irregular:** Carcinoma	Gummatous ulcer → Punched-out edge
Number	**Multiple ulcers:** Tuberculosis, venous ulcers. **Single ulcer:** Malignancy, trauma	Tuberculous ulcer → multiple lesions
Edge	**Undermined:** Tuberculosis. **Punched-out:** Syphilis. **Sloping:** Healing ulcer. **Everted:** Carcinoma	Epithelioma → everted edge
Floor	**Granulation tissue:** Healing ulcer. **Necrotic slough:** Malignant ulcer	Squamous cell carcinoma → necrotic floor
Surrounding skin	**Pigmented and Eczematous:** Venous ulcer. **Trophic Changes:** Neuropathic ulcer	Varicose ulcer → hyperpigmentation

GENERAL EXAMINATION

1. When the ulcer is suspected to be *syphilitic*, a thorough search should be made for presence of other syphilitic stigmas in the body as shown in **Figure 4.15**.
2. If the ulcer appears to be *tuberculous*, all the lymph nodes in the body should be examined along with other examination such as the chest, the neck, the abdomen, etc.
3. If the ulcer seems to be due to atherosclerotic or Buerger's disease (*ischemic*), the whole body must be examined for presence of atherosclerosis or its complication anywhere in the body. Moreover, Buerger's disease is a bilateral condition and the other limb should always be examined.
4. When the ulcer is a *trophic* (perforating) one general examination must be made to know the type of nervous disease present with this condition.

SPECIAL INVESTIGATIONS

1. **Routine examination of the blood,** e.g., total count and differential count of WBC, hemoglobin percentage, RBC count, erythrocyte sedimentation rate (ESR) should always be done in a patient with an ulcer. Blood sugar estimation may be performed to exclude diabetes. WR and Kahn test should be done to exclude syphilis. In tuberculous ulcers, lymphocyte count will be high and ESR will also be high. The patient may be anemic.
2. **Examination of the urine**—particularly sugar estimation, to exclude diabetes, is important.
3. **Bacteriological examination of the discharge** of the ulcer is particularly important in inflamed and spreading ulcers. This will not only give a clue as to the type of organism present

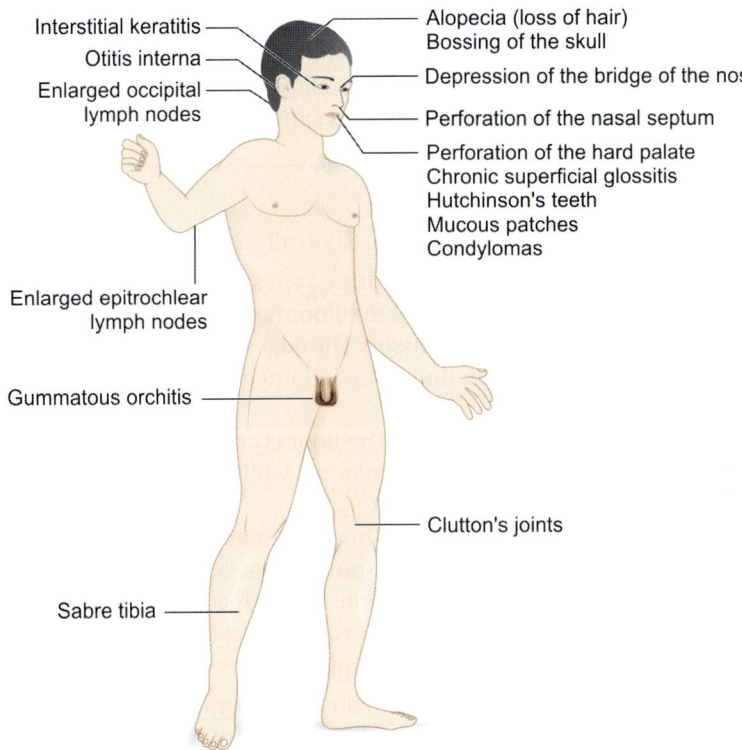

Fig. 4.15: Shows the common sites of syphilitic stigmas.

in the ulcer, but also its sensitivity to a particular antibiotic. 'In dark ground illumination' *Treponema pallidum* can be detected from the serous discharge of hard chancre. The chancre is first cleaned with saline, the serous discharge from the chancre is taken with a platinum loop and placed on a slide, which is seen under microscope 'in dark ground illumination'. Discharge from tuberculous ulcer will show acid fast bacilli and should be sent for guinea pig inoculation test.

4. **Skin test:** Mantoux test is more important in children to diagnose tubercular ulcer and in adults to exclude tubercular ulcer.
5. **Chest X-ray:** It is important in tuberculous ulcers to detect any primary focus in the lung. It is important to exclude metastatic deposit in the lungs in case of malignant ulcers.
6. **Biopsy:** It is very important in malignant ulcers. The biopsy is generally taken from the edge of the ulcer taking a portion of surrounding healthy tissue. Biopsy material is then examined histologically to know the type of tumor, its invasiveness and whether differentiated or anaplastic.
7. **X-ray of the bone and joint:** It is required when the ulcer is situated very near a bone or joint. In gummatous ulcer, it produces new bone formation and 'sabre tibia', which is discussed more elaborately in the chapter of 'Examination of bony lesion'.
8. **Contrast radiography:** Arteriography may be helpful to diagnose arterial or ischemic ulcer. Ascending functional phlebography is helpful to diagnose deep vein thrombosis in case of venous ulcer.

9. **Imaging technique:** (1) *Radioactive fibrinogen test* using ^{125}I-labeled fibrinogen is quite accurate (90%) in detecting deep vein thrombosis particularly in its formation stage. (2) *Technetium*^{99} clearance is used to know the blood flow of the calf muscle. More recently this isotope is used to take arterial imaging with gamma camera.

CLASSIFICATION OF ULCERS

Two types of classification of ulcers are possible: Clinically and pathologically.

1. CLINICALLY, an ulcer may be either of three types: **(a) Spreading ulcer,** when the surrounding skin of the ulcer is inflamed and the floor is covered with profuse and offensive slough without any evidence of granulation tissue. The edge is inflamed, edematous and ragged. It is a painful ulcer. The draining lymph nodes are inflamed, enlarged and tender and may be suppurated with abscess formation.
(b) **Healing ulcer** means the ulcer is healing. The floor is covered with pinkish or red healthy granulation tissue. The edge is reddish with granulation, while the margin is bluish with growing epithelium. The discharge is slight and serous.
(c) **Callous or chronic ulcer** means the ulcer shows no tendency towards healing. The floor is covered with pale granulation tissue. Sometimes it shows typical wash-leather slough in gummatous ulcer which is an example of this type. Discharge is scanty or absent. The base is considerably indurated and so is the edge and surrounding skin.

2. PATHOLOGICALLY, the ulcers can be classified into:
(a) **Nonspecific ulcers:** These ulcers can be further classified into the following categories—(1) *Traumatic*—can be either (i) mechanical, e.g., dental ulcer of the tongue from jagged tooth, from pressure of a splint, etc., or (ii) physical from electrical or X-ray burn or (iii) chemical from application of caustics. These types of ulcers heal quickly and do not become chronic unless supervened by infection or ischemia, which may turn this ulcer to chronicity.
(2) *Arterial*—as occurs in atherosclerosis, Buerger's disease, Raynaud's disease (primary and secondary), etc.
(3) *Venous*—e.g., varicose ulcer in postphlebitic limb.
(4) *Neurogenic (Trophic)*—e.g., bedsore and perforating ulcer.
(5) *Associated with malnutrition,* e.g., tropical ulcers, which occur in the legs and feet of the people in the tropical countries. Infection by Vincent's organisms *(Bacteroides fusiformis)* from a small abrasion may cause such ulcer. Wrongly, ulcers secondary to anemia, rheumatoid arthritis, diabetes, avitaminosis are sometimes included under this type of ulcer, but these ulcers should be classified separately.
(6) *Ulcers may be associated with certain other diseases* like gout, diabetes, anemia, avitaminosis, *Erythrocyanosis frigida*, rheumatoid arthritis, etc. In gout the skin over the gouty deposit (tophi) ulcerates and the chalky contents exude.

Clinical and pathological features of ulcers

Type	Subtype	Example
Clinical	Spreading	Pyogenic ulcer, Synergistic gangrene
	Healing	Post-traumatic ulcer
	Callous/Chronic	Venous ulcer, Marjolin's ulcer
Pathological	Infective	Tuberculosis, Syphilis, Actinomycosis
	Neoplastic	Squamous cell carcinoma, Basal cell carcinoma
	Neuropathic	Trophic ulcer in diabetes

In diabetes slight injury to the glucose laden tissue may cause chronic infection and subsequently ulcer develops, it can also occur from ischemia due to diabetic atherosclerosis and diabetic polyneuropathy. (7) *Certain other types of ulcers* require special mention, e.g., Bazin's ulcer, Martorell's ulcer, etc. Bazin's ulcer is found in fatty adolescent girls particularly on the calves as purplish nodules followed by indolent ulcers. Martorell's or hypertensive ulcer is found in people suffering from hypertension. It often affects legs where patches of skin necrosis are first noticed. It cannot be classified under arterial group as it is not generally associated with atherosclerosis.

(b) **Specific ulcers**—e.g., tuberculous, syphilitic, soft sores, actinomycosis (*see* Chapter 23 of this book and Meleney's ulcers.

(c) **Malignant ulcers**—e.g., epithelioma, Marjolin's ulcer, rodent ulcer (*see* page 60) and malignant melanoma (*see* page 61).

DIFFERENTIAL DIAGNOSIS

Differential diagnosis of ulcer

Type	Location	Key features	Example
Traumatic	Anywhere	Recent trauma, resolves with removal of irritant	Dental ulcer (sharp tooth)
Venous	Medial malleolus	Painless, sloping edge, pigmented surrounding skin	Varicose ulcer
Arterial	Toes, dorsum of foot	Painful, punched-out, cold periphery	Atherosclerotic ulcer
Neuropathic	Pressure points	Painless, deep, surrounded by callus	Diabetic foot ulcer
Malignant	Lip, tongue, breast, genitalia	Everted edges, hard base, slow-growing	Squamous cell carcinoma
	Neuropathic	Trophic ulcer in diabetes	

Traumatic ulcer: Traumatic ulcer can be either (i) *mechanical*, e.g., dental ulcer of the tongue from jagged tooth, from pressure of a splint, etc. or (ii) *physical* from electrical or X-ray burn or (iii) *chemical* from application of caustics. This ulcer heals quickly unless supervened by infection or ischemia, which may turn this ulcer to chronicity.

Ischemic or arterial ulcer: These ulcers are rare compared to venous ulcer. Arterial ulcers are due to peripheral arterial disease (atherosclerosis is the commonest followed by Buerger's disease and Raynaud's disease) and poor peripheral circulation. This condition is more often seen in older people and are episodes of trauma and infection of the destroyed skin over a limited area of the leg or the foot. When it occurs secondary to Buerger's disease, younger men between 20 and 40 years of age are affected. In this case patches of dry gangrene may be present alongwith arterial ulcer. Such ulcers tend to occur on the anterior and outer aspects of the leg, dorsum of the foot, on the toes or the heel (the parts exposed to trauma).

Unlike venous ulcer (which is painless) pain is the main complaint of this disease. When this ulcer occurs on the inner side of the ankle, possibility of venous ulcer should be excluded. Venous ulcer usually occurs above the medial malleolus, whereas arterial ulcer tends to occur below the medial malleolus. Moreover there is often a history of intermittent claudication and even rest pain in majority of cases of arterial ulcer. If the leg is kept elevated above the heart level, the ulcer shows no sign of healing and the patient will complain of pain in this position. *On examination,* these ulcers are punched out with destruction of the deep fascia (cf. venous ulcer). The tendons, bone or underlying joints may be exposed in the floor of the ulcer which is covered by minimal granulation tissue. Peripheral arterial pulses should always be felt. Pulse of dorsalis pedis artery is almost always either feeble or absent. Presence of ischemic changes can be detected in the foot, e.g., pallor, dry skin, loss of hair, fissuring of nails, etc. Arteriography is important to detect the arterial disease.

Venous ulcer: These ulcers are typically situated on the medial aspect of the lower third of the lower limb. Though these ulcers are often associated with varicose veins in the upper part of the limb yet the term 'varicose ulcer' will not be justified. These ulcers are not caused by the presence of varicose veins but these are complications of deep vein thrombosis. Eczema and pigmentation are often seen around these ulcers. The ulcer is slightly painful in the beginning but gradually the pain settles down and the main symptoms become discomfort, unsightliness and discharge.

Trophic ulcer (neurogenic): These ulcers have punched-out edge with slough in the floor thus resembling a gummatous ulcer. Bedsore and perforating ulcers are typical examples of trophic ulcers. These ulcers develop as the result of repeated trauma to the insensitive part of the body. So, some neurological disturbances in the form of loss of sensation is the cause behind this ulcer formation. These ulcers are commonly seen on the heel and the bail of the foot when the patient is ambulatory and on the buttock and on the back of heel when the patient is nonambulatory. These ulcers start with callosity under which suppuration takes place, the pus comes out and the central hole forms the ulcer which gradually burrows through the muscles and the tendons to the bone. The resulting is a callous ulcer with punched out corny edge. Floor is covered with offensive slough and tendons and even bone can be seen here. The base is slightly indurated. The surrounding skin has no sensation. The cause may be spinal or leprosy or peripheral nerve injury, diabetic neuropathy, tabes dorsalis, transverse myelitis or meningomyelocele.

Tropical ulcer: This ulcer may result from various diseases as it has been mentioned in the earlier section. The most important feature of this ulcer is its callousness towards healing. Its edge is slightly raised and exudes copious serosanguineous discharge. This ulcer practically retains the same size for months and years. In some cases, it destroys the surrounding tissue and thus spreads widely. Every effort should be made to detect the cause behind the ulcer and to treat accordingly. Otherwise, it may retain its existence or even spreads rapidly so as to require amputation.

Diabetic ulcer: Three factors play to produce diabetic ulcer. (i) Diabetic neuropathy. (ii) Diabetic atherosclerosis causing ischemia and (iii) Glucose laden tissue is quite vulnerable to infection and thus ulcer is formed.

When the ulcer is due to neuropathy a trophic ulcer results. The features are same as trophic ulcer with less sensation to the surrounding skin. When the ulcer is due to ischemia, an ischemic (arterial) ulcer results, but it is less painful than typical arterial ulcer. Infective ulcer is a type of spreading ulcer. Blood sugar estimation and urine examination should be performed to prove this diagnosis.

Tuberculous ulcer: This mostly results from bursting of caseous lymph nodes. This type of ulcer may also develop when cold abscess from bone and joint tuberculosis breaks out on the surface. The ulcer is slightly painful. Such ulcer is usually seen in the neck, axilla and groin according to frequency. The most characteristic feature of this ulcer is its edge which is thin, reddish blue and undermined. There is pale granulation tissue with scanty serosanguineous discharge in the floor and slight induration at the base, which indicates that this ulcer is a chronic one. The regional lymph nodes are enlarged, nontender and matted. Blood examination, Mantoux test, microscopic and guinea pig inoculation test of the discharge, chest X-ray are the investigations to be performed to diagnose such ulcer.

Lupus vulgaris (**Fig. 4.9**): It is a form of cutaneous tuberculosis, occurs commonly in the face and hand and the usual victims are the children and young adults. It starts very superficially as single or multiple cutaneous nodules which gradually turn into multiple superficial ulcerations of the skin. These ulcers remain active at the periphery and spread outwards whereas in the center they gradually heal. Due to its destructive nature at the periphery it is called 'lupus' which means 'wolf'. Squamous cell carcinoma may grow from the scar of lupus vulgaris to form Marjolin's ulcer.

Syphilitic ulcers: (i) *Hard chancre* appears on the external genitalia 3–4 weeks after infection in the first stage of the disease (**Fig. 4.16**). It is painless and possesses a characteristic indurated base, which feels like a button. In the penis chancre is found commonly in the coronal sulcus and frenum. Lymph nodes are enlarged, mobile, firm, discrete, painless and show no tendency towards suppuration. Extragenital chancres which are seen in the nipple, lip, tongue and anal canal are not often indurated and may be slightly painful. *Treponema pallidum* can be demonstrated in serous discharge of the ulcer.

(ii) *Mucous patches and condylomas* are the characteristic lesions of the secondary stage of syphilis.

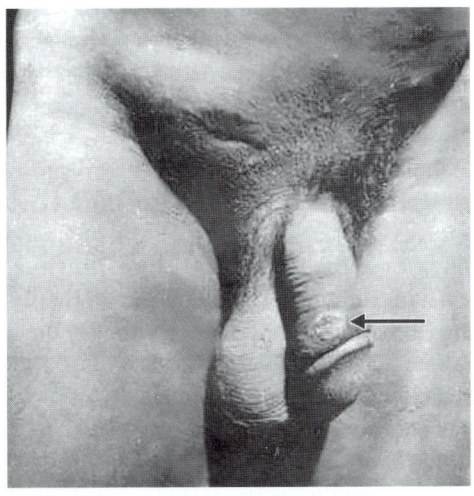

Fig. 4.16: Hunterian chancre on the penis with involvement of inguinal lymph nodes.

Mucous patches are white patches of sodden thickened epithelium. These are small, round, superficial, transient erosions particularly in the mouth which coalesce to form snail-track ulcer.

Condylomas are raised, flat, white and hypertrophied epithelium. Both these lesions usually occur at the mucocutaneous junctions, e.g., angles of the mouth, anus, vulva, etc. These are called *Condyloma lata* and should be clearly differentiated from *Condyloma acuminata* which are warts or papillomas often caused by a virus (HPV). In this stage of the syphilis there is generalized painless enlargement of the lymph nodes, particularly the epitrochlear and suboccipital groups which are diagnostic to some extent. There is also generalized coppery red rash, motheaten alopecia, iritis and arthritis in this stage.

(iii) *Gummatous ulcers* occur in tertiary (late stage) syphilis (**Fig. 4.17**). These ulcers are result of obliterative endarteritis, necrosis and fibrosis and are mostly seen over the subcutaneous bones (e.g., tibia, sternum, ulna and skull), in the scrotum in relation to the testis, upper part of the leg, etc. The most characteristic feature is punched-out indolent edge and yellowish gray gummatous tissue (wash-leather slough) in the floor. Pain and tenderness are totally absent. Lymph nodes are seldom involved unless secondarily infected as the lymphatics are early closed by perivascular inflammatory reaction. WR and Kahn tests are positive.

Soft chancre or sore (Ducrey's): These are multiple painful acute ulcers with edematous edge and yellowish slough on the floor. These are seen on external genitalia. These ulcers generally appear 3 days after infection and discharge copious purulent secretion. The regional lymph nodes show the picture of acute lymphadenitis with tendency towards suppuration. This leads to soft swelling in the inguinal region known as bubo.

Meleney's ulcer: These ulcers are seen in the postoperative wounds either after the operation for perforated viscus or for drainage of empyema thoracis. It is also found, though rare, on the dorsum of the hand. This type of ulcer is due to symbiotic action of microaerophilic nonhemolytic streptococci and hemolytic *Staphylococcus aureus*. Nowadays other synergistic pairs have been

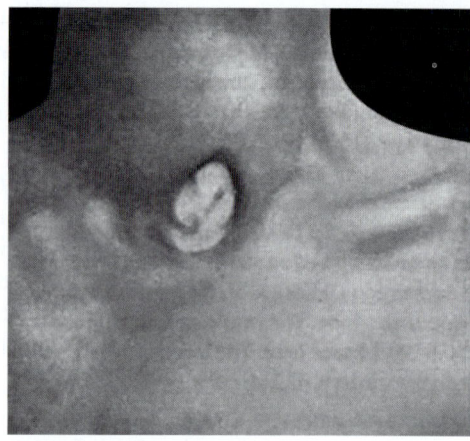

Fig. 4.17: Gummatous ulcer in the sternomastoid showing punched out edge and wash-leather slough in the floor.

isolated from such ulcer. This ulcer is most commonly seen in the abdomen as postoperative gangrenous wound following perforated viscus or in the thorax following drainage of empyema thoracis. Rarely, it is seen on the leg (more often associated with ulcerative colitis) or on the dorsum of the hand. It is a spreading ulcer which is very painful with signs of toxemia. It is an undermined ulcer as it destroys the tissues at the depth. The floor contains abundant foul smelling granulation tissue with copious seropurulent discharge. If not treated, the patient's general condition deteriorates and he will die ultimately. Clinically, it is an undermined ulcer with lot of granulation tissue in the floor. It is surrounded by deep purple zone, which in its turn is surrounded by an outer zone of erythema. This particular condition is painful, toxic and the general condition deteriorates without treatment.

Epithelioma (squamous cell or epidermoid carcinoma): It arises from prickle cell layer of the skin and hence may occur anywhere in the body. But it is more commonly seen on the lips, cheek, hands, penis, vulva and old scars. It may also occur in the internal organs, e.g., tongue, buccal cavity, pharynx, larynx and esophagus. In certain columnar cell area it may occur following metaplasia to squamous cells, e.g., cardiac end of stomach, gallbladder, etc. Similarly in certain transitional cell areas it may occur following metaplasia to squamous cells, e.g., pelvis of kidney, urinary bladder, etc. Histologically, this tumor presents 'structureless mass of keratin' surrounded by prickle cells in concentric manner as seen in 'onion skin'. This whole appearance is called 'cell-nest' or 'epithelial pearl'. This 'cell-nest' however is absent in rapidly growing tumor and in the mucous membrane, e.g., esophagus, urinary bladder, etc.

It is mostly seen after 40 years of age. It begins as a small nodule which enlarges and gradually the center becomes necrotic and sloughs out and thus ulcer develops. Such an ulcer is oval or circular in shape, but size varies considerably. The edge of the ulcer is raised and everted. Floor is covered by necrotic tumor, serum and blood. There may be some granulation tissue, but is pale and unhealthy. Base of the ulcer is indurated, which is the pathognomonic sign of epithelioma. In early cases epithelioma can be moved with the skin over the underlying structures. But later on it becomes fixed due to involvement of the deeper structures. Regional lymph nodes are almost always enlarged be it due to metastasis or secondary infection. When metastasized the nodes become hard, gradually matted and fixed. 'Kangri cancer' is also an example of epithelioma **(Fig. 4.18)**.

Marjolin's ulcer: This is a squamous cell carcinoma arising from a long-standing benign ulcer or scar. The commonest ulcer to become malignant is a long-standing venous ulcer. The scar which may show malignant change is the scar of an old burn. It is a slow-growing and less malignant squamous carcinoma. It is slight different from typical squamous carcinoma in the sense that its edge is not always raised and everted. Unusual nodules may develop as carcinoma.

Lymphatic metastasis is unusual as the lymphatics are already destroyed or occluded by previous chronic lesion of the skin. It is absolutely painless. Unlike squamous carcinoma it is radioresistant as it is relatively avascular and there is extensive fibrosis.

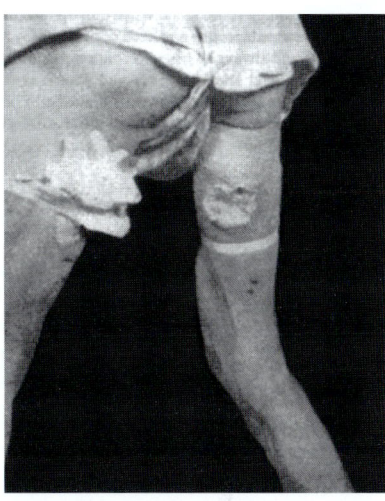

Fig. 4.18: 'Kangri Cancer' on the back of thigh. While being seated Kangri (portable charcoal brazier) is placed on the ground between the thighs. 45% of Kangri cancers are seen on the thighs. Other places where Kangri cancers can be seen are the abdominal wall (Fig. 1.1), the legs, the groins, etc. Majority lesions are ulcers, though one may find nodular growths or fungating growths.

ULCERS OF THE LEG

Ulcers of the lower part of the leg, the ankle and the foot are common problems faced by the surgeons all over the world. The followings are the common causes of ulcer peculiar to this place. Of course, the other types of ulcers discussed above can also occur in the leg.

Venous ulcer: The basic cause of the venous ulcer is abnormal venous hypertension in the lower third of the leg. The terms "varicose ulcer", "post-thrombotic ulcer" and "gravitational ulcer" are also used as synonyms of venous ulcer. When the calt pump and the main deep veins are normal, even the slightest movements empty the superficial veins lowering the superficial venous pressure. The main pathway of the venous drainage of the ankle skin in the erect posture is via the ankle perforating veins. When the valves of this vein are damaged there will be local venous hypertension. This condition is aggravated by obstructed main deep veins. Postcanalization of the thrombosed deep veins leads to destruction of the valves of the deep veins and this becomes the main contributing cause for ankle venous hypertension. The most important complication of this venous ulcer is the development of the carcinoma (Marjolin's ulcer) from the growing edge of the ulcer.

Majority of venous ulcers follow many years of venous disease, so the patients are usually of the age group of 40 to 60 years. Women are affected far more often than men. Discomfort and tenderness of the skin, pigmentation and eczema exist for months or years before a venous ulcer develops. The ulcer is painful in the beginning but once it settles down and becomes chronic it becomes painless.

Venous ulcers are mainly found in lower part of the leg on its medial side. These are never seen above the junction of the middle and upper thirds of the leg. Venous ulcer can be of any shape and size. The edge is sloping and pale purple-blue in color. The margin is thin and blue of growing epithelium. The floor is formed by pale granulation tissue. This ulcer is usually shallow and flat and never penetrates the deep fascia. The discharge is seropurulent with occasional trace of blood. The base of the ulcer is fixed to the deeper structures. The surrounding skin shows signs of chronic venous hypertension—pigmentation, induration and tenderness. There may be scars of previous ulcers. Varicose veins may or may not be seen in the proximal limb. Regional lymph nodes (inguinal group) are only enlarged if the ulcer becomes infected.

It must be remembered that squamous carcinoma can arise from the margin of a longstanding venous ulcer. When the edge of a longstanding venous ulcer is raised and everted or somewhat different from what described above should arouse suspicion of malignancy. The base of the ulcer becomes hard. This malignant ulcer is called *Marjolin's ulcer*. Biopsy should always be taken to confirm malignancy.

Arterial ulcer: These are rare compared to venous ulcer. Ulcers are due to peripheral arterial disease and poor peripheral circulation. These are often seen in older people and are episodes of trauma and infection of the destroyed skin over a limited area of the leg or the foot. The ulcers tend to be punched out and destroy the deep fascia (unlike the venous ulcer) and may expose the tendons at the base. When these ulcers occur at the inner side of the ankle the diagnosis is frequently overlooked, but a history of intermittent claudication with discoloration of one or more toes becomes the differentiating feature.

Ulcer from congenital arteriovenous fistula may be the rare cause of ulcer in the lower part of the leg. The peculiar feature of this ulcer is that it occurs at a comparatively early age and presence of venous encroachment around the ulcer.

Erythrocyanoid ulcer (Bazin's disease): These ulcers are associated with "erythrocyanosis frigida", which is an exclusive disease of young women. Abnormal amount of subcutaneous fat with thick ankles combined with an abnormally poor arterial supply are the predisposing factors. The blood supply of the lower third of the leg and the ankle are derived from a number of perforating arteries arising from the posterior tibial and peroneal arteries. In erythrocyanoid cases these arteries may be abnormally small and even absent causing low-grade ischemia of the whole ankle region. The patient finds that the ankle skin is abnormally sensitive to temperature changes. When the weather is cold, the ankle is blue, cold and often tender. In hot weather chronic reactive hyperemia becomes evident with the ankle becomes hot, edematous, swollen and painful. The patient is much troubled by chilblain. Palpation of the leg will reveal small, superficial and painful nodules which break down to form ulcers. These ulcers are small and multiple.

Gummatous ulcer: *See* page 79.

Martorell's ulcer (hypertensive ulcer): It is linked to atherosclerosis in old age, manifests as a punched-out ulcer on the calf's outer side, marked by intense pain and necrosis. Despite bilateral occurrence and intact peripheral foot pulses, the healing process may extend over several months.

Infective ulcers: The ulcers which are now coming in the limelight are the *Staphylococcus aureus*, present as small, red sores on the leg, often tied to poor hygiene and nutrition. "Footballer's ulcer" over the shin, a consequence of staphylococcal infection and repeated trauma, can become chronic and adhere to the bone without proper treatment.

Meleney's ulcer: It is initially linked to infected surgical wounds, can arise in the leg, especially with ulcerative colitis or pre-existing ulcers. Marked by burrowing and a deep purple zone surrounded by erythema, these painful ulcers, resulting from symbiotic streptococci and Staphylococcus aureus, may spread, causing systemic toxemia and deterioration without prompt treatment.

Ulcers associated with various diseases may arise spontaneously or worsen in venous ulcers, becoming more painful. Conditions like anemia, polycythemia, leukemia, rheumatoid arthritis, Paget's disease, and ulcerative colitis are often implicated. In rheumatoid arthritis, ulcers result from nodule breakdown, presenting as shallow, punched-out sores within subcutaneous tissue, characterized by pain and slow healing. Ulcers in Paget's disease, located over the anteriorly bowed tibia, exhibit dense adherence to the bone at their base.

Tropical ulcer: It is likely caused by Vincent's organisms (Bacteroides fusiformis), originates from skin trauma or insect bites, evolving from papule-pustules with inflammation and induration. Characterized by undermined edges, copious serosanguineous discharge, and persistent pain, the ulcer may become indolent, healing slowly with a parchment-like scar or, in rare cases, developing into squamous carcinoma.

Yaws: It is caused by Treponema pertenue, manifests as painless ulcers on the leg or foot, resulting from barefoot abrasions, and typically heals within a few weeks, leaving a tissue paper-like scar.

Algorithmic Approach to Patient with Ulcer

Patient presents with an ulcer

↓

History taking
- **Onset:** Sudden (trauma, infection) vs gradual (malignancy, vascular)
- **Duration:** Short-term (acute) vs long-standing (chronic)
- **Pain:** Present (infection, ischemia) vs absent (neuropathic, syphilitic)
- **Discharge:** Serous (healing), purulent (infected), bloody (malignancy)
- **Systemic conditions:** Diabetes, tuberculosis, syphilis, vascular disease

↓

Inspection
- **Size and shape:** Large (chronic ulcer), small and multiple (tuberculosis)
- **Edge type:** Undermined (TB), punched-out (syphilis), everted (carcinoma)
- **Floor:** Granulating (healing), Necrotic (malignant)
- **Discharge and surrounding skin:** Signs of infection or malignancy

↓

Palpation
- **Tenderness:** Painful (infective), nontender (neuropathic, malignancy)
- **Induration:** Present in **malignant, chronic** ulcers
- **Depth and base fixity:** Deeper ulcers may involve bones or vessels

↓

Determine likely etiology
- **Traumatic** (mechanical, chemical, physical)
- **Infective** (tuberculosis, syphilis, soft chancre, actinomycosis)
- **Vascular** (arterial, venous, diabetic)
- **Neuropathic** (trophic ulcers, leprosy)
- **Neoplastic** (squamous cell carcinoma, basal cell carcinoma)

↓

Order special investigations
- **Biopsy and FNAC** → Malignant ulcers
- **Doppler ultrasound** → Vascular ulcers
- **X-ray/MRI** → Bony involvement in chronic ulcers
- **Blood tests** → Syphilis (VDRL), tuberculosis (Mantoux, ESR)

↓

Confirm diagnosis and Initiate treatment
- **Medical management:** Antibiotics, wound care, lifestyle modifications
- **Surgical management:** Debridement, skin grafting, tumor excision

CHAPTER 5

Examination of a Sinus or a Fistula

Sinus: A sinus is a blind track leading from the surface down to the tissues. There may be a cavity in the tissue which is connected to the surface through a sinus. The sinus is lined by granulation tissue which may be epithelialized.

Fistula: It is a communicating track between two epithelial surfaces, commonly between a hollow viscus and the skin (external fistula) or between two hollow viscera (internal fistula). The track is lined with granulation tissue which is subsequently epithelialized.

Differences between sinus and fistula

Feature	Sinus	Fistula
Definition	Blind tract leading from the skin to deeper tissues	Abnormal communication between two epithelial surfaces
Cause	Foreign body, infection (osteomyelitis, tuberculosis), trauma	Postsurgical, inflammatory (Crohn's, diverticulitis), malignancy
Lining	Lined with granulation tissue, may epithelialize	Lined by epithelial tissue over time
Discharge	Usually purulent or serous	Contains irritant secretions (urine, feces, bile)
Natural healing	Can heal if the underlying cause is removed	Rarely heals spontaneously unless the underlying communication is corrected

Causes of persistence of a sinus are: (1) presence of foreign body or necrotic tissue (e.g., sequestrum or a suture material) in the depth; (2) absence of rest; (3) nondependent drainage or inadequate drainage of an abscess; (4) when a specific chronic infection (e.g., tuberculosis, actinomycosis, etc.) is the cause; (5) when the track becomes epithelialized; (6) sometimes there may be a dense fibrosis around the wall of the track and the cavity preventing their collapse, as occurs in chronic empyema.

Causes of persistence of a fistula are: once a true fistula has been formed, it seldom shows any intention towards healing. Moreover, irritant discharge such as urine, feces, bile, etc., are passed through the fistula and prevents its healing. But one thing should always be remembered that if the natural passage is made patent, all abnormal offshoots heal spontaneously.

■ HISTORY

Certain sinuses and fistulae are present since birth, e.g., *preauricular sinus*. When *a sinus is due to osteomyelitis* **(Fig. 5.1)**, the patient will give a history of high fever followed by swelling

Causes of sinus and fistula

Cause	Sinus	Fistula
Foreign body	Sequestrum, suture material, bullet fragments	Retained surgical material, fecal impaction
Chronic infection	Tuberculosis, actinomycosis	Crohn's disease, chronic abscess
Poor drainage	Nondependent drainage, inadequate abscess drainage	Continuous passage of irritants (urine, bile, feces)
Epithelialization	Track lined with epithelium prevents closure	Fistula tract fully epithelialized, preventing healing
Fibrosis	Prevents collapse of the sinus	Stenosed natural lumen causes persistence

and pain in the bone concerned. An abscess will develop, subsequently this will gradually move towards the surface and will burst resulting a discharging sinus. Sometimes a history of discharge of bone chips may be elicited. The sinus will persist so long as there will be necrotic bone (sequestrum) at the depth of the wound. In case of *tuberculous sinus* **(Fig. 5.2)**, a previous history of lymph nodes enlargement or tuberculous affection of the bone or joint may be elicited. Subsequently a cold abscess will develop which will burst (or be incised) leading to a sinus. In case of a sinus or fistula in the perianal region a previous history of perianal or ischiorectal abscess may be given by the patient. Intermittent contraction of the anal sphincter will prevent proper rest to the part and thus interfere with healing of the sinus or the fistula.

Pain: If pain is associated with, inflammatory nature of the sinus or blockage of the opening of the sinus or fistula is assured.

Fever and *redness of the surrounding skin* also suggest inflammatory origin of the sinus or fistula.

PAST HISTORY: This is important as a few diseases are prone to develop sinus or fistula later in life, e.g., tuberculosis, Crohn's disease, ulcerative colitis and actinomycosis. Colloid carcinoma of rectum may produce anal fistula in later stage. Sinus or fistula may develop as a complication of operation performed earlier.

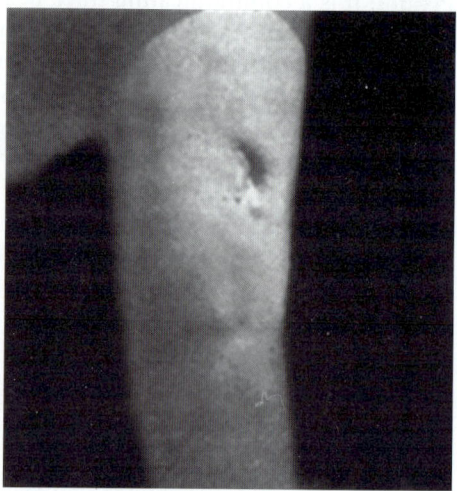

Fig. 5.1: Osteomyelitic sinus showing sprouting granulation tissue at the mouth of the sinus.

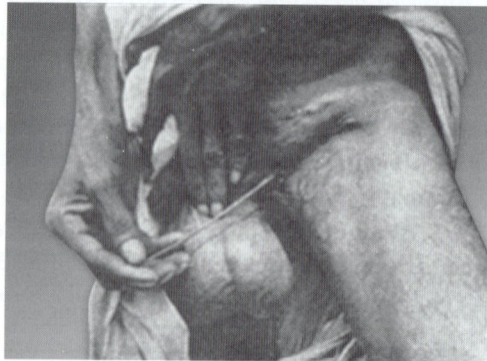

Fig. 5.2: Shows a tuberculous sinus following tuberculous lymphadenitis in the inguinal region.

FAMILY HISTORY: A few diseases often involve more than one member of the same family which may predispose sinus or fistula formation, e.g., tuberculosis, Crohn's disease, ulcerative colitis, etc. Even fistula-in-ano is often seen in more than one member in a family.

Examination of sinus and fistula

Aspect	Clinical significance	Key history taking questions
Onset and duration	Long-standing sinuses suggest **chronic infection or foreign body**	"How long have you had this condition?"
Pain	Painful → Inflammatory cause, painless → Tuberculous or malignant	"Is there pain? If yes, what is the nature of the pain?"
Discharge	Pus → Infection, serosanguineous → Tuberculosis, sulfur granules → Actinomycosis	"What does the discharge look like? Is it foul-smelling?"
Systemic symptoms	Fever → Infection, Weight loss → Malignancy	"Do you have any associated symptoms such as fever or weight loss?"
Previous surgeries/ injuries	Fistulae may form postsurgically or after trauma	"Have you had any past surgeries or injuries in this region?"

LOCAL EXAMINATION

A. **INSPECTION:** The following points are carefully noted:

1. **Number:** Though majority of the fistulae which occur in the body are single, yet a few are notoriously known for their multiplicity. These are 'Watering Can' perineum, Crohn's disease affecting the rectum and anal canal which produces multiple anal fistulae, actinomycosis always produces multiple sinuses and sometimes ulcerative colitis may produce multiple fistulae **(Fig. 5.3)**.

2. **Position:** Diagnosis of many sinuses and fistulae can be made only looking at the position of these sinuses and fistulae. *Preauricular sinus* (due to failure of fusion of the ear tubercles) is situated at the root of the helix or on the tragus of the pinna, the direction of sinus being upwards and backwards.

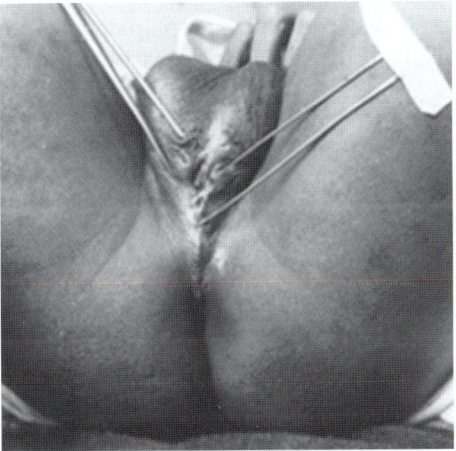

Fig. 5.3: 'Watering-can' perineum. Each opening is shown with a probe.

The *branchial fistula* (due to failure of fusion of the second branchial arch with the fifth) is almost always situated at the lower third of the neck just in front of the sternomastoid muscle. The *pilonidal sinus* is mostly seen in the middle behind the anus. Multiple indurated sinuses in the upper part of the neck suggest the diagnosis *of actinomycosis. Tuberculous sinus* often takes a peculiar position which by itself mentions the diagnosis. A single sinus over the lower irregular jaw is mostly due to *osteomyelitis*.

3. **Opening of the sinus:** Sprouting granulation tissue at the opening of the sinus suggests presence of foreign body at the depth, e.g., sequestrum, a drainage tube, bullet, etc. The opening of a tuberculous sinus is often wide and the margin is thin blue and undermined **(Figs. 5.4A and B)**.

4. **Discharge:** It is always advisable to look for the character of the discharge. In osteomyelitis it is often pus. In tuberculous ulcer it is often serosanguineous and most important is often presence of sulfur granules in the discharge of actinomycotic sinuses. In case of fistulae, urine, feces, bile, etc., may be seen coming out.

5. **Surrounding skin:** There may be a scar in the surrounding tissue which may indicate chronic osteomyelitis or previously healed tuberculous sinus, etc. There may be surrounding dermatitis and pigmentation which are characteristic features of Crohn's disease and actinomycosis.

B. **PALPATION:** While palpating a sinus or a fistula the following points should be noted:

1. **Tenderness:** Is the sinus tender? The sinus from inflammatory source will be tender (e.g., osteomyelitis).

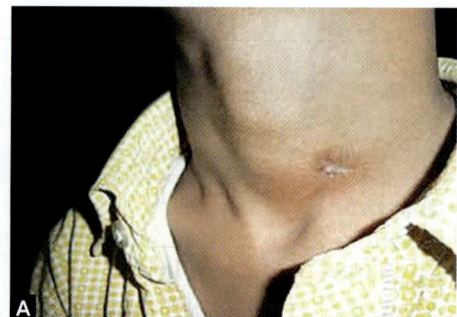
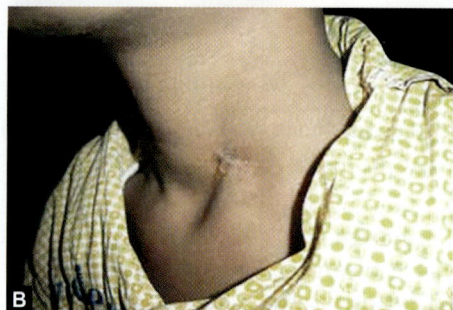

Figs. 5.4A and B: External opening of the branchial fistula at the anterior border of left sternocleidomastoid muscle, 2 cm above medical end of left clavicle.

2. **Wall of the sinus:** It is palpated to note any *thickening* there. Chronic sinuses will have thick wall due to presence of fibrosis surrounding the wall of the sinus.

3. **Mobility:** Is the sinus mobile over the deep structures? Sinuses resulting from osteomyelitis are fixed to the bone, which becomes irregular, thickened and tender.

4. **Lump:** Presence of lump in the neighborhood of a sinus often indicates tuberculous lymphadenitis.

C. **EXAMINATION WITH A PROBE:** This is important but should be performed with due precaution. This examination will inform the clinician about (i) the direction and the depth of the sinus **(Fig. 5.5)**, (ii) presence of any foreign body such as sequestrum, which will be moveable, at the depth of the wound, (iii) whether the fistula is communicated with a hollow viscus or not and (iv) whether fresh discharge comes out on withdrawal of the probe or not.

D. **EXAMINATION OF DRAINING LYMPH NODES:** This examination is always essential and should not be missed under any circumstances.

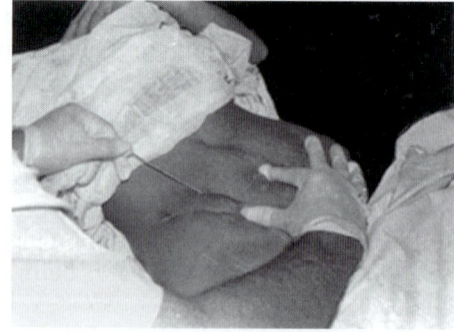

Fig. 5.5: A sinus in the appendicectomy scar is being examined with a probe.

Local findings in sinus and fistula

Feature	Findings and interpretation	Clinical example
Number	Multiple sinuses → Actinomycosis, Crohn's disease	Watering-can perineum in Crohn's disease
Position	Specific locations indicate cause	Branchial fistula → Lower neck, preauricular sinus → Ear
Discharge	Pus → Infection, Serous → Tuberculosis, Fecal → Enteric fistula	Bile-stained discharge → Biliary fistula
Surrounding skin	Pigmentation, scarring → Chronic condition	Crohn's disease → Perianal skin changes

GENERAL EXAMINATION

Depending on the site and cause of the sinus, examination of the particular system should be performed. In case of a sinus in the loin, the spine, ribs and the kidneys should be examined to know the exact cause of the lesion. In case of a sinus due to chronic empyema, the chest should be thoroughly examined. In case of a sinus due to osteomyelitis, the bone should be examined as described under 'Examination of diseases of bone'. In case of fistula around the anus a thorough examination not only of the anal canal and rectum both manually and proctoscopically should be called for but also sigmoidoscopic examination and examination of the whole abdomen should be performed. In case of multiple fistulae in the perineum and scrotum, the lower urinary track should be thoroughly examined. In case of a groin sinus the hip joint and the spine should be examined as it may be due to bursting of cold abscess originating from there.

SPECIAL INVESTIGATIONS

1. **Examination of the discharge**—is of utmost importance to come to a diagnosis. It should be examined macroscopically, physically, chemically, microscopically (e.g., for sulfur granules in case of actinomycosis) and bacteriologically.
2. **X-ray examination:** (a) Straight X-ray may show a sequestrum and osteomyelitic change of the bone concerned or presence of opaque foreign body.
(b) Injection of radio-opaque fluid (lipiodol or hypaque) into a sinus (sinogram) or a fistula (fistulogram) will indicate the cause of the sinus or fistula by delineating its course.
3. **Examination using colored solution:** (a) Sterilized methylene blue may be pushed through a catheter into the urinary bladder and if the color is detected in the vagina vesicovaginal fistula is confirmed. (b) Charcoal powder may be used in the food to confirm presence of upper gastrointestinal (GI) tract fistula by detecting charcoal particles in the discharge of the fistula after a few hours. (c) Colored drug, e.g., pyridium may be used to confirm presence of urinary fistula, as the colored drug is excreted through the urine.

CLASSIFICATION OF SINUSES

1. **CONGENITAL,** e.g., preauricular sinus.
2. **TRAUMATIC,** e.g., following trauma a foreign body may be implanted into deep tissues and following infection a sinus may persist.

3. **INFLAMMATORY,** e.g., osteomyelitic sinus, tuberculous sinus, actinomycotic sinus or sinus of a chronic abscess which discharges pus due to inadequate treatment of acute abscess.
4. **NEOPLASTIC,** e.g., sinus due to degenerative change of a malignant growth or due to secondary infection of a malignant growth which was incised for drainage.
5. **MISCELLANEOUS,** e.g., pilonidal sinus.

CLASSIFICATION OF FISTULA

1. **CONGENITAL,** e.g., branchial fistula, thyroglossal fistula, rectovesical fistula, vesicovaginal fistula, tracheo-oesophageal fistula, umbilical fistula.
2. **TRAUMATIC:** Such fistula may occur after operation or after accidental injury to certain viscera, e.g., salivary fistula, pancreatic fistula, biliary fistula, fecal fistula, urinary fistula, etc.
3. **INFLAMMATORY:** Abscess related to a viscus if bursts to the exterior may develop a fistula, e.g., appendicular fistula or external fistula following diverticulitis of colon.
4. **MALIGNANT:** Advanced carcinoma of one viscus may either infiltrate into the neighboring viscus to form a fistula (internal fistula) or may infiltrate into the parietes to form external fistula, e.g., carcinoma of the rectum may involve urinary bladder in males to produce rectovesical fistula. Carcinoma cervix may involve urinary bladder in females to produce uterovesical fistula. Extensive malignant lesion of abdominal viscus may involve umbilicus to produce umbilical fistula (fecal fistula).

Algorithmic Approach to Patient with Sinus or Fistula

Patient presents with a sinus or fistula

↓

History taking
- **Onset:** Congenital (since birth) vs acquired (post-trauma, infection, malignancy)
- **Pain:** Present (infection, inflammation) vs absent (tuberculous, malignant)
- **Discharge:** Purulent (infective), serous (tuberculous), fecal/bile-stained (enteric or biliary fistula)
- **Systemic conditions:** Diabetes, tuberculosis, Crohn's disease, malignancy
- **Previous surgery/trauma:** Postsurgical complications may cause fistula formation

↓

Inspection
- **Number:** Single (common) vs multiple (Crohn's, actinomycosis)
- **Position:** Perianal (fistula-in-ano), neck (branchial fistula), preauricular (congenital sinus)
- **Opening appearance:** Sprouting granulation → Retained foreign body
- **Surrounding skin:** Pigmentation, scarring → Chronic condition

↓

Palpation
- **Tenderness:** Painful → Infection; Painless → Tuberculosis, malignancy
- **Wall thickness:** Thickened wall → Chronic sinus/fistula
- **Mobility:** Fixed → Osteomyelitis; Mobile → Soft tissue pathology
- **Nearby lump:** Suggests associated lymphadenopathy or malignancy

↓

Probe test
- **Direction and depth:** Helps determine the extent of the tract
- **Foreign body:** Presence suggests osteomyelitis, actinomycosis
- **Communication with hollow organ:** If fecal/bile-stained discharge appears, suggests enteric or biliary fistula

↓

Evaluate likely etiology
- **Traumatic:** Postsurgical, foreign body-induced sinus/fistula
- **Infective:** Osteomyelitis, actinomycosis, tuberculosis
- **Neoplastic:** Malignant sinus/fistula due to infiltrating tumor
- **Congenital:** Preauricular sinus, thyroglossal or branchial fistula

↓

Order special investigations
- **X-ray:** Bone involvement in osteomyelitis-related sinus
- **Sinogram/Fistulogram:** Define sinus or fistula tract extent
- **FNAC/Biopsy:** Rule out malignancy
- **Blood tests:** CRP, ESR (infection), TB markers, Crohn's serology

↓

Confirm diagnosis and initiate treatment
- **Medical management:** Antibiotics, wound care, lifestyle modifications
- **Surgical management:** Sinus excision, fistulectomy, flap reconstruction

Examination of Peripheral Vascular Disease and Gangrene

CHAPTER 6

HISTORY

1. **Age and sex:** Atherosclerosis is obviously a disease of old age. It affects men more often than women. Buerger's disease (thromboangiitis obliterans) is commonly seen in men between 20 and 40 years of age. Raynaud's disease is a disease of young women. Diabetic arteriopathy is commoner in middle age.

2. **Limbs affected:** Buerger's disease and atherosclerotic gangrene commonly affect the lower limbs, but Raynaud's disease mainly affects the upper limbs. A patient who presents with superficial gangrene of the finger, the following causes should especially be considered: Raynaud's disease, the cervical rib, scalenus anticus syndrome, Morvan's disease—painless whitlow in syringomyelia.

3. **Bilateral or unilateral:** In Buerger's disease and Raynaud's disease the affection is usually bilateral. Atherosclerotic gangrene may be unilateral to start with but often ends as a bilateral disease. Gangrene due to embolism is mostly unilateral. Diabetic gangrene may be unilateral or bilateral.

4. **Mode of onset:** Gangrenes due to atherosclerosis, Buerger's disease and Raynaud's disease occur spontaneously and gradually. Embolic gangrene starts suddenly and the patient feels severe pain radiating down the course of the artery. Diabetic gangrene may start from slight trauma such as caused by careless paring of the toenail or mild infection.

5. **Pain:** Note its *site, character, radiation, whether it increases in walking or exercise, whether it disappears when the exercise stops and whether it becomes worse on application of warmth.* When circulation of the limb is impaired, two types of pain are noticed: (i) intermittent claudication and (ii) rest pain.

i. *Intermittent claudication:* Though literary 'claudio' means 'I limp', yet the term claudication is used here to describe the muscle pain due to accumulation of the excessive P-substance owing to inadequate blood flow. It is a pain in the muscles, *usually the calf* and it is described by the patient as a *cramp*. Of course the site of the pain depends on the level of arterial occlusion, e.g., in the foot in Buerger's disease in which the arterial occlusion is mostly in the lower tibial or plantar arteries; in the calf in case of arterial occlusion in femoropopliteal junction which is very common; in the thigh when the occlusion is at the opening of the superficial femoral artery and in the buttock in case of occlusion in the bifurcation of the common iliac artery or the aorta. The pain develops *only when the muscles are working*. The pain *disappears when the exercise stops.*

The patient often complains that after walking a distance, called the *'claudication distance*, the pain starts. Sometimes if the patient continues to walk the metabolites increase the muscles blood flow and sweep away the P-substances produced by exercise and pain disappears

(Grade I). More often the pain continues and the patient can still walk with effort (Grade II). But mostly the pain compels the patient to take rest (Grade III, Boyd's classification).

ii. *Rest pain:* This pain is *continuous and aching in nature.* This pain seems to be due to ischemic changes in the somatic nerves. *It is the cry of the dying nerves.* The pain is worse at night, gets aggravated by elevation of the leg above the level of the heart and is relieved by hanging the leg below the level of the heart. It usually affects the most distal part first that means the tip of the toes. The painful part becomes very sensitive and any movement or pressure causes an acute exacerbation.

6. **Effects of heat and cold:** Application of warmth will increase the symptoms of arterial occlusion. Raynaud's phenomenon, i.e., intermittent attack of pallor or cyanosis is often seen in Raynaud's disease and sometimes in Buerger's disease.

In Raynaud's disease a number of attacks can be seen—each attack is comprised of three stages viz. (i) *Local syncope,* in which the affected digits become cold and white with tingling and numbness. These changes are due to spasm of the digital arteries. (ii) *Local asphyxia,* in which the white digits turn blue with burning sensation; This change is due to slowing of circulation and accumulation of reduced hemoglobin. (iii) *Local recovery,* in which the bluish discoloration gradually disappears and the digits regain normal color due to release of spasm of digital arteries. Such attacks are repeated, till in the end patches of superficial ulceration and gangrene appear at the finger tips, which is known as *local gangrene* **(Fig. 6.1)**.

7. **Paresthesia:** When the muscle pain begins, the patient often feels numbness, pins and needles and other types of paresthesia in the skin of the foot. This is due to shunting of blood from the skin to muscle.

8. **History of superficial phlebitis:** This is characterized by swelling, redness and minor pain in the affected part. It occurs in high proportion of cases of Buerger's disease.

9. **Involvement of other arteries:** Enquiry must be made if there is complain *of fainting, transient black out, chest pain, weakness* or *paresthesia* in the upper limbs, *blurred vision, abdominal pain* to exclude occlusive arterial disease anywhere in the body.

10. **Impotence:** Due to failure in erection is not uncommon symptom in case of bilateral internal iliac artery occlusion.

11. **Past history:** The patient with arterial occlusion may give a history of previous cardiac attacks or embolic syndromes. The patient may be diabetic. There may be a history of exposure to cold (frost bite), etc.

12. **Personal history:** Excessive smoking has been incriminated as causing thromboangiitis obliterans and worsening atherosclerotic disease.

13. **Family history:** It is amazing to know that arterial disease particularly atherosclerosis is often familial and if you practice the habit of asking if other members of the family are affected with the same disease or not, you will find quite a few are or were suffering from this disease.

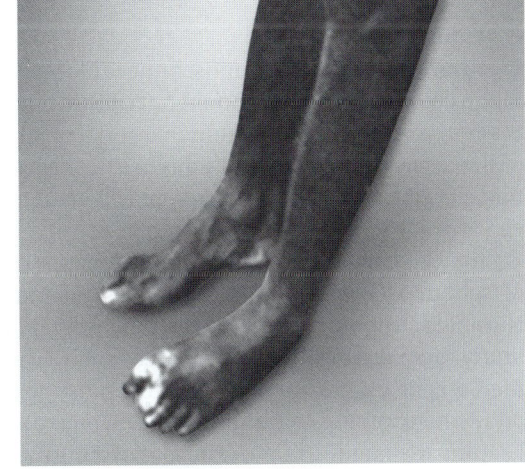

Fig. 6.1: Shows typical gangrene of the great and the middle toes of the left leg.

History in peripheral vascular diseases

Aspect	Clinical significance	Key history taking questions
Age and sex	Atherosclerosis affects elderly; Buerger's disease affects young male smokers; Raynaud's disease is common in young women	"When did the symptoms first appear? Do you have any known vascular conditions?"
Limb affected	Atherosclerosis and Buerger's affect the **lower limbs**; Raynaud's affects **upper limbs**	"Which limb is affected? Is it unilateral or bilateral?"
Mode of onset	**Acute** → Embolism; **Gradual** → Atherosclerosis, Buerger's disease	"Did the symptoms appear suddenly or develop gradually?"
Pain type	**Claudication** → Atherosclerosis; **Rest pain** → Severe ischemia	"Do you experience leg pain while walking or at rest?"
Smoking history	Strong association with **Buerger's disease and atherosclerosis**	"Do you smoke? If yes, how many cigarettes per day?"
Systemic conditions	Diabetes → Diabetic arteriopathy; Autoimmune disorders → Vasculitis	"Do you have diabetes, hypertension, or autoimmune diseases?"

■ PHYSICAL EXAMINATION

Considerable constitutional disturbances may be observed in severe acute ischemia from embolus and in gas gangrene. There may be lowering of the blood pressure and increase in the pulse rate in both these conditions. In chronic ischemia there is not much constitutional disturbances.

■ LOCAL EXAMINATION

A. INSPECTION

1. **Change in color** is the most noticeable feature of an ischemic limb. To detect minor change in the color the clinician should put the affected limb and its fellow side by side. Marked pallor is a remarkable feature of sudden arterial obstruction as seen in case of embolism or in spasm of the arterioles in Raynaud's disease. Congestion and purple-blue cyanosed appearance are the characteristic features of severe ischemia and pregangrenous stage. As soon as the limb is elevated it becomes pallor.

2. **Signs of ischemia:** While examining a case of arterial insufficiency, one must know the signs of ischemia. These are: thinning of the skin, diminished growth of hair, loss of subcutaneous fat, shininess, trophic changes in the nails which become brittle and show transverse ridges and *minor ulceration* in the pressure areas such as heel, malleoli, ball of the foot, tips of the toes, etc.

3. **Buerger's postural test:** This test must be carried out in broad day light. The patient lies on his back on the examining table. The patient is asked to raise his legs one after the other keeping the knees straight. The legs of a normal individual remain pink even if they are raised to 90°. But in case of an ischemic limb elevation to a certain degree will cause marked pallor and the veins will be empty and 'guttered'. The angle (between the limb and the horizontal

plane) at which such pallor appears is called 'Buerger's angle' or the 'Vascular angle'. A vascular angle of less than 30° indicates severe ischemia. If the feet do not become pallor and occlusive arterial disease is suspected the following addition may be performed. The elevated legs are supported by the examiner, while the patient flexes and extends his ankles and toes to the point of fatigue. If there is occlusive arterial disease the sole of the foot assumes cadaveric pallor and the veins on the dorsum of the foot become empty and guttered. The feet are now lowered so that the patient adopts sitting posture. Within 2 or 3 minutes a cyanotic hue spreads over the affected foot, whereas no change will be observed in case of healthy limb. This is due to cyanotic congestion.

4. **Capillary filling time:** After elevating the legs, the patient is asked to sit up and hang his legs down by the side of the table. A normal leg will remain pink as it was during elevated position. But an ischemic leg will first become pallor when elevated and gradually become pink in horizontal position. This change of color takes place slowly and is called 'the capillary filling time'. In severe ischemia it takes about 20–30 seconds to become pink. Then the ischemic limb again changes color and becomes purple-red quickly. This is due to the filling of the dilated skin capillaries with deoxygenated blood.

5. **Venous refilling:** After keeping the limb elevated for a while if it is then laid flat on the bed, there will be normal refilling of the veins within 5 seconds. But in ischemic limb it will be delayed. If a normal limb is raised to about 90° there will be gradual collapse or 'guttering of the veins'. But in ischemic limb the veins are seen collapsed either in the horizontal position or as soon as it is lifted to even 10° above the horizontal level.

In established gangrene the following points are noted: (1) **Extent and color** of the gangrenous area. This is important to ascertain the level of arterial occlusion. In gas gangrene, besides the typical odor of sulfurated hydrogen, the muscles also change their color to brick-red, green or even black according to the stage of the disease.

(2) **Type**—of the gangrene should be noted—whether *dry*, i.e., the part becomes mummified or *wet* and putrefying as seen in diabetic gangrene.

(3) **Line of demarcation**—is often seen between the dead gangrenous part and the normal living limb. In gangrene due to all the conditions this line of demarcation is poorly marked except in ainhum. In this condition there is a linear deepening groove at the base of the little or the fourth toe, which is the pathognomonic feature **(Figs. 6.2 and 6.3)**.

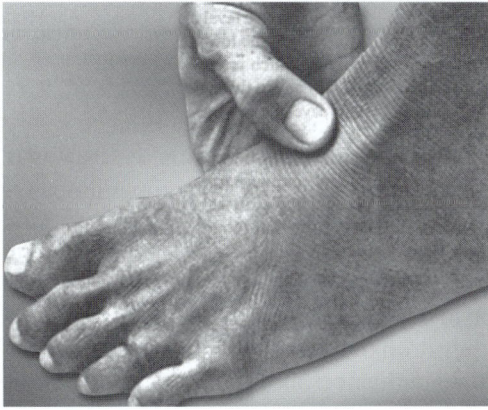

Fig. 6.2: Ainhum affecting the fourth toe. Note that the line of demarcation is grooved in.

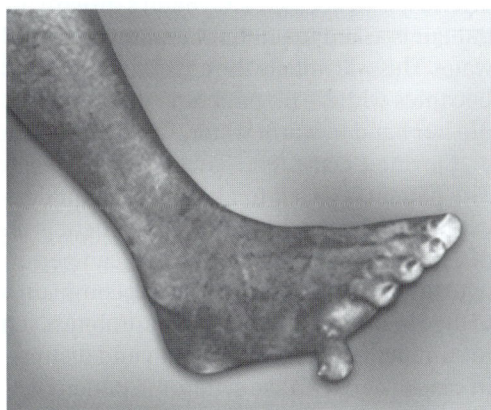

Fig. 6.3: Shows a typical case of ainhum where the 5th toe is affected and is almost shredding off.

(4) It is always advisable to observe the **limb above** the gangrenous area. This may be congested, edematous or pale, which indicates the possibility of later involvement of this area. There may be black patches, which indicate 'skip lesions'.

B. PALPATION

1. **Skin temperature:** The temperature is best felt with the back of the fingers. It is always essential to compare the two limbs and to feel the whole of the affected limb to find out the zone where the temperature changes from the normal warm temperature to cold skin of the ischemic site. It is wiser to feel for the temperature rather than to assess the temperature by looking at the color of the limb. The purplish-red and congested limb may be very cold.

2. **Capillary refilling:** The tip of the nail or the pulp of a toe or a finger is pressed for a few seconds and the pressure is released. The time taken for the blanched area to turn pink after the pressure has been released is a crude indication of capillary blood flow. This time will be definitely longer in case of ischemic limb.

3. **Venous refilling:** The two index fingers are placed side by side on a vein. The fingers are now pressed firmly and the finger nearer the heart is moved proximally keeping the steady pressure on the vein so as to empty the short length of the vein between the two fingers. The distal finger is now released. This will allow venous refilling to be observed. This is poor in ischemic limb and is increased in arteriovenous fistula. This is known as *Harvey's sign*.

4. **Crossed leg test** (Fuchsig's test): This is performed to detect popliteal pulsation **(Fig. 6.4)**. The patient is asked to sit with the legs crossed one above the other so that the popliteal fossa of one leg will lie against the knee of the other leg. The patient's attention is diverted by taking history. The crossed leg will show oscillatory movements of the foot which occur synchronously with the pulse of the popliteal artery. If the popliteal artery is blocked, this oscillatory movement will be absent.

5. **Cold and warm water test:** To provoke the arteriospasm in case of Raynaud's disease the patient is asked to put her hand into ice-cold water. This will initiate the attack and the hand becomes white. The patient is then asked to dip her hand in warm water. The hand will become blue due to cyanotic congestion.

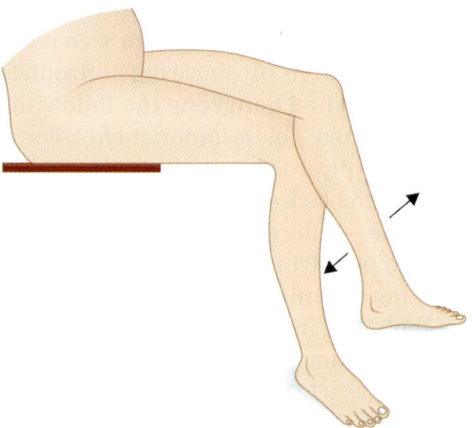

Fig. 6.4: Movements of the foot of the crossed leg are noticed only when the corresponding popliteal artery of the crossed leg is patent.

6. **Elevated arms test:** This test is performed when thoracic outlet syndrome is suspected. The patient is asked to abduct his shoulders to 90° and at the same time the upper limbs are externally rotated fully. Now the patient is instructed to open and close the hands for a period of 5 minutes. A normal individual can perform this without any difficulty. Whereas the patient with thoracic outlet syndrome will complain of fatigue and pain in forearm muscles, paresthesia of the forearm and tingling and numbness sensation in the fingers. Majority of these patients fail to complete this test due to pain and distress and they drop their arms. If this test is performed in case of cervical disc syndrome patient will feel pain in the neck and shoulders, though little distress is felt in the forearm and hand.

7. **Allen's test** to know the patency of radial and ulnar arteries: The patient is asked to clench his fist tightly. The surgeon presses on the radial and ulnar arteries at the wrist. After 1 minute

the patient is asked to open the fist. The palm appears white. Now pressure on the radial artery is removed and the change in color of the hand is noted. If the radial artery is blocked the color remains white, but if it is patent the palm assumes normal color. Now the pressure on the ulnar artery is removed. Now the test is repeated and the pressure on the ulnar artery is first removed keeping pressure on the radial artery. If the ulnar artery is blocked the hand remains white, but if it is patent the palm assumes normal color.

8. **Branham's sign or Nicoladonis sign:** This is performed when arteriovenous fistula is suspected. A pressure on the artery proximal to the fistula will cause reduction in size of swelling, disappearance of bruit, fall in pulse rate and the pulse pressure returns to normal.

9. **Costoclavicular compressive maneuver or test:** Patient's radial pulse is felt. The patient throws shoulders backwards and downwards as an exaggerated military position. This will compress the subclavian artery between the clavicle and the first rib leading to reduction or disappearance of the radial pulse. Simultaneously a subclavian bruit may be heard.

10. **Hyperabduction maneuver:** Patient's radial pulse is again monitored. The affected arm is now passively hyperabducted. This will cause reduction or disappearance of the radial pulse due to compression by the pectoralis minor tendon in pectoralis minor syndrome. An axillary bruit may be heard near the position where pectoralis minor tendon crosses the axillary artery.

11. **Gangrenous area (Figs. 6.5A and B):** By feeling the gangrenous area one can assess the type of gangrene. In case of dry gangrene the part will be hard and shriveled, whereas in case of wet gangrene the part will be edematous with or without crepitation.

12. **Crepitus:** Presence of crepitus is the characteristic feature of gas gangrene. This is due to presence of gas within the muscles.

13. **Limb above the gangrenous area:** It is always a good practice to palpate the limb above the gangrenous area as a routine. Tenderness along the line of the blood vessel indicates recent thrombosis. Pitting on pressure suggests edema which may be due to inflammatory condition and thrombophlebitis.

14. **Palpation of the blood vessels:** This is probably the most important part of the examination so far as an ischemic limb is concerned. Disappearance of arterial pulsation below the level of occlusion is the rule. The only exception is the presence of good collateral circulation when the pulse may be diminished but does not disappear.

An apparently normal peripheral pulse may disappear after exercising the patient to the point of claudication. This 'disappearing pulse' is a sign of unmasking the preliminary stage of

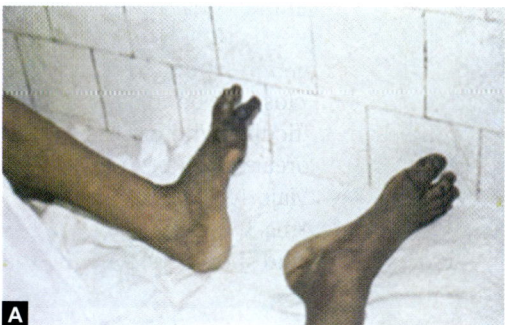
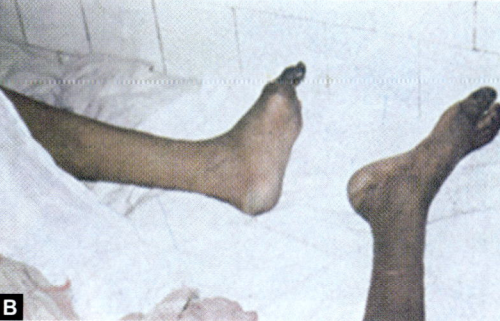

Figs. 6.5A and B: Bilateral gangrene of the toes encroaching feet in a case of diabetic.

arterial occlusion. The disappearing pulse reappears after a minute or two following cessation of exercise.

An expansile arterial pulsation indicates presence of aneurysm.

So much important is the feel of an artery. When there is embolus in an artery, the artery becomes firm and tender. Soft, non-tender, nonpulsatile artery means that the embolus has lodged higher up. In embolism, the pulse can usually be traced down to the point where it meets the obstruction. Here there is often a small tender swelling and the pulse is lost below.

The following arteries are often required to be examined: *The dorsalis pedis artery* (**Figs. 6.6A and B**)—is felt just lateral to the tendon of the extensor hallucis longus. It is absent in 10% of cases.

The posterior tibial artery—is felt just behind the medial malleolus midway between it and the tendo Achillis (**Figs. 6.7 and 6.8**).

The anterior tibial artery—is felt in the midway anteriorly between the two malleoli against the lower end of tibia just above the ankle joint and just lateral to the tendon of the extensor hallucis longus which is made prominent by asking the patient to extend his great toe (**Fig. 6.9**).

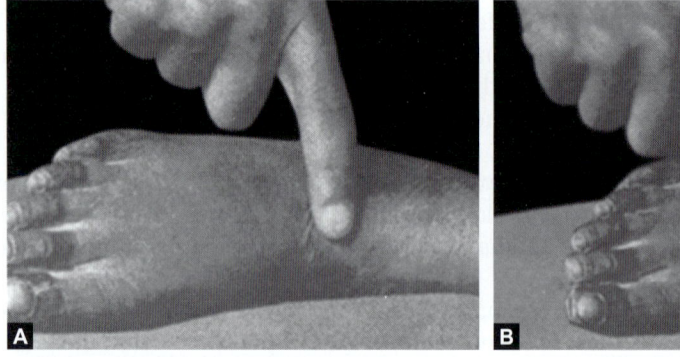
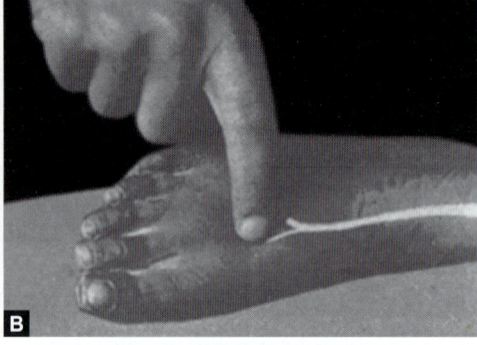

Figs. 6.6A and B: Showing the correct and incorrect methods of feeling the dorsalis pedis pulse. The white line in the second figure represents the artery and the palpating finger should be placed anywhere over this line as shown in the Figure A. The artery disappears through the proximal end of the first metatarsal space into the sole. Therefore searching for the pulse beyond this spot as shown in the Figure B is a wrong procedure.

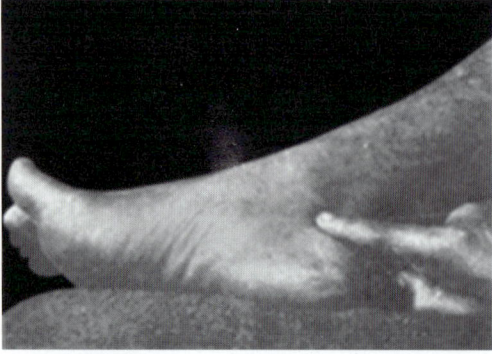
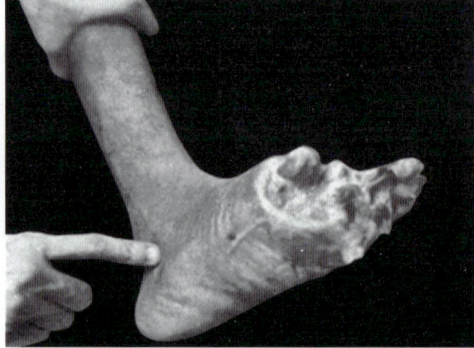

Fig. 6.7: Feeling for the posterior tibial pulse.

Fig. 6.8: Method of palpating the posterior tibial artery in a gangrenous foot.

The popliteal artery—is rather difficult to feel as it lies deep behind the knee. The knee is flexed to 40° with the heel resting on the bed, so that the muscles around the popliteal fossa are relaxed. The clinician places his fingers over the lower part of popliteal fossa and the fingers are moved sideways to feel the pulsation of the popliteal artery against the posterior aspect of the tibial condyles. It is rather impossible to palpate this artery in the upper part of the popliteal fossa as the artery lies between the two projecting femoral condyles.

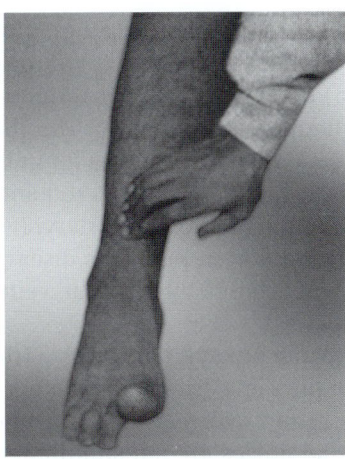

Fig. 6.9: Palpation of anterior tibial artery. Note that the extensor hallucis longus is made taut by extending the great toe and the artery is palpated just lateral to the tendon.

This artery can also be palpated by turning the patient into prone position and by feeling the artery with the fingertips after flexing the knee passively with another hand **(Fig. 6.10)**.

The femoral artery—is felt at the groin just below the inguinal ligament midway between the anterior superior iliac spine and the symphysis pubis **(Fig. 6.11)**.

The radial and ulnar arteries—are felt at the wrist on the lateral and on the medial sides of its volar aspect respectively.

The brachial artery—is felt in front of the elbow just medial to the tendon of biceps.

The subclavian artery—is felt just above the middle of the clavicle.

Common carotid artery—is felt in the carotid triangle just in front of the sternomastoid muscle against the carotid tubercle of the sixth cervical vertebra.

The superficial temporal artery—is felt just in front of the tragus of the ear.

When the pulse is feeble or absent, the pulsation of the examiner's own finger may be mistaken for that of the patient. In that case the clinician may palpate his own superficial temporal artery and compare the doubtful pulse of the patient. Otherwise, he can also compare the patient's radial artery with the doubtful pulse of the patient's lower extremity **(Fig. 6.12)**.

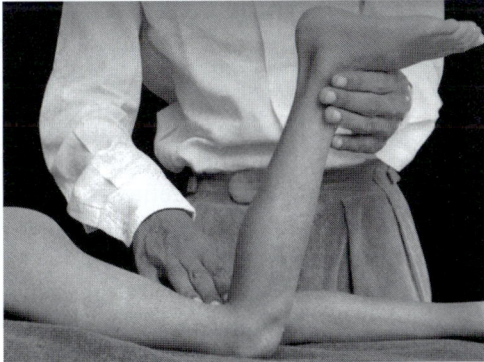

Fig. 6.10: Feeling for the popliteal pulse.

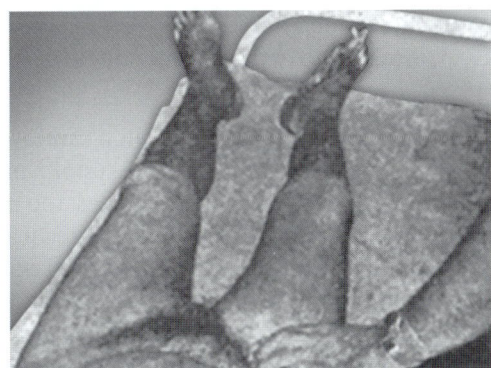

Fig. 6.11: Feeling for the femoral pulse.

While examining the artery the following points are noted: (a) Pulse—its volume and tension. (b) Condition of the arterial wall—whether atheromatous or not. (c) Thrombosis of the vessels—when the artery is thrombosed it feels midway between firm and soft and one can feel something within the artery. It must be remembered that in Buerger's disease not only the distal arteries but also the veins are thrombosed.

One should always compare with the pulsation of the same artery on the other side. In cervical rib and scalenus anticus syndrome, the two radial pulses are felt simultaneously after pulling both the arms downwards. This will cause diminution or obliteration of the pulse on the affected side.

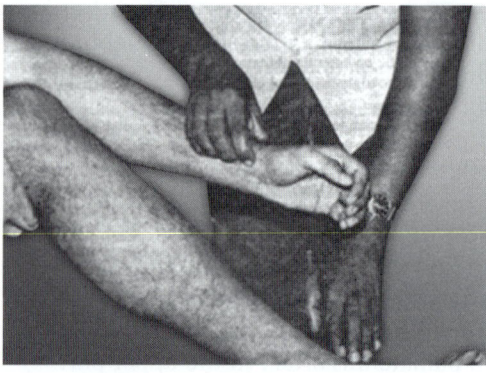

Fig. 6.12: When the dorsalis pedis pulse is very feeble or absent, the examiner's own arterial beat may be mistaken for that of the patient. Under such circumstances simultaneous palpation of patient's radial pulse eliminates the error.

15. **Neurologic examination:** Sensation of the gangrenous area is often lost. The patient is unable to move the part when the viability of the deeper tissues becomes at stake. On the border line of the gangrene the skin becomes hyperesthetic.

In case of superficial ulceration, one must exclude other disorders of the central nervous system, e.g., hemiplegia, transverse myelitis, syringomyelia, tabes dorsalis, etc.

16. **Adson's test:** This test is positive in presence of cervical rib and scalenus anticus syndrome due to compression of the subclavian artery. The patient sits on a stool. He is instructed to take a deep breath in and to turn the face to the affected side **(Fig. 6.13)**. The examiner examines his radial pulse, which is often obliterated due to compression of the subclavian artery.

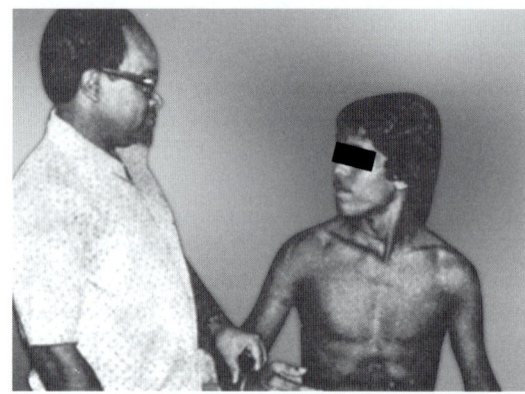

Fig. 6.13: Adson's test. See the text.

17. **Examination of the lymph nodes** (*see* Chapter 8).

C. AUSCULTATION

The importance of this examination cannot be overexaggerated. It is advisable to listen along the course of all major arteries. A systolic bruit over an artery is due to turbulent blood flow beyond stenosis. One should not exert too much pressure on the bell of the stethoscope, lest it should obliterate the artery and cause an artificial bruit. Systolic murmur can also be heard over an aneurysm. A bruit is also heard on the renal artery in case of hypertension due to renal artery stenosis. A continuous machinery murmur may be heard over an arteriovenous fistula. *Blood pressure of both the arms* are measured to exclude affection of subclavian, brachiocephalic or axillary artery. *Reactive hyperemia* test is performed to know the severity of arterial ischemia. This is done by inflating a sphygmomanometer cuff around the limb to

250 mm Hg for 5 minutes. Then the cuff is deflated and the time of appearance of red flush in the skin is noticed. It is 1–2 seconds in case of normal limb and it will be delayed in case of arterial occlusive disease and it may never appear in case of severely ischemic limb.

GENERAL EXAMINATION

1. Atherosclerosis is a generalized disease and the patient must be examined thoroughly to exclude ischemic heart disease, cerebrovascular disease, hypertension, renal artery stenosis, etc.
2. In embolic manifestation, the heart is examined for presence of cardiac murmur, which may indicate certain lesion to cause embolus formation.
3. Diabetes is often accompanied by atherosclerosis.
4. Peptic ulceration is sometimes found to be accompanied with these diseases.

SPECIAL INVESTIGATIONS

1. **Blood:** Routine examination of blood along with WR (for syphilitic endarteritis obliterans), sugar (for diabetes), urea and electrolytes will give a clue to the diagnosis. Estimation of serum lipoprotein, triglyceride and cholesterol should be performed when atherosclerosis is suspected.
2. **Urine:** Routine urine examination along with sugar will help the clinician to know whether the patient is diabetic or not and selective examination of urine from each kidney by ureteric catheterization will help the clinician to know whether there is renal vascular insufficiency or not.
3. **Straight X-ray:** This is helpful to diagnose: (i) arteriosclerosis with presence of arterial calcification (Monckeberg's degeneration); (ii) aneurysm with flecks of calcium to outline it; (iii) gas gangrene with presence of gas as dark spots in soft tissue and (iv) cervical rib.
4. **Arteriography (Fig. 6.14):** This is the most reliable method of determining the state of the main arterial tree. This procedure gives information about the size of the lumen of the artery, the course of the artery, constriction and dilatation of the arteries and the condition of the collateral circulation ('Run off'). Hypaque 45 (Sodium Diatrizoate) is the contrast medium often used. Either of the following two methods is generally used:

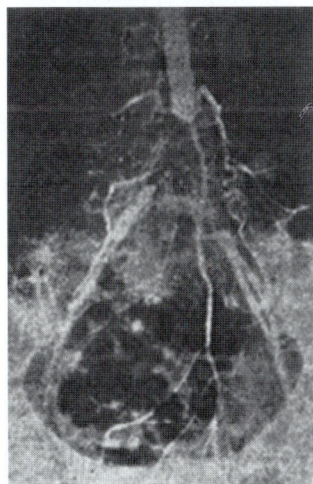

Fig. 6.14: Aortography showing an embolus obstructing the bifurcation of aorta.

A. **RETROGRADE PERCUTANEOUS CATHETERIZATION:** Under general or local anesthesia with proper aseptic precaution a special needle and a cannula are introduced into the femoral or brachial artery (Seldinger technique). The common femoral artery is used for aortoiliac, renal, mesenteric and femoropopliteal arteriography, whereas the brachial artery is used for subclavian, vertebral, carotid and thoracic angiography. The needle is now withdrawn and a flexible guide wire is threaded through the cannula. The cannula is withdrawn and a polythene catheter is passed over the guide wire into the artery for a distance.

To avert the dangers of arteriography namely: (a) iodine sensitivity and (b) dissection of the arterial wall if the tip of the needle is partly within the wall of the artery, a *trial injection* of 5–10 mL of 45% hypaque is made. This will ascertain the position of the tip of the needle.

Either a ***free flush arteriography*** or a ***selective angiography*** (Fig. 6.15) is done. In free flush arteriography the tip of the catheter lies in the main aorta and a 'bolus' of 30 mL of the same contrast medium is injected rapidly. Series of X-ray exposures are made to see particularly the whole length of the arterial tree, the origins and the adjacent part of its branches. In selective angiogram the tip of the catheter is introduced into the corresponding artery to delineate the artery and its branches precisely.

B. **DIRECT ARTERIAL PUNCTURE:** This method is used in carotid angiogram. Abdominal aorta (translumbar route) may be chosen for aortoiliac and femoropopliteal arteriography when the femoral arteries are occluded or the retrograde method has failed to produce necessary information.

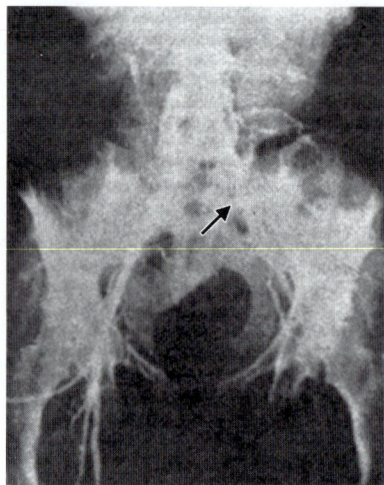

Fig. 6.15: Arteriography showing common iliac artery blockage.

5. **Determination of blood velocity by ultrasound Doppler effect:** By placing the probe of the apparatus over an artery, audible signals can be heard. Normal arterial sound consists of first, second and third sounds. In patients with occlusive lesion, abnormal signals can be obtained distal to the block and will be lost entirely over the site of the block. These abnormal sounds result from collateral flow and are of low pitch. The second and third sounds are absent when the flow signals are detected just below the stenotic lesion where high velocity flow is present, a single high-pitched continuous sound is present indicating turbulent flow.

This simple apparatus can be used to measure blood pressure at the ankle and at the arm. Normally the ankle systolic blood pressure is greater than the brachial (arm) systolic blood pressure by 5–15 mmHg. So, the ratio of the ankle blood pressure and arm blood pressure will also be greater than one and is known as 'pressure index'. If this pressure index becomes <1 it indicates some degree of arterial occlusion. When the ankle blood pressure goes down to 30 mmHg or less, it indicates severe ischemia and imminent gangrene.

6. **Isotope technique:** Xenon 133 dissolved in isotonic saline is injected intramuscularly and the clearance of which has been used to study the blood flow in the calf muscles. Recently technetium 99 has become the isotope of choice though the technique remains essentially the same. More recently intravenous injection of isotope has been used to get a direct arterial visualization. For this a gamma camera is used to picturize the blood flow in a limb.

7. **Electromagnetic flow meter:** When a column of blood moves an electric potential is produced which is proportional to the velocity of blood and the magnetic field strength. The electric potential is produced at right angles to the flow. It bears a linear relationship to the velocity of the blood flow. Two electrodes are placed diametrically opposite to each other in contact with the arterial wall. This is the 'cuff' type of electromagnetic flow meter. The electrodes on the surface of the artery pick up an electromotive force induced in the blood by its motion through the magnetic field and feed it back to suitable electronic amplification. Such a method can detect the change in the rate of the blood flow of 1%. But the greatest disadvantage of this technique is that the artery has to be exposed.

8. **Blood lipids:** Abnormal high level of blood lipids, e.g., blood cholesterol, lipoproteins, triglycerides, etc., is often found in atherosclerotic occlusion. Many of these patients are diabetic, though they may not show increased level of sugar in the blood. For this, glucose tolerance test should be performed.
9. **Investigation for vasospasm:** In early part of Raynaud's disease or Buerger's disease, vasospasm is the main cause of arterial obstruction. It is at this stage that sympathectomy plays its greatest role. Later on organic changes develop and sympathectomy does not do much good to the patient. So, importance of finding out the degree of vasospasm cannot be overemphasized to assess the value of sympathectomy. The method is nerve block with local anesthetic, e.g., the posterior tibial nerve behind the medial malleolus, the ulnar nerve behind the medial epicondyle or spinal anesthesia in case of whole lower limb. Any rise of skin temperature is recorded and is compared with the rise of mouth temperature.

$$\text{Brown's vasomotor index} = \frac{\text{Rise of skin temperature.} - \text{Rise of mouth temperature}}{\text{Rise of mouth temperature}}$$

Operation is only advisable when the index is 3.5 or more.

10. **Plethysmography:** This method is one of the earliest methods of measuring blood flow in human limbs. Venous outflow from a limb is briefly arrested while allowing arterial inflow to measure the volume change in the limb which is proportional to the arterial inflow. Three systems have been used, e.g., water-filled volume recorder, air-filled volume recorder and the mercury in a silastic strain gauze. This technique is still a good noninvasive method of measurement of blood flow. But it has rarely been found suitable for screening method for surgery, as the surgeon is more interested to know the site of the arterial block rather than to measure the blood flow as such. Recently **segmental plethysmography** has been introduced by placing venous occlusion cuffs around the thigh, calf and ankle. The cuffs are inflated to 65 mmHg and the pulsation is the quantitative measure of the arterial diseases.
11. **Oscillometry:** This is of particular value in detecting arterial pulsation at different levels of the limb. In embolism, a sudden decrease in the movement of its needle is obtained at the level of arterial occlusion. In thromboangiitis obliterans, if no pulsation is obtained in the leg, amputation should be performed in the thigh. But if oscillation can be seen in the leg a lower amputation should be advised.

SIGNS OF GANGRENE

1. Change of color—pale, bluish purple and finally black; 2. Loss of temperature; 3. Loss of sensation; 4. Loss of pulsation and 5. Loss of function.

CLINICAL TYPES

1. **Dry gangrene:** This results from gradual occlusion of arterial circulation, mostly seen in atherosclerosis. The affected part becomes dry, shriveled, hard, mummified and discolored from disintegration of hemoglobin.
2. **Moist (wet) gangrene:** This results when the artery is suddenly blocked, as by an embolus or when gangrene is superimposed on and associated with inflammation. Due to infection and putrefaction the affected part becomes edematous with blebs. Crepitus can be felt when there is presence of gas as seen in gas gangrene.

The term 'Pregangrene' is used to describe the changes in the tissue to indicate that its blood supply is so precarious that it will soon be inadequate to keep the tissue alive.

Causes of ischemia can be broadly classified as follows:

Large artery occlusion	Small artery occlusion
1. Atherosclerosis (chronic)	1. Buerger's disease
2. Embolism (acute)	2. Raynaud's disease
	3. Embolism
	4. Diabetes
	5. Scleroderma
	6. Physical agents: Trauma, radiation, electric burns, pressure necrosis

CAUSES OF GANGRENE

1. **Cardiovascular disease:** Senile gangrene (due to atherosclerosis); embolic gangrene; Raynaud's disease; Buerger's disease; cervical rib; syphilitic gangrene (due to endarteritis obliterans).
2. **Traumatic gangrene:** Direct (injury to the main artery) or indirect (crushing of the tissues).
3. **Infective gangrene:** (a) Acute, e.g., carbuncle, cancrum oris and postoperative progressive gangrene following drainage of empyema and appendicectomy, (b) Gas gangrene.
4. **Diabetic gangrene**.
5. **Nervous diseases:** Syringomyelia, tabes dorsalis, peripheral neuritis, leprosy, caries spine, fracture-dislocation of spine, etc.
6. **Physical gangrene:** Due to heat, cold (frost bite), corrosive, X-ray, etc.

DIFFERENTIAL DIAGNOSIS

SENILE GANGRENE

The usual victims are generally elderly persons above 50 years of age. The lower limbs are commonly involved. The patient will first complain of intermittent claudication. The claudication distance will gradually be reduced. There will be marked coldness of the feet and the patient will soon complain of 'rest pain'. Gradually dry gangrene will be developed with superficial ulceration. Various special investigations as stated above will help the clinician to diagnose the condition and the level of the block. Straight X-ray may reveal calcification of the arterial wall. Arteriography is also very helpful in detecting the site of block. Patients with bilateral internal iliac occlusion may complain of impotence, which is known as *Leriche's syndrome.*

BUERGER'S DISEASE (THROMBOANGIITIS OBLITERANS)

The usual victims of this disease are *young men* below 40 years of age. It is the inflammatory reaction in the arterial wall with involvement of the neighboring vein and nerve, terminating in thrombosis of the artery. The lesions in Buerger's disease are segmental and usually begin in arteries of small and medium size. Both upper and lower extremities are affected. In lower extremity, the disease generally occurs beyond popliteal artery, starting in tibial arteries extending to the vessels of the foot. The disease has also affected the arteries of the GI tract, lungs and heart. Early in the course of Buerger's disease the superficial veins are involved producing the characteristic migratory, recurrent superficial phlebitis. So far as etiology is concerned this disease has a striking association with cigarette smoking. Majority patients of Buerger's disease come from lower socioeconomic groups. An autoimmune etiology has been postulated and familial predisposition has been reported.

The pedal arteries are involved first and the patients complain of pain while walking at the arch of the foot (foot claudication), somewhat less often at the calf of the leg, but never at the thigh or buttock (which is common in atherosclerosis). Pain is typical of intermittent claudication, which progresses to 'rest pain'. Gradually postural color changes appear followed by trophic changes and eventually ulceration and gangrene of one or more digits and finally of the entire foot or hand may ensue. Buerger's test will be positive. Buerger's disease can be differentiated from Raynaud's disease by sex incidence, the extremity affected and disappearance of peripheral pulses. It is differentiated from senile gangrene by the age, by its association with superficial phlebitis and pitting edema. Characteristic arteriographic appearance of this disease is the smooth and normal appearance of larger arteries combined with extensive occlusion of the smaller arteries alongwith extensive collateral circulation.

RAYNAUD'S DISEASE

It is a disease of young women and commonly the upper limbs are affected specially the fingers (the thumb is generally escaped). The disease is characterized by Raynaud's phenomenon which is nothing but a series of attacks of local syncope, local asphyxia and local gangrene (see the text). Local syncope consists of tingling, numbness and blanching. Local asphyxia consists of pain and cyanosis. These two attacks are repeated until patches of anemic ulceration appear at the finger tips which is known as the stage of local gangrene. The *pulses remain unaffected,* as this is the disease which affects arterioles. Troublesome sweating is sometimes associated with this condition.

EMBOLIC GANGRENE

The onset is sudden with agonizing pain radiating down the course of the artery. Distal to the occlusion the limb becomes cold and numb. Superficial veins remain empty. Presence of localized tenderness at the site of embolus and complete disappearance of pulse below this level are the pathognomonic features of this disease. The heart when examined carefully often gives an indication of the source of the embolus.

THORACIC OUTLET SYNDROME

This syndrome is caused by compression of the brachial plexus or subclavian artery and/or vein in the region near the thoracic outlet. It may be caused by: (i) cervical rib, (ii) scalenus anticus muscle, (iii) costoclavicular syndrome, (iv) pectoralis minor syndrome, (v) wide first thoracic rib, and (vi) fracture of the first rib or clavicle.

Neurologic symptoms are pain, paresthesia and numbness in the fingers and hand in the ulnar nerve distribution. Symptoms of arterial compression include pain, numbness, paresthesia, coldness and weakness of the hand. Venous symptoms include edema, venous distension, pain and cyanosis. Costoclavicular compressive maneuver, hyperabduction maneuver and Adson's test will be positive.

CERVICAL RIB

Again young women are the usual victims. The symptoms gradually appear due to sagging down of the shoulder girdle with the advent of puberty. Sometimes symptoms appear later in life due to weakness of the muscles of the shoulder girdle. Presence of cervical rib does not always reveal symptoms or brings the patient to the surgeon. Symptoms of the cervical rib are mainly caused by angulation of the subclavian artery over the cervical rib and by the pressure irritation of the lowest trunk of the brachial plexus which contains the sympathetic nerve fibers to the upper limb. These symptoms will only appear when the muscles of the shoulder girdle will become weak and both the artery and the nerve trunk will be compressed on the cervical rib.

Symptoms of cervical rib can be described in three groups:

(1) **Local:** The patient presents with hard and fixed lump in the lower part of the posterior triangle of the neck. There may be local pain and tenderness in the supraclavicular region.

(2) **Neurogenic**: Symptoms are produced by pressure irritation of the lower trunk of brachial plexus. The symptoms can be divided into *sensory* (e.g., tingling, numbness and pain along the medial side of the forearm and hand), *motor* (e.g., loss of power of the hand with wasting of the thenar and hypothenar eminences leading ultimately to claw hand) and *vasomotor* (e.g., excessive sweating of the hand and circulatory impairment leading to gangrene).

(3) **Vascular:** Pain in the forearm is often complained of which becomes worse with exercise. The hand becomes colder than its fellow on the opposite side. When the hand is elevated it looks pale and it becomes blue on prolonged dependent position due to cyanotic congestion. Numbness of the fingers is complained of and the radial pulse becomes feeble on the affected side.

X-ray often reveals the cervical rib, though sometimes a fibrous band in its place causes the symptoms like cervical rib and will not be seen by X-ray.

The **scalenus anticus syndrome** is one in which the clinical pictures very much resemble those of the cervical rib. Here the pull of the scalenus anterior muscle, which compresses the subclavian artery and the lower trunk of the brachial plexus, is responsible for the symptoms. Adson's test is helpful to arrive at the diagnosis.

AINHUM

This condition is commoner in adult males, only occasionally found in women and children. Negroes, people of Central Africa, Central America and the East are more prone to be affected. It usually affects the little toe, sometimes the fourth and rarely the third, second or the great toe. Though it is rare in upper limbs yet cases are on the record when the terminal phalanx of the little finger has been involved. The disease starts as a linear groove in the skin on the inner and plantar side of the root of the toe. Frequently the involvement is bilateral affecting both the feet simultaneously or one after the other. The groove gradually deepens and extends round the whole circumference of the toe. The distal part becomes swollen as if the root of the toe has been tied with a ligature. The patient's main complaint is continuous and progressive pain. Rarely, this pain may be absent. In course of time the toe falls off.

INFECTIVE GANGRENE

A. **Carbuncle:** *see* page 53.

B. **Cancrum oris**—occurs in the mouth of the children usually in the terminal stage of typhoid fever, measles, kala-azar, etc. The disease starts as stomatitis and causes ulceration and extensive sloughing. The condition is toxemic manifestation of the severe diseases. This condition is more often seen in the undernourished. The affected area becomes ischemic and very much swollen and ultimately undergoes gangrenous changes. Large areas of the cheeks, lips and even jaws are destroyed.

C. **Gas gangrene:** The causative organisms are mainly *Clostridium welchii* and less commonly *C. septicum* and *C. oedematiens*. These organisms are present in the intestine and in soil. Gas gangrene is usually met with in street accident. Incubation period varies from a few hours to a few days. The onset is sudden accompanied by pain in the wound, swelling, fever, vomiting and toxemia. Characteristic odor of H_2S may be obtained. Gradually the whole limb becomes swollen and tense with crepitation on palpation over the muscles. The muscles if exposed are seen brick-red or green or black according to the stage of the disease. The toxins produced by the anerobic organisms exert a selective action on the adrenals and causes marked lowering of blood pressure. The diagnosis is confirmed by X-ray which reveals gas bubbles.

Types: (i) Local type—when a single muscle is affected. (ii) Subcutaneous type—is very confusing as the crepitus becomes well spreading for a considerable distance around the wound. But the muscles are not affected. The infection seems to be localized in the subcutaneous tissue plane. (iii) Gas abscess—is also confusing as it is not a true example of gas gangrene but indicates only presence of gas around foreign body which has been lodged within the muscle.
(iv) Group type—when a group of muscles is involved. (v) Massive type—when the whole limb is affected.

DIABETIC GANGRENE

This is quite commonly seen in diabetic individuals. There are three factors in causing diabetic gangrene: (i) atherosclerosis of the peripheral arteries; (ii) peripheral neuritis interfering with trophic function and (iii) diminished resistance to trauma and infection of the sugar-laden tissue. The gangrene is usually moist owing to infection (which is predominantly of fungal variety), unless atherosclerotic factor plays the major part when it becomes dry in nature.

SYPHILITIC GANGRENE

This condition is very rare and is caused by endarteritis obliterans and gummatous infiltration of the arterioles. The patient is usually of middle age when the gangrene is often of dry type. Other syphilitic stigmas and positive WR and Kahn test will clinch the diagnosis.

NEUROPATHIC GANGRENE

Such gangrene is not due to ischemia but due to lack of sensation. It is normally painless and progressive. Such gangrene occurs due to repeated trauma, compression and infection of the part which has lost sensation. The three features of such gangrene are—(i) it is painless, (ii) the surrounding skin has lost sensation and (iii) the surrounding tissues have normal blood supply.

CAROTID OCCLUSIVE DISEASE

It occurs due to atherosclerosis at the origin of the internal carotid artery or at the bifurcation of the common carotid artery. Carotid stenosis causes transient, recurrent and progressive strokes causing hemiplegia of the contralateral side. When anyone presents with brief episodes of weakness, tingling or pins and needles or loss of sensation on one side of the body, which last for a few minutes and then fully recover, remember the possibility of carotid artery occlusive disease and auscult over the carotid artery if there be any bruit heard. If such episodes are ignored, it may cause a major stroke.

SUBCLAVIAN STEAL SYNDROME

This is due to atherosclerotic stenosis of the subclavian artery proximal to the site of origin of the vertebral artery. Reduction in pressure in the subclavian artery beyond the stenosis results in retrograde flow from the brainstem down the vertebral artery to the arm (so blood is stolen from brain). Exercise of the upper arm produces syncopal attacks due to ischemia of the brainstem with visual disturbances alongwith decreased pulse and blood pressure in the symptomatic arm. There may be localized bruit in the supraclavicular space.

AORTIC-ARCH OCCLUSIVE DISEASE (TAKAYASU'S ARTERITIS)

Sometimes a nonspecific arteritis affects major branches of the aortic arch. This arteritis involves all layers of the aortic wall. It is particularly noticed among young Japanese women. It affects mainly the head, face and upper extremities in the form of transient fainting, headache, atrophy of the face, optic nerve atrophy and paresthesia and weakness of the upper limbs. There may be fever, malaise and general arthralgia.

ANTERIOR COMPARTMENT SYNDROME

Any condition which increases fluid in the anterior compartment of the leg, causes increase of pressure in this closed space surrounded by deep fascia. This causes obstruction of veins in the beginning which increases accumulation of fluid in this compartment, so that intracompartmental pressure gradually exceeds arterial pressure causing occlusion of arteries in this compartment leading to ischemia of the distal limb. Pain is the first and most important symptom. Gradually erythema of the skin over the anterior compartment is noticed and later on dorsalis pedis pulse becomes diminished or absent leading to ischemic changes in the toes.

ACROCYANOSIS

The basic pathology is the slow rate of blood flow through skin due to chronic arteriolar constriction may be due to constant spasm in response to an overactive vasomotor system. This results in a high percentage of reduced hemoglobin in the capillaries and this is the cause of cyanotic color. This condition affects young women. Coldness and blueness of the fingers and hands are persistently present for many years. It must be remembered that in this condition there is *persistent, painless* cold and cyanosis of the hands and *feet*. Though this condition mimics Raynaud's syndrome, yet the italic words in the previous sentence are the distinguishing features. The peripheral pulses are usually normal.

ACUTE ARTERIAL OCCLUSION

Sudden occlusion of a major peripheral artery can be due to: (A) Arterial embolus, (B) Trauma or (C) Acute arterial thrombosis.

A. **Arterial embolus:** 'Embolus' is a Greek word which means 'something thrown in'. Two types of embolization may occur—cardioarterial embolization or arterioarterial embolization. *Cardioarterial embolization* occurs in majority of cases of emboli in the lower extremity and such emboli originate in the heart either due to atrial fibrillation, mitral stenosis or myocardial infarction. *Arterioarterial embolization* originates from atherosclerotic plaque which has been ulcerated. In the lower extremity emboli usually lodge at the bifurcation of common femoral artery or at the bifurcation of popliteal artery or at the bifurcation of common iliac artery or at the bifurcation of aorta in order of frequency. In superior extremity the commonest site is at the bifurcation of the brachial artery followed by the axillary artery near shoulder joint.

The result of arterial embolization is the immediate onset of severe ischemia of the tissue supplied by the involved arteries. If untreated, gangrene occurs in 50% of cases. The peripheral nerves are very sensitive to ischemia and this leads to pain, paresthesia and paralysis.

B. **Arterial trauma** may also cause acute arterial occlusion. The causes of arterial trauma are— (a) Most arterial injuries result from *penetrating wounds* which partly or completely disrupt the walls of the arteries. (b) Pressure on a major artery by an angulated bone. (c) Intimal rupture of a major artery due to fracture or dislocation. (d) Injury to a major artery by a bone fragment. Followings are the fractures and dislocations which may cause acute arterial occlusion—(i) Supracondylar fracture of humerus; (ii) Supracondylar fracture of femur; (iii) Dislocated shoulder; (iv) Dislocated elbow; (v) Dislocated knee.

C. **Acute arterial thrombosis:** The most common site is the lower end of the femoral artery where it leaves subsartorial canal to enter the popliteal space. Commonly acute thrombosis occurs in an artery considerably narrowed by arterial disease. Moreover acute-on-chronic arterial thrombosis may occur in which case acute conditions develop on already existing chronic occlusion.

Pain in the limb is the most important and initial symptom which affects the limb distal to the acute arterial occlusion. Numbness and weakness are also present. The ischemic portion of the limb assumes a cadaveric pallor described as 'waxy' pallor. Within 1 hour or so the part becomes cyanosed. The prominent veins become emptied and guttered. Pulses distal to the obstruction are absent. The local temperature of the ischemic area is appreciably cold. There may be calf tenderness or pain on dorsiflexion of foot in an otherwise anesthetic limb. The clinical features of acute arterial occlusion are best described by 5 'P's—***Pain, Paralysis, Paresthesia, Pallor and absent Pulses***. Neurologic symptoms carry a prognostic value. If motor and sensory functions are intact, the extremity will survive. In majority of cases there may be some sensory disturbances only, which vary from paresthesia to anesthesia.

In **aortic embolism**, pain is felt in both the lower limbs, there is also loss of movements of hips and knees. Coldness and numbness and change of color affect the inferior extremities below the hip joints or midthighs.

In ***femoral embolism***, femoral pulse may be felt, but it affects the leg and foot. Numbness, coldness and change of color are seen below the knee joint.

In **popliteal embolism,** there is pain in the lower leg and foot, there is loss of movement of the toes. Coldness, numbness and change of color are seen only in the foot.

In **axillary embolism**, pain involves the whole of the upper arm. Numbness, coldness and change of color are noticed in the hands and distal forearm. There may be loss of movements in the wrist and fingers.

In **brachial embolism** pain is complained of in distal forearm and hand. Numbness, coldness and change of color are only seen in the fingers.

It is always advisable to examine the heart alongwith ECG. Though angiography is quite helpful in diagnosing the case it may delay operation. So in these cases clinical diagnosis is more considered before operation. Doppler ultrasound may be of some help.

ANEURYSM

Definition: Dilatation of a localized segment of arterial system is known as aneurysm.

Broadly, an aneurysm can be classified into three types—(1) True aneurysm, (2) False aneurysm and (3) Arteriovenous aneurysm.

(a) *True aneurysm* is one, which contains all the three layers of the arterial wall in the aneurysm. (b) *False aneurysm* is one, which has a single layer of fibrous tissue at the wall of the sac.

A true aneurysm, *according to shape,* may be fusiform, saccular or dissecting aneurysm **(Fig. 6.16)**. FUSIFORM ANEURYSM occurs when there is uniform expansion of the entire circumference of the arterial wall. SACCULAR ANEURYSM is an expansion of a part of the circumference of the arterial wall. This is usually traumatic. DISSECTING ANEURYSM occurs when tunica intima ruptures usually beneath an atheromatous plaque and the blood is forced through the intima to enter between the inner and outer courts of the tunica media.

An aneurysm can occur in any artery, though abdominal aorta, femoral and popliteal arteries are more commonly affected. However splenic, renal and carotid arteries have also undergone aneurysmal changes.

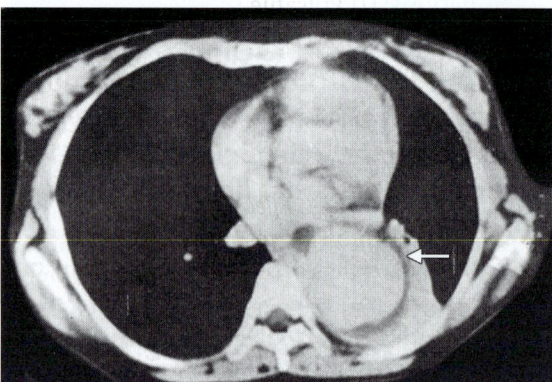

Fig. 6.16: Dissecting aneurysm of the thoracic aorta.

Causes: Aneurysm usually occurs due to weakening of the wall of the artery. Aneurysms can be: (I) Congenital or (II) Acquired.

I. *CONGENITAL:* (i) Congenital aneurysm may occur in the cerebral blood vessels particularly in the circle of Willis due to congenital deficiency of the elastic lamina at the sites of branching—this is known as *Berry aneurysm.* (ii) Cirsoid aneurysm **(Fig. 3.50)**. (iii) Congenital arteriovenous fistula. (iv) Congenital aneurysm may occur in Marfan's syndrome or Ehler-Danlos syndrome.

II. *ACQUIRED* varieties are further classified into (A) Traumatic, (B) Degenerative and (C) Infective.

A. *Traumatic* may be due to: (i) direct trauma such as penetrating wounds to the artery. (ii) Irradiation aneurysm. (iii) Arteriovenous aneurysm from trauma. (iv) Indirect trauma may cause aneurysm, e.g., at the subclavian artery distal to the point where it crosses the cervical rib.

B. *Degenerative* is by far the most common group and (i) atherosclerosis is the most common cause of aneurysm. (ii) A peculiar aneurysm of the abdominal aorta is noticed in young South African Negroes which is due to intimomedial mucoid degeneration.

C. *Infective:* (i) Syphilis. (ii) Acute infection may lead to formation of aneurysm. (iii) Mycotic aneurysm. (iv) Aneurysm may occur in an artery traversing tubercular cavity in the lung, (v) Infected embolus resting on peripheral artery may produce weakening of the wall forming aneurysm. (vi) Aneurysm may occur in an artery situated at the base of a peptic ulcer. (vii) Arteritis, particularly polyarteritis.

Symptoms: Aneurysm may be asymptomatic, when it is detected accidentally.
(i) Most common presenting symptom is a *dull aching pain.* (ii) *Acute pain* may occur when the vessel suddenly stretches. (iii) *Severe pain,* bursting in nature, is complained of when an aneurysm ruptures and a large hematoma forms. *Referred pain* is due to pressure on a nerve, e.g., patients with abdominal aortic aneurysm may present with sciatica. (iv) A common mode of presentation is a *pulsatile mass*—more often seen in femoral and popliteal aneurysm. (v) Sometimes patients may present with *severe ischemia of the lower limb* due to thrombosis of the aneurysm, which is more common in popliteal aneurysm. (vi) Patient may present with less severe ischemia caused by emboli originating in the aneurysm. (vii) Aneurysm may present with *venous obstruction* and *thrombosis* when enlargement of artery causes direct pressure on the neighboring vein. Presentation is painful swollen and blue limb.

Examinations: (i) Pulsatile swelling exhibiting expansile pulsation in the course of an artery should be suspected as aneurysm. (ii) Pulsation diminishes when pressure is applied proximal to the swelling. (iii) The swelling is compressible. (iv) A thrill may be palpable over the swelling. (v) On auscultation, a systolic bruit may be heard over the swelling. (vi) The swelling can be moved sideways but not along the course of the artery. (vii) Evidence of peripheral arterial insufficiency or venous obstruction may be present in the distal limb.

Effects of aneurysm: A. *Effects of pressure on neighboring structure:* (i) Pressure on veins—leads to edema of distal limb. (ii) Pressure on the nerves—leads to altered sensation, e.g., pain, numbness, tingling and paresthesia. (iii) Pressure on bones—leads to erosion of the bones. (iv) Pressure on adjacent organs—may cause dysphagia if esophagus is pressed by aortic aneurysm; aortic aneurysm may burst into stomach causing severe hematemesis. (v) Pressure on the skin—causes stretching of overlying skin which becomes red and edematous showing features of inflammation and thus aneurysm has been incised with the wrong diagnosis of an abscess with grave consequences.
B. *Thrombosis:* Laminated thrombus in an aneurysm may reduce the blood to the distal limb. Sometimes arteriography cannot diagnose an aneurysm as such thrombosis does not show dilated sac in arteriography.
C. *Emboli formation:* Multiple small emboli may originate from aneurysm and block very distal arteries leading to intermittent claudication, rest pain and even gangrene of the toes.

Complications of aneurysms: (1) *Pressure on adjacent structures:* See above. (2) *Thrombosis* and *emboli formation*—leads to circulatory *insufficiency* of the inferior extremity. (3) *Infection* may occur from organisms in the blood and signs of inflammation become evident. (4) *Rupture* is the gravest and ultimate complication of aneurysm. (5) *Spontaneous cure*—occasionally occurs particularly in saccular aneurysm due to gradual formation of clot.

Differential diagnosis
1. *Swellings over the arteries*—which yield 'transmitted pulsation'. Pseudopancreatic cyst is an example.
2. *Swelling beneath the artery,* e.g., cervical rib pushing up the subclavian artery.
3. *Pulsating tumors,* e.g., telangiectatic osteosarcoma, very vascular osteoclastoma, metastasis from hypernephroma and follicular carcinoma of thyroid, aneurysmal bone cyst.
4. *An abscess.*
Arteriography is the main diagnostic tool, though sometimes it cannot reveal dilatation of the artery due to presence of laminated thrombus inside the arterial sac.

ARTERIOVENOUS ANEURYSM

Communication between an artery and adjacent vein leads to arteriovenous aneurysm or arteriovenous fistula.
Causes are: (i) CONGENITAL, e.g., cirsoid aneurysm. (ii) ACQUIRED—mainly traumatic. (a) When the artery and the vein communicate through a short wide channel it is called *aneurysmal varix.* (b) When anastomosis becomes indirect through an intermediate sac lying in the soft tissues it is called *varicose aneurysm.* (iii) IATROGENIC: Arteriovenous fistula is created surgically for renal dialysis.

Manifestations
A. SYSTEMIC EFFECTS: (i) Cardiac output increases. (ii) Heart rate increases. (iii) Pulse pressure increases, i.e., diastolic pressure diminishes with increase in systolic pressure. (iv) Right and left

atrial pressures are increased with increase in pulmonary wedge pressure. (v) The blood and plasma volume increase. (vi) The heart size increases with cardiac hypertrophy. (vii) Congestive cardiac failure in case of arteriovenous fistula. (viii) Central venous pressure (CVP) is often increased. (ix) Sometimes bacterial endocarditis may associate with this condition.

B. LOCAL EFFECTS: (i) *Aneurysmal dilatation* at the site of fistula. (ii) Extensive collateral circulation with increase in temperature of the limb. (iii) The limb may be increased in length due to increase in bone growth from elevated local temperature. (iv) *A thrill* over the site of the lesion is quite characteristic. (v) The veins are enlarged and varicosed.

Clinical features: (1) A pulsatile swelling may be detected if the lesion is superficial. (2) There is increased temperature of the skin with port-wine discoloration due to increased collateral circulation. (3) Distended superficial veins. (4) Increased length of the limb is noticed particularly when the fistula is congenital. (5) On palpation, a thrill is detected at the site of the lesion. Pressure on the artery on the proximal of the fistula causes diminution of the swelling. (6) Below the fistula the limb is ill-developed and feels cooler. (7) Below the fistula muscle wasting may be noticed alongwith ischemic changes. Even indolent ulcer may be noticed—this is due to inadequate arterial supply below the fistula due to diversion of blood into the veins. (8) Auscultation reveals continuous bruit. (9) *Branham's sign*—in which if a finger is pressed on the artery proximal to the fistula there will be slowing of pulse rate and rise in diastolic pressure.

Algorithmic Approach to a Patient with Gangrene/Peripheral Vascular Diseases

Patient presents with limb pain, coldness, ulcer, or gangrene

↓

Is the onset acute or chronic?
- **Acute (hours to days):** Suggests **arterial embolism or thrombosis**
- **Chronic (weeks to months):** Suggests **atherosclerosis, buerger's disease, Diabetic arteriopathy**

↓

Are pulses present distal to the affected limb?
- **Absent pulses:** Suggests **severe arterial occlusion (atherosclerosis, thrombosis, embolism, vasculitis)** → proceed to step 4
- **Present pulses:** Suggests **venous or vasospastic disorder (raynaud's, chronic venous Insufficiency, diabetic neuropathy)** → Proceed to step 5

↓

Is there a clear line of demarcation between viable and necrotic tissue?
- **Yes:** Indicates **dry gangrene (mummified, black tissue, no infection)** → Proceed to step 6
- **No:** Proceed to step 5

↓

Does the affected tissue show swelling, wetness, and signs of infection?
- **Yes:** Suggests **wet gangrene (superimposed infection on ischemic tissue, foul smell, purulent discharge, edema)** → Proceed to Step 7
- **No:** Consider **nongangrenous ischemic ulcer or vasculopathy** → Proceed to step 9

↓

Is there any pain or systemic signs of infection (fever, sepsis, shock)?
- **Yes:** Suggests **early infection risk in dry gangrene** → monitor closely
- **No:** Stable dry gangrene → **conservative management (risk factor control, amputation if necessary)**

↓

Is there crepitus or gas formation in the tissue?
- **Yes:** Suggests **gas gangrene (clostridial myonecrosis, necrotizing fasciitis, surgical emergency)** → Proceed to step 8
- **No:** Proceed to step 9

↓

Order special investigations
- **Doppler ultrasound:** Assess arterial vs venous insufficiency
- **Ankle-brachial Index (ABI):** Assess severity of arterial occlusion
- **Arteriography/CT angiography:** Locate stenosis, embolism, or aneurysm
- **X-ray and MRI:** Detect gas in soft tissue (gas gangrene)
- **Blood Tests:** CRP, ESR (vasculitis), WBC count (infection), blood culture (sepsis)
- **Biopsy/FNAC:** Rule out malignancy (Marjolin's ulcer)

↓

Confirm diagnosis and initiate treatment
- **Medical management:** Anticoagulation (for embolism), vasodilators, smoking cessation, Antibiotics (for infection)
- **Surgical management:**
  – **Angioplasty or bypass surgery:** If salvageable ischemia
  – **Debridement and amputation:** If gangrene is extensive or septic

Examination of Varicose Veins

CHAPTER 7

A vein is called 'varicose' when it is dilated and tortuous. There are various places in the body where veins show tendency towards varicosity, e.g., veins of the lower limb, spermatic veins, esophageal veins and hemorrhoidal veins. In this chapter we shall only discuss the varicose veins of the lower limbs. The others will be discussed in appropriate chapters.

So far as the etiology is concerned varicose veins mostly occur due to incompetence of their valves. It is not found in other animals and seems to be a part of penalty of erect posture which the human beings have adopted. It occurs commonly in those whose works demand standing for long hours, e.g., conductors, drivers of the trams, etc. Yet it is not uncommon in women. So, some other etiologic factors seem to play major roles. These are tone and contractility of the muscles of the lower limb being encircled by a tough deep fascia. Incompetence of valves, which may be a sequel of venous thrombosis, seems to be the most important factor in initiating this condition. Varicosity may also be secondary, predisposed by any obstruction which hampers venous return, e.g., tumors (abdominal tumors, fibroid, ovarian cyst, abdominal lymphadenopathy), pregnancy, loaded colon, retroperitoneal fibrosis, ascites. A hormonal factor (progesterone?) gives an indication of occurrence of this disease in females. In younger age group congenital arteriovenous fistula may be the cause of varicose vein.

HISTORY

1. AGE: Though varicose vein can affect individuals of all age groups, yet middle-aged individuals are the usual sufferers.
2. SEX: Women are affected much more commonly in the ratio of 10 : 1.
3. ETHNIC GROUP: Varicose veins are less commonly seen in primitive civilizations—the poor in Africa and Far East.
4. OCCUPATION: Certain jobs demand prolonged standing, e.g., tram drivers, policemen, etc. and the persons involved in these jobs often suffer from varicose veins. Varicose veins may also occur in individuals involved in excessive muscular contractions, e.g., rickshaw-pullers and athletes. It is doubtful if these occupations cause the varicose veins or they just exacerbate the symptoms already present.

Symptoms: The most common symptom is the *pain* which is aching sensation felt in the whole of the leg or in the lower part of the leg according to the position of the varicose vein particularly towards the end of the day. The pain gets worse when the patient stands up for a long time and is relieved when he lies down. One thing the student must always remember that it is not the varicose veins which produce the symptoms, but it is the disordered psychology which is the root of all evils. So it is not impossible to come across asymptomatic varicose veins on one side and severe symptoms with very few visible varicose veins on the other side.

Patient may complain of bursting pain while walking, which indicates deep vein thrombosis. Night cramps may also be present. The ankle may swell towards the end of the day and the skin of the leg may be itching. Some patients complain of severe cramps at nights. Varicose ulcer may be seen on the medial malleolus.

A few questions should be asked: (i) Whether the patient is feeling difficulty in standing or walking, which indicates presence of deep vein thrombosis. (ii) The patient should be asked if he has any other complaint than varicose vein itself. He may feel such complaint as irrelevant. If the patient is suffering from constipation or a swelling in the abdomen, it may be a cause of secondary varicose vein.

Past history: Enquiry must be made if the patient had any injection treatment or operation for varicose veins. Any serious illness or previous complicated operation may cause deep vein thrombosis which is the cause of varicose vein now.

Personal history: Women should be asked about obstetric history, like details of previous pregnancies. Whether the patient suffered from 'white leg' during the previous pregnancies. If the patient had contraceptive pills for quite a long time, as this may cause deep vein thrombosis.

Family history: It is not uncommon to find varicose veins to run in families. Often patient's mother and sisters might have suffered from this disease.

History in varicose veins

Aspect	Clinical significance	Patient-friendly questions
Age and sex	More common in middle-aged individuals, higher in women due to hormonal influences	"How old are you? Have you noticed any changes in your legs as you've aged?"
Occupation	Jobs requiring prolonged standing lead to venous stasis and increased risk	"Do you have a job that requires standing or sitting for long hours?"
Leg symptoms	Aching, heaviness, and discomfort suggest venous insufficiency	"Do your legs feel heavy or achy, especially in the evening?"
Swelling	Leg swelling suggests venous hypertension or deep venous insufficiency	"Have you noticed swelling in your legs after standing? Does it go away overnight?"
Ulceration and skin changes	Skin pigmentation, eczema, and ulcers indicate advanced venous disease	"Have you noticed darkening of the skin, itching, or wounds that take longer to heal?"
Pain pattern	Pain worsens on standing, improves with elevation	"Does your leg discomfort get worse when standing and improve when you elevate your legs?"
Night cramps	Suggests poor venous circulation and calf muscle fatigue	"Do you experience leg cramps at night or after walking?"
Prior deep vein thrombosis (DVT)	Major risk factor for secondary varicose veins	"Have you ever had a blood clot in your legs?"

Contd...

Contd...

Aspect	Clinical significance	Patient-friendly questions
Surgical history	Previous vein surgery or lower limb procedures can affect venous competency	"Have you had any surgeries on your legs, including procedures for vein problems?"
Family history	Genetic predisposition to weak venous walls increases risk	"Do family members have similar leg problems or swollen veins?"
Lifestyle factors	Obesity, sedentary habits, and smoking worsen venous incompetence	"Do you exercise regularly? Have you gained weight recently?"
Pregnancy and hormonal influence (females)	Pregnancy increases intra-abdominal pressure, worsening venous reflux	"How many pregnancies have you had? Did you experience leg swelling during pregnancy?"

■ PHYSICAL EXAMINATION

A. INSPECTION

1. **Varicose veins:** Note, which vein has been varicosed—*long saphenous* or *short saphenous* or both. In case of the former a large venous trunk is seen on the medial side of the leg starting from in front of the medial malleolus to the medial side of the knee and along the medial side of the thigh upwards to the saphenous opening. This venous trunk receives tributaries in its course. In case of short saphenous vein varicosity the dilated venous trunk is seen in the leg from behind the lateral malleolus upwards in the posterior aspect of the leg and ends in the popliteal fossa.

2. **Swelling:** It may be (a) either *localized* as in case of varicose veins affecting a segment of superficial vein or the whole trunk of a venous system—either long or short saphenous vein. Localized swelling may also be due to superficial thrombophlebitis. (b) *Generalized* swelling of the leg is mostly due to deep vein thrombosis.

3. **Skin of the limb:** (i) **Color:** Local redness is usually due to superficial thrombophlebitis. Generalized change of color may be white *(phlegmasia alba dolens)* also known as 'white leg'. This is due to swollen limb from excessive edema or lymphatic obstruction. More important for this chapter is when the skin of the limb becomes congested and blue due to deep vein thrombosis and this condition is called *phlegmasia cerulea dolens.* In such severe venous obstruction the arterial pulses may gradually disappear and venous gangrene may ensue.
(ii) **Texture:** The affected limb should be carefully inspected to note: (a) if the skin is stretched and shiny due to edema following deep vein thrombosis. (b) If there is eczema or pigmentation of the skin affecting mostly the medial aspect of the lower part of the leg (around medial malleolus). (c) If there is any ulceration, often seen on the medial aspect of the lower part of the leg, which is known as the venous ulcer (See page 70 and **Fig. 4.5**). (d) *Scar* may be seen at the lower part of the leg which may be due to healed venous ulcer or previous operation for varicose veins. (e) One should also carefully inspect the toes to note if there is loss of hair or increased brittleness of the nails due to chronic varicosity which may indicate impending venous gangrene.

4. **Impulse on coughing:** The patient should be asked to cough and it is noted whether there is any *impulse on coughing* at the saphenous opening ('Saphena-varix'). This test is known as Morrissey's test which is more elaborately described in the section of palpation.

B. PALPATION

Examination of the varices is very important. The aim is to locate the incompetent valves communicating the superficial and deep veins.

1. **Brodie-Trendelenburg test:** This test is performed to determine the *incompetency of the saphenofemoral valve* and other communicating systems. This test can be performed in two ways. In both the methods, the patient is first placed in the recumbent position and his legs are raised to empty the veins. This may be hastened by milking the veins proximally. The saphenofemoral junction is now compressed with the thumb of the clinician or a tourniquet is applied just below the saphenofemoral junction and the patient is asked to stand up quickly. (1) In first method, the pressure is released. If the varices fill very quickly by a column of blood from above, it indicates incompetency of the saphenofemoral valve. This is called a positive Trendelenburg test. (2) To test the communicating system, the pressure is not released but maintained for about 1 minute. Gradual filling of the veins during the period indicates *incompetency of the communicating veins,* mostly situated on the medial side of the lower half of the leg allowing the blood to flow from the deep to the superficial veins. This is also considered as a positive Trendelenburg test and the positive tests are indications for operation **(Figs. 7.1 and 7.2A to C).**

In case of short saphenous vein same test is done by pressing the saphenopopliteal junction.

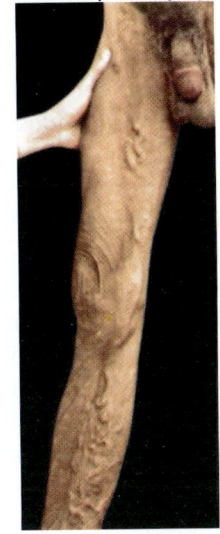

Fig. 7.1: Fine demonstration of long saphenous varicosity.

2. **Tourniquet test:** It can be called a variant of Trendelenburg test. In this test the tourniquet is tied round the thigh or the leg at different levels after the superficial veins have been made empty by raising the leg in recumbent position. The patient is now asked to stand up. If the veins above the tourniquet fill up and those below it remain collapsed, it indicates presence of incompetent communicating vein above the tourniquet. Similarly, if the veins below the

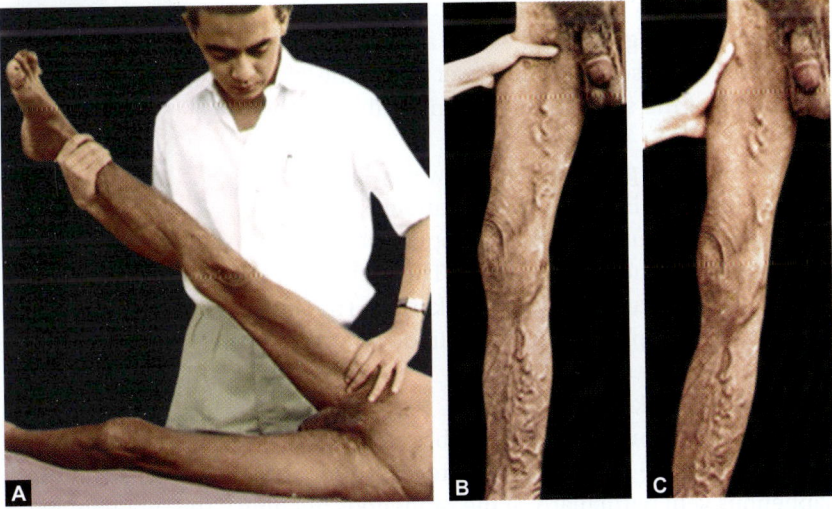

Figs. 7.2A to C: Show how to perform Trendelenburg test. See the text.

tourniquet fill rapidly whereas veins above the tourniquet remain empty, the incompetent communicating vein must be below the tourniquet. Thus, by moving the tourniquet down the leg in steps one can determine the position of the incompetent communicating vein.

The number of incompetent communicating sources in the lower limb in the long saphenous vein is the saphenofemoral junction (most important), the mid-thigh perforator, the lower-thigh perforator and the lower leg perforators on the medial side.

In case of short saphenous incompetence—application of the venous tourniquet to the upper thigh has the paradoxical effect of increasing the strength of the reflux, as shown by faster filling time. The sign, which has not been described before, is pathognomonic of varices of the short saphenous system. The mechanism is very simple—application of the upper thigh tourniquet blocks off the normal internal saphenous system which is carrying most of the superficial venous return and thus thrown into greater prominence the retrograde leak for the saphenous-popliteal junction. Final definite proof of short saphenous incompetence is obtained through following examination: The saphenopopliteal junction is marked with a pen with the patient standing. The short saphenous vein is emptied by elevation of the leg, firm thumb pressure is applied to the ink mark. The patient is made to stand. The pressure is released and the vein will be filled immediately. For all practical purposes that *there is no other incompetent perforating vein in the short saphenous system should be remembered.*

3. **Perthes' test:** The affected lower extremity is wrapped with elastic bandage. With the elastic bandage on the patient is instructed to move around and exercise. Severe crampy pain is complained of if there is deep vein thrombosis. Of course, arterial occlusive disease should be excluded.

4. **Perthes' test (modified):** This test is primarily intended to know whether the deep veins are normal or not. A tourniquet is tied round the upper part of the thigh tight enough to prevent any reflux down the vein. The patient is asked to walk quickly with the tourniquet in place **(Fig. 7.3)**. If the communicating and the deep veins are normal the varicose veins will shrink whereas if they are blocked the varicose veins will be more distended.

5. **Schwartz test:** In a long-standing case if a tap is made on the long saphenous varicose vein in the lower part of the leg an impulse can be felt at the saphenous opening with the other hand.

6. **Pratt's test:** This test is performed to know the positions of leg perforators. Firstly, an Esmarch elastic bandage is applied from toes to the groin. A tourniquet is then applied at the groin. This causes emptying of the varicose veins. The tourniquet is kept in position and the elastic bandage is taken off. The same elastic bandage is now applied from the groin downwards. At the positions of the perforators 'blow outs' or visible varices can be seen.

These are marked with a skin pencil.

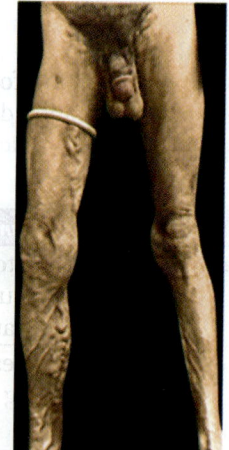

Fig. 7.3: Shows how to perform Perthes' test.

7. **Morrissey's cough impulse test:** The limb is elevated to empty the varicose veins. The limb is then put to bed and the patient is asked to cough forcibly. An expansile impulse is felt in the long saphenous vein particularly at the saphenous opening if the saphenofemoral valve is incompetent. Similarly, a bruit may be heard on auscultation.

8. **Fegan's method to indicate the sites of perforators:** In standing posture the places of excessive bulges within the varicosities are marked. The patient now lies down. The affected limb is elevated to empty the varicosed veins. The examiner palpates along the line of the marked varicosities carefully and finds out gaps or pits in the deep fascia which transmit the incompetent perforators.

9. One should look *for* **pitting oedema or thickening, redness or tenderness** at the lower part of the leg. These changes are due to chronic venous hypertension following deep vein thrombosis. Sometimes a progressive sclerosis of the skin and subcutaneous tissue may occur due to fibrin deposition, tissue death and scarring. This is known as *lipodermatosclerosis* and is also due to chronic venous hypertension. This may follow formation of venous ulcer.

C. PERCUSSION

If the most prominent parts of the varicose veins are tapped, an impulse can be felt by the finger at the saphenous opening. This is known as *Schwartz test* (**Fig. 7.4**). Sometimes the percussion wave can be transmitted from above downwards and this will imply absent or incompetent valves between the tapping finger and the palpating finger.

D. AUSCULTATION

The importance of auscultation is limited to the arteriovenous fistula, where a continuous machinery murmur may be heard.

E. REGIONAL LYMPH NODES (inguinal)

These are only enlarged if there be venous ulcer and this is infected.

F. OTHER LIMB

It should be examined for presence of varicose veins and different tests to exclude deep vein thrombosis, incompetent perforators and venous ulcer to plan treatment.

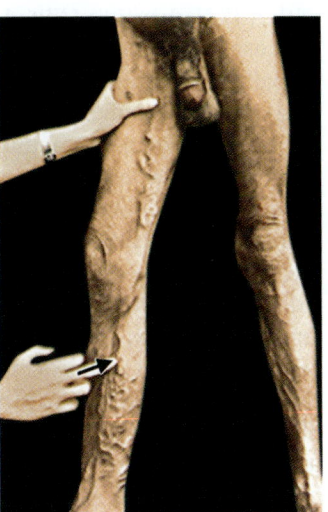

Fig. 7.4: Shows how to perform Schwartz test.

Examination in varicose veins

Step	Findings and interpretation	Clinical example
Inspection	Dilated, tortuous veins (long or short saphenous system), skin changes (eczema, pigmentation, ulcers)	Venous ulcer at medial malleolus
Palpation	Tenderness (phlebitis), impulse on coughing (saphenous varix)	Positive **Morrissey's Test**
Percussion	Tapping on varicose vein transmits impulse to saphenous opening	Positive **Schwartz Test**
Auscultation	Machinery murmur suggests **arteriovenous fistula**	Arteriovenous malformation

GENERAL EXAMINATION

EXAMINATION OF THE ABDOMEN

Of the general examinations, examination of the abdomen is probably the most important so far as a case of varicose vein is concerned. Sometimes a pregnant uterus or intrapelvic tumor (fibroid, ovarian cyst, cancer of cervix or rectum) or abdominal lymphadenopathy may cause pressure on the external iliac vein and becomes responsible for secondary varicosity.

Complications of varicose veins: (1) *Hemorrhage:* It may occur from minor trauma to the dilated vein. The bleeding may be profuse due to high pressure within the incompetent vein. Simple elevation of the leg does a lot to stop such bleeding. (2) *Phlebitis:* This may occur spontaneously or secondary to minor trauma. Mild phlebitis may be produced by the sclerosing fluid used in the injection treatment. In this condition varicose vein becomes extremely tender and firm. The overlying skin becomes red and edematous. Pyrexia and malaise may be associated with. (3) *Ulceration* **(Fig. 4.5)**: This is more due to deep venous thrombosis rather than varicose veins alone. The patients often give previous history of venous thrombosis suggested by painful swelling of the leg. After thrombosis has been recanalized the valves of the deep veins are irreparably damaged. The deoxygenated blood gets stagnated in the lower part of the leg particularly on the medial side where there are plenty of perforating veins. The superficial tissue loses its vitality to certain extent and a gravitational ulcer follows either spontaneously or following minor trauma. The majority of patients with venous ulcers have incompetent communicating veins. The arteries and nerves should be examined to exclude other causes of ulceration. These ulcers are commonly found at the lower third of the leg, usually on the medial side and even on the foot, but *never* above the junction of the middle and lower thirds of the leg. Venous ulcers are shallow and flat. The edge of the ulcer is sloping and pale purple-blue in color. The floor is usually covered with pink granulation tissue. In chronic ulcers white fibrous tissue are more seen than pink granulation tissue. The discharge is seropurulent with trace of blood. The surrounding tissues show signs of chronic venous hypertension, i.e., induration, tenderness and pigmentation. These ulcers have ragged edges. If the ulcer is healing, a faint blue rim of advancing epithelium may be seen at the margin. Rarely malignancy can develop at the edge of a long standing venous ulcer *(Marjolin's ulcer).* A patient when presents with long history of venous ulceration with edge raised and everted or different from the typical features of ulcer described above and when the inguinal lymph nodes are enlarged—it is suspicious of a Marjolin's ulcer (malignant change in a chronic ulcer). (4) *Pigmentation.* (5) *Eczema.* (6) *Lipodermatosclerosis:* This means the skin becomes thickened, fibrosed and pigmented. This is due to high venous pressure which causes fibrin accumulation around the capillary and it also activates white cells. (7) *Calcification of vein.* (8) *Periostitis* in case of long-standing ulcer over the tibia. (9) *Equinus deformity:* This only results from long-standing ulcer. When the patient finds that walking on the toes relieves pain, so he continues to do so and ultimately the Achilles tendon becomes shorter to cause this defect.

Causes of varicose veins in the lower limb:

Primary	Secondary
Cause is not known. The valves are incompetent both of the main vein or of the communicating veins. Venous walls may be weak which permit dilatation causing incompetence of valves. Very rarely there may be congenital absence of valves.	i. *Obstruction to venous outflow*—1. Pregnancy, 2. Fibroid, 3. Ovarian cyst, 4. Pelvic cancer (of cervix, uterus, ovary or rectum), 5. Abdominal lymphadenopathy, 6. Ascites, 7. Iliac vein thrombosis, 8. Retroperitoneal fibrosis. ii. *Destruction of valve*—from deep vein thrombosis. iii. *High pressure flow*—from arteriovenous fistula.

VENOUS THROMBOSIS

It must be said in the beginning that deep vein thrombosis is mostly an asymptomatic disease. Only one-fourth of the cases of deep vein thrombosis present with minor complaints. Various techniques have been introduced to detect asymptomatic deep vein thrombosis as they are dangerous and cause pulmonary embolism. Various preventive measures are also being practiced all over the world to reduce the incidence of deep vein thrombosis. But these are beyond the scope of this book and only the symptoms and signs of deep vein thrombosis, though rare, will be discussed here.

HISTORY

The patient may complain of pain and swelling of the leg. There may be slight fever. If the patient has already had pulmonary embolism he may complain of chest pain, breathlessness and hemoptysis.

PHYSICAL EXAMINATION

1. **INSPECTION:** Swelling of the leg is the most important feature which steals the show. The swelling is mainly found just around the ankle or little higher up. The swollen leg may become very much painful and is called **phlegmasia alba dolens**. When all the deep veins become blocked, the skin becomes congested and blue, which is called **phlegmasia cerulea dolens**.

2. **PALPATION: Homan's sign (Fig. 7.5A):** Passive forceful dorsiflexion of the foot with the knee extended will elicit tenderness in the calf. Gentle pressure directly on the calf muscles in the relaxed position will also elicit pain. Care must be taken to be gentle in manipulation test it may dislodge a clot and cause pulmonary embolism.

   Squeezing of the relaxed calf muscles from side-to-side is also painful as the thrombosed deep veins in the calf are always tender and this test is known as *Moses' sign* **(Fig. 7.5B)**.

   Direct palpation of the deep veins such as femoral or popliteal vein may become painful if they are thrombosed.

   Measurements—often reveal swollen calf muscles.

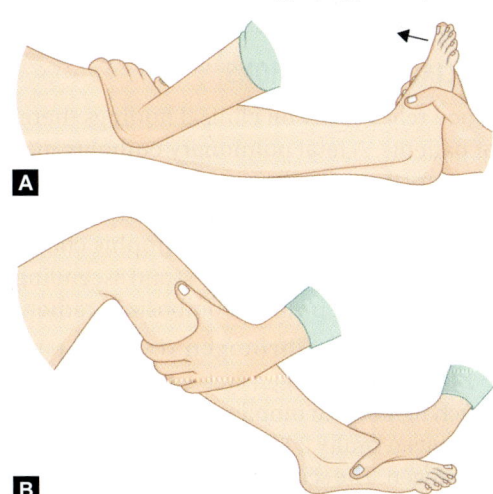

Figs. 7.5A and B: Showing two methods of eliciting calf tenderness; (A) indirectly by forcible dorsiflexion of the foot (Homan's sign) and (B) directly by squeezing the calf muscles from side to side (Moses' sign).

TYPES OF VENOUS THROMBOSIS

1. ***Deep vein thrombosis*** (Phlebothrombosis): This condition commonly occurs after operation under general anesthesia, when the calf muscles remain idle and fail to maintain the normal flow of blood within the deep veins, thus causing thrombosis. It also occurs following child birth, immobility or any debilitating diseases. As has already been mentioned this condition is mostly asymptomatic. Only about 1/4th of cases produce symptoms and signs.

   Pain and swelling of the calf or whole leg are the main symptoms. The onset of symptoms is often sudden. Sometimes it is severe enough to make walking difficult. If the patient has pulmonary embolism he may complain of breathlessness, hemoptysis and pleuritic pain.

Most important physical sign is *swelling of the leg*. This swelling may affect the thigh if the thrombosis is in the iliac vein or just around the ankle if the thrombosis is confined to the calf. The muscles which contain the thrombosed veins become *hard* and *tender*. Change in the texture of the muscle is more important than tenderness, as there are many conditions which make muscles tender, but there are very few conditions which make the muscle stiff and hard.

Forcible dorsiflexion of the foot which stretches the calf muscles will produce pain, which goes by the name of '**Homan's sign**' **(Fig. 7.5A)** and when pain is elicited with compression of calf against the tibia is known as **Mose's sign (Fig. 7.5B)**.

With obstruction of veins the lower limb gets swollen and edematous, which is called **phlegmasia alba dolens** or a 'white leg'.

When thrombosis of the veins obstruct outflow of blood from the limbs, the superficial veins dilate and the leg feels hot. With obstruction of all the main veins the skin becomes congested and blue, which is known as **phlegmasia cerulea dolens**. Later on arterial pulses may temporarily disappear and venous gangrene may develop.

2. ***Superficial vein thrombosis*** (Thrombophlebitis): This is an inflammatory condition and occurs after intravenous transfusion (most common cause) or in varicose veins. Pain is the main feature. The patient may run temperature. The skin appears inflamed. The vein feels hard and tender. The resulting thrombus is firmly attached to the vein, so incidence of pulmonary embolism is very much less in comparison to phlebothrombosis. Spontaneous thrombophlebitis may sometimes be migratory (thrombophlebitis migrans), which may be associated with Buerger's disease, polycythemia, polyarteritis and visceral carcinoma (bronchus, pancreas, stomach or lymphoma). Sometimes it may be idiopathic. It may also be iatrogenic (intravenous injection and injuries). Even if the patient has varicose veins, he should be thoroughly examined to exclude any occult cancer.

SPECIAL INVESTIGATIONS

If one relies solely on clinical findings there will be a failure to diagnose this condition in 50% of patients. A fatal pulmonary embolus may well be the first indication of thrombosis. To the contrary there may be extensive involvement of veins by the thrombotic process without clinical signs. In these cases destruction of venous valves with the sequelae of varicose veins, varicose eczema, ulceration and other trophic changes may result.

Radioactive fibrinogen test and ascending functional phlebography have gone a long distance to diagnose deep vein thrombosis in rather early stage **(Fig. 7.6)**.

1. **Radioactive fibrinogen test:** At first ^{131}I- labeled fibrinogen was used. Subsequently ^{125}I-labeled fibrinogen was employed due to its softer radioaction and its detectability with much lighter and mobile apparatus. The thyroid gland is firstly blocked by sodium iodide (100 mg) given orally 24 hours before the intravenous injection of 100 microcuries of ^{125}I-labeled fibrinogen. The scintillation counter is first placed over the precordial region and the radioactivity over the heart is measured. The machine is adjusted so that this reading represents 100%. The legs are elevated on an adjustable stand to decrease venous pooling and to give access to the calf for the scintillation counter. Counting is performed along the lower extremity at two inches

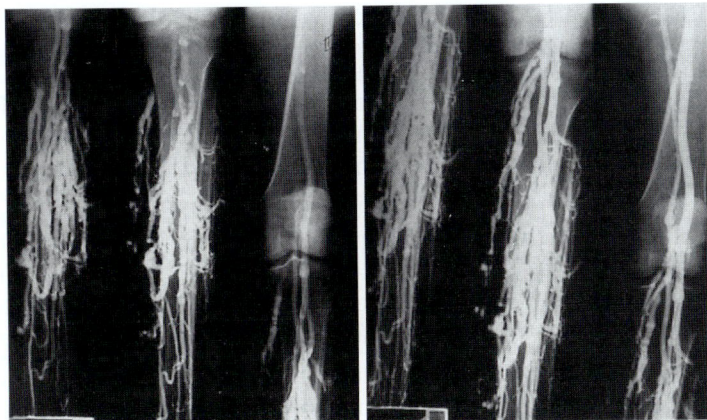

Fig. 7.6: Ascending functional phlebography showing deep venous thrombosis.

interval. Preoperative counting can be compared with the postoperative counting on the 1st, 3rd and 6th days after operation. An increase in the percentage value of 20 or more represents formation of thrombus in the deep veins of the legs.

2. **Phlebography:** The patient lies on a mobile table in horizontal position. 45% sodium diatrizoate is injected slowly into a vein on the dorsum of the great toe. A pneumatic cuff just above the ankle directs the contrast medium into the deep veins. Another cuff at the mid-thigh position confines the contrast medium initially to the lower leg. The amount and rate of injection of the contrast medium is controlled by the filling of the veins as viewed on the television screen. The patient is asked to dorsiflex and plantarflex his foot thus propelling the contrast medium into the tibial veins. When the veins are filled films are taken of the leg in two planes. At the end of the procedure the contrast medium is washed off the leg veins by injecting 100 mL of normal saline containing heparin.

Ascending functional cinephlebography can be obtained by continuous observation of the flow of the contrast medium on the television screen as it progresses through the tibial veins. Function of the valves can be particularly noticed. Similarly the popliteal and femoral veins can also be assessed. The valvular function is considered to be normal when both the valve cusps are seen to open and close with onward flow of blood and no retrograde flow occurs even with the Valsalva maneuver.

3. **Doppler ultrasonogram:** The sensing probe is placed over the femoral vein in the groin. This normally transmits a venous hum. If the calf is squeezed or the calf muscles contract, it changes hum into a roar due to increased blood flow. If there is deep vein thrombosis (femoral or popliteal) between the calf and the groin, the roar does not occur.

4. **Duplex imaging:** This technique involves the use of B mode ultrasound and a coupled Doppler probe. It allows direct visualization of the deep veins. It provides anatomical and physiological variations. Though it is costly, it is replacing venography.

5. **Ultrasound and CT scan**—should be performed when secondary varicose vein is suspected due to abdominal tumors.

Various tests in varicose veins examination

Test name	Purpose	Procedure	Interpretation
Trendelenburg test	Assess saphenofemoral valve competency	Leg elevated, veins emptied, tourniquet applied → patient stands	**Rapid refilling after release** = Incompetent valves
Tourniquet test	Locate incompetent perforators	Apply tourniquet at different levels, observe venous filling pattern	Filling above = perforator incompetence above tourniquet
Perthes test	Assess deep venous patency	Elastic bandage applied, patient asked to walk	Pain/cramping = Deep venous thrombosis
Schwartz test	Evaluate long saphenous vein incompetence	Tap on vein lower down, feel impulse at saphenous opening	Positive = Long saphenous vein incompetence

Algorithmic Approach to Patient with Varicose Veins

Patient presents with leg pain, swelling, visible veins, or ulcer

↓

Is there visible venous dilatation?
- Yes → Assess for **tortuous, dilated, or telangiectatic veins**
- No → Consider **deep venous insufficiency, lymphedema, or other causes**

↓

Is there leg swelling?
- Yes → Check if **swelling worsens with standing and improves with elevation**
  - Yes → Suggests **venous insufficiency**
  - No → Consider **lymphedema, deep vein thrombosis (DVT), or Systemic causes (cardiac/renal)**
- No → Move to skin changes assessment

↓

Are there skin changes (eczema, pigmentation, ulceration)?
- Yes → Suggests **chronic venous insufficiency**
- No → Could be **early-stage varicosities or another etiology**

↓

Perform special tests for venous competency
- **Trendelenburg test** → Assesses **saphenofemoral valve competency**
- **Tourniquet test** → Locates **incompetent perforators**
- **Perthes test** → Assesses **deep vein patency**

↓

Do special tests indicate valve incompetence?
- Yes → Suggests **primary varicose veins (idiopathic valve failure)**
- No → Consider **secondary causes (DVT, pelvic tumors, pregnancy, arteriovenous malformations)**

↓

Order investigations
- **Doppler ultrasound** → Evaluates venous reflux and valve function
- **Duplex venous scan** → Identifies incompetent perforators and deep venous obstruction
- **Venography (if required)** → Assesses deep venous involvement

↓

Confirm diagnosis and initiate treatment
- **Medical management:** Compression stockings, lifestyle modification, leg elevation
- **Surgical management:** Endovenous ablation, sclerotherapy, vein stripping

Examination of the Lymphatic System

CHAPTER 8

Lymphatic system includes lymph nodes and lymphatics. At first clinical features of the diseases of the lymph nodes will be described followed by diseases of the lymphatics.

HISTORY

The following points are particularly noted while taking the history of the patient.

1. **Age:** Tuberculous lymphadenopathy and syphilis are diseases of the young age. Acute lymphadenitis can occur at any age. Primary malignant lymphomas occur at young age, though secondary malignant lymphadenopathy occurs in old age.
2. **Sex:** Somehow or other females are more affected than males so far as primary lymphedema is concerned. Even secondary lymphedema is more common in women following radical mastectomy **(Fig. 8.1)** or due to involvement of the iliac and inguinal nodes from malignant tumors of the uterus or ovary.
3. **Distribution:** Lymphedema following filariasis **(Fig. 8.2)** is more common in tropical countries and Odisha seems to be the most affected state in India.
4. **Complaints:** Not many complaints are associated with this disease particularly the primary lymphedema. This is slowly progressive swelling of the limb and the genitalia which takes even years to develop.

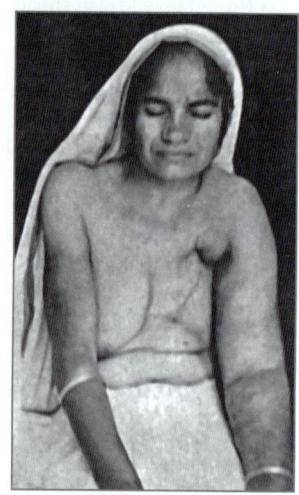

Fig. 8.1: Lymphedema of the arm following radical mastectomy.

To the contrary secondary lymphedema is often associated with some sort of complaints such as complaints of malignant growth, filariasis, etc. It often follows operation like extirpation of lymph nodes, e.g., radical mastectomy.

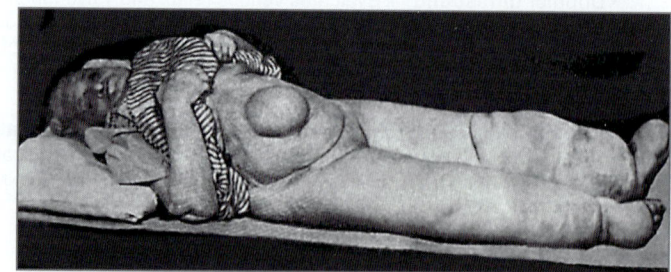

Fig. 8.2: Huge elephantiasis of both the legs.

5. **Duration:** In acute lymphadenitis the history is short, whereas it is long in chronic lymphadenitis, tuberculosis, etc.
6. **Which group was first affected?:** In case of generalized involvement of the lymph nodes, the clinician should know which group of lymph nodes was first affected. This may give a clue to the diagnosis. Cervical group of lymph nodes is first affected in many cases of Hodgkin's disease,

tuberculosis, etc.; to the contrary inguinal group of lymph nodes is first affected in filariasis, lymphogranuloma inguinale, etc. But too much stress should not be laid on this point.

7. **Pain:** Is the involvement of the lymph nodes painful? The nodes are painful in both acute and chronic lymphadenitis, but are painless in syphilis, primary malignant lymphomas and secondary carcinoma.

8. **Fever:** Evening rise in temperature is a characteristic feature of tuberculosis. In filaria a periodic fever (especially during the full or new moon) is very common. In Hodgkin's disease, intermittent bouts of remittent fever (Pel-Ebstein fever) is quite peculiar to this disease.

9. **Primary focus:** Whenever the lymph nodes are enlarged, it is the usual practice to look for the primary focus in the drainage area of the lymph nodes. This should be done particularly in acute and chronic septic lymphadenitis. An insignificant abrasion or inflammation in the drainage area may lead to lymphadenitis.

10. **Loss of appetite and weight:** This is often complained of in case of malignant lymphadenopathies.

11. **Pressure effects:** Patient may complain of pressure effects due to enlarged lymph nodes. Patient may complain of swelling of face and neck due to venous and lymphatic obstruction by the enlarged superior mediastinal group of lymph nodes or lymph nodes at the root of the neck. Enlarged retroperitoneal lymph nodes and para-aortic lymph nodes in Hodgkin's disease may cause oedema and venous congestion of lower limbs. Dyspnea may be complained of in case of enlargement of mediastinal group of lymph nodes due to pressure on trachea or bronchus. Dysphagia may be complained of when esophagus is pressured.

12. **Past history:** This should be particularly enquired into in syphilis, tuberculosis, secondary carcinoma etc. Enlargement of epitrochlear and suboccipital groups of lymph nodes may elude the clinician if he does not ask the past history of primary syphilis; as these lymph nodes may be enlarged in the secondary stage of syphilis. Similarly, a patient who presents with enlarged cervical group of lymph nodes may give a past history of tuberculosis and the diagnosis becomes easy without thorough clinical examination and costly special investigations. Sometimes a patient with penile cancer may present with lump in the abdomen, which is nothing but enlarged iliac group of lymph nodes. A patient with enlarged cervical lymph nodes may give history of previous lung tuberculosis if specifically asked for.

13. **Family history:** Sometimes tuberculosis runs in families and should be asked for. Lymphosarcoma and other types of lymphomas have also shown a tendency to run in families.

History in lymphatic disorders

Aspect	Clinical significance	Patient-friendly questions
Age and sex	Tuberculous lymphadenopathy and syphilis affect the young; lymphomas occur at all ages	"When did you first notice the swelling? Has it grown over time?"
Pain	Painful → Infection; Painless → Malignancy, Syphilis	"Do you feel any pain in the swollen area?"
Fever	Evening rise → Tuberculosis; Periodic → Filariasis; Pel-Ebstein → Hodgkin's Disease	"Have you experienced fever? Is it recurrent or associated with chills?"

Contd...

Contd...

Aspect	Clinical significance	Patient-friendly questions
Primary focus	Look for infections draining into lymph nodes	"Did you have a skin infection, wound, or sore before the swelling appeared?"
Loss of weight and appetite	Malignancies, Tuberculosis	"Have you unintentionally lost weight recently?"
Pressure symptoms	Mediastinal nodes → Dyspnea, Dysphagia	"Do you have breathing difficulty or trouble swallowing?"
Past history	Tuberculosis, syphilis, past malignancies	"Have you ever been treated for tuberculosis or had any cancers before?"
Family history	Genetic predisposition to lymphomas	"Has anyone in your family had a similar condition?"

■ PHYSICAL EXAMINATION

Investigations in lymphatic disorders

Investigation	Purpose	Findings in disease
Blood tests	Infection markers, autoimmune screening	↑ESR (TB, Malignancy), Eosinophilia (Filariasis)
FNAC and biopsy	Gold standard for lymph node evaluation	Reed-Sternberg Cells → Hodgkin's Disease
Chest X-ray	Detects mediastinal lymphadenopathy	Enlarged Hilar Nodes → Tuberculosis
CT scan and MRI	Advanced imaging for deeper lymph nodes	Abdominal and pelvic lymphadenopathy
Lymphangiography	Assesses lymphatic drainage	Obstruction in Malignancies

GENERAL SURVEY

Malnutrition, cachexia, anemia and loss of weight are often seen in cases of tuberculous lymphadenitis, primary and secondary malignant lymphadenopathies.

LOCAL EXAMINATION

A. **INSPECTION:** *Swellings at the known sites of the lymph nodes should be considered to have arisen from them* unless some outstanding clinical findings prove their origin to be otherwise **(Figs. 8.3 and 8.4)**.

Swellings: The swellings are examined in the same fashion as has been described in chapter 3 under "Examination of a lump or a swelling". That means the *number, position, size, surface,* etc., are noted. Of these

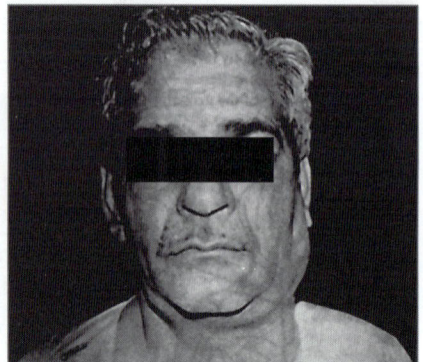

Fig. 8.3: Cervical lymph node swelling in tuberculosis.

the *position* is important, as it will not only give an idea as to which group of lymph nodes is affected, but also the diagnosis, e.g., Hodgkin's disease and tuberculosis affect the cervical group of lymph nodes **(Fig. 8.5)** in the beginning; filariasis and lymphogranuloma inguinale affect the inguinal group of lymph nodes **(Fig. 8.6)**; secondary stage of syphilis involves the epitrochlear and occipital groups. *Number* is important—whether single or multiple groups are involved. A few conditions are known to produce generalized involvement of lymph nodes. These are Hodgkin's disease, tuberculosis, lymphosarcoma, lymphatic leukemia, brucellosis sarcoidosis, etc.

Skin over the swelling: In acute lymphadenitis the skin becomes inflamed with redness, edema and brawny induration. In chronic lymphadenitis the skin over the swelling does not show such angriness. Skin over tuberculous lymphadenitis

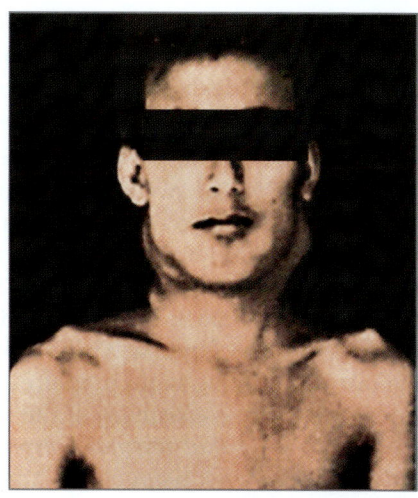

Fig. 8.4: Cervical lymph node swelling on both sides in Hodgkin's disease.

and cold abscess remains 'cold' in the true sense till they reach the point of bursting when the skin becomes red and glossy. Over a rapidly growing lymphosarcoma the skin becomes tense, shining, with dilated subcutaneous veins. In secondary carcinoma **(Fig. 8.7)**, though the skin remains free in the early stage, yet it becomes fixed to the swelling at later stage when the disease has gone beyond the scope of surgery. Not infrequently a scar, a sinus or an ulcer may be present by the side of or over the swelling. Scar often indicates previous bursting of cold abscess or a previous operation. So far as an ulcer or a sinus is concerned, the students are advised to examine them as described in chapters 4 and 5 respectively. Ulceration and sinus formation are not infrequent in lymphogranuloma inguinale.

Pressure effects: Careful inspection must be made of the whole body to detect any pressure effect due to enlargement of lymph nodes. Edema and swelling of the upper limb and lower limb may occur due to enlargement of axillary and inguinal groups of lymph nodes respectively. Swelling and venous engorgement of face and neck may occur due to pressure effect of lymph nodes at the root of the neck. Nearby nerves may be involved due to en-

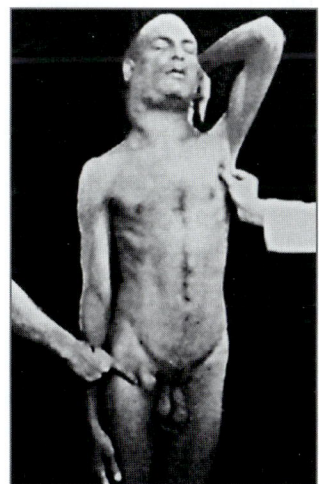

Fig. 8.5: Shows involvement of the cervical, axillary and inguinal lymph nodes in Hodgkin's disease.

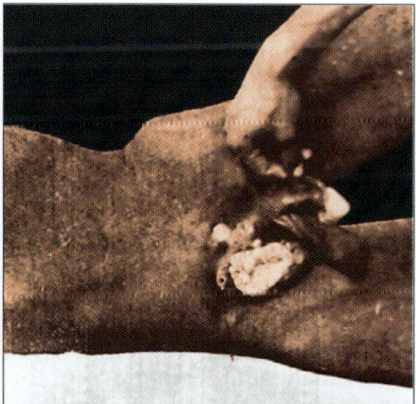

Fig. 8.6: Shows fungating inguinal lymph nodes from carcinoma of the penis. If the femoral vessels are involved by such lymph nodes fatal hemorrhage may result.

larged lymph nodes, e.g., hypoglossal nerve may be involved from enlarged upper group of cervical lymph nodes due to Hodgkin's disease or secondary carcinoma. Dyspnea and dysphagia may be complained of due to pressure on the trachea and esophagus respectively.

B. **PALPATION:** The swelling is palpated as discussed in Chapter 3 noting particularly, (i) the number, (ii) the situation, (iii) local temperature, (iv) tenderness, (v) surface, (vi) margin, (vii) **CONSISTENCY:** Enlarged lymph nodes should be carefully palpated with palmar aspects of the 3 fingers. While rolling the fingers against the swelling slight pressure is maintained to know the actual consistency of the swelling. *It must be remembered that normal lymph nodes without enlargement are not palpable.* Enlarged lymph nodes may be soft (fluctuating) or elastic and rubbery (Hodgkin's disease) or firm, discrete and shotty (syphilis) or stony hard (secondary carcinoma) or variable consistency—soft, firm and hard in places depending on the rate of the growth (lymphosarcoma). (viii) Whether the nodes are MATTED OR NOT?: If there be periadenitis, the adjoining nodes become matted.

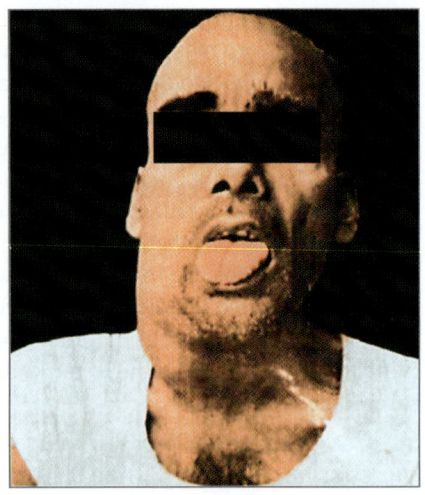

Fig. 8.7: Secondary carcinoma of the upper deep cervical lymph nodes on the right side has involved the hypoglossal nerve resulting in hemiparalysis of the right side of the tongue. This is evident by the fact that when the tongue is protruded out the tip of the tongue is deviated towards the side of lesion.

This can be diagnosed by careful palpation unless they are very painful. Lymph nodes are often matted in case of tuberculosis, acute lymphadenitis and metastatic carcinoma.

(ix) FIXITY TO SURROUNDING STRUCTURES: The enlarged lymph nodes should be carefully palpated to know if they are fixed to the skin, the deep fascia, the muscles, the vessels, the nerve, etc. Any primary malignant growth of the lymph nodes be it lymphosarcoma, reticulosarcoma, histiosarcoma or secondary carcinoma is often fixed to the surrounding structures—first with the deep fascia and underlying muscles followed by adjoining structures and ultimately the overlying skin if remain untreated. In many cases of carcinoma of the penis the secondarily involved inguinal group of lymph nodes infiltrates the femoral vessels and causes fatal hemorrhage. Upper deep cervical lymph nodes when involved secondarily from any carcinoma of its drainage area may involve the hypoglossal nerve and cause hemiparesis of the tongue which will be deviated towards the side of lesion when asked to protrude it out. Cases are not unknown when the patient complains of dyspnea or dysphagia due to pressure on the trachea or bronchus or esophagus by enlarged lymph nodes from Hodgkin's disease or lymphosarcoma or secondary carcinoma.

Drainage area: Whenever a patient comes with enlarged lymph nodes it should be the routine practice to examine its drainage area. This is particularly important in inflammatory and neoplastic lesion (carcinoma or malignant melanoma) of the lymph nodes. *The lymphatic drainage of the body may be discussed in the following way* (**Fig. 8.8**):

The cervical lymph nodes receive the lymphatics from the head, face, mouth, pharynx and neck, the left supraclavicular lymph node (Virchow's) receives lymphatics from left upper limb, left side of the chest including the breasts and also the viscera of the abdomen including both the testes.

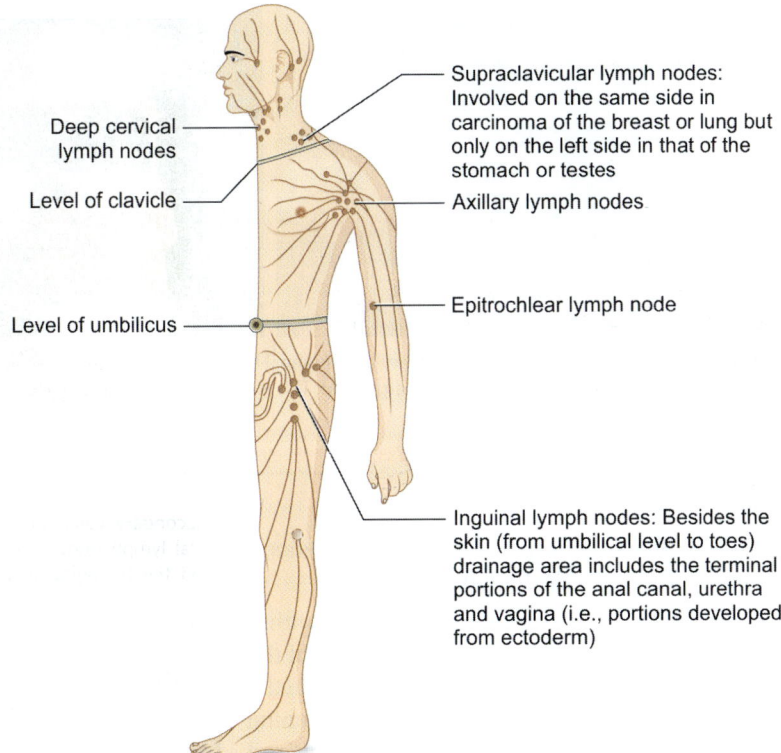

Fig. 8.8: Diagrammatic representation of the lymphatic drainage of the skin. The whole body has been broadly divided into three areas by two horizontal lines—one at the level of the clavicle and the other at the level of the umbilicus.

The axillary group of lymph nodes drains the upper limb of that side and the trunk which extends from the clavicle to the level of the umbilicus (including the breasts).

The inguinal lymph node drains the whole of the lower limb, the skin of the lower part of the abdomen below the level of the umbilicus, the penis, scrotum, perineum, vulva, anus, buttock, lower part of the back including the terminal parts of the anal canal, urethra and vagina (the portions which are developed from the ectoderm). That means the drainage area of the inguinal lymph nodes extends from the level of the umbilicus down to the toes.

GENERAL EXAMINATION

1. **Lymph nodes in other parts of the body**—should always be examined in any case of lymph node involvement. Not infrequently this examination reveals many cases of hidden generalized involvement of lymphatic system, e.g., Hodgkin's disease **(Figs. 8.9A and B)**, lymphosarcoma, lymphatic leukemia, tuberculosis, brucellosis, sarcoidosis, etc.
2. **Always examine: (a) spleen (Fig. 8.9C), (b) liver (Fig. 8.10), (c) mesenteric and iliac lymph nodes** (Hodgkin's disease).
3. **Examine the lungs for tuberculosis and secondary metastasis.**
4. **Syphilitic stigmas**—in syphilis (*see* **Fig. 4.15**).
5. **Parotid and lacrimal glands**—in sarcoidosis.

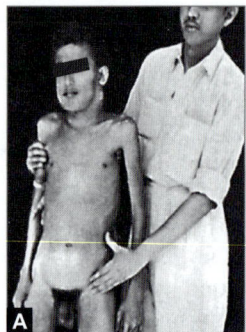 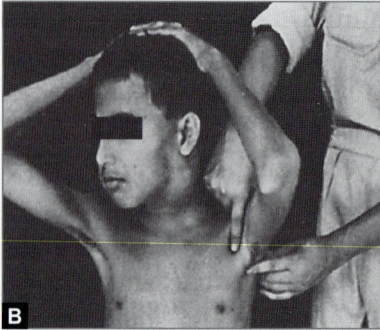 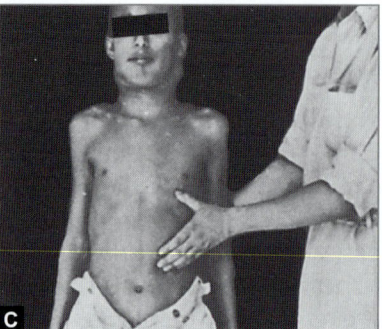

Figs.8.9 A to C: (A and B) Shows involvement of the axillary and inguinal lymph nodes besides the cervical group in Hodgkin's disease. (C) The spleen is being palpated for enlargement. This should be the routine practice in all cases of lymph node enlargement.

THE LYMPHATICS

Besides acute and chronic lymphangitis, lymphedema constitutes the major disease of the lymphatics.

Lymphedema—is caused by accumulation of lymph within the tissues. It mainly affects the subcutaneous tissues of the limbs **(Fig. 8.1)**. This is due to stagnation of lymph within the lymphatics. The causes may be classified into (A) Congenital malformation (primary lymphedema) and (B) Acquired obstruction (secondary lymphedema).

LOCAL EXAMINATION

One should look for prominent lymphatic vessels as red streaks progressing towards the regional lymph nodes. There may be brawny edema around. This is characteristic of acute lymphangitis. There may be subcutaneous nodules along the lymphatics as in case of malignant melanoma and carcinoma. In case of malignant melanoma these nodules are often of deep brown to black color.

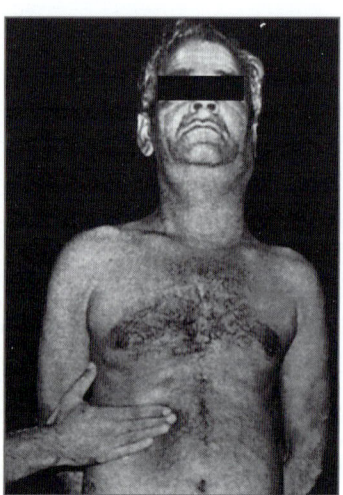

Fig. 8.10: One should also palpate the liver in case of enlargement of lymph nodes since liver is also involved in Hodgkin's disease.

In the early stage this edema pits on pressure, but gradually the subcutaneous tissue becomes fibrosed and the skin becomes keratotic (elephantiasis). In case of secondary lymphedema examination must include regional lymph nodes and general examination to find out the diagnosis.

SPECIAL INVESTIGATIONS

1. **Blood:** Routine examination of blood is essential for: (a) leukocytosis particularly polymorphs (acute lymphadenitis); (b) lymphocytosis (tuberculosis, lymphatic leukemia, etc.); (c) eosinophilia is often seen in case of filariasis; (d) raised erythrocyte sedimentation rate (ESR) (tuberculosis, secondary carcinoma and primary malignant lymphadenopathy);

(e) Wassermann reaction (WR) and Kahn test (syphilis); (f) microfilaria in the peripheral blood vessels when the patient is sleeping (filariasis). Complement fixation test should be performed for lymphogranuloma inguinale and syphilis.

2. **Aspiration**—of the abscess is essential for diagnosis be it a cold abscess or lymphogranuloma inguinale. In cold abscess one will look for acid-fast bacilli. In lymphogranuloma inguinale, pus from unruptured bubo is diluted ten times with normal saline and sterilized at 60° centigrade, 0.1 mL of the solution is injected intradermally. Appearance of a reddish papule within 48 hours at the site of injection indicates the test to be positive. This test is known as Frei's intradermal test, which is specific for lymphogranuloma inguinale.

3. **Mantoux test and Guineapig inoculation test**—are specific for tuberculosis.

4. **Gordon's biological test**—is specific for Hodgkin's disease. An emulsion of the affected lymph nodes is injected into a rabbit intracerebrally. This will initiate encephalitis within a few days.

5. **Biopsy:** This is probably the most important special investigation in this concern. Many cases may not be diagnosed clinically and with the help of the above special investigations. Biopsy should be called for in these cases. Under local and general anesthesia according to the circumstances, the isolated or matted lymph nodes are excised and examined both macroscopically and microscopically.

In TUBERCULOSIS, the lymph nodes on section show translucent, grayish patches in the early stage. As the disease advances these become opaque and yellowish, which is the result of necrosis and caseation. Microscopically, the tubercles will be found which consist of the epithelioid cells and giant cells having peripherally arranged nuclei in the early stage. After one week, lymphocytes with darkly stained nuclei and scanty cytoplasm make their appearance. By the end of the second week caseation appears in the center of the tubercle follicle. So in the center of the tubercle follicle lies eosin stained caseation surrounded by giant cells and epithelioid cells around which remains a zone of chronic inflammatory cells, e.g., lymphocyte and plasma cells, around which are the fibroblasts.

In HODGKIN'S DISEASE, the lymph nodes are firm and elastic and on section have a uniform gray translucent and moist appearance. Occasionally, yellow patches of necrosis may brake the homogeneity. Microscopically, its most important feature is cellular pleomorphism. There are lymphocytes, lymphoblasts and large mononuclear and multinucleated cells known as Reed-Sternberg cells which are the hallmark and pathologists always look for them to confirm the diagnosis. When the nucleus is single, it may be convoluted or ring shaped. In case of multinucleated forms generally there are two centrally placed nuclei, one of which is the mirror image of the other. Besides these giant cells there are also polymorphonuclears, eosinophils and plasma cells to add to pleomorphism. There are also reticular elements shown by silver staining.

In LYMPHOSARCOMA, the cut surface of the lymph node is grayish white and bulging. Microscopically, the normal structure of lymph node disappears and is replaced by diffuse arrangement of monotonously uniform large lymphoblast with hyperchromatic nucleus and scanty cytoplasm. The characteristic feature is that there is no increase of silver staining reticulum.

In RETICULUM-CELL SARCOMA—the microscopic picture shows abundance of reticulum cells with faintly acidophilic cytoplasm. The nucleus is double the size of lymphocytes and is commonly infolded to give a reniform appearance. Sometimes pseudopod-like processes may be seen in both the nuclei and the cytoplasms. Moreover the characteristic feature is the well distribution of silver staining reticulum, which has got intimate relation to the tumor cells.

In SECONDARY CARCINOMA, the tumor cells reach the nodes through the lymphatics by two methods—permeation or embolism. The carcinomatous cells first enter the peripheral lymph sinuses, gradually permeate the sinuses between the follicles and cords and finally destroy the normal architecture of the nodes. The microscopical structure of the secondary carcinoma very much resembles that of the primary one—whether epidermoid, adenocarcinoma, anaplastic, etc. Indeed, more often the secondary growth is more typical and characteristic than the primary one.

6. **Radiological examination:** In case of enlarged cervical lymph nodes, X-ray of the chest is essential, not only to find out enlargement of the mediastinal lymph nodes, but also to detect pulmonary tuberculosis or bronchogenic carcinoma as the cause of enlargement of cervical lymph nodes. Calcified tuberculous lymph nodes may easily be seen in X-ray film. But *tomography* will be essential to know particularly about the mediastinal lymph nodes.

7. **CT scan:** In case of abdominal and mediastinal lymph nodes enlargements, this investigation is extremely helpful.

8. **Mediastinal-scanning**—with Gallium 67 is sometimes performed to know whether the mediastinal lymph nodes are involved or not.

9. **Lymphangiography:** This test is of immense value in finding out the causes of lymphedema, lymph node enlargement and sites of lymph node metastasis in various carcinoma (particularly malignancy of the testis) and malignant melanoma.

Injection of patent blue dye into the web between the toes will show lymphatics on the dorsum of the foot. One of these lymphatics is cannulated and ultrafluid lipiodol (radio-opaque dye) is injected to visualize on X-ray the main lymphatic channels of the leg and subsequently the lymph nodes. Irregular filling defect in the lymph node means secondary metastasis. Soap bubble or foamy appearance is seen in Hodgkin's disease. Coarse nodular storage pattern is seen in lymphosarcoma and marginal sunburst appearance is the feature found in reticulum cell sarcoma.

In malignant melanoma, sometimes radioactive phosphorus is added to the radio-opaque dye for lymphangiography. This will destroy the malignant cells in the lymph nodes. This process is called 'endolymphatic therapy'.

Lymphadenography: Radio-opaque dye is injected directly into the lymph nodes either in vivo or during operation. After a few hours, X-rays are taken to delineate the lymph nodes **(Fig. 8.11)**. The various pathologies involving the lymph nodes are more clearly seen by this technique as mentioned above.

10. **Laparotomy:** This seems to be the last court of appeal in Hodgkin's disease. This is required not only to know the clinical staging of the disease by wedge biopsy of the liver and by biopsy of the aortic, mesenteric and iliac nodes and a small chip biopsy from iliac bone but also as treatment by splenectomy as the spleen is involved in about 90% of cases of the abdominally involved Hodgkin's disease and to obviate splenic irradiation due to its complications.

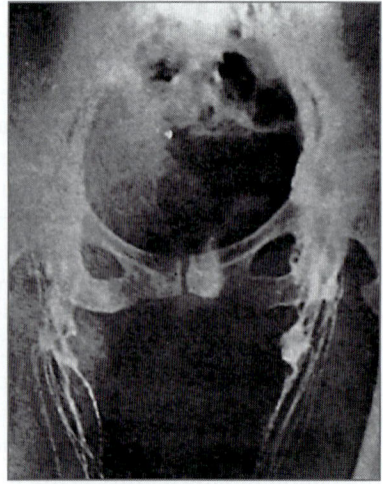

Fig. 8.11: Lymphangiography.

CAUSES OF ENLARGEMENT OF LYMPH NODES

A. INFLAMMATORY:
(a) ACUTE LYMPHADENITIS
(b) CHRONIC LYMPHADENITIS
(c) GRANULOMATOUS LYMPHADENITIS—the etiologic agents may be bacterial, viral or fungal. From BACTERIAL origin are tuberculosis, syphilis, tularemia, brucellosis, etc.; from VIRAL origin are lymphogranuloma venereum, cat-scratch disease, infectious mononucleosis; From PARASITOLOGICAL origin is filariasis due to infestation of *Wuchereria bancrofti* and toxoplasmosis; From FUNGAL origin are blastomycosis, histoplasmosis and coccidioidomycosis (not actinomycosis, as lymph node enlargement is unusual in this disease). In this group may be added condition like sarcoidosis, whose etiology is still controversial.

B. NEOPLASTIC:
(a) BENIGN—almost nonexistent
(b) MALIGNANT:
1. *Primary:*
OLD CLASSIFICATION:
(i) Giant follicle lymphoma
(ii) Lymphosarcoma
(iii) Reticulum cell sarcoma
(iv) Hodgkin's disease.
NEW CLASSIFICATION
The classification, which is currently used, is based on the classification of Rappaport et al. or Lukes et al. It is as follows:

Primary malignant lymphomas can be broadly classified into two groups—(i) Diffuse lymphomas (56%) and (ii) Nodular lymphomas (44%). The latter type is more prevalent in females but is distinctly rare in children and blacks. But these two groups are actually types of proliferation that any of the malignant lymphomas can exhibit at some points of their evolution. The natural history of the disease is primarily related to the cell type in which a nodular pattern indicates a slower evolution and a better prognosis than a diffuse one. It is also interesting to note that most nodular lymphomas change later to a diffuse pattern but maintaining the same cell composition.

The classification based on cell types are:
(i) Malignant lymphoma, undifferentiated type
(ii) Malignant lymphoma, histiocytic type
(iii) Malignant lymphoma, lymphocytic type (poorly differentiated)
(iv) Malignant lymphoma, lymphocytic type (well-differentiated)
(v) Malignant lymphoma, mixed type (histiocytic-lymphocytic)
(vi) Malignant lymphoma, Hodgkin's type: (a) lymphocytic predominance; (b) nodular sclerosis; (c) mixed cellularity; (d) lymphocytic depletion.

2. *Secondary*
Metastatic lymph node enlargement is often seen from carcinoma, malignant melanoma or rarely from sarcoma of the draining region.

C. LYMPHATIC LEUKEMIA
D. AUTOIMMUNE DISORDERS:

(i) Juvenile rheumatoid arthritis (Still's disease)
(ii) Other collagen diseases such as systemic lupus erythematosus, polyarteritis nodosa and scleroderma.

Causes of generalized lymph nodes enlargement:
1. Tuberculosis
2. Syphilis—secondary stage
3. Infectious mononucleosis
4. Sarcoidosis
5. Brucellosis
6. Toxoplasmosis
7. Hodgkin's disease
8. Lymphosarcoma
9. Lymphatic leukemia.

DIFFERENTIAL DIAGNOSIS

ACUTE LYMPHADENITIS

The nodes become enlarged and painful. The overlying skin becomes warm, red and brawny edematous. On palpation the nodes are extremely tender. This condition may subside with the primary focus or end in suppuration when fluctuation can be elicited in the center and pitting on pressure at the periphery. Finding of primary infective focus in the drainage area confirms the diagnosis.

CHRONIC NONSPECIFIC (PYOGENIC) LYMPHADENITIS

Clinically, it is often impossible to differentiate this condition from tuberculous lymphadenitis in its early stage. The nodes become moderately enlarged, slightly tender and elastic with or without matting. A history of acute lymphadenitis can be obtained which gradually attains chronicity. In the cervical group oral sepsis and lesions of the scalp are usually the common causes. In the groin, besides infected cuts and ulcers, walking on bare and cracked feet may lead to this condition amongst laborers.

HYPERPLASIA

Lymph nodes may respond to infection by enlarging. In various carcinomas the regional lymph nodes may be enlarged, due to inflammation rather than from spread of carcinoma. By palpation it is very difficult to know if the enlarged lymph nodes contain any malignant cells or not. Microscopically, the hyperplasia may be primarily located in the reactive centers, in the intervening lymphoid tissue or within the sinuses.

TUBERCULOUS LYMPHADENITIS

This is commonly found in children and young adults. The cervical lymph nodes are most frequently involved followed by mediastinal, mesenteric, axillary and inguinal groups according to the order of frequency. *Clinically three stages are discernible.* In the *first stage* the nodes become simply enlarged without matting. This is known as lymphadenoid type and differentiation from chronic septic lymphadenitis becomes difficult. In the *second stage* due to the advent of periadenitis the enlarged nodes become adherent to one another (matted). This is the most characteristic feature of tuberculous lymph nodes. Later on caseation takes place in the interior of the nodes so that the nodes become softer with gradual formation of cold abscess. This is the *third stage.* Gradually, the cold abscess makes its way towards the surface and ultimately bursts forming a typical tubercular ulcer or a sinus which refuses to heal.

SYPHILITIC LYMPHADENITIS

In the primary stage the lymph nodes in the groin become enlarged along with presence of genital chancres. The nodes are painless, discrete, firm and shotty. These nodes do not show any tendency towards suppuration. In extragenital chancres occurring in the lips, breasts, etc., the nodes may become inflamed, painful and matted. *In the secondary stage* generalized involvement of nodes may occur affecting particularly the epitrochlear and occipital groups. The characteristics are similar to those found in the primary stage. *In the tertiary stage* the lymph nodes are seldom involved. Other syphilitic stigmas (*see* **Fig. 4.15**), positive WR and Kahn tests along with presence of *Treponema pallidum* in dark ground illumination from the primary lesion confirm the diagnosis.

FILARIAL LYMPHADENITIS (FIG. 8.12)

The inguinal nodes are commonly affected and this condition is more often found in males. The lymph nodes become enlarged and tender. A history of periodic fever with pain (especially during the full or new moon) is very characteristic. Swelling of the spermatic cord with dilatation of lymphatic vessels (lymphangiectasis) is often found in filariasis. There may be thickening of the skin of the scrotum. Microfilaria can be demonstrated in the blood drawn at night. Eosinophilia is the rule. Biopsy of lymph nodes may reveal adult filaria within them.

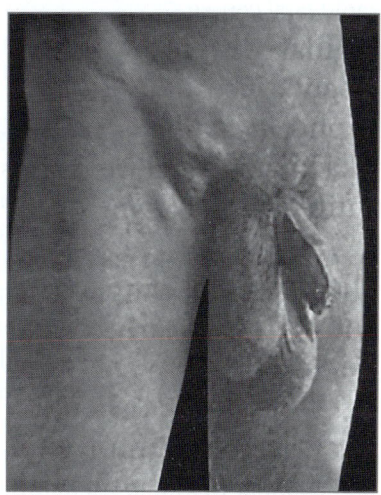

Fig. 8.12: Filarial lymphadenitis.

LYMPHOGRANULOMA INGUINALE

It is a type of venereal disease caused by a filtrable virus of the psittacosis-lymphogranuloma inguinale group which is transmitted through sexual intercourse. The primary lesion is often insignificant but the secondary lesion with enlarged lymph nodes in the medial part of one or both the groins is the presenting feature. The iliac lymph nodes may also be involved. Soon periadenitis occurs and the mass becomes brawny. Gradually the nodes suppurate and may break down to discharge thick yellowish-white pus. The resulting sinus persists for quite a long time. Biopsy, Frei's test and complement fixation test are confirmatory.

CAT-SCRATCH DISEASE

This is due to a virus of lymphogranuloma psittacosis group. This disease is characterized by fever, toxemia and malaise from localized inflammation around the lesion. The regional lymph nodes are enlarged and suppuration often occurs in due course.

INFECTIOUS MONONUCLEOSIS (GLANDULAR FEVER)

This causes generalized enlargement of lymph nodes which are firm, elastic and slightly tender. It is associated with sore throat, rash, splenic enlargement and irregular fever. Lymphocytosis and positive Paul Bunnell test help in the diagnosis.

SARCOIDOSIS

This may be due to tissue reaction against antigen or tubercle-like bacillus. Parotid and lacrimal glands enlargement, skin lesion like papule and nodule, bone cyst, hypercalcemia and above all generalized enlargement of lymph nodes are features of this disease. Kveim's test—a nodule develops within a month of intradermal injection of sarcoid tissue, is very much confirmatory.

NONHODGKIN'S LYMPHOMAS

1. **Undifferentiated lymphomas:** This is a malignant proliferation of primitive cells having scanty cytoplasm and a round or oval nucleus with delicate chromatin. Burkitt's lymphoma is regarded as specific variant of this type of lymphoma. It has a peculiar geographic distribution, mostly seen in tropical Africa and New Guinea. Typically, Burkitt's lymphoma affects children and young adults. It has a great tendency for extranodal involvement such as the jaws, ovaries, abdominal organ, retroperitoneum and the central nervous system. Untreated cases follow a rapid fatal course.

2. **Histiocytic lymphoma:** Lymph nodes involved by the histiocytic lymphoma (reticulum cell sarcoma) may be matted together and contain large necrotic areas. The lesion is composed of large cells with round to oval, sometimes pleomorphic vesicular nuclei and containing prominent nucleoli. Fibrosis with hyalinization of the stroma is sometimes prominent separating the tumor cells in clusters or cords.

3. **Lymphocytic lymphoma:** The individual nodes are not adherent. They appear highly cellular and occasionally contain areas of necrosis. *In poorly differentiated variant the* cells are large than matured lymphocytes but smaller than histiocytes. The nuclei are round, oval and irregular with focal chromatin clumping and a distinct nucleolus. Nuclear indentations are often present. *In well-differentiated lymphocytic lymphoma* the cells are similar to normal mature lymphocytes. It is very difficult to differentiate this type of lymphoma from chronic lymphocytic leukemia. The clinical history, the peripheral blood count and the bone marrow findings are required to make such distinction.

4. **Mixed lymphoma:** This designation should be restricted to tumors in which both histiocytes and lymphocytes are present in significant amounts. A nodular pattern of growth is common in the early stage, but majority however develop into a diffuse lymphoma of histiocytic type.

Clinically, one should be particular to stage the lymphomas. Stages I lesions have a good prognosis, but unfortunately, they comprise only 1/3rd of all the cases. Routine use of lymphangiography has demonstrated that most patients with nonHodgkin's malignant lymphoma have widespread disease at the time of diagnosis. In a series about 40% were in stage IV at the time of diagnosis. Malignant lymphoma involving a high cervical lymph node is the one most likely to be localized. Spread by involvement of contiguous lymph node groups is found in majority of the cases of nonHodgkin's lymphoma. In regard to the cell type the average survival is longer for the well-differentiated lymphocytic type, intermediate for the poorly lymphocytic type and shorter for the histiocytic variety. Involvement of mesenteric lymph nodes is exceptional in Hodgkin's disease, but quite common in other types of lymphoma. Among extranodal involvement the bone marrow and the spleen are the common sites.

HODGKIN'S DISEASE

The onset of this disease is about a decade earlier than lymphosarcoma and reticulosarcoma but it is not uncommon in young children. The symptoms are more local than constitutional except in acute cases. The most common presentation is painless and progressive enlargement of the lymph nodes, first detected in the cervical group on one side and then on the other. It may be that the deeper lymph nodes such as the mediastinal and mesenteric groups may have been involved earlier. The associated symptoms such as malaise, weight loss and fever are quite characteristic. Recurrent bouts of remittent fever is quite characteristic of this disease. Pressure effects by enlarged mediastinal lymph nodes such as venous engorgement, cyanosis of the head and neck and difficulty in respiration due to pressure on the bronchus are sometimes the presenting features. Bone pain with vertebral collapse secondary to bony metastasis, though rare, should be kept in mind. Root-pain, and even paraplegia may develop due to pressure on the spinal cord from deposits in the vertebrae or pressure by retroperitoneal nodes on the nerve roots while they come out of the intervertebral foramina. A peculiar feature of this disease is the complaint of enhanced pain at the sites of disease induced by drinking alcohol.

On examination, the lymph nodes are elastic and rubbery to feel. The nodes tend to remain discrete moveable with little tendency towards matting and softening. Splenic enlargement is a significant finding of this disease and is found in not less than 75% of the cases. Hepatomegaly is found in about 50% of the cases. Progressive anemia is more or less constant and may be due to splenomegaly or bony metastases. Occasionally, eosinophilia is associated with megakaryocytosis and increased platelet count. Sometimes jaundice is seen due to excessive hemolysis of red cells or involvement of liver. The course of the disease varies with the pathological type of the disease. Death may occur within a few weeks or the patient may survive longer without any treatment. The special investigations have already been discussed.

Clinical staging of the hodgkin's disease:

Stage I: Involvement of a single lymph node region or involvement of a single extralymphatic organ or site (IE).
Stage II: Involvement of two or more lymph node regions on the same side of the diaphragm alone or with involvement of limited contiguous extralymphatic organ or tissue (IIE).
Stage III: Involvement of lymph node regions on both sides of the diaphragm, which may include the spleen (III S) and/or limited contiguous extralymphatic organ or site (III E, III ES).
Stage IV: Multiple or disseminated foci of involvement of one or more extralymphatic organs or tissues with or without lymphatic involvement.

All stages are further subdivided on the basis of absence (A) or presence (B) of the following systemic symptoms, e.g., fever, weight loss more than 10%, bone pain etc.

PATHOLOGICALLY, Hodgkin's disease can be divided into four categories, which is important so far as the prognosis of the disease is concerned. The more numerous are the lymphocytes, the more favorable is the prognosis.
Type 1: Lymphocyte-predominant Hodgkin's disease.
Type 2: Mixed-cellularity—a diffuse infiltrate of lymphocyte, histiocytes, eosinophil and plasma cells that obliterate the normal architecture.
Type 3: Nodular sclerosis is often seen in clinical stage I and is associated with better prognosis.
Type 4: Lymphocytes depletion pattern—the most ominous form.

SECONDARY CARCINOMA

The nodes become enlarged, irregular and fixed to all the surrounding structures (including the skin) which are gradually pulled towards the mass. The most important characteristic feature is their stony hard consistency. Although painless to start with, continuous pain of varying severity will appear as the growth increases. Fungation into the skin occurs in neglected cases. Discovery of the primary growth confirms the diagnosis.

MALIGNANT MELANOMA (FIG. 8.13)

Affection is always secondary. The involved nodes grow much more rapidly and are less hard than those due to secondary carcinoma. When they break out or are divided after removal, black pigmentation becomes evident.

LYMPHATIC LEUKEMIA

This is characterized by a generalized involvement of lymph nodes with enlargement of the spleen. The most important diagnostic feature is marked increase in the number of lymphocytes and their precursors in the blood.

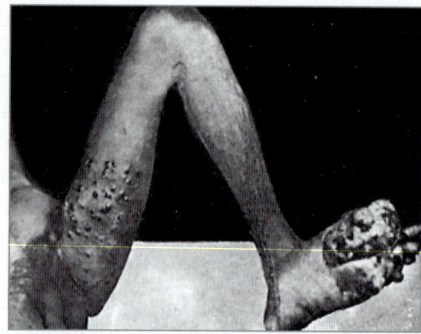

Fig. 8.13: Disseminated metastases in the lymph vessels from malignant melanoma of the foot.

Algorithmic Approach to Patient with Lymphatic Diseases

Patient presents with lymph node enlargement or lymphedema

↓

Is the lymph node enlargement localized or generalized?
- **Localized** → Consider **infection, malignancy, or reactive lymphadenopathy**
- **Generalized** → Consider **systemic disease (tuberculosis, lymphoma, autoimmune disorders, HIV)**

↓

Is the lymph node painful?
- **Yes** → Likely **infectious (acute lymphadenitis, tuberculosis, filariasis, syphilis, Cat-scratch disease)**
- **No** → Consider **malignancy (lymphoma, metastatic carcinoma, sarcoidosis)**

↓

What is the consistency of the lymph node?
- **Soft** → Suggests **benign/infectious causes**
- **Rubbery** → Suggests **hodgkin's or non-hodgkin's lymphoma**
- **Hard, fixed** → Suggests **metastatic carcinoma or lymphosarcoma**

↓

Is the node fixed or mobile?
- **Mobile** → Likely **benign, reactive lymphadenopathy**
- **Fixed** → Suggests **malignancy (metastases, lymphosarcoma, tuberculous lymphadenitis With matting)**

↓

Are there systemic symptoms (fever, weight loss, night sweats, fatigue)?
- **Yes** → Consider **tuberculosis, lymphoma, HIV, autoimmune disorders (SLE, RA, sarcoidosis)**
- **No** → Likely **benign, reactive lymphadenopathy or early-stage malignancy**

↓

Order special investigations
- **FNAC and biopsy** → Gold standard for lymph node evaluation
- **Blood tests** → CBC, ESR, CRP, LDH, peripheral blood smear
- **Imaging** → Chest X-ray (for mediastinal nodes), CT scan, MRI, lymphangiography
- **Mantoux test** → If tuberculosis suspected
- **Viral markers** → HIV, epstein-barr virus (EBV), cytomegalovirus (CMV)

↓

Confirm diagnosis and initiate treatment
- **Infectious causes:** Antibiotics, antitubercular therapy, antiviral drugs
- **Malignancies:** Chemotherapy, radiotherapy, surgery if necessary
- **Autoimmune causes:** Corticosteroids, disease-modifying agents

Examination of Peripheral Nerve Lesions

CHAPTER 9

HISTORY

History of present illness: History of trauma is usually associated with peripheral nerve lesion. Besides trauma, there is only other way of involvement of a peripheral nerve, and that is by infiltration of the nerve by malignant growth. The types of trauma which may injure a peripheral nerve may be a wound—either an incisional cut (e.g., by a broken glass) or a penetrating wound (e.g., a stab or a gunshot wound), or a fracture and/or dislocation, in which case the nerve is injured by the fractured segment or the dislocated bone rather than the trauma directly. Incisional wound or the penetrating wound may injure the nerve anywhere in the body but commonly seen at the wrist when the median or the ulnar nerve becomes the victim. Injury to the nerve caused by fracture or dislocation is commonly seen in the arm when the radial nerve is injured by the fractured shaft of the humerus, at the elbow in the supracondylar fracture of humerus when the median, the ulnar or the radial nerve may be injured. In fracture of the medial epicondyle the ulnar nerve is usually affected. In both the supracondylar fracture and the fracture of the medial epicondyle, there may be late paralysis of the ulnar nerve which is known as 'tardy ulnar palsy'—due to involvement of the nerve in callus formation. In fracture of the neck of fibula, the lateral popliteal nerve is often injured. In subcoracoid dislocation of the humerus and fracture of the neck of the humerus, the axillary nerve may be injured leading to paralysis of the deltoid. In posterior dislocation of the hip, subtrochanteric fracture and supracondylar fracture of the femur, the sciatic nerve may be injured. The most peculiar feature is that generally the common peroneal portion of the sciatic nerve is involved.

Lesion of the brachial plexus, though rare, is yet interesting anatomically. *The upper lesion* (Erb-Duchenne) is caused by the injury which causes forcible increase of the angle between the neck and shoulder thus stretching upper trunk of the brachial plexus. This type of injury may occur during difficult labor when a pull on the head of the fetus is made while the shoulder is arrested inside or due to fall of a load on the shoulder. *The lower lesion* (Klumpke) of a brachial plexus may occur when the arm is being forcibly hyperabducted. This can occur when a falling person tries to catch an object. This will stretch the lower trunk of the brachial plexus.

Sometimes the patient complains of a constant intense burning pain after an injury even after the wound has healed. This is called *causalgia* and is caused by partial nerve injury. This type of pain may commence immediately following the injury or more often after a month or so when the skin wound has healed.

Past history: Sometimes patients may present with peripheral nerve lesion without a history of trauma. The patient indicates the lesion to be spontaneous. In these cases, an enquiry must be made whether an injection has been made in the arm or in the thigh or any site near the nerve lesion. Irritating drug such as quinine when injected intramuscularly in the deltoid or in the thigh may affect the axillary nerve or the sciatic nerve respectively. Whether the patient is suffering from diabetes or leprosy. Often such patients present first with loss of sensation of a patch of skin. Is there any past history of diphtheria?

Sometimes the patients may not complain of nerve involvement immediately after injury but may complain of this later on when the wound has healed. In these cases enquiry must be made whether the wound was infected or not, as infection will lead to fibrosis and will not allow proper regeneration of the nerve.

Personal history: When the onset of the peripheral nerve lesion is spontaneous, an enquiry must be made whether the patient is diabetic, alcoholic or works with lead or arsenicals.

History in peripheral nerve diseases

Aspect	Clinical significance	Patient-friendly questions
History of trauma	Nerve injury due to direct trauma or fractures	"Have you had an injury, fracture, or surgery near the affected area?"
Onset and progression	Acute → Trauma, Chronic → Degenerative/Metabolic	"Did the weakness/sensation loss appear suddenly or gradually?"
Pain	Causalgia → Partial nerve Damage	"Do you feel burning pain in the affected area?"
Loss of sensation	Peripheral neuropathy vs focal nerve compression	"Do you feel numbness, tingling, or reduced sensation in any area?"
Muscle weakness	Nerve supply loss leads to atrophy and paralysis	"Do you feel weakness in specific muscles or difficulty moving a limb?"
Occupational exposure	Lead, arsenic poisoning can cause neuropathy	"Do you work with chemicals, metals, or repetitive hand movements?"
Diabetes, leprosy, alcoholism	Common causes of peripheral neuropathy	"Have you been diagnosed with diabetes or leprosy?"
Past medical history	Previous infections, surgeries, systemic diseases	"Have you had any nerve-related surgeries or infections in the past?"

LOCAL EXAMINATION

A. INSPECTION

1. Attitude and deformity: Many a diagnosis of the peripheral nerve injury can be made easily by the peculiar attitude and deformity of the limb concerned. Of these the followings are commonly seen and will be discussed.

Wrist drop (Fig. 9.1) is seen in paralysis of radial nerve, which supplies all the extensors of the wrist joint.

Foot drop is caused by paralysis of the lateral popliteal nerve which supplies the dorsiflexors and evertors of the foot.

Winging of the scapula (prominence of the vertebral border of the scapula) indicates paralysis of the long thoracic nerve of Bell **(Fig. 9.2)**.

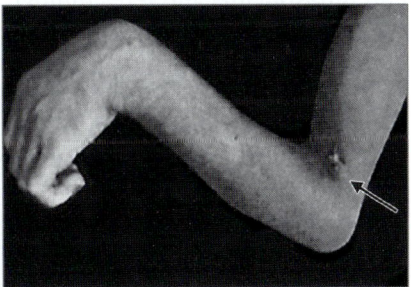

Fig. 9.1: Wrist drop. The arrow shows the scar of a compound supracondylar fracture of the humerus.

Clawhand (Main en griffe) means hyperextension of the metacarpophalangeal joints and flexion of the proximal and distal interphalangeal joints. This deformity is due to paralysis of the interossei and lumbricals, which are concerned with flexion of the metacarpophalangeal joints and extension of interphalangeal joints. The flexors of the fingers are unaffected. This deformity is seen in lesions of the ulnar nerve, more markedly in combined lesion of the ulnar and the median (this supplies first and second lumbricals) nerves and in Klumpke's paralysis. The extensor digitorum is mainly concerned with extension of the metacarpophalangeal joints and has little action in extension of the interphalangeal joints. Those muscles being unopposed by the interossei in the metacarpophalangeal joints and the flexors of the fingers act unopposed by the interossei on the interphalangeal joints. This causes the deformity **(Figs. 9.3 and 9.4)**.

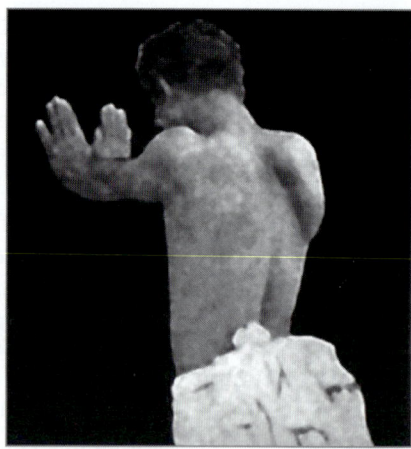

Fig. 9.2: Winging of the scapula.

'*Ape-thumb*' deformity and the '*pointing index*' are due to lesion of the median nerve. The former deformity is due to paralysis of the opponens pollicis and the latter deformity is due to paralysis of the lateral half of the flexor digitorum profundus, both supplied by the median nerve.

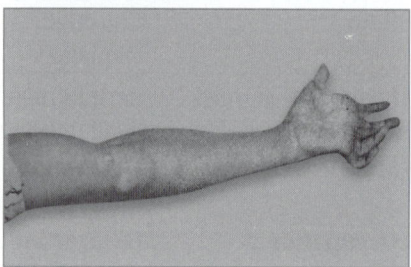

The typical '*policeman receiving the tip*' deformity is due to upper lesion of the brachial plexus (Erb-Duchenne). Since this lesion affects the Erb's point, which is the commencement of the upper trunk of the brachial plexus from the 5th and 6th cervical nerves and the point of emergence of the suprascapular nerve and the nerve to the subclavius, the abductors and lateral rotators of the shoulder (deltoid, supra- and infraspinatus and teres minor) and the flexors and supinators of the elbow (biceps, brachialis, brachioradialis and supinator) are mainly paralyzed. In this deformity the arm hangs by the side of the body and internally rotated with forearm extended at the elbow and fully pronated **(Fig. 9.5)**.

Fig. 9.3: One can see the clawhand due to injury to ulnar nerve, the wound scar at elbow is clearly seen.

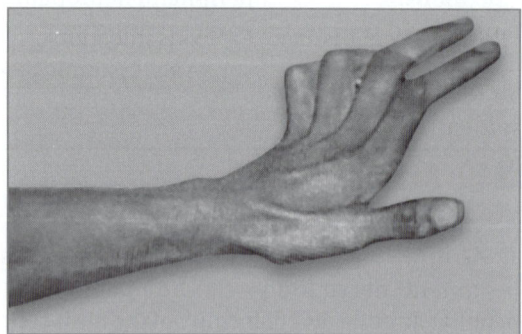

Fig. 9.4: Clawhand.

2. **Wasting of the muscles (Fig. 9.6):** This will be always obvious in long standing paralysis. So it is the rule to compare with the sound side always. Wasting of the deltoid, thenar and hypothenar eminences, hollows between the metacarpals due to atrophy of the interossei should be looked for and when the corresponding nerve is damaged this becomes obvious. Sometimes measurement of the circumference may be required to establish definitely muscular wasting.

3. **Skin:** The skin becomes dry (no sweating due to involvement of the sympathetic nerve), glossy and smooth with disappearance of cutaneous folds and subcutaneous fat in complete paralysis. In partial lesion, there may be causalgia. Vasomotor changes in the form of pallor, cyanosis, excessive sweating and trophic disturbances such as ridged and brittle nails, scaly skin, etc., may become evident. Sometimes trophic ulcers may be seen.

4. **Scar or wound:** Scar indicates previous wound and by looking at the scar one may guess whether the wound was infected or not. Presence of scar or wound will also give an indication as to which nerve may be injured **(Fig. 9.1)**.

B. PALPATION

1. The **temperature** of the affected limb should always be compared with that of the normal side. The paralyzed parts are usually cold.

2. **Muscles:** Paralyzed muscles are generally wasted in long standing cases. They are softer and more flabby. The function of the muscles will obviously be hampered.

3. **Skin:** Whether any part of the limb is anesthetized or not? This is very important as this will give a clue as to which nerve has been affected. As for example in case of lesion of the axillary nerve (due to dislocation of shoulder or fracture of the neck of the humerus) the deltoid muscle will be paralyzed, but cannot be tested as the dislocation or fracture will itself prevent abduction of the shoulder. In this case if the students remember that the axillary nerve is also concerned in supplying cutaneous twigs to the skin over the lower part of the deltoid, that part will automatically be anesthetized and the diagnosis of injury to the axillary nerve will be established.

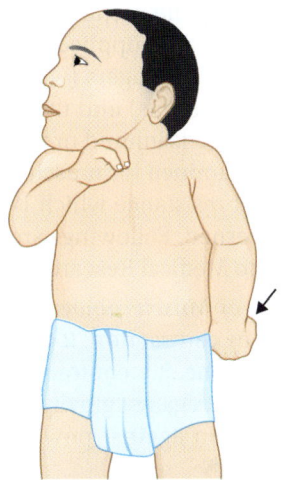

Fig. 9.5: Erb's paralysis.

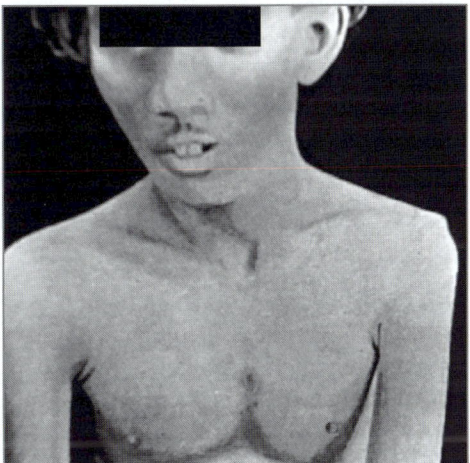

Fig. 9.6: Note the wasting of the deltoid on the left side. It has been caused by intramuscular injection of quinine which has affected the axillary nerve.

If the skin of the affected side is seriously palpated an area of hyperesthesia can be detected which is the site of nerve regeneration. By the shifting of this site of hyperesthesia one can assess the speed of regeneration of the nerve.

4. **Scar:** If present, should be palpated for tenderness, which indicates adhesion of the nerve to the scar.

C. MUSCLES POWER

While investigating for muscle power, one must have a clear conception about the anatomy as to which nerve supplies which muscle. It may so happen that the muscle concerned is supplied by more than one nerve. In that case, the clinician will not be able to assess the severity of the nerve injury by investigating the muscle power. As for example, the flexor muscles of the fingers are supplied by the median nerve mostly except for the medial half of the flexor digitorum profundus which is supplied by the ulnar nerve. So the patient with median nerve injury will be able to flex the fingers (with the help of lumbricals, interrossei and medial half of flexor digitorum profundus) and the wrist (with the help of flexor carpi ulnaris). To test whether a particular nerve is injured or not, the muscle which is exclusively supplied by the same nerve should be examined for muscle power. The patient is asked to carry out the movement of the joint against resistance which is performed by the same muscle supplied exclusively by the nerve concerned. Followings are the gradations of the muscle power which has been quoted according to Medical Research Council, London.

Gradation of Muscle power: 0 = complete paralysis, 1 = flicker of contraction, 2 = contraction with gravity eliminated alone, 3 = contraction against gravity alone, 4 = contraction against gravity and some resistance and 5 = contraction against powerful resistance (normal power).

The muscles to be tested for individual nerves are described below:

ACCESSORY NERVE

Trapezius: This muscle is tested by asking the patient to elevate the shoulder against resistance **(Fig. 9.7)**.

HYPOGLOSSAL NERVE

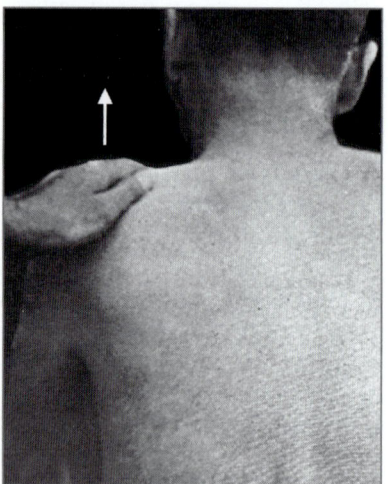

Fig. 9.7: Trapezius muscle is being tested against resistance to know intactness of the accessory nerve.

Muscles of the tongue: The patient is asked to protrude his tongue. In case of hemiparesis of the tongue due to involvement of the hypoglossal nerve of one side the tip of the tongue will be deviated towards the side of lesion.

LONG THORACIC NERVE

Serratus anterior: The patient is asked to push against a wall with his outstretched hand. If the muscle is paralyzed, the vertebral border and the inferior angle of the scapula will stand out from the chest wall—which is known as "winging of the scapula" **(Fig. 9.8)**.

AXILLARY NERVE

Deltoid: The patient is asked to abduct his shoulder with the elbow flexed at right angle against resistance **(Fig. 9.9)**. With another hand the clinician palpates the muscle to know if it is contracting or not.

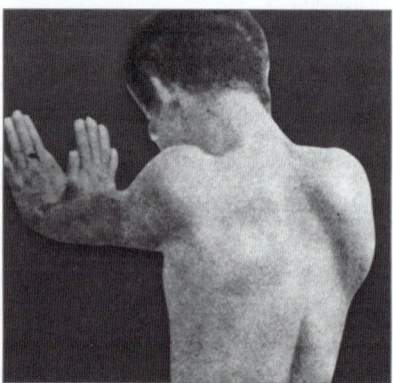

Fig. 9.8: Note the winging of the right scapula as the patient pushes against the wall. It indicates paralysis of the muscle due to involvement of the long thoracic nerve.

RADIAL NERVE

1. **Brachioradialis:** The muscle is tested by asking the patient to flex the elbow joint keeping the forearm in midprone position against resistance. The muscle will stand out as a prominent band as shown in **Figure 9.10**.
2. **Extensor muscles of the wrist joint:** Except the extensor carpi radialis longus which is supplied by the radial nerve itself, all the other extensor muscles of the wrist joint are supplied by the posterior interosseous branch of the radial nerve. There will be "wrist drop" **(Fig. 9.1)** and inability to extend the wrist joint when these muscles are paralyzed. To know the muscle power of these muscles the patient is asked to extend the wrist joint against resistance.
3. **Extensor digitorum:** This muscle is mainly concerned with extension of the metacarpophalangeal joint. It also extends the interphalangeal joints along with the corresponding interossei and lumbricals. So when this muscle is paralyzed the patient will not be able to extend the metacarpophalangeal joints *but will be able to extend the interphalangeal joints to some extent* **(Fig. 9.11)**, the students must not forget this.

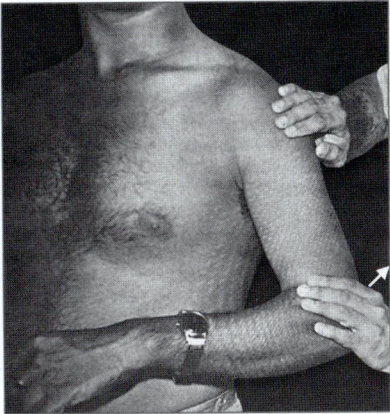

Fig. 9.9: The patient is asked to abduct the shoulder against resistance at the elbow. The other hand at the shoulder palpates the deltoid muscle to know if it is contracted or not.

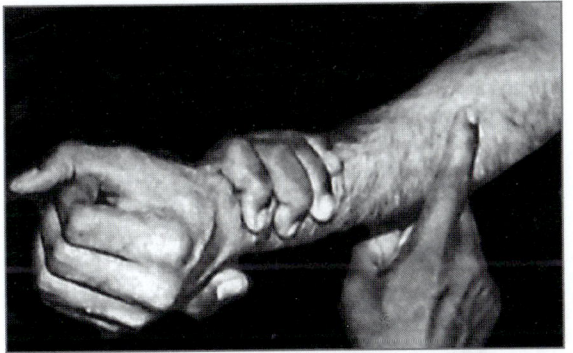

Fig. 9.10: The brachioradialis muscle is made to contract to know the intactness of the radial nerve.

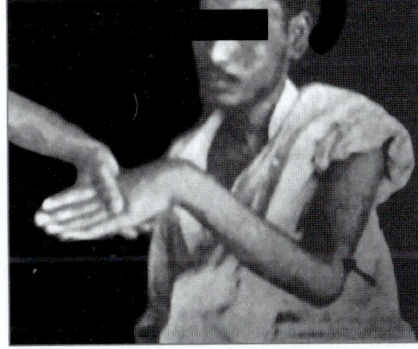

Fig. 9.11: In case of radial nerve paralysis note that the fingers can be extended with the help of the interossei.

MEDIAN NERVE

1. **Flexor pollicis longus:** The patient is asked to bend the terminal phalanx of the thumb against resistance while the proximal phalanx is being steadied by the clinician. This muscle is only paralyzed when the median nerve is injured at or above the elbow **(Fig. 9.12)**.
2. **Flexor digitorum superficialis and profundus (lateral half):** In case of injury to the median nerve if the patient is asked to clasp the hands, the index finger of the affected side fails to flex and remains as a "pointing index". This test is known as ***Ochsner's clasping test*** **(Fig. 9.13)**.

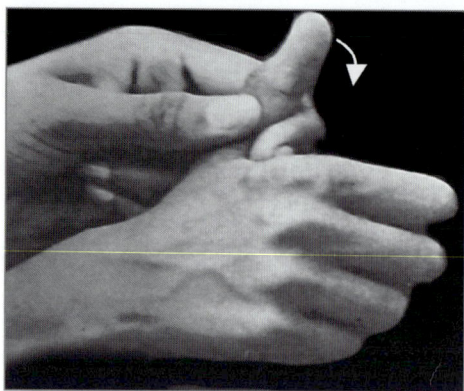

Fig. 9.12: The terminal phalanx of the thumb is bent when the proximal phalanx is being steadied to know the power of the flexor pollicis longus.

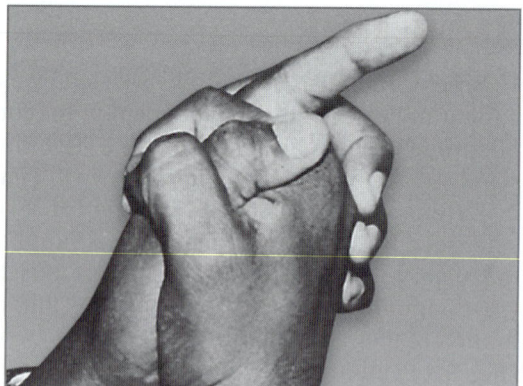

Fig. 9.13: Ochsner's clasping test.

3. **Abductor pollicis brevis:** This muscle is concerned in abduction of the thumb that means the thumb moves upwards at right angle to the palm of the hand when the hand is laid flat on the table. This is done by asking the patient to touch the pen which is kept at a slight higher level than the palm of the hand with the thumb. This is known as *pen test* (**Fig. 9.14**).

4. **Opponens pollicis:** This muscle swings the thumb across the palm to touch the tips of the other fingers. The patient with paralysis of this muscle will be unable to do this movement. The students must not forget that a vicarious movement short of proper opposition movement is possible by adductor pollicis supplied by the ulnar nerve (**Fig. 9.15**).

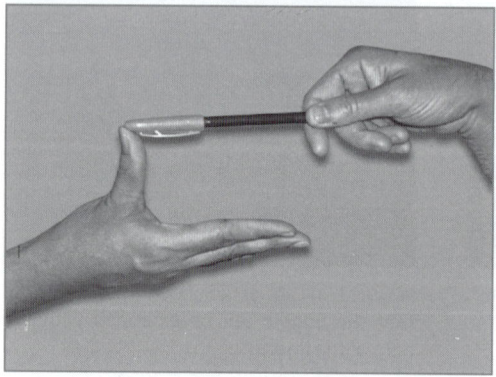

Fig. 9.14: Pen test is being performed to know the muscle power of abductor pollicis brevis.

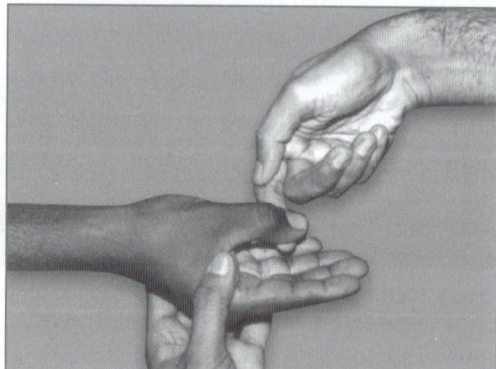

Fig. 9.15: Testing the opponens pollicis against resistance of the clinician's fingers. During the test the thumb nail must remain in a plane parallel to the palm.

ULNAR NERVE

1. **Flexor carpi ulnaris:** When the wrist joint is flexed against resistance, the hand tends to deviate towards radial side.
2. **Interossei:** The dorsal interossei are concerned with abduction of the fingers, while the palmar interossei adduct the fingers. Besides this, interossei along with the lumbricals flex

the metacarpophalangeal joints and extend both proximal and distal interphalangeal joints.

(i) The patient is asked to abduct his fingers against resistance. This will give an idea about the muscle power of the dorsal interossei.

(ii) A card is inserted between the two fingers, which are kept extended. The patient is asked to hold the card by adducting these two fingers as tightly as possible. The clinician will try to pull the card out of his fingers. This will give an idea about the strength of the palmar interossei. This test is known as—*the card test* (Fig. 9.16).

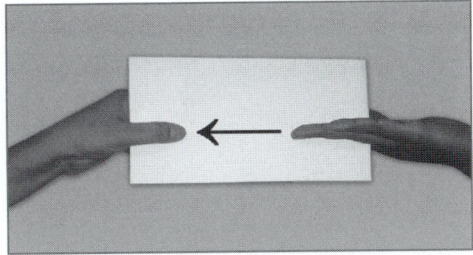

Fig. 9.16: The card test to note the strength of interossei.

(iii) Flexion of the metacarpophalangeal joints cannot be tested, as this movement is also brought about by the flexor digitorum superficialis and profundus.

(iv) While extension of the metacarpophalangeal joint is mainly the function of extensor digitorum, extension of the proximal and the terminal interphalangeal joints is mainly performed by the interossei along with the lumbricals through extensor expansions. The clinician steadies the proximal phalanx and the patient is instructed to extend the middle and terminal phalanges against resistance (Fig. 9.17). This will give an idea about the strength of the interossei and lumbricals (Fig. 9.18).

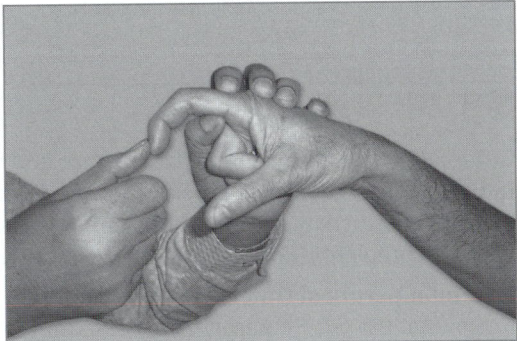

Fig. 9.17: Interossei along with the lumbricals are concerned with extension of the interphalangeal joints. This is being tested while the proximal phalanx is being steadied.

3. **First palmar interosseous and adductor pollicis:** The patient is asked to grasp a book between the extended thumb and the other fingers. If the ulnar nerve is intact the patient will grasp the book with extended thumb taking full advantage of the adductor pollicis and the first palmar interosseous muscles. But if the ulnar nerve is injured these two muscles will be paralyzed and the patient will hold the book by flexing the thumb with the help of flexor pollicis longus. This sign is known as "Froment's sign" (Fig. 9.19). This test can be performed with a card by asking the patient to hold the card firmly between the extended thumb and the other fingers (Fig. 9.20).

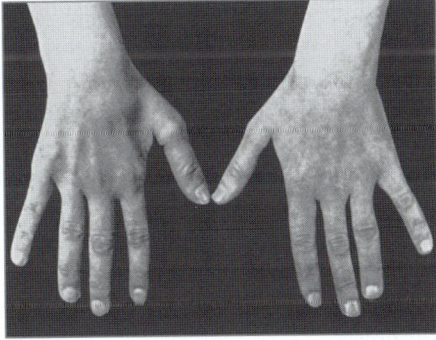

Fig. 9.18: Shows wasting of interosseous muscles in the right hand in case of cervical rib.

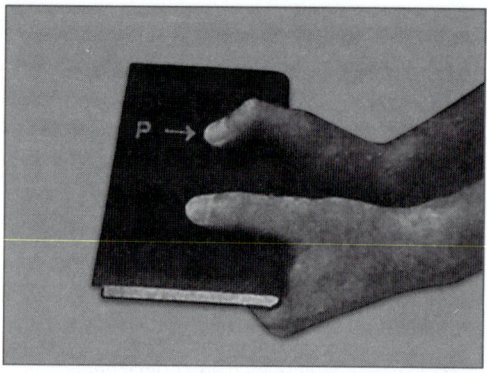

Fig. 9.19: Froment's sign. 'p' indicates the paralyzed side.

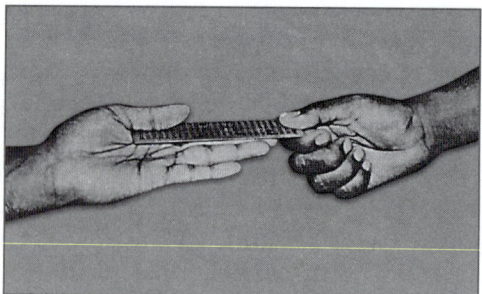

Fig. 9.20: Testing adductor pollicis and first palmar interosseous with a card.

SCIATIC NERVE

Complete lesion of this nerve is very rare and will cause complete paralysis of the hamstring muscles and all the muscles below the knee. What is more common is incomplete lesion of this nerve by subtrochanteric fracture of femur or posterior dislocation of the hip. The peculiar feature of this incomplete lesion is that it almost always involves the common peroneal part of the nerve.

Common peroneal (lateral popliteal) nerve: This nerve supplies the extensor and peroneal muscles of the leg. So paralysis of these muscles will lead to a deformity of the foot known as "talipes equinovarus". The patient will be unable to dorsiflex and evert the foot. He will walk with undue lifting of the foot to clear the "dropped foot" off the ground.

Tibial (medial popliteal) nerve: This nerve supplies the plantar flexors of the ankle joint. In paralysis of these muscles the patient will be unable to plantar flex the joint. This will lead to a deformity known as "talipes calcaneovalgus". The muscles are tested by asking the patient to plantar flex the ankle joint against resistance.

D. SENSATION (Figs. 9.21 to 9.25)

The different forms of sensation are usually tested:
(1) *Tactile sensitivity:* This includes light touch, tactile localization, pressure and discrimination.
(2) *Pain.*
(3) *Temperature.*
(4) *Recognition of the size, shape and form of the object.*
(5) *Position*—the appreciation of passive movement.
(6) *Appreciation of vibration.*

To know the sensory loss and the type of sensory changes, patient's cooperation is absolutely essential. It largely depends on the patient's intelligence. It is the usual practice

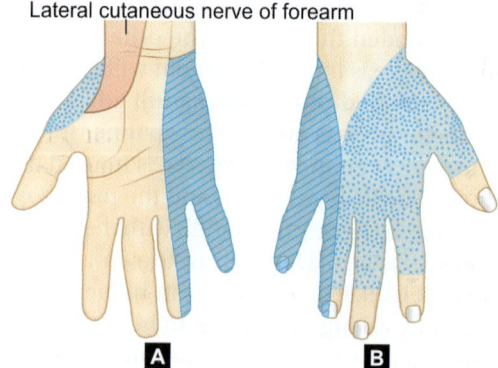

Figs. 9.21A and B: Sensory distribution of the median nerve (shown as orange), radial nerve (shown as blue dotted area) and ulnar nerve (shown as blue striped area) of the hand is shown: (A) Shows palmar aspect of the hand; whereas; (B) Shows dorsal aspect of the hand.

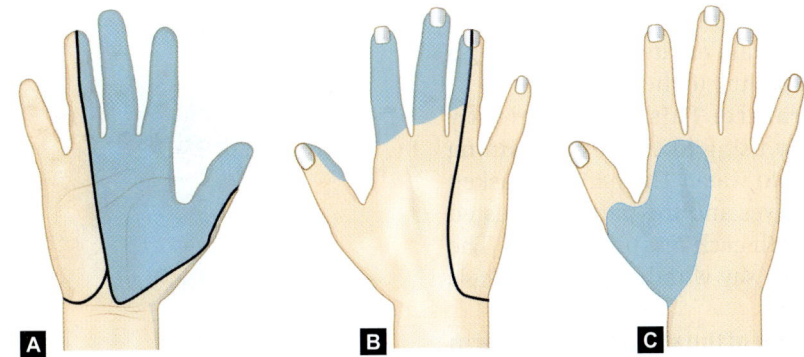

Figs. 9.22A to C: (A and B) Showing the sensory loss in the median nerve (blue shaded area), ulnar nerve (the area demarcated by the black line in A and B); (C) Radial nerve (blue shaded area) injury.

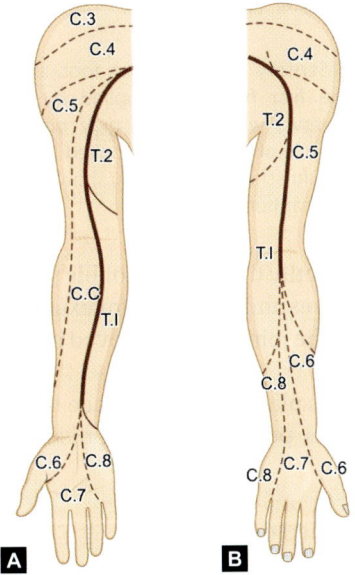

Figs. 9.23A and B: It is a diagrammatic representation of the cutaneous supply of the various spinal nerves in the superior extremity.

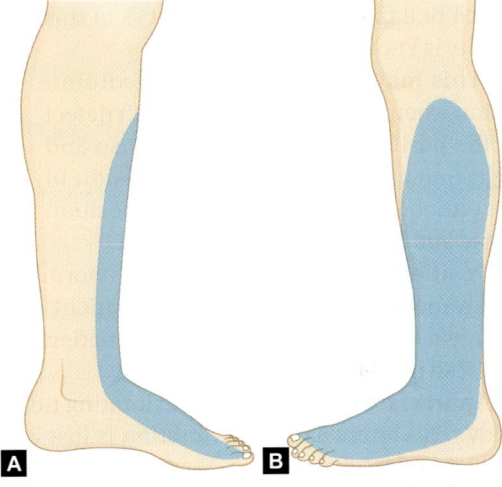

Figs. 9.24A and B: Sensory loss in lesions of the lateral popliteal nerve (blue shaded area).

to apply the sensory stimulus first to an area of impaired sensation and its borders are made out *from the abnormal to normal area of sensation.*

1. **Tactile sensitivity:** This can be differentiated into *protopathic sensation*, which is appreciation of gross touch and *epicritic sensation*, which is appreciation of light touch and accurate localization. A wisp of cotton wool is used for the latter sensation and the tip of the finger for the former sensation. The patient is asked whether he can feel the sensation and should be compared with that of the other side to know whether the sensation appreciated by the patient in the affected area is normal or not.

To discriminate between the two points is another test in this category and a compass is used for this purpose. Normally one should appreciate 2 mm of separation of points but will definitely be impaired in peripheral nerve lesion. This type of sensation is carried by the posterior column of the spinal cord to the parietal sensory area of the brain.

2. **Pain:** Pain may be of two varieties—a superficial cutaneous stimulation as the prick of a pin and a deep pressure sensation from muscles or bones. Care must be taken to elicit the difference

between the sharpness of the point of a pin and a diffuse pain elicited by squeezing a muscle or an injury to the bone.

3. **Temperature:** This is conveniently examined by using test tubes containing warm and cold water. The patient is asked to close his eyes and the part to be tested is touched with each test tube in turn. The patient has to say whether the tube feels warm or cold.

4. **Recognition of the size, shape and form of the object:** Commonly one should be able to identify a familiar object which is kept on one's palm with closed eyes, e.g., a coin or a pencil or a pair of scissors, etc. Loss of this faculty is known as astereognosis.

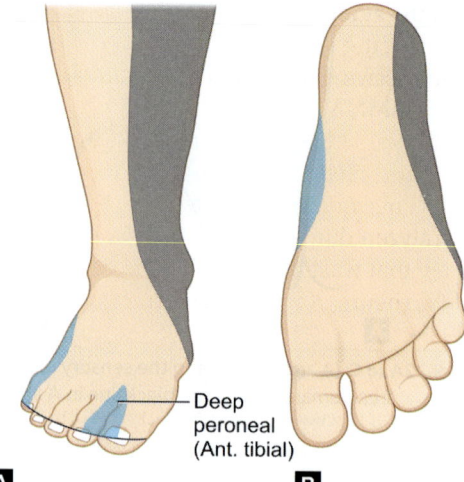

Figs. 9.25A and B: Sensory supply of the foot. Light gray portion of the first figure is supplied by the musculocutaneous nerve, whereas light gray portion of the second figure (sole of the foot) is supplied by the posterior tibial nerve. Blue shaded area in (A) shows sural nerve and in (B) shows saphenous nerve.

This may occur in posterior column lesion when it will be associated with defect in the position sense, vibration sense and light touch. It may also occur in lesion of the parietal lobe of the brain when position sense and light touch may be normal.

5. **Position sense:** With closed eyes a normal person should identify the position of his joints or any movements there about. The patient is asked to close his eyes and a joint (as for example the great toe) is moved *passively*. The patient has to say whether the joint is being moved or not and if so in which direction.

6. **Appreciation of vibration:** A vibrating tuning fork of 128 Hz is placed on the surface of the body. This appreciation of vibration is lost in peripheral neuritis, posterior column disorder and tabes dorsalis.

E. REFLEXES

In peripheral nerve injury the respective reflexes will be diminished or abolished.

F. NERVE

When a peripheral nerve injury is suspected, one should always examine the whole course of the nerve. There may be evidence of injury such as displaced bone fragments or a scar to suggest an old injury.

The nerve should be palpated, as in many cases of leprosy there may be thickening of the involved nerve.

Moreover after injury to the nerve or suturing of the nerve, signs of regeneration can be assessed by the palpation. Regeneration starts after a couple of months and if gentle tapping over the course of the nerve *from distal to the proximal side* is made, a sensation of "pins and needles" or hyperesthesia will be felt at the site of regeneration. This is known as **Tinel's sign**.

G. MOVEMENTS

Movements of the joints are of two types—*active* and *passive*. Normally the range of active movement is similar to that of the passive movement of the same joint. But when the muscles, which are concerned in the movement, are paralyzed or their tendons are torn, the passive movement will by far exceed the active movement of the same joint. So in case of peripheral nerve lesion one must note the extent of active as well as passive movements of the joint. In this context the students should remember that matting together of the muscles in the scar tissue, adhesion of the tendons with their sheaths or ankylosis of the joints will impair both the active and the passive movements of the joints.

H. DEFORMITY

In peripheral nerve lesion paralysis of one group of muscles and unopposed action of the active group of muscles will definitely lead to deformity of the limb—whether it is wrist drop or foot drop or "Policeman taking the tip", etc. Deformity may also be from wasting of the muscles which are paralyzed due to peripheral nerve lesion. In this respect the students should remember a fallacy that wasting of the muscles may be due to affections of the joints, e.g., tuberculous arthritis, rheumatoid arthritis, etc.

GENERAL EXAMINATION

In peripheral nerve lesion, one must exclude the general diseases like diabetes, leprosy, beriberi, syphilis, lead and arsenic poisoning etc. Besides these, alcoholism may be the cause of peripheral nerve lesion such as "Saturday night palsy".

In Klumpke's paralysis, there is every possibility that the cervical sympathetic supply may be affected which may produce Horner's syndrome. This syndrome is comprised of (i) myosis, i.e., contraction of the pupil due to paralysis of the dilator pupillae, (ii) ptosis, i.e., drooping of the upper eyelid due to paralysis of the levator palpebrae superioris, (iii) enophthalmos,, i.e., regression of eye-ball due to paralysis of the Muller's muscle and (iv) anhidrosis,, i.e., absence of sweating of the face and neck of that side.

SPECIAL INVESTIGATIONS

1. **Blood**—for sugar to exclude diabetes and for Wassermann reaction and Kahn test to exclude syphilis are important investigations in peripheral nerve lesion.
2. **Urine** is also tested for sugar to exclude diabetic peripheral neuritis.
3. Nasal scrapping should be examined when leprosy is suspected.
4. **Electrical responses:** Denervated muscles will show 'reaction of degeneration', i.e., no response in Faradic stimulation and weak Galvanic response with reversal of polarity, that means ACC becomes stronger than KCC (normally KCC or Kathodal closure contraction is stronger than ACC or Anodal closure contraction). The reaction of degeneration starts to appear from the fourth day after lesion and becomes fully established in about a fortnight.
5. **Nerve conduction study** is useful to detect site of nerve lesion and evidence of regeneration.

TYPES OF INJURY OF THE PERIPHERAL NERVES

According to extent of damage, injury to the peripheral nerves can be divided into three categories—1. Neuropraxia, 2. Axonotmesis and 3. Neurotmesis.

1. NEUROPRAXIA

This condition is equivalent to concussion, in which there is no organic damage to either the nerve fiber or its sheath, but there is a temporary physiological paralysis of conduction through the nerve fibers. It may occur due to minor stretching or torsion or vibratory effect of a high-velocity missile passing near the nerve. Clinically, it is manifested by temporary loss of sensation, paresthesia or weakness of the muscles supplied by the nerve. There is no reaction of degeneration. Recovery is complete, which may take a period of a few hours to even a few weeks.

2. **AXONOTMESIS (Incomplete division)**

In this condition there is division or rupture of nerve fibers or axons though the nerve sheath remains intact. Wallerian degeneration occurs in the distal portion of the broken axons. Recovery takes place slowly by down growth of the axons into the empty distal nerve sheath. There may be some loss of nerve fibers due to blockage of down growing axons by intraneural fibrosis. The relative positions of the axons are preserved and hence the quality of regeneration is quite good. Regeneration rate is 2 mm per day, which diminishes to 1 mm per day after a couple of months. Recovery is almost complete, though partial paralysis, slight sensory loss or causalgia may persist. Nerve conduction test is helpful to know the rate of regeneration. Axonotmesis usually results from a stress, traction or compression of the nerve in closed fracture and dislocations or from excessive zealed manipulation to reduce such injuries.

Clinically there is loss of sensation, tone and power of muscles with diminished reflex activity of the limb. Later on area of anesthesia and paralysis of muscles will be restricted to those which are supplied by the damaged nerves only. Usually the total area affected is less than the known anatomical distribution of the nerve due to the fact that a few fibers within the nerve usually escape. There may be impaired circulation due to disuse which makes the affected portion cold and blue. There may be trophic changes, e.g., the nails becomes brittle and the skin becomes thin. Reaction of degeneration appears, so that ACC becomes greater than KCC.

3. **NEUROTMESIS**

In this condition there is complete or partial division of the nerve fibers as well as their sheaths. Wallerian degeneration is noticed both in the distal segment and in the proximal segment. In the proximal segment retrograde degeneration takes place up to the first node of Ranvier. After fortnight the distal ends of the axons in the proximal segment start grow downwards. But, as there is a gap between the divided ends which is replaced by organic clots and fibrous tissue further downgrowth of the axons is not possible, so suturing is the only treatment if restoration of function is to be achieved. In the distal end typical Wallerian degeneration takes place, in which axis cylinder becomes fibrillated, medullary sheath breaks up into droplets of myelin and the cells of the sheath of Schwann are converted into phagocytes which remove remnants of axis cylinder and medullary sheath. The cells of Schwann proliferate forming a slight bulb at the commencement of the distal end from which sprouts of Schwann cells grow proximally towards the downgrowing axons of the proximal segment by chemotaxis.

There will be complete loss of motor, sensory and reflex functions of the limb supplied by the nerve. Secondary pathological changes may occur in the skin and joints of the affected part. Quality of regeneration is less perfect even after accurate nerve suturing. This is due to maldistribution of axons into the distal fragment. A motor nerve may grow down a sheath previously occupied by a sensory nerve, so it cannot function. Moreover a few axons will be wasted in the scar tissue at the suture line. So recovery of function will be worse in mixed motor and sensory nerves, whereas it will be better if the nerve is pure motor or sensory nerve. So recovery of the radial nerve injury at the elbow will be better than the ulnar nerve or median nerve injury at the wrist.

CAUSES OF PERIPHERAL NERVE LESION

Causes of peripheral nerve lesions

Category	Cause	Examples
Traumatic	Direct injury	Fractures (humerus, fibula, medial epicondyle), dislocations, lacerations
	Compression	Crutch palsy (axilla), saturday night palsy (radial nerve), carpal tunnel syndrome (median nerve)
Inflammatory	Infection	Leprosy, diphtheria, herpes zoster
Metabolic	Systemic disease	Diabetes mellitus, alcoholism, beriberi
Neoplastic	Tumors	Neurofibromas, metastatic compression
Toxic	Heavy metal poisoning	Lead, arsenic

These can be divided into two primary groups.

A. **Causes of single nerve involvement**
1. TRAUMATIC: It may be due to: (a) *closed injury* which usually causes either neuropraxia or axonotmesis lesion of the nerve or (b) *open injury* which usually causes neurotmesis.
2. INFLAMMATORY: Herpes zoster, leprosy, diphtheria.
3. NEOPLASTIC: Neurofibroma, neurofibrosarcoma.
4. MISCELLANEOUS: Tunnel syndrome, lead poisoning, arsenical poisoning, diabetes, etc.

B. **Causes of multiple nerves involvement.—**
1. INFLAMMATORY: Herpes Zoster, leprosy, diphtheria.
2. METABOLIC DISORDERS: (a) Vitamin B complex deficiency (particularly Bl). (b) Diabetes mellitus. (c) Alcoholism. (d) Porphyria.
3. IDIOPATHIC.
4. MISCELLANEOUS: Lead poisoning, arsenical poisoning.

Leprosy: It is an infectious disease caused by *Mycobacterium leprae*, an acid-fast bacillus almost similar to tubercle bacillus. The source of infection is mainly from nasal secretions of patients with lepromatous leprosy. According to resistant of the host two external varieties of leprosy are noticed—lepromatous leprosy and tuberculoid leprosy. In *lepromatous leprosy* there is least resistant from the host and the bacteria multiply with little cellular response. In *tuberculoid leprosy* there is resistance from the host and the tissue responses are strong. There are localized lesions where bacilli are present alongwith epithelioid cells, foreign body giant cells and many lymphocytes almost like a tubercle.

Clinically, it is a systemic infection and mainly involves the skin, upper respiratory tract and peripheral nerves. Certain superficial nerves, e.g., great auricular, superficial temporal and ulnar nerve at the elbow become swollen and tender. Common peroneal nerve at the neck of the fibula and median nerve at the wrist may also be affected. Tibial nerve above the flexor retinaculum and behind the medial malleolus may be affected. Patches of anesthesia from involvement of cutaneous nerves is an important sign of this disease. Disfigurement of hands and feet which are seen in leprosy are not due to disease itself, but to the damage and misuse which follows loss of pain sensation.

DIFFERENTIAL DIAGNOSIS OF INDIVIDUAL NERVE LESIONS

BRACHIAL PLEXUS

Lesion in brachial plexus may be either complete or partial. COMPLETE LESION is rare and occurs only after severe accidents. It damages all the roots of the plexus. There will be anesthesia of the whole of the upper limb except the upper part of the arm which is supplied by C3, 4 and 5. There will be complete paralysis of the arm, though long thoracic nerve supplying the serratus anterior or the nerve supplying the rhomboid may escape.

Incomplete lesion may be due to stabs or cuts which involve any of the roots. But common injury is either upper brachial plexus lesion (Erb-Duchenne paralysis) or lower brachial plexus lesion (Klumpke's paralysis).

Upper brachial plexus lesion (Erb-Duchenne paralysis) **(Fig. 9.5)**: This injury occurs due to excessive depression of the shoulder or displacement of the head opening out the angle between shoulder and the neck. In adult it may occur due to fall of weight on the shoulder or motorcycle accident where the head is moved away from the shoulder. It may occur after difficult labor when the angle between the shoulder and the neck is opened out. It involves injury to C5 and C6 nerve roots. The muscles affected are the deltoid, the biceps, brachialis, brachioradialis and supinator. The affected limb becomes internally rotated, extended at the elbow and pronated in the well-known position of 'Policeman taking a tip'. There may be sensory loss over the outerside of the arm and upper part of the lateral aspect of the forearm.

Lower brachial plexus lesion (Klumpke's paralysis): Such injury occurs due to forceful abduction of the shoulder, which may occur during breech presentation with arms above the head. In adult this injury may occur when a falling person clutches at an object or a person failing to obtain a foot hold on a passing bus may forcefully hyperabduct his arm. The C8 and T1 nerve roots may be affected, though T1 is more often involved. The result is paralysis of the intrinsic muscles of the hand (with clawhand and features of combined median and ulnar nerve palsy) with anesthesia of the innerside of the forearm, hand and inner 1½ fingers. It is usually associated with Horner's syndrome which includes ptosis, enophthalmos, contraction of the pupil and anhidrosis of the affected side of the face.

ACCESSORY NERVE

This nerve passes downwards and backwards at right angle to the center of the line connecting the angle of the jaw and the mastoid process. After supplying the sternomastoid muscle, it emerges from the posterior border of the same muscle at its junction of the upper third and lower two thirds. It then runs across the floor of the posterior triangle and disappears under cover of the trapezius muscle which it supplies. This nerve is rarely damaged by injury, but it is often involved during bloc dissection of the cervical lymph nodes or during removal of tuberculous lymph nodes. Very occasionally this nerve may be injured before it supplies the sternomastoid muscle. Even in these cases, complete paralysis of the sternomastoid muscle may not result due to the additional supply from second and third cervical roots, which this muscle derives. More often this nerve is injured during its course through the posterior triangle. In this case, the trapezius muscle will lose its nerve supply. In case of this muscle also there is additional supply from the third and fourth cervical nerves. On examination there will be drooping of the shoulder and the patient will be unable to elevate the shoulder against resistance **(Fig. 9.7)**.

Wasting of the trapezius will also be obvious. The sternomastoid muscle is tested by asking the patient to turn his head to the side *opposite* to the muscle against resistance. The muscle will stand out as a rigid band.

HYPOGLOSSAL NERVE

This nerve comes out of the skull through the hypoglossal or anterior condylar canal in the occipital bone. At first the nerve lies at a deeper plane behind the internal carotid artery, the internal jugular vein, the ninth, tenth and eleventh cranial nerves. Gradually it gains the interval between the internal carotid artery and the internal jugular vein and takes a half-spiral turn crossing the internal and the external carotid arteries and the loop of the lingual artery a little above the tip of the greater cornu of the hyoid bone, being itself crossed by the facial vein. It then passes deep to the tendon of the digastric, the stylohyoid and the posterior border of the mylohyoid to gain the interval between the hyoglossus and the mylohyoid, where it comes in relation with the deeper part of the submandibular salivary gland, the submandibular duct and the lingual nerve.

This nerve is liable to be damaged during dissection for bloc resection of cervical lymph nodes, during surgical removal of tuberculous lymph nodes in the submandibular region and during operative removal of the submandibular salivary gland.

Injury to the twelfth nerve will cause paralysis of that half of the tongue leading to hemiatrophy and diversion of the tip of the tongue to the same side when it is protruded out.

LONG THORACIC NERVE (NERVE OF BELL)

This nerve, which is comprised of the fifth, sixth and seventh cervical nerve roots, mainly supplies the serratus anterior muscle. This nerve may be injured along with the cervical nerve roots in a severe accident involving the brachial plexus. This nerve is also injured accidentally during operation on the chest wall or on the breast.

Paralysis of serratus anterior muscle will cause "winging" of the scapula, i.e., the vertebral border and the inferior angle of the scapula stand out when the patient is asked to push against a wall with extended arm **(Fig. 9.26)**.

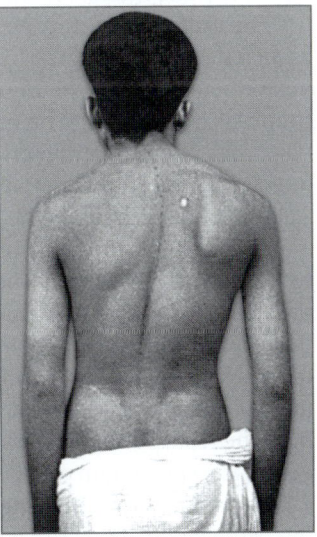

Fig. 9.26: A typical example of "winging of the scapula".

RADIAL NERVE

This nerve receives twigs from the fifth, sixth, seventh, eighth cervical nerves and from the first thoracic nerve. This nerve is a branch of the posterior cord of the brachial plexus. It descends behind the third part of the axillary artery and in front of the subscapularis and the tendons of the latissimus dorsi and teres major. It then passes obliquely across the back of the humerus, first between the lateral and the medial heads of the triceps being accompanied by the arteria profunda brachii to reach the lateral side of the humerus where it pierces the lateral intermuscular septum and enters the anterior compartment of the arm. It then descends between the brachialis on one side and the brachioradialis above and the extensor carpi radialis longus below on the other side. In front of the lateral epicondyle it divides into its two terminal branches the *superficial* and the *deep*.

The *superficial branch* descends in front of the lateral epicondyle and lies in front of the supinator and behind the brachioradialis. It now runs in front of the pronator teres, the radial head of the flexor digitorum superficialis and the flexor pollicis longus. About 7 cm above the wrist the nerve turns back round the lateral side of radius, pierces the deep fascia and divides into five dorsal digital nerves to supply the skin on the radial side of the thumb, adjoining part of the thenar eminence, the medial side of the thumb, the index finger, the middle finger and the lateral half of the ring finger. It must be remembered that these digital nerves do not supply up to the tip of the fingers, but they stop as far as the root of the nail in the thumb, as far as the middle phalanx in the index finger and up to the proximal interphalangeal joints in case of the middle and the ring fingers. The remaining distal areas of the skin are supplied by the palmar digital branches of the median and the ulnar nerves.

The deep branch (posterior interosseous nerve) winds round the lateral side of the radius between the two planes of fibers of the supinator to reach the back of the forearm. Before it enters the supinator muscle it gives a branch to the extensor carpi radialis brevis and another to the supinator. After it comes out of the supinator, it gives off three short branches—to the extensor digitorum, extensor digiti minimi and extensor carpi ulnaris and two long branches one to the extensor pollicis longus and the extensor indicis and another to the abductor pollicis longus and the extensor pollicis brevis.

The radial nerve itself, before it divides into its terminal branches, gives off the muscular branches to the triceps, anconeus, brachioradialis, extensor carpi radialis longus and lateral one-fourth of the brachialis. It must be remembered that it sends off the twigs to supply the three heads of triceps before it reaches the groove at the back of the humerus. It gives off the three cutaneous branches—the posterior cutaneous nerve of the arm, which arises in the axilla, the lower lateral cutaneous nerve of the arm to supply the skin of the lateral part of the lower half of the arm and the posterior cutaneous nerve of the forearm which supplies back of the forearm and wrist. The radial nerve also sends articular branches to the elbow joint.

The radial nerve may be injured: (a) *in the axilla* by the use of a crutch, which is not properly adjusted (crutch palsy) or fracture dislocation of the upper end of the humerus or by attempts for reduction. It may be injured: (b) *in the radial groove* either by fracture of the shaft of the humerus or by pressure on the arm at the edge of the operating table or at the edge of a chair or a pavement after a deep sleep being drunk (Saturday night palsy) or by inadvertent intramuscular injection on the radial nerve at this region. The posterior interosseous nerve may be injured by fracture or dislocation of the upper end of the radius or during operations involving this region.

According to the site of the injury the various muscles will be paralyzed. As for example when the radial nerve is injured in the axilla all the muscles supplied by the radial nerve will be paralyzed and the cutaneous sensation of the regions supplied by the cutaneous branches of the radial nerve will be abolished. When injury affects the radial nerve at the radial groove the triceps muscle escapes, similarly the posterior cutaneous nerve of the arm. When the posterior interosseous nerve is injured, all the muscles supplied by the radial nerve itself and the cutaneous branches escape as also the supinator and the extensor carpi radialis brevis which are supplied before the site of injury.

The radial nerve through its posterior interosseous nerve is mainly concerned in supplying the extensors of the wrist joint. So, the most common complaint after radial nerve injury is inability of the patient to extend the wrist (wrist drop) and metacarpophalangeal joints of the fingers. The students must remember that extension of interphalangeal joints is done by interossei through the extensor expansions. These interossei are supplied by the ulnar nerve and hence unaffected by radial nerve injury. If this knowledge of anatomy is lacking, extension of interphalangeal joints may be erroneously interpreted as signs of regeneration.

Brachioradialis is supplied by the radial nerve before it divides into the superficial and the deep branches. So by testing this muscle one can assess the level of the radial nerve injury. The muscle is tested by asking the patient to put the forearm in mid-prone position and flexing the elbow against resistance. The muscle will stand out prominent as shown in **Figure 9.10**. Bilateral wrist drop may occasionally be due to lead palsy, in which case the brachioradialis may escape and the paralysis of the other muscles is often incomplete.

MEDIAN NERVE

This nerve arises by two roots, one from the lateral cord (C5,6,7) and the other from the medial cord (C8 and T1) of the brachial plexus. The median nerve descends into the arm lying at first lateral to the brachial artery and at the level of the middle of the arm it crosses in front of the artery and descends on its medial side to the cubital fossa. The nerve enters the forearm between the two heads of the pronator teres crossing from medial to the lateral side the ulnar artery being separated by the deep head of this muscle. It then passes deep to the tendinous bridge that connects the humeroulnar to the radial head of the flexor digitorum superficialis and descends through the forearm deep to but adherent to the flexor digitorum superficialis and in front of the flexor digitorum profundus. 5 cm above the wrist it emerges at the lateral edge of the flexor digitorum superficialis and becomes superficial just above the wrist, where it lies between the tendons of the Flexor digitorum superficials and the Flexor carpi radialis. The nerve then passes deep to Flexor retinaculum to gain the palm of the hand. At this place the nerve may be compressed in the fibro-osseous canal to produce "carpal tunnel syndrome". A short and stout muscular branch comes out of the median nerve in the palm and supplies the abductor pollicis brevis, the opponens pollicis, the flexor pollicis brevis and rarely the first dorsal interosseous muscle. It ends as palmar digital branches which are 4 to 5 in number and provide digital branches to the thumb, the index finger, the middle and lateral half of the ring finger. These palmar digital branches also supply the first and the second lumbrical muscles.

The branches of the median nerve in the arm are only vascular branches to the brachial artery and a muscular branch to the pronator teres.

The branches in the forearm are the *muscular branches* to all superficial flexor muscles, e.g., the pronator teres, flexor carpi radialis, palmaris longus and flexor digitorum superficialis. *Anterior interosseous* nerve, which comes off the median nerve when it passes between the two heads of the pronator teres, supplies the lateral half of the Flexor digitorum profundus, Flexor pollicis longus and Pronator quadratus. *Articular branches* supply the elbow joint and the proximal radio-ulnar joint. The *palmar cutaneous branch* supplies the skin over the thenar eminence and the central part of the palm.

According to the level of the median nerve injury, the various muscles will be affected. The median nerve may be injured at the elbow by the supracondylar fracture, dislocation of the elbow joint or inadvertent use of the tourniquet. At the wrist, the median nerve is more commonly injured by cut injury and accidents as the nerve is comparatively superficial here.

1. **Flexor digitorum superficialis and profundus (lateral half):** These muscles are paralyzed when the median nerve is injured at the elbow or above. When the patient is asked to clasp the

hands, the index finger of the affected side fails to flex. Other fingers are flexed by the medial half of the profundus muscle, which is supplied by the ulnar nerve. This test is called *Ochsner's clasping test* and the index finger, which fails to flex is called the "pointing index".

2. **Flexor pollicis longus:** This muscle is also affected when the median nerve is injured at or above the elbow. When this muscle is paralyzed, the patient is unable to flex the terminal phalanx of the thumb. This is tested by holding the thumb at its base and the patient is asked to bend the terminal phalanx as shown in **Figure 9.12**.

3. **Flexor carpi radialis:** The hand deviates to the ulnar side when it is flexed against resistance.

4. **Muscles of the thenar eminence:** These muscles are paralyzed and ultimately become wasted when the median nerve is injured anywhere at or above the wrist joint. The wasting of these muscles will be obvious on inspection as the eminence is flattened and the thumb apparently comes to the same plane as the other metacarpal bones. This is called **"Simian"** or **"Ape-like hand".**

Abductor pollicis brevis: The action of this muscle is to draw the thumb forwards at right angle to the palm of the hand. The patient is asked to lay his hand flat on the table, a pen is held above the palm and the patient is asked to touch the pen with his thumb—the "pen test". In median nerve injury the muscles will be paralyzed and this test will be negative.

It must be remembered that the first metacarpal bone is placed at right angle to the other metacarpal bones. So its flexion and extension occurs in the plane of the palm slight in front of it, whereas abduction and adduction occur at right angle to this plane.

Opponens pollicis: This muscle brings the tip of the thumb towards the tips of other fingers. While testing this muscle it must be noted that the real opposition movement is a swinging movement of the thumb across the palm and not a simple adduction movement of the thumb brought about by the adductor pollicis supplied by the ulnar nerve.

ULNAR NERVE

This nerve arises from the medial cord of brachial plexus comprising of C8 and T1. It runs downwards through the axilla on the medial side of the axillary artery, between it and the vein of the same name up to the middle of the arm. Here it pierces the medial intermuscular septum and reaches the posterior compartment of the arm in front of the triceps upto the elbow where it lies behind the medial epicondyle accompanied by the superior ulnar collateral artery. It enters the forearm between the two heads of the flexor carpi ulnaris and descends along the medial side of the forearm lying *in front of* the flexor digitorum profundus. At the wrist, it passes in front of the flexor retinaculum on the lateral side of the pisiform bone and on the medial side of the ulnar artery and ends by dividing into *superficial* and *deep* terminal branches.

The branches of the ulnar nerve are:

The muscular branches are two in number which supply the flexor carpi ulnaris and the medial half of the flexor digitorum profundus.

The palmar cutaneous branch—arises from the middle of the forearm, descends in front of the ulnar artery and supplies the ulnar artery, the skin of the medial aspect of the palm and sometimes Palmaris brevis.

The *dorsal branch*—supplies the medial side of the little finger and the posterior aspect of the adjacent sides of the ring and the little fingers and occasionally the adjoining sides of the middle and the ring fingers.

The *articular branch*—supplies the elbow joint.

The *superficial terminal branch* supplies the skin of the medial side of the hand, and through the palmar digital nerves the medial side of the little finger and the adjacent sides of the ring and little fingers. It also supplies the palmaris brevis.

The *deep terminal branch*—passes between the abductor digiti minimi and flexor digiti minimi and then perforates the opponens digiti minimi and supplies all these three muscles. It then crosses the hand and supplies branches to the interossei and to the third and the fourth lumbricals. It ends by supplying the two heads of the adductor pollicis.

Ulnar nerve may be injured at the elbow or at the wrist.

At the elbow this nerve may be injured (i) in supracondylar fracture either in recent injury by the fractured segments or in late cases (Tardy ulnar palsy) by the callus formed at the fractured site or by the cubitus valgus deformity as a sequel of malunion. (ii) In fracture of the medial epicondyle of the humerus this nerve is often injured. In all cases of open reduction of this fracture the ulnar nerve should be transposed anteriorly to prevent further damage to the nerve by friction or by involvement of the nerve in callus formation. *Anterior transposition* of the ulnar nerve should always be performed wherever there is possibility of the ulnar nerve involvement.

At the wrist the ulnar nerve may be damaged by the same injury as described under the median nerve. As this nerve is more superficially placed than the median nerve the possibility of injury to this nerve is more in this region.

Ulnar nerve injury will cause loss of sensation of the medial side of the hand, the whole of the little finger and a small part on the medial side of the ring finger.

The muscles which are involved in ulnar nerve injury anywhere above the wrist are muscles of the hypothenar eminence, the interossei, the third and fourth lumbricals and the adductor pollicis. When the ulnar nerve is injured at the elbow, besides the muscles mentioned above, the flexor carpi ulnaris and the medial half of the flexor digitorum profundus will be paralyzed.

The muscles are tested as follows:
1. **Flexor carpi ulnaris**: When the wrist joint is flexed against resistance, the hand tends to deviate towards the radial side.
2. **Interossei:** These muscles extend the middle and the terminal phalanges of the fingers through the extensor expansions. These are also concerned in flexion of the metacarpophalangeal joints along with the lumbricals. Besides these, the dorsal interossei abduct the fingers and the palmar interossei adduct the fingers. So far as the flexion of the metacarpophalangeal joint is concerned, it cannot be tested as this joint is also flexed by the continued action of the flexor digitorum superficialis and profundus. (i) These muscles can be tested for their *power of extension of the middle and the terminal phalanges.* This is tested by holding the proximal phalanx and asking the patient to straighten his finger against resistance **(Fig. 9.17)**. The patient is asked to abduct his fingers against resistance. This test will reveal the *power of abduction of the dorsal interossei.* (iii) The patient is asked to adduct his fingers keeping straight. A card may be inserted between the two fingers for grasping. The card is now pulled out against the adducted fingers to see the *power of adduction of palmar interossei.* This test is known as the "card test".

SCIATIC NERVE

As has already been discussed the common peroneal part of the sciatic nerve is more often affected than the medial tibial part in injury to the sciatic nerve.

Common peroneal nerve: This nerve itself is liable to be injured in fracture neck of fibula. This nerve supplies the extensor and peroneal groups of muscles of the leg as also through its musculocutaneous branch it supplies the anterior and lateral aspects of the leg and whole of the dorsum of the foot and toes except the skin between the great and the 2nd toe which is supplied by its deep peroneal (anterior tibial) nerve. So injury to this nerve will result in the foot drop and talipes equinovarus deformity. The sensory loss will affect the anterior and lateral aspect of the leg, dorsum of the foot and the toes.

Medial popliteal nerve: This nerve is rarely injured except in open wounds. This nerve supplies the muscles of the calf, e.g., the soleus, the gastrocnemius, the popliteus, the plantaris, the tibialis posterior, the flexor digitorum longus and the flexor hallucis longus. Through sural nerve it supplies the lateral part of the leg and sole and through plantar nerves it supplies the sole. So, injury to this nerve will make the patient unable to plantar flex his ankle with loss of sensation of the whole of the sole. As it supplies the plantar muscles through the plantar nerves, there will be claw foot.

Chapter 9: Examination of Peripheral Nerve Lesions

Algorithmic Approach to Patient with Peripheral Nerve Lesions

Patient presents with weakness, numbness, deformity, or loss of function

↓

History of trauma or surgical injury?
- Yes → Consider **traumatic nerve injury (fracture, laceration, dislocation, crush injury, postsurgical injury)**
- No → Consider **metabolic (diabetes, alcoholism), infectious (leprosy, diphtheria), toxic (lead poisoning), or autoimmune causes (GBS, CIDP, Vasculitis)**

↓

Is the weakness localized or generalized?
- Localized → Suggests single peripheral nerve involvement (radial, median, ulnar, sciatic, common peroneal, tibial nerve)
- Generalized → Suggests polyneuropathy (diabetes, alcoholism, leprosy, autoimmune disorders like Guillain-barré syndrome)

↓

Is sensory loss present?
- Yes → Assess sensory distribution:
  – Dermatomal pattern → Suggests **radiculopathy (Spinal nerve root involvement)**
  – Peripheral nerve pattern → Suggests **mononeuropathy or polyneuropathy**
- No → Indicates **pure motor neuropathy (ALS, polio, nerve compression without sensory fibers affected)**

↓

Is there a specific deformity?
- **Wrist drop** → Radial nerve palsy (midshaft humerus fracture, crutch palsy)
- **Foot drop** → Common peroneal nerve palsy (fibular head fracture, compression)
- **Claw hand** → Ulnar nerve palsy (elbow or wrist injury, tardy ulnar palsy)
- **Ape thumb** → Median nerve palsy (carpal tunnel, supracondylar fracture)
- **Erb's palsy (Waiter's tip)** → Upper brachial plexus lesion (birth injury, shoulder trauma)
- **Winging of scapula** → Long thoracic nerve palsy (serratus anterior weakness, postsurgical)

↓

Perform special tests to confirm nerve involvement
- **Tinel's sign** → Nerve regeneration (Tapping along nerve produces tingling)
- **Phalen's test** → Carpal tunnel syndrome (Wrist flexion produces numbness)
- **Froment's sign** → Ulnar nerve dysfunction (Thumb flexion while holding paper)
- **Ochsner's clasping test** → Median nerve lesion (Pointing index finger sign)
- **Pen test and Card test** → Tests for interossei muscle weakness in ulnar nerve palsy

↓

Assess reflexes to differentiate upper vs lower motor neuron lesion
- **Absent reflexes (LMN lesion)** → Peripheral nerve injury, polyneuropathy
- **Hyperreflexia (UMN lesion)** → Spinal cord injury, stroke, ALS
- **Babinski sign positive** → Upper motor neuron lesion

↓

Order investigations to confirm diagnosis
- **Nerve conduction study and electromyography (EMG)** → Localize nerve injury and severity
- **MRI/CT of nerve or plexus** → Identify tumor, compression, inflammation
- **Blood tests for metabolic and autoimmune causes** (diabetes, B_{12}, lead, autoimmune markers)
- **Skin biopsy for leprosy** (If sensory loss with thickened nerve)

↓

Confirm diagnosis and initiate treatment
- **Conservative treatment:**
  – Splinting, physiotherapy, pain management
- **Medical treatment:**
  – Neuropathic pain management (gabapentin, pregabalin, amitriptyline)
  – Diabetic control, infection management (antibiotics, MDT for leprosy)
- **Surgical treatment:**
  – Nerve decompression (carpal tunnel release, ulnar nerve transposition)
  – Nerve grafting or repair (If neurotmesis confirmed)

Diseases of Muscles, Tendons and Fasciae

CHAPTER 10

In this chapter the nonspecific diseases such as nonarticular rheumatism, pathological tendon ruptures, tenosynovitis (simple, suppurative and stenosing), Dupuytren's contracture and ganglia will be discussed. These conditions affect more or less whole of the body.

Classification of muscle, tendon and fasciae disorders

Category	Disorder	Key features
Tendinopathies	Supraspinatus tendinitis	Shoulder pain, painful arc (60–120°), stiff shoulder
	Tennis elbow (lateral epicondylitis)	Pain over lateral epicondyle, worsens with wrist extension
	Golfer's elbow (medial epicondylitis)	Pain over medial epicondyle, worsens with wrist flexion
	Achilles' tendinitis	Pain at the Achilles tendon, worse on tiptoes
Fasciopathies	Plantar fasciitis	Heel pain, worst in the morning or after rest
	Dupuytren's contracture	Palmar fascia thickening, flexed ring and little fingers
Tenosynovitis	De quervain's disease	Pain at the radial wrist, Finkelstein's test positive
	Trigger finger	Finger locking in flexion, painful snapping
Tendon ruptures	Supraspinatus tendon rupture	Loss of abduction initiation, shoulder pain
	Biceps tendon rupture	Popeye sign, biceps bulge with elbow flexion
	Achilles' tendon rupture	Sudden pain, inability to plantarflex, Thompson's test positive
Ganglia	Wrist ganglion	Tense, cystic swelling over wrist, transilluminates

■HISTORY

The following points should be particularly noted while taking history:
1. **Pain:** This is the most important complaint in the above conditions. Pain at the elbow, particularly while extending the wrist and fingers, is come across in "Tennis elbow". Similarly

localized pain on the medial epicondyle of the humerus which is aggravated by flexing of the wrist against resistance is seen in Golfer's elbow. Pain during abduction of the shoulder particularly in the middle of the arc is the regular feature of supraspinatus tendinitis. Pain on the ligamentum patellae particularly during active extension of the knee indicates the diagnosis of patellar tendinitis. Similarly, pain in the sole just in front of the calcaneum tuberosity is seen in plantar fasciitis. In Achilles' tendinitis pain is felt on the attachment of the Achilles' tendon and it is aggravated by plantar flexion of the ankle, more so when the patient tries to stand on his toes.

Pain is also a regular feature of tenosynovitis when the affected tendon is being used, be it a simple tenosynovitis or a stenosing tenosynovitis. In de Quervain's disease the patient complains of pain when the thumb is extended or abducted. In carpal tunnel syndrome the patient complains of a rest pain along the distribution of the median nerve.

2. **Deformity:** It is the first complaint in conditions like Dupuytren's contracture, ganglia, rupture of the tendons, e.g., long head of the biceps, Achilles' tendon, etc. In the first two conditions deformity is obvious whereas in the rupture of tendons deformity becomes obvious only when the muscles concerned contract.

History taking in muscular disorders

Aspect	Clinical significance	Patient-friendly questions
Pain onset	Acute → Rupture, Trauma; Chronic → Tendinitis, Overuse	"When did the pain start? Was it sudden or gradual?"
Pain aggravating factors	Movements that stress affected tendons worsen pain	"Does your pain worsen with specific movements or activities?"
Location of pain	Helps localize the affected tendon or fascia	"Can you point to where it hurts the most?"
Swelling or deformity	Suggests **rupture (biceps, Achilles) or chronic pathology (ganglia, Dupuytren's)**	"Have you noticed any swelling, lumps, or deformity in the area?"
Morning stiffness	**Tendinitis, Fasciitis** may be worse in the morning	"Is your pain and stiffness worst when you wake up?"
Occupation and activities	Repetitive movements increase risk	"Does your job or hobby involve repetitive hand or foot use?"
History of trauma or injury	Acute ruptures or chronic strain-related injuries	"Have you had any recent injuries or surgeries in the area?"

EXAMINATION

A. INSPECTION

1. **Deformity:** In Dupuytren's contracture inspection is all that is necessary for the diagnosis. Localized thickening of the fascia, which affects the palmar fascia much more often than the plantar fascia, is a characteristic feature. Contracture of the fascia causes flexion of the fingers or toes. Most commonly this disease affects the ring finger first and then the little finger.

2. **Swelling:** Abnormal swelling of a muscle particularly when it contracts is a feature of rupture of the tendon or the muscle concerned. A little thickening of the flexor sheath of the tendon of the finger is the feature of a "trigger finger".

B. PALPATION

1. **Tenderness:** Localized tenderness on the particular point of the attachment of the tendon is diagnostic of any type of tendinitis, e.g., supraspinatus tendinitis, patellar tendinitis, Achilles' tendinitis and plantar fasciitis. Similarly, localized tenderness on the attachment of the extensor muscles of the forearm to the lateral epicondyle or the flexor muscles of the forearm to the medial epicondyle indicates 'Tennis elbow" or Golfer's elbow respectively.
2. **Deformity:** Palpation of the deformity, which is come across in conditions like Dupuytren's contracture and ganglia, is more informative about the type of operation and the extent of dissection rather than diagnosis. Diagnosis is easy in these cases.
3. **Swelling:** In stenosing tenovaginitis as seen in de Quervain's disease or trigger finger, palpation of the swelling of the sheath of the tendon is important. Gradually as consequence of constriction caused by the tendon sheath the tendon distal to the constriction may bulge out to form a swelling. In carpal tunnel syndrome a careful palpation will yield thickening of the flexor retinaculum and will reveal the neurological deficits of the median nerve due to this condition. In rupture of the tendon and muscles while the muscles concerned are contracting against resistance palpation of the swelling of the muscle will immediately make the diagnosis as to which muscle has been involved in rupture. As ganglion is a tense cystic swelling, fluctuation test may not be performed, but the swelling is softest at its center.

Examination of muscular disorders

Feature	Finding and interpretation	Clinical example
Inspection	Visible deformity, swelling, thickened fascia	Dupuytren's Contracture, Biceps rupture (Popeye Sign)
Palpation	Tenderness over tendon insertions	Tennis elbow (lateral epicondyle), Achilles tendinitis
Pain with movement	Worsens with specific muscle activation	Painful Arc in supraspinatus tendinitis
Special tests	Finkelstein's (De Quervain's), Thompson's (Achilles rupture)	Positive tests confirm the diagnosis

DIFFERENTIAL DIAGNOSIS

SUPRASPINATUS TENDINITIS

Degenerative process of the supraspinatus tendon following deficient blood supply seems to be the cause of this condition. It commonly affects the middle aged and old people and males are predominantly sufferer than the females. The main complaint is the *pain* in the shoulder particularly felt during abduction and external rotation movements. Pain becomes very much aggravated during the middle third of the abduction arc when the head of the humerus comes very close to the acromion process and the degenerated supraspinatus tendon becomes compressed between the two bones. This condition is popularly known as "painful arc syndrome". That means when the patient abducts his arm, the first 60° is painless. The pain starts henceforth and continues till the arm reaches an angle of 120°. After this the pain subsides as the shoulder is further abducted. The second complaint of the patient is *stiffness* of the shoulder, which is popularly known as "frozen shoulder". The natural sequence is that the pain gradually subsides and the stiffness increases. Up to 3 months stiffness remains static, after which stiffness also gradually subsides in next 3 months.

The main sign is the localized tenderness over the insertion of the supraspinatus tendon. Sometimes degenerative calcification of the tendon may develop which becomes obvious radiologically. Degenerative process may proceed further as to cause spontaneous rupture of the tendon.

TENNIS ELBOW

In this condition the patient complains of pain on the lateral epicondyle of the humerus where the extensor group of muscles of the forearm is attached. The pain is aggravated when the patient tends to extend the wrist and the fingers, more so against resistance. On examination localized tenderness is felt on the lateral epicondyle where the extensor muscles of the forearm are attached.

GOLFER'S ELBOW

This condition is more or less similar to the tennis elbow, but on the medial side. Pain and tenderness are localized on the medial epicondyle of the humerus, where the flexor muscles of the forearm take origin. Patient complains of pain when asked to flex the wrist and fingers against resistance.

ACHILLES' TENDINITIS

The patient complains of pain at the attachment of the Achilles' tendon to the bone. The condition is sometimes attributed to the unaccustomed prolonged walking or sometimes due to ill-fitting shoes.

PLANTAR FASCIITIS

In this condition the patient experiences unbearable pain under the heel particularly during walking when the weight of the body is carried by the heel. The cause seems to be a small tear in the attachment of plantar fascia to the os calcis. Nonspecific infection from nonspecific urethritis or from specific gonococcal infection may develop this condition. Sometimes a bony spur may be seen at the attachment of the plantar fascia. This may or may not be the cause of pain.

FIBROSITIS OR FIBROSITIC NODULE

This condition is also a type of nonarticular rheumatism and a common cause of low back pain. The pain and tenderness is localized at the attachment of the erector spinae muscle or the fascia covering it.

RUPTURE OF THE SUPRASPINATUS TENDON

Spontaneous rupture of the supraspinatus tendon may occur due to degenerative change in the tendon in elderly individuals. The patient complains of sudden pain in the shoulder while involved in normal activities. The most important physical sign is *inability to initiate abduction.* So, the patient leans to the affected side making an angle of abduction between his body and the arm initiated by gravity. After this he can continue the movement of abduction in a normal way. Thus, the diagnosis may be escaped by the inexperienced.

RUPTURE OF THE LONG HEAD OF THE BICEPS BRACHII

This condition also affects elderly individual and also a sequel of degenerative process. The rupture commonly takes place in the bicipital groove and mostly spontaneous. The patient sometimes complains of a sudden pain in the upper arm, but it is often neglected. More commonly the patient complains of an abnormal swelling when he flexes his elbow due to bunching of the biceps muscle.

RUPTURE OF THE ACHILLES' TENDON

This is due to vascular insufficiency of the tendon and may occur due to violence on the contracted muscle while playing football, etc. The presenting complaint and the signs are similar to the rupture of the biceps tendon described above.

STENOSING TENOVAGINITIS

The cause of this condition is rather unknown, but it involves mostly the common sheath of the abductor pollicis longus and extensor pollicis brevis (de Quervain's disease) and the fibrous sheath of the flexor tendons of the fingers and the thumb (Trigger finger).

De Quervain's disease: Women between 40-50 years are the usual victims. In this condition the patient complains of pain and difficulty in abducting and extending the thumb. On examination a bulge is detected on the said tendons over the radial styloid process. Pain is felt if the thumb is adducted across the palm.

Trigger finger: In this condition the tendon just distal to the constriction becomes swollen and can only be forced down through the constricted sheath by the powerful flexor muscle but the patient finds difficulty in extending the finger with rather weak extensor muscle. With continued effort he suddenly becomes successful in forcing the swollen tendon through the constricted sheath and as soon as it is done the finger becomes extended quickly and abruptly like a trigger of a pistol.

CARPAL TUNNEL SYNDROME

This condition is also an example of stenosing tenovaginitis. The only difference is that the cause is not only thickening of the flexor retinaculum but also some other pathology such as rheumatoid arthritis involving the synovial sheaths of the flexor tendons or dislocation of lunate bone which compresses on the contents of this osseofibrous canal, mainly the median nerve, also exits. The main complaint of the patient is some sort of difficulty in flexing fingers with pain and neurological deficits of the median nerve, e.g., paresthesia or numbness or incoordination or weakness of the muscles innervated by median nerve. On examination, slight tenderness can be elicited on the carpal tunnel. There will be neurological signs along the distribution of the median nerve. Flexion movement of the fingers will be painful and conduction studies on the median nerve will demonstrate a delay at the carpal tunnel.

DUPUYTREN'S CONTRACTURE

This condition mainly affects the palm and very occasionally the plantar fascia There is localized thickening and contracture of the palmar fascia. There may be nodules in the fascia or in the subcutaneous tissue indicating excessive fibrous tissue activity. This condition mostly affects the medial part of the palmar fascia in which the ring finger and less often the little finger become flexed. This is due to the fact that the extensions of the palmar fascia are attached to the proximal as well as middle phalanges.

The etiology of this condition is not clearly known. Repeated trauma which was previously incriminated as the cause of this condition has been discarded due to the fact that it often involves the persons who do not inflict trauma so repeatedly in the palm. Its peculiar association with cirrhotic patients, epileptics who are having sodium hydantoin and Peyronie's disease add more to its intricacy.

On examination, there is thickening of the medial aspect of the palmar fascia with firm nodules within the fascia or in the subcutaneous tissue. The overlying skin is more or less fixed to the fascia and there is flexion deformity of the ring and the little fingers.

GANGLION (FIG. 10.1)

This is a tense and cystic swelling containing gelatinous material in it. This mostly originates from the capsule of a joint or a tendon sheath. It may be due to a leakage in the capsule or the tendon sheath following trauma and subsequent encapsulation with fibrous tissue or it may be due to mucoid degeneration of the fibrous sheath. Ganglia are commonly seen on the dorsum of the wrist or the palm of the hand.

On examination, a tense and cystic swelling will be revealed in relation to a capsule of the joint or a tendon sheath. When it originates from a tendon sheath it can be moved sideways slightly but not at all along the length of the tendon particularly when the tendon is made taut.

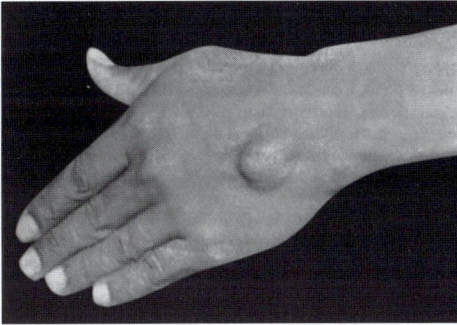

Fig. 10.1: A ganglion on the dorsal aspect of the wrist in relation with the extensor tendon of the finger.

Algorithmic Approach to Patient with Muscle, Tendon, and Fascia Disorders

Patient presents with pain, swelling, deformity, or movement limitation

↓

Where is the pain localized?
- Shoulder → Consider **rotator cuff tear, suraspinatus tendinitis, frozen shoulder, biceps tendinitis**
- Elbow → Consider **tennis elbow (lateral epicondylitis), golfer's elbow (medial epicondylitis), olecranon bursitis**
- Hand/Wrist → Consider **carpal tunnel syndrome, de quervain's tenosynovitis, trigger finger, dupuytren's contracture**
- Knee → Consider **patellar tendinitis (jumper's knee), prepatellar bursitis, meniscus tear, osteoarthritis**
- Ankle/Foot → Consider **achilles tendinitis, plantar fasciitis, ankle sprain, morton's neuroma**

↓

Is the pain acute or chronic?
- Acute → Suggests **trauma, tendon rupture, overuse injury, acute bursitis**
- Chronic → Suggests **degenerative, overuse, or inflammatory causes (tendinitis, fasciitis, bursitis, fibrosis)**

↓

Is there swelling or deformity?
- Yes → Suggests **tendon rupture (biceps, achilles), ganglion cyst, dupuytren's contracture, inflammatory bursitis**
- No → More likely **tendinitis or fasciitis**

↓

Is the pain aggravated by specific movements?
- Yes → Proceed to **special tests** to confirm diagnosis
- No → Consider **neurological or systemic causes** (e.g., rheumatoid arthritis, neuropathy, fibromyalgia, autoimmune disease)

↓

Perform special tests for clinical confirmation
- Shoulder:
  - **Painful arc test** → Supraspinatus tendinitis
  - **Drop arm test** → Rotator cuff tear
  - **Speed's test** → Biceps tendinitis
- Elbow:
  - **Cozen's test** → Tennis elbow
  - **Medial epicondylitis test** → Golfer's elbow
- Hand/Wrist:
  - **Finkelstein's test** → De quervain's tenosynovitis
  - **Phalen's test** → Carpal tunnel syndrome
  - **Ochsner's clasping test** → Median nerve dysfunction
- Knee:
  - **McMurray's test** → Meniscus tear
  - **Patellar grind test** → Patellar chondromalacia
- Ankle/Foot:
  - **Thompson's test** → Achilles tendon tupture
  - **Windlass test** → Plantar fasciitis

↓

Does the special test indicate a specific disorder?
- Yes → Confirm diagnosis and move to treatment
- No → Consider a broader **differential diagnosis** (e.g., autoimmune disorders, neuromuscular diseases, chronic pain syndromes)

↓

Order imaging for confirmation
- Ultrasound or MRI → Identify **tendon tears, fasciopathy, or ganglia**
- X-ray → Rule out **calcifications, bone spurs, or fractures**
- Electromyography (EMG) → If neuropathy or nerve compression suspected

↓

Confirm diagnosis and Initiate treatment
- Conservative management:
  - Physiotherapy, activity modification, NSAIDs, corticosteroid injections (if needed)
- Surgical management:
  - Tendon repair (if ruptured), fascia release (dupuytren's contracture), ganglion excision (if symptomatic)

Examination of Diseases of Bone

CHAPTER 11

A bony lesion or a swelling is always fixed to the bone and cannot be moved apart from the bone. Various sites and types of bone lesions are shown in **Figure 11.1**.

HISTORY

1. **Age:** Solitary cyst of a bone is seen in children up to the age of puberty and after that it becomes increasingly rare. Monostotic fibrous dysplasia, though rare, is chiefly a disease of adolescents but may remain symptomless till the bone breaks. Osteogenesis imperfecta (brittle bones) congenita presents with multiple fractures, dwarfism and deformities since birth; whereas osteogenesis imperfecta tarda presents later near 10 years of age. Acute osteomyelitis is common in children. Tuberculous osteomyelitis may be seen at any age. Paget's disease (osteitis deformans) is a disease of old age. Nearly all benign bone tumors occur in adolescent and in young adults; osteoclastoma occurs between 20 and 30 years of age. Primary malignant bone tumors mainly occur in young people; osteosarcoma occurs between 15 and 30 years of age; multiple myeloma occurs late—30–50 years. Secondary carcinoma of bone is seen in old age above 40 years.

2. **Onset and progress:** History *of trauma* is frequently obtained in many bone diseases particularly in acute osteomyelitis and osteosarcoma. *Spontaneous development of swelling* is most likely to be seen in cases of bone tumors. But even in these cases the patients may give a history of trauma, which has probably drawn the attention of the patient towards a small swelling which was so long unnoticed. Acute onset with high rise of temperature and toxemia is a feature of acute osteomyelitis. In chronic osteomyelitis the onset is usually insidious, but acute exacerbation of chronic osteomyelitis is not uncommon. Malignant tumors grow very rapidly and the history is relatively short since the patient had discovered the swelling.

3. **Pain:** Pain is always associated with inflammation. But in bone the peculiar feature is that the malignant growth *osteosarcoma* presents *with pain first and swelling later on.* Otherwise the tumors whether they are benign or malignant are painless to start with. One must note the

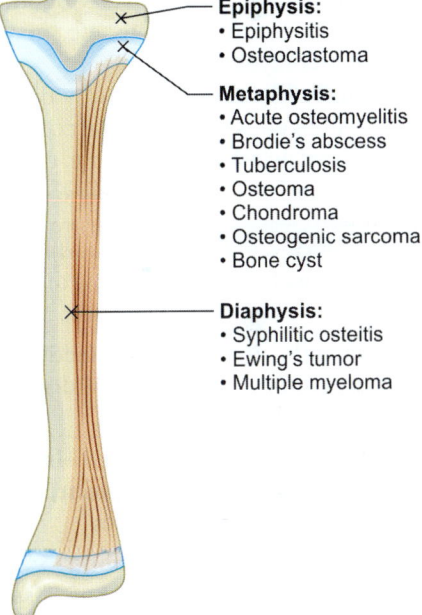

Fig. 11.1: Characteristic sites of various types of bone diseases.

- **Epiphysis:**
  - Epiphysitis
  - Osteoclastoma
- **Metaphysis:**
  - Acute osteomyelitis
  - Brodie's abscess
  - Tuberculosis
  - Osteoma
  - Chondroma
  - Osteogenic sarcoma
  - Bone cyst
- **Diaphysis:**
  - Syphilitic osteitis
  - Ewing's tumor
  - Multiple myeloma

character of the pain—whether it is *throbbing* (characteristic of inflammation) or dull *aching* (characteristic of tumors in their late stages barring osteosarcoma).

4. **Duration:** In acute osteomyelitis the duration is very short whereas chronic osteomyelitis resents healing for months and even years. In malignant bony tumors the duration is relatively short in comparison to the benign bony swellings.

5. **Sinuses:** This may be present in chronic osteomyelitis (**Fig. 11.2**) either pyogenic or tuberculous. History of extrusion of bone chips strongly suggests pyogenic osteomyelitis.

6. **Similar swellings:** An enquiry must be made if there is any similar swelling anywhere else in the body. In diaphyseal aclasis there will be multiple swellings arising from the metaphyses of different bones affecting a young boy.

7. **Past history:** A past history of otitis media, pneumonia, typhoid fever, multiple boils, etc., may be obtained in case of acute osteomyelitis.

8. **Family history:** A few bony disorders run in families, e.g., osteogenesis imperfecta congenita, achondroplasia, diaphyseal aclasis, marble bone, cleidocranial dysostosis, Marfan's syndrome, etc.

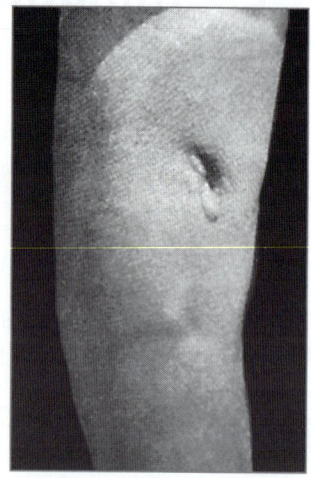

Fig. 11.2: A typical sinus following chronic osteomyelitis. Sprouting granulation tissue at the mouth of the sinus suggests presence of sequestrum underneath.

History in patients with bone diseases

Aspect	Clinical significance	Patient-friendly questions
Age of onset	Helps narrow diagnosis (e.g., Osteosarcoma in adolescents, Multiple Myeloma in adults)	"At what age did the swelling or pain start?"
Onset and progression	Acute → **Infection, Trauma**, Gradual → **Benign or Malignant Tumor**	"Did the pain/swelling appear suddenly or grow slowly over time?"
Pain characteristics	Throbbing → Infection, Dull-Aching → Benign Tumor, Severe, Night Pain → Malignancy	"Is the pain dull, sharp, or throbbing? Is it worse at night?"
Swelling fixity	Fixed to bone → Tumor or Infection, Mobile → Soft Tissue Mass	"Does the swelling move, or is it fixed?"
Systemic symptoms	Fever → **Infection**, Weight Loss → Malignancy	"Have you had fever, night sweats, or weight loss?"
Family history	Genetic Bone Disorders (Osteogenesis Imperfecta, Achondroplasia)	"Does anyone in your family have similar bone problems?"

GENERAL SURVEY

(1) Anemia, cachexia and malnutrition are come across in secondary carcinomas and a few primary malignant conditions of bone. (2) Toxic features with fever and malaise are noticed in acute osteomyelitis.

LOCAL EXAMINATION

INSPECTION

1. **Swelling:** The swelling is examined as has been described in Chapter 3. *All swellings arising from the bone will be fixed to it.*
2. **Skin overlying the swelling:** In acute osteomyelitis the skin overlying the swelling will be red, edematous and congested. In osteosarcoma the skin over the swelling remains tense, glossy with dilated veins **(Fig. 11.3)**. In tuberculous osteomyelitis cold abscess will lead to a swelling in the beginning and later on *sinus* formation. Chronic pyogenic osteomyelitis also presents with sinuses. The tuberculous sinus will reveal its characteristic features like undermined edge and bluish margin, whereas in chronic pyogenic osteomyelitis there will be sprouting granulation tissue which indicates presence of sequestrum at the depth. But both these sinuses will be fixed to the bone. Sometimes there may be scar on the skin overlying the lesion. Depressed, puckered *scar* indicates previous suppuration and abscess formation.

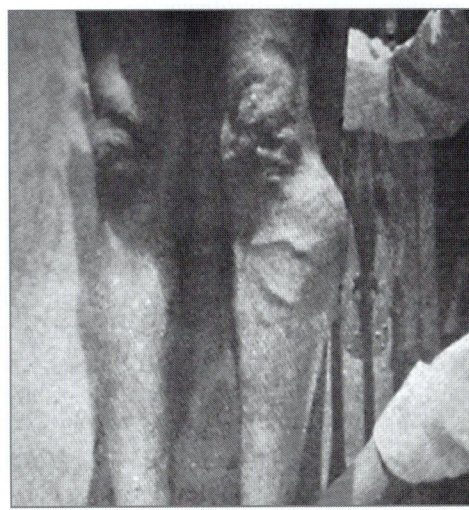

Fig. 11.3: Dilated subcutaneous veins in case of osteosarcoma.

3. **Pressure effects:** It is always essential to have a look at the limb distal to the swelling. There may be edema due to pressure of the bony swelling on the veins. There may be paresis due to involvement of the nerves by the bony swellings.
4. **Neighboring joints:** Sympathetic effusion of the neighboring joints is a common feature in acute osteomyelitis. Sometimes acute osteomyelitis may destruct the epiphyseal cartilage thereby hampering the growth of that particular bone. This may lead to deformities like manus valgus, i.e., outward deviation of the hand due to the destruction of lower epiphysis of the radius and its deficient growth which is out grown by the normal development of the ulna. Genu valgum or genu varum may be the result of asymmetrical destruction of the lower epiphyseal cartilage of the femur. Deformed joints are also encountered in diaphyseal aclasis.
5. **Muscular wasting:** This becomes prominent and obvious in probably one bony lesion, i.e., tuberculous osteomyelitis.
6. **Shortening or lengthening of the bone—**may sometimes be seen following infection of the bone which either provokes the growth of the bone or destroys the epiphyseal cartilage and hence retards the growth of the bone.

PALPATION

1. **Local temperature:** This is best palpated by the back of the fingers and local temperature is raised in acute pyogenic inflammatory conditions and in osteosarcoma.
2. **Tenderness:** Inflammatory swellings are always tender. Tumors are generally nontender.
3. **Swelling:** It has already been emphasized that *all bony swellings will be fixed to the bone* and cannot be moved. Assessment must be made from which part of the bone the swelling has originated. The following points should be noted with details.

(i) **Situation:** A swelling arising from the epiphysis is probably an osteoclastoma. Acute osteomyelitis, Brodie's abscess, tuberculous osteomyelitis, bone cyst, osteoma and osteosarcoma commonly start in the metaphysis. Ewing's tumor, multiple myeloma and syphilitic osteomyelitis are diseases of the diaphysis.

(ii) **Size and shape:** A swelling, which is diffuse and very difficult to get at the margins probably due to extreme pain and tenderness, is an inflammatory swelling. Pedunculated swellings are generally exostoses. Spherical, ovoid and irregular swellings are generally tumors of the bone.

(iii) **Surface:** Smooth and lobulated surface are features of benign growth. Irregularity are features of malignant growth and chronic infection.

(iv) **Edge:** Ill-defined edge is the feature of inflammatory swelling and well-defined edge is the feature of new growth. As osteosarcoma is a very rapidly growing tumor it loses its well-defined edge.

(v) **Consistency:** It is bony hard in osteoma. In osteoclastoma, the outer bony shell may be very thin as to yield or break during palpation ('egg-shell crackling'); otherwise when the outer covering is thick, it is also bony hard in consistency. In osteosarcoma the consistency varies—somewhere bony hard, somewhere firm and may be even soft at places. This is a diagnostic feature of osteosarcoma. In acute osteomyelitis, it will pit on pressure. Being a bony swelling its consistency should also be bony hard, but the condition is so painful and tender that the clinician hardly reaches the bone during palpation and can only palpate the soft tissues overlying the bone which pits on pressure.

(vi) **Pulsation:** Is the swelling pulsatile? Some pathological condition of the bone may be pulsatile, e.g., telangiectatic osteosarcoma, aneurysmal bone cyst, occasionally highly vascular osteoclastoma, very rarely hemangioma of bone and highly vascular metastatic carcinomas from thyroid cancer and renal adenocarcinoma.

4. **Bony irregularity:** A careful palpation of the affected bone is very essential. In chronic pyogenic osteomyelitis, syphilitic osteomyelitis and even tuberculous osteomyelitis the affected bone may be irregular. This irregularity will also be present in Brodie's abscess.

5. **Ulcers and sinuses:** Whenever there is an ulcer or a sinus, it is good practice to hold the base of the ulcer or the sinus and to move it against the bone. Fixity to the bone indicates its relation with the bony lesion. These are commonly seen in chronic pyogenic osteomyelitis and tuberculous osteomyelitis. In case of the former there will be sprouting granulation tissue at the orifice of the sinus indicating presence of sequestrum in the depth and in case of the latter the ulcer will be undermining with bluish newly growing epithelial edge.

6. **Presence of fracture:** Not infrequently patients with metastatic carcinoma present with pathological fracture. In fact sometimes this fracture becomes the first presenting symptom of the primary carcinoma which may be in the lung, kidney, breast, prostate, thyroid, etc.

7. **Neighboring structures:** While examining a case of bony lesion one must examine the neighboring structures, i.e., the muscles—their power and mobility over the bony lesion, the nerves and the blood vessels. These structures may be involved by the lesion.

PERCUSSION

Localized tenderness of chronic osteomyelitis, Brodie's abscess, etc., may be well elicited by percussion. In case of spine and pelvis this can be elicited by gently striking with a fist.

AUSCULTATION

In case of pulsatile swellings, this examination will be required to detect the presence of a murmur and to note its character.

MEASUREMENTS

(i) *Length of the long bone:* In osteomyelitis the bone may be shortened or lengthened. Shortening will be found when the epiphyseal cartilage is destroyed and the bone may be lengthened when the metaphysis is included within the zone of hyperemia. (ii) Circumference of the limb is measured if muscular wasting is suspected.

Examination of the neighboring joints: The neighboring joints may be sympathetically effused in acute osteomyelitis. Osteoclastoma generally starts in the epiphysis and may involve the joint. Osteosarcoma, which mainly starts from the metaphysis, does not invade the epiphyseal cartilage until late and hence the joint remains unaffected.

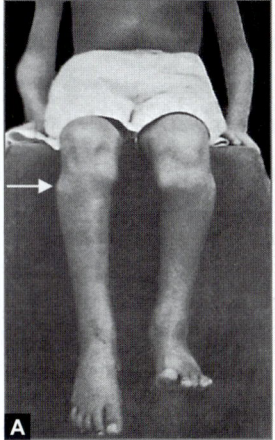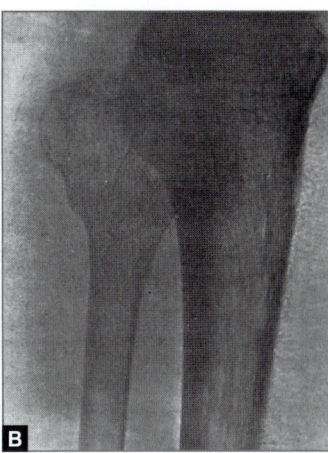

Figs. 11.4A and B: The patient is asked to dorsiflex both ankle joints. Note the foot drop on the right side due to involvement of the lateral popliteal nerve by an osteoma at the head of the fibula.

Examination of the lymph nodes: See Chapter 8.

Pressure effects: Different swellings of the bone may press on the neighboring blood vessels and the nerves to cause respective symptoms. Swellings of the distal limb and venous engorgement may be due to pressure on the neighboring veins. Nerves may also be affected due to pressure effect of the bony swellings and 'foot drop' due to paralysis of the external popliteal nerve may be seen in case of a tumor of the upper end of the fibula **(Figs. 11.4A and B)**.

GENERAL EXAMINATION

1. In tuberculous osteomyelitis general examination must be made to exclude pulmonary tuberculosis and lymphadenitis. Enquiry must be made whether the patient had cough, evening rise of temperature, pain in the chest, hemoptysis, etc. Neck, axilla and groin must be palpated to exclude lymph node enlargement.
2. In syphilitic osteitis, one should look for other syphilitic stigmas in the body (*see* **Fig. 4.15**). One must try to elicit the history of syphilitic contact.
3. In osteomyelitis a search should be made for infective foci in the skin, tooth, tonsil, ear, air sinuses, etc.
4. Certain bony lesions involve more than one bone at a time. Diaphyseal (metaphyseal) aclasis **(Fig. 11.5)**, generalized osteitis fibrosa, multiple myeloma are the examples of this condition. So the patient must be asked if there is any other bony swelling in his body or not.

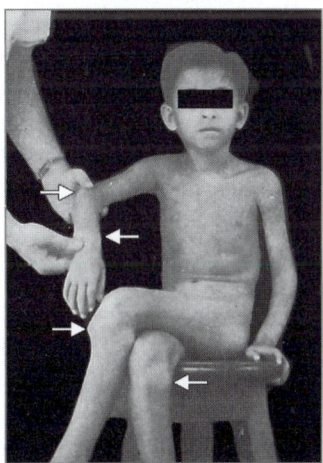

Fig. 11.5: Diaphyseal (metaphyseal) aclasis. Arrows indicate the exostoses.

5. In secondary carcinoma a thorough examination must be made to exclude primary carcinoma in the thyroid, kidneys, lungs, prostate, breasts, uterus, gastrointestinal tract, testis, etc.

SPECIAL INVESTIGATIONS

1. **BLOOD:** (a) Leukocytosis is the feature of bony inflammation, particularly acute osteomyelitis. (b) In multiple myeloma the serum calcium level will be raised. There will be hyperproteinemia, the globulin (particularly gamma globulin) being raised. (c) A rise in serum calcium indicates generalized osteolysis (which is seen in cases of hyperparathyroidism, metastatic bone tumors, multiple myeloma, sarcoidosis, etc.). (d) A rise in serum alkaline phosphatase suggests osteoblastic activity as occurs in osteitis deformans and some sarcomas. (e) Higher level of serum acid phosphatase serves to distinguish prostatic metastasis in bone from other skeletal metastasis. (f) Reduced serum phosphorus and increased alkaline phosphatase with high erythrocyte sedimentation rate (ESR) are seen in osteomalacia. (g) Wassermann reaction (WR) and Kahn tests will be positive in cases of syphilitic osteitis.

2. **URINE:** (a) Albumin may be present when amyloid disease has affected the kidneys in long continued suppuration as in osteomyelitis. (b) Presence of Bence Jones protein (a globulin) can be demonstrated in the urine of the patient by appearance of coagulation when the urine is heated to 55°C, its disappearance by further heat to 80°C and its reappearance again on cooling. But this appears in only 50% of multiple myeloma cases. Bence Jones protein may also be found in cases of skeletal carcinomatosis, leukemia and rarely in nephritis.

3. **X-RAY EXAMINATION:** It goes without saying that this examination is probably the most important special investigation, which clinches the final diagnosis. X-ray examination of the affected bone will reveal local pathology, whereas that of the other bones will reveal generalized involvement of the bones.

A. **Affected bone:** In the first instance it must be noticed whether the bone is rarefied (i.e., of reduced density) as is often seen in tuberculous affection or is sclerosed (i.e., of increased density) as seen in syphilis, Paget's disease, marble bone or chronic osteomyelitis (sequestrum or involucrum).

In **Osteomyelitis**, it must be remembered that there is practically no place of X-ray examination in acute cases and diagnosis must be made clinically. In chronic osteomyelitis, a dense sequestrum and surrounding involucrum may be noticed **(Figs. 11.6A to C)**. Density of the sequestrum is due to decreased mobilization of calcium from decreased blood supply, whereas in involucrum calcium deposition has just commenced.

In **Brodie's abscess** an osteolytic cavity will be seen surrounded by dense or sclerosed bone. There is hardly any sequestrum inside the cavity **(Fig. 11.7)**. Similar cavity is seen in **bone cyst**, but surrounding sclerosis is conspicuous by its absence **(Fig. 11.8)**.

An **osteoma** is seen as a pedunculated bony outgrowth from the metaphysis. The growth of the osteoma continues so long the bone grows in length **(Fig. 11.9)**.

Osteoid osteoma is seen as a radiolucent nidus with a surrounding zone of bony sclerosis.

In **diaphyseal aclasis** multiple exostoses are seen **(Fig. 11.10)**.

In **chondroma**, whether enchondroma or ecchondroma, X-ray shows an osteolytic lesion with demarcated outline **(Figs. 11.11 to 11.13)**.

X-ray features of **osteoclastoma** are characteristic **(Fig. 11.14)**. The metaphysio-epiphyseal areas are seen to be enlarged and occupied by a cystic tumor. The cortex is thin with a sharp line of demarcation between the tumor and the unaffected shaft in contradistinction to the sarcomas.

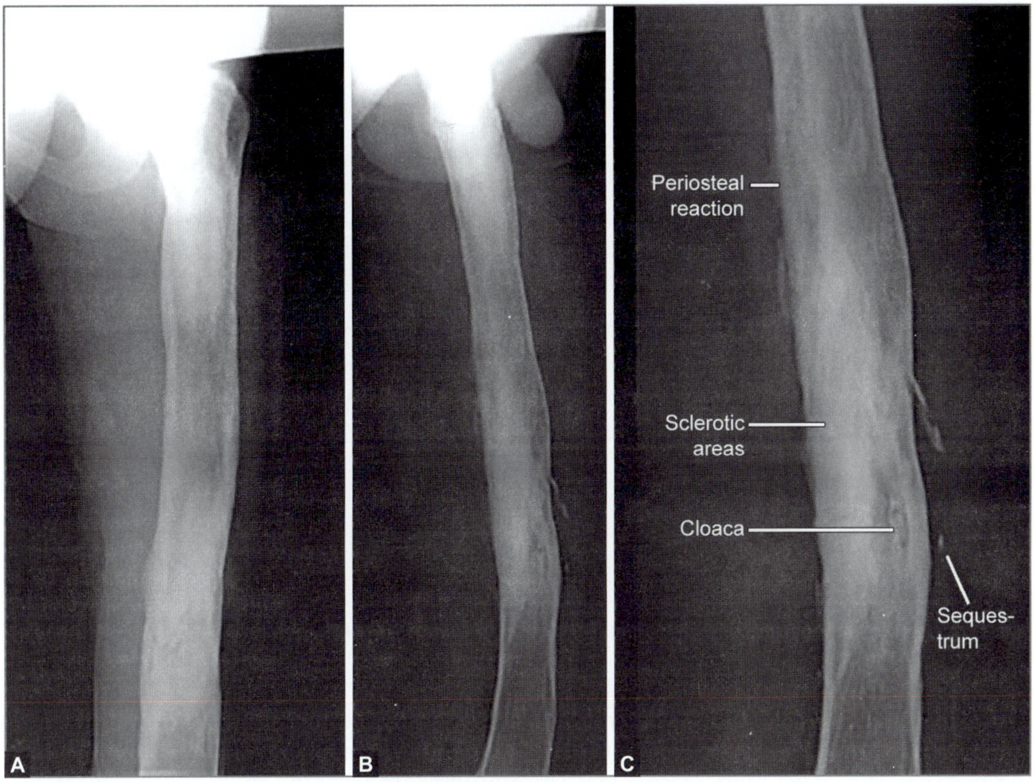

Chapter 11: Examination of Diseases of Bone   177

Figs. 11.6A to C: Chronic osteomyelitis.

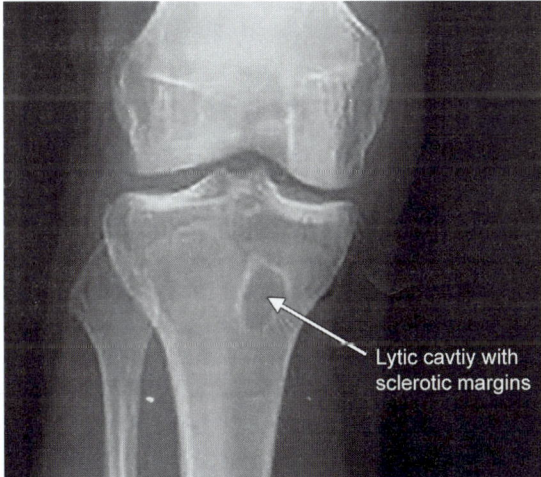

Fig. 11.7: Brodie's abscess.

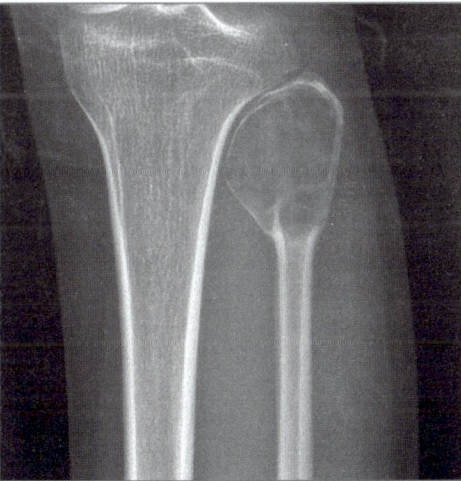

Fig. 11.8: Bone cyst. Note that the expansion occurs along the long axis of the bone (cf. osteoclastoma).

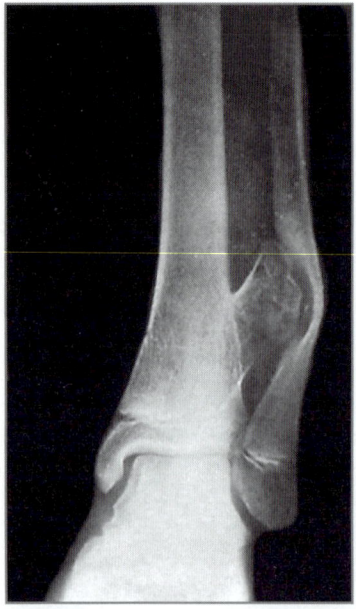

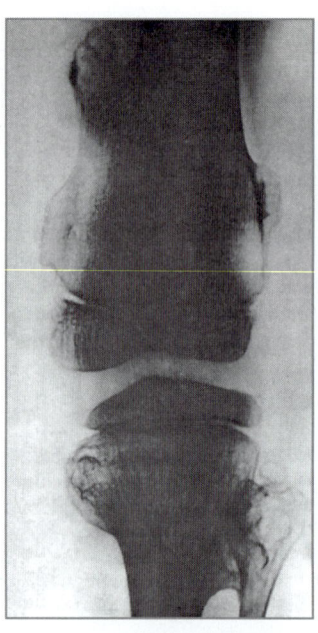

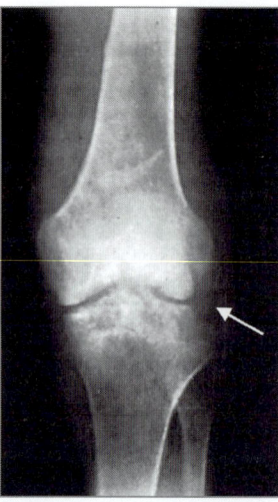

Fig. 11.11: Chondroma at the lateral aspect of the knee joint. This is revealed in X-ray by an osteolytic lesion affecting the lateral condyle of the tibia (indicated by an arrow).

Fig. 11.9: Osteoma at the lower end of the tibia.

Fig. 11.10: Multiple exostoses are seen in diaphyseal aclasis.

The expanding osteolytic lesion can continue to destroy the cortex, although usually it leaves some external rim. The cavity is traversed by bony trabeculae giving mosaic or soap-bubble appearance. Mostly the tumor grows eccentrically, often destroys the epiphyseal cartilage and it may penetrate the articular cartilage. Pathological fractures may occur. This tumor expands transversely whereas a bone cyst expands along the long axis of the bone.

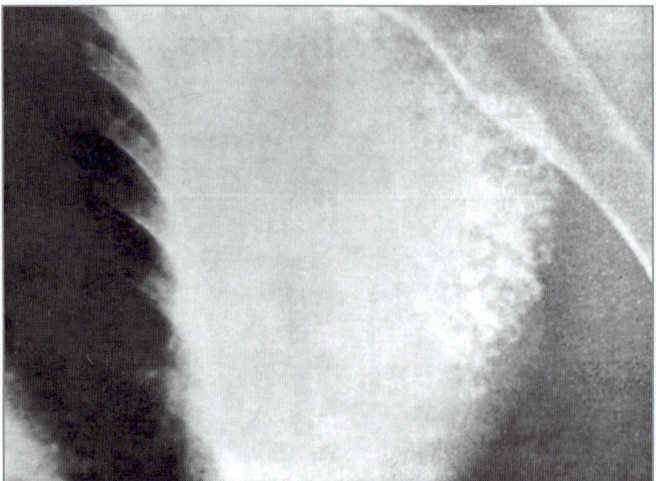

Fig. 11.12: A huge osteochondroma.

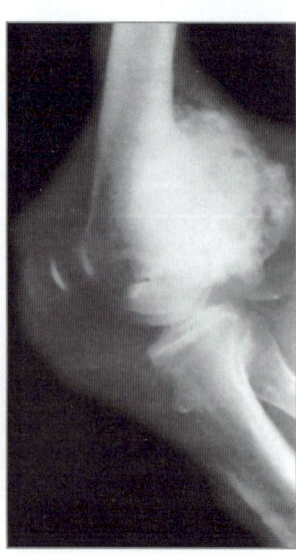

Fig. 11.13: Osteochondroma.

X-ray appearance of **osteosarcoma** shows a combination of bone destruction and bone formation **(Figs. 11.15 and 11.16)**. The tumor has an ill-defined junction with the rest of the shaft. Three types are commonly seen—(i) Sclerotic type, usually found at puberty, shows dense new irregular bone with a few spicules projecting from its surface in the metaphysis. (ii) Osteolytic type shows an eccentric translucent gap and at its edges a gradual increase of density compared to that of the normal bone is seen. (iii) The radiating spicule type. The cortex is almost always perforated. A small wedge-shaped area of ossification (Codman's triangle) is seen at the spot where the periosteum is elevated from the shaft. The periosteum may show sunray spicules due to calcification along the blood vessels supplying the raised periosteum. As the tumor spreads into the soft tissues its outline becomes indefinite. In bone sarcoma there is always the soft tissue shadows in the skiagram due to increased vascularity of the tumor.

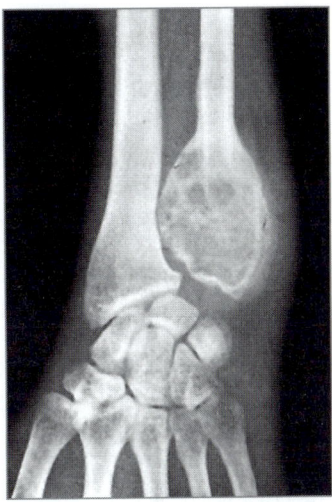

Fig. 11.14: Osteoclastoma affecting the lower end of the ulna. Note that the expansion occurs transversely (cf. bone cyst).

Chondrosarcoma in skiagram shows frank destruction of the trabecular bone and cortex with an expanding lesion which contains irregular flecking and the mottling of calcified tissue. There may be new bone formation which extends outward.

Ewing's tumor grows from the diaphysis **(Fig. 11.17)**. There is widespread diffuse rarefaction with subperiosteal deposition of bone longitudinally—the so-called 'onion effect'.

X-ray is not reliable for early detection of **secondary carcinoma** in the bones **(Fig. 11.18)**. At least 50% of medulla must be destroyed before a lesion will be seen radiologically. Tomograms are more sensitive. Osteolysis without formation of new bone is the feature except in carcinoma of the prostate where osteosclerosis is observed. This is due to high level of alkaline phosphatase.

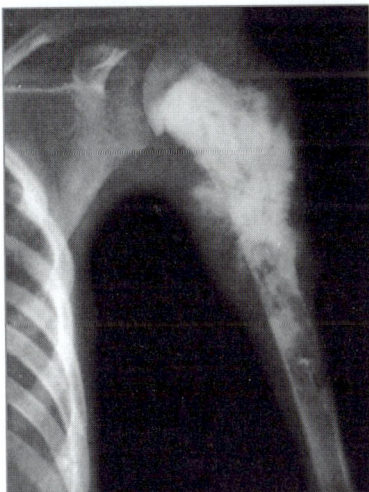

Fig. 11.15: Osteosarcoma showing the typical radiating spicule type.

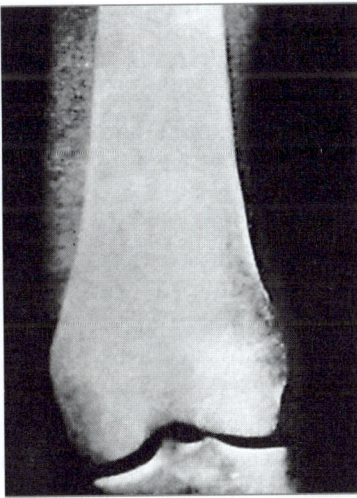

Fig. 11.16: Osteosarcoma affecting the lower end of the femur with typical sunray appearance.

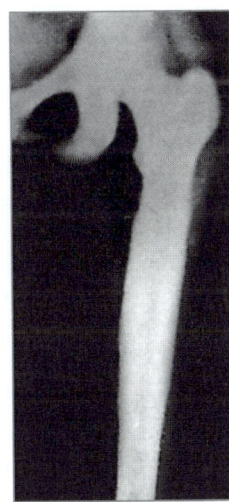

Fig. 11.17: Ewing's tumor affecting the femur.

B. **X-ray examination of the other bones** should be taken in generalized affections of bones. In **Ricket**, X-ray will show general decalcification. The epiphysis is widened with delay in appearance of centers of ossification. The growth discs are too deep. The metaphysis is splayed out.

In **Paget's disease** the bone as a whole is thick and bent; its density in the vascular stage is decreased and in the sclerotic stage increased. The trabeculae are coarse and widely separated. This gives honeycomb appearance. Striated appearance is seen in the pelvis, sacrum and calcaneum. True cystic areas can be seen in the pelvis or long bones.

In **Osteitis fibrosa (Hyperparathyroidism; Von Recklinghausen's disease)** skiagram shows a mixture of osteoporosis, cystic changes and coarsening of the trabecular pattern. Cysts may extend beyond the confines of the long bones and there may be subperiosteal erosions of the cortex. There may be even disappearance of the terminal outline with only longitudinal trabeculae remaining.

In **Multiple myeloma** circumscribed areas of rarefaction affect the different bones, which may mimic secondary metastasis.

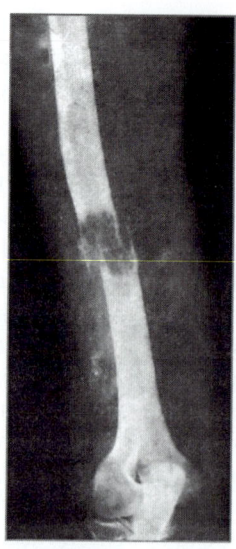

Fig. 11.18: Secondary carcinoma affecting the shaft of the humerus which leads to pathological fracture.

C. **Lungs** must be X-rayed to exclude secondary deposits in the lungs in cases of osteosarcoma, chondrosarcoma, fibrosarcoma or suspected malignant osteoclastoma **(Fig. 11.19)**.

4. **ARTERIOGRAPHY:** The changes of the character of the blood vessels supplying the tumor vary characteristically in all malignant tumors. The vessels become aimless, tortuous and engorged. Sometimes they end abruptly or terminate in pools of contrast which empty slowly. Early venous filling is also seen. But the most important feature is the presence of *'Contrast blush',* which delineates the extent of the tumor. All these features may not be present simultaneously in all primary malignant tumors, but one or the other change will be obvious. But there are fallacies, e.g., a few malignant tumors do not show the characteristic arteriographic changes. Conversely some benign osteoclastomas can show these features. But there are two distinct places where its value is undebatable—(i) to define the extent of the tumor and (ii) to detect malignant change in Paget's disease, which may be difficult on an ordinary X-ray film.

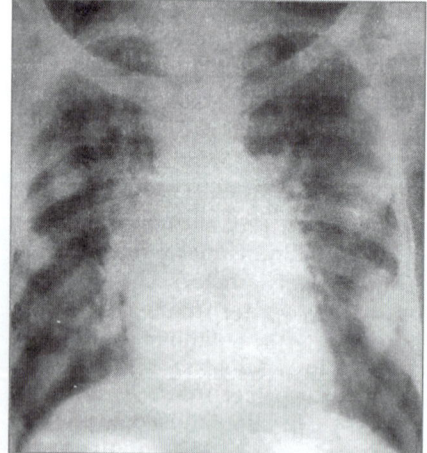

Fig. 11.19: Secondary deposits in the lungs (canon ball metastasis) in a case of osteosarcoma.

5. **RADIOACTIVE SCANNING:** This method depends upon the relatively high uptake of the radioisotope in areas of bone with high mineral turnover and reflects the metabolic state of the bone. It can indicate the presence of local infection in the same fashion as a primary or metastatic bone tumor. So the scan reflects the metabolic process and a change in mineralization. Thus positive bone scan is seen before X-ray changes. *Only very anaplastic tumors and quiescent, longstanding lesions fail to show positive results.*

Scanning is performed 1–4 hours after the intravenous injection of 5–10 mci of 99 Tcm-phosphates complex. The patient must empty his bladder before the pelvis is scanned as about 40% of the injected dose is excreted in the urine within first 4 hrs after injection.

The gamma camera detects, records and displays the activity within its total field of view (about 25 cm diameter). Using a gamma camera and taking multiple overlapping views, it can detect a far greater number of counts leading to much better statistical quality than the whole body scanner in a similar time. The great potential value of bone scanning lies in its ability to detect early active lesions in bone before they are visible on X-ray. It might possibly be of value in clinical practice in the early detection of primary osteosarcoma, although usually they are already clearly visible on X-ray when the patient is first seen. But it is probably more valuable in detecting bone secondaries to know the spread of the disease, suitability of radical operation, differentiation between simple and pathological fracture, to find out the site suitable for biopsy and for staging reticulosis. It has been claimed that some 20% bone secondaries which are not visible on X-ray could be detected by radioisotope scanning.

6. **BIOPSY:** To know the exact pathology of the bony lesion, biopsy is very essential. It gives a clear picture of the disease and the cellular pattern. It is essential in all cases, for one cannot with certainty make the diagnosis on clinical or radiological ground alone. The only exception to this can be in Paget's sarcoma in the elderly, when the signs and X-rays alone may occasionally suffice, *Open biopsy* is still the popular method. The risk of dissemination which was supposed to be great, is now found to be absolutely theoretical. To give clear decision on frozen section biopsy is difficult and only a few institutions in the world can have the privilege to get pathologists of that grade. There is hardly any place of prophylactic small dose irradiation before taking biopsy. *Aspiration biopsy* though unrivalled in surgically difficult regions such as spine (where open biopsy is not possible), biopsy of limb tumors by means of wide-bore needle has never become popular in this country. This is partly due to reluctance on the part of pathologists to give opinion on small cores of tissues. *Marrow biopsy* is helpful in diagnosing multiple myeloma in which numerous plasma cells will be present.

7. **BACTERIOLOGICAL EXAMINATION** of the pus obtained by aspiration in cases of acute osteomyelitis is of immense value to determine the causative organism and the most effective antibiotic by sensitivity test. Blood culture may be of use when septicemia is suspected.

8. **HISTOPATHOLOGICAL EXAMINATION** of the tumor, either from *biopsy* or from curettage as done in osteoclastoma and bone cyst, is of great value in determining the diagnosis and to exclude possibility of malignant change. *Marrow biopsy* should be performed in case of multiple myeloma which reveals presence of numerous plasma cells.

CLASSIFICATION OF BONY SWELLINGS

A. Traumatic
(i) Excess of callus formation from fractured bone; (ii) Malunited fracture; (iii) Myositis ossificans; (iv) Subperiosteal hematoma and its ossification.

B. Inflammatory
(i) Acute osteomyelitis; (ii) Chronic osteomyelitis; (iii) Brodie's abscess; (iv) Typhoid osteomyelitis; (v) Tuberculous osteomyelitis; (vi) Syphilitic osteitis; (vii) Pneumococcal osteomyelitis.

C. Developmental disorders
(i) Achondroplasia; (ii) Osteogenesis imperfecta (brittle bone); (iii) Mucopolysaccharide disorders: (a) Morquio-Brailford disease; (b) Hurler's disease; (c) Hunter's disease, etc.; (iv) Diaphyseal aclasis (Multiple exostoses); (v) Multiple chondromas (Ollier's disease); (vi) Marble

bones (osteopetrosis); (vii) Candle bones, spotted bones and striped bones; (viii) Cleidocranial dysostosis; (ix) Fibrous dysplasia.

D. Nutritional, metabolic and endocrine disorders
(i) Rickets; (ii) Osteomalacia; (iii) Scurvy; (iv) Hyperparathyroidism (Von-Recklinghausen's disease); (v) Osteoporosis.

E. Malformation syndromes
(i) Nail-Patella syndrome; (ii) Marfan's syndromes; (iii) Paget's disease (osteitis deformans).

F. Cyst
(i) Solitary cyst; (ii) Cyst associated with generalized osteitis fibrosa; (iii) Hydatid cyst; (iv) Aneurysmal bone cyst.

G. Tumors
(a) Benign tumors: (i) Osteoma; (ii) Osteochondroma; (iii) Osteoblastoma; (iv) Osteoid osteoma; (v) Chondroma; (vi) Chondroblastoma; (vii) Periosteal fibroma; (viii) Fibroma; (ix) Chondromyxoid fibroma; (x) Hemangioma; (xi) Lipoma; (xii) Neurofibroma.
(b) *Locally malignant:* Osteoclastoma (giant cell tumor).
(c) *Malignant: Primary*—(i) Osteosarcoma; (ii) Chondrosarcoma; (iii) Ewing's tumor; (iv) Multiple myeloma; (v) Reticulum cell sarcoma; (vi) Plasmacytoma; (vii) Fibrosarcoma; (viii) Liposarcoma; (ix) Angiosarcoma.

Secondary carcinoma of bone by (i) primary carcinomas metastasis from thyroid, bronchus, breast prostate, kidney, uterus, gastrointestinal tract, testis, etc.; or by (ii) direct infiltration from adjacent growth, e.g., carcinoma of the tongue involving the lower jaw.

DIFFERENTIAL DIAGNOSIS

Differential diagnosis of bone disorders

Category	Condition	Key features
Traumatic	Callus formation	History of fracture, irregular hard swelling
	Malunited fracture	Previous fracture, deformity, pain with stress
	Myositis ossificans	Follows trauma, calcified mass in muscle
Infectious	Acute osteomyelitis	High fever, localized tenderness, swelling, systemic toxemia
	Chronic osteomyelitis	Sinus formation, sequestrum on X-ray, recurrent infections
	Tuberculous osteomyelitis	Cold abscess, chronic course, joint involvement
Developmental	Achondroplasia	Short stature, disproportionate limb shortening
	Osteogenesis imperfecta	Brittle bones, blue sclera, multiple fractures
Metabolic	Rickets	Bowing of long bones, widened growth plates
	Osteomalacia	Bone pain, Looser's zones on X-ray
Neoplastic	Osteosarcoma	Aggressive growth, pain, Codman's triangle on X-ray

Contd...

Contd...

Category	Condition	Key features
	Chondrosarcoma	Slow-growing, calcifications, occurs in older adults
	Multiple myeloma	Bone pain, lytic lesions on X-ray, Bence Jones protein in urine
Cystic lesions	Bone cyst	Fluid-filled, metaphyseal, no sclerosis
	Aneurysmal bone cyst	Blood-filled cavities, soap-bubble appearance

ACUTE OSTEOMYELITIS

The patients are usually children and the bones are affected mainly in the metaphyseal region. Generally, the children of the first decade are involved by this disease and the incidence considerably comes down after the age of twelve. The symptoms and signs can be both local and general.

High pyrexia, intense toxemia with high pulse rate and leukocytosis are the general signs found in acute fulminating type of osteomyelitis. In chronic type, which is most common in the adult, there will be malaise, fever, headache and backache.

Locally there will be swelling, extreme tenderness, local erythema, limitation of joint movement and effusion of the nearest joint (10% of cases). Later on, subperiosteal pus may find its way superficially and then fluctuation test will be positive. In more chronic cases the pus will find its way out through a sinus and may lead to chronic osteomyelitis.

Polymorphonuclear leukocytosis is constant with raised ESR pus may be sent for culture and sensitivity tests. It must be emphasized that radiography, which plays an important role in the diagnosis of bone diseases, is practically valueless in the detection of early stage of this condition.

COMPLICATIONS: A. *General*: Toxemia and Septicemia. B. *Local*: (i) Suppurative arthritis when the metaphysis is included partly or wholly within the joint; (ii) Deformity—either shortening or lengthening of the limb due to destruction or better nourishment to the epiphyseal cartilage; (iii) Pathological dislocation when the joint is very much involved and destroyed.

This condition is mainly diagnosed on clinical examination. Superficial edema, localized swelling, temperature, extreme tenderness with general signs of toxemia will tell the diagnosis by themselves.

The clinician must *differentiate this condition from* (i) *Rheumatic fever,* in which the joint pain is flitting in nature and the tenderness is maximum at the joint line and (ii) *Acute suppurative arthritis* in which again tenderness is mostly found in the joint line with great effusion and tremendous pain affecting the joint.

CHRONIC OSTEOMYELITIS

This condition is actually an aftermath of acute osteomyelitis. A piece of bone becomes dead (sequestrum) and remains within the cavity which is formed by destruction of the bone due to the infection. This cavity is generally connected outside through a sinus. The cavity contains serous fluid and pus, which may be discharged through the sinus. The mouth of the sinus shows sprouting granulation tissue, which indicates presence of the sequestrum in the depth. On palpation, the bone becomes thick and irregular. X-ray shows areas of bony rarefaction surrounded by dense sclerosis and sometimes sequestrum within the cavity of the bone. In long standing cases amyloid degeneration may occur.

BRODIE'S ABSCESS

It is a localized form of infection, which is usually situated at the metaphysis of the long bone. This condition is usually caused by the Staphylococcus of low virulence. The patients are usually between 10 to 20 years of age. The most common sites are the upper end of the tibia, the lower end of the femur, the lower end of the tibia and the upper end of the humerus according to the frequency. This condition may remain silent for years or present with recurrent attacks of pain. During an attack the bone becomes tender with a little swelling. Typically, the pain becomes worse at night, but in some instances it is worse on walking and relieved by rest. Skiagram shows translucent area with a well defined margin and surrounding sclerosis, beyond which the bone looks normal.

TYPHOID OR PNEUMOCOCCAL OSTEOMYELITIS

This condition is very rare nowadays. It may occur during the later period of prolonged suffering from this disease or may even occur months or years after one has suffered from this disease. The disease runs a mild course with poor bone formation which is observed in X-ray. Diagnosis is mainly confirmed by clinical observations, but discovery of causative organisms in the pus collected by aspiration wipes away any suspicion about the diagnosis.

TUBERCULOUS OSTEOMYELITIS

This condition is also becoming rare day by day. The ends of the long bones and short bones of the hand and foot are usually affected. The onset is insidious and may remain silent. Swelling and pain of the affected area of the bone, sympathetic effusion of the neighboring joint, formation of the cold abscess and sinus with undermining edge are the clinical features of the condition. X-ray shows rarefaction of the affected bone with bone destruction, i.e., thinning and disappearance of the bony lamellae and cavity formation. Recalcification occurs at the healing stage.

SYPHILITIC OSTEOMYELITIS

It is another rare condition and manifestation of the tertiary stage of syphilis. Mainly the subcutaneous bones are affected, e.g., the tibia, sternum, clavicle, skull, ulna, etc. The pathology may be either diffuse periostitis or localized gumma. The patient experiences a deep boring pain particularly at night. The gumma may soften and break down to form a typical syphilitic ulcer. X-ray shows periosteal thickening or punched out translucent areas in the midst of dense sclerosis. The lesions are often multiple. Positive WR and Kahn tests reiterate the diagnosis.

Achondroplasia: This is an autosomal dominant inheritant disease. The cartilage cells produced by the epiphysis fail to line up properly and undergo degeneration. The individual becomes dwarf with normal intelligence and often with excellent muscles. The limbs are grossly short, particularly the proximal segments, so that the hands fail to reach the buttocks. The spinal canal becomes narrow. The X-ray shows relative shortness of the limb-bones. The metaphyses at the knee are splayed out. The pelvis is too small for normal delivery.

OSTEOGENESIS IMPERFECTA (BRITTLE BONES)

There are two types of this condition: (i) *Congenita* (of recessive inheritance)—reveals itself soon after birth with dwarfism, deformities and multiple fractures. (ii) *Tarda* (of dominant inheritance)—reveals itself later in life nearing puberty. Both these conditions present with broad skull (with Wormian bone), blue sclera, scoliosis, ligament laxity, coxa vara, knock knee, bowing of the femur and the tibia, etc. X-ray shows marked osteoporosis with cystic appearance. The shafts of the long bones are bent and slender. Multiple fractures are frequently associated with this condition which may lead to tremendous periosteal reaction with hyperplastic callus formation which may mimic a bone sarcoma.

MUCOPOLYSACCHARIDE DISORDERS

These include a group of conditions with inborn defects in mucopolysaccharide metabolism. Dwarfism is again the main feature of these conditions. The three common diseases which are included in these disorders are:
(i) Morquio-Brailsford disease, which is manifested by too flat vertebrae, grossly distorted hip, marked ligamentous laxity and presence of Keratan sulfate in urine.
(ii) Hurler's disease, which is manifested by early mental retardation, absence of ligament laxity, cardiopulmonary complications and presence of dermatan sulphate and heparan sulphate in urine.
(iii) Hunter's disease, which is a X-linked recessive inheritant disease, more or less similar to Hurler's disease in its manifestations.

MULTIPLE EXOSTOSES (DIAPHYSEAL ACLASIS)

This is an autosomal dominant inheritant disease with failure of bone remodeling, in which excess of the metaphyseal bone is not absorbed and forms irregular exostoses, Multiple lumps **(Fig. 11.5)** are found on the upper humerus, lower ends of the radius and ulna, around the knee joint, above the ankle and very occasionally on flat bones. Some deformities and complications may be expected from these exostoses. X-ray shows presence of sessile or pedunculated exostoses projecting from the surface.

MULTIPLE CHONDROMAS (OLLIER'S DISEASE)

This rare disease is not familial like the previous conditions. The main defect is the ossification of cartilage at the growth discs. One limb or even one bone may be involved in this condition. The affected limb becomes short. The fingers and toes frequently contain multiple enchondromata, which are characteristics of this condition. Malignant change may be seen in 1% of these chondromata. X-ray shows multiple translucent islands mainly in the metaphyses of the long bones and diaphyses of the short bones.

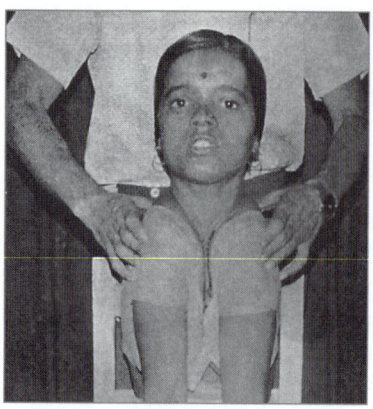
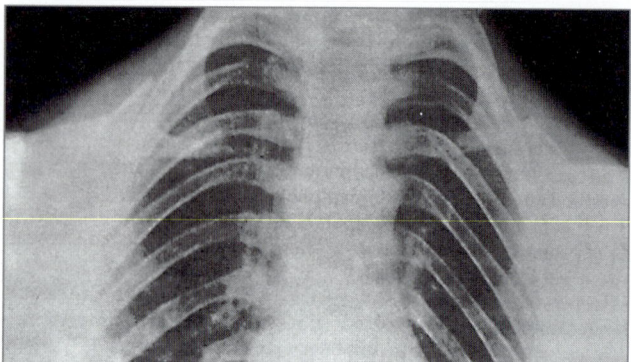

Fig. 11.20: Shows a typical case of cleido-cranial dysostosis. The shoulders can be easily brought in front of the chest.

Fig. 11.21: X-ray picture of the patient shown in Fig. 11.20. Note that the outer half of the clavicle has not been developed.

CLEIDOCRANIAL DYSOSTOSIS

This autosomal dominant inheritant condition mainly affects the membrane bones, chiefly the clavicles and the skull. The patient is somewhat short, with a large head and drooping shoulders. Because the clavicles are partly absent, the two shoulders of the patient can be brought in front of the chest **(Fig. 11.20)**. X-ray shows nondevelopment of outer half of each clavicle **(Fig. 11.21)**. Wormian bones may be present in the skull.

FIBROUS DYSPLASIAS (FIBROCYSTIC DISEASE)

It is the last and probably the most important in the group of developmental disorders. The condition may affect one bone (monostotic), one limb (monomelic) or many bones (polyostotic). A solitary bone cyst is most common. In all varieties the cellular fibrous tissue in the medullary cavity proliferates destroying the trabeculae; the bone may be expanded and the cortex may be eroded. The resulting cavities contain fluid or fibrous tissue and the walls contain giant cells.

Solitary cyst: This usually affects the upper humerus, femur or tibia, but may occur in other bones. Usually, the victims are children up to the age of puberty, after which this condition becomes increasingly rare. This disease presents with local pain, slight swelling with or without tenderness. Very rarely a pathological fracture may complicate this condition. X-ray shows a translucent area at the metaphysis. The bone becomes expanded and the cortex is thinned out. The cyst has a clear cut edge without any surrounding sclerosis.

Monostotic fibrous dysplasia: This rare condition occurs chiefly in adolescents and remains symptomless until the bone breaks. The lamellar pattern of the affected bone is replaced by multiple cysts and fibrous bands which may be calcified to give the X-ray appearance a mixture of "bubbles and stripes" **(Figs. 11.22A and B)**.

Polyostotic fibrous dysplasia: The long bones are generally affected either in one limb or in one half of the body or scattered throughout the skeleton. The patients present with deformity, irregular bony swellings, pain or fracture. X-ray shows cystic areas with patches of calcification in the shaft of the bone. The short bones may show uniform ground-glass appearance. The skull

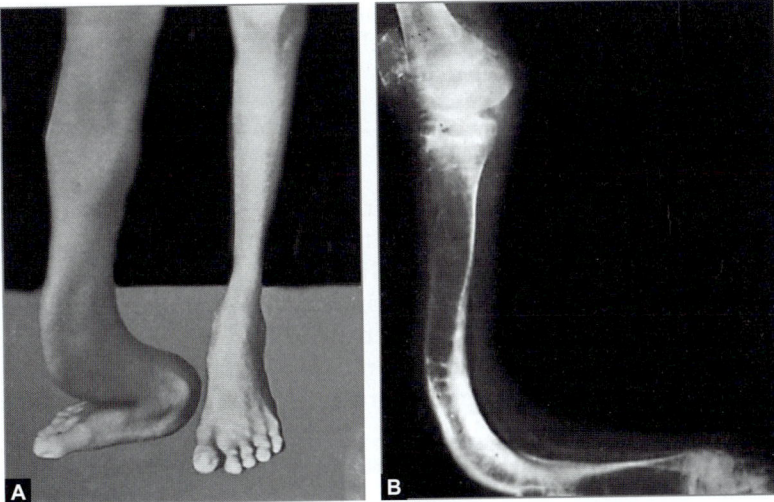

Figs. 11.22 A and B: (A) A typical case of monostotic fibrous dysplasia. (B) Note the presence of multiple cysts and fibrous bands to give the typical picture of bubbles and stripes.

may be irregularly thickened. Otherwise the bones are normal and not osteoporotic as seen in cases of hyperparathyroidism.

Albright's disease is a combination of polyostotic fibrous dysplasia, pigmentation in the skin and sexual precocity in girls.

RICKETS

This condition occurs due to insufficient vitamin D, which results from inadequate diet or insufficient exposure to sunlight. Because of lack of vitamin D, calcium and phosphorus absorption is reduced. Compensatory parathyroid secretion increases, calcium is not deposited in bones and may even be withdrawn. The growth disc produces abundant cartilage but this is not converted to bone. Growth becomes retarded and the soft bones bend. There are various types of rickets, of which the infantile ricket is most common.

Infantile ricket: This condition is common in infants below 4 years of age. The limbs show enlargement of the bone ends with deformities due to bending of the soft bones. The soft bones may crack by trivial injury. The skull is bossed ('Hot-cross-bun head'), dentition becomes delayed and the costochondral junctions are enlarged (rickety rosary). There may be kyphosis. X-ray shows general decalcification. The growth discs are too deep and the metaphyses are too wide.

Renal ricket: In this condition the kidneys are unable to excrete phosphorus properly due to developmental defect of the renal tubules or some organic disease affecting the kidney. The blood phosphate level increases and the excess phosphorus is excreted in the gut where it combines with calcium, so the serum calcium level falls and consequently excess of parathormone is secreted resulting in the rickety condition. Again the children are more often affected. They become dwarf and anemic. X-ray changes are similar to those of infantile rickets.

Renal tubule ricket: In this condition the glomeruli excrete phosphorus, but the tubules fail to reabsorb resulting in a fall in serum phosphorus level. Consequently serum calcium increases, calcium being withdrawn from the bones. The children become dwarf with polyuria. Presence of sugar, amino acid and cystine in the urine helps to make the diagnosis. X-ray changes are more or less similar to those of infantile ricket.

OSTEOMALACIA

This condition is the adult counterpart of the ricket. The bones lose calcium due to gross malnutrition either in pregnancy or after gastrectomy or after prolonged treatment with anticonvulsants. The patients present with general ache especially at the back. Muscle tenderness is common. Weakness is felt on walking for a distance and more so while climbing up the stairs. X-ray shows loss of bone density with characteristic bands of translucency, called Looser's zones, particularly seen in the upper humerus, femoral neck, ribs, pubis, etc. The serum alkaline phosphatase is increased and the serum phosphorus level becomes reduced. The sedimentation rate of the erythrocytes is also raised. Diagnosis becomes confirmed by generalized osteoporosis and may require bone biopsy which shows excessive uncalcified osteoid tissue.

HYPERPARATHYROIDISM (VON RECKLINGHAUSEN'S DISEASE)

In this condition, oversecretion of the parathormone is the main pathology commonly associated with parathyroid adenoma. The kidneys excrete excess phosphorus which lowers the serum phosphorus level. To restore the calcium-phosphorus balance, calcium is withdrawn from the bone raising the serum calcium level. This may lead to formation of renal calculi. Adults are mainly affected and women outnumber men in this condition. The patients present with aches all over which may make the patient bedridden. The bones may bend and fractures are not uncommon. X-ray shows osteoporosis with cystic changes in the medulla and the trabecular pattern becomes coarse. The skull becomes granular and ground-glass. Subperiosteal erosions of the cortex are common. In the hand, disappearance of the outline with presence of only longitudinal trabeculae in the phalanges, are the characteristic features.

OSTEOPOROSIS

This is the response of the bony skeleton to a variety of factors—(i) *Mechanical factors* are those of prolonged immobilization of the part concerned, anterior poliomyelitis, rheumatoid arthritis and paraplegia. (ii) *Nutritional factors* in the form of severe protein deficiency resulting from malnutrition or failure in absorption or abnormal protein excretion may lead to osteoporosis. Senile osteoporosis may be included in this group. Scurvy due to vitamin C deficiency is also an example of this group. (iii) *Endocrinal factors* include Cushing's syndrome, hyperparathyroidism, ovarian insufficiency which leads to postmenopausal osteoporosis, thyrotoxicosis, etc. (iv) *Miscellaneous* factors, which include myelomatosis, tumor invasion, etc.

Most of the patients, who present with osteoporosis, are included in the senile or postmenopausal group. The main complaints are general aches which are aggravated by movement or jarring. Sudden onset of pain with localized tenderness is suggestive of pathological fracture. Thoracic kyphosis is a common accompaniment of this condition. X-ray shows ground glass appearance with loss of definition of the trabeculae in the different bones. The vertebral bodies become flattened with increase in the intervertebral spaces. Varying degrees of collapse and wedging may be seen. Healing of the pathological fracture is usually accompanied by little callus formation. Biopsy may be taken by trephining the iliac crests or the spinous processes. This is significant so far as the diagnosis is concerned. This shows a reduction in the number and size of the trabeculae and in the number of osteoblasts present.

MARFAN'S SYNDROME

This is an autosomal dominant inheritant disorder with a defect in elastin or collagen formation or both. The patients are usually tall with scoliosis, the limbs are unduly long especially the distal segments. The fingers become long and narrow, which are called arachnodactyly (spider fingers). Other features include a high arched palate, presence of hernias, dislocation of ocular lens and aortic aneurysm. If this condition is associated with presence of homocysteine in the urine a condition called *"homocystineuria"* should be thought of. This condition is more or less similar to Marfan's syndrome except for the fact that this condition is of autosomal recessive inheritance.

PAGET'S DISEASE (OSTEITIS DEFORMANS)

The main pathology of this condition is high rates of bone resorption and formation. Resorption of the existing bone is brought about by the osteoclasts and bone formation is performed by the osteoblasts. The first stage is the vascular stage when the spaces left by bone absorption are filled with vascular fibrous tissue. On both sides of the cortex new osteoid tissue forms but this is not converted to mature bone, so the bone becomes thick but soft and bends under pressure. The second stage is the sclerotic stage in which the new lamellae are formed which become thick and sclerosed, so that the bone can be broken easily.

The disease is rare under the age of 40 and becomes progressively commoner as the age advances. Males are more often affected and even the disease may be localized to a part or whole of one bone for many years. The pelvis and the tibia are the most common sites. The femur, skull, spine and the clavicle are next involved. When a single bone is affected, the pain is the most important symptom. Its character is dull and constant ache, which becomes worse at night. The affected bone may be bent. Pain becomes severe when the condition is complicated by fracture or sarcoma. On palpation the bone feels thick and looks bent. The overlying skin becomes unduly warm. In case of generalized involvement, the patients present with headache, deafness, limb pain, pathological fractures, deformities and even heart failure. The skull enlarges and otosclerosis is the cause of deafness; occasionally pressure on the optic nerve may produce blindness. There is considerable kyphosis. Backache and root pain are not uncommon. A slight coxa vara may be expected with considerable anterolateral bowing of the legs.

X-ray shows that the bone involved becomes thick and bent. The normal clear line of demarcation between the cortex and the medullary cavity becomes blurred. The trabeculae are coarse and widely separated giving rise to a honeycomb appearance. In the vascular stage areas of osteoporosis may be expected in different parts of the cortex. Later on, the cortex becomes thick and the whole bone is bent. Fine subperiosteal cracks may be seen if carefully noted. In the special investigations, very high alkaline phosphatase and hydroxyproline in the plasma are noted features. Hydroxyproline is also excreted in the urine in high quantity. But the serum calcium and phosphorus levels remain within normal limits.

COMPLICATIONS include general and local complications. Of the *general complications,* high rate of cardiac failure, deafness, optic atrophy and paraplegia are worth mentioning. Of the *local complications* pathological fracture and osteosarcoma are very important. The frequency of osteosarcoma may vary from 1 to 10% (average is 5%). This condition is suspected if the patient already suffering from Paget's disease, complains of more pain, tenderness and swelling of a particular region. Osteosarcoma complicating Paget's disease is extremely malignant and death is almost invariable once this complication has developed. Pathological fractures complicating Paget's disease are common in the femur, of which subtrochanteric fracture is most common.

ANEURYSMAL BONE CYST

This is a lesion which contains cavities filled with blood. This condition is commonly seen in the ends of growing long bones. X-ray shows a rarefied area which may contain lamellae within it to give the appearance of a honeycomb. The lesion may expand to destroy the inner aspect of the cortex which becomes thin and may slightly bulge out. Pathological fracture may occasionally complicate this condition.

TUMORS

OSTEOMA

Two varieties of osteomas are commonly come across.

(i) **Cancellous osteoma (exostosis):** This is nothing but a conical lump of bone with a cap of cartilage which arises from the metaphysis of a long bone. It stops enlarging when the bone growth ceases. This condition mainly affects the adolescents. The presenting feature is a painless bony lump which gradually increases in size. Occasionally, it may interfere with the tendon action and may cause injury to a nerve giving rise to secondary symptoms. X-ray shows the exostosis obviously **(Fig. 11.23)**, whose medullary cavity and the cortex are continuous with those of the parent bone.

(ii) **Compact osteoma (ivory exostosis):** Generally, the membrane bones are affected and the tumor is sessile. The most common site is the outer surface of the skull; very occasionally this tumor may originate from the inner surface of the skull when it may give rise to focal epilepsy. Adolescents or young adults are again the common victims. The presenting symptom is the hard painless lump. X-ray shows a dense sessile well-circumscribed bulge from the involved bone.

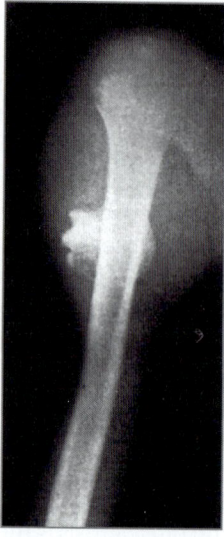

Fig. 11.23: Exostosis at the upper end of the humerus.

OSTEOID OSTEOMA

Usually, the boys of second decade are affected. Any bone except the skull may be affected, the commonest being the femur or the tibia. The only presenting symptom is the pain which is very rarely severe and is not relieved by rest. This boring pain may continue for many months before the patient comes to doctor. X-ray shows a small radiolucent area, which may or may not contain a tiny dense opacity (the nidus). There may be slight surrounding sclerosis which becomes obvious in lesions affecting the medullary cavity. This condition is difficult to differentiate from Brodie's abscess without biopsy.

CHONDROMA

This tumor is nothing but a lobulated mass of cartilage. The tumor may affect any bone, but most frequently the short long bones, e.g., the metacarpals, the phalanges and metatarsals. When this tumor remains entirely within the medullary cavity, the cortex is bulged out and thinned, it is called *enchondroma*. When this tumor protrudes on the surface it is called *ecchondroma*. The matrix of the tumor may be calcified or even ossified, when it is called *osteochondroma*. Enchondromas may be multiple but ecchondromas are generally solitary tumors. Malignant change, though rare, may be seen in multiple enchondromas.

FIBROMA

This tumor is an island of fibrous tissue in the bone. It is commonly seen in adolescents. X-ray shows an oval gap in the cortex of the metaphysis of a long bone.

CHONDROMYXOID FIBROMA

The patients are usually between 10 to 30 years of age. Lower limbs are mostly involved. The patients present with chronic boring pain. X-ray shows a round or oval radiolucent area in the metaphysis. Malignant change, though rare, has been recorded.

HEMANGIOMA

This condition is very rare in bone but may occasionally involve the spine.
The patients present with persistent backache. If it involves the long bones, it may cause elongation of the bone. X-ray shows radiolucent trabeculated tumors expanding the bone. Pathological fracture is not uncommon in this condition.

OSTEOCLASTOMA (GIANT CELL TUMOR)

This "treacherous" tumor mainly affects individuals between 20 and 40 years of age. It nearly always affects the very end of a long bone. The tumor probably originates from the metaphysis and very quickly destroys the epiphysis. This tumor most commonly affects the bones around the knee joint, but tumors of the radius, ulna, and humerus are not uncommon. The usual presenting symptom is vague discomfort with a swelling. A history of trauma is sometimes elicited, but this probably has only drawn attention of the patient towards the tumor. On palpation, egg-shell crackling may be elicited. X-ray shows a rarefied area towards the end of the long bone due to destruction of the bone by osteolytic process. The bone may be destroyed irregularly so that the tumor is traversed by remnants of the original bone which is heavily trabeculated. This gives rise to a typical 'soap-bubble' appearance in X-ray. So long the tumors remain benign, there is a sharp well-defined line of junction with the rest of the bone. As soon as the tumor becomes malignant, this delineation disappears. The cortex is sometimes destroyed or may be very thinned and ballooned. When becomes malignant this tumor shows a low grade malignancy. Metastasis may occur to the lungs via the bloodstream. More common is the recurrence following local removal. Such recurrences are more malignant than the original tumor.

OSTEOSARCOMA

This is a highly malignant tumor. The tumor originates from the medulla of the metaphysis. Gradually, the cortex is eroded and the periosteum is first pushed away from the shaft. At this time one may find "Codman's triangle" at the region where the periosteum is elevated from the bone and "Sunray spicules" due to new bone formation along the periosteal blood vessels. Eventually the periosteum is also penetrated and the soft tissues around the bone are involved. The tumor metastasis mainly through the bloodstream to the lungs and also to other bones commonly to skull, femur, pelvis, etc. The incidence of osteosarcoma is highest between the age of 10 to 20 years. Thereafter the incidence falls rapidly. The most common site is the metaphysis of the long bone and around the knee joint. A history of trauma may be present but this again has no relation with the etiology of the condition. Pain is usually the first symptom which is followed very soon by a swelling. Pain is of constant boring nature, which becomes worse at night and gradually becomes severe as the tumor grows rapidly. The overlying skin becomes shiny with prominent veins. The lump feels warm and tender and lacks a definite edge. Varying consistency may be felt in different regions of the tumor. Sometimes the tumor may be pulsatile. This is called "telangiectatic osteosarcoma". X-ray shows area of rarefaction in the medulla with bone formation in the form of sunray spicules, Codman's triangle, etc. A definite opacity may be noticed along the extent of the tumor even in the soft tissues.

Old people may suffer from osteosarcoma but this is mostly a complication of Paget's disease.

CHONDROSARCOMA

In this condition cartilage cells predominate. A true chondrosarcoma affects people between the ages of 35 and 50 years. It may arise in any bone with a predilection towards the flat bones, such as ilium and ribs etc. The presenting symptom is again a constant ache with a swelling which has very recently increased in size. X-ray appearances are variable but mostly osteolytic. This tumor is slightly less malignant than the previous one. It also metastasizes mainly through blood vessels.`

FIBROSARCOMA

This tumor contains spindle-shaped fibroblasts. It may originate in the medullary cavity or periosteally (when it is called periosteal fibrosarcoma). The patients are usually 30 to 50 years of age and present with pain, swelling and even pathological fractures. X-ray shows an osteolytic lesion which may be surrounded by reactive subperiosteal new bone. This also produces blood-borne pulmonary metastasis.

SYNOVIAL SARCOMA

This condition may affect individual of any age. This tumor usually arises close to a major joint either the knee or the ankle or the wrist. But it may occasionally occur in connective tissue or muscle. Metastasis occurs by blood, the lymphatics and by migration of cells through the tissue planes. Microscopically, it is a tumor, composed of both synovial cells and malignant fibroblasts. This tumor is extremely malignant.

EWING'S TUMOR

This tumor arises from the reticulum cells of the medullary cavity of the diaphysis of the long bones. The tumor gradually lifts the periosteum, which appears to resist the spread of the tumor and may lay down layers of bone formation giving rise to an onion-like appearance in X-ray. Distant spread is mainly via the bloodstream to the lungs also to other bones. Lymphatic spread is rare.

The tumor mainly affects the young between 10 and 20 years of age. Long bones are mainly affected of which the tibia is most common. The patients present with the pain, which is of throbbing nature and becomes worse at night. A history of trauma may be present. The patient is sometimes ill with fever which makes this tumor so often mistaken for osteomyelitis. The swelling is warm and tender and has an ill-defined margin. X-ray appearances are a rarefied area in the medulla, the cortex may be perforated and there may be the onion layers of calcification. That the tumor melts by radiotherapy as the snow in sunshine is the pathognomonic feature of this condition.

MULTIPLE MYELOMA

The tumor arises from the plasma cells of the bone marrow. The tumors are found wherever there is red marrow in the bone, e.g., the skull, the trunk bones and the ends of the longs bones. The tumor is usually multiple.

Mostly individuals between 45 to 65 years of age are affected. The patients present with bone pain, which is root pain from collapse of a vertebra and occasionally nephritis contribute to the general ill-health of the patient. X-ray shows multiple small areas of rarefaction in the affected bones which are usually osteoporotic.

Special investigations of the urine will show the presence of Bence Jones protein in 50% of cases. Electrophoretic analysis of the plasma and urine will show presence of excessive protein mostly albumin. Sternal marrow puncture will reveal typical myeloma cells. High erythrocyte sedimentation rate is also a feature of this condition. As the disease advances, general lymphadenopathy together with enlargement of the liver and spleen and bleeding tendency with epistaxis, hemoptysis or hematemesis may be found.

PLASMACYTOMA

This is an example of solitary myeloma. The patient presents with pain, swelling or a pathological fracture. Radiologically, an area of translucency at the tumor site may be observed.

SECONDARY CARCINOMA OF BONE

Bony metastasis mainly occur by blood streams and the primary sites are mainly the thyroid, breast, the prostate, kidney, bronchus, uterus, GI tract and testis. About 2/3rd of cases of secondary bone deposits, the primary is seen either in the breast or in the prostate. The bones, commonly affected, are the vertebrae, ribs, sternum, pelvis and upper ends of the humerus and femur. The patients are usually more than 40 years of age. The patients present either with mild bony pain, backache or root pain or even pathological fracture. X-ray may show either osteolytic (when the primary carcinoma is in any viscus other than prostate) or osteoblastic (when the primary carcinoma is in the prostate) lesion. Bone scan shows the metastatic lesion much earlier than the skiagraphy **(Figs. 11.24A and B)**.

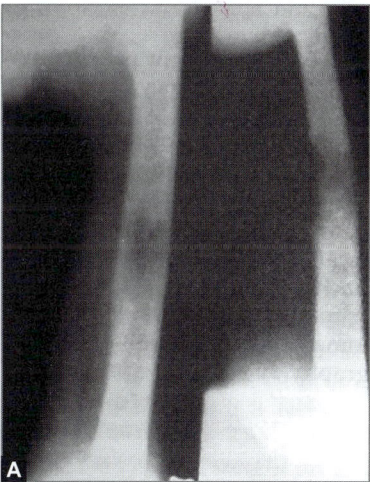 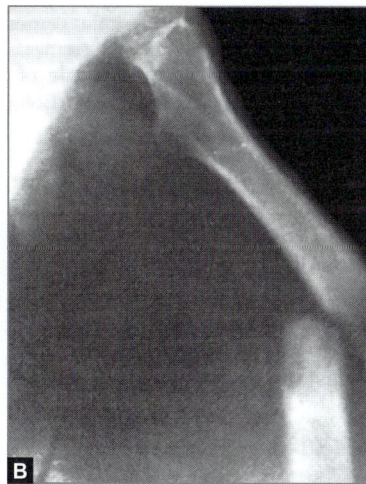

Figs. 11.24A and B: (A and B) A typical case of osteolytic lesion of secondary carcinoma affecting the shaft of femur: (A) The bone is not yet fractured and in the; (B) A few weeks shows that the femur is fractured.

Algorithmic Approach to Patient with of Bone Lesions

Patient presents with bone pain, swelling, or deformity

↓

Is the swelling fixed to bone?
- Yes → Suggests **bone lesion (tumor, infection, cyst)**
- No → Suggests **soft tissue mass (lipoma, ganglion cyst, hematoma)**

↓

Is the pain acute or chronic?
- Acute → Suggests **trauma, fracture, or infection (acute osteomyelitis, septic arthritis)**
- Chronic → Suggests **bone tumor, bone cyst, or metabolic bone disease (paget's, osteomalacia)**

↓

Are there systemic symptoms (fever, weight loss, night sweats)?
- Yes → Consider **infection (osteomyelitis, tuberculosis) or malignancy (osteosarcoma, multiple myeloma, metastases)**
- No → More likely **benign tumor (osteoid osteoma, chondroma) or cyst (aneurysmal bone cyst, solitary bone cyst)**

↓

Perform X-ray imaging to characterize the lesion
- Osteolytic lesion (bone destruction) → Consider **multiple myeloma, osteosarcoma, metastatic carcinoma**
- Osteoblastic lesion (bone formation) → Consider **prostate cancer metastasis, osteoid osteoma, paget's disease**

↓

Is the lesion well-demarcated or ill-defined?
- Well-demarcated → Suggests **benign lesion (bone cyst, osteochondroma, enchondroma)**
- Ill-defined with periosteal reaction → Suggests **malignancy (osteosarcoma, ewing's tumor)**

↓

Perform biopsy to confirm diagnosis
- Histopathology to differentiate benign vs malignant lesions
- Bacteriological culture if infection suspected

↓

Confirm diagnosis and initiate treatment
- **Conservative management:** Benign bone tumors, nonsurgical cases
- **Surgical management:** Tumor excision, curettage for cysts, amputation in malignancies
- **Oncologic treatment:** Radiotherapy and chemotherapy for malignant tumors

Examination of Bone and Joint Injuries

CHAPTER 12

HISTORY

1. **Age:** Epiphyseal separation is only seen in children before the epiphysis unites. Greenstick fracture is also common in children. Dislocation is common in adults. Fractures may occur at any age.
2. **The amount and nature of violence:** The clinician must enquire about the details of the accident—'how did it occur?' 'what was the mechanism of force?' and 'how forceful was the injury?' If the violence is not severe enough to cause fracture, one should suspect that the bone was diseased before and this type of fracture is called ***pathological fracture***. The causes which may lead to pathological fracture are discussed later in this chapter. At the present moment the students should remember that a trivial fall in old subjects may cause fracture of the femoral neck due to senile osteoporosis, similarly subtrochanteric fracture may result from Paget's disease or femoral shaft fracture may be due to secondary carcinoma.

    The nature of violence, which may cause a fracture, may be of three types—(1) direct, (2) indirect and (3) muscular.
    - **Direct** violence may be of (i) *tapping* in nature which will cause a transverse fracture with minimum skin damage or (ii) *crushing* in nature in which there will be multiple fragments which is known as 'comminuted fracture' and a good amount of soft tissue injury.
    - **Indirect** violence may be of: (i) *twisting* in nature which will lead to a spiral fracture, (ii) *bending force* which will lead to a transverse or oblique fracture, (iii) *a bending force with axial compression* leading to double oblique fractures with separation of a 'butterfly' fragment and (iv) a combination of twisting, angulation and axial compression will cause a short oblique fracture.
    - **Muscular** violence, in which the muscle contracts against resistance, may lead to a fracture which is come across in case of patella, olecranon and lesser trochanter of the femur.

    Sometimes there is no history of one severe violence but the bone is fractured. This is most commonly seen in the neck of the second metatarsal bone and due to repeated stress as for example when a soldier marches for a long distance or unaccustomed repeated stress. This is known as 'march fracture'.
3. **Pain:** It is interesting to note that in case of fracture pain is felt only during movement of the fractured site. In contradistinction to the common belief, a fracture is less painful than a sprain or a strain. Pain is the least in impacted and greenstick fractures. In dislocation, pain is constant and unbearable till it is reduced.
4. **Loss of function:** The patient will obviously be unable to move the fractured limb due to pain. He cannot put weight on it. In case of dislocation the patient is unable to move the joint even slightly.

5. **Deformity or swelling:** A fracture or a dislocation often presents with a swelling or deformity. Sometimes a swelling from hematoma or callus may attract the attention of the patient, which may be the sequel of fracture. This is commonly seen in march fracture.

History in fracture cases

Aspect	Clinical significance	Patient-friendly questions
Age of onset	Helps identify fracture risk factors (e.g., Greenstick fractures in children, hip fractures in elderly)	"How old are you? Have you had fractures before?"
Nature of trauma	Identifies type of injury (high vs. low energy)	"How did the injury happen? Was it a fall or a direct hit?"
Pain characteristics	**Fracture** → Pain increases with movement, **Dislocation** → Severe and constant	"Is your pain worse when moving, or is it there all the time?"
Loss of function	**Fracture** → Movement painful but possible, **Dislocation** → Movement impossible	"Can you move the limb at all?"
Swelling and deformity	Indicates fracture displacement or joint injury	"Have you noticed any abnormal swelling or changes in shape?"
History of previous injury	Recurrence common in ligament injuries	"Have you injured this joint before?"
Systemic symptoms	Fever → Infection (osteomyelitis, septic arthritis)	"Do you have fever or chills?"

■ LOCAL EXAMINATION

The injured side should always be compared with the sound side.

A. INSPECTION

1. **Abnormal swelling and deformity:** In fracture the first thing which attracts the clinician's eye is the deformity and/or swelling. The deformity is mostly due to displaced fractured segments and the swelling is mostly due to hematoma and edema. If the fracture is very near a joint, effusion will lead to an obvious swelling.

   In dislocation again the deformity is the main feature in inspection which often by itself indicates the diagnosis.

2. **Attitude:** In certain fractures the patients adopt particular attitudes which are very diagnostic. As for example in fracture neck of femur the patient lies helpless with the lower limb externally rotated. In posterior dislocation of the hip the thigh assumes the attitude of flexion, adduction and internal rotation. These are elaborately described under 'Examination of injuries about individual joints'.

3. **Shortening:** A little amount of shortening is almost always expected in fractures due to overlapping of the segments. This is more obvious in case of lower limb than in case of upper limb.

4. **Overlying skin:** This is an important point in inspection of a case of fracture. If there is a wound which communicates with the fracture site, the fracture is said to be *compound* or *open* and it runs the risk of being infected. Wound must be carefully inspected to know its size and actual depth. In gas gangrene the muscle may peep out through the wound which will be brick red, green or black in color, there will be serosanguineous discharge and the characteristic odor. In *simple* or *closed* fracture the skin is intact. Edema, blebs and bullae are quite common due to interference with venous return. Ecchymosis also appears within a few days after a fracture or dislocation.

B. PALPATION

Before palpation is actually started the patient should be asked to point out the site of injury. This will reduce beating about the bush, unnecessary discomfort to the patient and will definitely save time. It has got another greater advantage of not missing any injury.

1. **Tenderness:** Local *bony* tenderness is a valuable sign of a fracture. This tenderness should be elicited in relation with the bone and not with the soft tissue. So palpation to elicit tenderness should be made through a healthy soft tissue, otherwise damaged soft tissue will mislead the clinician by its own tenderness. Bony tenderness due to fracture is called local bony tenderness. All throughout the length, the bone is palpated through comparatively healthy tissue. In joint injuries a careful examination should be made to elicit the maximum point of tenderness to know which structure is affected. As for example tenderness on the medial side of the medial condyle of the femur means the upper attachment of the tibial collateral ligament of the knee joint has been sprained. Similarly tenderness on the attachment of the anterior horn of the medial meniscus of the knee joint along with other definite signs indicate torn medial semilunar cartilage. Sometime a joint has to be moved in different directions to elicit tenderness by passive stretching of the injured ligament. This is also a sign of sprain.
2. **Bony irregularity:** The whole length of the injured bone should be palpated to note if there is any irregularity such as a sharp elevation, a gap, etc. This is a definite sign of a fracture.
3. **Abnormal movements:** This is also a definite sign of fracture and can be elicited by moving one fragment against the other. Utmost gentleness is expected from the clinician while eliciting this physical sign. In fact it should be used only to exclude the presence of a fracture. This physical sign is however necessary in old fractures to know if they have been united or not.
4. **Crepitus:** It is a sensation of grating which may be felt or heard, when the bone ends are moved against each other. It should never be sought deliberately since its demonstration adds nothing to the diagnosis and nearly always causes pain. The students should remember the other conditions which may produce crepitus to avoid fallacy. These are hematoma, surgical emphysema, gas gangrene, osteoarthritis, tenosynovitis and Charcot's joint.
5. **Pain elicited by manipulation from a distance:** This is sometimes required to find out the possibility of a fracture. It may be done (a) by *rotating* the bone in case of humerus or the femur, (b) by *squeezing* both the bones of the leg or the forearm, which is popularly known as "springing" of the fibula or the radius, (c) by making *axial pressure* in the line of the bone as can be applied in case of metacarpals or metatarsals.
6. **Absence of transmitted movements:** When the continuity of the bone is broken, transmitted movement will obviously be absent. This can be tested by rotating humerus or femur with flexed elbow or knee respectively and by palpating the tubercle of the humerus or the trochanter of the femur with another hand.
7. **Swelling:** If there is a swelling its characteristic should be noted—whether it is a bony swelling or a swelling arises from the neighboring joint. A bony swelling may be either a displaced

fragment of a fracture or the callus or the articulate end of the bone of a dislocated joint. A swelling of the joint is mainly due to effusion.

8. **Wound:** Under aseptic ritual the wound should be explored to note the position of the broken fragments, the presence of a foreign body and the color of the muscles to exclude any possibility of gas gangrene. The neighboring muscles and the subcutaneous tissue of the wound are also palpated to exclude the presence of surgical emphysema which is a sign of gas gangrene.

C. MEASUREMENT

In examination of bone injuries two types of measurement should be taken—(i) longitudinal, to know if there is any shortening and (ii) circumferential, to know if there is any wasting due to injury.

(i) **Longitudinal:** Before taking measurement of the affected limb, the clinician must make sure that there was no pre-existing shortening of the limb. *While taking measurement, the sound limb should be kept in the same position as the affected limb.* If this simple instruction is not remembered there may be a great difference in measurements in different positions of the limb. The bony points, which are considered in measurement, should be marked with skin pencil before the use of measuring tape. *It is always a good practice to measure the healthy limb first.*

(ii) **Measurement of the circumference of the limb:** It takes sometimes for muscular wasting to develop after a bone or joint injury. While measuring the circumference of the limb two things should be borne in mind—(a) the healthy limb should be measured first and (b) the measurements should be made at the same level in both the limbs.

D. MOVEMENTS

Both active and passive movements should be tested. When the diagnosis is already established this part of the examination should be omitted as this will not give any additional information but will simply hurt the patient. This examination is more essential to exclude any bone or joint injury than anything else. Good active and passive movements mean there is no bone or joint injury. In dislocation of a joint both active and passive movements become nil and an abnormal rigidity with elastic recoil is encountered with any attempt to passive movements.

Stiffness of the joint is a complication of the fracture and may be due to—(i) intra-articular and periarticular adhesions, (ii) myositis ossificans, (iii) Sudeck's osteodystrophy and (iv) muscular adhesion which leads to inability of the muscle to lengthen during movement—as is seen most commonly after fracture of the shaft of the femur where quadriceps muscles are affected by adhesion and prevent flexion of the knee joint.

E. COMPLICATIONS

These are elaborately discussed in later part of this chapter. At this stage it will be sufficient to mention that one should exclude any other associated injury which may be accompanied with bone or joint injury. These are injury to the nerve, injury to the blood vessels and injury to the internal organs within the thorax or abdomen which is more dreadful and may be fatal.

GENERAL EXAMINATIONS

Look for evidence of shock. This is mainly due to good amount of blood loss in major fractures. Some amount of neurogenic shock may be associated with this.

It is of immense importance to exclude any other injury which may be associated with the bone or joint injury. In this context one must remember that thoracic and abdominal injuries, which tend to be overlooked, are more dangerous.

When a **pathological fracture** is suspected, an attempt should be made to know the cause of the pathological fracture. In this respect **age** of the patient is an important guide. *In infants,* multiple fractures may be seen in cases of osteogenesis imperfecta (brittle bones), which is characterized by dwarfism, broad skull, blue sclera, scoliosis, ligament laxity, otosclerosis (although deafness may not appear until adult life) and various deformities. Marble bones (osteopetrosis) are also brittle and fracture easily at this age. *In children,* acute osteomyelitis and solitary bone cysts are usually the causes. *In young adults,* osteoclastoma and osteosarcoma are responsible. *In adults,* generalized fibrocystic disease (hyperparathyroidism) and multiple myeloma are the causes of multiple fractures. *In the elderly,* besides senile osteoporosis, Paget's disease and secondary carcinoma are the main causes. In case of secondary carcinoma a thorough search should be made to get at the primary focus either in the breast or thyroid or bronchus or kidney or prostate, etc.

SPECIAL INVESTIGATIONS

1. **X-ray examination:** This is by far the most important investigation so far as the bone and joint injuries are concerned. At least two views *anteroposterior* and *lateral* should be taken to determine which bone has been fractured, the line of fracture and the type of displacement. Two views are essential to note exactly the above points. The anteroposterior view shows sidewise displacement—external or internal whereas the lateral view reveals anterior or posterior displacement. The three points are mainly noted while reading X-ray plate: (i) *Situation*—which bone is broken and which part of it? Whether any other bone has been fractured or not? Has the fracture involved the joint surface? (ii) *Line of fracture:* It may be transverse or small oblique or spiral or double oblique with a butterfly segment, etc. A careful assessment of the line of fracture is very important to know the mechanism of the injury and the treatment to be instituted. *(iii) Displacement:* It is best described by three components—(a) *shift* forwards, backwards or sideways. There may not be any shift as the fragments may be impacted or overlap each other. (b) *Tilt*—may be again forwards, backwards and sideways. (c) *Twist* (rotation) which may be in any direction.

Sometimes X-ray picture should be taken from different positions to locate the sites of fracture which are difficult to be revealed in classical anteroposterior and the lateral views **(Figs. 12.1 and 12.2)**. These are *oblique view* in scaphoid fracture, *stereoscopic views* in fracture of the skull and pelvis, *special axial radiograph* in fracture of the calcaneum.

In skiagram, one should look for any pathology in the bone which may be the cause of fracture.

In old fractures, one should look for the following points—(i) Signs of union—callus formation which appears in X-ray as early as on the tenth day after fracture. Consolidation and bone remodeling take quite a long time and one should not wait

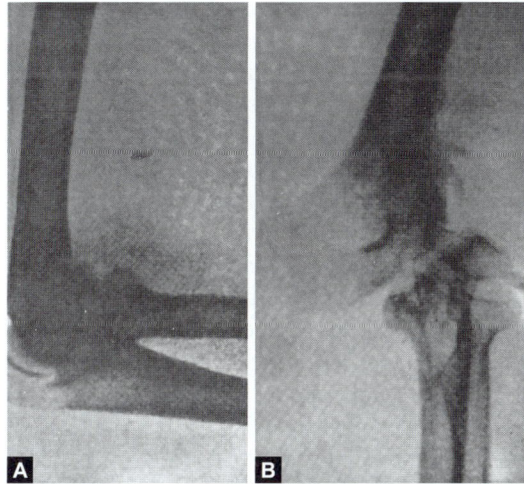

Figs. 12.1A and B: Showing the importance of taking two views. Note that there is hardly any evidence of fracture in the lateral view, but the anteroposterior view reveals fracture dislocation with considerable displacement.

for these signs as the signs of union. In fact union occurs long before these signs develop and clinical test is better evidence of union than the radiological evidence. If there is no local tenderness at the site of fracture and attempt at abnormal movement between the fracture fragments fails to produce any pain or movement, it should be taken into granted that the fracture has been united (clinically) though X-ray shows a small gap between the fragments. (ii) *Sclerosis at the fractured ends with a gap in between them* indicates non-union and differentiates it from the delayed union. (iii) Myositis ossificans traumatica (*see* **Fig. 13.19**). (iv) Avascular necrosis, etc.

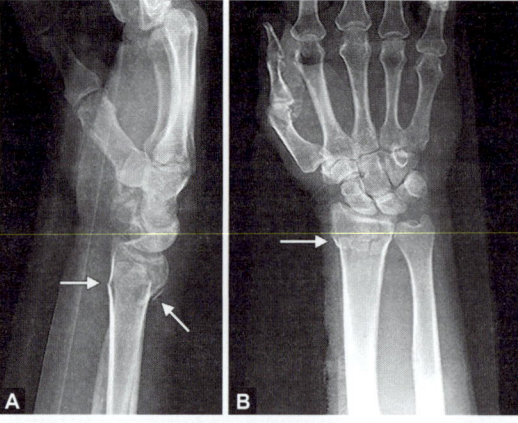

Figs. 12.2 A and B: Show the lateral and anteroposterior views of a typical Colles' fracture. Note that the lower fragment is shifted upwards, slightly laterally and tilted posteriorly.

2. **Serum:** Calcium should be estimated when there is a slightest doubt about the possibility of hyperparathyroidism . Alkaline phosphatase will be high in Paget's disease. Acid-phosphatase is high in bony metastasis from carcinoma of prostate.

3. **Urine:** In multiple myeloma, presence of Bence Jones proteins can be demonstrated by heating the urine. Hydroxyproline excretion in urine will be high in Paget's disease.

4. **Bone scan:** Skeletal scanning with a variety of bone-seeking isotopes has been used in clinical practice and it is now well established that when properly applied this technique is more effective than skeletal X-rays in delineating focal bone diseases, especially metastasis. The increased blood flow and increased osteoid tissue formation, which are the processes of tumor-cell invasion, can be demonstrated by locally increased concentration of the gamma-emitting radioisotope. The increased radioactivity is displayed either as a number of counts on a scaler or pictorially as a "hot-spot" on a scintiscan. Infrequently, in case of very anaplastic carcinoma, indolent tumors such as thyroid cancer or some cases of myeloma, there may be little or no "hot-spot" seen.

Many radioisotopes have been used for bone scanning. Of these strontium (85 Sr.), which is taken up by bone in a similar manner as calcium and which is a pure gamma emitter and more recently radioactive technitium ($^{99}Tc^m$) have become popular. Scanning is performed 1 to 4 hours after the intravenous injection of 5 to 10 mCi of $^{99}Tc^m$-phosphate complex. The bladder must be emptied before the pelvis is scanned as about 40% of the injected dose is excreted through the urine within first 4 hours after injection and pelvic lesions are liable to be obscured by overlying bladder activity.

It should be remembered that the simple radiograph shows no abnormality until more than 50% of bone mineral has been destroyed and obvious metastasis may be present even in the absence of X-ray changes. 24% of preoperative patients with clinically and radiologically early disease have metastases demonstrable by scanning. Bony metastasis from cancer of prostate may be present despite normal acid and alkaline phosphatase levels. Bone scan sometimes demonstrates "silent" metastasis which has produced fracture, which was initially thought to be simple.

Bone scan may be usefully employed in the study of nonmalignant conditions, e.g., abscesses, aseptic necrosis, Paget's disease and arthropathies.

5. **Arthroscopy** is extremely helpful to detect joint injuries and particularly the semilunar cartilage (meniscus) injuries of the knee.

6. **Arthrography** with opaque contrast medium (Conray, urografin, etc.), gas or both (double contrast) is helpful to detect precisely the internal structure damage in injuries particularly of the knee joint.

DIAGNOSIS

FRACTURE

Diagnosis is made by: (i) history of trauma, (ii) localized pain, (iii) swelling and deformity, (iv) local bony tenderness, (v) local bony irregularity, (vi) crepitus and (vii) X-ray. Of the above symptoms and signs local bony tenderness, local bony irregularity, crepitus and X-ray are the most important points to be remembered.

Types of fracture

Type	Description	Examples
Closed fracture	Skin intact over fracture	Colles' fracture, tibial shaft fracture
Open (compound) fracture	Fracture communicates with skin	Open tibial fracture
Transverse fracture	Perpendicular to bone axis	Direct blow injuries
Oblique fracture	Angled across bone	Fall on outstretched hand
Spiral fracture	Twisting force	Skiing injuries
Comminuted fracture	Multiple bone fragments	High-velocity trauma
Greenstick fracture	Incomplete fracture in children	Pediatric long bone fractures
Impacted fracture	Bone fragments driven into each other	Femoral neck fracture

DISLOCATION

This is a condition in which one bony component loses its contact completely with the other bony component of the joint. If it retains partial contact, the term subluxation is applied. Dislocation is diagnosed by: (i) the deformity, (ii) abnormal swelling near a joint, (iii) rigidity of the joint in passive movements and X-ray.

SPRAIN

It means ligamentous injury. This condition gives rise to tremendous pain. Diagnosis is made by: (i) presence of tenderness on the ligament particularly at its bony attachment, (ii) passive stretching of the ligament will cause excruciating pain, (iii) there is no local bony tenderness or local bony irregularity and (iv) X-ray shows no bony injury.

COMPLICATIONS OF FRACTURES AND DISLOCATIONS

GENERAL COMPLICATIONS

Shock, venous thrombosis and pulmonary embolism, fat embolism, 'fracture fever', delirium tremens following alcoholism, accident neurosis, hypostatic pneumonia and tetanus in compound fracture.

Complications of fractures and dislocations

Category	Complication	Clinical significance
General	Shock	Blood loss in major fractures (pelvic fracture)
	Fat embolism	Risk in long bone fractures
	Deep vein thrombosis	Prolonged immobilization increases risk
Local—immediate	Nerve injury	Axillary nerve (shoulder dislocation), radial nerve (humerus fracture)
	Vascular injury	Brachial artery (supracondylar humerus fracture)
	Soft tissue injury	Muscle entrapment in fractures
Local—late	Nonunion	Failure of fracture healing
	Malunion	Improper healing leading to deformity
	Avascular necrosis	Femoral head (neck fracture), scaphoid bone
	Joint stiffness	Postfracture immobilization

LOCAL COMPLICATIONS

These can be classified into: (A) *recent complications,* e.g., injury to the neighboring joint, nerve, blood vessels, muscles or tendons, viscera of the abdomen or thorax and infections in compound fracture; and (B) *late complications,* e.g., delayed union, non-union, malunion, avascular necrosis. Volkmann's ischemic contracture, myositis ossificans traumatica, joint instability and stiffness.

1. **Joint injury:** Dislocation, subluxation and/or ligamentous injury of the neighboring joint may be associated with the fracture.

2. **Nerve injury:** This should be diagnosed at the time of injury to the bone. Usually, the lesion is a neuropraxia which heals automatically. Sometimes severe traction on the nerve during injury or during overzealous manipulation may lead to axonotmesis. Neurotmesis is hardly associated with closed fractures.

   Immediate nerve injuries which are seen with different bone and joint injuries are—
   (i) The spinal cord or cauda equina injury in fracture-dislocation of the spine,
   (ii) The axillary nerve in shoulder dislocation or fracture neck of the humerus,
   (iii) The radial nerve in fracture shaft of the humerus,
   (iv) Ulnar, median and/or radial nerve in supracondylar fracture of the humerus,
   (v) Sciatic nerve in posterior dislocation of the hip and subtrochanteric fracture of the femur and
   (vi) The common peroneal nerve in fracture of the neck of the fibula.

   Late nerve injury is sometimes seen as a late complication of fracture. The most common example is the "tardy ulnar palsy" in supracondylar fracture of the humerus which has been malunited with cubitus valgus deformity and in fracture of the medial epicondyle of the humerus where the ulnar nerve is involved in callus and gradual injury to the nerve by bony irregularity if anterior transposition of the ulnar nerve has not been performed.

3. **Injury to blood vessels:** The blood vessels that are likely to be damaged in different fractures and dislocations are: (i) the middle meningeal vessels in fracture of the skull, (ii) the brachial

artery in supracondylar fracture of the humerus and (iii) the popliteal artery in supracondylar fracture of the femur. Mostly the vessels are either thrombosed or occluded by spasm or edema. Sometimes they are pressed upon by the displaced fragment and very rarely they are completely divided. Impairment of circulation following fracture or dislocation should be diagnosed as early as possible. If the impairment is due to displaced fragment, prompt reduction of the fracture or dislocation should be called for. Sometimes the impairment of circulation is due to incorrect application of plaster of Paris and these cases should be treated by immediate removal of the plaster and bandages till the pulsation of the artery comes back. If these procedures fail to bring about improvement in circulation, there is a place for immediate arteriography with a view to possible excision and grafting.

Vascular injury may lead to gangrene in severe cases and late ischemic contracture of muscles in less severe cases.

4. **Muscle complications:** The adjoining muscle fibers are often *torn* in fracture. The torn fibers may become adherent to the intact fibers, fractured site or capsule of the neighboring joint. This may lead to stiffness of the joint and may require lengthy rehabilitation after the fracture has been consolidated. So every attempt should be made to keep the muscles active when the fracture is kept immobilized.

Another complication of the muscle following fracture is *disuse atrophy.* Active movement is again the treatment of this condition.

5. **Tendon complications:** *A torn tendon* is rare in association with closed fracture. It is seen in fracture of patella where the tendinous expansion of the quadriceps tendon is torn.

Late rupture of tendon is sometimes seen in certain fractures, e.g., the extensor pollicis longus tendon in fracture of the lower end of the radius and the long head of the biceps in fracture neck of the humerus.

Tendinitis is a very rare complication of a fracture and occasionally affect the tibialis posterior tendon following fracture of the medial malleolus.

6. **Injury to viscera:** Injury to internal organs are often seen in various fractures of bones lying near to them. Such examples are injury to the urinary bladder and urethra in fracture of the pelvis, rectum in the fracture of the sacrum, lung, liver or spleen in fracture of the ribs and the brain in fracture of the skull.

7. **Infection:** This is quite common in compound fracture and a dreadful complication of the fracture. It may give rise to osteomyelitis with formation of sequestrum and sometimes absorption of bone overwhelms leading to disappearance of some part of the bone. However simple may be the infection, nonunion may be the sequel. The most dreadful complications of a compound fracture are the gas gangrene and tetanus.

8. **Delayed union:** The students must have clear conception about what is meant by the term "delayed union". When a fracture takes an unduly longer time than is expected for union of the particular fracture, the term 'delayed union' is used.

The causes are: (i) inadequate immobilization; (ii) internal fixation which always delays union as the hematoma between the fracture ends which acts as a scaffold for union is disturbed and because the periosteum is stripped off and (iii) intact fellow bone—when one bone of the forearm or the leg remains unbroken, the fractured bone always takes longer time for union.

9. **Nonunion:** The term "non-union" means bony union of the fracture is not possible without operative intervention. The fragments are joined by fibrous tissue. To know whether the fracture

concerned is a case of delayed union or nonunion, X-ray is very much essential. In nonunion there will be presence *of sclerosis* at the bone ends and a gap between them.

Causes of nonunion are: (i) infection; (ii) interposition of soft tissue either periosteum or muscle between the bone ends; (iii) inadequate blood supply, e.g., fracture of lower half of tibia; (iv) wide separation of fragments, e.g., fracture of patella, fracture of the olecranon process or excessive traction; (v) inadequate treatment of delayed union that means adequate immobilization for a long period was not maintained in a case of delayed union.

10. **Malunion:** This means union of fragments in a defective position. Most common deformity is angulation, besides this there may be overlapping with shortening and malrotation. The causes of malunion are: (i) fracture was not reduced properly; (ii) after reduction redisplacement occurs within the plaster, for this a check X-ray after a week is advisable in certain fractures anticipating redisplacement, e.g., fracture of both bones of the forearm; (iii) growth disturbance due to injury to the epiphyseal cartilage may lead to malunion. Fracture-separation of an epiphysis does not lead to growth disturbance as the fracture occurs through the metaphyseal plate keeping the epiphyseal cartilage intact.

Sites of malunion are those where the bone is cancellous so union occurs as a rule, but malunion complicates due to imperfect position of the bone ends. These sites are fracture neck and the supracondylar fracture of the humerus, Colles' fracture, fracture through the condyles of the tibia, etc.

11. **Avascular necrosis (Fig. 12.3):** It means necrosis of the bone due to inadequate blood supply. It complicates fracture when the blood supply of one fragment was derived from the other fragment when the bone was intact. So after fracture the blood supply of one fragment becomes completely deficient and undergoes avascular necrosis. This avascular necrosis will lead to nonunion and osteoarthritis of the involved joint. Diagnosis is made by X-ray and the change takes about 1 to 3 months to develop. The avascular bone shows greater density due to the fact that it does not share in the general osteoporosis due to deficient blood supply.

The common sites of fracture which are liable to undergo this complication are the fracture neck of the femur, fracture of the scaphoid, fracture of the neck of the talus where the body undergoes avascular necrosis and dislocation of the lunate bone when the whole bone becomes necrosed.

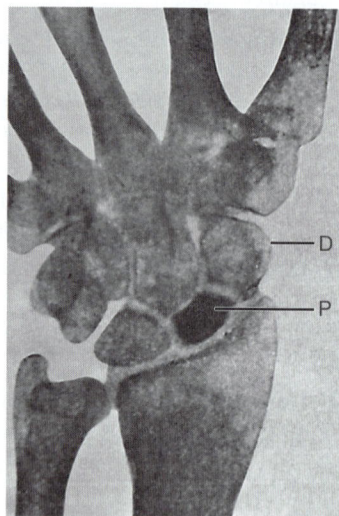

Fig.12.3: Avascular necrosis of the proximal fragment 'P' of the scaphoid bone. The distal piece 'D' remains unaffected. This is a complication of fracture of the scaphoid which so commonly takes place through its waist.

12. **Volkmann's ischemic contracture:** This condition occurs when the arterial obstruction is not complete and not too long lasting otherwise gangrene would have developed. Though muscles can survive 6–8 hours ischemia in contradistinction to the nerve tissue which can survive only a short period of ischemia, yet the muscles cannot regenerate whereas the nerves can regenerate. So the damage to the muscle is replaced by fibrosis which leads to contracture.

This condition is commonly seen in the forearm following supracondylar fracture of the humerus which leads to occlusion of the brachial artery either by thrombosis or spasm or by the displaced lower end of the upper fragment. The flexor muscles of the forearm are more often affected. Nerves are also affected by ischemia suggested by pain, weakness and numbness of the finger, but the nerves regenerate.

In the early stage *diagnosis* is made by impaired circulation of hand and fingers, absence of the radial pulse and inability of the patient to extend the fingers fully with complaint of pain in full passive extension. The treatment at this stage is relatively easy and the cure is guaranteed. In the established stage there will be obvious flexion deformity of the wrist and the fingers.

13. **Myositis ossificans traumatica:** This term is rather confusing as by 'myositis' one may consider to be one of inflammation of the muscle. But it has got no connection with inflammatory condition of the muscle and it should better be called *'post-traumatic ossification.'* Actually this condition develops when the hematoma under the stripped periosteum is invaded by osteoblasts and becomes ossified. This condition is commoner in children and young adults in whom the periosteum is loosely attached to the bone. Diagnosis is made by X-ray.

This condition is more commonly seen in elbow after supracondylar fracture or fracture of the head of the radius. It is also seen in some cases of fracture neck of the femur after operative fixation.

14. **Joint complications:** Stiffness of the neighboring joint is one of the most common complications of fracture. The causes are:

(i) *Adhesion:* Intra-articular adhesion results from organization of blood poured into the joint. More commonly periarticular adhesions occur from effusion into the ligaments and the capsules. Stiffness following fracture occurs mostly in the knee joint, the elbow joint, the wrist joint and the finger joint. In the shoulder joint the synovial fold on the inferior aspect of the joint is redundant and becomes adherent causing limitation of abduction movement. Adhesions of the injured muscle can also cause stiffness of the joint. The most common example is the stiffness of the knee following fracture of the shaft of the femur due to adhesion of the quadriceps muscles. In these cases quadriceps-plasty does a lot to increase the movement of the knee joint.

(ii) *Myositis ossificans:* This has already been discussed.

(iii) *Malunion*

(iv) *Osteoarthritis:* This is a late complication of a fracture which has involved the joint surface. After union the joint surface becomes irregular and thus results in osteoarthritis. Malunion may be the cause of osteoarthritis particularly in weight bearing joints where the direction of stress transmission becomes abnormal. Avascular necrosis is another potential factor which may lead to osteoarthritis.

(v) *Unreduced dislocation:* This will definitely cause stiffness of the joint and closed reduction often fails. The only treatment is open reduction or osteotomy.

(vi) *Sudeck's osteodystrophy:* Though this condition may affect the foot, yet it is more common in the hand and wrist injury. Pain and stiffness of the fingers, hyperesthesia and moistness of the ankle is diagnostic of this condition. X-ray shows patchy rarefaction of the bones in the region of the fracture.

Algorithmic Approach to Patient with Bone and Joint Injuries

Patient presents with pain, swelling, or deformity in a bone or joint

↓

Is there a history of trauma?
- Yes → Consider **fracture, dislocation, ligamentous injury, or contusion.**
- No → Consider **pathological fracture (osteoporosis, tumor), arthritis, or joint infection.**

↓

Is the pain sudden or gradual?
- Sudden → Suggests **fracture, dislocation, ligamentous tear, or acute joint effusion.**
- Gradual → Suggests **osteoarthritis, rheumatoid arthritis, bone tumor, or osteomyelitis**

↓

Is there loss of function?
- Yes → Suggests **fracture, dislocation, or severe ligamentous injury**
- No → Consider **contusion, sprain, or overuse injury**

↓

Is there visible deformity?
- Yes → Suggests **dislocation, fracture with displacement, or joint subluxation**
- No → More likely **soft tissue injury or incomplete fracture (greenstick in children)**

↓

Perform X-ray to confirm diagnosis
- Fracture present?
  - Yes → Classify as **simple, comminuted, open, impacted, or pathological fracture**
  - No → Consider **soft tissue or ligamentous injury (e.g., ACL tear, rotator cuff injury)**

↓

Perform additional imaging (MRI, CT) if needed
- MRI → Best for **soft tissue and ligamentous injuries**
- CT scan → Best for **complex fractures, joint injuries, and bone tumors**
- Bone scan → Best for **occult fractures, stress fractures, and metastatic bone disease**

↓

Confirm diagnosis and initiate treatment
- **Fractures:** Immobilization, casting, surgery (if needed)
- **Dislocations:** Closed reduction, immobilization, physiotherapy
- **Soft tissue injuries:** RICE protocol (rest, ice, compression, elevation), NSAIDs, rehabilitation
- **Pathological fractures:** Treat **underlying condition (osteoporosis, tumor, infection)**

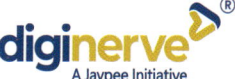

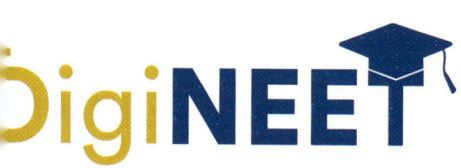

mplify your undergraduate studies and NEET PG preparation h this comprehensive program covering all 19 subjects. fted by India's top faculty, it includes video lectures, printed es, OSCEs, a QBank, test series, and the innovative Dr. Wise Chatbot.

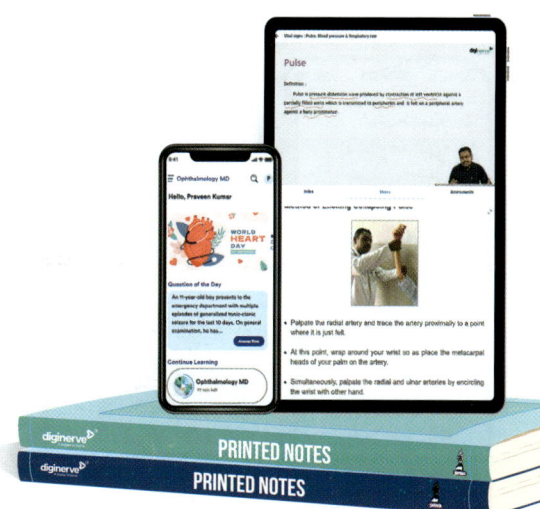

Course Features

1400+ hrs Video Lectures

1500+ Topics in Notes

15000+ Questions in QBank

1800+ GEMS

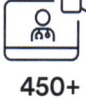

450+ OSCEs

Test Series

Dr. Wise AI Chatbot

Drug Chart

Regular Webinars by Esteemed Faculty

Access Anytime, Anywhere

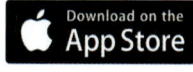
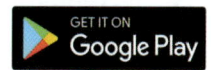

+91-8800-418-418   marketing@diginerve.com

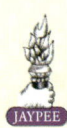
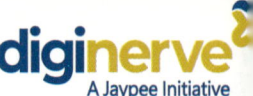

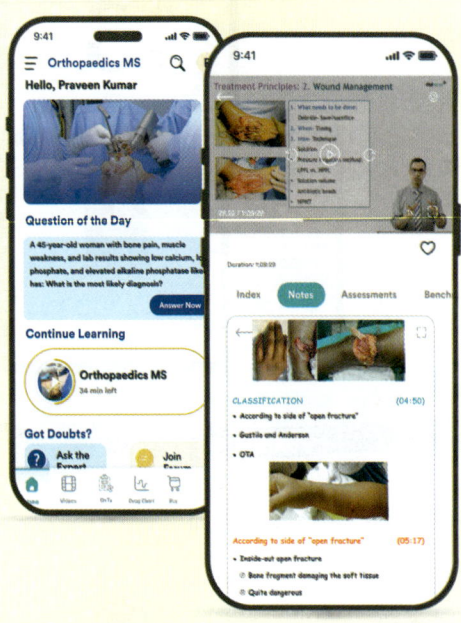

Premium Medical Content Anytime, Anywhere

Trusted by 150K+ Users

20+ Courses | **3600+** Hrs of Video Content | **790** Mentors

A host of features for UnderGrads, PostGrads and Professionals

Available on

 **Video Lectures**

 **Notes**

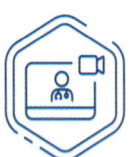 **OSCEs**

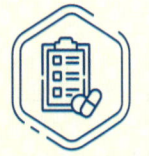 **Drug Chart**

 **Question Bank**

 **Dr. Wise AI Chatbot**

 +91-8800-418-418   marketing@diginerve.com

CHAPTER 13

Examination of Injuries about Individual Joints

The students must go through the previous chapter to make a clear conception about the general scheme of examination of injuries of bone and joint. In this chapter only those particular points of clinical examination are mentioned which will be required for a particular joint.

History in bone injuries

Aspect	Clinical significance	Patient-friendly questions
Age of onset	Helps differentiate conditions (e.g., hip fractures in elderly, ligament injuries in young adults)	"How old are you? Have you had joint injuries before?"
Mechanism of injury	Identifies **fracture vs dislocation vs ligamentous injury**	"How did the injury happen? Did you fall on an outstretched hand?"
Pain characteristics	Sudden Pain → Dislocation/Fracture Dull Pain → Soft tissue injury	"Was the pain immediate or did it start later?"
Loss of function	Fracture → Pain with movement Dislocation → Unable to move	"Can you move the joint at all?"
Swelling and deformity	Indicates **fracture displacement or joint injury**	"Did you notice any swelling or change in shape?"
Systemic symptoms	Fever → **Infection** Weight loss → **Chronic disease**	"Have you had fever or weight loss recently?"

■ EXAMINATION OF INJURIES ABOUT THE SHOULDER

A. INSPECTION

The patient must be stripped up to his waist and must stand against good daylight before the examination is actually started. One should always compare the injured side with the sound side.

1. **Attitude:** By noting the attitude of the patient while he is entering the clinic one can diagnose certain fractures. *With fracture of the clavicle* the patient often supports the flexed elbow of the injured side with the other hand. Similarly with *anterior dislocation of the shoulder* the patient supports the flexed elbow of the injured side with the other hand.

2. **Deformity or swelling:** An abnormal swelling on the line of the clavicle at its middle or more commonly at the junction of the lateral one-third and medial two-third should at once arouse the suspicion of *fracture clavicle* in the mind of the clinician. If there is any undue prominence at the acromial or the sternal end of the clavicle, the case is probably nothing but *dislocation of*

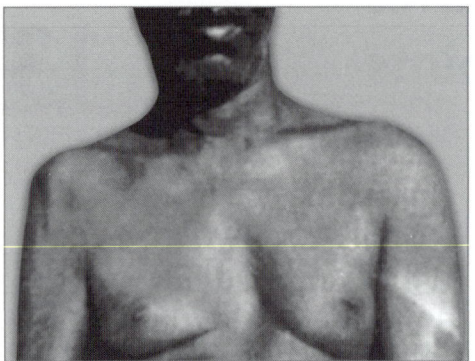

Fig. 13.1: Another case of flattening of the right shoulder due to subcoracoid dislocation of the humerus.

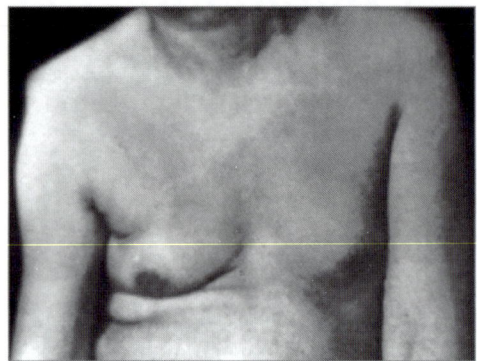

Fig. 13.2: Note obvious flattening of the right shoulder which indicates dislocation of the shoulder joint.

acromioclavicular or sternoclavicular joint respectively. In *subcoracoid dislocation* **(Fig. 13.1)** of the shoulder an abnormal swelling can be seen in the deltopectoral groove, there will be undue prominence of the acromion process with flattening of the shoulder **(Figs. 13.2 and 13.3)**. There will be drooping of the shoulder with undue lengthening of the arm *in fracture neck of the scapula.*

3. **Contour of the shoulder:** Inspection of the shoulder must be performed from all aspects—anterior, posterior and lateral to know fully about any defect in the contour of the shoulder. Undue flattening and loss of roundness of the shoulder just below the acromion process occur in *dislocation of the shoulder.* The most common type of dislocation of the shoulder is the *subcoracoid dislocation,* in which the head of the humerus lies below the coracoid process. In this condition there is also lowering of the anterior axillary fold. In contrast to this, considerable swelling of the shoulder just below the acromion process occurs in *fracture neck of the humerus,* without any loss of roundness of the shoulder.

4. **Bony arch** of the shoulder which is formed by the clavicle in front, the acromion process laterally and the spine of the scapula posteriorly, should be carefully inspected for any irregularity or abnormal swelling which may suggest fracture at that site.

B. PALPATION

All the bones which take part in the formation of the shoulder girdle should be palpated systematically to know if there is any bone or joint injury.

1. **Clavicle:** The surgeon stands behind the patient, who remains seated on the stool. The surgeon places his hands on the sternal ends of the clavicles of the both sides. Firstly, he palpates the sternoclavicular joints and then proceeds laterally on both sides to palpate the entire length of the two clavicles simultaneously. Any break in the line or

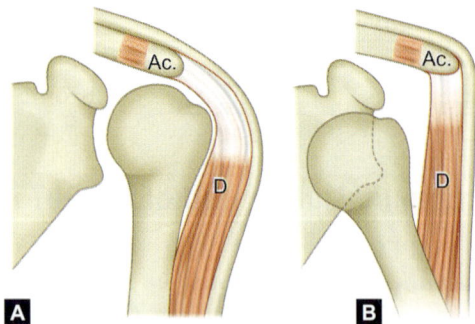

Figs. 13.3A and B: Roundness of the shoulder is mainly formed by the outward projection of the greater tuberosity beyond the acromion 'AC' and the thickness of the deltoid 'D'. Flattening in case of dislocation of the shoulder is due to inward displacement of the upper end of the humerus. It may also occur to certain extent in fracture of the neck of the scapula. Remember, apparent flattening of the shoulder is observed in wasting of the deltoid. Here, of course prominence of the greater tuberosity can be felt.

abnormal prominence suggests fracture of this bone. The two joints on two sides of the clavicle are also examined in this process to exclude any dislocation there. The sternal end of the clavicle is mostly anteriorly displaced in sternoclavicular dislocation, whereas the acromial end of the clavicle is subluxated upwards in acromioclavicular joint dislocation. It must be remembered that the conoid and trapezoid ligaments are almost always torn in acromioclavicular joint dislocation.

2. **Upper end of the humerus:** At first, one must ascertain that the head of the humerus is in normal position within the glenoid socket. The surgeon again stands behind the patient, who remains seated on a stool. The surgeon first palpates the acromion processes of both sides with the fingers of his two hands. He now gradually slides his fingers downwards to palpate the greater tuberosity of the humerus on both sides. Disappearance of the greater tuberosity of the humerus and loss of resistance here indicate dislocation of the shoulder **(Fig. 13.4)**. He now gradually slides his fingers downwards along the line of the humerus on both sides. Local bony tenderness and bony irregularity at the surgical neck of the humerus suggest fracture neck of the humerus. Similarly if the surgeon goes down to palpate the shaft of the humerus, he may exclude the fracture at this site by absence of local bony tenderness and bony irregularity **(Fig. 13.5)**. It must be remembered that in an unbroken bone the medial epicondyle shows the direction of the head of the humerus, whereas the lateral epicondyle shows the direction of the greater tuberosity. If this relation is disturbed, one must suspect the possibility of fracture either at the neck of humerus or at the shaft. In case of dislocation of shoulder one can try to rotate the arm by rotating the flexed elbow. If there is no transmitted rotation of the head of the humerus and a crepitus and pain are felt at the neck of the humerus, the diagnosis of fracture-dislocation is established.

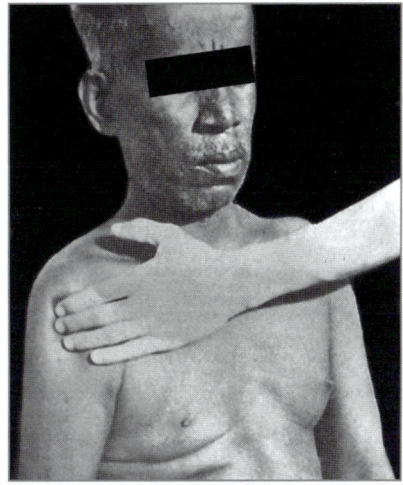

Fig. 13.4: Note loss of resistance by deeping the fingers below the acromion. This should be compared with the other side.

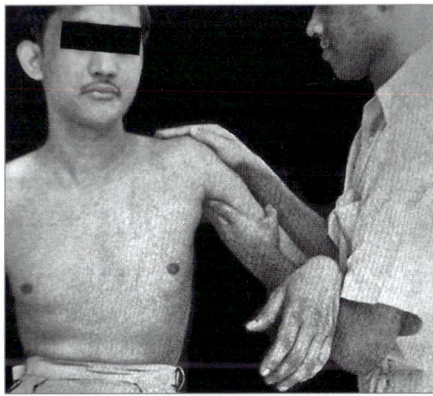

Fig. 13.5: Bimanual palpation of the upper end of the humerus through the deltoid and axilla. It is better felt by the hand in the axilla.

Marked tenderness just below the acromion process indicates *fracture of the greater tuberosity or rupture of the supraspinatus tendon.*

3. **Palpation of the scapula:** At first the subcutaneous portions of the bone are palpated. These are the spine of the scapula and the acromion process. The vertebral border of the scapula and the inferior angle though covered by muscles can be easily palpated. The axillary border of the scapula is more difficult to palpate, yet localized bony tenderness and swelling on this border which suggest fracture of the scapula can be elicited. The coracoid process is situated ½ inch below the clavicle at its junction between the medial 2/3rd and lateral 1/3rd. This process can be felt easily though it remains under cover of the medial margin of the deltoid. Probably the most difficult fracture of scapula so far as the diagnosis is concerned is the fracture of the neck

of the scapula. It is often confused with the fracture of the upper end of the humerus as diffuse swelling in the shoulder region is the common finding. Drooping of the shoulder with tenderness and crepitus by axial pressure upward through the flexed elbow remain the diagnostic feature of the fracture neck of the scapula. Very careful palpation of the upper end of the humerus will reveal no tenderness, whereas palpation medial to the glenoid cavity will elicit tenderness.

4. **Relative position of 3 bony points**, viz. the tip of the coracoid process, the acromial end of the clavicle and the greater tuberosity of the humerus are compared with those of the healthy side. Any deviation from the normal should be recorded. In acromioclavicular dislocation the acromial end of the clavicle becomes prominent and comes closure to the greater tuberosity of the humerus. But the distance between the tip of the coracoid process and the acromial end of the clavicle becomes increased.

C. **MEASUREMENTS**

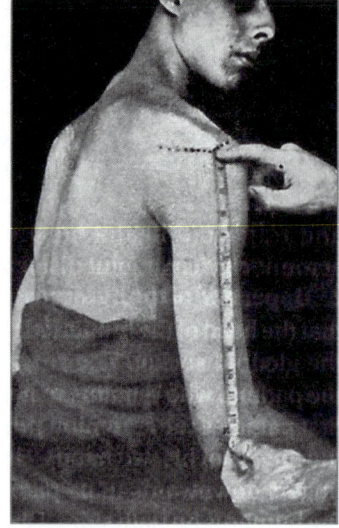

Fig. 13.6: Showing how to measure the length of the arm from the angle of the acromion to the lateral epicondyle of the humerus. The former point is slightly posteriorly placed in comparison to the latter point.

1. The length of the arm (Fig. 13.6): This is measured from the angle of the acromion to the lateral epicondyle of the humerus. The angle of the acromion is the point where the spine of the scapula bends forward to become the acromion process. This angle lies more posteriorly than the longitudinal axis of the arm. So in subcoracoid dislocation of the shoulder as well as in fracture neck of the humerus and shaft of the humerus the *length of the arm will be shortened.* In subglenoid dislocation of the shoulder and fracture neck of the scapula the length of *the arm will be longer.*

It must be remembered that any damage to the upper epiphysis of the humerus will shorten the length of the arm.

2. Vertical circumference of the axilla: This will be increased in any dislocation of the shoulder. But this measurement will also be increased in conditions like fracture of the upper end of the humerus and fracture neck of the scapula. The test to know lowering of anterior or posterior axillary fold is known as *Bryant's test.*

3. Hamilton's ruler test (Fig. 13.7): Normally a straight ruler cannot be made to touch the acromion process and the lateral epicondyle of the humerus. This is because of the presence of the greater tuberosity of the humerus which pushes the ruler away from the acromion process. But this becomes possible in dislocation of the shoulder where the greater tuberosity of the humerus is displaced medially.

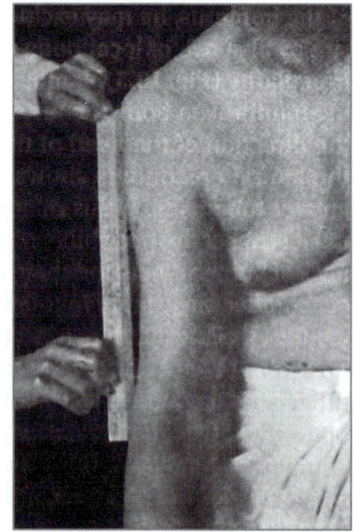

Fig. 13.7: Hamilton's ruler test.

D. **MOVEMENTS**

A full movement of the shoulder joint excludes the possibility of any bony injury near this joint.

Dugas' test: In dislocation of the shoulder the patient is unable to touch the opposite shoulder with the hand of the affected side while the arm is kept in contact by the side of the chest. After reduction of the dislocation in a muscular patient this test helps to be definite about the reduction and this position is maintained during the postreduction period.

Complications: In any injury around the shoulder joint examination cannot be complete without a search for any complication which might have been caused by such injury. The most important complication at this region is injury to the axillary nerve. This nerve besides supplying the deltoid muscle gives off a cutaneous twig which supplies the skin over the lower part of the deltoid muscle. Any injury at this region will limit the abduction of the shoulder joint by itself and it is of no use asking the patient to abduct the shoulder to test for the integrity of the axillary nerve. For this it is better to test the sensation of the skin supplied by the cutaneous branch of the axillary nerve.

SPECIAL INVESTIGATIONS

X-RAY

No doubt this is the only and most important investigation so far as the injury around the shoulder joint is concerned. Both anteroposterior and lateral views are essential. Even when the diagnosis is almost certain by clinical examination, X-ray is essential to know more precisely the line of fracture, the type of displacement (e.g., adduction or abduction type in case of fracture of the neck of the humerus) and the type of dislocation (e.g., whether subglenoid or subcoracoid or posterior dislocation of the shoulder). These are of utmost importance in treatment of the injury. In abduction type of fracture of the neck of the humerus the shaft is abducted in relation to the humeral head that means the outer half of the fracture is impacted.

In adduction type of fracture the shaft is adducted in relation to the head of the humerus that means the inner half of the fracture is impacted. In dislocation of the shoulder the position of the head of the humerus indicates the type of dislocation. When the head lies below the glenoid cavity the dislocation is said to be 'subglenoid' type; when the head of the humerus lies below the coracoid process the dislocation is called 'subcoracoid' type and when the head of the humerus lies posterior to the glenoid cavity in the infraspinatus fossa it is called the 'posterior' dislocation of the shoulder joint.

When the diagnosis is in doubt due to excessive swelling around the shoulder region, X-ray becomes the mode of diagnosis.

Different conditions which may develop due to injury around the shoulder joint:
1. Fracture of the clavicle.
2. Sternoclavicular dislocation.
3. Acromioclavicular dislocation.
4. Fracture of the scapula.
5. Dislocation of the shoulder joint.
6. Fracture of the neck of the humerus and the greater tuberosity.
7. Dislocation of the shoulder joint with fracture of the upper end of the humerus **(Fig. 13.8)**.

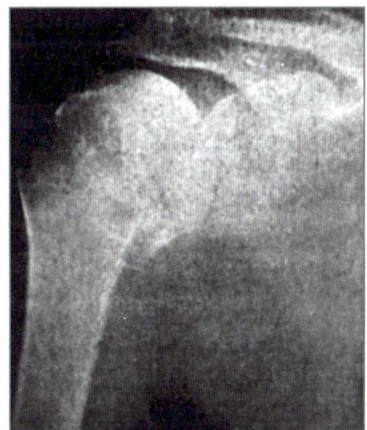

Fig. 13.8: Fracture of the upper end of the humerus.

Injuries of individual joints

Joint	Injury	Key clinical features	Diagnostic tests
Shoulder	Clavicle fracture	Swelling at midshaft, arm supported by opposite hand	X-ray (AP and lateral views)
	Shoulder dislocation	Flattening of shoulder, arm held in abduction	X-ray (check for subcoracoid, subglenoid dislocation)
Elbow	Supracondylar fracture	Swollen elbow in flexed position, olecranon displacement	X-ray (AP and lateral views)
	Posterior elbow dislocation	Prominent olecranon, severe movement restriction	X-ray (check for associated coronoid fracture)
Wrist	Colles' fracture	Dorsal displacement, dinner-fork deformity	X-ray (AP and lateral views)
	Scaphoid fracture	Snuffbox tenderness, high risk of avascular necrosis	X-ray (oblique and scaphoid views)
Hip	Neck of femur fracture	Shortened, externally rotated leg, unable to bear weight	X-ray (pelvis AP view)
	Posterior hip dislocation	Internally rotated, flexed, and adducted leg	X-ray (check for femoral head displacement)

DIFFERENTIAL DIAGNOSIS

FRACTURE OF THE CLAVICLE

The history is usually a fall on the outstretched hand. The fracture usually takes place at the junction of the middle third and the outer third of the clavicle. Very often the lateral fragment is pulled down by the weight of the arm and the medial fragment is displaced upward by the pull of the sternomastoid muscle. On examination there is an obvious swelling by the displaced medial fragment and localized tenderness at the fracture site. The diagnosis is confirmed radiologically **(Fig. 13.9)**.

STERNOCLAVICULAR DISLOCATION

This is a rare injury and is caused by the fall on the shoulder which forces the inner end of the clavicle forwards and upwards. On examination an abnormal swelling becomes obvious at the inner end of the clavicle with localized tenderness at that region. Movements of the shoulder become painful and restricted. The diagnosis is confirmed by X-ray.

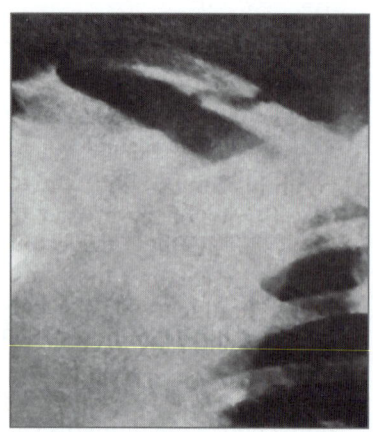

Fig. 13.9: Fracture of the clavicle.

ACROMIOCLAVICULAR DISLOCATION

History of a sudden traction on the arm or a fall of a weight on the point of the shoulder is often elicited. It must be remembered that rupture of the acromioclavicular ligaments will only cause subluxation of the acromioclavicular joint. For complete dislocation to occur there must be rupture of the conoid and the trapezoid ligaments which constitute the coracoclavicular ligament. On examination, an obvious prominence is present at the outer end of the clavicle by the upward pull of the sternomastoid muscle and the acromion process is dislocated downwards by the weight of the arm. Movements of shoulder will be restricted. X-ray is confirmatory.

FRACTURE OF THE SCAPULA

This usually occurs by direct injury on this bone. Swelling, bruising, local tenderness and bony irregularity are elicited on examination. Movement of the shoulder will be very much restricted. A careful examination and radiological investigation will confirm the exact site of fracture.

DISLOCATION OF THE SHOULDER JOINT

This is not uncommon injury caused by a fall on the outstretched hand. Forced extension along with lateral rotation will drive the head of the humerus forward tearing the capsule or avulsing the glenoid labrum **(Fig. 13.10)**. Nearly always the head takes the position just below the coracoid process and attains the name of *subcoracoid dislocation.* Rarely, the head may lie below the glenoid cavity when it is called the *subglenoid dislocation.* It may so happen that the whole dislocation process occurs in the abducted position of the arm and the acromion process levers the head downwards to attain a position called *luxatio in erecta. Posterior dislocation* is a very rare occurrence and caused by a forced internal rotation on the abducted arm. Very occasionally is the dislocation complete and what is more common is subluxation with fracture of the head of the humerus.

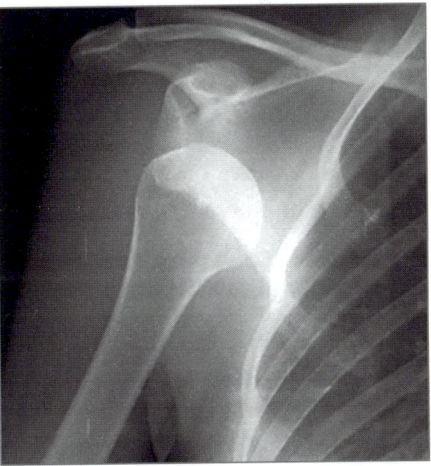

Fig. 13.10: X-ray right shoulder showing anterior shoulder dislocation (of humeral head) and empty glenoid.

Of the four varieties of dislocation which have just been described the subcoracoid is by far the commonest. The patient enters the clinic by supporting the flexed elbow of the affected side with his sound hand. The round contour of the shoulder joint is lost and it becomes flattened due to absence of the greater tuberosity at its normal position. On careful inspection one may find a bulge at the deltopectoral groove caused by the head of the humerus which is easily confirmed by rotating the arm with flexed elbow. The patient would not be able to touch the opposite shoulder with the hand of the affected side. The tests of academic interest such as Dugas' test and Hamilton's ruler test will help to come to the diagnosis.

RECURRENT DISLOCATION OF THE SHOULDER

Repeated dislocation of the shoulder by trifle injury is considered to be recurrent dislocation of the shoulder. When the anterior capsule is stripped from the anterior margin of the glenoid rim but attached to the neck of the scapula, there remains a chance of recurrent dislocation as the head of the humerus always remains within the capsule but outside the glenoid cavity. This condition may also occur when the glenoid labrum is detached along with the capsule and when there is a bony defect gouged out at the posterolateral aspect of the humeral head.

The history is diagnostic. If the patient's arm is abducted to right angle and externally rotated the patient will show immediate resistance due to apprehension. This is the position of the arm in which a trifle force will result dislocation. This test is pathognomonic of this condition.

FRACTURE OF THE NECK OF THE HUMERUS AND THE GREATER TUBEROSITY

The mechanism is usually a fall on the outstretched hand. The surgical neck breaks and the upward thrust may shear off the greater tuberosity. A direct injury on the point of the shoulder may cause fracture at the anatomical neck of the humerus.

FRACTURE THROUGH THE SURGICAL NECK: This fracture can be classified into abduction and adduction varieties. The greater tuberosity may be avulsed in abduction type of fracture. In adduction type of fracture the inner half of the fractured ends are impacted whereas in abduction type of fracture the outer half of the fractured ends are impacted and the shaft remains abducted against the head of the humerus.

FRACTURE THROUGH THE ANATOMICAL NECK: This condition is very difficult to diagnose from outside without X-ray. This may be in association with anterior dislocation of the shoulder.

FRACTURE OF THE GREATER TUBEROSITY: This mostly occurs by direct injury on the greater tuberosity or by a fall on the abducted arm where the greater tuberosity impinges against the acromion process. It may occur in association with dislocation of the shoulder and fracture neck of the humerus.

EXAMINATION OF INJURIES AROUND THE ELBOW

A. INSPECTION

A careful inspection of the patient when he enters the clinic gives to certain extent a clue to the diagnosis. A young child with swollen flexed elbow supported by his other hand is probably a case of supracondylar fracture of humerus.

1. **Attitude:** Patients with injury to the elbow often present with swollen elbow in *flexed position*. Attitude of the elbow joint has to be observed from in front, behind and from side.

In FRONT, note: (i) *the position of the joint*—whether extended or flexed, pronated or supinated. In majority cases of injury to the elbow the joint is held in the position of flexion. (ii) *Carrying angle:* This angle is the normal outward deviation of the extended and supinated forearm from the axis of the arm. This angle is normally 10°–15°, but in case of females this angle is more. To note the carrying angle the patient is asked to stand in the anatomical position, i.e., the forearm is extended and supinated. This angle should be noted on both the sides. The angle disappears on pronation or on full flexion of the forearm. When the carrying angle is abnormally increased the condition is called cubitus valgus and when it is abnormally decreased the condition is called cubitus varus **(Fig. 13.11)**.

From BEHIND, note the *position of the olecranon*—does it appear to be unduly prominent? If it is so it does not always mean posterior dislocation of the elbow, to the contrary in children it is more likely due to supracondylar fracture of the humerus. Note also whether the olecranon is displaced sideways. In large number of supracondylar fractures, the lower fragment, besides being displaced backwards and upwards, is often shifted either laterally or medially. This will be

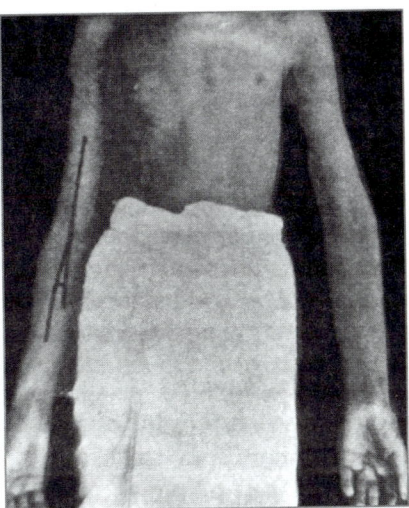

Fig. 13.11: The normal carrying angle is seen on the right side whereas cubitus varus deformity is obvious on the left side.

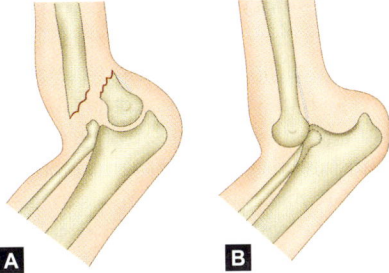

Figs. 13.12A and B: Showing how olecranon becomes unduly prominent in supracondylar fracture and posterior dislocation of elbow.

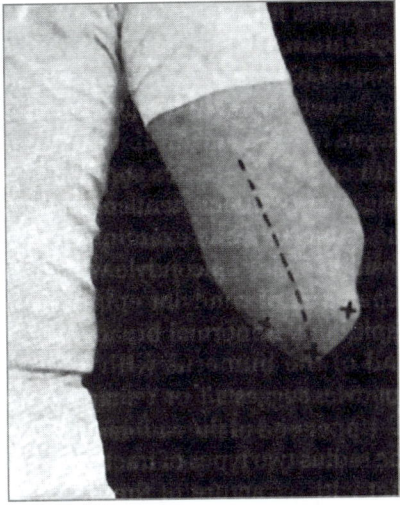

Fig. 13.13: A midposterior line of the arm is drawn. This line passes through the olecranon process. Any deviation of the olecranon sideways can thus be demonstrated.

evident by the position of the olecranon which moves along with the lower fragment (Figs. 13.12A and B).

From *THE SIDE*, note if *there is anteroposterior broadening of the elbow*. This is evident in posterior dislocation and supracondylar fracture (Fig. 13.13).

2. **Swelling:** Any injury to the elbow will give rise to tremendous amount of swelling. So much so that at times the diagnosis becomes difficult to make without X-ray examination. Sometimes localized swelling near the head of radius is probably due to fracture at this site.

Similarly, a swelling wholly confined to the posterior aspect of the elbow around the olecranon process is probably due to fracture of the olecranon process.

3. **Deformity:** Sometimes an obvious deformity can diagnose the type of injury. An abnormal swelling in front of the upper part of the ulna with surrounding generalized swelling is probably due to Monteggia fracture. An abnormal protrusion of the olecranon process backwards in an adult is probably a case of posterior dislocation of the elbow. Similar deformity with an undue anterior prominence just above the elbow in children is probably caused by supracondylar fracture.

B. PALPATION

Bones around the elbow are palpated systematically to look for any (i) local bony tenderness; (ii) local bony irregularity; (iii) displacement if any; (iv) unnatural mobility; (v) crepitus; (vi) referred tenderness, etc. The bones to be palpated are the lower part of the humerus, the head of the radius, upper part of the ulna, the olecranon process and the relative positions of 3 bony points viz. the two epicondyles of the humerus and the olecranon process.

1. **Lower third of the humerus:** The most important fractures in this group are the supracondylar fracture in case of children and T-or Y-shaped supracondylar fracture in case of adult. Besides these there are fracture-separation of the lateral condylar epiphysis and separation of medial epicondylar epiphysis in case of children and fractured capitulum in case of adult which should also be kept in mind. While examining the lower end of the humerus first one should palpate both the epicondyles of the humerus with the thumb and the four fingers of the clinician. If it seems that there is no condylar fracture or separation, the clinician with his other hand should hold the upper part of the humerus and the lower fragment is made to move with the fingers of this hand. An abnormal mobility along with crepitus indicates supracondylar fracture **(Fig. 13.14)**. Utmost gentleness is expected from the clinician while examining this. Abnormal position of any epicondyle will suggest fracture separation of condylar epiphysis or fractured capitulum. Abnormal broadening of the lower end of the humerus with distortion of the condyles suggests T-or Y-shaped fracture.

2. **Upper end of the radius:** In the upper end of the radius two types of fractures are commonly met with—fracture of the head of the radius (adults) and fracture of the neck of the radius (children). In both these circumstances there is no generalized swelling of the elbow, but there is localized swelling at the upper end of the radius.

The head of the radius can be best palpated in the lower part of the dimple just below the lateral condyle of the humerus when the forearm is pronated and supinated. This examination should be done in the flexed elbow **(Fig. 13.15)**. In case of fracture of the radial head there will be tenderness and irregularity during rotation of the radius. Sometimes a referred pain can be elicited at the fracture site particularly at the neck and the upper part of the shaft of the radius by springing the radius **(Fig. 13.16)**. This is done by squeezing the radius and ulna together at the lower part of the forearm, when the patient will complain of pain in the upper end of the radius.

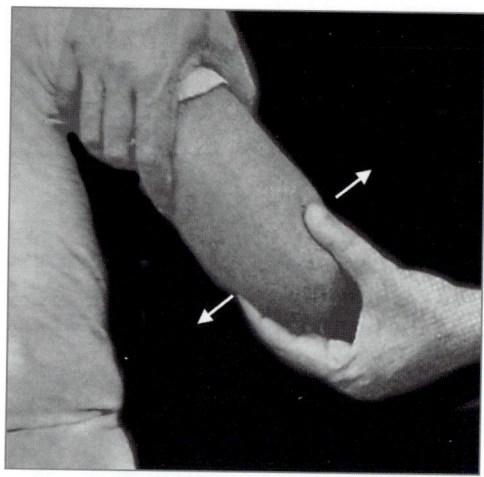

Fig. 13.14: Showing how to test for abnormal mobility in a suspected case of supracondylar fracture. The arm is steadied with one hand while with the other hand two epicondyles are held and moved sideways with utmost gentleness.

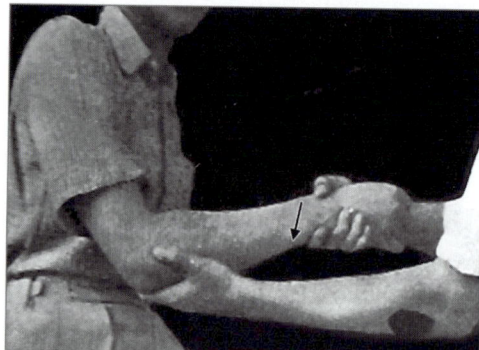

Fig. 13.15: Note how to palpate the head of the radius. The forearm is pronated and supinated to feel that the head of the radius rotates.

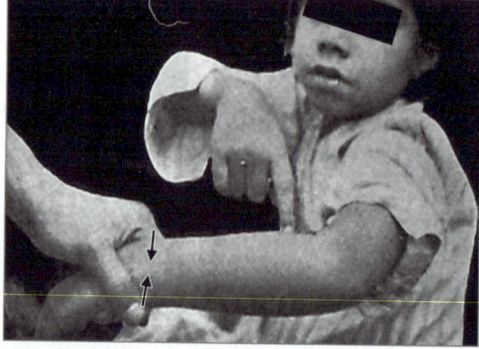

Fig. 13.16: Springing the radius. The patient shows the site of pain.

While palpating the upper end of the radius one must also keep in mind the possibility of *dislocation of the head of the radius*. It may occur alone or may be associated with fracture-displacement of the upper third of the ulna either forwards (Monteggia fracture) or backwards (reversed Monteggia) The palpation of lateral humeral epicondyle in relation to head of radius is shown in **Figure 13.17**.

3. **Upper part of the ulna:** Palpation of ulna is rather easier as its one border is subcutaneous. The clinician should move his finger along the subcutaneous border of the ulna to detect any local bony irregularity or local bony tenderness to suggest a crack fracture of the ulna. Any obvious deformity in the ulna and an abnormal prominence of the displaced fragment suggest fracture of the upper end of the ulna with displacement. In these cases one must not forget to palpate the head of the radius as this is very often dislocated along with displaced fracture of the upper end of the ulna which is popularly known as Monteggia fracture if the displacement is anteriorly.

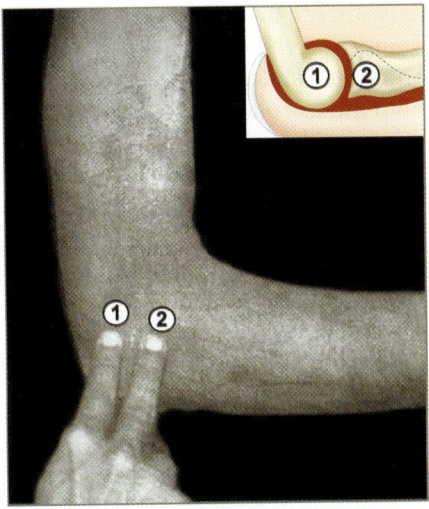

Fig. 13.17: By the index finger the lateral humeral epicondyle (1) is being felt and by the middle finger the head of the radius (2) is being felt. In the inset the relative position of these two bony points are being shown.

4. **Olecranon process:** Importance of examining this process cannot be overemphasized. Local bony irregularity with bony tenderness suggests a crack fracture of the olecranon. When the fracture is associated with separation, there will be gap in between the two fragments. Abnormal projection of the olecranon process posteriorly suggests posterior dislocation of the elbow in adult and supracondylar fracture in children.

5. **Relative positions of three bony points:** The two epicondyles of the humerus are palpated with the thumb and the middle finger and the tip of the olecranon process is palpated with the index finger **(Figs. 13.18A and B)**. In extended elbow these three bony points lie on a straight horizontal line but in flexed elbow they form a triangle which is neither isosceles nor equilateral but has the shortest side between the medial epicondyle and the olecranon and the longest

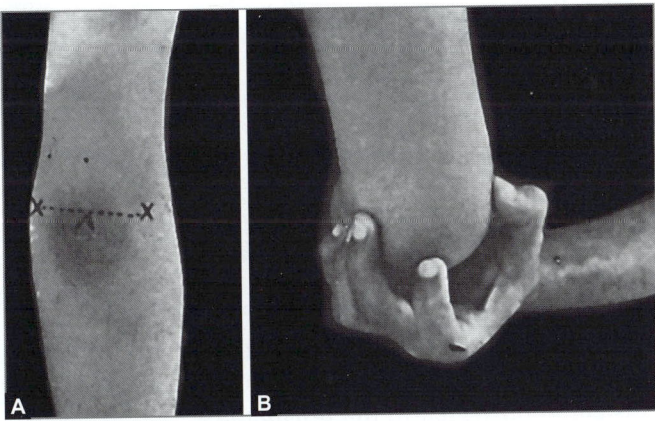

Figs. 13.18A and B: Show that the three bony points of the elbow viz. the two epicondyles and the olecranon lie in a line when the elbow is extended but form a triangle when the elbow is flexed.

between the two epicondyles. *One should always compare the relative positions of these bony points with those of the sound side.* When the olecranon process is pushed more posteriorly and a little above its usual position the case is one of posterior dislocation of the elbow. When both the epicondyles are more widely separated one should suspect a T-or Y- shaped fracture of the condyles.

C. MEASUREMENTS

While taking measurement, the forearm should be held at a right angle to the arm so that the epicondyles become prominent.

1. The length of the arm is measured from the angle of the acromion to the lateral epicondyle of the humerus. The arm will be shortened in supracondylar fracture.
2. The length of the forearm is measured from the lateral epicondyle of the humerus to the tip of the radial styloid process. The forearm will be shortened in posterior dislocation of the elbow.
3. The three bony points, i.e., the two epicondyles and the tip of the olecranon process are first marked with skin pencil before the three sides of the triangle are measured.

D. MOVEMENTS

Unhindered movements of the elbow which include flexion, extension, pronation and supination suggest that there is no bony injury around the elbow joint. Except injury to the upper end of the radius, which will only cause pain during pronation and supination movements, all other injuries around the elbow will cause pain and limitation of movements of flexion and extension. While testing the movements of pronation and supination, one should always keep the elbow of the patient flexed otherwise *in extended elbow rotation of the humerus will give a false impression of these movements.*

Complications: Complications of fracture have already been dealt with generally. In injury around the elbow the fracture which causes maximum complications is the supracondylar fracture of the humerus. The complications are injury to the blood vessels, injury to the nerves, Volkmann's ischemic contracture, Myositis ossificans traumatica, etc.

1. One should always *feel the radial pulse* while examining a case of an injury around the elbow joint.
2. All the three main nerves which cross the elbow joint run the risk of being damaged by the supracondylar fracture. Even if there is no recent injury to any of these nerves, there remains a chance of late (tardy) ulnar palsy. *So one must examine for any neurological deficits* that might be caused by such injury around the elbow.
3. *Volkmann's ischemic contracture* is a sequel of inadequate blood supply to the forearm muscles. The brachial artery is commonly the victim either by thrombosis or spasm or kinking. This condition should be suspected if the patient complains of pain down the forearm after the fracture has been reduced and plastered. An attempt to extend the flexed fingers with extended wrist will cause pain.
4. In no other condition is the *myositis ossificans traumatica so* common as after injury around the elbow **(Fig. 13.19)**. This is commonly seen in the brachialis muscle as a bony-hard mass. It is often a sequel of forcible massage and passive stretching of the elbow.

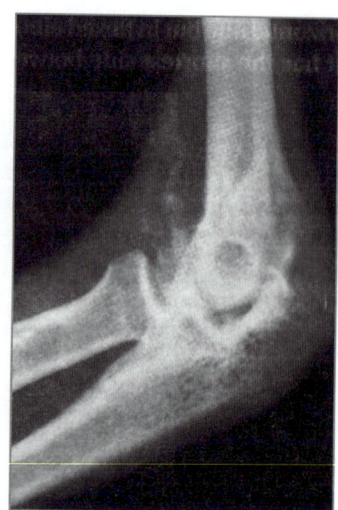

Fig. 13.19: Myositis ossificans traumatica.

SPECIAL INVESTIGATIONS

X-RAY EXAMINATION

Both anteroposterior and lateral views are essential to diagnose a bony injury around the elbow. Only anteroposterior view may not be able to detect such injuries as fracture of olecranon, posterior dislocation of the elbow and even the supracondylar fracture without lateral displacement. Similarly lateral view may fail to detect a fracture head or neck of the radius.

While interpreting a skiagram of the elbow joint after injury one must have a clear conception of time of appearance, the size, the shape, the position and time of fusion of all the epiphyses in the region of the elbow. Cases are not uncommon when epiphyseal line was erroneously diagnosed as fracture line and there was no real bony injury. The first center of ossification appears in the capitulum in the first year and extends medially to form the chief part of the articular surface. In the fourth year in case of females and in the sixth year in case of males ossification begins in the medial epicondyle. At the same age the disc-like center of ossification appears at the upper end of the radius. The center for the medial part of the trochlea appears in the ninth year in females and tenth year in males. At about the same age or a year later a thin scale-like epiphysis appears on the top of the olecranon process. The center of ossification in the lateral epicondyle appears at about the twelfth year in both sexes. The centers for the lateral epicondyle, capitulum and trochlea fuse around puberty and the large epiphysis thus formed unites with the shaft of the humerus in the fourteenth year in the females and the sixteenth year in the males. The upper epiphysis of the radius fuses with the shaft at the same age as the previous one (14th to 16th year). The upper epiphysis of the ulna also joins with the shaft at the same age. An additional center sometimes appears in the tuberosity of the radius at about the fourteenth or fifteenth year. One more anatomical peculiarity has to be noted that the lower epiphysis of the humerus after it has fused with the shaft is bent anteriorly. This fact can be verified by drawing a line which is drawn downwards along the anterior surface of the humerus which divides the circular trochlea into anterior 1/3rd and posterior 2/3rd in the lateral X-ray film **(Fig. 13.20)**. This anterior bent is more prominent in case of females.

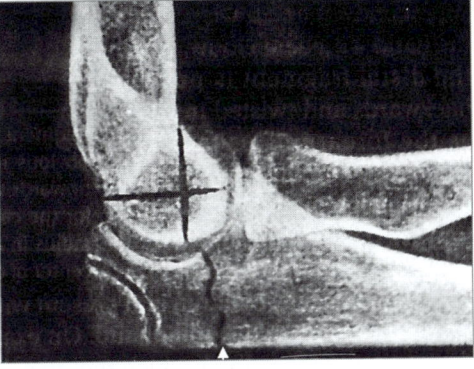

Fig. 13.20: Shows that a line drawn downwards along the anterior surface of the humerus divides the circular trochlea into anterior 1/3rd and posterior 2/3rd in the lateral X-ray film. This is due to the fact that the lower epiphysis of the humerus after it has fused with the shaft is bent anteriorly. Note also the position and shape of the epiphysis forming the olecranon. This must not be mistaken for a fracture which usually occurs at the base of the olecranon as shown by the arrow.

The following conditions are to be considered in injury around the elbow:
1. Supracondylar fracture.
2. T-and Y-shaped fractures.
3. Fracture-separation of the lateral condylar epiphysis.
4. Fracture-separation of the medial epicondyle.
5. Fractured capitulum.
6. Fracture neck of the radius.
7. Fracture head of the radius.

8. Fracture of the olecranon process.
9. Posterior dislocation of the elbow with or without fracture of the coronoid process.
10. Subluxation of the head of the radius in children (pulled elbow).
11. Monteggia fracture and reversed Monteggia.

DIFFERENTIAL DIAGNOSIS

SUPRACONDYLAR FRACTURE

Though *backward supracondylar fracture* that means the lower fragment is displaced backward is much commoner, *yet forward supracondylar fracture* is occasionally seen with forward displacement of the lower fragment **(Figs. 13.21A and B)**. The mechanism of backward supracondylar fracture is a fall on the hand with bent elbow, when the distal fragment is pushed backwards and twisted inwards as the forearm is usually full pronated. The displacement of the distal fragment is backwards, upwards, backward angulation with a slight internal rotation. The victims are usually children and present with a gross swelling at the elbow which is supported by the patient with his other hand. On examination there may be bruising and the posterior prominence of the elbow which requires differentiation from the posterior dislocation of the elbow. The possibility of an injury to the brachial artery as well as three main nerves should be foreseen and properly examined to exclude such possibility. An immediate reduction of the displaced fracture is essential and the elbow joint is kept flexed in collar and cuff in such a position as the radial pulse is well palpated.

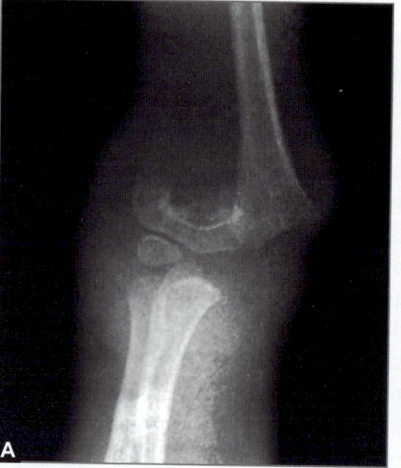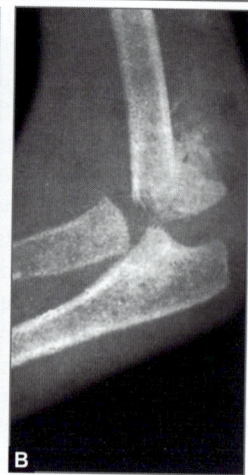

Figs.13.21A and B: Supracondylar fracture of the humerus. The lower fragment is displaced laterally for a considerable distance which is obvious in anteroposterior film. It is also displaced backwards and upwards which is evident in the lateral film. The center of ossification for the capitulum is likely to be mistaken for that of the head of the radius in anteroposterior view but not in the lateral view. In fact the center of ossification for the head of the radius has not yet appeared.

The mechanism of forward supracondylar fracture which is very much rarer than its previous counterpart is caused by a fall on the stretched hand with fully extended elbow so that the lower fragment is tilted forward. The patient presents with a more extended elbow than its previous counterpart and swelling around the elbow. A careful palpation will reveal the forwardly tilted distal fragment.

Complications of supracondylar fracture are—(i) Malunion; (ii) Cubitus valgus or varus; (iii) Myositis ossificans traumatica; (iv) Injury to the brachial vessels; (v) Volkmann's ischemic contracture; (vi) Injury to the nerves—ulna, median and/or radial.

T- AND Y-SHAPED FRACTURES

These fractures are more commonly seen in adults and are caused by falls on the points of the elbows which drive the olecranon processes upwards splitting the two condyles apart. The patient presents with a grossly swollen elbow which is very much wide. The elbow remains slightly flexed supported by the other hand and movement is extremely painful and restricted. X-ray confirms the diagnosis.

FRACTURE-SEPARATION OF THE LATERAL CONDYLAR EPIPHYSIS

The history is that the child has fallen on the hand and a large fragment including the lateral condylar epiphysis and a portion of the metaphysis break off. Swollen elbow and tenderness on the lateral condyle are the usual clinical features. X-ray is diagnostic.

FRACTURE-SEPARATION OF THE MEDIAL EPICONDYLE

The mechanism of injury is usually a severe abduction force and young children between ten and fifteen years of age are the usual victims (before the medial epicondylar epiphysis fuses with the shaft). The epiphysis is pulled distally by the attached flexor muscles. Sometimes it may be associated with lateral dislocation of the elbow. The peculiar feature of this fracture is that besides slight rotational displacement the medial epicondyle may be included into the joint by the forced abduction which momentarily opens up the medial side of the joint and thus sucks in the fractured medial epicondyle. The possibility of injury to the ulnar nerve has already been emphasized. X-ray picture will detail the fracture and the displacement.

FRACTURED CAPITULUM

This is an adult injury and is caused by fall on the hand with the straight elbow. The anterior half of the capitulum and the trochlea are broken off and displaced proximally. The patient presents with fullness of rather an extended elbow. On examination, tenderness on the fracture site is without question. Flexion movement is extremely painful and limited. X-ray is diagnostic.

FRACTURE NECK OF THE RADIUS

This commonly affects the children and is caused by a fall on the outstretched hand while the elbow is in slightly valgus position. It is actually an epiphyseal separation with a triangular metaphysis attached to it. The patient can usually flex and extend the elbow but rotation, i.e., pronation and supination is painful and restricted. There is tenderness at the upper end of the radius with a lateral projection of the head of the radius which can be palpated. X-ray shows fracture of the neck of the radius with the head tilted forwards, outwards and distally.

FRACTURE HEAD OF THE RADIUS

While the previous fracture is mainly a fracture of children, this fracture mostly affects the adults and the mechanism is more or less similar to that of the previous one that means a fall on the outstretched hand with the elbow on the valgus position so that the radial head is crushed against the capitulum. On examination there will be localized tenderness on the head of the radius and rotation of the forearm, i.e., supination and pronation is painful and restricted though the patient may be able to flex or extend the elbow with a little pain. X-ray will confirm the diagnosis by showing either a vertical split in the radial head or a lateral major fragment of the head broken off and displaced laterally or a comminuted fracture with multiple fragments.

FRACTURE OF THE OLECRANON PROCESS

A direct fall on the point of the elbow is probably the cause of fracture of olecranon. The fracture line is at the narrowest point of the olecranon almost where it joins with the shaft of the ulna and must not be confused with the epiphysial line which lies near the tip of the olecranon process. If the triceps muscle goes in action during the injury a gap is expected between the two fragments of the olecranon process.

If there is just a crack fracture, slight swelling, bruising, localized bony tenderness and bony irregularity will be the clinical features. The patient may be able to extend the elbow. Whereas in more severe injury with separation of fragments there will be more swelling, oedema and bruising at the fracture site. Palpation will reveal an obvious gap between the fragments. X-ray examination is obligatory not only to know the details of the fracture and displacement but also to assess the type of treatment which would be best suited for the particular case.

DISLOCATION OF THE ELBOW

While there are possibilities of anterior and lateral dislocations yet the posterior dislocation is by far the commonest. The mechanism of posterior dislocation is a fall on the outstretched hand with the elbow in slightly flexed position. The coronoid process may pass posteriorly below the distal end of the humerus intact or may be fractured by the thrust against this part of the humerus. Very often the posterior dislocation is associated with lateral displacement of varying range.

Clinically, this condition may mimic the supracondylar fracture and the *differentiating points between these two conditions* should be borne in mind. They are in dislocation of elbow (i) the patient is frequently an adult; (ii) palpation will reveal an abnormal posterior displacement of the olecranon process which will be obvious by palpating the three bony points; (iii) absence of abnormal mobility and crepitus while an attempt is made to move the lower end of the humerus; (iv) there will be shortening of the forearm as measured from the lateral epicondyle of the humerus to the tip of the radial styloid process and (v) X-ray examination is probably the most important.

SUBLUXATION OF THE HEAD OF THE RADIUS IN CHILDREN (PULLED ELBOW)

Very often when a child is pulled suddenly by his forearm in the position of supination, there is a chance of the head of the radius being dislocated from the grip of the annular ligament. Generally, such a history can be elicited and the patient presents with a complaint of pain at the elbow. The elbow is more or less fixed in slight flexion and pronation; more flexion of the elbow and supination become painful and limited. On palpation one may find the head of the radius a little below and lateral to its normal position.

MONTEGGIA FRACTURE AND REVERSED MONTEGGIA

Fracture of the upper third of the ulna with displacement is often associated with dislocation of the head of the radius. When the displacement of the ulnar fracture is anteriorly and the head of the radius is dislocated anteriorly this is known as Monteggia fracture-dislocation **(Fig. 13.22)**. When the displacement of the ulnar fracture is posteriorly and the head of the radius also dislocates backwards—this is known as reversed Monteggia.

Monteggia fracture is much commoner than reversed Monteggia. Mechanism is usually a fall on the hand and the body twists

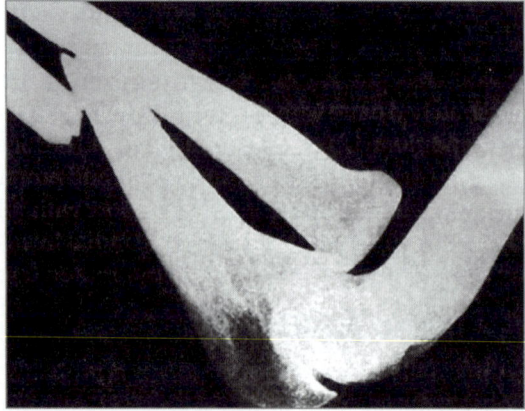

Fig. 13.22: Monteggia fracture.

at the moment of impact thus forcibly pronating the forearm. The ulnar deformity is obvious on inspection. A careful palpation will reveal radial dislocation besides rather easy detection of ulnar fracture-displacement. Movement of the elbow joint is completely restricted in both extension and flexion as well as supination and pronation. X-ray is the final court of appeal to settle the diagnosis.

EXAMINATION OF INJURIES AROUND THE WRIST AND HAND

A. INSPECTION

1. Deformity: (a) The characteristic "dinner-fork" deformity of *Colles' fracture* do not require any detailed discussion. But two points deserve mentioning—(i) that the dorsal prominence is *not* at the level of the wrist but about one inch above it and (ii) that there is also a slight radial deviation which makes the head of the ulna more prominent. (b) An abnormal slight anterior projection at the wrist following a fall on the dorsiflexed hand is due to *dislocation of the lunate bone*. (c) Fracture of the lower third of the radius with inferior radioulnar dislocation which is known as Galeazzi fracture is sometimes quite obvious on inspection.

(d) In *Madelung's deformity* or *manus valgus* there is dorsal subluxation with prominence of the lower end of the ulna in an adolescent girl. The hand is deviated laterally **(Figs. 13.23A and B)**.

(e) In *Bennett's fracture-dislocation* the typical abnormal lateral projection at the base of the first metacarpal bone is quite obvious.

(f) In *metacarpal fractures* abnormal bony projections almost make the diagnosis obvious. When the patient is asked to make a fist, the line of knuckles may not be on the normal line.

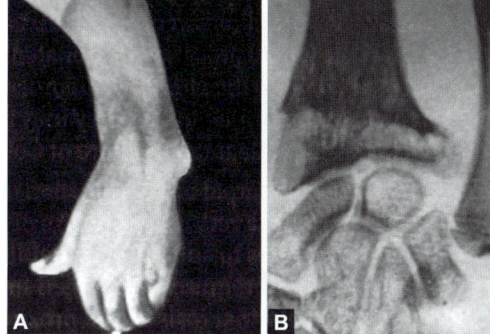

Figs. 13.23 A and B: Manus valgus (made—lung's deformity), resulting from injury to the lower radial epiphysis six years ago. The growth of the radius has been stopped and the normally growing ulna (shown in the skiagram) pushes the hand outwards.

(g) In case of fracture of the phalanges the finger becomes unduly swollen and deformed. In *"mallet finger"*, which is caused by rupture of the extensor tendon at its insertion at the base of terminal phalanx, there is persistent flexion of the terminal phalanx.

(h) In dislocation of the interphalangeal and metacarpophalangeal joint anterior projection of the head of the phalanx or the head of the metacarpal as the case may be becomes obvious.

B. PALPATION:
In injury around the wrist one should palpate the neighboring bones systematically to elicit (i) Local bony tenderness; (ii) bony irregularity; (iii) displacement; (iv) unnatural mobility and (v) crepitus.

1. Lower third of the radius: In suspected fracture of the lower third of the radius, one should follow the outer border as well as the dorsal aspect of the bone for any irregularity and tenderness. It must be remembered that normally the lower third of the radius is smoothly concave in front. Feel whether this concavity is preserved or not. In Colles' fracture there is posterior displacement of the lower fragment which becomes obvious on palpation.

Springing the radius may be of help to diagnose fracture of the lower third of the radius above the typical site of Colles' fracture, which is surrounded by muscles and tendons and not so available for direct palpation. In this case squeezing of the upper part of the radius and ulna together will elicit pain at the site of fracture.

2. **Lower third of the ulna:** It must be borne in mind that in Colles' fracture as well as in the fracture of lower third of the radius it is of immense importance to palpate the head of the ulna. In Colles' fracture very often the styloid process of the ulna is also fractured and in fracture of the lower third of the radius very often the head of the ulna is dislocated (Galeazzi).

Otherwise palpation of the ulna is easy being a subcutaneous bone. Fracture of the ulna as such will elicit tenderness and bony irregularity.

3. **Relative position of the two styloid processes** (radial and ulnar): Normally, the radial styloid process is about half an inch lower than the ulnar styloid process **(Fig. 13.24)**. In order to demonstrate this, the clinician uses his two index fingers to locate the tips of the styloid processes in pronated forearm of the patient. In Colles' fracture the radial styloid process will remain at a higher level than normal, in fact they may remain on the same line. This is also a diagnostic feature of Colles' fracture.

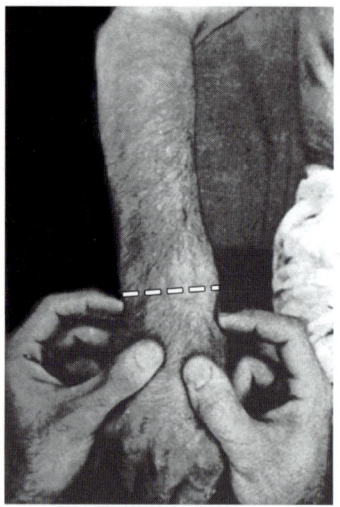

Fig. 13.24: Normally the tip of the radial styloid process is about 1 cm lower than the tip of the ulnar styloid process. The dotted line represents the horizontal level at the tip of the ulnar styloid process.

4. **Carpal bones:** Of the carpal bones palpation of the scaphoid bone is most important as very often fracture of the scaphoid is misdiagnosed as simple sprain and the patient continues to suffer from disability and painful wrist for a long time. Moreover fracture of the scaphoid requires prolonged immobilization as this fracture is notorious for nonunion and avascular necrosis of the proximal fragment. The scaphoid is palpated at the anatomical snuff-box with the wrist bent medially to expose the bone for palpation. If there is any fracture of the scaphoid bone, the patient will complain of pain as soon as a pressure is made over the anatomical snuff-box.

Another important carpal bone which should be considered here is the lunate bone. This bone may be dislocated anteriorly and requires careful palpation for the diagnosis of this condition.

5. **Metacarpals and phalanges:** To feel for fracture or dislocation of the metacarpals and phalanges one should palpate the full length of the metacarpal bone or the phalanx. For this, the examiner should run his finger along the length of the said bone to find out any gap, bony irregularity, bony tenderness or abnormal projection. In Bennett's fracture, i.e., fracture-dislocation of the base of the first metacarpal, a traction along the axis of the bone often elicits tenderness at the site of fracture.

A careful palpation of the metacarpophalangeal joints and inter phalangeal joints should be a must to exclude subluxation or dislocation of the said joints which are often missed.

C. **MOVEMENTS:** Movement of the affected part will obviously be painful and limited. As for example in Colles' fracture movement of the wrist will be restricted. In case of metacarpal fractures movement of the metacarpophalangeal joints will be restricted. Similarly in fractures of the phalanges movement of the interphalangeal joints will be painful and restricted.

D. **COMPLICATIONS:** These have been discussed in details in the previous chapter. In differential diagnosis complications of the important fractures around the wrist will be discussed in nutshell.

X-ray examination: As in any other bony injury importance of X-ray examination cannot be re-emphasized here. In all fractures, not only the fracture is diagnosed but also a careful study of the displacement of the fractured fragments will help the clinician in reduction of the fracture concerned. As for example in Colles' fracture, the lower fragment is displaced backwards, upwards and laterally and is also tilted backwards so that the articular surface of the lower end of the radius looks more posteriorly than anteriorly (which is normal). In this case, to reduce the fracture a pull is directed downwards, slightly medially and anteriorly holding the thumb and the heads of the metacarpals of the patient simultaneously, while with the two thumbs of the clinician the upper edge of the lower fragment is pushed anteriorly so that the normal alignment of the radius is restored.

After discussing the general points, the peculiarity of the X-ray examination of the scaphoid requires special mention. Very often the orthodox anteroposterior and lateral views fail to detect a minor crack fracture of the scaphoid. For this *an oblique view* and views from different angles are very much essential to diagnose fracture of the scaphoid bone. Even a negative X-ray finding does not exclude the presence of fracture. If clinical findings go very much in favor of the diagnosis of fracture of the scaphoid, one should treat the case according to that and take another X-ray after ten days, as by that time the fracture line often delineates itself.

The following conditions are to be considered in injury around the wrist:
1. Colles' fracture with or without fracture of the ulnar styloid process.
2. Smith's fracture or reversed Colles'.
3. Chauffeur's fracture of the radius just above the radial styloid process, caused by the backward jerk of the starting handle of a car.
4. Galeazzi fracture.
5. Scaphoid fracture.
6. Lunate and perilunate dislocation.
7. Bennett's fracture-dislocation.
8. Fractures and dislocations of the metacarpals and phalanges.
9. Mallet finger.

DIFFERENTIAL DIAGNOSIS

COLLES' FRACTURE

This injury is caused by a fall on the palm of the outstretched hand with a supination force. The victims are usually elderly ladies, which is attributed to the osteoporosis in postmenopausal women. The fracture line lies about 2 cm proximal to the distal articular surface of the radius. The distal fragment is displaced dorsally, proximally, slightly laterally and angulated backwards **(Fig. 13.25)**.

The patients present with swelling and dinner-fork deformity of the wrist. On examination, there is tenderness and bony irregularity of the lower end of the radius. The normal anterior concavity of the radius is lost. The radial styloid process does not remain lower than the ulnar styloid process which is normal. On the

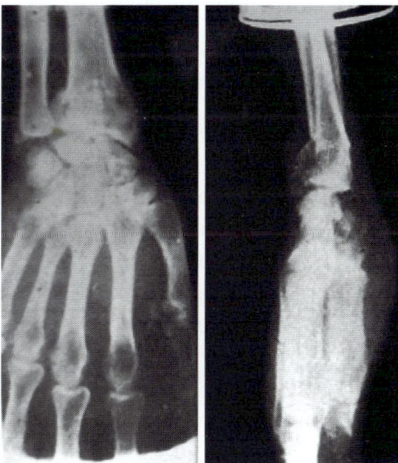

Fig. 13.25: Colles' fracture.

contrary it remains at the same level or a little higher than the ulnar styloid process. Malunion, manus valgus and stiffness of the wrist, are the usual complications. The complications which are peculiar to this fracture are Sudeck's osteodystrophy, causalgia and spontaneous rupture of the extensor pollicis longus tendon which may be due to friction over the ridge of the bone at the site of fracture or due to degeneration of the tendon following insufficient blood supply.

SMITH'S FRACTURE (REVERSED COLLES')

A true reversed Colles' fracture, that means a transverse fracture of the lower end of the radius with anterior displacement of the lower fragment is very rare. Again the usual victims are the elderly women and diagnosis both clinically by anterior projection of lower fragment and radiologically is not very difficult. The mechanism is due to a fall on the dorsum of the palmar-flexed wrist and not to a fall on the palm of the outstretched hand. A commoner injury at this region with anterior displacement is the fracture dislocation of the lower end of the radius. In this case the radial fracture is obliquely vertical extending upwards and forwards from the wrist joint and separated anterior fragment of the radius shifts proximally carrying the hand with it.

CHAUFFEUR'S FRACTURE

The typical history is that the patient wanted to start his vehicle with a starting handle and ultimately injured his wrist by the kick back. The fracture line is usually transverse extending laterally from the articular surface of the radius and the fracture is more often undisplaced.

GALEAZZI FRACTURE (FIG. 13.26)

This is in fact a fracture-dislocation of the lower end of the radius with dislocation of the inferior radioulnar joint. The mechanism seems to be fall on the hand with a rotational force superimposed on it. On examination there is undue swelling of the lower end of the forearm due to displaced fracture of the radius and an abnormal prominence of the head of the ulna due to dislocation of the inferior radioulnar joint. The most important test which most clinicians forget to perform is to look for ulnar nerve lesion—a common associate with this condition. X-ray examination is confirmatory.

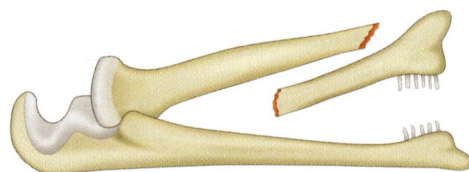

Fig. 13.26: Diagrammatic representation of Galeazzi fracture.

MADELUNG'S DEFORMITY

There is dorsal subluxation of the lower end of the ulna. The patient is usually an adolescent girl who complains of weakness of the wrist. On inspection there is a very prominent dorsal displacement of the lower end of the ulna. Palpation reveals a grossly unstable inferior radioulnar joint. Controversy still exists whether this condition is congenital or acquired. While majority favor congenital theory, yet the advocates of acquired theory postulate that repeated minor injuries may delay growth of the radius while the ulna continues to grow forcing the lower end of the ulna to subluxate.

SCAPHOID FRACTURE

The history is usually a fall on the outstretched hand and the force is the combination of dorsiflexion and radial deviation in which the waist of the scaphoid is impacted against the radial styloid process. Young adults are usually the victims. The appearance of the wrist is deceptively normal most of the time with little impairment of the function of the wrist. Sometimes there may be slight fullness of the anatomical snuff box. The main help to the diagnosis is suspicion of such a fracture. Tenderness at the anatomical snuff box, while the wrist is deviated medially adds more to the suspicion. X-ray is confirmatory, but the first X-ray may not show any fracture and typical 'scaphoid views' are to be taken to exclude such fracture. Repeated X-ray after a week or so is essential when the suspicion still remains even after the negative first X-ray.

The importance of this fracture is mainly due to the fact that it is notorious for two complications—(i) nonunion for which a prolonged immobilization is required and (ii) avascular necrosis of the proximal fragment which may later on cause osteoarthritis of the wrist joint.

LUNATE AND PERILUNATE DISLOCATIONS

The mechanism is again a fall on the dorsiflexed hand which displaces the whole of the carpus backwards leaving only the lunate in contact with the radius (perilunar dislocation). Usually the hand immediately snaps forward again but while doing so the lunate is displaced forwards out of position (lunate dislocation). Sometimes the lunate bone may be dislocated without prior perilunar dislocation and this is probably due to forced dorsiflexion of the wrist which throws away the lunate bone forwards. These dislocations may be associated with fracture of the scaphoid.

On examination, the displacement of the lunate may be obscured by swelling of the wrist. A careful palpation may diagnose the condition. Median nerve compression in the carpal tunnel occurs almost always with this condition and a particular examination in this regard is very much essential. X-ray examination is again confirmatory and a lateral view is more essential for the diagnosis of this condition. The anteroposterior view is important to exclude the associated fracture of the scaphoid. The most important complication of lunate dislocation, besides the median nerve injury, is avascular necrosis *(Kienbock's disease).*

BENNETT'S FRACTURE-DISLOCATION

The usual history is an attempted punch to the point of the thumb. It is an oblique fracture at the base of the first metacarpal bone extending distally and medially from its articular surface. So a triangular piece of bone remains in its position whereas the main shaft dislocates proximally and laterally on the trapezium. On examination there is abnormal swelling at the base of the first metacarpal bone and if the clinician pushes the projection distally and medially with his thumb the dislocated shaft moves causing a great pain to the patient.

FRACTURES AND DISLOCATIONS OF THE METACARPALS AND PHALANGES

The fractures of the shaft and neck of the metacarpals are diagnosed by localized swelling, deformity, bony irregularity and bony tenderness. Fractures of phalanges are also diagnosed clinically in the same way. Dislocation of the metacarpophalangeal joint is diagnosed by careful palpation at the metacarpophalangeal joint where the head of the metacarpal bone is dislocated anteriorly most of the time. A careful palpation will also diagnose dislocation of the interphalangeal joint. X-ray is confirmatory in all these conditions.

MALLET FINGER

This is due to rupture of the terminal slip of the extensor tendon to the distal phalanx or avulsion-fracture of a small piece of bone where the extensor tendon is inserted at the base of the distal phalanx. The cause is usually a forced flexion of the terminal phalanx when the extensor is contracting. On examination, the typical flexion deformity of the terminal phalanx to a position of 30° flexion is obvious. The patient is unable to extend the distal interphalangeal joint to the full extent. Of course passive extension is possible. Radiological investigation is of value in case of chip fracture of the terminal phalanx.

EXAMINATION OF INJURIES TO THE PELVIS

History of severe violence directly to the pelvis or indirectly through the thigh is usually obtained. Patient complains of severe pain in the region of the pelvis, which gets worse on moving the legs or the body.

On examination, bruising and swelling over the injured site can be easily revealed. A careful palpation of the whole pelvis is required to know the exact type of fracture. In multiple injuries one can exclude the possibility of any bony injury to the pelvis by pressing two iliac bones and the greater trochanters medially by the two hands of the clinician (**Fig. 13.27**).

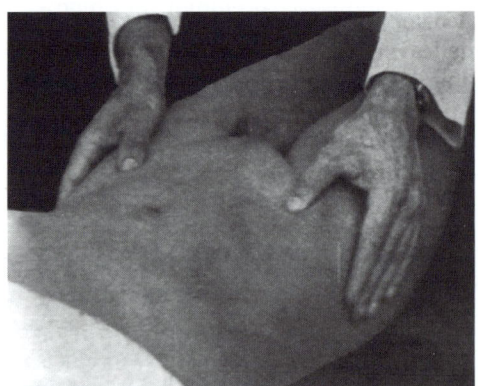

Fig. 13.27: In case of injury to the pelvis patient complains of pain when the two iliac bones are pressed medially by two hands of the clinician.

Fracture of the pelvis can be classified into four groups:
(a) *Isolated pelvic ring fractures,* i.e., the pelvic ring is broken at one place and the displacement is naturally slight. Chance of complication is rare. In this group are the fracture of the blade of the ilium, fracture of the floor of acetabulum with central dislocation of the hip and fracture of ischiopubic ramus.
(b) *Pelvic ring disruption,* i.e., the pelvic ring is broken at two places with considerable displacement and disruption.
(c) *Avulsion fracture* commonly occurs at the anterior superior iliac spine (sartorius avulsion), anterior inferior iliac spine (rectus avulsion) and ischial tuberosity (hamstring avulsion).
(d) *Injuries to the sacrum and coccyx.* One must be very methodical in palpating the parts of the pelvis one by one to elicit the fracture which might have occurred.

X-ray examination is confirmatory and besides anteroposterior and lateral views, stereoscopic views are also required to diagnose fracture which may not be evident in these views.

Examination of visceral complications: Fracture of the pelvis is notorious for visceral complications, of which damage to the urethra and/or bladder is important. Injury to both these structures occurs commonly in fracture of the pubic bone.

Injury to the urethra is diagnosed by the three classical signs—blood per urethrum, perineal hematoma and distended bladder.

Injury to the bladder are of two varieties—*extraperitoneal* (commoner) and *intraperitoneal*. Extraperitoneal rupture is sometimes difficult to differentiate from the rupture of the posterior urethra. Of course the diagnosis of these conditions are discussed more elaborately in the chapter of "Examination of a urinary case", yet it is sufficient to narrate at this stage that a straight X-ray with ground glass appearance of fluid in the lower abdomen and intravenous pyelography with descending cystography may confirm a leak in the bladder.

EXAMINATION OF INJURIES AROUND THE HIP

History of severe violence, e.g., motor car collision (dashboard dislocation), a fall from a height or falling of a heavy weight on the back of a stooping workman is usually obtained in dislocation of the hip. A direct impact on the greater trochanter medially may drive the head of the femur through the floor of the acetabulum into the pelvis causing central dislocation of the hip. Minor injuries such as stumbling or missing a step or a fall on slippery surface may cause fracture of the femoral neck in elderly persons. So adequate emphasis should be laid on elicitation of the history to come to a proper diagnosis. Even an enquiry should be made in a case of suspected fracture neck of femur. Whether the patient was able to get up after the fall (which indicates the fracture to be impacted) or he was on the floor helpless and was unable to move his leg (unimpacted fracture).

A. INSPECTION

1. **Attitude (Figs. 13.28 and 13.29):** The attitude of the patient on the bed after the injury will itself indicate the diagnosis. An elderly patient lying helplessly on the bed with *externally rotated,* lower limb indicates fracture of the neck of the femur. Young patient lying with similarly *externally rotated, slightly abducted and flexed* lower limb indicates anterior dislocation of the hip which is not very common in comparison to the posterior dislocation. In the latter condition young patient lies with *flexed, adducted and internally rotated lower limb.*

2. **Swelling:** Abnormal swelling and bruising will be evident in the injured hip either due to hematoma in case of fracture neck of femur or due to abnormal position of the head of the femur.

3. A note should be made whether the injured limb appears to be shortened or lengthened (see under "Measurement").

B. PALPATION

1. **Greater trochanter:** Palpation of the greater trochanter and its relation with other bony points are the key-stones for diagnosis of injuries around the hip.

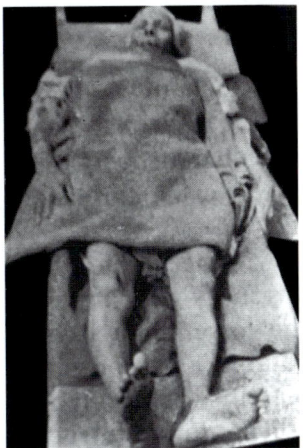

Fig. 13.28: Note the typical attitude of external rotation of the left lower limb due to fracture of the femoral neck.

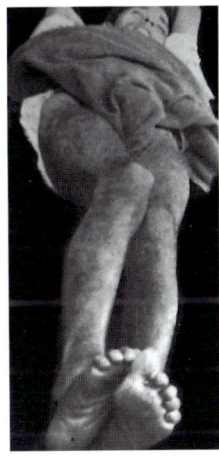

Fig. 13.29: Posterior dislocation of right hip. Note the characteristic attitude of flexion, adduction and internal rotation of the thigh.

   A triangle formed by the anterior superior iliac spine, the greater trochanter and a line drawn vertically downwards from the anterior superior iliac spine is called the *Bryant's triangle* (Fig. 13.30). When the shortest side of the triangle, i.e., the distance between the tip of the greater trochanter and a point on the imaginary line drawn vertically downwards from the anterior superior iliac spine, becomes shortened, it indicates a fracture of the femur, posterior dislocation of the hip and separation of the upper femoral epiphysis. This indicates upward displacement of the greater trochanter.

   In posterior dislocation of the hip, the greater trochanter moves towards the anterior superior iliac spine due to internal rotation of the limb. In anterior dislocation or fracture of the neck of

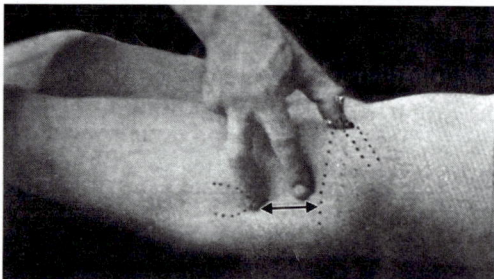
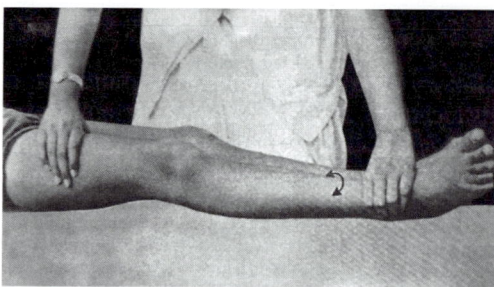

Fig. 13.30: Showing the method of palpation of the greater trochanter and how to determine Bryant's triangle.

Fig. 13.31: In fracture below the trochanters, the greater trochanter will remain immobile while the shaft of the femur is being rotated.

the femur the greater trochanter recedes from the anterior superior iliac spine due to external rotation of the femur.

If the greater trochanter lies in its normal position but the lower limb is externally rotated, the possibility of fracture below the greater trochanter (subtrochanteric fracture) should be kept in mind. This is confirmed by absence of transmitted movement, i.e., the greater trochanter fails to move while the leg is rotated **(Fig. 13.31)**.

2. **Head of the femur:** A search should be made to find out the position of the head of the femur. In different types of dislocation the position of the head of the femur will vary. It may be on the dorsum ilii (posterior type), in the groin (pubic type) or rarely in the perineum (obturator type). Confirm the identity of the head by noting that it moves with rotation of the shaft. In this context one must remember that *medial surface of the medial condyle looks to the same direction as the head of the femur.*

Another important point in this regard is the palpation of the femoral artery at the base of the femoral triangle. Normally it is well palpated as the artery is being supported from behind by the head of the femur. In posterior dislocation due to the absence of the head of the femur in its normal position the artery cannot be palpated so easily.

3. **Tenderness:** Bony tenderness on the site of fracture will be obvious particularly in trochanteric fracture. In transcervical and subcapital fractures, tenderness can only be elicited when an attempt is made to rotate the shaft of the femur.

C. MEASUREMENTS

Various types of measurement can be tried in injuries around the hip.

1. **Bryant's triangle (Fig. 13.32):** The patient lies in the dorsal position. A line is drawn vertically downwards from the anterior superior iliac spine. Another from the tip of the same spine to the tip of the greater trochanter and lastly a horizontal line is drawn from the tip of the greater trochanter to the first line. Diminution in the length of the last line or the horizontal line in comparison to the other side denotes an upward elevation of the greater trochanter, the most common cause

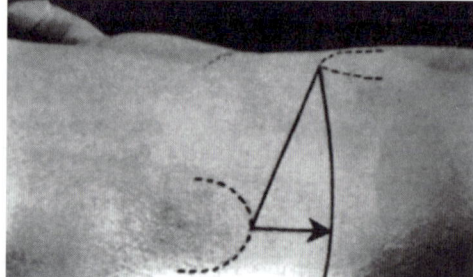

Fig. 13.32: Bryant's triangle. Elevation of the greater trochanter is determined by comparing the horizontal line (shown by arrow) with that of the normal side.

of which being the transcervical or subcapital fracture of the neck of the femur or separation of the upper femoral epiphysis. Diminution or increase in the length of the second line indicates the anterior or posterior displacement of the greater trochanter accordingly (which occurs in posterior dislocation and anterior dislocation of the hip respectively).

2. **Nelaton's line:** The patient lies on his sound side. A line is drawn or a measuring tape is placed from the most prominent part of the ischial tuberosity to the tip of the anterior superior iliac spine. Normally, this line touches the tip of the greater trochanter and therefore any upward displacement of the trochanter can be easily demonstrated without comparing it with the other side **(Fig. 13.33)**.

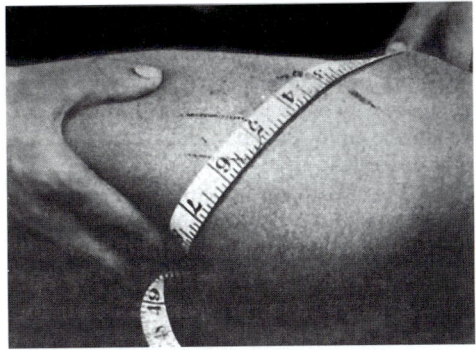

Fig. 13.33: Shows how to draw Nelaton's line with a measuring tape from the most prominent part of the ischial tuberosity to the tip of the anterior superior iliac spine. See that this line normally touches the tip of the greater trochanter.

3. **Schoemaker's line:** The line from the tip of the greater trochanter to the anterior superior iliac spine if prolonged anteriorly will reach the umbilicus of the patient. This is called Schoemaker's line. If the greater trochanter is elevated the line will cross the midline below the umbilicus.

4. **Morris' bitrochanteric test:** The distance between the outer border of the greater trochanter to the symphysis pubis is measured on both sides by means of a pair of calipers and is compared with the other side. It will reveal any medial (posterior and central dislocation) or lateral (anterior dislocation of hip) displacement of the trochanter.

5. **Chiene's test:** Normally, a tape joining the tips of the greater trochanters is parallel to another joining the two anterior superior iliac spines. When a trochanter is raised, these two lines converge towards the affected side.

6. **Length of the lower limb:** Before taking measurement of the affected limb, the normal limb must be placed in the identical position and there should not be tilting of the pelvis as determined by the line joining the two anterior superior iliac spines. The length of the lower limb is measured from the anterior superior iliac spine **(Fig. 13.34)** to the medial malleolus. The thigh alone is measured from the anterior superior iliac spine to the joint-line of the knee which can be easily felt in the flexed position of the knee. It was customary to make the upper border of the patella or more commonly the adductor tubercle as the lower landmark instead of the joint line. But the former is moveable and the latter is difficult to locate particularly in obese individuals. It is always advisable to mark the bony points first and then measured with the measuring tape. Shortening is expected in all the fractures and dislocation with the sole exception of the obturator type of anterior dislocation in which slight lengthening may be present.

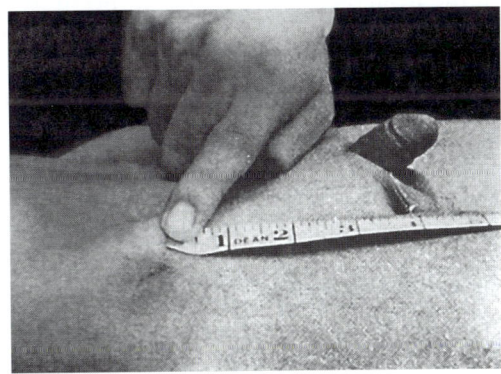

Fig. 13.34: Shows how to hold the metal end of the measuring tape against the anterior superior iliac spine.

D. MOVEMENTS

All movements of the hip joint to the full extent exclude possibility of any bony injury. If the patient is able to lift his leg off the bed keeping the knee straight, it indicates no bony injury around the hip. It must be remembered that some use of limb is possible in an impacted fracture of the neck of femur. In posterior dislocation, there is complete limitation of abduction and lateral rotation whereas slight adduction and internal rotation may be possible.

Complications: (a) Excessive bleeding at the fracture site and shock after fracture neck of femur is not unusual. Blood transfusion is often required at the time of operation. (b) Sciatic nerve injury may occur in posterior dislocation of the hip and subtrochanteric fracture. Femoral nerve may be rarely injured in pubic type of dislocation and the obturator nerve in the obturator type of dislocation.

Rectal examination is essential in central dislocation of the hip joint where the head of the femur lies within the pelvis. While doing rectal examination if the limb is rotated, the head of the femur can be felt rotating by the finger in the rectum. Central dislocation very much resembles fracture neck of femur. By the medial displacement of the greater trochanter, shortening and pain down the course of the obturator nerve this rare condition can be diagnosed.

E. X-RAY EXAMINATION

This is again the most important investigation which will not only indicate the type of injury but also will give a clue to the line of fracture, the type of displacement, the type of treatment to be required for the particular case and the probable outcome of the treatment.

So far as the **fracture neck of the femur** is concerned, there are five types of fractures according to the site of fracture which will be evident in skiagram. The fracture may be situated at: (i) high in the neck (subcapital), (ii) low in the neck (basal) **(Fig. 13.35)**, (iii) in the middle of the neck (transcervical), (iv) in the trochanteric region and (v) just below the trochanter (subtrochanteric). The angle of the fracture line is also important, as more vertical it is, the less favorable is the prognosis. In this context one may draw *Pauwel's angle* **(Fig. 13.36)** which is formed between the fracture line and an imaginary horizontal line. How much rotation the shaft has undergone after the fracture can be assessed by looking at the lesser trochanter. It is normally situated at the posteromedial aspect of the femur and is partly visible in X-ray. When the femur is externally rotated it is clearly visualized and when the femur is internally rotated it becomes concealed by the superimposed shadow of the femur. In trochanteric fracture, it is often comminuted with three or four pieces and indicates difficulty in fixation.

So far as the **dislocation of hip** is concerned, the orthodox anteroposterior and lateral views will give a clue to the position of the head of the femur—whether the dislocation is an anterior one or central or posterior one. There will be definite distortion of the Shenton's line.

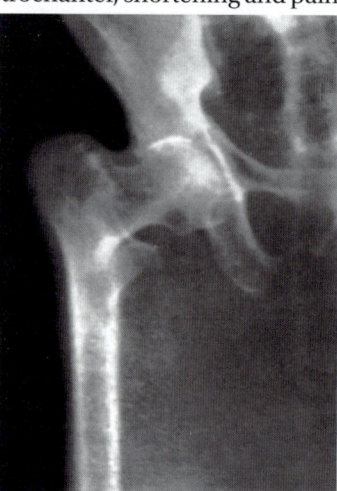

Fig. 13.35: Fracture neck of the right femur at its base (intertrochanteric).

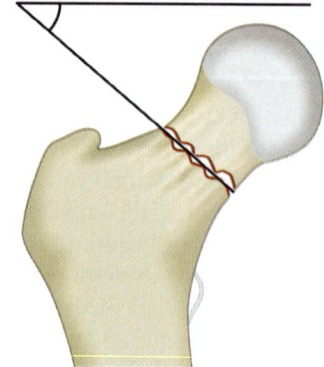

Fig. 13.36: Shows Pauwel's angle formed by the fracture-line with the horizontal plane.

In injuries about the hip the followings are important and worth mentioning:

1. **Fracture of the neck of the femur:** Classically, an old patient after trivial injury such as missing a step or falling down on the ground sustains an injury to the hip for which he neither moves his limb nor finds himself capable of getting up. On examination there will be swelling and bruising in the region of the greater trochanter. The limb will be seen externally rotated and there is definite shortening of the limb. There is tenderness near the greater trochanter. Relative elevation of the greater trochanter will be evident by Bryant's triangle and Nelaton's line. X-ray is confirmatory.

   Complications are: (i) Avascular necrosis of the head of the femur, (ii) malunion, (iii) non-union and (iv) late osteoarthritis.

2. **Dislocation of the hip:** The *posterior dislocation* is by far the commonest. This is diagnosed by: (i) history (see above), (ii) the attitude of flexion, adduction and internal rotation of the limb, (iii) shortening, (iv) rigidity of the hip towards the movements of abduction and external rotation and (v) difficulty in feeling the pulsation of the femoral artery. X-ray will show the displaced head on the dorsum ilii.

   Anterior dislocation, which results from a classical accident in which a man stands with one foot on the river bank and the other on a boat which is gradually moving away from him, so that the limb concerned is gradually abducted until it dislocates anteriorly. The lower limb takes an attitude of flexion, abduction and external rotation. The head of the femur is easily palpated by the side of the symphysis pubis in the pubic type and under the adductor muscles in the obturator type in which the limb appears to be lengthened.

   Central dislocation is rare accident in which the femoral head is forced through the broken acetabulum. When this is suspected a finger in the rectum will feel the head of the femur in the pelvis and will be moving on rotation of the thigh. More often the condition is not recognized until an X-ray is taken **(Fig. 13.37)**.

3. **Avulsion fracture of the lesser trochanter:** Classically, it occurs at school boy age by a violent contraction of the iliopsoas muscles. The pathognomonic sign is inability to flex the stretched leg when the patient is seated (Ludloff's sign).

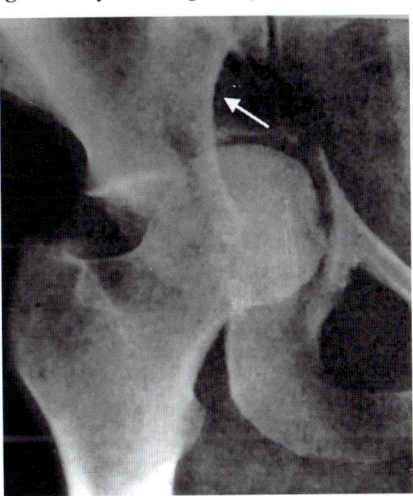

Fig. 13.37: Central dislocation of the hip. Note that the head of the femur has been pushed through the broken acetabulum into the pelvis.

EXAMINATION OF INJURIES IN THE THIGH

HISTORY

(i) **Age:** Fracture of the shaft of the femur may occur at any age. An enquiry should be made regarding the severity of the injury. Though slightly oblique or transverse fracture of the shaft of the femur in young age is very common in motor cycle accident, yet this type of fracture in older age group with minor trauma should raise the suspicion of malignancy.

(ii) **Mechanism of injury:** Direct injury of angulation force will cause slightly oblique or transverse fracture. When the foot is anchored to the ground a twisting force transmitted to the femur will cause a spiral fracture.

LOCAL EXAMINATION

A. INSPECTION

Abnormal swelling and deformity in the thigh after an injury are probably due to fracture of the shaft of the femur. The **attitude** that the patient is lying helplessly also goes in favor of fracture of the shaft of the femur.

B. PALPATION

Bony irregularity, local tenderness and **crepitus** are the diagnostic features, as in case of other fractures. So far as the **displacement** is concerned, it depends on the site of fracture. In fracture of the *upper third* of the femur, the proximal fragment is flexed by the iliopsoas muscle, abducted by the gluteal muscles and everted by the external rotators, but the lower fragment is adducted by the adductor muscles and overlapped proximally by the hamstrings and quadriceps and everted by the weight of the limb. In case of fracture of the *middle third and lower third of* the femur the deformity is the backward angulation and overlapping of the distal fragment by the action of the gastrocnemius and quadriceps respectively.

C. MEASUREMENTS

Shortening of the length of the femur measured from the tip of the greater trochanter to the joint line of the knee joint is the marked feature of the fracture of the shaft of the femur. **X-ray** is confirmatory.

EXAMINATION OF INJURIES AROUND THE KNEE JOINT

HISTORY

To come to a diagnosis about the type of injury the knee has sustained one must take a thorough history. Most emphasis should be laid on the following points:

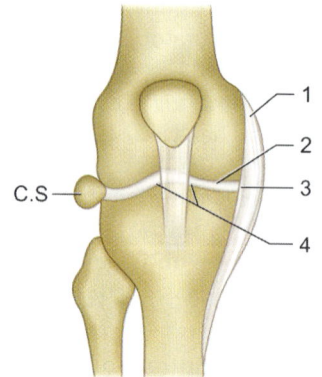

Mechanism (Fig. 13.38): The details of the type of injury and the position of the knee joint in respect to the body as a whole at the time of injury should be considered. A blow on the lateral side of the knee when the patient is bearing weight on the leg will stress the medial collateral ligament. If the violence is relatively weak and only some fibers but not the whole of the ligament give way, it is called a simple *sprain*. If the violence is very severe, the ligament may be ruptured in its entirety usually at its femoral attachment. A blow on the medial side of the knee, which is very rare may cause injury to the lateral collateral ligament. When a backward thrust is given to the anterior aspect of the tibia with the knee joint flexed an injury to the posterior cruciate ligament may be expected. This may occur to the front-passenger in a motor car if he is thrown violently forwards against the dashboard during sudden break or accident. Isolated injury to the anterior cruciate ligament is rather uncommon and only occurs when the knee is forcible hyperextended. *Injury to the menisci* is very important and peculiar to the knee joint. It occurs commonly to the footballers and coal miners. Tears of degenerated menisci also occur in the osteoarthritic knees. The medial meniscus is more often damaged than its lateral counterpart. The mechanism is

Fig. 13.38: Points of tenderness 1: sprain of the medial collateral ligament, 2: injury to the medial semilunar cartilage, 3: sprain of deep fibers of the medial collateral ligament and injury to the semilunar cartilage, 4: injury to the infrapatellar pad of fat. C.S: cyst of the semilunar cartilage (common on the lateral side).

rotation of the tibia on the femur when the knee is flexed and carrying weight of the body. The medial meniscus is damaged when the femur is internally rotated on the tibia and the lateral meniscus is damaged when the femur is externally rotated on the tibia. Just after injury the joint gives way and becomes swollen due to effusion. Sometimes the joint becomes 'locked', i.e., it cannot be extended after a limit. At times after a period of temporary inactivity the footballer stands up and continues the game for the rest of the period. But he gradually realizes that his knee is giving way in minor injuries and may be swollen and even 'locked'. Locking of the knee joint, unlike locking of the door, means the joint can be flexed freely but cannot be extended beyond certain degree.

Locking of the knee joint may also occur due to presence of loose bodies the causes of which are discussed later in this chapter. The bony injuries around the knee joint may occur from direct injuries or indirect injuries such as muscular violence which may cause fracture of the patella of the other knee joint when one leg slips.

LOCAL EXAMINATION OF KNEE

A. INSPECTION
The patient should lie down on the examining table with the two lower limbs *completely exposed* and placed in *identical position*. Inspection should be made from all aspects *including the popliteal fossa.*

1. **Attitude:** This is particularly important when the knee is locked in flexed position. The joint should be carefully inspected whether it is abducted or adducted, hyperextended or displaced backward.
2. **Swelling:** After many injuries the knee joint is effused. In ligamentous injuries the effusion is mostly serous or serosanguineous. In bony injuries affecting the articular surfaces the effusion is mostly hemorrhagic. Any effusion of the knee joint will give rise to a characteristic horse-shoe shaped swelling around the superior and lateral aspects of the patella. Dislocation of the patella mostly occurs on the lateral condyle of the femur giving rise to an abnormal swelling at that region. Recurrent dislocation of patella after trifle injury to the knee joint is not uncommon.
3. **Muscular wasting:** It occurs in old injury to the knee joint leading to muscular wasting of quadriceps muscles. Very often it is seen after an old injury to the meniscus. But this may not occur if the patient continues quadriceps exercise after such injury.

B. PALPATION
In palpation particular care is taken to elicit the exact point of tenderness around the knee joint. This will give a clue as to the diagnosis of the condition. Palpation of all the bones around the knee joint is also important. This includes palpation of the patella, lower part of the femur and upper ends of the tibia and the fibula. In case of effusion in the knee joint 'patellar tap' and fluctuation tests are important.

1. **Exact point of tenderness:** In lesion of the medial collateral ligament tenderness is characteristically present at its femoral attachment. Tenderness over the ligament at the level of the joint without any tenderness at its bony attachments is suggestive more of an injury to the medial semilunar cartilage and less of the sprain of the deep fibers of the medial collateral ligament. Tenderness at the joint level midway between the ligamentum patellae and the tibial collateral ligament indicates torn anterior horn of the medial semilunar cartilage. Tenderness posterior to the tibial collateral ligament is diagnostic of a torn posterior horn. Tenderness

just on both the sides of the ligamentum patellae indicates nipped infrapatellar pad of fat. *The best method of eliciting tenderness for the torn anterior horn of the medial meniscus is as follows:* The knee is flexed at right angle. Gentle pressure is exerted by the tip of the thumb at the midpoint between ligamentum patellae and the tibial collateral ligament **(Fig. 13.39)**. This often elicits tenderness. If not, the thumb is kept pressed over the same region while the knee joint is gradually extended. The patient will complain of pain which he has not done previously.

2. **Palpation of the patella:** In any injury to the knee joint it is a good practice to palpate the patella as a whole as it is very vulnerable to fracture in injuries of the knee joint particularly with effusion. While palpating the patella the fingers should run along the borders of the patella to find out any gap therein. Various types of fracture of patella are come across in surgical practice. In case of a transverse fracture, a considerable gap is always felt between the two fragments. In case of comminuted fracture irregularity of the bone will be obvious. In case of simple crack fracture the diagnosis is sometimes difficult and may be missed. Local bony tenderness and slight bony irregularity are the diagnostic features. The diagnosis may only be unveiled by X-ray of the knee joint.

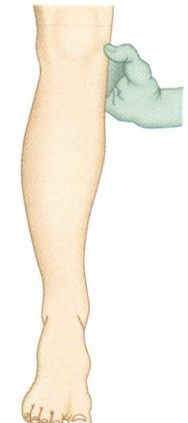

Fig. 13.39: Method to elicit tenderness by pressure of clinician's thumb at the mid point between ligamentum patellae and the tibial collateral ligament when the anterior horn of the medial meniscus is torn.

Sometimes quadriceps tendon or the ligamentum patellae is torn from the patella. The diagnosis of this condition is also not very difficult by palpation. In any injury to the patella or the extensor mechanism of the knee joint viz. the quadriceps tendon and the ligamentum patellae, the patient will be unable to lift the extended limb from the bed.

3. **Palpation of the lower end of the femur:** In supracondylar fracture, the lower fragment is tilted *backwards* by the pull of the gastrocnemius. So during palpation the lower end of the upper fragment becomes projected forwards and easily palpated In separation of the lower epiphysis, on the other hand, the epiphysis is displaced forwards over the lower part of the shaft. A word of caution will not be out of place here that the pulse in the foot should always be felt during this type of injury as the popliteal artery runs the risk of being damaged by the displaced fragment. Injury to the femoral condyles can be easily suspected by careful palpation which will elicit bony irregularity and local bony tenderness.

4. **Palpation of the upper ends of the tibia and fibula:** Usually the lateral condyle of the tibia is more frequently fractured than the medial one. Palpate carefully the tibial tubercle and the upper end of the fibula for bony tenderness and irregularity.

Springing the fibula **(Fig. 13.40)**: In fracture of the upper end of the fibula tenderness at the fracture site can be elicited by squeezing the lower parts of the tibia and fibula.

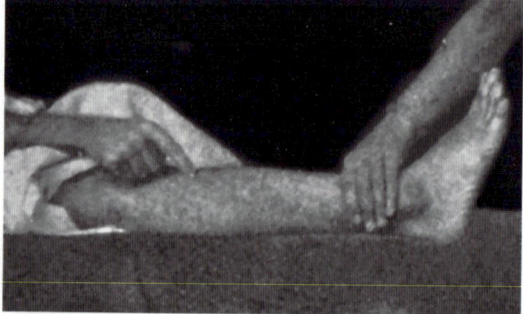

Fig. 13.40: Shows how springing the fibula is being performed.

5. **Swelling:** Besides the fracture around the knee joint which will cause abnormal swelling, effusion of the knee joint is by far the most common cause of swelling after injury to the knee. It must be borne in mind that besides fracture extending into the joint hemorrhage may be due to hemophilia in which the affection is often bilateral. The tests for fluctuation and "patellar tap" are discussed in Chapter 15.

C. MEASUREMENTS

In injury to the knee joint the following measurements may be of necessity :

(i) Breadth of the lower end of the femur and upper end of the tibia can be measured with the help of a pair of calipers.

(ii) Circumference of the thigh and calf at fixed points from the joint-line of the knee will indicate if there is any muscular wasting following injury.

D. MOVEMENTS

As has already been discussed derangement of the extensor mechanism of the knee joint which may be brought about by fracture of the patella or rupture of the quadriceps tendon or ligamentum patellae will make the patient unable to lift the extended lower limb above the bed. The clinician must not try to flex the knee joint in such type of injury as it will cause further damage to the extensor apparatus of the knee joint. When the joint cannot be fully extended (locked) the possibility of a bucket handle tear of the medial meniscus or presence of a loose body within the knee joint should be kept in mind.

McMurray's test (Fig. 13. 41): This is a very popular test to detect any tear either in the medial or lateral semilunar cartilage. In making the examination the patient must be recumbent and relaxed, the surgeon standing at the side of the injured limb. He grasps the foot firmly with one hand and the knee with the other hand. The knee joint is completely flexed that means the heel touches the buttock. The foot is now rotated externally and the leg abducted at the knee. This twisting movement is done for a few times and then the joint is slowly extended keeping the foot externally rotated and abducted. If the posterior end of the medial semilunar cartilage is torn the patient will complain of

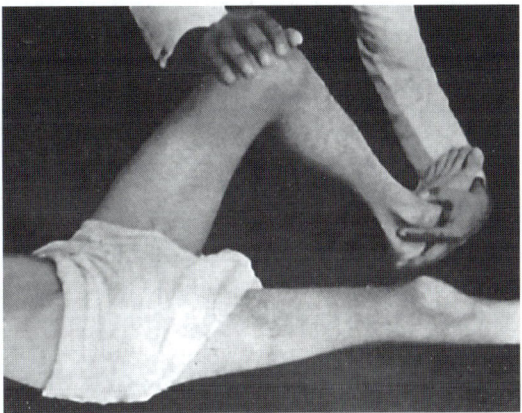

Fig. 13.41: Demonstration of McMurray's test. See the text.

pain at this stage as the torn cartilage will be caught between the femur and the tibia. At the same time a definite 'click' will be felt by the hand at the knee and the patient will experience a feeling of giving way of the knee joint simultaneously. The angle at which this occurs, indicates the position of the cartilaginous lesion. When middle of the cartilage is torn the click is felt at the middle of extension and when the anterior horn is torn click is felt almost at the end of extension.

Similar exercise with the foot rotated internally and the knee adducted, if elicits pain and a 'click' as discussed in the previous paragraph, indicates tear in the lateral semilunar cartilage. Similarly the angle of the knee at which the pain and 'click' will be experienced will give a clue as to the position of the tear.

Apley's grinding test: The patient lies prone on the table. The clinician places his knee on the patient's thigh in order to fix the femur. The knee joint is flexed to the right angle. Now the clinician applies compression and lateral rotation to the leg from the foot, i.e., grinding. If the patient complains of pain by the maneuver, there is a tear in the medial semilunar cartilage. If the patient complains of pain while the clinician compresses and internally rotates the leg, there is a tear in lateral semilunar cartilage.

Apley's distraction test: If the patient complains of pain while the leg is pulled upwards and rotated laterally a tear of the medial collateral ligament is diagnosed. Similarly, if the pain is elicited by pulling the leg upwards and rotating it internally, a tear of the lateral collateral ligament, which is very rare, is diagnosed.

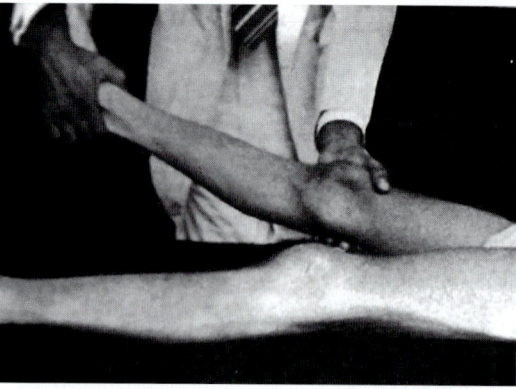

Fig. 13.42: The knee is being abducted to detect any sprain or rupture of the medial collateral ligament.

Test of stability: The two collateral ligaments and cruciate ligaments are mainly responsible for the stability of the knee joint. If any of these ligaments is ruptured the stability of the joint is jeopardized. The integrities of these ligaments are tested as follows:

1. **Abduction and adduction tests (Fig. 13.42):** The knee joint is held in full extension lifting the foot up with one hand from the bed and the other hand is kept at the knee. Using the hand at the side of the knee as the fulcrum the leg is first abducted to test the integrity of the medial collateral ligament, which is more frequently injured than its lateral counterpart and next adducted to test the integrity of lateral ligament. If the ligament is torn the joint will be abnormally opened at that side. But if the ligament is sprained the joint will remain stable but the patient will complain of excruciating pain during the exercise.

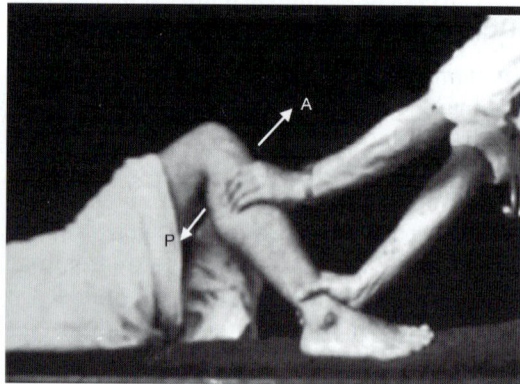

Fig. 13.43: Shows how to demonstrate Drawer sign. Excessive anterior 'A' or posterior 'P' mobility of the tibia indicates tear of the anterior or posterior cruciate ligament respectively.

2. **Drawer sign (Figs. 13.43 and 13.44):** This is diagnostic of injury to the cruciate ligaments. The patient lies in the supine position and the knee joint is flexed at right angle keeping the foot on the bed. The clinician sits on the foot of the patient to fix the lower limb. The upper part of the tibia is pulled forward and pushed backward. If the anterior cruciate ligament is ruptured there will be increased anterior mobility and if the posterior cruciate ligament is ruptured there will be increased posterior mobility of the joint.

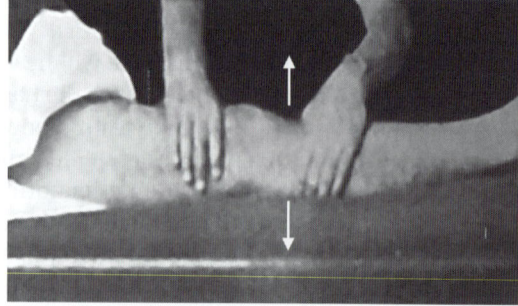

Fig. 13.44: Testing for integrity of the cruciate ligaments. An attempt is being made to move the upper end of the tibia on the femur.

Complications: The lateral popliteal nerve is liable to be injured in fracture of the upper end of the fibula particularly the neck. The popliteal vessels are liable to be injured in supracondylar fracture of the femur and separation of the lower epiphysis of the femur. When the artery is pressed upon there will be diminution or absence of pulsation of the dorsalis pedis and the posterior tibial arteries. When the vein is pressed upon there will be edema of the leg.

E. X-RAY EXAMINATION

Besides the usual anteroposterior and lateral views, the knee joint should also be X-rayed in forced abduction and adduction positions. The latter skiagram will show the degree of joint laxity due to rupture of the ligaments concerned. Pneumoarthrography, i.e., taking X-ray picture of the knee joint after injecting air may prove useful in detecting doubtful lesion of the meniscus.

In injuries about the knee joint the following conditions are to be remembered:
1. Fracture and dislocation of the patella.
2. Fracture and epiphyseal separation of the lower end of the femur.
3. Fracture of the upper end of the fibula.
4. Dislocation of the knee (very rare).
5. Injury to the collateral ligaments (the internal ligament is more often affected).
6. Injury to the semilunar cartilage or the meniscus (commonly medial).
7. Injury to the cruciate ligaments.
8. Injury to the infrapatellar pad of fat.
9. Fracture of the tibial spine.
10. Traumatic loose bodies.

DIFFERENTIAL DIAGNOSIS OF INJURIES AROUND KNEE

FRACTURE OF THE PATELLA

While direct violence results in comminuted fracture of the patella, transverse fracture is caused by indirect muscular violence. In case of muscular violence the man slips on one leg, automatically the other knee gradually flexes until he falls down. In order to avert the fall, his quadriceps contracts violently when the patella is situated at its highest point on the femoral condyle. This results in transverse fracture of the patella which is forced against the femoral condyle by violent contraction of the quadriceps.

The diagnosis is made by the history of trauma (as discussed above), swelling of the knee joint due to effusion of blood, irregularity and bony tenderness which becomes obvious on careful palpation and grating sensation during movement of the knee joint.

INJURY TO THE COLLATERAL LIGAMENTS

The medial collateral ligament is more often injured than its lateral counterpart due to the fact that it is adherent to the capsule of the knee joint, whereas the lateral collateral ligament is free from the capsule being intervened by the tendon of the popliteus.

The patient complains of pain on the medial side of the knee joint and points out the site of pain at the femoral attachment of the medial collateral ligament. Very occasionally the patient shows tenderness over the medial aspect of the joint line due to torn deep fibers of this ligament. But this type of tenderness is more often due to injury to the medial semilunar cartilage. Forced abduction of the extended leg will open out the joint at its medial aspect indicating complete rupture of the medial collateral ligament. This opening out of the medial aspect of the joint in the forced abduction position of the knee joint in X-ray confirms the diagnosis.

INJURY TO THE SEMILUNAR CARTILAGES

This is by far the most important injury and peculiar to the knee joint. The medial semilunar cartilage is more often injured being fixed to the collateral ligament, whereas the lateral semilunar cartilage enjoys the advantage of being more mobile as it is not attached to the lateral collateral ligament and it gives origin to the tendon of popliteus which pulls it backwards and does not give any chance of being nipped between the two condyles of femur and the tibia. The **mechanism** of injury to the semilunar cartilage is that the knee joint must be primarily *flexed* since rotation cannot occur when the knee joint is extended. A *rotational strain* (either internal rotation of femur on the tibia or external rotation of the tibia on the femur) a*nd forceful abduction* are necessary as the latter tends to open up the inner side of the joint and exerts a suctional influence on the cartilage, which is drawn inwards and then nipped between the condyles of the femur and the tibia during the rotational strain causing longitudinal tear of the medial semilunar cartilage. There are three types of tear. (i) Anterior horn tear, (ii) Bucket-handle tear and (iii) Posterior horn tear. A transverse tear, if at all occurs, is always an artefact. Usually the footballers and the workers in mines are the victims of this type of injury. After injury to the knee joint, the mechanism of which has already been described, the joint becomes locked generally followed by sudden unlocking and giving way. The joint becomes effused. On examination a definite point of tenderness can be elicited at the joint-line between the patellar ligament and the medial collateral ligament in tear of the anterior horn. Very often this injury is ignored and the footballer continues to play. Similar injury even of a milder variety will cause locking and effusion of the knee joint. In "Bucket-handle" tear generally locking persists. In tear of the posterior horn, the joint may be locked, often gives way and effused **(Fig. 13.45)**. *McMurray's test* is of great help in diagnosing tear of the semilunar cartilages. In an old lesion, there will be marked wasting of quadriceps and laxity of the joint. X-ray pictures are mainly required to exclude any bony lesion particularly fracture of the tibial spine.

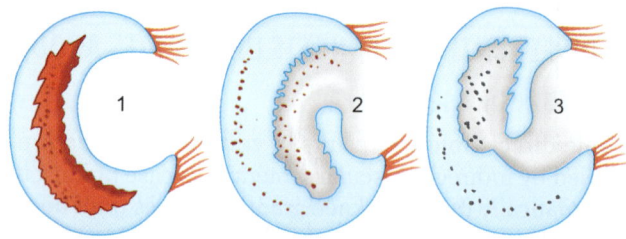

Fig. 13.45: Three types of tear of medial meniscus. 1: Bucket handle tear. 2: Anterior horn tear and 3: Posterior horn tear.

Though the lateral semilunar cartilage is rarely injured yet two distinct types of pathology—(i) congenital discoid cartilage and (ii) cyst of the cartilage are commonly met with this cartilage. These are discussed in the chapter of "Examination of Individual Joint Pathologies".

INJURY TO THE CRUCIATE LIGAMENTS

This generally results from severe injury to the knee joint as the cruciate ligaments are placed interiorly and are very strong. The diagnosis of tear of the anterior or posterior ligament is made by Drawer's sign, i.e., abnormal forward or backward mobility of the tibia on femur respectively. In case of torn anterior ligament the knee joint can be hyperextended.

INJURY TO THE INFRAPATELLAR PAD OF FAT

This injury is by far less common than the previous entities. When the infrapatellar pad of fat becomes hypertrophied, it may be nipped between the femur and tibia during extension of the knee joint. Diagnosis is made by the history of sudden pain with or without locking. On examination tenderness can be elicited on both sides of the ligamentum patellae. Signs and symptoms of osteoarthritis are frequently present.

FRACTURE OF THE TIBIAL SPINE

After an injury to the knee joint there will be locking with a feel of bony block and effusion. There may or may not be any localized tenderness which can be elicited from outside. Only X-ray is confirmatory.

LOOSE BODIES OF THE KNEE JOINT

This itself forms a chapter and there are numerous causes of forming loose bodies inside the knee joint (**Fig. 13.46**).

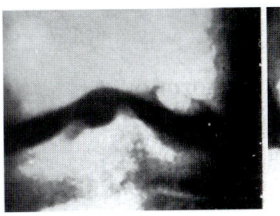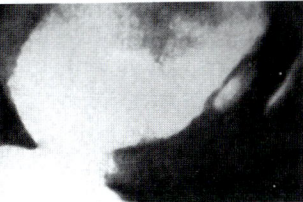

Fig. 13.46: Skiagram of a typical case of loose body of the knee joint due to osteochondritis dissecans.

CLASSIFICATION OF LOOSE BODIES

A. **FIBROUS LOOSE BODIES:** *Traumatic,* i.e., organization from hemorrhage into villus and *pathological*—in association with (i) tuberculosis, (ii) syphilis and (iii) osteoarthritis.
B. **FIBRINOUS LOOSE BODIES:** *Traumatic*—after hemorrhage and *pathological* in association with (i) tuberculosis and (ii) chronic synovitis.
C. **CARTILAGINOUS LOOSE BODIES:** *Traumatic*—separation of whole or part of an intra-articular fibrocartilage, e.g., meniscus.
D. **OSTEOCARTILAGINOUS LOOSE BODIES:** *Pathological*—it may be from (i) osteochondritis dissecans, (ii) detachment of osteophytes in osteoarthritis, (iii) separation of sequestrum in acute osteomyelitis, (iv) synovial chondromata, etc. *Traumatic*—fracture of the tibial spine.
E. **MISCELLANEOUS LOOSE BODIES**—(i) introduced foreign body, (ii) lipoma and (iii) secondary carcinoma.

Diagnosis of presence of loose body inside the knee joint is made by history of recurrent locking at different angles. There will be associated findings according to the cause of loose bodies. The most difficult part is to differentiate injury to the meniscus with the presence of loose bodies inside the joint. This difference is easier when the loose body is radio-opaque, i.e., bony or osteocartilaginous or radio-opaque foreign bodies. This requires only X-ray for diagnosis. Two conditions should be kept in mind which are often misdiagnosed as bony loose bodies in the knee joint. They are: (a) **Fabella**—a sesamoid bone in the lateral head of the gastrocnemius and (b) **Pellegrini-Stieda's disease** in which calcification occurs in the tibial collateral ligament after partial avulsion from the medial condyle of the femur.

EXAMINATION OF INJURIES ABOUT THE ANKLE AND FOOT

HISTORY

The *mechanism* of injury around the ankle is usually violence. The foot is everted, externally rotated or internally rotated on the tibia. Actually the foot is anchored to the ground while the momentum of the body drives the tibia. This usually occurs when the foot is fixed by a hole in the ground or in a ski, while the body moves forwards. It may occur when the patient stumbles over an unexpected obstacle or stair. To these may be added an upward thrust if the patient falls from a height. The injuries are generally of three types—(i) external rotation, (ii) internal rotation and (iii) vertical compression.

A. INSPECTION

The **deformity** of the foot is carefully observed whether it is displaced laterally, medially or forwards or backwards in comparison to the tibia. Excessive broadening of the ankle suggests inferior tibiofibular diastasis, i.e., the inferior tibiofibular ligament is torn and the talus is wedged between the tibia and fibula.

B. PALPATION

1. All the bones forming the ankle, i.e., the lower ends of the tibia and fibula including the two malleoli, the calcaneus and the talus are carefully palpated. Similarly in injury to the foot, the bones concerned, i.e., the tarsal bones, the metatarsals, the phalanges, etc. are examined. (i) **Local bony tenderness**, (ii) **local bony irregularity**, (iii) **displacement**, (iv) **unnatural mobility** and (v) **crepitus** are the findings which one should look for to diagnose if any bone concerned has been fractured or not.

   Palpation of the lower end of the tibia and fibula and the two malleoli are not very difficult. The calcaneum is palpated from posterior aspect while the talus is palpated by deep pressure with the thumb in front and just below the ankle. To palpate the tarsal bones is not also very difficult. The metatarsals and the phalanges are palpated along their length.

2. Sprain of ankle is also very common. Tenderness just below a malleolus suggests *sprain of the ankle.* If the foot is turned to the opposite direction to stretch the ligament concerned the patient will complain of pain. This suggests sprain of the ankle.

3. *Springing the fibula:* By squeezing the upper ends of the tibia and fibula pain will be elicited at the lower part of the fibula if it is fractured.

4. Lastly one must palpate tendo Achilles to find if there is any gap or tenderness at its attachment with the os calcis. Palpation of injuries around the ankle remains incomplete if this examination is missed.

C. MOVEMENTS

In fracture around the ankle, obviously there will be restriction in movements of the ankle joint. By holding the ankle joint with one hand, slight active or passive movement of the ankle with the other hand will give an indication about the type of fracture that has probably occurred.

D. MEASUREMENTS

(i) The length of the leg, which is not so vital has already been discussed in page no. 230. (ii) The distances between the medial malleolus to the head of the first metatarsal bone and the point of the heel are important. Similarly the distances between the lateral malleolus to the head of the 5th metatarsal bone and the point of the heel are important. These measurements should be compared with those of the sound side. In fracture of the calcaneus the distances between the malleoli and the point of the heel are shortened if there is upward displacement of the tuberosity. (iii) Broadening of the ankle as measured by means of calipers, is often seen in inferior tibiofibular diastasis.

X-RAY EXAMINATION

Usual anteroposterior and lateral views are quite useful in determining different fractures around the ankle and the foot. Only in cases of suspected fracture of the calcaneus axial X-ray may be needed to detect displacement in vertical fractures involving the joint. In case of a fracture of the calcaneus *tuber-joint angle* must be noted. This angle is formed at the back of the ankle by two lines—one passing over the nonarticular surface of the calcaneus and the other along the articular surface of the same bone for the talus. Normally, this angle is about 40°. In fractures when the tuberosity is displaced upwards lifting the posterior nonarticular surface, *this angle is reduced* (*see* **Fig. 13.50**).

In complete tear of any collateral ligament of the ankle joint an anteroposterior X-ray is taken with the foot forcibly tilted towards the opposite direction. Such *strained positional skiagram* shows an unusual increased gap between the malleolus and the talus in complete tear of the collateral ligament.

DIFFERENT FRACTURES AROUND THE ANKLE AND THE FOOT

1. **External rotation injury (Figs. 13.47A to C):** This will cause a spiral fracture of the fibula. With continuing force the medial malleolus may be avulsed or fractured transversely. Further rotation will lead to avulsion of the posterior fragment of the tibia to which the tibiofibular ligament is attached leading to tibiofibular diastasis.
2. **Abduction injury (Fig. 13.48):** Abduction force fractures the fibula transversely approximately 2 inches above the ankle joint. A continuing force may also avulse the medial malleolus and later on avulsion of the posterior fragment of the tibia with tibiofibular diastasis.
3. **Adduction injury (Fig. 13.49):** This will cause a vertical fracture of the medial malleolus extending upwards along its lateral margin. This is the most important differentiating feature from the external rotation or abduction injury in which the medial malleolus is fractured transversely. A continuing adduction force will avulse the tip of the fibula.

Vertical injury with an upward thrust will split the tibia vertically. It may shears off the anterior or posterior corner of the lower tibia. Sometimes this vertical fracture may join a transverse fracture of the lower end of the tibia about 2–3 inches above the ankle joint. In adolescents this type of injury will cause fracture-separation of the lower tibial epiphysis.

Fracture of the calcaneum: This usually results from a fall from height. The calcaneum is driven up against the talus and subsequently split or crushed.

Split fracture: The calcaneum is split into two segments by vertical fracture and usually extends from the medial aspect near the back of the bone to the lateral aspect in front. The larger lateral segment is usually shifted laterally and the smaller medial segment is displaced upwards. The fracture usually extends into the subtalar joint.

Crush fracture (Fig. 13.50): In this type of injury the calcaneum is crushed and the talus is driven downwards into the body of the calcaneum grossly damaging the subtalar joint. The

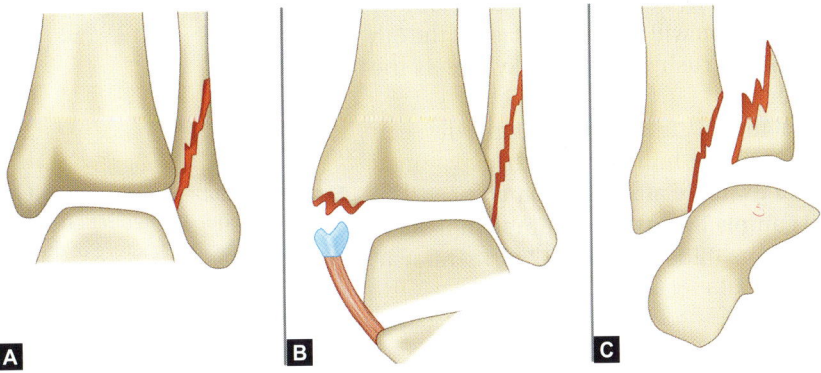

Figs. 13.47A to C: Diagrammatic representation of the three stages of external rotation injury.

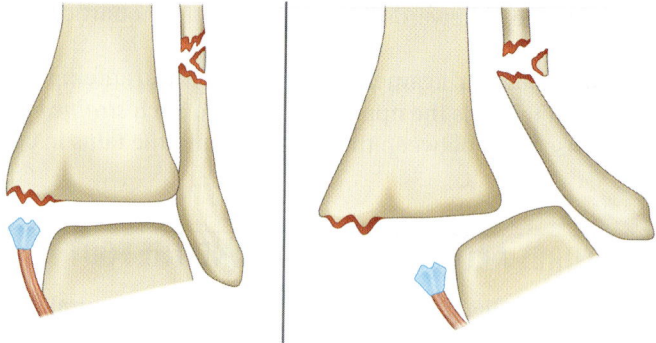

Fig. 13.48: Diagrammatic representation of abduction injury to the ankle.

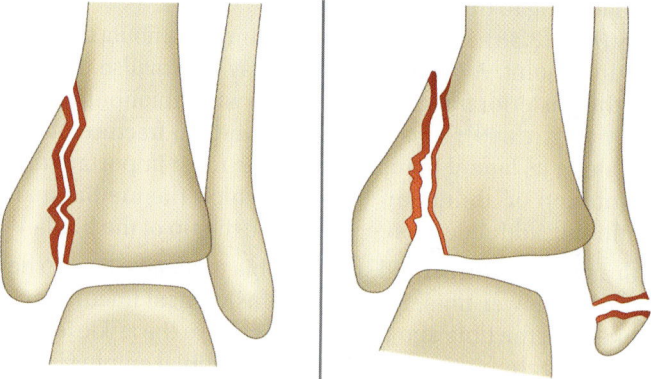

Fig. 13.49: Diagrammatic representation of adduction injury of ankle.

tuber-joint angle is considerably reduced from 40° (normal) to about 20°.

Fracture of metatarsal bone: Metatarsal bone may be fractured either by rotational injury or by crush injury. In rotational injury with eversion and plantar flexion commonly the first metatarsal bone is injured near its base. The typical rotational injury with forced inversion will avulse the base of the 5th metatarsal bone. Crush injury usually affects the metatarsal necks.

March fracture or stress injury is typically seen at the 2nd metatarsal bone due to unaccustomed overuse as for example after long march past. The patient will complain of a tender lump palpable at the neck or at the midshaft of the 2nd metatarsal bone.

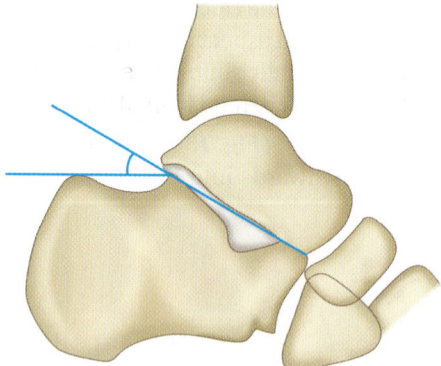

Fig. 13.50: Tuber-joint angle which normally measures about 40°. Reduction of this angle may be evident in crush fracture of the calcaneum.

Chapter 13: Examination of Injuries about Individual Joints

Algorithmic Approach to Patient with Joint Injuries

Patient presents with joint pain, swelling, or deformity

↓

Is there a history of trauma?
- Yes → Consider **fracture, dislocation, ligamentous injury**
- No → Consider **arthritis, infection (septic arthritis), neuropathy, or autoimmune disorders**

↓

Is there visible deformity?
- Yes → Suggests **dislocation, fracture with displacement, or joint subluxation**
- No → More likely **soft tissue injury or ligament sprain**

↓

Is the joint stable on passive movement?
- Yes → Suggests **soft tissue injury or minor ligament sprain**
- No → Suggests **ligament rupture or severe dislocation**

↓

Perform X-ray imaging to confirm diagnosis
- Fracture present?
  - Yes → Classify as **simple, comminuted, open, or impacted fracture**
  - No → Consider **soft tissue or ligamentous injury (MRI required)**

↓

Perform MRI or ultrasound if ligament/tendon injury suspected
- MRI → Best for **ligament and meniscal tears (ACL, rotator cuff, meniscus)**
- Ultrasound → Best for **dynamic joint assessment (tendon tears, bursitis, effusions)**

↓

Confirm diagnosis and initiate treatment
- **Fractures:** Immobilization, casting, surgery (if needed)
- **Dislocations:** Closed reduction, immobilization, physiotherapy
- **Soft tissue injuries:** RICE protocol (rest, ice, compression, elevation), NSAIDs, rehabilitation
- **Joint infections:** Antibiotics, joint aspiration, surgery if abscess formation

Examination of Pathological Joints

CHAPTER 14

HISTORY

1. **Age and sex:** Rheumatoid arthritis occurs more commonly in young adult women and osteoarthritis is a disease of old age. Acute arthritis is commonly seen in young children. Tuberculous arthritis is commonly seen in children and adolescents.
2. **Occupation:** Manual workers, e.g., blacksmiths and coolies are more often the victims of osteoarthritis.
3. **Mode of onset and progress:** Acute onset with constitutional disturbances is found in acute arthritis. This is more common in the hip or knee joint rather than the shoulder. Insidious onset is the feature of chronic arthritis including tuberculous variety, rheumatoid arthritis and osteoarthritis.
4. **Pain:** This is the main complaint of a patient with arthritis. This is conspicuous by its absence in Charcot's joint (due to tabes dorsalis or syringomyelia) and Clutton's joint (due to congenital syphilis). The clinician should take a proper history of the pain regarding its site, its character, its relation to movements of the joint and its relation with the new and full moon.
(a) *Site:* Whether the pain is localized to the affected joint or referred to some other joint, e.g., to the knee in case of hip diseases or fleeting type from one joint to the other as seen in rheumatic fever.
(b) *Character:* Whether the pain is of dull aching in nature which is commonly seen in chronic arthritis including the tuberculous variety or throbbing in nature which is a feature of acute arthritis. In tuberculous joint when the articular cartilages are destroyed the child often cries at night during sleep; commonly known as 'night cry'. This is due to the fact that when the patient is awake during the day the joint is kept immobilized by the muscles spasm, but during sleep the muscles relax and allow friction between the eroded articular surfaces giving rise to 'night-cry'.
(c) *Relation to movements:* In any affection of a joint, movement aggravates the pain. But in osteoarthritis pain is first felt in the early morning when the patient gets up from the bed. With gradual movement of the joint the pain is eased off due to increase in synovial secretion.
(d) *Its relation to weather and new or full moon:* The pain becomes aggravated during new or full moon in rheumatoid arthritis and gout. The pain also gets worse in rainy season.
5. **Locking:** This is due to presence of loose bodies within the joint.
6. **Deformity:** Sometimes a pathological joint may present with deformity of course at late stage, when its early stages have been ignored. Such deformity is seen in late stage of rheumatoid arthritis, osteoarthritis and tuberculous arthritis. These are discussed in the differential diagnosis in this chapter and in the next chapter 'Examination of Individual Joint Pathologies'.
7. **Past history:** Enquire whether the patient suffered from tuberculosis, gonorrhea, syphilis, typhoid fever or pneumonia in the past. This gives a clue to the diagnosis. Previous trauma is

sometimes responsible for subsequent osteoarthritis. So careful history should be taken to know the details of past injury, X-ray findings and any other investigations performed.

8. **Family history:** Hemophilia, tuberculosis, gout, rheumatism, etc., often run in families.

History in joints examination

Aspect	Clinical significance	Patient-friendly questions
Age of onset	Helps differentiate conditions (e.g., RA in young adults, OA in elderly)	"At what age did your joint pain start?"
Pain characteristics	Morning Stiffness >1 hour → RA, Worse with Activity → OA	"Is your pain worse in the morning or after movement?"
Swelling and warmth	Hot, swollen joint → Septic arthritis	"Is your joint swollen, warm, or red?"
History of trauma or infection	Identifies **post-traumatic arthritis, infectious arthritis**	"Did you have an injury or infection before the joint pain started?"
Systemic symptoms	Fever → **Infection**, weight loss → TB or RA	"Do you have fever, weight loss, or other symptoms?"

PHYSICAL EXAMINATION

GENERAL SURVEY
In acute suppurative arthritis evidence of toxemia is frequently present. Generalized wasting and cachectic features are noticed in tuberculosis of joints.

Fever: High rise of temperature is an important diagnostic feature of acute suppurative arthritis. Evening rise of temperature is a feature of tuberculous arthritis.

LOCAL EXAMINATION

A. INSPECTION
The affected joint and the corresponding healthy joint should be fully exposed and placed in the same position. The affected joint is compared with the sound side. The joint should be inspected from all sides, particularly the posterior aspect which is often overlooked. In the case of the lower limb the patient's *gait* must be watched.

1. **Swelling:** Very often a pathological joint is swollen and can be noticed very easily. A careful watch must be made to differentiate between generalized swelling of the joint due to effusion and a localized swelling from a bursa or a ganglion. A bursa often communicates with the joint and may become prominent in presence of effusion in the joint. The best example of this condition is Baker's cyst which is often associated with effusion of the knee joint due to osteoarthritis or tuberculosis.

2. **Deformity and position of the joint:** The joint is sometimes deformed in the position of abduction or adduction, popularly known as valgus or varus deformity respectively. This can be found in any joint which is pathologically involved to produce such deformity. After the Latin names they are called coxa (hip) valgus or varus, genu (knee) valgus or varus, cubitus (forearm) valgus or varus and manus (hand) valgus or varus. There may be rotational deformity which should also be noticed. When a joint is distended with fluid, it takes up an *'optimum position'* or *'position of ease,'* in which capacity within the joint is maximum. This position is adduction,

slight flexion and internal rotation for the shoulder joint; slight flexion, abduction and external rotation for the hip joint; flexion and slight pronation for the elbow joint; slight flexion for knee joints; slight flexion for wrist joint and slight plantar flexion and inversion for the ankle joint. If the joint is not held in the 'optimum position' or in the 'position of rest', deformity is likely to develop.

3. **Skin over the joint:** Red and glossy skin suggests acute inflammation of the joint. Scar, sinus, ulcer and deformities of the joint are the late features of tuberculous arthritis.

4. **Muscular wasting:** When the joint is diseased the muscles concerned in movement of the joint will be wasting. In case of the knee joint the quadriceps muscles waste first, similarly in case of hip the glutei waste first.

B. PALPATION

1. **Local temperature:** An acute inflamed joint will be warm. The backs of the fingers are mainly used to assess the temperature of the joint. The temperature of the diseased joint must be compared with that of the healthy joint. The teaching is that always feel the joint of the sound side first and then the diseased joint.

2. **Tenderness:** An acutely inflamed joint will be highly tender. This tenderness will be present all round the joint line. The bones in the vicinity of the joint and the bony attachments of various ligaments are carefully palpated for tenderness, as the former will be tender in fracture and the latter will be tender in sprain.

3. **Bony components**: This must be palpated to exclude the possibility of previous osteomyelitis or old fracture.

4. **Swelling:** An effusion of the joint will make the fluctuation test positive. Moreover the swelling takes the form of the joint. An enlarged bursa will be soft and cystic and will correspond with the anatomical position of the bursa. Communicating bursa may be associated with effusion of the joint. Synovial thickening will feel elastic and spongy or 'boggy'. Occasionally, a swelling at the joint may not be due to effusion but due to swelling like subcutaneous lipoma or cyst. Sometimes loose body may be felt within the joint.

5. **Muscular wasting:** During palpation this is corroborated with the findings of inspection. Of course, measurement will follow.

C. MOVEMENTS

Both active (the movements made by the patient's effort) and passive (the movements made by the surgeon and the patient remains passive) movements should be examined. The ranges of the movements are noted on both the sound and the affected sides. It is always advisable to examine the sound side first so that the patient knows what is to be done with the affected joint and his fear and muscle spasm can be greatly eliminated.

During the movement a few things should be noted: (a) Does the movement cause pain to the patient? If so, when does the pain start and when does it disappear. (b) Is there any restriction of the movements? At what angle the movements become restricted? In certain diseases certain types of movements are restricted whereas the other movements remain normal. (c) Is there any protective muscular spasm? To demonstrate, a short sharp movement is made and the muscle will be seen to go into spasm. Muscular spasm is almost always associated with active stage of arthritis. (d) Is there any crepitus felt during movement of the joint? This suggests osteoarthritis. For this, the joint must be palpated during its movements. *Limitation of movements in all directions* is an important feature of acute arthritis.

One thing must be borne in mind during examination of movements of different joints that a few joints, e.g., the shoulder, the hip and the ankle exhibit some range of movements even though the joints concerned are completely ankylosed. This is due to the movements of the neighboring joints, as for example in case of shoulder joint the movement of the scapula, acromioclavicular and sternoclavicular joints; in case of the hip such movements occur at the lumbar spine; in case of the ankle movements may occur at the subtaloid and midtarsal joints.

D. MEASUREMENTS

Though one can take the measurements of the length of the limbs and relation of the different bony points as has been described in the hip, elbow, shoulder, etc., yet the most important measurement so far as the pathological joint is concerned is the *circumference of the limb* above the joint at the same level on both the sides to detect muscular wasting.

Auscultation: As has already been discussed crepitus is the feature often accompanied by osteoarthritis. In early cases of osteoarthritis fine crepitation may be missed by the palpating fingers. Auscultation is of immense value in detecting these fine crepitations.

Examination of the lymph nodes: The regional lymph nodes are often enlarged in different arthritis. But the clinicians often forget to examine these lymph nodes. In case of the hip joint the external iliac group of lymph nodes are affected, whereas in case of the knee joint the inguinal group of lymph nodes are affected.

GENERAL EXAMINATION

1. The lungs and the cervical lymph nodes should be examined in case of suspected tuberculous arthritis.
2. Signs of syphilitic stigmas should be looked for in case of syphilitic affection of the joint (*see* **Fig. 4.15**).
3. Gonococcal infection also involves the joints in chronic stage. History of urethral discharge and examination of the smear obtained from prostatic massage will help to diagnose the condition.
4. In rheumatic fever one should examine the heart.
5. Search for septic foci in teeth, tonsils, air sinuses and even cervix uteri in case of acute arthritis, rheumatic fever and rarely in rheumatoid arthritis.
6. **Neurological examination** is important in Charcot's joint, affected by tabes dorsalis and syringomyelia. Ask the patient if he had 'lightening' pain down the leg or 'girdle' pain around the trunk.

The jerk will be gradually losing and the ankle jerk will be lost earlier than the knee jerk **(Fig. 14.1)**. Loss of sensation, Argyll Robertson pupil (i.e., presence of accommodation reflex but loss of light reflex) **(Fig. 14.2)**, the Romberg's sign (i.e., the patient sways or even falls if he stands with his feet close together and the eyes shut) etc., are the features of Charcot's joint (neuropathic joint).

In the upper limb syringomyelia is the common lesion and this is diagnosed by dissociation of sensations (i.e., loss of pain and temperature sense but presence of tactile sensation), inequality of accommodation reflex, etc.

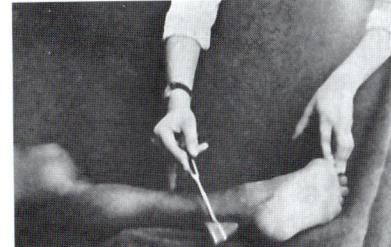

Fig.14.1: Testing the ankle jerk. Note that this is lost earlier than the knee jerk in Charcot's joint.

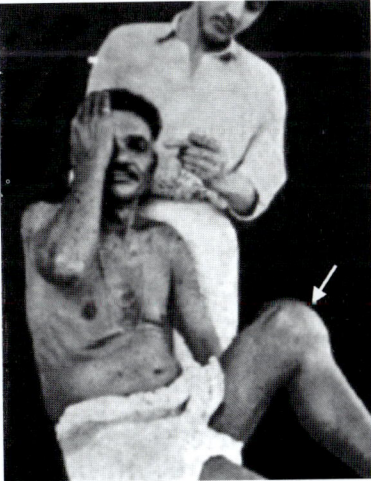

Fig.14.2: Testing for the Argyll Robertson pupil in Charcot's knee joint. The other eye is closed to prevent consensual light reflex.

7. **Examination of neighboring joints** is of immense importance in case of certain joints. The patients may complain of knee joint when the pathology lies in the hip joint. This is referred pain due to common nerve supply of these two joints (femoral, obturator and sciatic nerves).

SPECIAL INVESTIGATIONS

1. **Blood:** This is examined for: (i) leukocytosis (suppurative arthritis), lymphocytosis (tuberculous arthritis); (ii) increased erythrocyte sedimentation rate (ESR) (tuberculosis and rheumatoid arthritis); (iii) wassermann reaction (WR) and Kahn test (Clutton's joint); (iv) uric acid (gout); (v) coagulation time and bleeding time (hemophilia) and (vi) immunological tests—**venereal disease research laboratory (VDRL)** and Kahn test (syphilis), widal (typhoid), Rose-Waaler and latex (rheumatoid).

2. **Aspiration:** The aspirated fluid is examined for physical, microscopical and bacteriological characteristics.

3. **X-ray examination:** This is the most useful special investigation so far as a pathological joint is concerned. Both the anteroposterior and the lateral views of the pathological joints are taken and may be compared with those of the sound side. The following findings should be noted:
(i) *Bony components* of the joint should be carefully examined for any localized or generalized rarefaction (tuberculosis), gross destruction (Charcot's joint, tuberculosis and occasionally in septic arthritis) or pathological dislocation (commonly seen in late stages of tuberculous arthritis and rarely seen in septic and typhoid arthritis). In tuberculous arthritis appearance of sclerosis in the rarefied area is considered to be a definite sign of recovery.
(ii) *Articular ends:* Normally the articular ends are distinct and continuous in outline. Haziness or loss of definition is a positive sign of any form of arthritis. Peripheral lipping of the articular surface is characteristic of osteoarthritis.
(iii) *Joint space:* This is nothing but the space occupied by the articular cartilages and shows as a gap between the articular ends of the bones in X-ray. Increase in this space indicates effusion in the joint and denotes the first stage of arthritis. Diminution of this space indicates erosion of the articular cartilage and signifies the second stage of arthritis.
(iv) *Abnormal bone shadows:* These may be loose bodies or disorganized bone in Charcot's joint.
(v) *Abnormal soft tissue shadow:* This may be seen when an abscess is formed either in acute arthritis or a cold abscess in tuberculosis. Evidence of periostitis may be seen in neighboring bones.

4. **Mantoux test:** This is done in suspected cases of tuberculosis. Its negative result is more important as it excludes the presence of this disease.

5. **Biopsy** of the lymph nodes may be done, though occasionally practiced, in suspected cases of tuberculous arthritis. Biopsy of the synovial membrane besides its diagnostic value possesses a therapeutic advantage in rheumatoid arthritis particularly when it affects a single joint.

6. In gonococcal arthritis, demonstration of **gonococci in urethral discharge** after prostatic massage will confirm the diagnosis.

7. **Arthroscopy** is particularly helpful in detecting the pathology of the joint.

8. **Arthrography** is more helpful in detecting internal derangement of joint due to injury than due to pathology. Both arthrography and arthroscopy are contraindicated in acute suppurative arthritis.

9. **Isotope scan** with ^{67}Ga or ^{99m}Tc is helpful in the diagnosis of inflammatory lesion of the joint due to high uptake.

DISEASES OF THE JOINT

1. **Acute suppurative arthritis:** Though staphylococcal and streptococcal infections by far outnumber the other varieties of acute arthritis, yet pneumococcal, gonococcal and typhoid arthritis should be borne in mind under this heading.
2. **Chronic arthritis:** Four main varieties are included under this heading. They are: (a) tuberculous arthritis; (b) rheumatoid arthritis; (c) osteoarthritis and (d) gout.
3. **Neuropathic joints:** In this group are included: (a) Charcot's joint due to tabes dorsalis, syringomyelia and peripheral neuritis from diabetes and (b) hysterical joint.
4. **Osteochondritis:** This is a separate entity and includes 3 distinct types—(a) crushing osteochondritis; (b) splitting osteochondritis (dissecans) and (c) pulling osteochondritis (traction).
5. **Hemophilic joints:** These may present like acute arthritis, but presence of the history of bleeding tendency suggests the diagnosis.
6. **Loose bodies.**
7. **Miscellaneous group:** This group includes Clutton's joint, a manifestation of congenital syphilis and subacute arthritis which occasionally complicates bacillary dysentery and brucellosis.

Causes of joints disorders

Category	Condition	Key features
Inflammatory	Rheumatoid arthritis	Chronic, symmetric joint involvement, morning stiffness, positive rheumatoid factor
	Gout	Acute, severe pain, big toe involvement, elevated uric acid
	Pseudogout	Calcium pyrophosphate crystals, chondrocalcinosis on X-ray
Infectious	Septic arthritis	High fever, red, hot swollen joint, leukocytosis
	Tuberculous arthritis	Gradual onset, cold abscess formation, positive Mantoux test
Degenerative	Osteoarthritis	Asymmetric joint space narrowing, osteophytes, pain worsens with activity
Neuropathic	Charcot's Joint	Painless destruction, seen in diabetes, syphilis, syringomyelia
Metabolic	Hemophilic arthropathy	Recurrent hemarthrosis, seen in hemophilia

DIFFERENTIAL DIAGNOSIS

ACUTE SUPPURATIVE ARTHRITIS

The causative organisms are usually *Staphylococcus* and occasionally *Streptococcus*. The joint is affected either by penetrating wound or secondary to acute osteomyelitis when the metaphysis is included within the joint or by blood spread from a distant site. Infection affects the articular cartilage and the synovial membrane in the beginning. Pus is formed which may burst out of the joint to form abscesses and sinuses **(Fig. 14.3)**. Later on, with healing, the opposing bony surfaces may adhere by fibrosis (fibrous ankylosis) and sometimes bony trabeculae grow between the opposing bones to form 'bony ankylosis'.

The patients are usually children and the condition reveals itself with severe throbbing pain, swelling and redness of the affected joint, high temperature, rapid pulse and a very toxic outlook. The patient often does not allow to touch the affected joint. On inspection the joint is held slightly flexed, swollen and red. On palpation, the joint is warm with diffuse tenderness and fluctuation. Active movement is absolutely nil and passive movement is very painful. When the articular cartilages are affected, the patient gets 'night pain' as the muscles become relaxed and allow movement between the eroded articular cartilages. Without treatment the end result is fibrous or bony ankylosis according as the articular cartilage is partially or completely destroyed.

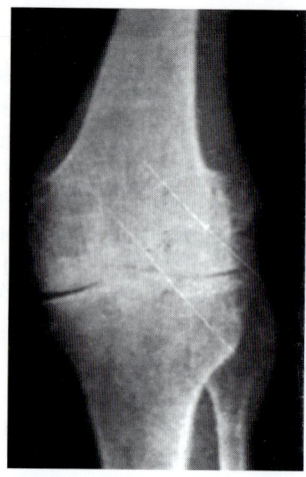

Fig.14.3: Acute pyogenic arthritis. Note that the joint space is absolutely diminished due to erosion of the articular cartilages.

X-ray shows normal appearance with increased joint space for the first two weeks. Gradually, the joint space becomes narrowed indicating erosion of the articular cartilages with widespread patchy rarefaction of the neighboring bones. With healing the bone recalcifies and may show trabeculae across the joint indicating bony ankylosis.

PNEUMOCOCCAL ARTHRITIS

As the name suggests, arthritis is secondary to pneumococcal infection of the throat, ear or lung. The common victims are the children and the knee joints are mainly affected. Arthritis is characterized by painless purulent effusion. Aspiration will bring out creamy greenish pus containing pneumococci, which clinches the diagnosis.

GONOCOCCAL ARTHRITIS

The joint is involved after about 3 weeks of primary infection and when the urethral discharge has ceased. The infection is mainly blood-borne. The condition is manifested by joint pain and acute arthritis. It may affect one large joint as for example the elbow or the knee or many joints—both small and large (polyarticular). The outstanding features of gonococcal arthritis are (i) sudden onset with fever, (ii) severity of pain, (iii) redness and edema of the joint, (iv) hemorrhagic vesicopustular rash and (v) demonstration of gonococci in urethral discharge after prostatic massage.

REITER'S DISEASE

This is characterized by multiple arthritis commonly affecting the knee, the ankle, the foot and sacroiliac joints. The joints are hot, red, swollen, tender and painful. *This condition is associated with nonspecific urethritis and conjunctivitis.*

TYPHOID ARTHRITIS

This is a rare disease nowadays. Joints are affected, if at all, at the 3rd week of the typhoid fever.

TUBERCULOUS ARTHRITIS

Tuberculosis of the joint is merely the local manifestation of the generalized disease. The onset is insidious with a history of poor appetite, loss of weight, slight evening pyrexia, malar flush, etc. Generally, the children are affected and the lower limbs are more often involved than the upper limbs. The diagnostic features are: (i) Indication of presence of tuberculosis by the history has already been mentioned. Tuberculosis of the urogenital tract may be the presenting feature. (ii) Pain is not so prominent as in acute arthritis. 'Night pain' wakes the child with a cry when the articular cartilages are involved and when the protective muscular spasm becomes nil during sleep. (iii) Muscular wasting. (iv) Restriction of movements *in all directions* with protective muscular spasm. (v) Formation of cold abscess and sinus. (vi) X-ray shows diminution of the joint space due to erosion of the articular cartilages, recalcification with or without bony focus and at the last stage pathological dislocation. Recalcification indicates beginning of the healing process. (vii) Special investigation like Mantoux test, culture of *M. tuberculosis* from the aspirated fluid and biopsy, positive guinea-pig inoculation test are all suggestive of this condition. If the condition remains untreated end result is fibrous ankylosis. Bony ankylosis is possible only when the joint is secondarily infected. In tuberculous spine osseous ankylosis can occur spontaneously without secondary infection.

RHEUMATOID ARTHRITIS

The usual victims are the women between the ages of 30 and 50 years. The disease is gradual in onset affecting small joints of the hand and foot. Pain is the main symptom followed by stiffness, swelling and deformity. The tendency is to spread slowly and symmetrically up the limbs involving the larger joints. Occasionally, the onset of the course is rapid and rarely a single large joint may be affected (monoarticular).

Sometimes the condition is associated with fever and loss of weight. Sedimentation rate is raised, anemia is common and lymph nodes may be enlarged. Sometimes this disease is seen in children and is called Still's disease. It is a polyarticular rheumatoid arthritis. The joint changes are similar to those of the adult disease but are usually preceded by severe general illness, skin rashes, lymphadenopathy, splenomegaly and pericarditis.

On examination the skin overlying the joint is shiny and atrophic. The joint is swollen and muscle wasting becomes obvious. Various deformities in different joints are characteristic features of this disease, e.g., **ulnar drift** is common at the metacarpophalangeal joints, **swan-neck deformity** (hyperextension at the proximal interphalangeal joint and the flexion at the distal joint), **boutonniere deformity** (flexion at the proximal interphalangeal joint and hyperextension at the distal), **finger drop** following rupture of the extensor tendon at the level of the wrist, etc.

Movements are restricted by pain and spasm. During quiescent period a good range may return. Gradually stiffness due to fibrous ankylosis may result.

X-ray shows diffuse rarefaction of the neighboring bones as an early feature. Cysts may be seen in the bones. Later on the joint space becomes decreased and may completely disappear. At the last stage some sort of deformity may become obvious. In most patients with rheumatoid arthritis the Rose-Waaler and latex serum tests for rheumatoid factor are positive, but some 25% of patients are seronegative and the prognosis in them is better.

OSTEOARTHRITIS

The nomenclature does produce some confusion as this condition has got no relation with inflammation of the joint and should better be called "osteoarthrosis". The etiology of this condition remains still in doubt. Probably increased mucopolysaccharide in articular cartilage and diminished hyaluronic acid in the synovial fluid which develops with increasing age may be the causative factor. Of the **general causes:** (a) a *genetic background* seems to play its role as it is often seen in a few members of the same family and (b) *metabolic disorders* like alkaptonuria and gout may lead to premature cartilage degeneration. Of the **local factors**—(a) injury in the form of *repeated minor injuries* as seen in certain occupations, recurrent subluxation of the patella, undue joint laxity, torn meniscus and loose bodies are examples; (b) *incongruent joint surfaces* as seen in congenital subluxation of the hip, pseudocoxalgia, etc.; (c) *malalignment* of the joints such as coxa vara, genu valgum, genu varum, etc.; (d) *inflammatory diseases* such as rheumatoid arthritis, septic arthritis, etc. and (e) *inadequate blood supply* with avascular necrosis of the bone ends are important.

The changes start in the articular cartilage, which becomes soft, irregular and pitted. Minute flecks of cartilage are set into the joint. In the non-stress area, the subchondral vessels become hypertrophied and invade the cartilage which calcifies and later ossifies forming osteophytes. The hyperemia spreads into the bone underneath the stress area. The cartilage continues to be rubbed away and the bone becomes exposed and dense. Subchondral cysts may develop as the sinusoidal distension damages the trabeculae and also because the synovial fluid is forced into the bone through minute cracks in the cartilage.

Generally, the patients are men above 50 years of age. One joint, occasionally two or even three may be involved. But this is not a true polyarticular disease like rheumatoid arthritis. The main symptom is the pain. In the beginning the pain is felt particularly in the early morning when the patient gets up. There may be some stiffness associated with it. Pain and stiffness gradually pass off on continued use of the limb owing to increased synovial secretion. This is the pathognomonic feature. Deformity is the late feature due to capsular shrinkage and muscular imbalance, e.g., flexion and adduction deformity at the hip joint. On examination some limitation of the movements and grating sensation are frequently obtained. Restriction of movements is characteristically asymmetrical, thus at the hip extension, abduction and internal rotation are more limited than their opposites.

X-ray shows diminution of the joint space at the pressure areas only and presence of osteophytes, i.e., peripheral lipping of the articular ends. Sclerosis and presence of cysts are noticed in subjacent bones.

GOUT

It is a metabolic disorder with abnormal high level of serum uric acid due to excessive production or inadequate excretion or both. The joints mainly affected are the toe joints (especially the metatarsophalangeal joint of the hallux), the finger joints, the wrists and the ankles. The victims are usually the middle aged and elderly people. Urate crystals are actually irritating and this results in acute painful arthritis. The skin overlying the joint becomes red, warm, edematous. Crystals of sodium biurate may be deposited in the bone, in cartilage and in joints. X-ray shows normal features in early stages but in late cases bone deposits are revealed as punched-out translucent areas under the cartilage. Later on the joint becomes osteoarthritic.

The diagnosis is confirmed by the family history, a history of previous similar attacks, the raised uric acid level (this level may be increased in nongouty patients who are taking aspirin), X-ray appearance and probably the most important is the presence of "tophi" (i.e., chalky deposits in different parts of the body and around the joints).

PSEUDOGOUT
In this condition the attacks are similar to those of the gout. The only difference is that this condition affects the spinal joints and the proximal joints. The condition is associated with chondrocalcinosis, i.e., calcification in hyaline and in fibrocartilage.

CHARCOT'S JOINT
Tabes dorsalis, syringomyelia and peripheral neuritis are the common causes. Tabes affects the inferior extremity whereas syringomyelia affects the superior extremity. The condition is characterized by little pain and marked destruction of bone leading to abnormal mobility of the joint associated with coarse crepitus.

HYSTERICAL GOUT
The common victims are the women. The affected joint is kept rigid in some deformed position. Any attempt to move the joint is resisted. Clinical examination fails to reveal any organic disease of the joint and the joint assumes normal attitude when the muscles are made relaxed.

OSTEOCHONDRITIS
Three distinct varieties are included under this heading.
1. *Crushing osteochondritis:* The examples of this condition are Perthes' disease in the hip joint, Freiberg's disease in the second metatarsal, Kohler's disease in the navicular bone, Kienbock's disease in the lunate bone and Scheuermann's disease in the thoracic spine. Mostly children between 5 and 15 years are affected. Of these Freiberg's disease is commoner between the ages of 15 and 25 years and Scheuermann's disease is a disease of the adolescents. The common problem is the pain of the affected joint with irritability and some deformity, i.e., adduction and internal rotation in Perthes' disease of the hip, kyphosis in Scheuermann's disease, etc. The main problem is avascular necrosis of the epiphysis of unknown etiology which makes the bone dense on X-ray. The nomenclature suggests that the affected bones are under pressure and may be the cause of avascular necrosis.
2. *Splitting osteochondritis (dissecans):* In this condition trauma seems to play a major role and gradually leads to formation of an avascular fragment which split off. On X-ray a line of demarcation first appears and avascular segment becomes gradually detached and forms a loose body inside the joint **(Figs. 14.4A and B)**. This will ultimately lead to osteoarthritis.

The affected individuals are generally adolescents. The knee is the most common joint to be affected followed by the elbow and rarely the ankle. In the *knee joint* generally the articular surface of the medial femoral condyle is involved and the patient complains of vague aching, swelling and tenderness in the affected area. The patient may present with locking and giving way, which are features of loose body in the joint. *In the elbow* generally the capitulum or radial head is affected, and the signs and symptoms are similar to the knee joint. *In the ankle* commonly one corner of the upper surface of the talus is affected. The symptoms are again similar to those of the knee joint.
3. *Traction osteochondritis:* This condition occurs only in those places where the tendon is attached to an epiphysis or apophysis. The possible exception is probably Johansson-Larsen's disease in which this condition affects the lower pole of the patella (a sesamoid bone) at the attachment of ligamentum patella.

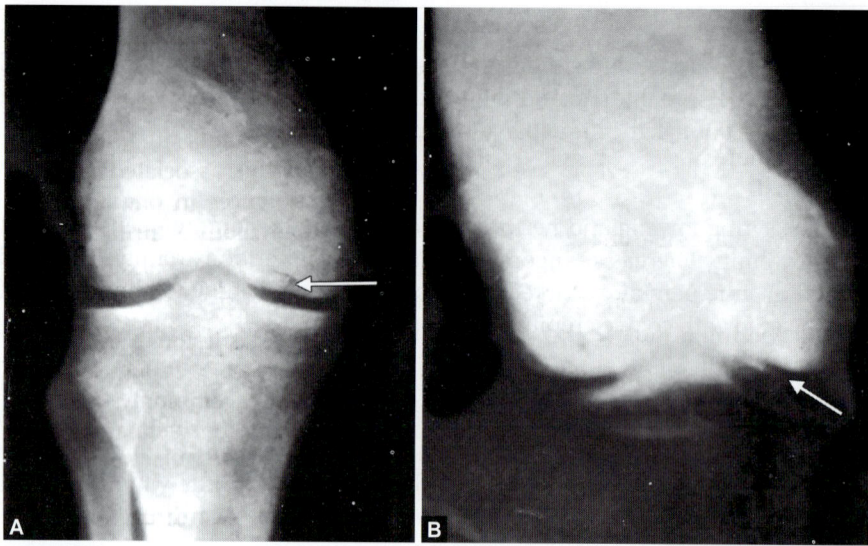

Figs. 14.4A and B: Osteochondritis dissecans affecting the medial condyle of the right femur shown by arrow. In the second figure axial skiagram is taken in extreme flexion of the knee joint.

In this condition also the adolescents are affected and the two places are notoriously involved by this condition. These are the *knee joint* where the ligamentum patellae is attached to the tibial (Osgood-Schlatter's disease) tubercle and at the heel where the tendo-Achillis is attached to the calcaneum (Sever's disease). In both these conditions the patient presents with swollen and tender spots. When the tendons are made taut against resistance the pain increases. On X-ray the affected bone looks more dense and fragmented.

HEMOPHILIC JOINT

Hemophilic patients sometimes present with sudden bilateral effusion of the knee joints, without very suggestive cause. That the patient is a bleeder will confirm the diagnosis.

LOOSE BODIES

They may arise (1) *from the synovial fluid,* e.g., fibrinous loose bodies resulting from hemorrhagic or inflammatory effusion—'melon-seed' bodies found in tuberculous joints belong to this group, (2) *from the synovial membrane* numerous cartilaginous loose bodies developing within villous synovial processes (osteochondromatosis), (3) *from the bone* resulting from injury, e.g., fracture of the tibial spine, detached osteophytes in the case of osteoarthritis, sequestra from acute arthritis secondary to acute osteomyelitis, but most important in this group is loose body from osteochondritis dissecans.

CLUTTON'S JOINT

This is a manifestation of the congenital syphilis. Symptomless and symmetrical synovitis with boggy fluid distension of both the knee joints suggests this condition. Moreover there will be wasting of muscles of the thighs and this associated with interstitial keratitis will confirm the diagnosis. This condition often commences in one joint and at this stage it is very difficult to differentiate this condition from tuberculous arthritis.

ANKYLOSIS

This condition means stiffness of a joint either by intra-articular lesions (true ankylosis) or by extra-articular involvement (false ankylosis).

A. **True ankylosis:** (i) *Fibrous variety:* Fibrous ankylosis is commonly seen as a sequel of tuberculous arthritis, acute arthritis, gonococcal arthritis and rarely rheumatoid arthritis. As the name suggests this condition signifies fibrosis between the two articular surfaces following damage to the cartilages leading to limitation of movements.

(ii) *Bony variety:* Bony ankylosis occurs following suppurative arthritis and occasionally after tuberculous arthritis becomes secondarily infected. This condition signifies formation of bony trabeculae between the two articular ends following severe destruction of the articular cartilages.

B. **False ankylosis:** This means extra-articular structures are involved in such a way as to cause limitation of movements of the joint. From superficial to deep, the causes are:

(i) *Skin and subcutaneous tissue*—in burns following contracture.

(ii) *Muscles and tendons*—due to adhesion to the bone following fracture (e.g., commonly seen after fracture of the shaft of the femur when quadriceps adhere to the fractured site resulting in limitation of extension of the knee joint), Volkmann's ischemic contracture, etc.

(iii) *Fascia*—in Dupuytren's contracture and occasionally in gonococcal fibrofascitis, ankylosis of the joints will result.

(iv) *Capsules and ligaments*—in prolonged immobilization, which is a common cause of limitation of movements following trauma. Contracture of these structures are held responsible.

(v) *Bone*—myositis ossificans traumatica is probably the most common condition of this group. Rarely excessive callus formation and displaced fragments may be responsible for the false ankylosis.

Algorithmic Approach to Patient with Pathological Joints

Patient presents with joint pain, swelling, or deformity

↓

Is the joint pain acute or chronic?
- Acute → Suggests **septic arthritis, gout, trauma, or hemarthrosis (bleeding disorder)**
- Chronic → Suggests **rheumatoid arthritis, osteoarthritis, or tuberculosis**

↓

Is the joint warm and red?
- Yes → Suggests **septic arthritis (infection), gout, or pseudogout**
- No → More likely **osteoarthritis, neuropathic joint, or metabolic joint disease**

↓

Is morning stiffness present for more than 1 hour?
- Yes → Suggests **rheumatoid arthritis or other inflammatory arthritis**
- No → Suggests **osteoarthritis or mechanical joint disease**

↓

Perform X-ray imaging to confirm diagnosis
- Joint space narrowing present?
  - Yes → Classify as **osteoarthritis (asymmetric narrowing)** or **rheumatoid arthritis (symmetric narrowing, joint erosions)**
  - No → Consider **soft tissue or autoimmune cause (MRI needed)**

↓

Perform special investigations
- Rheumatoid factor (RF) and anti-CCP → Positive in **rheumatoid arthritis**
- Serum uric acid → Elevated in **gout**
- ESR, CRP → Elevated in **inflammatory arthritis or infection**
- Joint aspiration and synovial fluid analysis:
  - WBC >50,000 and bacteria → **septic arthritis**
  - Monosodium urate crystals → **gout**
  - Calcium pyrophosphate crystals → **pseudogout**

↓

Confirm diagnosis and initiate treatment
- **Septic arthritis:** Antibiotics, joint drainage
- **Rheumatoid arthritis:** DMARDs (methotrexate, biologics), NSAIDs
- **Gout:** NSAIDs, colchicine, Urate-lowering therapy
- **Osteoarthritis:** Pain management, physiotherapy, joint replacement if needed

CHAPTER 15

Examination of Individual Joint Pathologies

SHOULDER JOINT AND SHOULDER GIRDLE

HISTORY: In diseases of the shoulder joint the patients usually complain of pain—either localized in the shoulder joint or radiating from the acromion process down the outer side of the arm up to its middle. The students must remember a fallacy in this respect that pain in the shoulder joint may be referred from the neck, chest or the abdomen (from irritation of the diaphragm which is supplied by the same segments, i.e., C3, 4 and 5).

History in individual joint pathologies

Aspect	Clinical significance	Patient-friendly questions
Pain onset	Sudden → Trauma, Rotator cuff Tear	"Did your pain start suddenly or gradually?"
Pain localization	Lateral pain → Rotator cuff, **Top of shoulder** → AC joint arthritis	"Where exactly do you feel the pain?"
Night pain	Frozen shoulder, Rotator cuff tear	"Is your pain worse at night?"
Stiffness vs weakness	Stiffness → Frozen shoulder, Weakness → Rotator cuff tear	"Do you have trouble moving your shoulder or does it feel weak?"
History of trauma	Fractures, Dislocations, Rotator Cuff Injuries	"Did you have a fall or accident before the pain started?"

Causes of major joint pathologies

Category	Condition	Key features
Inflammatory	Rheumatoid arthritis	Chronic, symmetric joint involvement, morning stiffness, positive rheumatoid factor
	Gout	Acute, severe pain, big toe involvement, elevated uric acid
	Pseudogout	Calcium pyrophosphate crystals, chondrocalcinosis on X-ray
Infectious	Septic arthritis	High fever, red, hot swollen joint, leukocytosis
	Tuberculous arthritis	Gradual onset, cold abscess formation, positive Mantoux test
Degenerative	Osteoarthritis	Asymmetric joint space narrowing, osteophytes, pain worsens with activity

Contd...

Contd...

Category	Condition	Key features
Neuropathic	Charcot's joint	Painless destruction, seen in diabetes, syphilis, syringomyelia
Metabolic	Hemophilic arthropathy	Recurrent hemarthrosis, seen in hemophilia

■ LOCAL EXAMINATION

A. INSPECTION

The patient must be stripped up to the waist and stand in front of the surgeon for proper inspection not only of the affected joint but also to compare with the sound side.

1. **Position:** In affection of the shoulder joint the arm is held by the side of the chest, medially rotated and slightly flexed. Very often the arm is being supported by the other hand and kept slightly raised.

2. **Contour:** This is important. It may be *flattened* due to wasting of the deltoid muscles from tuberculous arthritis, rheumatoid arthritis, osteoarthritis, rotator cuff* lesions, etc. It may be *prominent* with rounded fullness seen in subdeltoid bursitis or effusion of the joint. In effusion of the shoulder joint, which is not very common, the swelling extends beyond the anterior and posterior margins of the deltoid and along the long tendon of the biceps due to existence of synovial sac. But in subdeltoid bursitis fullness is only seen just beneath the deltoid muscle and does not go beyond the margins of this muscle.

B. PALPATION

1. **Tenderness:** The shoulder joint is best palpated by keeping the arm by the chest wall with one hand and with the other hand to palpate the shoulder joint from all aspects. In supraspinatus tendinitis pressure just below the acromion process will elicit tenderness. In painful arc syndrome pressure just below the acromion will elicit tenderness if the arm is adducted, but not if the arm is abducted as the tender spot will disappear under the acromion process. Similarly in front just below the coracoid process one can feel the anterior aspect of the joint and note if there is any tenderness. Posteriorly also the joint is palpated similarly. In osteoarthritis if the arm is made to sway a little the palpating hand at the shoulder joint will feel the crepitus. Three bony joints are important to palpate in the shoulder joint—(a) Tip of coracoid, below which is the anterior aspect of the shoulder, (b) Tip of the acromion, below which lies the superior aspect of shoulder and (c) Greater tuberosity, its prominence.

    It is a good practice to feel the acromioclavicular as well as the sternoclavicular joints to exclude any organic disease there.

2. **Codman's method:** This is another method of palpating the shoulder joint. The left hand is used to palpate the right shoulder of the patient. The thumb lies along the depression below the spine of the scapula to palpate the posterior aspect of the shoulder joint. The tip of the index finger is placed just anterior to the acromion to feel the superior aspect (at the insertion of the supraspinatus) and slightly anterior aspect of the joint and other three fingers are placed on

---

* 'Rotator cuff' is a cuff comprised of tendons of the four muscles which fuse with the capsule of the shoulder joint to give additional strength to it. These four muscles are—anteriorly subscapularis, superiorly supraspinatus and posteriorly infraspinatus and teres minor.

the clavicle to hold it. Examiner's right hand grasps the patient's flexed elbow and the patient's arm is moved gently backwards (extension) and forwards (flexion) and the shoulder joint is carefully palpated. The examiner's right hand is used to palpate patient's left shoulder **(Fig. 15.1)**.

3. **Swelling:** Effusion in the joint is difficult to palpate through the deltoid. Fullness, however, can be discovered in the axilla. Subdeltoid bursitis may give rise to swelling and tenderness just beneath the acromion process.

The corresponding axilla should be always palpated while examining the affected shoulder. This palpation should be deep high in the axilla to detect any fullness there to indicate joint effusion. As the inferior aspect of the joint is lax and redundant accumulation of fluid starts here in case of joint effusion.

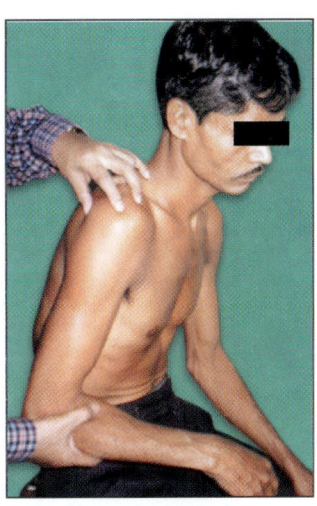

Fig. 15.1: Codman's method of palpation of the shoulder joint. Note the placement of the clinician's fingers on the shoulder joint. See the text.

MOVEMENTS: The shoulder joint is a very mobile joint and the bony configuration is such as to sacrifice the stability of the joint to certain extent to compromise with greater ranges of movement.

While examining for the ranges of different movements of shoulder joint **(Figs. 15.2A to F)**, *firstly*, the patient must be stripped up to the waist and these movements should be examined not only from in front but also from behind (particularly during abduction to see the scapular movement). This is because of the fact that an ankylosed glenohumeral joint will show some range of movement due to the movement of the scapula as also the acromioclavicular and sternoclavicular joints. *Secondly,* the different movements must be compared with those of the normal side to exactly assess the differences. *Thirdly,* the clinician must have a clear idea about the plane of the body of the scapula along which the abduction and adduction movements occur. This is not in the coronal plane of the body but is slightly inclined forwards about 30° with this plane **(Fig. 15.3)**. So during abduction the arm is carried forwards and outwards while during adduction the arm is carried backwards and inwards. Flexion and extension take place at a right angle to this plane, i.e., in flexion the arm is carried forwards and medially and in extension backwards and laterally. *Fourthly* in the movement of abduction the shoulder joint itself moves for 100°–120°, the additional 60°–80° is obtained by the forward rotation of the scapula and some movement of the clavicle. But these movements occur almost simultaneously except in the initial 25°–30° when the whole of the movement takes place at the shoulder joint. For every subsequent 15° of elevation of the arm, the glenohumeral joint contributes 10° and the scapular movement 5°. To note exactly how much movement is contributed by the glenohumeral joint, the scapula is fixed by the clinician from behind and the patient is asked to abduct the shoulder.

The range permitted in each movement is as follows:

Abduction—180°; flexion—90°; extension—45°; rotations—both medial and lateral—one quarter of a circle about a vertical axis; circumduction—results from succession of the foregoing movements.

Active movements: The patient is asked to carry out all the movements simultaneously on both sides (for comparison) one after another and the difference from the normal side is noted. The

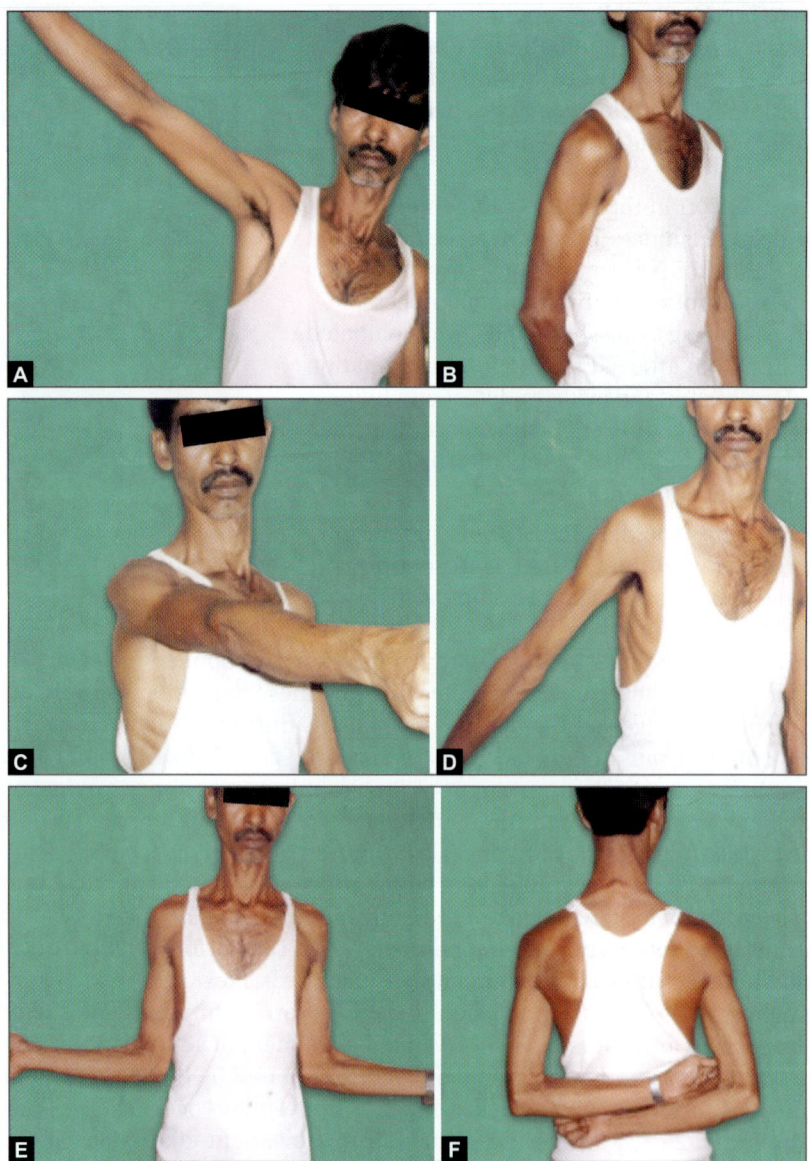

Figs. 15.2A to F: Showing movements of the shoulder joint: (A) Abduction; (B) Adduction; (C) Flexion; (D) Extension; (E) External rotation and (F) Internal rotation.

important movements are abduction and external rotation which are often affected in different diseases of the shoulder joint.

During abduction it is noted whether the patient shrugs his shoulder at the beginning of the act or not. This indicates complete rupture of supraspinatus tendon. This muscle is concerned in starting the movement of abduction. In chronic supraspinatus tendinitis (painful arc syndrome), pain is felt at the midrange of abduction (60°–120°), the extremes of the range are painless **(Fig. 15.4)**. The whole range of abduction is painful in acute supraspinatus tendinitis and

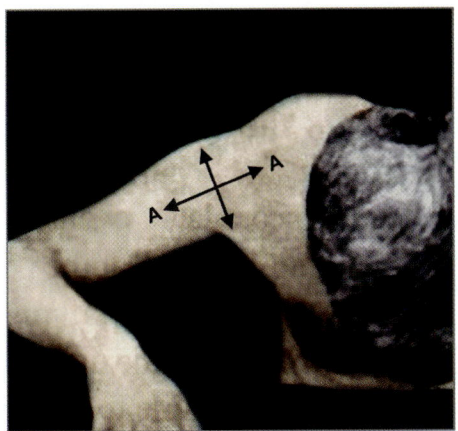

Fig. 15.3: Note that the plane of the scapula is not in the coronal plane of the body but is slightly inclined forwards (about 30°). Abduction and adduction take place in the plane of the body of the scapula (A-A) whereas flexion and extension occur at right angles to that plane.

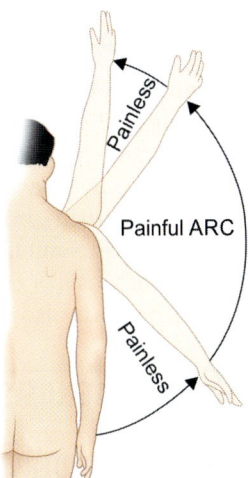

Fig. 15.4: In painful arc syndrome, the midrange abduction is painful, the extremes are painless.

any arthritis of the shoulder joint. In arthritis of acromioclavicular joint sharp pain is felt when the arm is raised above right angle. Determine how much of the shoulder movement occurs at the shoulder joint proper (glenohumeral joint) and how much is contributed by rotation of the scapula and the clavicle. In frozen shoulder proper abduction is very much limited and this is practically nil in bony ankylosis. Yet a good range of abduction is possible because of the rotation of the scapula and the clavicle.

Rotation of the shoulder joint is restricted, particularly the external rotation in different arthritis of the joint and in frozen shoulder.

Passive movement (Fig. 15.5): The importance of this movement is not much except in complete rupture of supraspinatus tendon. In this condition if the patient is made to abduct his shoulder for the initial 30°, he will be able to complete the whole range of abduction with the help of the deltoid muscle.

Acromioclavicular and sternoclavicular joints: These joints are best examined from the front. The patient must be stripped up to the waist. The joints are inspected for any redness, swelling and deformity. The joints are palpated for local tenderness, temperature and to assess the swelling. The patient is asked if the joints become painful in different movements of the shoulder joint. It is useful to note that the movements of these joints occur during elevation of the arm and when the shoulders are braced backwards or drawn forwards.

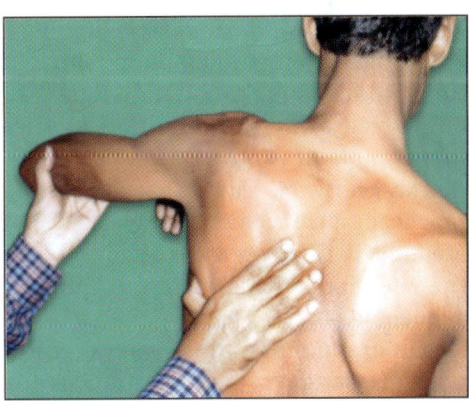

Fig. 15.5: Testing passive movements of the shoulder joint. Note that the scapula is fixed with one hand.

SPECIAL INVESTIGATIONS

1. **Blood**—is examined for hemoglobin, total count, differential count and erythrocyte sedimentation rate (ESR) in acute arthritis and tuberculous arthritis of the joint.
2. **X-ray examination**—provides most of the required informations regarding diseases of the shoulder joint. It not only shows whether the joint is involved by acute or tuberculous arthritis, rheumatoid or osteoarthritis, but also shows calcification above the greater tuberosity in acute supraspinatus tendinitis. Sometimes the patients complain of referred pain in the shoulder joint due to cervical spondylosis or cervical rib or irritation of the diaphragm following gallstone or splenic rupture. These are also revealed in X-ray.

DIFFERENTIAL DIAGNOSIS

ARTHRITIS OF THE SHOULDER JOINT

Acute arthritis rarely affects a shoulder joint, but occasionally seen in children. *Rheumatoid arthritis* is also occasionally seen in shoulder joint and usually the young adult females are the victims. Similarly, *osteoarthritis* is also not commonly seen in the shoulder joint. *Tuberculous affection* of the joint is occasionally seen and the disease starts as a synovitis or osteomyelitis. In this condition cold abscess and sinus formations (florid type) are not uncommon, but "Caries Sicca", i.e., without abscess formation is often confused with "frozen shoulder". Previously many cases which were diagnosed as "Caries Sicca" were nothing but "frozen shoulders". X-ray examination is confirmatory as destructive lesions of tuberculosis will be obvious in "Caries Sicca".

ACUTE SUPRASPINATUS TENDINITIS (FIG. 15.6)

Localized degeneration of the supraspinatus tendon with or without deposition of calcium is the main underlying pathology of this condition. Degeneration leads to rapid swelling and tension with often calcium deposition which leads to tremendous pain. Young individuals between 25–45 years are the common victims. The first complaint is obviously a dull ache which quickly gets worse leading to agonizing pain and practically all movements—especially abduction are limited. After a few days pain subsides once the calcified substance has erupted into the subdeltoid bursa.

On examination there is tenderness at the point of insertion of the supraspinatus on greater tuberosity just beneath the acromion process. Skiagram will reveal calcification of supraspinatus tendon which later on bursts into the subdeltoid bursa relieving pain.

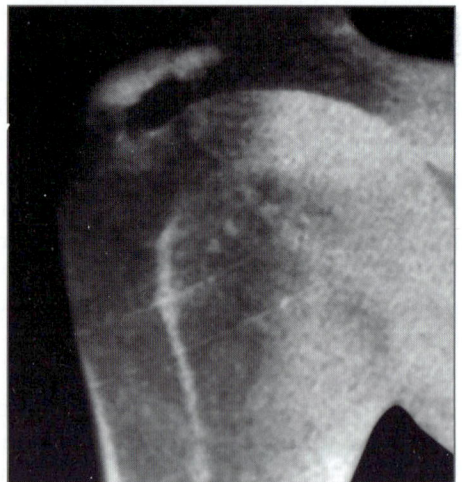

Fig. 15.6: Shows calcification in the tendon of supraspinatus following degeneration. This is a case of acute supraspinatus tendinitis.

CHRONIC SUPRASPINATUS TENDINITIS (PAINFUL ARC SYNDROME)

This condition is also due to a process of degeneration of the supraspinatus tendon which is probably triggered by an injury or by overuse. The swelling of the tendon is again the underlying pathology and is so situated that on abduction (during the middle of the range) it impinges upon the under surface of the acromion process. Commonly older men in the age group of 45–60 years are the victims. The most important finding is that the mid-abduction (60°–120°) is painful. This is the range of abduction in which there is very little space between the greater tuberosity and the acromion and the thickened supraspinatus tendon becomes nipped between these two bones. The beginning and the end of abduction remain painless.

The painful arc syndrome is definitely the pathognomonic feature of chronic supraspinatus tendinitis but is sometimes come across in conditions like (a) subdeltoid bursitis, (b) incomplete rupture of the supraspinatus tendon and (c) crack fracture of the greater tuberosity of the humerus.

FROZEN SHOULDER

The underlying pathology is that an exudate causes the layers of the infra-articular synovial membrane (inferior aspect of the synovial membrane) and the capsule to adhere to one another. Patients between 45 and 60 years are commonly affected. Females seem to outnumber the male patients. The patient sometimes gives a history of trauma. The patient first experiences a pain which becomes worse at night and prevents the patient from sleeping on the affected side. Gradual stiffness of shoulder follows. In a matter of months all movements especially abduction and external rotation are restricted. As the process continues the pain abates. By this time the muscles around the shoulder show signs of disuse atrophy. Months later stiffness gradually lessens and the disease recovers spontaneously. Thus there are three phases of this disease: (i) increasing pain and increasing stiffness, (ii) decreasing pain with persistent stiffness and (iii) disappearance of stiffness with return of all the movements. Each phase lasts from 4 to 8 months and the whole process takes about 2 years.

X-ray appearance is widely *accepted as normal,* which differentiates this condition from others.

RUPTURE OF THE SUPRASPINATUS TENDON

Degeneration of the supraspinatus tendon is again the cause of this condition. The injury which causes tear is rather trifle in that way. Usually elderly men between 45 and 65 years are affected. The patient usually gives a history of trauma in the way of lifting weight or protecting himself from falling. The pain is felt immediately radiating from the shoulder to the middle of the outer side of the arm. The patient soon discovers that he is unable to lift the arm or abduct his shoulder. But if he bends to the affected side a little to make an angle of 20°–30° when the deltoid muscle takes over the process of abduction and completes the full range of abduction. The supraspinatus muscle is concerned to begin the process of abduction which is later carried on by the deltoid muscle. Palpation will reveal a gap just beneath the acromion process. Straight X-ray will not give much information, but arthrography will reveal the tear.

SUBDELTOID (SUBACROMIAL) BURSITIS

Fluid in the subdeltoid bursa will present as cystic and fluctuating swelling beneath the acromion process. In this condition the humeral head can be distinctly palpated below the acromion process which differentiates this condition from the effusion of the shoulder joint.

BRACHIAL NEURALGIA

This term signifies pain extending over a large part of the upper limb. There are numerous causes of this condition and careful examination will reveal the exact cause in a particular case. The common causes are—(A) *In the neck:* (i) Disc prolapse commonly seen at the level between C6 and C7. Patient will complain of pain radiating from the neck towards the shoulder and down the arm with painful and restricted neck movements. X-ray will show diminished disc space. (ii) Tuberculosis of the cervical vertebrae. (iii) Vertebral body tumor. (iv) Cord or root tumor. (B) *In the neck-arm junction*: (i) Cervical rib, (ii) Pancoast's syndrome, i.e., bronchial carcinoma affecting the apical lobe of the lung giving rise to Horner's syndrome and a hard lump at the root of the neck. (C) *In the shoulder*— (i) Musculotendinous cuff lesions. (ii) Arthritis—any arthritis of the joint, be it rheumatoid, osteoarthritis, tuberculosis, etc.

RUPTURE OF THE BICEPS TENDON

This condition is a sequel of avascular degeneration of the biceps tendon or may be due to rubbing against osteophytes in an osteoarthritic shoulder. The patients are usually over 50 years of age. A history of trauma is almost inevitable in the form of lifting weight or saving himself from a fall. The clinical picture is unmistakable, i.e., whenever the bicep muscle is made to contract, belly of the biceps looks prominent and rounder with a gap proximal to it.

■ THE ELBOW JOINT

A. HISTORY

Patients with elbow disorders mostly complain of pain, stiffness, deformity and occasionally locking. One thing must be noted that pain in the elbow may be referred from the neck or shoulder disorders.

B. INSPECTION

1. **Position:** The patient is asked to stand straight with his arm at the side of the body with the palms looking forwards that means in anatomical position. Observe the carrying angle (normally it is 10° in case of males and 20° in case of females) and compare it with that of the sound limb. This angle is the outward deviation of the extended and supinated forearm from the axis of the arm. This angle disappears when the forearm is flexed or pronated. It must be noted that varus or valgus deformity of the elbow is only obvious when this joint remains straight. This deformity disappears when the joint is flexed. In case of effusion of the elbow joint, this joint is held in semiflexion position—the position of ease or greatest capacity.

2. **Swelling:** Any swelling near about the elbow joint is noted. Normal hollows on either side of the olecranon and obliterated in effusion of the joint. Olecranon bursitis (miner's or student's elbow) will give rise to swelling over the olecranon process. Great effusion of the elbow joint will also show fullness in the antecubital fossa. Sometimes a bursa beneath the tendon of the biceps near its insertion may become inflamed giving rise to a condition known as bicipitoradial bursitis. This condition also gives rise to a slight swelling in front of the elbow joint which may be missed.

3. **Muscular wasting:** This will be obvious in any affection of the elbow joint which will limit its function.

C. PALPATION

1. **Local temperature:** This will be increased in acute arthritis, olecranon bursitis and bicipitoradial bursitis.

2. **Localized tenderness:** This is an important part of examination which will often indicate the diagnosis by itself. In tennis elbow a localized tenderness will be elicited in the region of origin

of the common extensor muscles at the lateral epicondyle. In Golfer's elbow the tenderness is situated on the common flexor origin from the medial epicondyle.

3. **Bony components** of the joint viz. the lower part of the humerus and the upper parts of the ulna and the radius are carefully palpated for any thickening or irregularity—the evidence of previous osteomyelitis. The three bony points—the tip of the olecranon, the medial epicondyle and the lateral epicondyle—form a triangle when the elbow is flexed. But these three bony points come to a straight horizontal line when the elbow is extended.

4. **Swelling:** Swellings around the elbow joint are palpated along the usual lines of the examination. Fluctuant swelling will be seen in effusion of the elbow and in all bursitis. In case of *effusion of the elbow joint* first there is filling up of the concavity on each side of the olecranon, as the synovial cavity is nearest to the surface at this region and the posterior ligament is thin and lax. When more fluid accumulates, a swelling is noticed on the posterolateral aspect of the elbow joint over the radiohumeral joint. Crossed fluctuation can be elicited between this area and swelling over the medial aspect of the olecranon. This sign distinguishes an effusion of the elbow joint from enlargement of bursa beneath the triceps tendon.

5. **Examination of the supratrochlear lymph node:** To examine for enlarged supratrochlear or epitrochlear lymph nodes one must flex the elbow to the right angle to relax the surrounding structures. The node will be palpated on the anterior surface of the medial intermuscular septum 1 cm above the base of the medial epicondyle. When enlarged, the node will be found slipping beneath the finger and thumb. If the elbow is kept extended the enlarged lymph node may not be palpated. While unilateral enlargement of this lymph node indicates some infective lesions of the hand, wrist and forearm, but bilateral enlargement suggests a generalized disease, e.g., syphilis and calls for biopsy of the gland.

D. MOVEMENTS

The elbow joint has got two components—humeroulnar and superior radio-ulnar joints. The humeroulnar joint permits flexion and extension. The full range of extension means when the elbow joint becomes straight. The full range of flexion is 180° from this position that means when the soft tissues of the anterior aspect of the joint come to approximation. The radioulnar joint permits pronation and supination movements and *these movements are best examined when the elbow joint is kept flexed at 90°* and the arm is kept by the side of the chest. When the elbow joint is extended these movements will be mixed with rotation of the humerus.

DIFFERENTIAL DIAGNOSIS

ACUTE ARTHRITIS

Acute arthritis often leads to effusion of the elbow joint. The joint becomes very painful and is always held in semiflexion position (optimum position). On both sides of the olecranon normal concavity will disappear. Effusion of the elbow joint will elicit transmitted fluid impulse between the two sides of olecranon posteriorly and at the bent of the elbow anteriorly.

CHRONIC ARTHRITIS

All the usual forms of chronic arthritis may be seen in the elbow joint. But these are uncommon. Tuberculosis occurs in adults more often than in children.

OSTEOCHONDRITIS DISSECANS

This condition, though more often seen in the knee joint, yet it does occasionally affect the elbow joint. The capitulum is generally involved. The head of the radius is also affected (**Fig. 15.7**). The patient complains of aching pain and recurrent effusion. On X-ray there will be a dense spot in the capitulum affecting its articular surface. Later on this portion may be detached forming loose body in the joint.

CHARCOT'S JOINT

This condition occasionally affects the elbow.

TENNIS ELBOW (LATERAL EPICONDYLITIS)

This is more often seen among the tennis players and hence the name. But quite a number of the sufferers of this condition have never played tennis. Probably, the common extensor origin is damaged and subsequent adhesion binds torn to untorn fibers and to the joint capsule. Tendinitis, nipping of a synovial fringe and entrapment of a branch of the radial nerve may be the other explanations which the students should keep in mind.

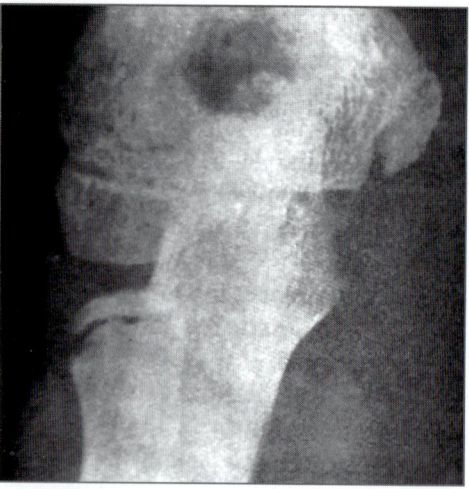

Fig. 15.7: Osteochondritis dissecans affecting the head of the radius. Note the dense epiphysis of the radial head.

Patients complain of pain on the lateral aspect of the elbow, accentuated by dorsiflexion of the wrist when the extensor muscles are put in action, such as during pouring out tea in a cup or turning a door handle.

Palpation will reveal considerable tenderness over the lateral epicondyle of the humerus where the extensor muscles originate. *Cozen's test*, i.e., when the patient is asked to extend his clenched fist against resistance, considerable pain is experienced at the lateral epicondyle (**Fig. 15.8**). *Mill's maneuver*, i.e., the patient's wrist is passively flexed when his forearm is pronated. This gives rise to tremendous pain on the attachment of the common extensor tendons (**Fig. 15.9**).

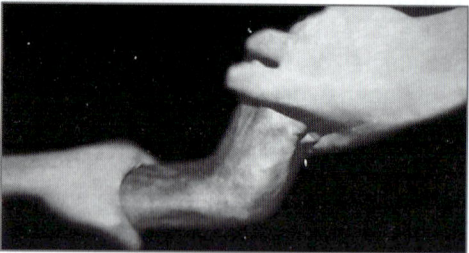

Fig. 15.8: Cozen's test. See the text.

GOLFER'S (OR BASEBALLER'S) ELBOW (MEDIAL EPICONDYLITIS)

This condition is quite uncommon in comparison to the previous one. It is the medial counterpart of the previous condition, i.e., the tenderness is situated in the common flexor origin at the medial epicondyle.

STUDENT'S (OR MINER'S) ELBOW

The bursa over the olecranon process sometimes gets infected and leads to effusion in it. This is nothing but olecranon bursitis and is caused by repeated movement of the skin over the olecranon

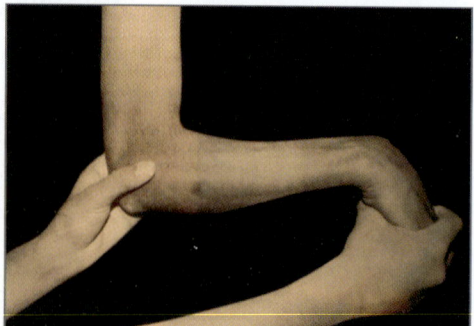

Fig. 15.9: Mill's maneuver. Note that the clinician's left thumb is palpating the origin of the common extensor tendons where the patient is experiencing severe pain due to the maneuver.

bursa. This condition mainly affects the students and the friction is caused while writing between the skin over the olecranon and the table.

BICIPITORADIAL BURSITIS

This is a very rare condition in which the bursa beneath the tendon of biceps becomes inflamed and effused. This is caused by repeated throwing of a ball. The patient complains of pain over the insertion of the biceps tendon which is accentuated by flexion and supination (movements caused by the biceps muscle at the elbow).

THE ELBOW TUNNEL SYNDROME

This condition is by far rarer than carpal tunnel syndrome. This condition affects the ulnar nerve whereas the latter condition affects the median nerve. The involvement of the ulnar nerve occurs when it passes between the two heads of the flexor carpi ulnaris. This condition may be due to osteoarthritis of the elbow joint and the ulnar nerve is injured by the osteophytes.

THE WRIST AND OTHER JOINTS OF THE HAND

A. HISTORY

The patients with the problems of the wrist may present with either pain, swelling such as caused by ganglion or deformity such as tuberculous affection of the wrist or more commonly of the joints of the fingers.

B. INSPECTION

1. **Position:** In all affections of the wrist joint this joint will remain in flexed position and characteristic ulnar deviation is noticed in wrist and the finger joints particularly in rheumatoid arthritis.
2. **Swelling:** Swelling may be due to effusion of the wrist joint which is rather uncommon and should be differentiated from effusion of the tendon sheaths. In the latter condition the effusion extends upwards and downwards beyond the extent of the joint and along the corresponding tendon sheath, while the former is limited within the extent of the joint and is seen both anteriorly and posteriorly. In *rheumatoid arthritis* the metacarpophalangeal joints become swollen with prominent knuckles. *In tuberculous tenosynovitis of the ulnar bursa* (compound palmar ganglion), a swelling is present on the palmar aspect and extends both proximally and distally beyond the flexor retinaculum. A small circumscribed swelling either on the dorsal (more common) or on the ventral aspect of the wrist is nothing but a *ganglion* (Fig. 15.10).
3. **Deformity:** Obvious deformities of the wrist are rare and barring rheumatoid arthritis they are mostly congenital deformities, e.g., radial club hand, Madelung's deformity, etc.
4. **Sinus:** In tuberculosis of the wrist joint sinus formation is not uncommon.

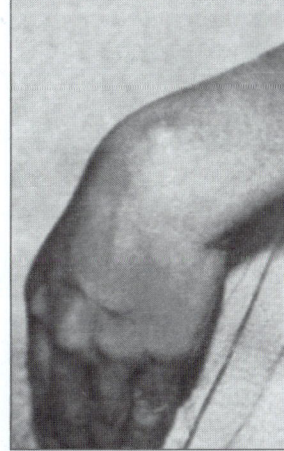

Fig. 15.10: The ganglion on the dorsal aspect of the wrist (the most common site).

C. PALPATION

1. **Swelling:** Is the swelling fluctuant? Effusion of the wrist, ganglion and the compound palmar ganglion are all fluctuant swellings. In *effusion* of the wrist joint cross fluctuation on both anterior and posterior aspects of the joint can be elicited. Similarly in *compound palmar ganglion* cross fluctuation can be elicited above and below the flexor retinaculum. In *ganglion*, which is often a tense swelling fluctuation can be seldom elicited. Sometimes it is felt as hard as a bone. The ganglion becomes fixed as soon as the concerned tendon is made taut due to its intimate connection with the tendon sheath.
2. **Tenderness:** Tenderness exactly on the joint line indicates arthritis. Tenderness along the tendon sheath indicates tenosynovitis.
3. **Deformity:** By palpation the actual deformity is noted.

D. MOVEMENTS

The wrist joint, like the elbow has got two components : (i) the radiocarpal and (ii) the inferior radioulnar joint. Pronation and supination movements occur at the inferior radioulnar joint. All other movements, i.e., flexion, extension, adduction and abduction occur in both the radiocarpal and the midcarpal joints. Extension and adduction mostly occur in radiocarpal joint, whereas flexion and abduction take place in midcarpal joint. Normal range of flexion is about 60°, that of extension is about 70°, adduction about 35° and abduction about 25°.

Flexion and extension can be tested in the following way **(Figs. 15.11A and B)**: to determine *the range of extension* the patient is asked to place his palms and fingers of both the hands in contact (Indian method of salutation). Now he is asked to lift both the elbows gradually as far as he can keeping the hands firmly in apposition. The angle formed by the hand and the forearm of the affected side is compared with that of the sound side. This angle is the range of extension movement. To determine the *range of flexion* the backs of the hands are placed in contact and the elbows are lowered as far as possible. The angle between the hand and forearm is the range of flexion movement.

In arthritis of the wrist joint all the movements of the wrist are painful and limited.

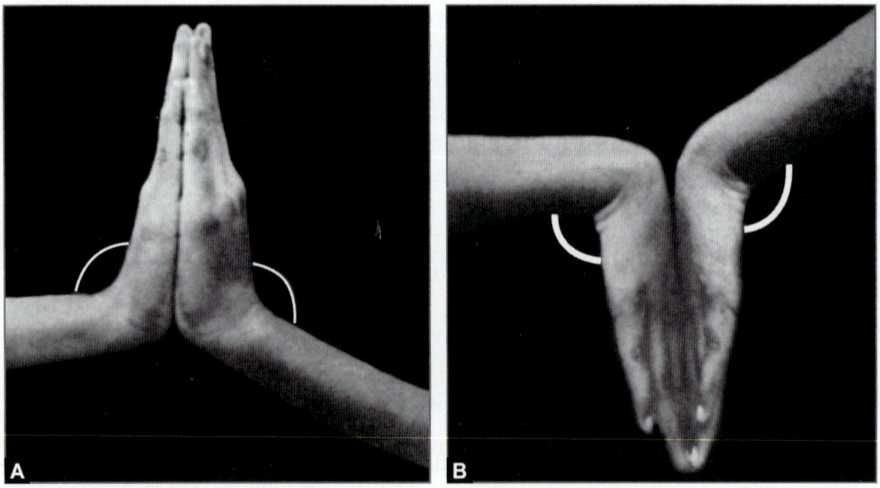

Figs. 15.11A and B: Showing the methods of testing the ranges of extension and flexion of the wrist joint. Note that there is restriction of both the movements on the affected left side.

DIFFERENTIAL DIAGNOSIS

ACUTE ARTHRITIS
This will lead to pain, tenderness and effusion of the joint.

TUBERCULOSIS
This is rarely seen in the wrist. The patient complains of gradual aching, stiffness and the hands feel weak. The wrist becomes swollen with wasting of the forearm, thenar and hypothenar muscles. The joint is kept flexed a little, later on cold abscess and sinus formation may result. X-ray shows narrowing and irregularity of the radiocarpal and midcarpal joints with rarefaction of the adjacent bones.

GANGLION
This is a cystic swelling caused by mucoid or myxomatous degeneration of the connective tissue of the joint capsule or the tendon sheath. Usually young adults are affected. The patients present with painless lump which may give rise to slight ache and weakness. This is commonly seen at the back (dorsal aspect) of the wrist but may occur in front of the joint, when it may compress the median nerve leading to symptoms simulating carpal tunnel syndrome. The cyst contains crystal-clear gelatinous fluid. When on dorsal aspect of the wrist, the swelling becomes tense and prominent when the wrist is flexed. The gelatinous fluid is filled so tight that it feels solid.

COMPOUND PALMAR GANGLION
This is nothing but chronic inflammation of the common sheath of the flexor tendons leading to swelling of this sheath (ulnar bursa) above and below the flexor retinaculum. Rheumatoid arthritis and tuberculosis are incriminated for this condition. The synovial membrane becomes thick and villous. The fluid contains fibrin particles and melon seeds. The patient presents with the swelling mostly without pain but with some wasting of the thenar and the hypothenar muscles. There may be some interfering with the movements of the fingers. Paresthesia due to median nerve compression may occur. The swelling shows cross fluctuation above and below the flexor retinaculum.

DEQUERVAIN'S DISEASE (STENOSING TENOSYNOVITIS) (FIG. 15.12)
This is a condition in which the common sheath of the tendons of abductor pollicis longus and extensor pollicis brevis becomes chronically inflamed, thickened and later on stenosed as a result of degenerative changes or unaccustomed overuse. The patients are usually women in their forties. The main complaint is pain on the radial styloid process where the sheath enclosing the said two tendons exists. On examination there is

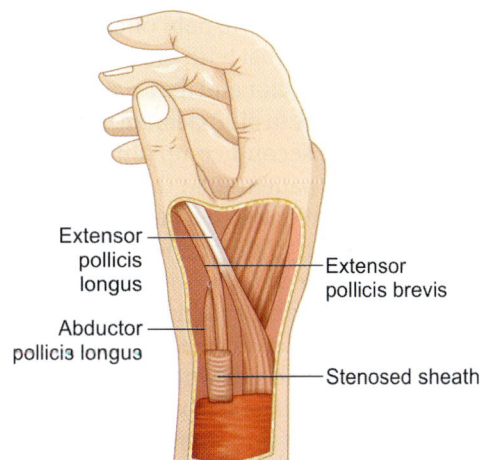

Fig. 15.12: Diagrammatic representation of the positions of the tendons of the abductor pollicis longus and extensor pollicis brevis alongwith their common sheath which becomes thickened and stenosed in stenosing tenosynovitis (De Quervain's disease).

local tenderness and a localized swelling may or may not be present. The pain is aggravated when the patient extends her thumb against resistance. If the wrist is passively adducted or the thumb is ulnar deviated, the patient winces with pain. With the thumb in the palm, the patient is asked to make a fist by superimposing the fingers over the thumb. The hand is then pushed passively to the medial (ulnar) side. Pain is experienced at the radial styloid process which shoots down to the thumb or upwards towards the elbow (Finkelstein's test).

CARPAL TUNNEL SYNDROME

This is nothing but a type of compression neuropathy of the median nerve as it passes beneath the flexor retinaculum. This is due to narrowing of the osseofibrous tunnel (carpal tunnel) either due to rheumatoid arthritis or pregnancy or as a complication of Colles' fracture or idiopathic (which by far outnumbers the other conditions). The majority of the patients are women between the ages of 40 and 60 years. This condition may be bilateral but more often the more active side is affected. The main complaint is progressive weakness and impairment of fine movements. Pain, tingling and numbness along the sensory distribution of the median nerve are also the presenting features. Occasionally, the pain may shoot upwards and may mislead the clinician. On examination there will be some sensory changes and motor impairment of the nerve (median nerve) concerned. In late cases there may be wasting of the thenar eminence. When the patient is asked to flex the wrist there will be exacerbation of the symptoms particularly paresthesia within 1 minute and the symptoms will disappear as soon as the wrist is straightened. This is known as the *'Wrist flexion Test' (Phalen's sign)*. Electrical nerve conduction study will elicit a delay in motor conduction of the median nerve at the wrist.

THE HIP JOINT

A. HISTORY

The most common symptom of the hip disorders is *pain,* which is mostly felt in front rather than in the buttock. The pain often radiates to the knee thus misleading the clinician. This is because of the fact that both the hip and the knee joints are supplied by the common nerves viz. the femoral, obturator and the sciatic. With destruction of the articular cartilages pain becomes worse at night due to disappearance of the protective muscular spasm. This is called "night pain".

Limp is the second complaint and this is more often discovered by the clinician or the relatives of the patient than the patient himself. The gait of the patient must be noticed very carefully. If a patient with a painful hip is using stick, he usually holds it in the opposite hand. Is he lurching on to the sound side or to the affected side? In arthritis the patient lurches on the sound side because he tries to take the weight off the affected side as quickly as possible to avoid pain. On the other hand the patient lurches on the affected side (Trendelenburg's gait) in unilateral congenital dislocation and coxa vara. This is to counteract the tendency of the pelvis to sink on the sound side when the leg of that side is raised off the ground. In bilateral congenital dislocation and bilateral coxa vara the characteristic *waddling gait* is seen.

Age of onset of symptom often suggests the diagnosis. From birth to 5 years—congenital dislocation; 5–10 years—Perthes' disease; 10–15 years—slipped epiphysis (adolescent coxa vara); 20–40 years—osteoarthritis due to previous disorders; over 40 years—osteoarthritis (idiopathic). Tuberculosis of the hip may occur at any age.

Preparation for examination: A child is completely stripped for examination of hip joints. A man can only keep his shirts on. In case of females some cover for genitals is provided with.

B. INSPECTION

The patient is first inspected in the standing posture both from front and behind. Observe the gait carefully.

1. **Attitude:** The clinician must not concentrate on the hip joint alone so far as the attitude of the patient is concerned. Any fixity of the hip joint either by muscular spasm or by fibrosis is made good by the mobility of the lumbar spine and the pelvis as a whole. In standing position it should be noted that the patient with arthritis of the hip joint tends to bear most of his weight on the sound leg. Thus the patient lurches on the sound side with slight flexion of the affected hip joint. A good look is made to detect any muscular atrophy which may result from long standing disease of the hip. Lastly, one should look for any scar or sinus near the hip joint.

Trendelenburg's test (Figs. 15.13 and 15.14): Normally each leg bears half of the body weight. When one leg is lifted, the other leg takes the entire weight and the trunk inclines towards the weight bearing leg and the pelvis tilts raising that side of the pelvis which is not taking the weight. This is due to the pull exerted by the abductors of the hip. When the mechanism fails, Trendelenburg's sign becomes positive. The test is performed in the following way: The patient stands on the unaffected lower limb first, the buttock on the affected side automatically rises. Next the patient stands on the affected side, the pelvis on the opposite (normal) side sinks as shown by gluteal folds and iliac crest. It indicates a defect in the osseomuscular mechanism between the pelvis and the femur. This test becomes positive (i) when the abductors are weak as in poliomyelitis, muscle dystrophies or motor neurone disease; (ii) in congenital or pathological dislocation of the hip where the muscles do not have stable fulcrum to act on; (iii) in fracture neck of femur, coxa vara, Perthes' disease, etc., when the lever system loses its intactness; (iv) when it hurts the patient as in different arthritis of the hip. Presence of fixed deformities are usually demonstrated with the patient lying on the bed.

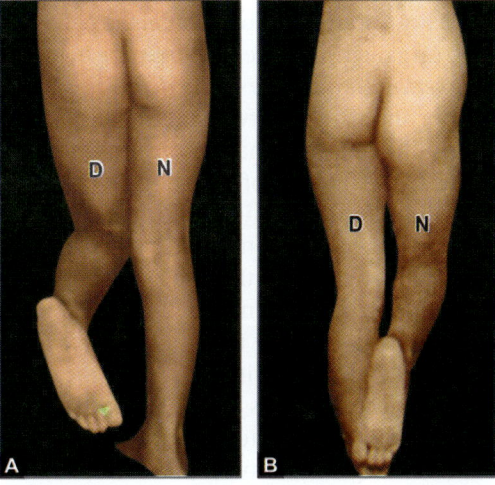

Figs.15.13A and B: Trendelenburg's test. Normally when the weight of the body is taken on one leg the pelvis rises on the other side. The test is positive if the pelvis drops on the other side. N and D indicate normal and diseased sides respectively.

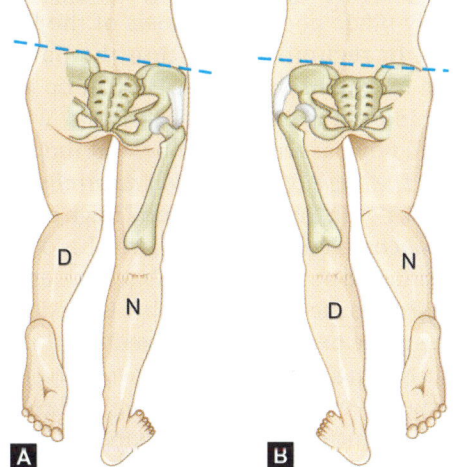

Figs. 15.14A and B: Diagrammatic representation of Trendelenburg's test.

Fixed abduction or adduction deformity (Figs. 15.15A and B): A limb when fixed in abduction position is brought to the ground by lateral flexion of the lumbar spine, i.e., scoliosis with convexity towards the affected side, the pelvis being tilted down causing apparent lengthening of the limb. Similarly, a fixed adducted limb is brought parallel to its fellow by scoliosis with convexity towards the sound side, the pelvis being tilted up causing apparent shortening of the limb. *To ascertain the nature of the deformity,* a line is drawn connecting the two anterior superior iliac spines. This line is normally horizontal and at right angles to the midline of the body. In presence of abduction and adduction deformities it will no longer be horizontal. In the former, the anterior superior iliac spine on the affected side will be at a lower level, whereas in the latter it will be found at a higher level. Now the *angle of deformity* is estimated in the following way:

The affected limb is held just above the ankle and is gradually adducted or abducted according to the existing deformity till the interspinous line becomes horizontal. Now the *angle of deformity* is estimated by the amount of abduction or adduction made in relation to the normal vertical to bring interspinous line horizontal.

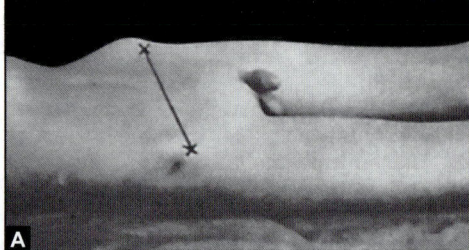
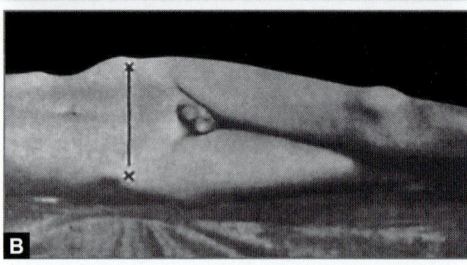

Figs. 15.15A and B: (A) fixed adduction deformity has been concealed by raising the left anterior superior iliac spine. (B) The angle of fixed adduction deformity is measured by adducting the affected limb till the interspinous line becomes horizontal.

Fixed flexion deformity (Fig. 15.16): This is usually made good by lordosis of the lumbar spine. In recumbent position the patient is asked to extend the limbs. He will be able to do so in expense of lumbar lordosis, which is detected by passing a hand behind the lumbar spine.

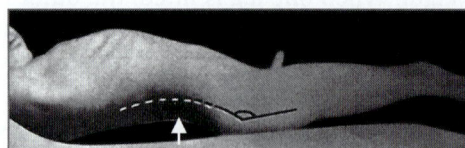

Fig. 15.16: It is shown that even with the 'fixed flexion' deformity the patient can extend his hip joint fully by bending the lumbar spine forwards.

The angle of fixed flexion deformity is accurately measured by Hugh Owen **Thomas' test** **(Fig. 15.17)**. In this test the sound thigh of the patient is bent with the flexed knee till the lumbar lordosis completely disappears, which is detected by the fact that the hand of the clinician cannot be insinuated between the lumbar spine and the bed. This maneuver will automatically bend up the hip up to the angle in which it is fixed flexion. So the angle between the affected thigh and the bed is *the angle of fixed flexion deformity.* It must be remembered that the sound thigh is flexed only upto the point to obliterate the lumbar lordosis and this maneuver should not be forcibly continued as this will simply increase the flexion of the affected hip showing an exacerbated deformity.

Fixed lateral or medial rotation deformity: This deformity cannot conceal itself by compensation at the lumbar spine. It always remains revealed and *is determined by noting the direction of the anterior surface of the patella or* of the toes when

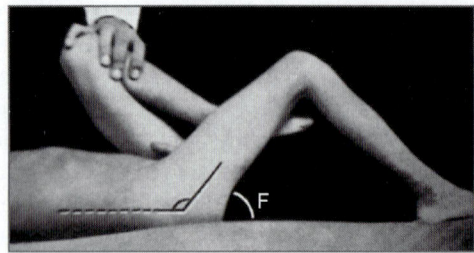

Fig. 15.17: Thomas' test is demonstrated. The normal hip is flexed to the limit to obliterate the compensatory lordosis. This will flex the affected thigh to the extent of 'fixed flexion' deformity. 'F' shows the angle of fixed flexion deformity.

the foot is held at right angle to the leg. Normally, the lower limb remains with a slight lateral rotation. So in recumbent position if the patella or the toes point up to the ceiling, it indicates slight medial rotation. In presence of marked rotation deformities there will be corresponding change in the direction of the anterior surface of the patella or the tips of the toes.

Is the affected limb shortened? This is easily demonstrated in case of children by flexing both the hip joints as well as the knees. The levels of the knees are compared (**Fig. 15.18**). The details of taking measurements of the limbs are discussed later in this chapter.

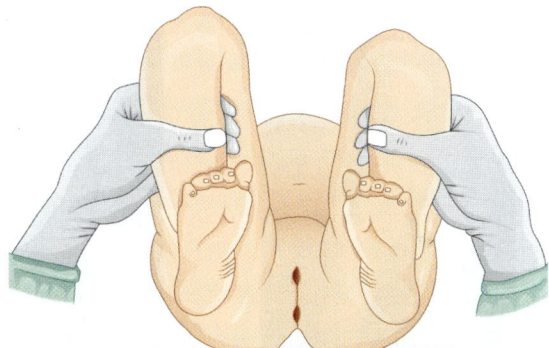

Fig. 15.18: Demonstration of how shortening of the affected limb is measured in case of children.

In tuberculous arthritis of the hip joint, the attitude is typical and differs according to the stage of the disease. *IN STAGE 1* (synovitis)—there is effusion into the joint which demands maximum capacity within the joint and is obtained by the optimum position, i.e., slight flexion, slight abduction and lateral rotation **(Fig. 15.19)**. Flexion is concealed by lumbar lordosis and by tilting the pelvis forwards. Abduction is corrected by tilting the pelvis downwards and scoliosis of the lumbar spine with convexity towards the affected side. This is called *the stage of apparent lengthening,* as the pelvis is tilted downwards and the affected limb looks longer than its fellow. *IN STAGE 2* (arthritis)—the effusion subsides and the articular cartilage is involved. This leads to spasm of the powerful adductors and flexors of the hip to protect its movements, which is very painful. So the attitude becomes one of the slight flexion, slight adduction and medial rotation **(Fig. 15.20)**. Flexion is concealed as discussed earlier. Adduction is corrected by tilting the pelvis upwards resulting in scoliosis of the lumbar spine with convexity towards the sound side. This is called the *stage of apparent shortening,* as the pelvis is tilted upwards and the affected limb looks shorter than its fellow. *IN STAGE 3* (erosion)—there will be erosion of the upper part of the acetabulum and the femoral head becomes dislocated by the spasm of the adductors (wandering acetabulum or pathological dislocation). This is the *stage of real shortening.* The attitude is more or less similar to that of stage 2 except for the fact that deformities are exacerbated at this stage. In this context one should remember the *various causes of pathological dislocation.* Besides tuberculosis which is by far the most common cause, septic arthritis and very occasionally typhoid arthritis may sometimes give rise to this type of dislocation.

In adolescent coxa vara (Fig. 15.21), the attitude is one of marked external rotation with slight adduction possibly due to eversion of the femur resulting from upper epiphyseal separation.

In congenital dislocation of the hip, the attitude is one of lordosis, which is particularly marked in bilateral cases with undue protrusion of the abdomen anteriorly and the buttock posteriorly. The space just below the perineum is broadened. In unilateral cases the grooves between the labia (girls are more often affected) and the thigh are asymmetrical and an additional skin crease on the medial side of the thigh can be noticed.

2. **Muscular wasting:** In any long standing disease of the hip joint there will be obvious muscular wasting mainly affecting the glutei and adductors. This becomes obvious in tuberculosis. Circumference of the thigh should be measured to know about wasting. It must be remembered

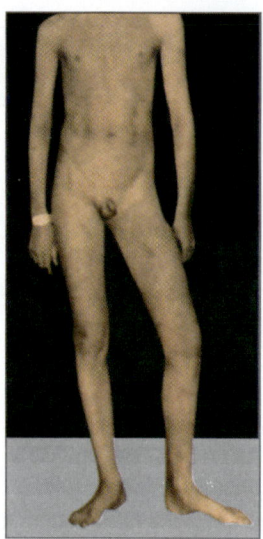
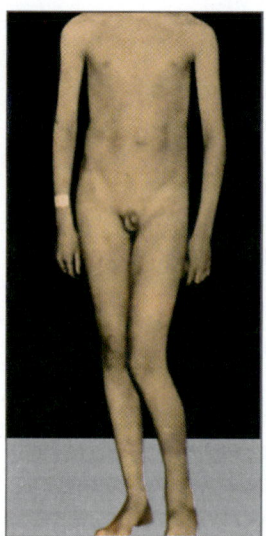
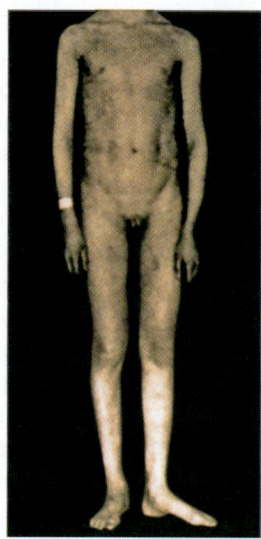

Fig. 15.19: First stage of tuberculosis of the left hip joint. The deformity is one of flexion, abduction and external rotation with apparent lengthening.

Fig. 15.20: Second stage of tuberculosis of the left hip joint. Note the deformity of flexion, adduction and internal rotation with apparent shortening.

Fig. 15.21: Note the characteristic attitude of adolescent coxa vara. The deformity is one of marked external rotation with slight adduction.

that flattening of the buttock and loss of gluteal fold may be brought about by flexion of the limb besides muscular wasting.

3. **Swelling:** This is occasionally seen in tuberculous arthritis of the hip joint when a cold abscess is formed either in the femoral triangle or in the gluteal region.

C. **PALPATION**

1. **Tenderness**—of the hip joint is elicited by applying steady pressure inwards over the two greater trochanters **(Fig. 15.22)**. Tenderness over the joint a little below the midinguinal point can be elicited in any arthritis.

2. Palpation of the **greater trochanter** is important to note whether it is broadened or tender and whether it is displaced upwards or not.

3. **Palpation of hip joint:** As the hip joint lies in its socket and is heavily clothed with strong muscles all around, this joint is almost inaccessible. Only a small part of the neck which lies outside the socket but inside the capsule may be palpated to know if the joint is diseased or not. To palpate this part a finger is placed just below the inguinal ligament and lateral to the femoral artery. The finger is pressed deep to detect if there is any tenderness or not. Tenderness indicates arthritis of the joint.

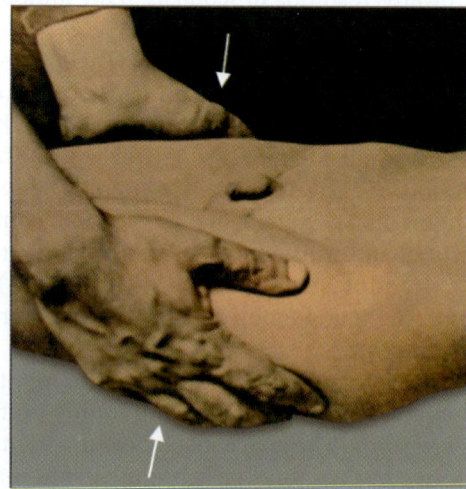

Fig. 15.22: Method of eliciting tenderness in the hip joint. Simultaneous steady pressure inwards over the two greater trochanters elicits pain on the affected side.

4. **Swelling:** Effusion of the hip joint, when considerable, as in suppurative arthritis in children, presents itself as a fluctuating swelling just below the midinguinal point. For *cold abscess* one should search the following regions: (a) in front of and medial of the greater trochanter, (b) on the medial side of the femoral vessels, (c) posteriorly in the gluteal region and (d) rarely in the pelvis from perforation of acetabulum. Such abscess may gravitate towards the ischiorectal fossa and may burst to form fistula-in-ano.

5. **The femoral artery** is felt particularly in congenital dislocation of the hip. This artery passes over the head of the femur and this bony support helps its palpation. In congenital dislocation the head of the femur is dislocated and this bony support is missing. So there will be great difficulty in feeling this artery. This is known as 'Vascular sign' of Narath **(Fig. 15.23)**.

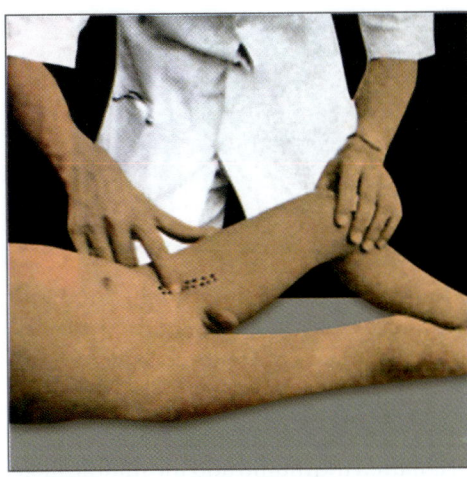

Fig. 15.23: Femoral artery is difficult to feel in congenital dislocation of hip because of loss of bony support.

D. **MOVEMENTS:** Flexion, extension, abduction, adduction, rotations and circumduction are the different movements of the hip joint. During examination the clinician must always compare the range of a certain movement of the affected joint with that of the sound counterpart. This is because of the fact that the range of each movement varies according to the individuals. The average ranges of movements are as follows:

Flexion—with the knee extended cannot be done more than 90° due to the tension of the hamstring muscles which prevents full flexion; but with the bent knee the hip joint can be flexed up to 120° or more till the front of the thigh comes in contact with the front of the abdomen.

Extension—is permitted to about 15°; *Abduction*—to about 40°; *Adduction*—to about 30°, that means the limb can be made to cross the middle third of the other thigh. *Internal rotation*—is possible to about 30° and *external rotation*—to about 45°.

During **testing the movements** (both active and passive movements) one must make sure that the pelvis does not move. For this, the pelvis is steadied by the clinician.

1. **Flexion:** Firstly, the pelvis is grasped and the patient is asked to flex the hip as far as possible. The amount of flexion possible without causing any movement of the pelvis is noted. When there is a *"fixed flexion deformity"*, the exact range of free flexion present can be demonstrated in the following way: The Thomas test is first performed. The thigh of the sound side is held and the patient is asked to make an attempt to flex the affected hip. Any bending of the thigh beyond the position of "fixed flexion" is the range of free flexion permissible to the joint.

2. **Extension:** In fixed flexion deformity, extension of the joint is not possible at all. This is demonstrated by applying a downward pressure on the thigh after the affected limb has been kept in the position of fixed flexion deformity by Thomas' test. When there is no fixed flexion deformity, extension of the hip joint is best tested by lying the patient in prone position on the table and asking him to lift affected limb **(Fig. 15.24)**. The range of extension is not more than 15° and is first restricted in arthritis of the hip joint.

3. **Abduction:** The range of abduction can be tested in two ways. *In the first method* the patient lies supine on the table. The pelvis is steadied by holding the iliac crest of the affected side. In case

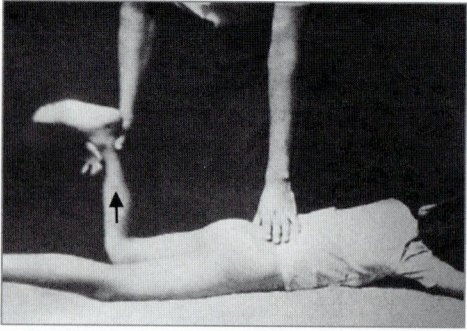

Fig. 15.24: Method of testing extension when there is no 'fixed flexion' deformity.

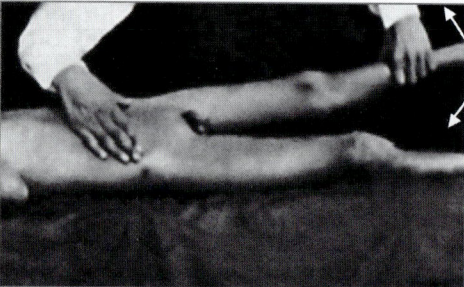

Fig. 15.25: Shows the method of testing abduction and adduction of the hip with the knee extended. Note that the clinician touches the two anterior superior iliac spines to detect any movement of the pelvis.

of children the thumb and the middle finger of the left hand of the clinician are used to touch the two anterior superior iliac spines so that any movement of the pelvis will be detected at once **(Fig. 15.25)**. Keeping the pelvis at right angle to the limbs the patient is asked to abduct the affected limb. It can be compared with that of the sound side. The *second method* is to make the patient lying on the table in supine position. Flexing his both hips and the knees the soles of the feet are placed together. The knees are now bent outwards simultaneously on both sides. The range of abduction on both the sides can be measured. It may be noted that the abduction is the first movement to be restricted in tuberculous arthritis **(Fig. 15.26)**.

4. **Adduction:** The pelvis is first steadied and the patient is asked to lift the affected limb and then cross it over its fellow. It is noted whether the limb crosses the sound thigh at its upper third or middle third or lower third.

5. **Rotation:** The patient lies supine on the table. The clinician places the flat of his hand upon the thigh and moves the limb to and fro observing the foot as an index of the degree of rotation

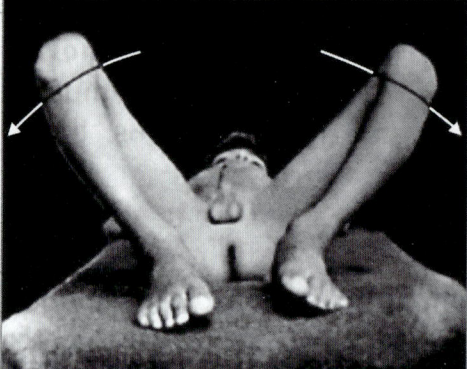

Fig. 15.26: Shows the second method of testing the abduction movement with acutely flexed knees.

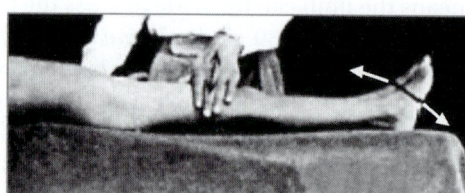

Fig. 15.27: Easiest method of testing rotations of the hip joint keeping both the hip and knee joints extended.

(Fig. 15.27). Rotatory movement can also be tested by flexing both the hip and the knee joints of the affected side to the right angles and then rotating the thigh internally and externally by holding the foot **(Fig. 15.28)**. These movements are also tested by asking the patient to lie on his face to flex the knee to the right angle and moving the whole leg sidewise **(Fig. 15.29)**.

The restriction of different movements depends upon the nature of affection of the hip joint. *In any arthritis,* including tuberculous variety, restriction of all the movements is the characteristic feature. *In adolescent coxa vara,* there will be limitation of abduction and internal rotation, but adduction and external rotation are not only be free but often exaggerated. *In Perthes' disease,*

Chapter 15: Examination of Individual Joint Pathologies

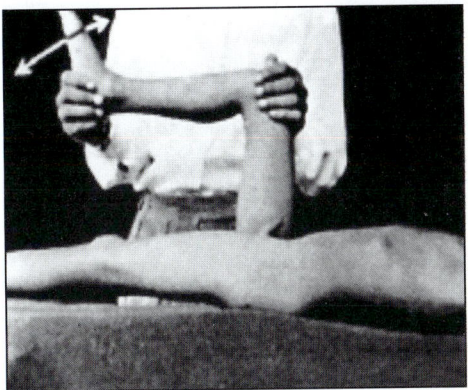

Fig. 15.28: Shows the method of testing the rotation movement of the hip joint keeping the hip and knee flexed. This test can be performed in 'fixed flexion' deformity of the hip.

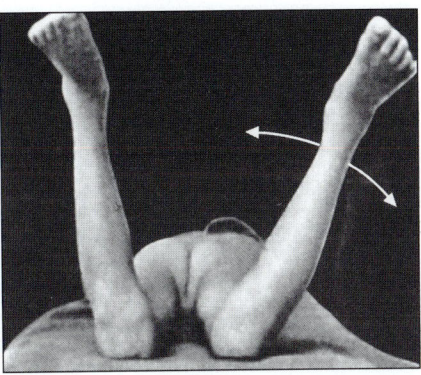

Fig. 15.29: Shows another method of testing rotations of the hip. Note that this test cannot be performed in 'fixed flexion' deformity of the hip.

again abduction and internal rotation are restricted. *In congenital dislocation of the hip,* abduction and rotations are limited to varying degree, flexion and extension are free whereas adduction is excessive.

6. **Examination for stability:** Stability of the hip joint is mainly jeopardized in congenital dislocation of the hip. So the following three tests are performed when this condition is suspected.

1. **Telescopic test (Fig. 15.30):** The pelvis is fixed with one hand touching the greater trochanter. The hip is now flexed to 90° and the knee is grasped

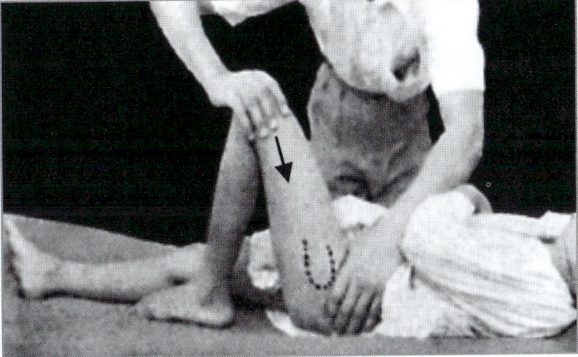

Fig. 15.30: Telescopic test. The femur can be moved on to the dorsum ilii in congenital and pathological dislocation of the hip.

with the other hand of the clinician, who pushes the thigh downwards along the axis of the thigh with this hand, while the other hand notes whether the greater trochanter is moving downwards. This "positive telescopic test" is seen in congenital as well as pathological dislocations of the hip and in Charcot's joint.

2. **Ortolani's test (Fig. 15.31):** Both the hips and knees are flexed by holding the limbs. Now the thigh of the affected side is gradually abducted. A 'click of entrance' will be felt as the femoral head slips into the acetabulum and a 'click of exit' as it quits the acetabulum when the pressure is released.

3. **Barlow's test (Fig. 15.32):** The surgeon holds both the lower extremities in such a way that the hips are flexed at 90° and the knees are fully flexed. The lower limbs are now completely adducted and pressure is exerted downwards along the bony axis of the femur while the little fingers of both the hands are placed on the greater trochanters. If the hip is dislocatable, the femoral head will be heard to roll over the posterior rim of the acetabulum as a distinct 'cluck'. The hip is dislocated. The second phase of the test is started. The hip is now gradually

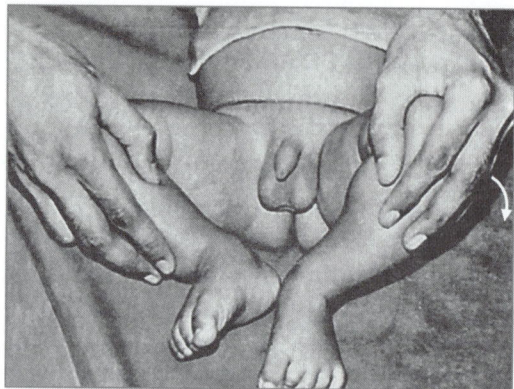

Fig. 15.31: Ortolani's test.

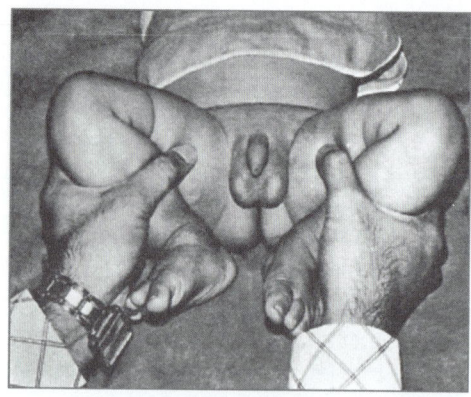

Fig. 15.32: Barlow's test. See the text.

abducted from the position of full adduction. The little fingers on the greater trochanter are now pushed inwards simultaneously. The head can now be felt to reduce with a soft cluck into the acetabulum.

E. MEASUREMENTS

1. **Length (Figs. 15.33 and 15.34):** The length of the whole limb is measured from the anterior superior iliac spine to the tip of the medial malleolus. When only length of the thigh is measured, measurement is taken from anterior superior iliac spine to the joint line of the knee. It must be remembered before taking the measurement that the interspinous line is brought to the horizontal level by abducting or adducting the affected limb. While comparing the length of the affected limb with that of the sound limb, the sound limb must be placed in the same position as the affected one. That means, if there is adduction deformity of the affected limb, the normal limb must also be adducted *to the similar extent* before the measurements. The bony points which are considered for measurement must be marked with skin pencil first before taking the measurements.

2. **Girth of the limb:** This is measured to find out the presence or absence of muscular wasting. When there is considerable muscular wasting, it can be assessed by inspection only. The importance of this measurement remains only in cases of slight muscular wasting which may not be obvious on inspection. A mark is made on the affected limb at a convenient distance from the anterior superior iliac spine. This mark is made on both the limbs and circumferences of the limbs at that level are compared.

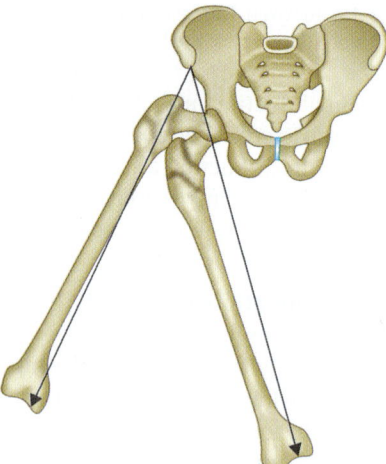

Fig. 15.33: Shows that the distance from the anterior superior iliac spine to the joint line of the knee is shorter when the limb is abducted and longer when adducted.

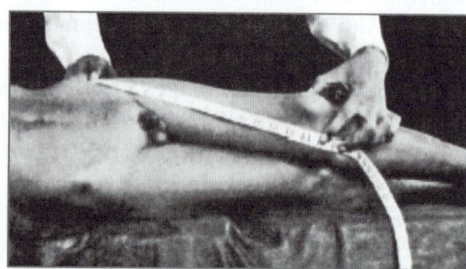

Fig. 15.34: Shows the method of taking measurement of the thigh from the anterior superior iliac spine to the joint-line of the knee. The thigh of the normal side has been adducted the affected hip is deformed in adduction.

3. **Shortening above the greater trochanter:** This is determined by drawing the Bryant's triangle, Nelaton's line, etc., as discussed in 'Injuries around the hip' (see page 229). The greater trochanter is raised in dislocation of the hip, separation of the upper femoral epiphysis (adolescent coxa vara) and to a slight extent when the head of the femur eroded, e.g., in Perthes' disease, suppurative arthritis, etc.

Lymph nodes: Palpation of lymph nodes is important in inflammatory conditions, be it acute or chronic of the hip joint. The external iliac group of lymph nodes are palpated by deep palpation.

Other joints: Examination of the hip joint remains incomplete until other major joints like lumbosacral spine, sacroiliac joints and especially the knee joints are examined.

Rectal examination should be undertaken in tuberculous arthritis if an intrapelvic abscess is suspected.

SKIAGRAPHY

The general points discussed in Chapter 12 should be borne in mind. In pathology of the hip *Shenton's line* (**Fig. 15.35**) which extends from the upper curved border of the obturator foramen on to the lower border of the neck of the femur is important and is a continuous arched line. In Perthes' disease or in slightly distorted; but in pathological dislocation this line will be grossly distorted.

In congenital dislocation of the hip, X-ray picture will show that the upper epiphysis of the femur of the affected side is usually smaller than the normal side. The neck is anteverted and is not properly seen in X-ray due to superimposition. There will be distortion of the Shenton's line. When the dislocation is of mild nature, the following lines are drawn to detect the pathology. These lines are known as *Perkin's lines* (**Fig. 15.36**). A horizontal line is drawn through the triradiate cartilage and a vertical line is drawn down from the outer edge of the acetabulum tuberculous arthritis where destruction of the head of the femur becomes obvious this line will be on both sides. The upper femoral epiphysis normally lies medial to the vertical line and below the horizontal line. But in congenital dislocation of the hip the epiphysis will lie on the outer aspect of the vertical line and above the horizontal line. An idea of the development of the acetabular roof may be obtained by drawing the *acetabular angle.* The normal inclination of the roof is about 22° from the horizontal plane, but

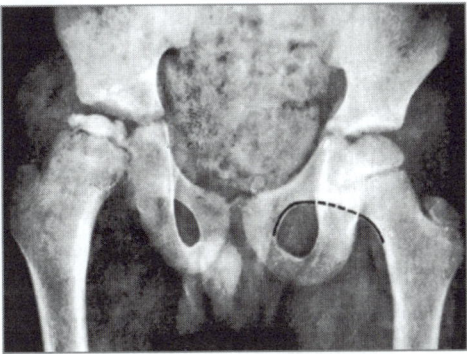

Fig. 15.35: Shenton's line has been drawn on the normal left side. On the right side which is affected by Perthes' disease, if this line is drawn it will not correspond with the upper curved border of the obturator foramen.

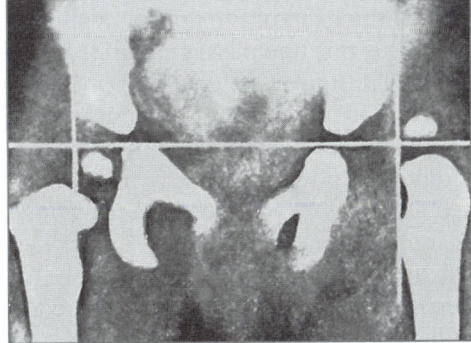

Fig. 15.36: Perkin's lines are drawn. See that on the left side, which is affected by congenital dislocation the upper femoral epiphysis lies above the horizontal line and outside the vertical line.

in congenital dislocation of the hip it is increased to 40–45° **(Fig. 15.37)**. Another maneuver was advocated by Von Rosen. A film is taken with both the hips abducted to 45° and internally rotated. If the line of the femoral shaft is extended upwards, it will touch the acetabular roof on the normal side; on the dislocated side it will strike the pelvis above the top of the acetabulum. An *arthrogram* is essential before advocating the type of treatment required for the particular case. Lateral views may be taken to measure anteversion of the neck.

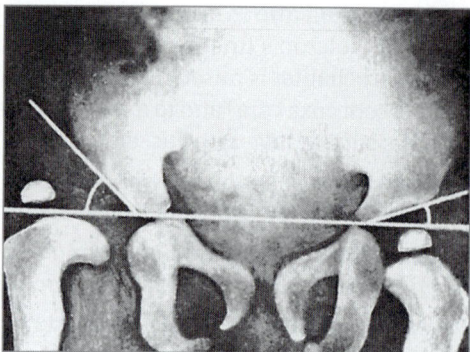

Fig. 15.37: Normal inclination of the acetabular roof is about 22° from the horizontal plane, but in congenital dislocation of the hip it is increased to 40°–45°.

In Perthes' disease (Figs.15.38 and 15.39), early stage will be evident in X-ray, with increased joint space (this is a differentiating point from tuberculous arthritis) and the head of the femur will stand away a little laterally. With the onset of ischemia the femoral head will show increased density—at first granular and later on uniform. As the condition advances flattening of the head with patchy fragmentation becomes obvious. The neck of the femur becomes wide with a band of rarefaction and even a cystic appearance with surrounding sclerosis will be seen at the metaphysis.

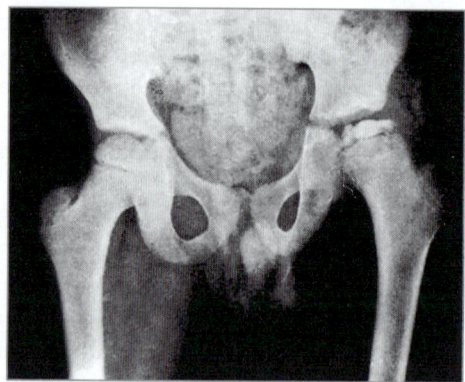

Fig. 15.38: Perthes' disease. See the text.

In slipped epiphysis (adolescent coxa vara) even a trivial change becomes apparent in antero-posterior film **(Fig. 15.40)**. The epiphyseal cartilage becomes wider and "wooly" on its metaphyseal side. A line drawn along the upper surface of the neck of the femur normally passes through the superior part of the head of the femur. In slipped epiphysis this line passes superior to the head (Trethowan's sign). The posterior acetabular margin normally cuts across the medial corner of metaphysis. But in slipped epiphysis the entire metaphysis remains lateral to the posterior acetabular margin (Capener's sign). In the lateral view the deformity is usually obvious from the beginning. The upper epiphysis of the femur is displaced backwards and downwards. The neck-shaft angle is reduced to a varying extent from the normal (about 150° in a child and 127° in an adult). The neck is pushed up and externally rotated causing the lesser trochanter to be more prominent.

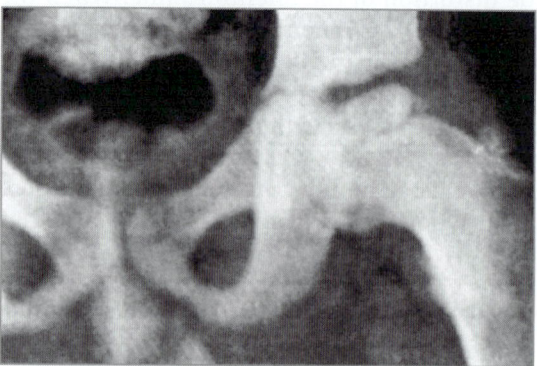

Fig. 15.39: X-ray of a typical case of Perthes' disease involving left hip.

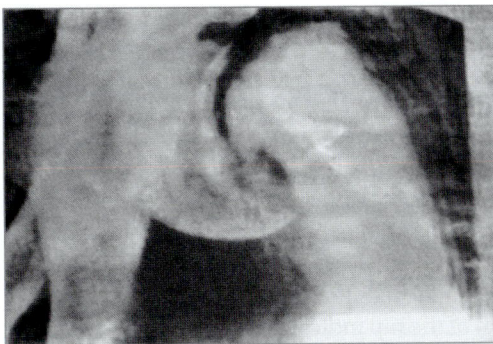

Fig. 15.40: X-ray of a case of adolescent coxa vara showing the typical displacement of capital epiphysis.

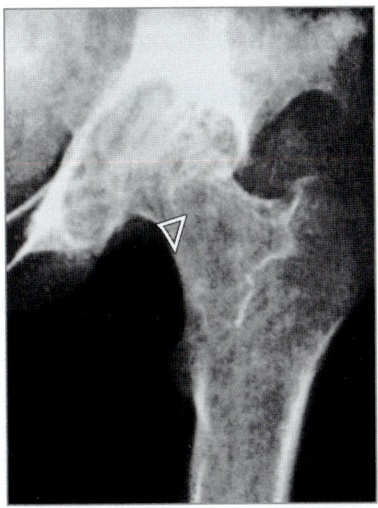

Fig. 15.41: Tuberculous arthritis showing destruction of the femoral head. Triangle at the inferior aspect of the femoral neck indicates the position of Babcock's triangle.

In **tuberculosis of the hip joint** the earliest sign is general haziness of the bones as seen in a bad film, with or without an area of rarefaction in the Babcock's triangle **(Fig. 15.41)** or in the upper part of acetabulum. The joint space may be increased due to effusion. In the next stage, destruction of the articular surfaces will lead to loss of distinct outline of the articular ends with diminution of the joint space. In the final stage further destruction of the upper part of the acetabulum allows the deformed head to be dislocated on to the eroded dorsum ilii, which is then called the "traveling or wandering acetabulum" **(Figs. 15.42 and 15.43)**. Such dislocation can be easily demonstrated in X-ray and by drawing the Shenton's line.

Ultrasound: It can confirm clinical suspicion, may be used as a screening tool and also to monitor early treatment.

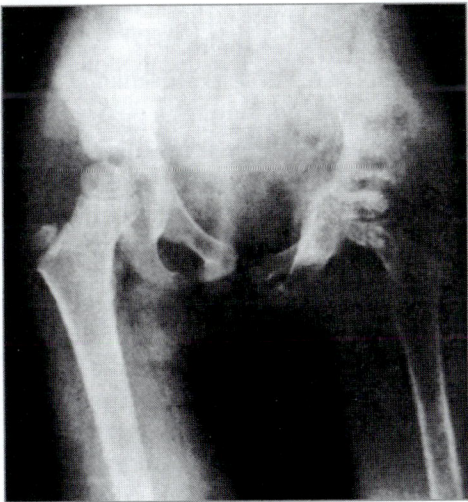

Fig. 15.42: Shows the typical wandering acetabulum on the left side.

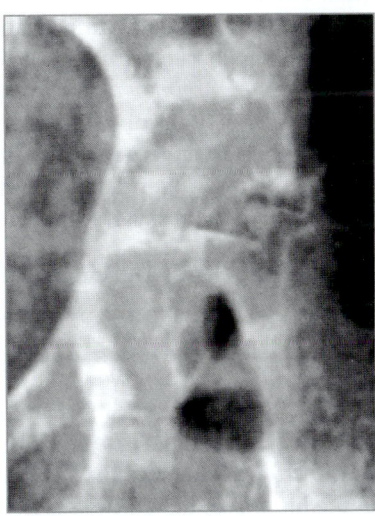

Fig. 15.43: X-ray of an advanced case of tuberculosis of hip. Note the wandering acetabulum.

DIFFERENTIAL DIAGNOSIS

CONGENITAL DISLOCATION OF THE HIP OR DEVELOPMENTAL DYSPLASIA OF THE HIP (DDH)

This condition is commonly seen among girls and about 4 times more frequently seen than the boys. This is more commonly seen in European countries and in Japan, but a rare occurrence in Chinese and Negro races probably due to the fact that the latters carry their babies on their backs with the hips abducted. The earlier the diagnosis is made, the easier will be the treatment and more will be the chance of cure.

In *the neonate and the infant,* this condition is diagnosed firstly by Barlow's test, Ortolani's test and telescopic test. Limited abduction in flexion of the hip indicates actual dislocation. Extra skin crease along the medial aspect of the thigh in unilateral case and widening of the perineum in bilateral case will be noticed by an observant mother. Lastly delayed walking and a limp when the child begins to walk should arouse suspicion of this condition.

In *childhood,* that means when weight bearing has already been started, typical Trendelenburg's gait, i.e., the patient lurches on the affected side becomes obvious. In bilateral cases typical waddling gait may be missed by the clinician but will not be missed by an observant mother. There will be obvious lordosis and prominence of the hips. Movements are painless, but abduction and rotations are limited in completely dislocated hip. The "vascular sign" of Narath becomes positive. The findings in X-ray have already been discussed in the earlier section. Arthrography, i.e., injection of diodone (3 mL) into the joint is helpful in determining the presence of limbus or hour-glass constriction of the capsule. Ultrasound helps in diagnosis.

PERTHES' DISEASE (PSEUDOCOXALGIA, OSTEOCHONDRITIS JUVENILIS)

The underlying pathology is deficient blood supply to the head of the femur, which undergoes aseptic necrosis resulting in collapse. The cause is still to be known. Unlike the previous condition the boys are more affected by this condition and about 4 times commoner than the girls. The boys are mainly between the ages of 5–10 years. The most constant early sign is a comparatively painless limp. In the beginning, when the joint becomes rather irritable, more or less all movements are slightly restricted. Later on in the established stage *there is limitation of abduction and internal rotation.* Other movements are full and painless. Muscular wasting of the limb becomes obvious and there may be moderate flexion and adduction deformity. In established cases there may be a little real shortening of the limb. In 10% of cases the condition may be bilateral. Trendelenburg's sign may or may not be positive. The diagnosis cannot be confirmed without skiagraphy, the findings of which have been discussed in the earlier section.

SLIPPED EPIPHYSIS (ADOLESCENT COXA VARA)

Boys and girls are affected by this condition in the ratio of 3 : 2 with the average age of onset is 15 in case of boys and 12 (rarely seen after menstruation has started) in case of girls. The majority of the patients are overweight and sexually underdeveloped. There may be a history of trauma in which case this condition suddenly appears, otherwise the majority of cases are gradual in onset. The earliest symptom is a painful limp and pain may be referred to the knee joint. Continued weight bearing will lead to more pain and limp with shortening and external rotation of the limb. Trendelenburg's sign is mostly positive. The patient stands with leg adducted and externally rotated limb. As regards movements the most constant and diagnostic are *limitations of abduction and internal rotation.*

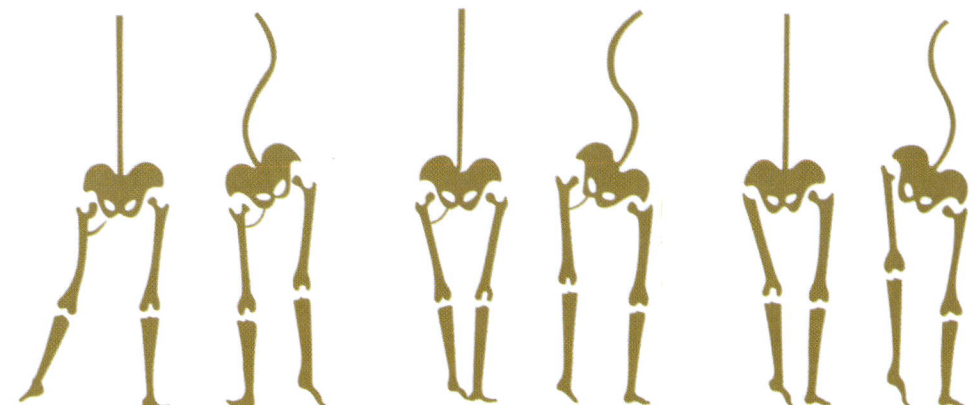

Fig. 15.44: Diagrammatic representation of the various stages of tuberculosis of the hip. See page 276 and Figures 15.19 and 15.20.

On examination the greater trochanter is higher and more posteriorly placed than the unaffected side. Muscular wasting is little present. X-ray is confirmatory and discussed earlier.

TUBERCULOSIS OF THE HIP (FIG. 15.44)

No sex or age is exempt from this disease. The hip joint is second only to the vertebral column so far as the sites of tuberculosis of the bones and the joints are concerned. The disease starts as synovitis or as a bony focus in the acetabulum or in the femoral head (more frequently in Babcock's triangle). The earliest sign is the *limp,* which in the beginning comes on after the patient has walked some distance. Later on it becomes evident even in the early morning. *Pain* is probably the first symptom which is more often referred to the thigh or to the knee than to the hip. The general signs and symptoms such as malaise, pallor, loss of weight, evening rise of temperature, night sweat, etc., may be noticed. Muscular wasting becomes obvious very soon. "Night cry", i.e., pain starting at night is very important and this indicates the movement between the inflamed joint surfaces allowed by disappearance of protective muscular spasm during sleep. On examination, the characteristic deformities of different stages have already been discussed in details under the heading of "attitude". Limitation of movements occurs *in all directions.* X-ray is confirmatory.

ACUTE SUPPURATIVE ARTHRITIS

This condition is more common in children. A child with high pyrexia, a limp, pain in the hip with redness and brawny edematous swelling, should be considered as suffering from acute suppurative arthritis. The hip joint is kept in position of flexion, slight abduction and external rotation—'optimum position' to accommodate more fluid. Gentle pressure over the joint will cause the child to scream. Diagnosis is confirmed by aspirating the hip joint with a needle under anesthesia.

IRRITABLE HIP

The patient usually presents with pain and limp. Both become evident following activity. The pain is felt in the groin and may be referred to the knee joint. There will be slight wasting, but the cardinal sign is the *limitation of all movements at their extremes.* The patient is immediately put to bed and a skin traction is applied to the affected leg. Investigations like examination of the blood and X-ray are essential to come to a diagnosis. The followings are the causes of this condition.

(i) *Transient synovitis:* Minor trauma is the presumed cause and there will be effusion of the hip joint. The symptoms may mimic acute suppurative arthritis, but absence of toxemia, high pyrexia, localized redness and edema will differentiate this condition from acute suppurative arthritis. X-ray will reveal a normal joint and the investigations will be normal. A few days' bed rest will absorb the effusion and normal ranges of movement will be restored.

(ii) *Chronic synovitis:* A chronic synovitis from rheumatoid arthritis is very difficult to distinguish and sometimes indistinguishable from tuberculosis in the early stage.

Besides these conditions, (iii) Perthes' disease, (iv) slipped epiphysis and (v) tuberculosis are sometimes the causes of irritable hip.

PATHOLOGICAL DISLOCATION OF HIP

Acute arthritis following acute osteomyelitis of the femoral head or neck seems to be the most common condition which leads to pathological dislocation of the hip. The inflammatory process leads to destruction of the head and neck of the femur and pathological dislocation may result from it. *Tuberculosis of the hip* is the second cause of the pathological dislocation. Besides these infective destructive lesions, *spastic paralysis, poliomyelitis* may also lead to pathological dislocation of the hip.

OSTEOARTHRITIS

In adult life this is the most common condition which brings the patient to a surgeon. *Pain* is the usual presenting symptom which is of boring character, mainly localized to the hip but may be referred to the knee joint. In the beginning the pain is complained of when movement follows a period of rest, later on it is more constant and disturbing. *Stiffness*, especially after rest, is common. After a period of rest on a chair, it is difficult to get up. *Limp* may be noticed early, but more often than not it comes later than pain and stiffness. The limp is due to either pain or stiffness or apparent shortening due to adductor spasm. Muscle wasting (chiefly glutei) is detectable but not severe. There may be apparent shortening but there is hardly any true shortening. Some limitation of all movements is detectable but abduction, extension and medial rotation are restricted early. X-ray shows decreased joint space particularly at the pressure areas. Elsewhere the joint space is not decreased. The bone becomes sclerosed with lipping and osteophytes at the margins of the joint. There may be cyst in the femoral head.

■ THE KNEE JOINT

A. HISTORY

The common symptoms, with which a patient generally presents, are pain, swelling, stiffness, mechanical disorders (e.g., locking, giving way, click, etc.) and limp.

B. INSPECTION

Both the lower limbs are fully exposed for proper inspection. The patient is first examined in the standing position both from front and behind, secondly in the seated position, thirdly in the supine position and lastly in the prone position. During these examinations the hip is also examined, as very often a patient with the pathology in the hip will complain of pain in the knee. In the conclusion the students must not forget to examine the *popliteal fossa* both in the standing position and in the prone position **(Fig. 15.45)**.

Note the wasting of the muscles (compare with the left thigh). There are flexion, lateral rotation and posterior subluxation (triple displacement) of the affected knee.

1. **Gait:** The patient is carefully observed while he enters the clinic. With the stiff knee the affected leg will swing outwards during walking. In other conditions the patient will limp mostly lurching on the sound side to avoid weight bearing through the affected knee.

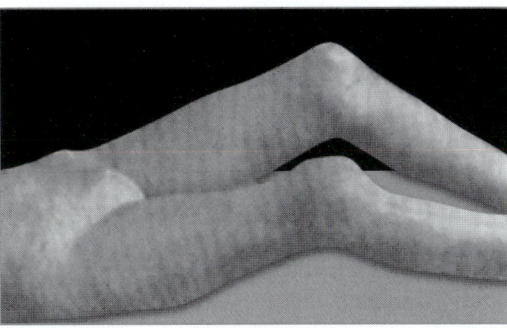

Fig. 15.45: Tuberculous arthritis of right knee.

2. **Attitude:** In arthritic joint, be it the first stage of tuberculous arthritis or acute arthritis, the joint will assume a position of moderate flexion—the 'optimum position' of the knee joint to accommodate maximum fluid within the joint cavity. As the arthritic process continues, the joint surfaces are destroyed so are the ligaments resulting in "triple displacement", i.e., flexion, posterior subluxation and lateral rotation of the tibia due to the contraction of the hamstring muscles. This indicates destruction of the cruciate and collateral ligaments. Abnormal abduction (genu valgum) **(Fig. 15.46)**, abnormal adduction (genu varum) or abnormal hyperextension (genu recurvatum) **(Fig. 15.47)** are carefully noted. In case of locking the patient fails to extend the joint beyond a certain angle and the knee is kept in flexed position with limping. *Always note the anterior surface and the position of patella.* This often gives some idea about the nature of existing deformity.

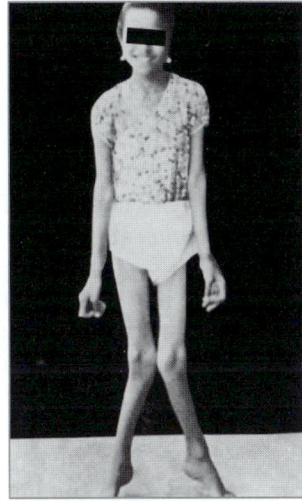

Fig. 15.46: Genu valgum.

3. **Swelling:** An *effusion* of the knee joint gives rise to a horse-shoe swelling above the patella and on both sides of the patella and the ligamentum patellae obliterating the normal depressions. This condition may be confused with superficial cellulitis, but the latter will extend over the patella and its ligament which is never the case in effusion of the joint. Bilateral effusion of the joint is uncommon and may occur in bilateral injury to the knee, in syphilitic affection (Clutton's joints) **(Fig. 15.48)** or in hemophilia.

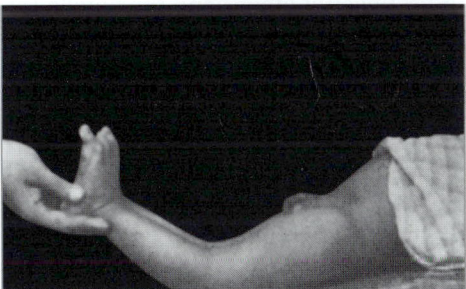

Fig. 15.47: Genu recurvatum.

Extra-articular swellings are quite common around the knee due to enlargement of the different *bursae* around the joint. The semimembranosus bursa is seen behind the knee on its medial aspect and slightly above the joint line. It becomes more prominent and tense on extension of the knee. Prepatellar bursa which is situated just in front of the lower part of the patella and ligamentum patellae may be inflamed and enlarged in prepatellar bursitis (housemaid's knee). Infrapatellar bursa (lying deep to the ligamentum patellae), bicipital bursa (lying under the biceps tendon) may occasionally be enlarged. The suprapatellar bursa almost always communicates with the knee joint and becomes swollen in effusion of the joint. Morrant Baker's cyst which is a herniation of the synovial membrane posteriorly through the fibers of the oblique popliteal ligament forms a swelling in the middle of the posterior aspect of the knee slightly below the joint line (*see* **Fig. 15.55**). This condition also gives rise to a swelling on the posterior aspect of the knee joint in its middle and becomes prominent on extension and disappears on flexion of the joint. This condition is often associated with tuberculosis or osteoarthritis of the joint.

4. **Muscular wasting:** This should be looked for both above and below the joint. But in affections of the knee joint if there be any muscular wasting, it is more obvious in the thigh.

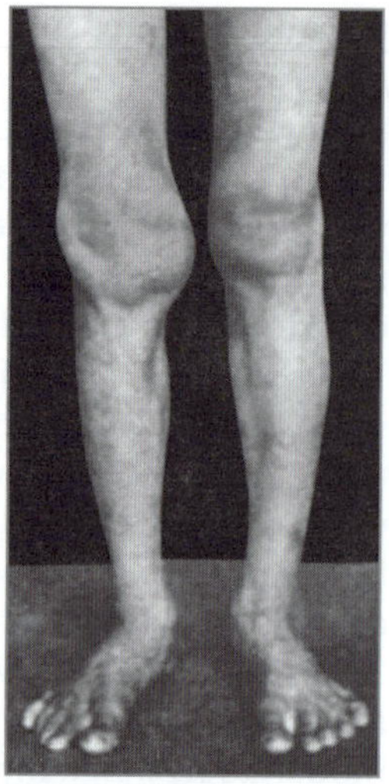

C. **PALPATION**

1. Firstly one should examine for **local temperature** with the back of the hand and compare it with that of the other side. Look for **local tenderness**.

2. **Swelling:** So far as the effusion of the joint is concerned, two important tests may be performed—fluctuation and "patellar tap".

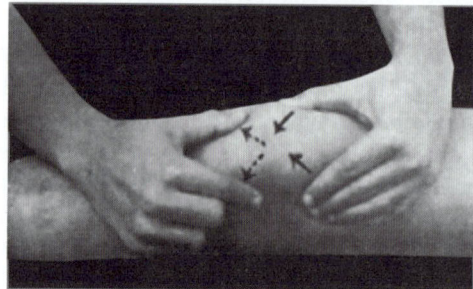

Fig. 15.48: Clutton's joint—bilateral serous syphilitic synovitis of the knee joints.

Fluctuation (**Fig. 15.49**) is demonstrated by pressing the suprapatellar pouch with one hand and feeling the impulse with the thumb and the fingers of the other hand placed on either side of the patella or the ligamentum patellae.

"Patellar tap" which is a pathognomonic sign of effusion of the knee joint, is elicited by pressing the suprapatellar pouch with one hand driving whole of its fluid into the joint proper so as to float the patella in front of the joint. With the index finger of other hand the patella is pushed backwards towards the femoral condyles with a sharp and jerky movement. The patella can be felt to strike on the femur, which is known as "patellar tap" (**Fig. 15.50**). A moderate amount of fluid must be present in the joint to make this test positive.

Fig. 15.49: Showing how to demonstrate fluctuation test in effusion of the knee joint.

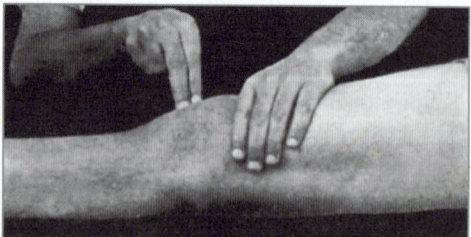

For demonstration of small amount of fluid in the knee joint two tests can be performed. The patient keeps standing and gentle pressure is applied over one of the obliterated hollows on either side of the ligamentum patellae (in order to displace fluid) and now the pressure is released. The hollow will be refilled slowly. The second method is to elicit 'patellar tap' with the patient standing.

Fig. 15.50: Showing how to demonstrate 'patellar tap' in effusion of the knee joint.

A thickened synovial membrane may also present a fluctuating swelling in the joint line, on either side of the patella and just above the patella. Its "spongy" or "boggy" feel and absence of patellar tap differentiate it from effusion of the joint. The edge of the thickened synovial

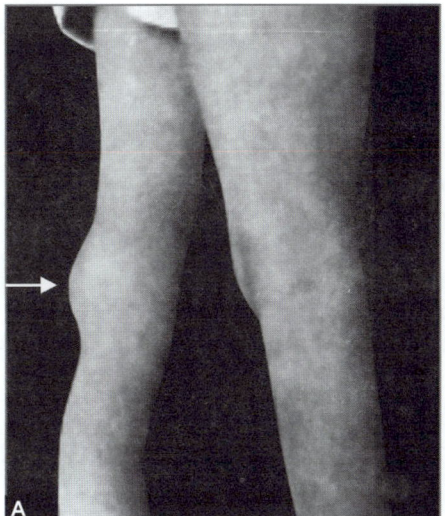
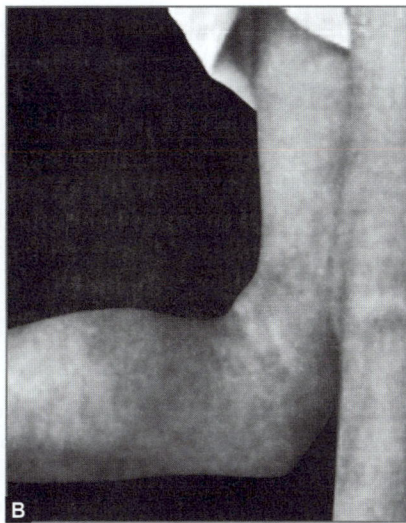

Figs. 15.51A and B: Enlarged semimembranosus bursa which becomes obvious on extension and disappears in flexion of the knee joint.

membrane can be rolled under the finger as in a lipoma, but there is no edge felt in effusion as in a cyst.

When a swelling appears to be an *enlarged bursa*, its relation with the tendon (by making the appropriate tendon taut), its consistency, its mobility and translucency are ascertained. Whether the bursa communicates with the joint or not is also assessed **(Figs. 15.51 and 15.52)**. In case of bursae in the popliteal fossa, these are examined in the prone position keeping the knee joint flexed for proper palpation.

A swelling in the joint line on the lateral side of the ligamentum patellae is probably a *cyst of the lateral semilunar cartilage*.

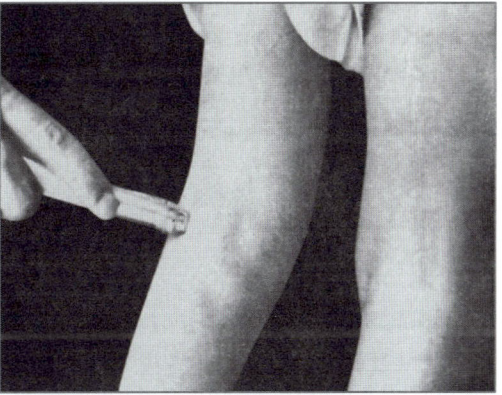

Fig. 15.52: Demonstration of translucency test in an enlarged semimembranosus bursa.

Any swelling in the popliteal fossa (particularly in the midline) should be examined for expansile pulsation. *Popliteal aneurysm* is not uncommon.

Transillumination test should always be performed in case of swellings around the knee joint. This test will be positive when swelling is an enlarged bursa or any cystic swelling, e.g., Morrant-Baker cyst (*see* **Fig. 15.57**, page 294). In case of swellings containing blood (aneurysm) or pus, this test will be negative.

Examine whether the swelling is *compressible* or not. For this uniform gentle pressure is applied over the swelling and the reduction in size of the swelling is noted. This is due to displacement of fluid. This test is positive in case of Morrant-Baker cyst or popliteal aneurysm.

3. **Palpation of popliteal fossa:** It must be remembered that examination of the knee joint is incomplete without examination of the popliteal fossa. The patient lies down prone on the table.

The knee joint is flexed and the popliteal fossa is palpated **(Fig. 15.53)**. The knee joint, the popliteal artery, the areolar tissue, the vein and nerves and the tendons in and around the popliteal fossa are all palpated carefully to detect any pathology there.

4. **Bony components:** The femoral condyles above the joint and the tibial condyles below the joint are very carefully palpated for any tenderness, irregularity and swelling. The patella is also carefully palpated and crepitus during movement of patella indicates osteoarthritis. Bones are also examined for any pathology or tumor there.

5. Patients may sometimes point out the presence of a loose body. This should be palpated properly, but X-ray is more informative in this respect.

6. Lastly the muscles are palpated for evidence of **wasting** or adhesion to the bone.

7. **Significance of a click:** Often patients present with a click in the knee joint. If the click is painless, it has hardly any significance. If the click is associated with discomfort or pain, one should carefully examine to detect pathology. The patella is examined, particularly its margins and its mobility—whether this is giving rise to pain to the patients or not. An intra-articular click may simulate extra-articular sounds, e.g., the sound of a snapping tendon such as produced by the semitendinosus slipping around and becoming hitched over the medial condyle, or the tendon of biceps over the head of the fibula, or the edge of the iliotibial tract over the lateral condyle, or any tendon becoming hooked over an exostosis. Such extra-articular sound is a dull thud. The most common cause of intra-articular click is osteoarthritis. Sometimes in childhood a painless click may occur as the patella moves over the condyle in a normal joint.

8. **Palpation of the joint:** The knee joint is comprised of 2 components—patellofemoral component and femorotibial component. Often the clinicians forget to examine the patella and the patellofemoral component of the knee joint and thus miss cardinal informations regarding intra-articular pathology and also the pathologies like chondromalacia patellae. Palpate the patella and its margin for tenderness. Next, push the patella medially and laterally. This may produce crepitus in case of chondromalacia patellae. For tibiofemoral component the joint line is thoroughly palpated to detect any tenderness or irregularity or swelling.

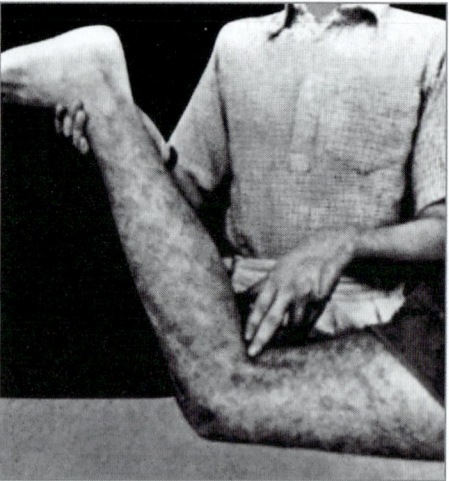

Fig. 15.53: It must be remembered that examination of the knee joint is incomplete without examination of popliteal fossa. Flexion of the knee greatly facilitates palpation of the popliteal fossa.

D. MOVEMENTS

The movements permitted in the knee joint are mainly flexion and extension. Minor degrees of abduction, adduction and rotations may be permitted when the joint is partly flexed. Both active and passive movements should be examined.

Flexion and extension: Normally, the knee can be flexed until the calf touches the back of the thigh and can be extended till the thigh and leg form a straight line.

Abduction and adduction: These movements are virtually absent with the knee straight, but slight degrees of abduction and adduction are possible when the knee is semiflexed.

Rotation: This movement is also not possible when the knee is straight. When the hip and knee are flexed to 90° some degree of rotation is possible.

During active or passive movement the palm of one hand is placed over the patella, crepitus will be felt if osteoarthritis has involved the patellofemoral joint. Abnormal passive movement in any direction is possible in Charcot's joint.

E. MEASUREMENTS

In any affection of the knee joint there will be wasting of the quadriceps. Though many a time it becomes obvious on inspection, yet measurement of the thigh along its circumference at a level same distance from the anterior superior iliac spine should be considered. Length of the limb is not so important in affection of the knee joint. But the students must remember that a line from the anterior superior iliac spine to the middle of the patella if extended downwards, strikes the medial malleolus. This of course cannot be the fact in case of genu valgum (abnormal abduction of the knee joint) or genu varum (abnormal adduction of the knee joint). In case of genu valgum or knock knee, the degree of deformity can be estimated by the intermalleolar separation present when the inner sides of the knees are kept in apposition.

Lymph nodes: In arthritis of the knee joint the popliteal group of lymph nodes will be enlarged in the beginning and later on the inguinal group of lymph nodes. The popliteal lymph nodes are not very accessible to the examining fingers and may often be missed. So it is wiser to palpate the inguinal lymph nodes to detect arthritis of the knee joint.

General examination: In Charcot's joint neurological examination is carried out.

X-ray examination: *Tuberculosis of the knee joint* (**Figs. 15.54A and B**): General or localized decalcification of the bones becomes obvious. There may be increased joint space due to effusion. When the articular cartilages are damaged the joint space will be diminished and the joint line becomes irregular. In late cases, a triple deformity with flexion, posterior subluxation and lateral rotation of the tibia becomes evident with practically no joint space in between. In most of the pathologies of the knee joint X-ray fail to show any abnormality, as the cartilaginous pathologies out number the bony pathologies.

In *chondromalacia patellae* the patellofemoral joint space becomes narrowed and tomograms may reveal small patellar cysts. Later on osteoarthritic changes appear. Yet in all affections of the knee joint one should advise X-ray to exclude a minor fracture or loose bodies. Osteochondritis dissecans affecting the medial condyle of the femur becomes very much obvious in X-ray as a dense spot with a clear demarcating margin.

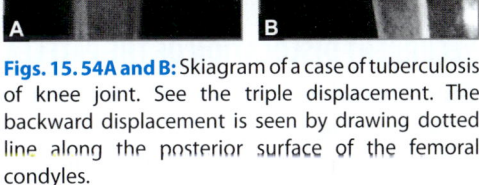

Figs. 15.54A and B: Skiagram of a case of tuberculosis of knee joint. See the triple displacement. The backward displacement is seen by drawing dotted line along the posterior surface of the femoral condyles.

Arthrography with contrast medium (conray or urografin) or air is particularly helpful in the knee joint to detect any internal derangement here.

Arthroscopy—is of particular help in diagnosing tear in the meniscus as also chondromalacia patellae.

The students are again reminded that in *every case of pain in the knee joint,* if there is no evidence of pathology in the joint, the *hip joint of that side must be examined thoroughly,* as pain may be referred to the knee from the hip.

DIFFERENTIAL DIAGNOSIS

ACUTE PYOGENIC ARTHRITIS

This condition commonly affects the children. The knee becomes swollen, the overlying skin becomes red and warm compared to the opposite side. The joint is kept in flexed position and even a slight movement will be very much painful. The joint is very much tender. The general signs are more or less similar to those of acute arthritis of the hip.

TUBERCULOSIS OF THE KNEE

This is a part of the generalized affection and infection is mainly blood-borne and settles in synovium or in the metaphysis or epiphysis of the femur or the tibia. Limp and aching are early symptoms. Soon there will be a swelling in the joint with a slight flexion deformity. At this stage one or more enlarged lymph nodes in the groin can be felt. Later on stiffness will be obvious. Without antitubercular treatment, cold abscess and sinuses are not uncommon. Muscular wasting will be obvious. In the early stage examination of the aspirated effusion or synovial biopsy will clinch the diagnosis. In the second stage (Arthritis), the patient will complain of 'night pain'. In the last stage 'triple deformity' may be noticed. X-ray findings have already been discussed.

OSTEOARTHRITIS OF THE KNEE

This is a disease of old age. The knee and hip joints are very often affected. An old bony injury, a long standing internal derangement, recurrent dislocation of the patella, genu valgum or varum are the predisposing factors.

Pain is the leading symptom, which becomes worse after use. The joint feels stiff after rest and it hurts the patient to 'get going'. Swelling is not uncommon and the joint may 'give way' or be 'locked'. Crepitus may be easily elicited if the clinician puts his hand on the sides of the patella during movement of the knee joint. X-ray shows diminution of the joint space at the pressure areas, osteosclerosis, small cysts near the articular surfaces and osteophytes at the margins of the joints.

RECURRENT DISLOCATION OF THE PATELLA

There are various causes which may be incriminated for recurrent dislocation of the patella. Of these *anatomical abnormalities* such as genu valgum and poor development of the ridge on the lateral femoral condyle should be cited first. Of the other causes, weakness of the vastus medialis and lax ligaments may lead to recurrent dislocation of the patella. The most important clinical feature is the "apprehension test", in which the patient resists the maneuver of displacing the patella laterally with the knee joint flexed for fear of pain and dislocation of the patella.

CHONDROMALACIA PATELLAE

This is characterized by fissures and softening of the articular surface of the patella. Not infrequently a "kissing" lesion may be found on the femoral condyle opposite the affected area of the patella. Young adults, especially females, are affected. The main complaint is the pain particularly at the time of climbing the stairs. Occasional swelling is also complained of. The knee tends to give way. True locking is only possible when there is a loose body within the joint. Tenderness at the patellar margin and that the patient complains of pain when the patella is pressed and moved against the femoral condyles are the main diagnostic features. X-ray findings have already been discussed.

OSTEOCHONDRITIS DISSECANS

Repeated trauma has been incriminated as the likeliest cause of this condition. Possibly impingement of the spine of the tibia against the femoral condyle is the type of trauma in this condition. Young adult males are mostly affected. The convex lower aspect of the medial femoral condyle is the most common region, the lateral condyle is the second and the patella is very occasionally affected. Ischemic necrosis and partial detachment are the main pathological processes. This is the most common source of the loose bodies in the knee joint in young persons.

This condition sometimes runs in families and may be bilateral. The main complaint is intermittent ache and swelling. The knee becomes unreliable and often gives way. Locking may occur when the ischemic area has been detached to form a loose body. After an attack of giving way and locking, there may be hemarthrosis. The most pathognomonic sign is the localized tenderness on the medial aspect of the medial femoral condyle. X-ray shows a dense area on the medial condyle of the femur which is separated from the rest of the femur by a clear zone. Later on the fragment may be hinged on one side and projected into the joint on the other side. Still later a loose body will be seen in the joint whose site of origin will be obvious.

PELLEGRINI-STIEDA'S DISEASE

Due to incomplete rupture of the medial collateral ligament calcification near its femoral attachment is the main pathology of this condition. The patient complains of pain on the medial aspect of the joint. On examination there is localized tenderness at the femoral attachment of the ligament and thickening at this region. Full extension of the joint is resisted and is extremely painful. After a year a bony prominence can be felt on the medial aspect of the femoral condyle, but by this time pain has very much subsided. Radiography confirms the diagnosis.

CYSTS ABOUT THE KNEE

The clinical features of these swellings are similar to those of cyst anywhere in the body. These can be classified according to their positions.

ANTERIORLY: (i) *Prepatellar bursitis* (Housemaid's knee)—results from friction between the skin and the patella while cleaning the floor in kneeling posture. This cyst covers the lower half of patella and upper half of the ligamentum patellae, (ii) *Infrapatellar bursitis* (clergyman's knee) also results from repeated kneeling and the bursa lies on the lower half of the ligamentum patellae.

MEDIALLY: (i) The *bursa anserina* is interposed between the tendons of the sartorius, gracilis and semitendinosus superficially and the medial ligament deep to it. (ii) *Cyst of the medial meniscus* is rarer than its lateral counterpart and the most important finding is that it disappears on acute flexion of the joint and reappears on extension till the knee joint is nearly fully extended.

LATERALLY: (i) *Cyst of the lateral meniscus* is commoner than that of the medial meniscus. The cyst is quite tense and its tendency towards disappearance on flexion is more or less similar to that of the cyst of the medial meniscus.

POSTERIORLY: (i) *Semimembranosus bursitis* is the most common and lies between the medial head of the gastrocnemius and the semimembranosus tendon, i.e., slightly more medial and higher than the Baker's cyst **(Fig. 15.55)**. The cyst becomes tense and prominent when the knee is extended and becomes flaccid when the joint is flexed. It hardly communicates with the knee joint. The patient is usually young or middle aged. The skin over the swelling and the knee joint are normal. It fluctuates and transilluminates. (ii) *Morrant Baker's cyst* lies centrally in the popliteal space and is often bilateral **(Figs. 15.56 and 15.57)**. The victims are usually over 40 years of age. It is nothing but a pressure (pulsion) diverticulum of the synovial membrane so that it can be compressed. It also stands out with extension of the knee and tends to disappear with flexion. It is usually secondary to osteoarthritis or rheumatoid arthritis of the knee joint. The swelling is soft and fluctuant, but does not transilluminate due to density of muscles covering it. It is a compressible swelling. Arthritis of the joint is evident by crepitus, limited movement and effusion.

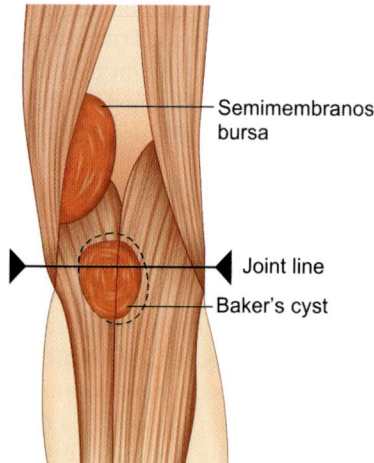

Fig. 15.55: Typical positions of the semimembranosus bursa and Baker's cyst. Note that the semimembranosus bursa lies above the knee joint line whereas the Baker's cyst lies in or slightly below the joint line.

SWELLINGS IN THE POPLITEAL FOSSA

In the beginning it must be emphasized that examination of the knee joint remains incomplete if the popliteal fossa on the posterior aspect of the knee is not properly examined. The swellings which deserve mention in this region are: (i) popliteal aneurysm, (ii) subcutaneous and nerve tumors which may occur anywhere in the body and (iii) the popliteal abscess, (iv) of course one

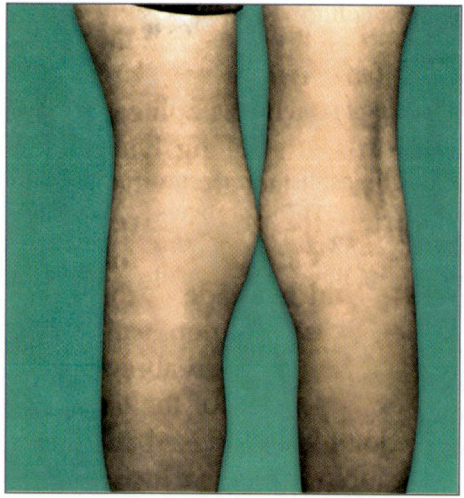

Fig. 15.56: Morrant-Baker's cyst affecting the left knee.

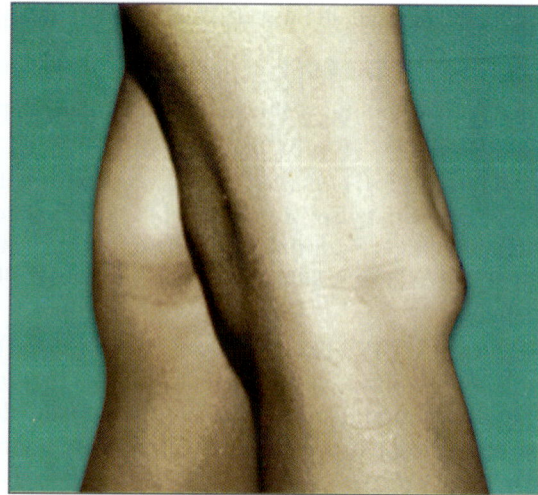

Fig. 15.57: Morrant Baker's cyst in the left knee. Note that it is being better seen with extended knee.

must remember the different bursae which may be noticed in this region (these are discussed in the earlier section).

(i) **Popliteal aneurysm:** A swelling in the midline of the popliteal space should always be examined whether it is pulsatile or not. In elderly person popliteal aneurysm is not uncommon which will give rise to an expansile pulsating swelling. One should examine the other arteries for atherosclerotic lesion.

(ii) **Swelling arising from the skin, subcutaneous tissue, popliteal lymph nodes, nerves and bones** may be seen in the popliteal fossa as anywhere in the body. These swellings can be classified into: (a) *solid swellings;* (b) *cystic swellings,* e.g., in connection with bursae on the posterior aspect of the knee (already been discussed), lymphangiectasis (from lymph vessels), varicosity of the vein mainly the short saphenous, etc. and (c) *pulsatile swellings* in which popliteal aneurysm tops the list, of course transmitted pulsation may be present in any swelling lying over the popliteal artery and can be differentiated from an aneurysm by the fact that when they are grasped from both the sides and lifted up from the popliteal artery the pulsation ceases.

(iii) **Popliteal abscess:** This is an acute condition with redness and brawny edematous swelling on the posterior aspect of the knee. A careful search should be made in the foot and the same leg for presence of an infected focus, as the most common cause of a popliteal abscess is infection of the popliteal lymph nodes. Infection of cellular tissue from a small abrasion in that region and acute osteomyelitis of the lower end of the femur or upper end of the tibia are the other causes of inflammatory condition in this region. The knee joint is kept flexed and slightest effort to extend the knee will give rise to tremendous pain. Before making an incision on the abscess one must exclude the presence of popliteal aneurysm otherwise disaster will be imminent.

EXAMINATION OF THE ANKLE AND OTHER JOINTS OF THE FOOT

A. INSPECTION

1. **Attitude:** In arthritis of ankle joint a position of plantar flexion is assumed.
2. **Swelling:** In effusion of the ankle joint there will be fullness on either side of the tendo Achilles and a bulge across the front of the joint. An effusion of the tendon sheath will produce a swelling which extends along the long axis of the leg and foot far beyond the joint-level.
3. **Muscular wasting** will be obvious in tuberculous affection of the ankle joint.

B. PALPATION

1. One should look for **local temperature** and **tenderness** in arthritis of the ankle joint.
2. **Swelling:** Fluctuation between the swelling on either side of the tendo Achilles may be obtained in effusion of the joint. With the other hand an impulse can be felt in front of the joint simultaneously.
3. Palpation of the **bones** for tenderness and irregularity is important. The two malleoli are the most obvious landmarks in the body. The lateral is less prominent and descends 1 cm lower and behind the medial malleolus.

C. MOVEMENTS

The ankle joint, being a hinge joint, permits movements in one plane, i.e., dorsiflexion and plantarflexion. In the position of plantarflexion slight rotational rocking movements are possible owing to the narrower posterior part of the talus being then engaged with the tibiofibular mortice. The range of dorsiflexion is about 25° and that of plantarflexion is 35°. *Inversion and eversion take place at the subtaloid joint and abduction and adduction occur at the midtarsal joints.*

The normal ranges of inversion and eversion or abduction and adduction are about 20° from the normal position.

In testing the passive movements of the ankle joint the leg is held with one hand and the foot is grasped with the other hand in such a manner as to include the head of the talus in the grip **(Fig. 15.58)**. This will exclude the possibility of any movement at the subtaloid and the midtarsal joints. In ankylosis of the ankle joint, movements of the subtaloid and midtarsal joints may give a false impression as the movements being occurred at the ankle joint.

The movement at the subtaloid joint can be tested by holding the leg with one hand and everting and inverting the foot by grasping the calcaneous with the other hand. The movements of the midtarsal joint are tested by holding the calcaneous with one hand and adducting and abducting the forefoot with the other hand.

It is always advisable to feel for the popliteal and inguinal groups of lymph nodes.

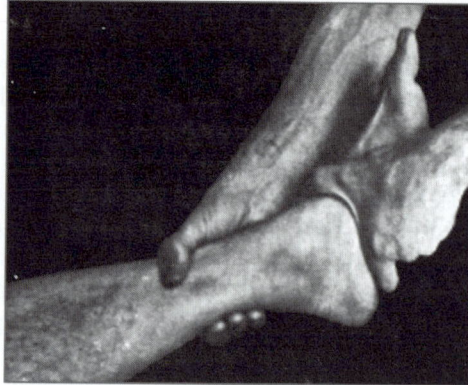

Fig. 15.58: Testing the passive movements of the ankle joint. See the text.

DIFFERENTIAL DIAGNOSIS

TUBERCULOSIS OF THE ANKLE JOINT

This is a rare condition. In the early stage the pain is slight, limping is a little and there is some wasting of the calf muscles. When the bones are affected, the pain increases. The patient tends to avoid weight bearing. The flexion and extension, the only movements of the ankle joint are greatly restricted. In the late stage there may be formation of cold abscess and sinus formation. X-ray shows rarefaction of the bone with narrowed joint space with irregularity of the articular surfaces. Primary focus may be detected in the lower end of the tibia or the talus.

SWOLLEN ANKLE

This is a very common condition which the general practitioners often confront. Bilateral ankle swelling is mainly due to systemic causes, e.g., cardiac or renal insufficiency, endocrine diseases or lymphatic origin.

Unilateral edema of the ankle is more of a surgical problem and recent bony or ligamentous injury must be excluded first. Instances of phlebothrombosis are not uncommon and Sudeck's atrophy resulting from injury should be borne in mind as a possible cause of this condition.

TAILOR'S BURSA

On the lateral surface of the lateral malleolus an adventitious bursa may become enlarged rarely in tailors or others who work with sitting cross-legged.

CHRONIC STENOSING TENOSYNOVITIS OF THE PERONEAL TENDON SHEATH

It may present itself with tenderness and localized swelling in the course of this tendon below and behind the lateral malleolus. This condition very much mimics the De Quervain's disease. The patient will complain of pain on inversion of the foot.

Algorithmic Approach to Patient with Pain, Weakness, and Deformity in Major Joints

Patient presents with pain, weakness, or deformity in a joint

↓

Which joint is affected?
- Shoulder → Proceed to **shoulder assessment**
- Elbow → Proceed to **elbow assessment**
- Wrist → Proceed to **wrist assessment**
- Hip → Proceed to **hip assessment**
- Knee → Proceed to **knee assessment**
- Ankle → Proceed to **ankle assessment**

↓

Shoulder joint assessment
Is there a history of trauma?
- Yes → Consider **fracture, dislocation, rotator cuff tear**
- No → Consider **inflammatory (RA, bursitis), degenerative (OA, calcific tendinitis), or referred pain (cervical radiculopathy, gallbladder, cardiac pain)**

↓

Perform special tests
- Neer's and hawkins-kennedy test → Subacromial impingement
- Drop arm and empty can test → Rotator cuff tear
- Apprehension and relocation test → Shoulder instability
- Cross-body adduction test → AC joint pathology

↓

Confirm diagnosis and initiate treatment
- Rotator cuff tear → Physiotherapy, NSAIDs, surgery if needed
- Frozen shoulder → Stretching exercises, NSAIDs, manipulation
- Osteoarthritis → Pain management, joint replacement if needed
- Recurrent shoulder dislocation → Rehabilitation or surgery

↓

Elbow joint assessment
Is there a history of trauma?
- Yes → Consider **fracture, dislocation, ligament injury, olecranon bursitis**
- No → Consider **arthritis, tendinopathy, nerve compression**

↓

Perform special tests
- Cozen's test → Tennis elbow
- Mill's test → Lateral epicondylitis
- Tinel's sign at elbow → Cubital tunnel syndrome

↓

Confirm diagnosis and initiate treatment
- Tennis elbow → Rest, brace, physiotherapy
- Arthritis → NSAIDs, joint injections, surgery if severe
- Cubital tunnel syndrome → Splinting, nerve decompression surgery if needed

↓

Wrist joint assessment
Is there a history of trauma?
- Yes → Consider **scaphoid fracture, Colles' fracture, lunate dislocation**
- No → Consider **arthritis, carpal tunnel syndrome, Kienbock's disease**

↓

Perform special tests
- Finkelstein's test → De Quervain's tenosynovitis
- Phalen's and Tinel's test → Carpal tunnel syndrome
- Watson's test → Scaphoid instability

↓

Confirm diagnosis and initiate treatment
- Fracture → Casting, surgery if displaced
- Carpal tunnel syndrome → Wrist splint, steroid injection, surgery if persistent
- Arthritis → NSAIDs, physiotherapy, surgery if severe

↓

Hip joint assessment

Is there a history of trauma?
- Yes → Consider **fracture of femur, dislocation, acetabular injury**
- No → Consider **osteoarthritis, AVN, rheumatoid arthritis, infections**

↓

Perform special tests
- Trendelenburg test → Gluteus medius weakness
- FABER test → Hip joint pathology
- Log roll test → Femoral neck fracture

↓

Confirm diagnosis and initiate treatment
- Fracture → Surgery (hip replacement, ORIF)
- Osteoarthritis → NSAIDs, joint replacement
- AVN → Core decompression, joint preservation surgery

↓

Knee joint assessment

Is there a history of trauma?
- Yes → Consider **ACL tear, meniscal injury, fracture, patellar dislocation**
- No → Consider **osteoarthritis, rheumatoid arthritis, infection**

↓

Perform special tests
- Lachman test → ACL tear
- McMurray's test → Meniscus injury
- Patellar apprehension test → Recurrent dislocation

↓

Confirm diagnosis and initiate treatment
- ACL tear → Physiotherapy, surgery if active lifestyle
- Meniscus tear → Physiotherapy, surgery if locked knee
- Osteoarthritis → Pain management, knee replacement if needed

↓

Ankle joint assessment

Is there a history of trauma?
- Yes → Consider **sprain, fracture, achilles tendon rupture**
- No → Consider **arthritis, flat foot, tarsal tunnel syndrome**

↓

Perform special tests
- Anterior drawer test → ATFL sprain
- Thompson test → Achilles rupture
- Tinel's sign → Tarsal tunnel syndrome

↓

Confirm diagnosis and initiate treatment
- Sprain → RICE protocol, rehabilitation
- Achilles rupture → Surgical repair or cast immobilization
- Arthritis → NSAIDs, orthotics, surgery if needed

CHAPTER 16

Examination of Head Injuries

HISTORY

As the patients with head injuries are frequently unconscious, detailed history of the accident can only be obtained from one who was present during the accident. So only in these cases outsiders should be allowed at the time of taking the history.

1. **Type of accident:** Elaborate history should be taken regarding the type of accident—whether road accident or fall from a height, whether acceleration injury or deceleration injury during driving a motor car. If injured with a weapon, the type of weapon used should be noted—whether sharp or blunt (lathi). The exact *site* of head injury should be noted.

2. **Level of consciousness:** When the patient was brought to the hospital, what was his level of consciousness? Was he conscious or semiconscious or fully unconscious? If the patient is conscious he can give a history of the type of accident occurred, the site of head injury and the sites of other injuries in the body. If the patient is unconscious, a careful history should be taken from the attendant that whether the patient became unconscious as soon as the accident occurred or he was conscious at the time of accident, but became unconscious afterwards. *The time of onset of unconsciousness* should be noted—whether appeared with the accident or a little later. *The duration of unconsciousness* should be noted. When unconsciousness appears immediately after the injury and is maintained, it is primarily due to injury to the brain and may be perpetuated by a secondary cerebral compression (as occurs in subdural hemorrhage). If the patient becomes unconscious with the accident, but regains consciousness for a while (lucid interval) and again becomes comatose, it indicates injury to the middle meningeal vessel (extradural hemorrhage). *Lucid interval* is the short period of consciousness between initial unconsciousness which occurs immediately after accident and unconsciousness at later stage after the lucid interval. It must be remembered that if the patient remains conscious following head injury (absence of unconsciousness) does not always exclude a serious head injury.

3. **Post-traumatic amnesia (PTA) and retrograde-traumatic amnesia (RTA)**
Post-traumatic amnesia (PTA) is the time between the head injury and return of continuous memory. PTA commonly persists for a while after return of consciousness. This can conveniently be assessed by asking the patient how long he was 'out' since the accident. If it is less than an hour, the injury can be regarded as slight. If it is between 1 and 24 hours, the injury is moderate. If it is between 1 to 7 days, the injury is severe and if it is more than 1 week, the injury is almost fatal. So PTA is a good guide to assess the severity of head injury.

Retrograde-traumatic amnesia (RTA) means loss of memory for events before the occurrence of the accidents. So far as severity of head injury is concerned, it is less reliable than PTA.

4. **Vomiting:** Enquire whether the patient vomited since the accident or not. If the patient has vomited, note the usual points including the type of vomitus. If it is blood mixed it may indicate fracture of the middle cranial fossa of the skull. It should be realized that *vomiting is often a sign of recovery* from cerebral concussion. But persistent vomiting may indicate increased intracranial pressure.

5. **Epileptic fits or seizures:** Patient may have epileptic fits earlier. Epileptic fit however may occur following head injury and its nature may give a clue to localization of the site of trauma. It is usually bilateral in case of hemorrhage from the superior longitudinal sinus. Jacksonian epilepsy (unilateral fit) may be due to middle meningeal hemorrhage. Occasionally, convulsive seizure or fit may be the first sign that something more serious than simple concussion is present. It is hardly to be fortunate enough to observe a 'fit'. Usually clinician may have to rely on description given by a relative or a nurse.

6. **Swelling and pain in the head:** Following head injury the patient may complain of a swelling in the head due to hematoma or fracture of the skull. Pain in the head (headache) is a very common symptom following head injury when the patient is conscious. Ask about the nature of headache. Persistent and localized headache following head injury may be due to a slowly progressive extradural hematoma or subdural hematoma or a postconfusional state.

7. **Other complaints:** Bleeding with or without watery discharge from ear, nose and mouth indicates injury to the base of the skull. For detailed description see later part of this chapter.

8. **Past history:** Enquiry must be made whether the patient had fits or similar type of head injury in the past. It should also be noted whether the patient is suffering from high blood pressure, renal disease or diabetes.

9. **Personal history:** When an unconscious or comatose patient is brought in, the clinician has to decide whether the unconsciousness is the result of head injury or the patient became unconscious due to some other cause (e.g., alcohol, apoplexy, uraemia, diabetic coma, opium poisoning, etc.) and then sustained head injury. So enquiry must be made whether the patient is alcoholic or opium addicted or having epileptic fits earlier.

10. **Family history:** It should be noted that epilepsy, diabetes, hypertension often run in families.

History in head injuries

Category	Clinical significance	Patient-friendly questions
Mechanism of injury	Determines **blunt vs. penetrating trauma, acceleration-deceleration forces**	"Can you describe exactly how the injury happened?"
Loss of consciousness (loc)	**Immediate LOC → Severe trauma, DAI; Lucid interval → Extradural hemorrhage**	"Did you lose consciousness at any point? If yes, for how long?"
Post-traumatic amnesia	**Retrograde amnesia → More severe injury**	"Do you remember what happened before and after the injury?"
Headache	**Persistent, worsening → Raised ICP**	"Do you have a headache? Has it been getting worse?"
Vomiting	**Multiple episodes → Raised ICP, hemorrhage**	"Have you vomited after the injury? If yes, how many times?"

Contd...

Contd...

Category	Clinical significance	Patient-friendly questions
Seizures	Early seizures → Cortical injury, hemorrhage	"Did you have any unusual body movements or fits after the injury?"
Vision changes	Blurred vision → ICP rise, optic nerve damage	"Have you noticed any changes in your vision or double vision?"
Hearing issues	Basal skull fracture → Hemotympanum, CSF otorrhea	"Do you have ringing in your ears or hearing loss?"
Nasal or ear bleeding	CSF leak → Basilar skull fracture	"Have you noticed any fluid or blood leaking from your nose or ears?"
Weakness or numbness	Focal deficit → Contusion, hemorrhage, spinal injury	"Do you feel weakness or numbness in any part of your body?"
Behavioral or mood changes	Frontal lobe damage → Irritability, agitation	"Have you been feeling confused, irritable, or unusually sleepy?"
Past head injuries	Repeated trauma → Chronic subdural hematoma risk	"Have you had any previous head injuries or concussions?"
Use of blood thinners	Increased risk of hemorrhage (Warfarin, aspirin, DOACs)	"Are you on any blood thinners like aspirin or warfarin?"
Alcohol/drug use at injury time	Intoxication can mask neurological deficits	"Had you consumed alcohol or any drugs before the injury?"

PHYSICAL EXAMINATION

The patient should be completely stripped. If the patient is bleeding from the scalp, this must be immediately controlled since scalp bleeding seldom stops by itself. The vessels of the scalp are prevented from normal contraction by fixation of their walls to the fibrous stroma of the scalp. It must be assured that an *adequate airway* is maintained. If the patient is vomiting, his face should be turned to one side to prevent aspiration of blood or vomitus. Jacksonian epilepsy (unilateral fit) is sometimes seen in cases of middle meningeal hemorrhage. It starts in the fingers or toes, one forearm or leg or one side of the face depending on the site of irritation of the cerebral cortex. In hemorrhage from the superior longitudinal sinus, the fits are usually bilateral. The following points should be carefully noted to come to a diagnosis:

1. **Head:** The patient must be shaved fully. The area of injury should be examined thoroughly to know if there is any fracture of the skull. If present, the type of fracture should be noted. Depressed fracture is invariably compound in case of adults but may remain simple in case of children. Sometimes a hematoma simulates a depressed fracture owing to its softened center and hard periphery (due to clotted blood). If an indentation can be produced by applying steady pressure on the rim it is a hematoma. When there is a wound in the scalp its extent and depth are carefully examined. When a wound gapes, it indicates division of the galea aponeurotica.

When a hematoma is present, it is ascertained whether (i) it is confined to an area over one cranial bone and fixed (subpericranial), or (ii) it extends beyond such limits but remains confined within the attachments of the galea aponeurotica (subaponeurotica), or (iii) it is situated superficially and moves with the scalp (subcutaneous).

It must be remembered that a boggy swelling at the temporal region often indicates a fracture affecting the temporal bone which has probably caused extradural hemorrhage from the anterior or the posterior branch of the middle meningeal artery. These cases, even if they remain conscious, should be admitted to the hospital and observed for no less than 24 hours. The cases are on record that these patients, during the lucid period of consciousness, may drink and may be arrested, only to be found dead in the next morning in the cell. The site of injury often gives a valuable indication about the diagnosis of the condition. Injury to the front or back of the head, particularly in an old man, with signs of cerebral compression, should immediately rouse the suspicion of subdural hemorrhage.

2. **Position of the patient:** Note whether the patient is lying flaccid with his jaw relaxed (a serious condition) or is curled up on his side and resents all interferences (cerebral irritation, a favorable sign).

3. **Depth of unconsciousness:** It must be assessed by applying pressure on the supraorbital nerve or pushing the angle of the jaw forcibly forwards and noting the facial expression. In complete unconsciousness, the patient cannot be roused by any kind of painful stimuli such as pricking the finger tips. There will be absence of corneal reflex and presence of incontinence of urine and feces. Level of consciousness is very important. In this respect, vague words like 'semicoma' or 'stupor' should be avoided and simple description of the responses should be noted. Is he oriented with time and place, does he answer the questions accurately or obey the command appropriately? There are different grades in responding to painful stimulus. First grade is to repel the stimulus with coordinated attempt. Second grade is a simple grunt and third grade is reflex decerebrate posturing. A baseline must be drawn so far as the consciousness of the patient is concerned. This will help to find out subsequent changes. Further deterioration of the state of consciousness may be due to cerebral compression.

4. **Bleeding from the nose, ear or mouth:** This is a sign of fracture of the base of the skull. It should be remembered that it may be due to laceration of soft tissues concerned. If the bleeding is profuse and the blood is more watery due to dilution with the cerebrospinal fluid or is mixed with brain matter, a diagnosis of fracture becomes unquestionable. *Bleeding from the nose occurs in fracture of the anterior fossa* **(Fig. 16.1)**, *whereas bleeding from the ear or mouth indicates fracture of the middle cranial fossa.* The importance of this sign lies in the fact that it indicates that the fracture, particularly in the anterior and middle cranial fossa, has become compound. The question of possibility of meningitis comes in. Very occasionally it may so happen that the ear drum remains intact with a middle cranial fossa fracture in which cases escaping CSF may trickle down the Eustachian tube and present as cerebrospinal rhinorrhea. Fracture of the middle cranial fossa may give rise to facial palsy and/or deafness.

In fracture of the posterior fossa behind the foramen magnum, a patch of ecchymosis appears within 3 or 4 days near the tip of the mastoid process (Battle's sign). The patient may vomit a quantity of swallowed blood.

Fracture of the posterior cranial fossa is more dangerous as the venous sinuses on the occipital bone may be torn.

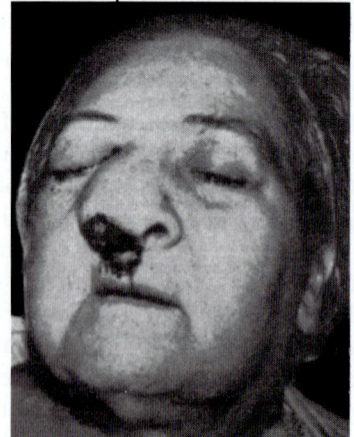

Fig.16.1: A case of head injury showing bleeding from the nose indicating probable fracture of the anterior cranial fossa. One can also find ecchymosis and edema of the eyelids.

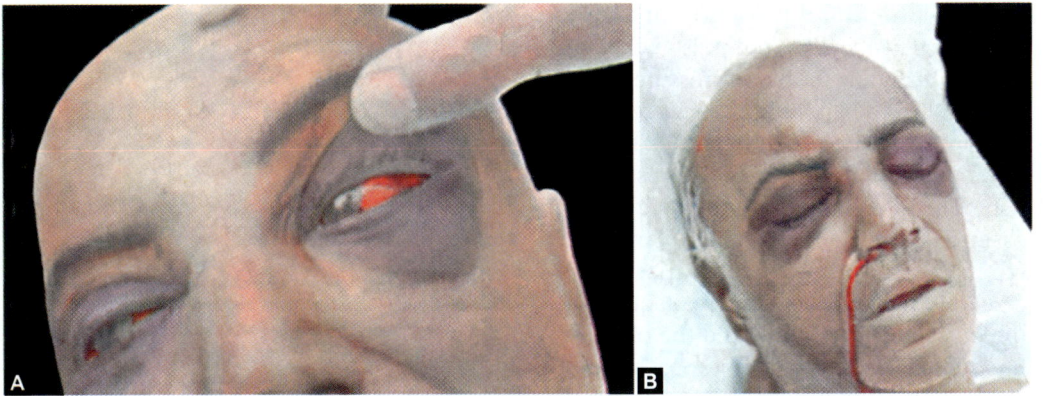

Figs.16.2A and B: Signs of fracture of the anterior cranial fossa. (A) subconjunctival hemorrhage and (B) bleeding from the nose.

So the coma persists and soon the pupils become dilated and do not react to light. Normal respiratory rhythm is lost culminating in Cheyne-Stokes' respiration. Pulse may be irregular which indicates a lesion in the brainstem and is more dangerous.

5. **Eyes:** In the eyes two things are to be noted—(i) If there is any evidence of hemorrhage in and around the eyes and (ii) the condition of the pupil.

(i) In case of fracture of the anterior cranial fossa, a few signs of hemorrhage will be noted in the eye. Similarly in case of local injury a 'black eye' will be noticed.

In fracture of the anterior cranial fossa **(Figs. 16.2A and B)**, (a) ecchymosis due to extravasated blood is seen later, usually after 24 hours. (b) It appears first in the lower eyelid due to gravitation and then in the upper. (c) It cannot go beyond the orbital margin due to attachment of the palpebral fascia to the orbital margin. (d) If the conjunctiva is examined, it will be evident that the hemorrhage is sub-conjunctival and does not move with the conjunctiva. (e) This subconjunctival hemorrhage will point towards the cornea and its posterior limit cannot be seen as it is coming from the back of the eye. (f) There will be edema of the conjunctiva. (g) If there is excessive bleeding, the eyeball will be pushed forwards and will lose its mobility.

In local injury or 'blackeye', (a) the ecchymosis appears early. (b) It may spread beyond the eyes, on to the cheek, forehead or side of the nose. (c) There will be signs of local injury around the orbit. (d) If the conjunctiva is examined, there may be conjunctival hemorrhage which will be moved with the conjunctiva. Its posterior limit will always be seen as it is a superficial hemorrhage.

(ii) The examination of pupils is very important in a case of head injury. In case of *cerebral concussion*, the pupils will be slightly dilated, equal and react to light. In case of *cerebral compression* **(Fig. 16.3)**, Hutchinson's pupils will be seen—(a) In the first stage, the pupil on the side of injury contracts due to irritation of the oculomotor nerve, the pupil of the other side remains normal. (b) In the second stage, the pupil of the injured side becomes dilated due to paralysis of the oculomotor nerve, whilst the pupil of the other side contracts since the nerve of that side becomes irritated. (c) Finally, the pupils of both sides become dilated and fixed, not reacting to light. This is a grave sign.

Pin-point and fixed pupils, pyrexia and paralysis (i.e., three 'P's) are the characteristic features of pontine hemorrhage. If the pupil was dilated when the patient was first seen, the possibility of either injury to the optic nerve or traumatic mydriasis should be considered.

6. **Pulse and blood pressure:** In case of *cerebral concussion,* the pulse will be rapid, thready and the blood pressure falls down. With the appearance of *cerebral compression,* the pulse becomes slow and bounding and the blood pressure rises. This is an attempt to maintain the essential cerebral circulation. Finally when this compensation fails, the cerebral circulation becomes inadequate, the pulse becomes rapid and the blood pressure falls for the last time. So a rapid pulse in one who is deeply unconscious heralds impending death. In *cerebral contusion,* in the beginning, the pulse will be rapid and when cerebral compression will be added on it, the pulse will be slow and bounding. But in the last stage again the pulse becomes low in volume and rapid. In *cerebral irritation,* an irregular pulse may indicate a serious prognostic sign.

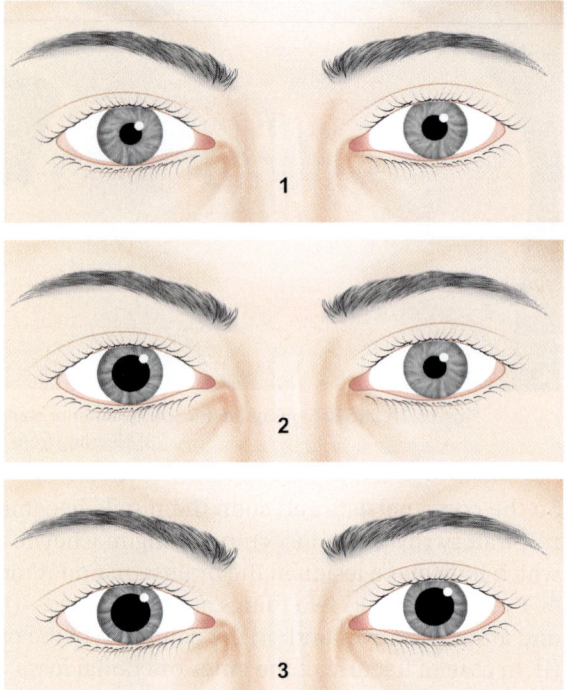

Fig.16.3: Shows the pupillary changes in cerebral compression. See the text.

7. **Respiration:** In *concussion,* respiration becomes slow and shallow. With the advent of *cerebral compression* the respiration becomes slow and deep. Later on Cheyne-Stokes' respiration will indicate grave prognosis. Stertorous breathing in which the lips and cheeks blow in and out with each breathing and there is loud snoring noise (caused by obstruction to airway by the relaxed soft palate and falling back of the tongue) is of grave prognosis as it indicates increasing medullary compression.

8. **Temperature:** In cerebral concussion and contusion in the initial stage, the temperature remains subnormal. With the appearance of cerebral compression, the temperature may rise up to 100°F. Occasionally, a difference of 1° to 2°F of temperature between the two sides of the body may be found, being higher on the paralyzed side (Victor Horsley's sign). In pontine hemorrhage a very high pyrexia is expected. In case of intraventricular hemorrhage again a high temperature may be noted.

9. **Presence of neurological deficits:** It must be noted whether the limbs are paralyzed or not. A thorough examination of the whole nervous system should be carried out to know if there is any loss of power or reflexes which may be a localizing sign and indicates the area of cerebral compression. This is of great importance since Burr-hole will be made at that region to relieve compression.

10. **Rigidity of the neck:** This is seen in case of irritation of the meninges by blood in subarachnoid hemorrhage. It must be remembered that this is also present in case of fracture-dislocation of the cervical spine. But in the first condition, there will be presence of pyrexia, but in the second condition there will be no fever. This condition must not be confused with decerebrate rigidity which may be noted in case of cerebral contusion or cerebral laceration at the midbrain.

11. **Cranial nerves:** These should be examined one after the other to know if there is any neurological deficit in one of the nerves. In an unconscious patient only a few of them can be examined. Of these the most important is the third nerve, i.e., the oculomotor nerve. In the early stage of cerebral compression the medial aspect of the temporal lobe presses upon the oculomotor nerve and this becomes irritated causing constriction of the same side of the pupil. Further pressure against the tentorium cerebelli will cause paralysis of this nerve leading to dilatation of the pupil. Different cranial nerves are injured in fracture of the different cranial fossae of the skull. These are discussed under the heading of the 'Injury to the base of the skull' in Differential Diagnosis. Supraorbital nerve is sometimes pressed very hard to know the reaction of the patient. In deeply unconscious patient, he will not react to this pressure.

12. **Other CNS manifestations:** Jacksonian epilepsy is evident in lesion of the cerebral hemisphere. Ataxia and nystagmus are features of cerebellar lesion and these focus the attention to the posterior fossa. Primary midbrain damage, which may occur from even cerebral compression due to herniation of the medial aspect of the temporal lobe through the hiatus of the tentorium cerebelli and inflict trauma to the contralateral crus of the mid brain, will produce decerebrate rigidity and pupillary dilatation. In case of hemiplegia in unconscious patients, one should look for absent abdominal reflexes, increased knee jerk, biceps jerk, triceps jerk and a positive Babinski's sign on the side of hemiplegia.

GENERAL EXAMINATION

It is extremely important to search for other injuries of the body since an unconscious patient will not indicate their presence. Examine: (1) The **chest** for fracture of the ribs, surgical emphysema, hemothorax and pneumothorax; (2) The **spine**, the **pelvis** and the **limbs** for presence of fracture; (3) The **abdomen** to exclude rupture of any hollow viscus and internal hemorrhage from injury to any solid viscus, e.g., the liver, the spleen, etc. So one should look for rigidity, sluggish or absent bowel sound, obliteration of the liver dullness, shifting dullness, presence of extravasation of urine to exclude such injuries.

REPEATED EXAMINATION

It cannot be emphasized too strongly that repeated examination of the patient is essential to know the clinical stage of the patient. In this, the level of unconsciousness must be carefully assessed, as deepening unconsciousness is a very valuable sign of cerebral compression, which requires immediate operation to save the patient from impending danger.

SPECIAL INVESTIGATIONS

Blood: Blood should be examined for diabetes and grouping and cross-matching.

X-ray pictures are taken to know if there is any fracture of the skull. It should be borne in mind that it is harmful to move the head in different positions for the purpose of taking plates. In case of middle meningeal hemorrhage it gives useful information by indicating the fracture line crossing the arterial groove. Besides the traditional anteroposterior and lateral views, stereoscopic pictures of the skull are of great value in exact localization of a fracture. In case of depressed fracture skiagram should be taken tangentially to show the amount of depression. One may find air in the subdural space or in the brain substance (aerocele).

Lumbar puncture: In the beginning, the students are cautioned to carry out this examination very carefully, as in cerebral compression there is always a risk of pressure-cone being formed by the impaction of the medulla into the foramen magnum while draining the cerebrospinal fluid. The pressure of the CSF is measured by means of a manometer. In cerebral compression the pressure will be raised and the fluid will be crystal clear in case of hemorrhages outside the membranes. In case of cerebral contusion or laceration, the fluid will be blood stained and the pressure will be high. The pressure may be normal or low with high protein content in case of chronic subdural hematoma. In serious brainstem lesion the pressure is abnormally low.

Carotid angiography: This also plays an important role to demonstrate the site of the lesion. The technique consists of an injection of the dye (10 mL of 35% diodone) into the common carotid artery followed by skiagraphy immediately. Carotid angiography can only be performed when the patient's condition is not so acute as it takes no less than two hours to complete taking pictures. This will indicate the presence of subdural hematoma by displacement of the cortical vessels away from the inner table of the skull. In case of extradural hemorrhage the middle cerebral artery will be displaced inward and the anterior cerebral artery will also be displaced across the middle line. While there is subtemporal hematoma or subcortical bleeding in the temporal lobe, the middle cerebral artery will be displaced upward.

Electroencephalography (EEG): This investigation will show areas of suppressed activity of the cortex due to injury or pressure by hemorrhage.

Echoencephalography: This will indicate the presence of hematoma by indicating a shift of the midline structure. It is not of much help in subdural hematoma as half of the cases are bilateral with no midline shift.

Ultrasonography—is also useful in locating the site of hemorrhage.

Brain scan: This has now occupied a very important position so far as the investigations of the head injury and space occupying lesions are concerned. It has almost replaced the air studies and even arteriography. The head is scanned in a very systemic manner from above downwards in a series of transverse planes. The information is fed to a computer and produces a record in which the brain substance appears gray, the ventricular fluids black and the blood clot or the tumor appears white. This is particularly important in chronic subdural hematoma.

Magnetic resonance imaging (MRI): This has superseded all previous investigations in accuracy. It gives a clear picture of brain injury and injury of the skull, subdural and extradural hematoma.

Ventriculography—is not very often used but may be of value in diagnosing chronic subdural hematoma.

Inspection holes—are often made in the skull to establish the diagnosis in doubtful cases. These holes are placed at points determined by neurological signs and are made with a trephine so that the disc of bone may be replaced if nothing abnormal is found.

■ CLASSIFICATION OF HEAD INJURIES

1. **Injury to the scalp:** Mostly this is an open injury whose depth may vary involving various layers of the scalp. When the wound gapes it is obvious that the injury has involved the galea

aponeurotica. Sometimes, though rare, scalp injury may be closed. This may lead to hematoma which may be subcutaneous, subaponeurotic and subpericranial. Osteomyelitis may develop after closed injury following infection of a subpericranial blood clot. This is *Pott's Puffy tumor.*

2. **Injury to the vault of the skull:** This may lead to fracture of the skull and is often associated with wound of the sclap. Fracture of the skull may be broadly classified into two varieties—*simple* fracture, i.e., the fracture is not exposed outside through a wound and *compound*, i.e., the fracture is exposed outside through the wound of the scalp. According to the type of the fracture it can be classified into linear, fissure, depressed fracture, comminuted fracture or avulsion fracture.

3. **Injury to base of the skull:** This may affect either the anterior cranial fossa or middle cranial fossa or posterior cranial fossa.

4. **Injury to the duramater:** This is often associated with injury to the scalp and skull. The type of fracture of the skull which causes laceration of the duramater is the depressed compound fracture.

5. **Injury to the brain:** This is by far the most important part so far as head injury is concerned. Of course very little can be done by a surgeon to improve the condition of the patient or treat the patient with such injuries. Mainly three types of injury to the brain are come across in head injury. They are cerebral concussion, cerebral contusion and cerebral laceration. All these injuries to the brain are produced by one mechanism namely displacement and distortion of the cerebral tissues occurring at the moment of impact. Brain is slightly capable of anteroposterior riding movement within the spaces of the cerebrospinal fluid. Blows on the front or back of the head lead to the maximum displacement of the cerebral hemisphere in relation to the brainstem and hypothalamic region. One hemisphere may be distorted in relation to the other with the resulting stretch and strain on the junctional tissues. So this type of injury may inflict trauma to the midbrain and is often very fatal. The different types of injury which have been discussed in the name of cerebral concussion, contusion or laceration may not be limited to the cerebral hemispheres, on the contrary they may involve midbrain, cerebellum or very rarely medulla. When the neurones of the reticular activating system in the midbrain are sufficiently damaged, consciousness is lost. Neuronal damage may be minor and transient and is often followed by recovery. To the contrary the damage may be severe and permanent. The remaining neurones may take over the function of the destroyed ones, which depends upon the quantity of cells remaining, the age of the patient and the previous intellectual capabilities of the patient. So primary brain damage will be followed by a steady improvement towards normality which depends on the amount of normal remaining brain tissue.

Concussion, contusion and laceration of the brain occur directly beneath the blow. The other type of brain injury occurs by mass movement of the cerebral hemispheres allowing shearing forces to be generated within the brain and is focused mainly to the relatively fixed midbrain. *Contrecoup injury* to the surface of the brain opposite to the side of the blow may be seen in odd cases.

6. **Injury to the blood vessels:** This is important due to the fact that injury to the blood vessels will cause cerebral compression leading to deterioration in level of consciousness and impending danger of death. The detection and treatment of which will considerably reduce the mortality rate of head injuries. Three types of intracranial hemorrhages are seen—(i) Subcortical, (ii) Extradural and (iii) Subdural.

7. **Escape of cerebrospinal fluid:** Cerebrospinal fluid may be drained due to open fracture of the anterior and middle cranial fossae through the nose, mouth and ear. From the treatment point of view the importance of this condition lies in the fact that there remains the chance of

intracranial infection from these open injuries, which should be treated prophylactically with high dose of broad spectrum antibiotic. Very rarely CSF may be leaked into the subdural space producing subdural hygroma.

8. **Injury to the cranial nerves:** Head injury may be associated with the injuries to different cranial nerves, of which the 3rd cranial nerve is the most important as it is involved even by cerebral compression besides direct injury. The different cranial nerves are injured in fracture of the different parts of the base of the skull. This is discussed later in this chapter.

DIFFERENTIAL DIAGNOSIS

INJURY TO THE VAULT OF THE SKULL

Whenever a patient comes with head injury, the patient must be shaved completely and thorough examination of the injury must be made to know if it is associated with the fracture of the skull or not. Fractures of the vaults of the skull are mainly caused by: (i) compression of the sphere, (ii) by local indentation and (iii) by tangential injury. When the head is compressed against a hard flat surface, it renders the spherical skull more ovoid and a *linear fracture* starts from the point of maximum convexity through the thin areas of the bone. The fracture line often deflects from the bony buttresses towards the base of the skull. So it must be remembered that many fractures of the base are produced by extension of fissures starting in the vault. Local indentation may produce *closed pond depressed fracture* caused by a large round object in which the scalp may be bruised but remains intact and the skull becomes indented but not indriven so the underlying dura remains intact. There may be bruising of the underlying brain surface but is not penetrated. Local indentation of the skull may also be produced by small round object which produces *compound depressed fracture*. The scalp is lacerated, the fractured bone is depressed and indriven, lacerating both the dura and the subjacent brain. There is immediate risk of infection and a later risk of epilepsy resulting from the contracting fibrous scar of the healing brain. Fracture of the vault of the skull by tangential injury is rare and is caused by tangentially directed violence which may secure a grip on the skull and lift it up producing a *horse-shoe shaped fracture* surrounding the calvarium.

INJURY TO THE BASE OF THE SKULL

A. **FRACTURE OF THE ANTERIOR CRANIAL FOSSA:** In this fracture there will be hemorrhage from the nose (epistaxis) and/or escape of cerebrospinal fluid (traumatic rhinorrhea) and even brain matter through the nose. There will be evidence of hemorrhage in the orbital cavity by the presence of ecchymosis starting in the lower eyelid and gradually involving the upper eyelid, subconjunctival hemorrhage the posterior limit of which cannot be seen and excessive hemorrhage will push the eye forwards. The olfactory nerve (first cranial nerve) is frequently torn and unless its fellow of the other side is also damaged, partial anosmia may pass unrecognized. The optic nerve usually escapes injury. The 3rd, 4th, the 1st division of the 5th and 6th cranial nerves may be injured at the sphenoidal fissure. 3rd nerve palsy produces a dilated pupil in a conscious patient.

B. **FRACTURE OF THE MIDDLE CRANIAL FOSSA:** Hemorrhage and escape of cranial contents (including CSF and brain matter) may be expected from the ear and mouth only. Occasionally, there may be epistaxis when the nasal sinuses are affected. Of the cranial nerves the 7th nerve (facial), the 8th nerve and occasionally the 6th nerve may be injured. Facial nerve injury will cause paralysis of the facial muscles which may occur late due to compression by blood clot or pressure from fibrous tissue or callus. Injury to the 8th nerve will cause deafness and injury to the 6th nerve will result in internal strabismus.

C. **FRACTURE OF THE POSTERIOR CRANIAL FOSSA:** Extravasation of blood may be seen in the suboccipital region producing a swelling at the back of the upper part of the neck and ecchymosis posterior to the mastoid process. The 9th, 10th, and 11th cranial nerves are occasionally injured at the jugular foramen. The 12th nerve usually escapes as it is protected by strong bony buttresses.

INJURY TO THE BRAIN

A. **CEREBRAL CONCUSSION:** This is a temporary physiological paralysis of function without any organic structural damage. The patient becomes unconscious for a short period, followed by complete and perfect recovery. It is a condition of shock and develops immediately after the injury. The pulse becomes rapid and is of low volume. The blood pressure is reduced slightly. The respiration is quick and shallow. The temperature remains subnormal. The muscles become flaccid. A deep or prolonged stupor means something more than pure concussion.

B. **CEREBRAL CONTUSION:** In this condition there will be rupture of white fibers of the brain causing petechial hemorrhages. Ring hemorrhages are produced by bleeding into the perivascular spaces of Robin-Virchow. Some hemorrhages are also noticed in the corpus callosum in the 3rd ventricle and in the substantia nigra of the brainstem. A low intracranial pressure is noticed. Unconsciousness is more prolonged. The initial recovery is imperfect as degeneration following rupture of axons leads to a postcontusional state associated with defective memory and change of personality. So the patient recovers with confusion, irritability, delirium, etc. When the patient remains unconscious, the pulse rate is increased and it is of low volume. The blood pressure is reduced, respiration remains shallow. The muscles remain relaxed. This is followed by recovery when the patient survives. At this stage the respiration becomes deeper, the pulse increases in volume and the face becomes flushed from the previous condition of pallor. The patient complains of headache and photophobia, becomes irritable and often vomits.

C. **CEREBRAL IRRITATION:** It develops about 2-3 days after head injury and is mainly caused by cerebral edema. The patient is not unconscious but takes no interest in the surroundings. He remains curled up with knees drawn up and arms flexed *(an attitude of flexion)* and interference of any kind is resisted. Recovery is apparently complete, but in majority of cases headache, irritability, depression, lack of concentration, defective memory and a change of personality are expected.

D. **CEREBRAL LACERATION:** In this condition the brain surface is torn with effusion of blood into the cerebrospinal fluid leading to subarachnoid hemorrhage. This is mainly caused by injury of the brain surface against bony ridges and the edges of the dural septa. So lacerations are common on the inner aspect of the hemisphere under surface of the frontal lobe and tip of the temporal lobe. These may lead to anosmia and change of personality. Lacerations may occur on the opposite side to the site of impact. This is known as contracoup injury. Signs and symptoms are more or less similar to those of cerebral contusion.

INJURY TO THE BLOOD VESSELS

Hemorrhage from any intracranial vessel may occur above or below the tentorium cerebelli and will be responsible for causing brain compression. It requires sometime to develop cerebral compression. In this period the patient remains conscious and is typically known as the 'lucid interval'. Of course this time varies according to the type of the vessel (whether artery or vein) and the caliber of the vessel injured.

The hemorrhage may be *supratentorial* or *infratentorial*.

Of these, **SUPRATENTORIAL HEMORRHAGES** is by far much commoner and includes subcortical hemorrhage, subdural hemorrhage and extradural hemorrhage.

Subcortical hemorrhage is produced by arterial bleeding from an area of surface laceration or from rupture of a central artery. This bleeding becomes fatal when it ruptures into the ventricle causing *intraventricular hemorrhage,* the main symptom of which is hyperthermia. Epileptic fits may be seen with localized paralysis. The symptoms and signs develop from 1 to 10 days time after head injury. Old blood clots in the brain may produce the signs and symptoms which may mimic those of cerebral tumors.

Subdural hemorrhage: This condition is about 6 times commoner than extradural hemorrhage and is mainly caused by the rupture of the superior cerebral vein within the subdural space. Injury to the front or back of the head, particularly in elderly individuals, may lead to subdural hemorrhage. The cerebral hemispheres move while the superior cerebral veins draining from the cerebral hemispheres to the lower part of the superior sagittal sinus remain fixed (*See* **Fig. 31.1** in author's 'A Concise Textbook of Surgery'). About 50% of cases are bilateral. The acute form of this condition produces cerebral compression which is fatal and demands immediate surgical interference. In subacute or chronic varieties, the symptoms are less dramatic and consist of headache which is unduly severe and prolonged, mental apathy, slowness to respond to questions; the patient may go into coma when the midbrain pressure-cone is developed.

Extradural hemorrhage (Fig. 16.4): The classical syndrome of extradural hemorrhage results from injury to the anterior or posterior branch of the middle meningeal artery. The injury in force is generally a blow from the lateral side which may cause fracture of the temporal bone and injury to the said artery. The anterior branch bleeding is more significant and occurs mostly at a point when it leaves the bony canal at the pterion. Immediately after the injury the patient goes into concussion and then a period of 'lucid interval' during which the hemorrhage collects. The next change is the level of consciousness. The patient becomes confused and irritable. Confusion changes to drowsiness and the hematoma gradually presses on the motor cortex causing twitching which is quickly followed by paralysis of the face, then the arm and then the leg on the opposite side of the body. At this time the temporal lobe is displaced medially and its inner portion presses on the 3rd nerve above the edge of the tentorium causing contraction, rapidly followed by dilatation of the pupil on the side of hemorrhage. Gradually, the opposite crus of the brainstem is pressed against the opposite rim of the tentorium (*See* **Fig. 31.3** in author's 'A Concise Textbook of Surgery') leading to hemiplegia and this time on the side of the hemorrhage. Finally impaction of the

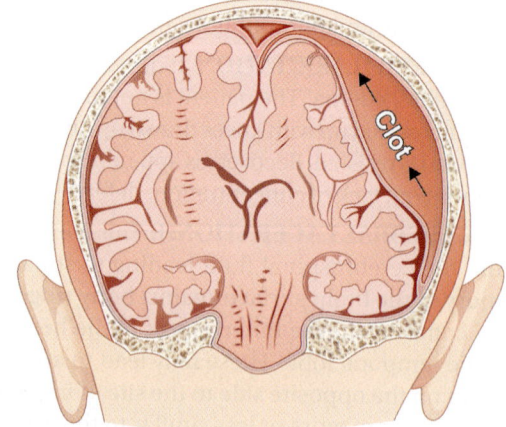

Fig.16.4: Shows clot at the extradural space in extradural hemorrhage. Middle meningeal hemorrhage usually takes place at the bony tunnel where the artery of the same name enters the skull. The arrow shows how the clot gradually spreads from below upwards involving successively the area for the face, arm and leg.

midbrain cone leads to decerebrate rigidity and fixed dilatation of both the pupils. The side of the middle meningeal hemorrhage is diagnosed by:

(i) The side of skull fracture; (ii) The side of boggy swelling under the temporal muscle and (iii) The side of the initial dilatation of the pupil.

Extradural hemorrhage can also occur from internal maxillary or anterior meningeal vessels by fracture of the anterior fossa.

Supratentorial hemorrhage produces its effect partly by local pressure on the brain underlying the hematoma, but more importantly by herniation of the uncus of the temporal lobe through the tentorial hiatus causing midbrain compression. The midbrain compression leads to: (i) deterioration in the level of consciousness by damaging the reticular activating system; (ii) pupillary changes due to the effect of pressure on the oculomotor nerves and lastly (iii) hemiplegia due to compression on the opposite crus of the midbrain with continuing pressure. *Signs of damage to the pons* may develop, which are (i) elevation of the blood pressure, (ii) slowing of the pulse and (iii) irregular respiration. The cerebral compression as a whole is discussed below :

Cerebral compression: The patient after being conscious or irritable for a while, passes into profound unconsciousness. Progressive deterioration in level of unconsciousness is the main feature. The pulse becomes slow and bounding (of high volume). Respiration remains slow and deep, frequently stertorous. The patient's cheeks flap with respiration. His face becomes flushed. The temperature may be unequal, being higher on the paralyzed side. The pupil on the side of the lesion dilates after initial contraction with poor reaction to light. In the last stage both the pupils become dilated and fixed without reacting to light.

Cerebral compression mainly results from hemorrhage from intracranial vessels or edema from local injury to the brain.

INFRATENTORIAL HEMORRHAGES causes compression to the cerebellum, pons and the medulla. The midbrain is not initially compressed, therefore consciousness is not impaired. The effects of this hemorrhage are: (i) elevation of blood pressure, (ii) slowing of the pulse, (iii) irregular respiration, (iv) ataxia, (v) nystagmus and (vi) lower cranial nerve palsies. It must be remembered that infratentorial hemorrhage is by far less common than its supratentorial counterpart.

DIFFERENTIATION BETWEEN EXTRADURAL AND SUBDURAL HEMORRHAGES

1. **Incidence:** Subdural hemorrhage is about 6 times commoner than extradural hemorrhage.
2. **Onset:** In extradural hemorrhage signs of compression appear later than those of subdural hemorrhage.
3. **Lucid interval:** In extradural hemorrhage after a period of initial unconsciousness (stage of cerebral concussion), there will be a stage of consciousness in which the patient behaves normally (lucid interval). During this lucid interval the duramater is slowly stripped off the skull by the accumulating blood, but the intracranial pressure continues to be normal by displacement of the cerebrospinal fluid into the spinal canal. When this compensation fails, intracranial pressure increases and the medial aspect of the temporal lobe herniates through the tentorial hiatus to compress on the midbrain. This damages the activating reticular system in the brainstem with deterioration in the level of consciousness. Gradually, the patient passes into deep coma. In subdural hemorrhage, on the other hand, blood accumulates more quickly and does not allow much time for compensation to take place. Therefore lucid interval is much less or even absent in subdural hemorrhage.

4. ***Paralysis:*** In case of hemorrhage from the anterior branch of the middle meningeal artery, the extradural hematoma will press on the motor cortex from below upwards. This causes paralysis on the other side of the body starting from the face, then the arm, trunk and gradually towards the leg. When the medial aspect of the temporal lobe herniates through the tentorial hiatus by increasing intracranial pressure, the contralateral crus of the midbrain is pressed against the edge of the tentorial hiatus causing hemiplegia of the same side as the lesion. This occurs late in extradural hemorrhage but occurs earlier in cases of unilateral subdural hemorrhage.

5. ***X-ray of the skull***—may reveal fracture line in the temporal bone across the groove for middle meningeal vessels in case of extradural hemorrhage. This may not be evident in case of subdural hemorrhage.

6. ***Echoencephalography*** will indicate a shift of the midline structures towards the opposite side in case of extradural hemorrhage and unilateral subdural hemorrhage. 50% of the subdural hemorrhage is bilateral. *Brain scan* will also reveal extradural or subdural hemorrhage.

COMPLICATIONS OF HEAD INJURIES

Post-traumatic headache, insomnia, infection like osteomyelitis, meningitis, encephalitis, etc., post-traumatic epilepsy, hydrocephalus, metabolic disorders like uremia, diabetes insipidus, etc., caroticocavernous fistula, fat embolism are the various complications which may occur after head injury.

Of these complications, post-traumatic headache and epilepsy deserve special mention. One thing must be remembered that headache may be due to injury to upper cervical vertebrae pressing on the great occipital and posterior auricular nerves supplying the vertex, the temple and the forehead. In this condition the patient will complain of pain during flexion of the cervical spine and tenderness can be revealed at the upper cervical spines.

A type of early post-traumatic epilepsy may be seen in the first 24 hours and is mainly caused by bruising and edema of the brain near the site of injury. True post-traumatic epilepsy due to the scar tissue formation in the brain or between the brain and the membranes will take no less than 6 months to develop. Post-traumatic epilepsy is mainly Jacksonian type, uncontrollable twitching may affect the thumb or the hand in the beginning. Gradually, the muscles of the arm, shoulder or even face will be affected. The convulsion may become generalized. Typical aura may be seen before a generalized fit.

Algorithmic Approach to Patient with Head Injuries

Patient presents with head injury

↓

Is the patient conscious?
- Yes → Proceed with **history-taking and neurological examination**
- No → Assess **airway, breathing, circulation (ABC)** and stabilize immediately

↓

Check for skull fracture or scalp injury
- Depressed skull fracture → Urgent neurosurgical referral
- Linear skull fracture → Observe and monitor neurological status
- Open skull fracture → Risk of infection, Broad-spectrum antibiotics, Neurosurgical intervention

↓

Assess level of consciousness (Glasgow coma scale – GCS)
- Mild (GCS 13–15) → Concussion, Observe, Symptomatic treatment
- Moderate (GCS 9–12) → Perform CT scan, Admit for observation
- Severe (GCS ≤8) → Immediate intubation, Neurosurgical evaluation

↓

Look for signs of intracranial hemorrhage
- Lucid interval present?
  - Yes → Suggests **extradural hemorrhage**
  - No → Consider **subdural hemorrhage, subarachnoid hemorrhage, or contusion**

↓

CT scan to confirm diagnosis
- Extradural hemorrhage → Urgent hematoma evacuation
- Subdural hemorrhage → Consider burr hole drainage (if large and symptomatic)
- Subarachnoid hemorrhage → Neurosurgical consultation, BP control, ICP monitoring
- Diffuse axonal injury → Supportive care, ICP control, prognosis guarded

↓

Determine surgical vs conservative management
- Surgical intervention required → Emergency craniotomy for mass lesions
- Conservative management → Monitor for neurological deterioration, repeat CT scan

↓

Admit and monitor for signs of deterioration
- Worsening GCS → Urgent neurosurgical reevaluation
- New-onset seizures → Antiepileptics, EEG monitoring
- Persistent vomiting, headache → Increased ICP, consider mannitol or surgery

Investigation of Intracranial Space-occupying Lesions

CHAPTER 17

Chronic space-occupying lesions include the tumors, chronic hematomas and intracranial abscesses.

HISTORY

Age and sex: *Medulloblastoma* is a tumor of childhood (between the ages of 5 and 15 years), boys outnumber the girls. *Spongioblastoma polare* usually affects young subjects. *Glioblastoma multiforme* occurs in adult males. *Astrocytomas* occur at any age—in the frontal lobes in adults and at other sites of the hemispheres in young subjects. *Acoustic neurofibroma* is uncommon before the age of 30.

Previous history of trauma: In presence of history of head injury, one should always consider the possibilities of intracranial abscess and chronic subdural hematoma.

Infected frontal air sinus and otitis media: Previous history of these conditions should make the surgeon to think in the line of intracranial abscesses. The patient may forget that he once suffered from these conditions.

Complaints: A chronic space-occupying lesion produces symptoms after an initial period of silent growth. These are of the following types: Focal or localizing symptoms, symptoms due to raised intracranial pressure and due to cone formation.

a. **Focal or localizing symptoms are:**
(i) *Epileptic fits* arising for the first time in adults should always be suspected as being due to tumors unless proved otherwise. Tumors commencing in the cerebral hemisphere will produce this symptom. When this symptom is associated with hallucination of taste or smell, the uncinate process is probably involved with the tumor.
(ii) *Attacks of twitching*, paresis and/or loss of sensation commencing in both the feet and lower limbs, subsequently spreading to one side of the body is suggestive of parasagittal meningioma of the opposite side. In cerebellar hemisphere tumors there will be in coordination of the corresponding side of the body (deviation to the affected side on walking). Nystagmus may or may not be present in case of such tumors.
(iii) *Mental symptoms* such as change of personality, loss of memory, loss of power of concentration, etc., are commonly associated with tumors affecting the frontal lobe.

b. **Symptoms due to raised intracranial pressure** vary in their appearance according to the situation of the tumor. These symptoms appear earliest in cases of tumors arising from the midline and posterior fossa and later on in temporal and parietal lobe tumors as these tumors partially obstruct the outflow of the cerebrospinal fluid (CSF) from the ventricles and produce internal hydrocephalus. Tumors of the frontal lobe generally push the ventricles back and the symptoms of raised intracranial pressure appear late. Intracranial tumors increase the intracranial pressure due to their own bulk and due to retained ventricular fluid. These symptoms are:

(i) *Headache:* This is the most constant of all the symptoms in this group. It is most marked in the early morning on getting out of the bed. Of course, in the terminal stage it becomes continuous and intense. Headache on one side of the head may indicate tumor of that side of the head. Occipital headache with a tendency towards radiation down the neck is commonly encountered in subtentorial growth. Bitemporal headache is often a feature of pituitary tumor.

(ii) *Vomiting:* This is also mostly experienced in the early morning, usually before breakfast. This type of vomiting is usually not preceded by nausea and may sometimes become aggravated by coughing and straining which increase cerebral congestion.

(iii) *Deamness of vision:* This is due to papilloedema. It occurs early in the subtentorial growth and growth affecting the inferior aspect of the frontal lobe or temporal lobe.

(iv) *Slow pulse rate* and retarded cerebration with loss of concentration, loss of memory and even stupidity are also features of increased intracranial pressure.

c. **Symptoms due to cone formation** appear as the last stage of an intracranial tumor when the temporal lobe is forced down through the tentorial hiatus or the cerebellar vermis is pushed up through the same opening or the cerebellar tonsil is forced downward through the foramen magnum. These symptoms are: (i) Drowsiness, (ii) Slow pulse rate, (iii) Neck stiffness, (iv) Paroxysmal headache and (v) Pupillary dilatation.

History in space-occupying lesions

Aspect	Clinical significance	Patient-friendly questions
Age and sex	Helps identify **age-specific tumors** (e.g., medulloblastoma in children, glioblastoma in adults)	"How old are you?"
History of trauma	Chronic hematoma, post-traumatic abscess	"Have you had a recent or past head injury?"
Headache	**Raised ICP, tumor compression**	"Do you have headaches? when are they most severe?"
Seizures	First-time adult seizure → Think tumor	"Have you ever had a seizure before?"
Vision problems	Papilledema (Raised ICP), bitemporal hemianopia (pituitary tumor)	"Have you noticed any changes in vision?"
Hearing loss/ringing in ears	Acoustic neuroma	"Do you have hearing loss or ringing in one ear?"
Memory/behavioral changes	Frontal lobe tumors, chronic hematomas	"Have you noticed personality changes or forgetfulness?"
Nausea and vomiting	Raised ICP, hydrocephalus	"Do you feel nauseous or vomit in the morning?"
Neurological deficits	Localizing signs (hemiparesis, ataxia, cranial nerve palsies)	"Have you noticed weakness, numbness, or difficulty speaking?"

PHYSICAL EXAMINATION

GENERAL APPEARANCE

Gigantism in the lower age group and acromegaly in adults are features of hyperpituitarism. Round face, excess of hair, purple striae are features of basophil adenoma of the pituitary (Cushing's syndrome).

PULSE AND BLOOD PRESSURE

Bradycardia is a common feature of raised intracranial pressure. Tachycardia may be seen in subtentorial growths. Blood pressure, contrary to expectation, is seldom high. In Cushing's syndrome blood pressure becomes raised.

LOCAL EXAMINATION OF THE HEAD

Local examination of the head is not much informatory so far as intracranial tumors are concerned. Occasionally, localized tenderness may be present over the underlying tumor, particularly the meningiomas. In meningioma there may be local thickening in scalp with engorged veins. Sometimes a bruit may be heard over the tumor.

EXAMINATION OF THE NERVOUS SYSTEM

A general scheme of examination of the nervous system is set out below. This is not specific for intracranial tumors which may not show any neurological deficit. Special investigations are more helpful in diagnosing intracranial tumors. Examination of the whole nervous system is more carefully taught in the department of medicine. Yet a textbook on clinical surgery cannot be made complete without describing in nutshell the points of examination of the nervous system.

1. **Mental state and intellectual functions:** (a) Ascertain if the memory is good or impaired by asking questions about known events in the patient's past history. (b) Next investigate the speech functions. Is the patient right-handed or left-handed ? Speech functions are localized in the left cerebral hemisphere in the right-handed person and vice versa. Test for motor aphasia, i.e., loss of power of speech (without paralysis of muscles of speech); agraphia, i.e., loss of power of writing (without paralysis of muscles of writing); word-deafness, i.e., inability to understand spoken questions as evident by failure to touch the nose or to smile on being asked to do so (when there is no defect of hearing); and word-blindness, i.e., inability to understand written questions (with no defect of vision).

2. **Examination of the cranial nerves:**

❖ **Olfactory nerve:** Can the patient smell? Anosmia or loss of sense of smell is due to meningioma in the olfactory groove or tumor at the base of the frontal lobe. Parosmia or perversion of sense of smell may be present in a lesion of the uncinate gyrus.

❖ **Optic nerve:** The degree of loss of vision is tested by asking the patient to read different letter-types or to count fingers. In suitable cases ophthalmoscopic examination and perimetry for the visual field must be undertaken by an expert. The field of vision can be roughly estimated by asking the patient to gaze straight ahead at a fixed object and then moving a small object, e.g., a white pin head, from the periphery to the center of the visual field first horizontally and then vertically.

Blindness in one-half of each visual field is known as hemianopia. If it affects the same half of each field, it is called homonymous hemianopia. This occurs in lesions of the optic tract and optic radiation. If the outer half of each field is affected, it is called bitemporal hemianopia, which indicates a chiasmal lesion, e.g., pituitary tumor, suprasellar cyst, etc. Since the pituitary tumor exerts pressure on the chiasma from below, the hemianopia is upper quadrantic at the beginning, whereas in the case of a suprasellar cyst the hemianopia starts as a lower quadrantic defect because the upper aspect of the chiasma is first pressed upon.

❖ **Oculomotor, trochlear and abducent nerves:**
a. Look at the pupils and note their size and shape—whether abnormally dilated (oculomotor paralysis) or contracted (pontine lesion); determine whether they react normally to light and accommodation. The reaction to light is tested by throwing light on to the pupil and the reaction to accommodation, by asking the patient to look first, at some distant object and then at the finger held in front of the eyes. Normally, the pupils contract in each case.
b. Test the ocular movements: The patient with his head held fixed is asked to move the eyes in turn to the right, to the left, upwards and downwards as far as possible in each direction. Any limitation of movement is noted. Ask the patient if he has seen double (diplopia) in any direction. Note also if there is squint, ptosis (drooping of the upper eyelid) of nystagmus (involuntary oscillation of the eyeball). Nystagmus indicates a lesion of the cerebellum or the vestibular apparatus. Is there conjugate deviation (i.e., eyes persistently turned towards one side)? If so, note the direction. In lesions of the cerebral hemisphere, the eyes are directed towards the side of a paralytic lesion but away from the side of an irritative lesion. In lesions of the pons, on the other hand, the eyes look towards the irritative lesion and away from the paralytic lesion. In some cerebellar lesions, skew deviation, i.e., one eye looking upwards and the other looking downwards, is often seen.

Oculomotor nerve paralysis: Complete paralysis of this nerve leads to: (i) Ptosis—due to paralysis of the levator palpebrae superioris; (ii) Externoinferior squint—due to unopposed action of the external rectus (abducent nerve) and inferior oblique (trochlear nerve); (iii) Inability to move the eyeball inwards or upwards; (iv) Dilatation of the pupil with loss of light and accommodation reflexes; and (v) Diplopia.

Trochlear nerve paralysis: Downward and outward movement of the eyeball is impaired and diplopia occurs when such movement is attempted.

Abducent nerve paralysis: There is internal squint and inability to move the eye outwards. When such movement is attempted diplopia occurs.

❖ **Trigeminal nerve:**
▶ **Motor function:** (a) Feel the masseter and the temporalis muscles of both sides simultaneously while the patient clinches the teeth. (b) On asking the patient to open his mouth, the jaw will deviate towards the affected side owing to paralysis of the pterygoids.
▶ **Sensory function:** (a) All sensations over the face supplied by the three divisions of the trigeminal nerve will be lost. The sensation of the conjunctiva, nasal mucosa and anterior two-thirds of the tongue will also be lost. The patient should not speak but write down what he tastes.
▶ **Reflexes:** Test for the reflex sneezing (by tickling the nasal mucosa) and the corneal reflex. These will be absent if the nerve is paralyzed.

❖ **Facial nerve:** Observe that the nasolabial fold and the furrows of the brow are less marked on the affected side. The angle of the mouth is drawn to the sound side.
▶ **Motor function:** (1) Ask the patient to show his teeth when the angle of the mouth will be drawn to the healthy side. (2) Ask the patient to puff out the cheeks, the paralyzed side bellows out more than the normal side. (3) Ask the patient to shut his eyes. He will not be able to close the eye on the affected side and on attempting to do so the eyeball will be seen to roll upwards. (4) Ask the patient to move his eyebrows upwards; the paralysis side remains immobile **(Figs. 17.1A to D).**

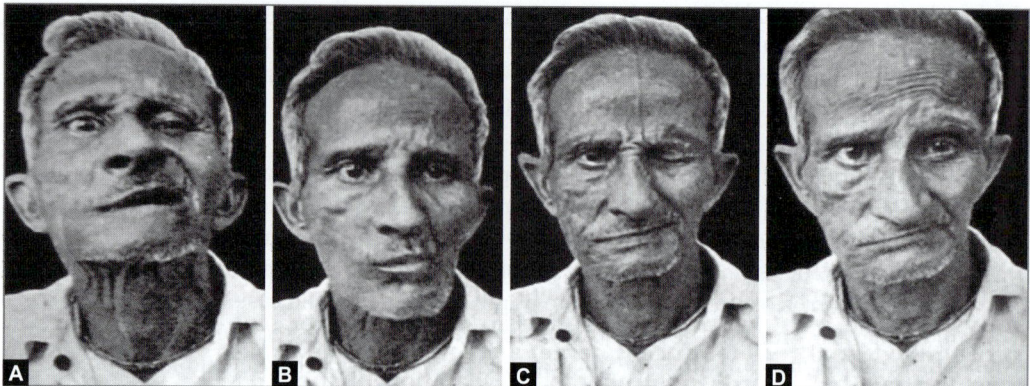

Figs. 17.1A to D: Testing for the facial nerve. The patient is asked (A) to show his teeth, (B) to puff out the cheeks, (C) to close his eyes and (D) wrinkle the forehead. Note that the right side is paralyzed.

In supranuclear paralysis (upper motor neuron lesions) the upper part of the face escapes owing to bilateral cortical representation.

❖ **Auditory nerve:** Test the patient's power of hearing by means of a watch which is gradually brought to the ear with the eyes closed; note the distance at which he can hear. As the power of hearing may be lost due to affections other than involvement of the auditory nerve, Rinne's test should be employed.

❖ **Glossopharyngeal nerve:** Test for the loss of sensation of the posterior third of the tongue and the back of the pharynx with a probe, first on one half, then on the other and note if there is any difference.

❖ **Vagus nerve:** Ask the patient to open the mouth, depress the tongue with a spatula and watch the movements of the palate as the patient says 'Aah'. In paralysis, the affected half of the palate will remain immobile.

❖ **Accessory nerve:** The sternomastoid muscle should be tested for paralysis by asking the patient to turn his face to the other side, while resistance is offered to the act by the hand over the chin. The paralyzed muscle will not stand out prominently (*see* 'Examination of the Neck"). Test also for paralysis of the trapezius (*see* "Examination of Peripheral Nerve Lesions").

❖ **Hypoglossal nerve:** Ask the patient to put out his tongue. In paralysis the tip of the tongue at once points to the paralyzed side. The patient is also unable to move the tongue to the other side. In long-standing cases atrophy of the affected half of the tongue becomes evident.

3. **Investigation of motor functions:**

a. A patient, who can walk and move his upper limbs freely, is not suffering from any gross paralysis. Investigation for paralysis or weakness of different groups of muscles should be made, when necessary, as described under 'Examination of Peripheral Nerve Lesions.'

b. The degree of coordination of muscular action is next determined: The patient is asked (i) to extend his arm and then to bring his forefinger to the tip of his nose keeping his eyes closed; in the presence of incoordination, he will not be able to do this. (ii) Walking along a straight line is difficult if there is incoordination. (iii) Rapid movements of pronation and supination of the forearm with the elbow at a right angle are either not possible or slow in cases of cerebellar lesions (adiadochokinesia). (iv) The patient is asked to stand with his feet close together and to shut the eyes. Note any tendency to fall (Romberg's sign). (v) The recumbent patient feels difficulty in placing his heel on the opposite knee with his eyes shut, if there is incoordination. Nystagmus is also a sign of incoordination.

c. Estimate the muscle tone. Wasted and flabby muscles can be easily distinguished from the spastic muscles by noting the amount of resistance offered to passive movements. Rigidity of the neck muscles is present in cerebellar lesions, e.g., medulloblastoma.
d. Note the presence of involuntary movements, e.g., tics, athetosis, tremor, etc.

4. **Investigation of sensory functions:**
a. Cutaneous sensations are tested as described under "Examination of Peripheral Nerve Lesions" (Chapter 9).
b. Joint sense: Can the patient, with the eyes carefully shut, say whether the joint is being flexed or extended? Or can he recognize the position in which the joint is finally kept after moving it in several directions?
c. Absence of stereognostic sense, i.e., failure to recognize the size, shape and form of different objects in common use such as coin, a match box, knife, etc., is significant of lesions of the sensory cortex.

5. **Reflexes:**
a. **Plantar reflex (S1):** The inner or the outer border of the foot is scratched with a pin. Normally, the great toe is flexed (flexor response) but in lesions of the pyramidal tract and in infants (in whom the tract is not yet myelinated) the great toe will be extended (Babinski's sign).
b. **Ankle jerk (S1, 2):** The foot is dorsiflexed slightly so as to put the tendo Achillis on the stretch. A gentle stroke on the back of the tendon leads to a momentary contraction of the calf muscles as evidenced by a sharp plantar flexion of the foot **(Fig. 17.2)**.
c. **Ankle clonus (S1, 2):** The patient's knee is slightly flexed and the leg is supported with one hand while the other hand over the sole of the forefoot makes sudden dorsiflexion of the foot. The foot will be set oscillating if slight pressure on the sole is maintained **(Fig. 17.3)**. This is pathognomonic of lesions of pyramidal system.
d. **Patellar clonus (L2,3,4):** Keeping the knee straight the patella is suddenly pushed downwards with the clinician's thumb and the index finger from its upper border and the pressure is maintained. When the test is positive there will be clonic movement of the patella due to clonic contraction of the quadriceps.
e. **Knee jerk (L2, 3, 4):** The patient should sit with one knee crossed over the other or if he is unable to sit, the flexed knee is allowed to rest on the clinician's hand. Now a sharp blow on the ligamentum patellae with the edge of the hand or with a percussion hammer will elicit a brisk contraction of the quadriceps, the leg being extended with a jerk **(Fig. 17.4)**.

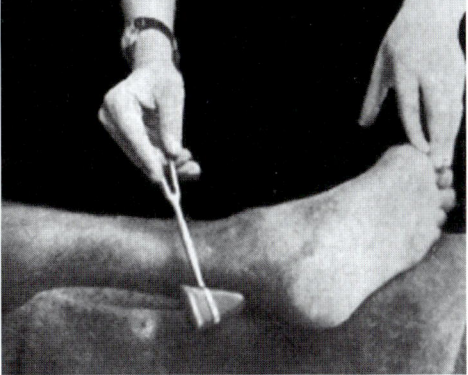

Fig.17.2: Shows how to elicit ankle jerk.

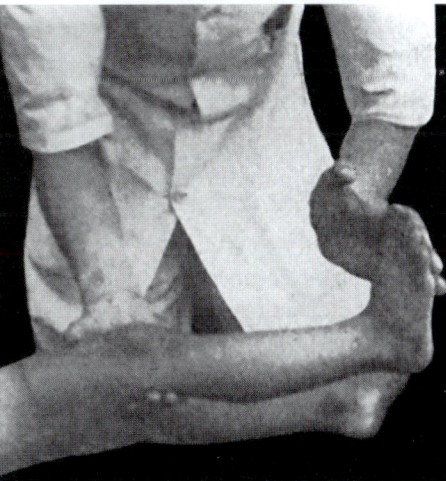

Fig.17.3: Shows how to elicit ankle clonus.

f. *Cremasteric reflex (T12):* This is elicited by scratching the skin at the upper and inner part of the thigh when the testis will be drawn upwards.

g. *Abdominal reflexes (T7 to 11)* are elicited by stroking the abdominal wall parallel to the costal margins and iliac crests and observing the movements of the umbilicus which indicate contraction of the abdominal muscles. These reflexes are abolished in lesions of the pyramidal tract.

h. *Triceps jerk (C7):* A tap just above the olecranon with the elbow flexed will bring about contraction of the triceps.

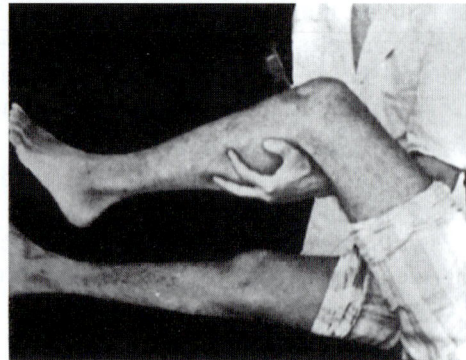

Fig.17.4: Shows how to elicit knee jerk.

i. *Biceps jerk (C5, 6):* Grasp the patient's elbow with the left hand so that the thumb rests on the biceps tendon. A tap on the examiner's thumb elicits contraction of the biceps.

It is useful to remember that in lesions of the pyramidal system, all deep or tendon reflexes are exaggerated, sometimes so much that a clonus can be elicited; the superficial or skin reflexes are diminished or absent (e.g., abdominal reflexes) or altered as in plantar reflex (Babinski's sign).

GENERAL EXAMINATION

1. **Examine the ears and nose.** Cerebral and cerebellar abscesses may develop during the course of chronic otitis media.
2. Presence of cutaneous **naevi** on the face often indicates a similar affection in the brain.
3. **Chest:** The lungs should be thoroughly examined for bronchiectasis, lung abscess, bronchial carcinoma, etc., since dissemination from the lungs into the brain is very common. An enquiry should also be made about hemoptysis, chronic cough and loss of weight.
4. **Abdomen** should also be examined for the presence of a primary growth, since the cerebral lesion may be secondary.
5. **Rectal examination** is necessary with particular attention to the condition of the prostate in the case of males.

SPECIAL INVESTIGATIONS

Besides examination of the urine and blood [including Wassermann reaction (WR), urea, nonprotein nitrogen (NPN) and erythrocyte sedimentation rate (ESR)] the following special investigations are essential.

1. **Lumbar puncture:** One should not do lumbar puncture in case with papilledema. This is mainly indicated to exclude nontumorous conditions.

a. *Pressure* should be measured by a manometer. Normally, it is about 120 mm of water. Any pressure above 160 mm would mean a raised intracranial pressure. If the pressure is high only a very small quantity of fluid should be drained since there is always the danger of herniation of the temporal lobe through the tentorium cerebelli and of the medulla through the foramen magnum. Although brain tumors are usually associated with increased pressure, yet a normal or even low pressure as measured by lumbar puncture is not unusual.

b. *The cellular content is* not markedly increased in the majority of cases, but in 10% of cases it is raised. In glioma it is more seen. Generally less than 50 cells are found, but one may find up to 100 cells due to necrosis of malignant glioma close to the ventricle.

c. *Protein content:* Considerable increase in protein content is sometimes found in neurofibromas of the auditory nerve and in meningiomas; in the latter condition it may rise up to 500 mg or even more. Normally, the protein content of the cerebrospinal fluid is 20–30 mg %. Protein content is generally increased in cases of tumors. Site of tumor is important in this respect and intraventricular or paraventricular tumors produce more protein level in CSF. Increase in number of cells and protein content (approximately 80 mg/100 mL) are seen in acute stage of cerebral abscess. Gradually the number of cells is reduced but the protein content increases to even 120 mg/100 mL.

d. *Wassermann reaction* of the cerebrospinal fluid should also be tested.

2. **Skiagraphy:** Straight X-ray films of the skull reveal many facts:

a. When the *intracranial tension is increased,* note the following points: (i) separation of all the sutures of the vault in children; (ii) hammer markings or 'beaten silver' appearance of the skull **(Fig. 17.5)**; (iii) simple dilatation of pituitary fossa with thinning of the posterior clinoid processes.

b. In *meningioma* (i) The skull shows three types of involvement: erosive, hypertrophic and sclerotic—the first type is frequently encountered in the vault and the last one at the base of the skull, whilst hyperostosis is found in either place: (ii) Enlarged vascular grooves caused by engorged meningeal veins; (iii) Calcification in the tumor.

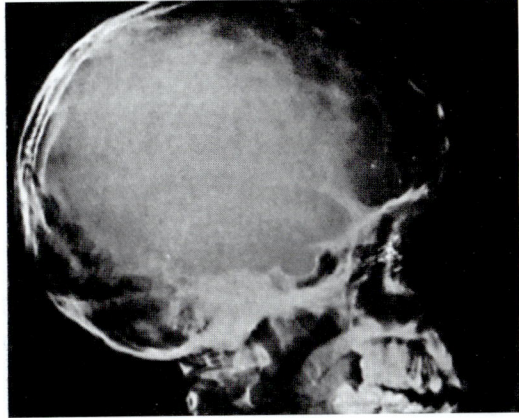

Fig.17.5: Note the 'beaten silver' appearance of the skull suggesting increased intracranial pressure. Note also the thinning of the posterior clinoid processes.

c. *Astrocytoma* also shows calcification. About 40% oligodendroglioma calcify.

d. In *suprasellar cyst,* patchy calcification is characteristic. Widened but shallow sella turcica with erosion of the clinoid processes is often evident.

e. *Pituitary adenoma* causes enlargement of the pituitary fossa; the enlargement is great and rarely regular—a fact that differentiates extrapituitary causes of enlargement of the pituitary fossa (internal hydrocephalus, suprasellar cyst).

f. Displacement of the calcified pineal body—*'pineal shift'*—is indicative of a large tumor in the opposite hemisphere.

g. Over half of the cases of *craniopharyngioma* and some tuberculomas show *calcification.*

X-ray of the **chest** should be taken for primary focus in the lungs since 30% of bronchial carcinoma comes with cerebral symptoms before any chest symptoms.

3. **Ventriculography** is done by passing a brain cannula into each lateral ventricle through a hole bored in the skull 7 cm above the external occipital protuberance and 3 cm from the middle line. The direction of the cannula will be so guided as to aim at the pupil of the same side. The ventricle will be found at a depth of about 5 cm from the surface. 5 mL of fluid is slowly withdrawn and a little less than 5 mL (to allow expansion at body temperature) of air is introduced. Skiagrams are taken immediately after. By means of ventriculography any alteration of the size, shape and

position of the ventricular system can be clearly visualized. Myodil ventriculography can be done by pushing 1.5 mL of myodil through anterior horn of the lateral ventricle.

4. **Encephalography** is the skiagraphy taken after replacing the cerebrospinal fluid by air or oxygen through a lumbar or cisternal puncture. First a lumbar puncture is performed and the operation table is tilted to about 45°, so that the head is uppermost, then for every 11 mL of fluid withdrawn 10 mL of oxygen is injected until about 45 mL has been introduced. This is immediately followed by skiagraphy. X-ray pictures will show gas in the basal cisternae, over the cortex and in the ventricles. This investigation is dangerous in cerebral tumors and should be reserved for low pressure cases with symptoms of epilepsy.

5. **Carotid angiography** is the skiagraphy taken immediately after the injection of 8–12 mL of 45% hypaque into the carotid artery. Three lateral films are exposed at intervals of two seconds. This is followed by further injection to obtain anteroposterior vessels. This method is helpful to demonstrate the presence or absence of an aneurysm or of an angiomatous tumor such as a meningioma.

6. **Vertebral angiography:** 30 mL of 50% hypaque is used for this. Either retrograde method through the brachial or femoral artery or horizontal approach just above the atlas is made.

7. **Electroencephalography** (EEG) is a modern method of localizing brain tumor. A cerebral tumor is electrically dead compared with the normal cortex. Tumors produce delta or theta waves on the surface. Occasionally, it gives a clue as to which side carotid angiography is to be carried out.

8. **Cerebral puncture:** If secondary carcinoma or malignant glioma or cyst is suspected cerebral puncture is very valuable investigation. A burr-hole is made on the site of the cyst or a tumor and aspirating needle or ventricular cannula is introduced into the cyst or the tumor for aspiration. A cyst produced by astrocytoma contains golden yellow colored fluid. A malignant cyst contains muddy nonclotting fluid. *Meningiomas* provide resistance to the aspirating cannula. After aspiration, air or thorotrast is injected into the cavity in order to produce a picture of the cyst.

9. **Biopsy:** A sample of the tumor may be obtained by the brain cannula during ventriculography or by means of a special punch such as that designed by Jackson.

10. **Echoencephalography:** Displacement of the midline structures above the tentorium can be detected by reflecting the sound waves from both sides of the skull off those structures. A shift of more than 0.5 cm will be revealed by this technique.

11. **Scintillation-encephalography**: Radioactive iodinated human serum albumin is used for this. On the third day after giving this isotope the scanning is done.

12. **Brain scan:** Intracranial tumor and other space-occupying lesions can now be diagnosed with no morbidity by brain scanning with a certainty of 80–90%. A locally increased concentration of injected radioisotope substance may be found. It can be visualized by an external scanner or camera, which produces a map of the radioactive distribution in the head. Its usefulness is immense and to narrate in short the main points are: (i) detection and localization of primary brain tumors; (ii) detection of cerebral metastases; (iii) differentiation between diffuse and focal inflammatory diseases, i.e., between diffuse meningoencephalitis and localized brain abscess; (iv) in the assessment of head injury, i.e., differentiation among simple concussion, contusion, extradural and subdural hemorrhages; (v) assessing the effect of carotid stenosis on cerebral blood flow and how it improves after endarterectomy.

In case of brain tumors, arteriography, ventriculography, pneumoencephalography can be used but they are complex and not without morbidity. Electroencephalography is not precise in localizing a brain tumor. Ultrasonic encephalography is more recent and quite safe, but indicates only lateral shift of the midline structure of the anterior half of the cranium. To the contrary radioisotope scanning is simple and free from risk. Even when angiography or ventriculography has revealed the site of lesion, scanning may give additional information which will be of great diagnostic value. The most commonly used isotopes are ^{131}I, ^{99m}Tc, etc. The optimum time for scanning in ^{131}I is about 24–48 hours whereas in ^{99m}Tc the optimum time for scanning is about 1–3 hours. Brain tumors are demonstrated as areas of increased activity on the scan or camera pictures. Intracranial non-malignant cystic lesions do not show significant uptake. The overall accuracy of detection of brain tumors by scanning varies between 65%–93%.

13. **CT scan:** When available, this has become the major method of diagnosis of intracranial space-occupying lesions. It indicates presence of the tumor with or without ventricular displacement or distension. It is also possible to know the type of the tumor. Meningioma and pituitary adenomas appear dense white, whereas glioma shows variable pattern of enhancement but usually appears less dense. Astrocytoma with cyst formation shows dark shadow. Secondary metastasis appears as multiple shadows. But sometimes exact nature of the tumor cannot be assessed by this investigation.

14. **Magnetic resonance Imaging (MRI) or nuclear magnetic resonance (NMR):** It presents excellent anatomical details of the brain. It is more sensitive than CT in detecting cerebral space-occupying lesions. It also helps in early detection of cerebral metastasis. For more detail the students are referred to the author's 'A Concise Textbook Of Surgery', in the section of 'Intracranial Tumors', in the chapter of 'The Head'.

CLASSIFICATION OF INTRACRANIAL TUMORS

This can be best classified under two headings—(A) Extracerebral and (B) Intracerebral.

A. **EXTRACEREBRAL Tumors** may be: (1) Meningioma, (2) Acoustic neuroma, (3) Pituitary adenoma, (4) Craniopharyngioma, (5) Teratoma, (6) Cholesteatoma, (7) Pinealoma, (8) Chordoma and (9) Retinoblastoma.

B. **INTRACEREBRAL Tumors** may be : (1) Glioma, (2) Metastatic carcinoma, (3) Hemangioma, (4) Colloid cyst, (5) Sarcoma and (6) Tuberculoma.

1. **Gliomas (43%):** They are subdivided according to the stage of development of the glial cells into (a) *Astrocytoma:* It is benign growth composed of star-shaped adult neuroglial tissue. It may occur at any age. In children it affects the cerebellum, whereas in adults it affects the frontal lobe most commonly. (b) *Oligodendroglioma:* It is also an adult cell tumor, the cells having short stunted processes. It affects the deep parts of the cerebrum in adults. (c) *Spongioblastoma Polare:* It arises from primitive unipolar or bipolar cells. It usually affects the optic chiasma, third ventricle and hypothalamus in young subjects. (d) *Medulloblastoma:* It is a highly malignant growth and affects the vermis of the cerebellum in children. It grows rapidly and gives rise to seeding metastases throughout the cerebral hemisphere and spinal meninges. (e) *Glioblastoma multiforme:* It arises as a result of malignant degeneration in a pre-existing astrocytoma and therefore occurs in the cerebrum of adult males. It contains all varieties of glial cells including giant cells. (f) *Ependymoma:* It is an uncommon tumor found mostly in fourth ventricle. Age of predilection is 2nd and 3rd decades. These tumors are slow growing and of low malignancy.

2. **Meningiomas (18%):** These tumors are essentially benign growths originating in the arachnoid villi. According to their situations, they are called *parasagittal,* when occurring along the superior longitudinal sinus; *frontobasal,* when occurring on the cribriform plate, sphenoid

wing and tuberculum sellae; and *posterior,* when occurring at the cerebellopontine angle and jugular foramen.

3. **Pituitary adenoma:** There are three types: chromophobe, acidophil and basophil. (a) *Chromophobe adenoma* affects usually women between the ages of 20 and 50. Headache and bitemporal hemianopia are the characteristic features. (b) *Acidophil adenoma* gives rise to gigantism in children and acromegaly in adults, owing to excessive production of growth hormone by the acidophil cells and inhibition of basophil sex secretion. (c) *Basophil adenoma* gives rise to Cushing syndrome. Females are mostly affected. There is accumulation of fat on the trunk, neck and face.

4. **Acoustic neurofibroma:** It is the most frequent variety of subtentorial tumor occurring in adult life.

5. **Metastatic tumors:** Most common primary site is the lung. Breast cancer, adenocarcinoma of kidney, intestinal carcinoma, carcinoma of prostate, neuroblastoma, malignant melanoma, etc., are known to metastasize in the brain.

6. **Tuberculoma:** It is quite common in this country. It occurs usually in children and frequently it is multiple. It affects cerebellum more often than cerebrum. It forms a well defined firm, spherical mass producing signs and symptoms of a tumor.

Classification of intracranial tumors

Type	Examples	Key clinical features
Primary brain tumors	Glioma, astrocytoma, medulloblastoma, pituitary adenoma	Progressive headache, focal neurological deficits, seizures
Secondary (metastatic) tumors	Lung, breast, melanoma, renal cell carcinoma	Rapid neurological deterioration, multiple lesions on imaging
Vascular lesions	Chronic subdural hematoma, cavernous angioma, AV malformation	Gradual onset confusion, headache, focal signs
Infective lesions	Brain abscess, tuberculoma	Fever, headache, signs of raised ICP
Cystic lesions	Colloid cyst, epidermoid cyst, craniopharyngioma	Hydrocephalus, headache worsened by position changes

■ DIAGNOSIS OF INTRACRANIAL TUMORS

Clinically, the diagnosis is made by the general and localizing symptoms.

❖ **General symptoms** due to increased intracranial pressure, are *headache, vomiting, dimness of vision, bradycardia* and *retarded cerebration.* They occur earliest in midline and posterior fossa tumors, early in temporal and parietal lobe tumors, and late in frontal lobe tumors. In a meningioma, their onset may be delayed for several years. *Hence the absence of these symptoms does not exclude an intracranial tumor.*

❖ **Localizing syndromes** depend upon the site of the tumor.

In frontal lobe tumors, there may be: (i) changes in personality, (ii) weakness of the opposite side of the face, and (iii) inability to count correctly due to involvement of Broca's area on the left side in right-handed persons.

In parietal lobe tumors, there are: (i) astereognosis, i.e., failure to recognize the size, shape and form of different objects, (ii) exaggerated deep reflexes, (iii) weakness on the opposite side.

In temporal lobe tumors, there may occur: (i) aphasia, (ii) hemianopia and (iii) uncinate fit with hallucination of smell in lesions of the uncinate gyrus.

In cerebellar tumors, there are: (i) ataxic gait with Romberg's sign, (ii) asthenia with absence of tendon reflexes, (iii) strabismus, (iv) nystagmus, (v) stiffness of the neck, etc.

DIAGNOSIS OF INTRACRANIAL ABSCESS

Acute stage presents with pyrexia and persistent headache. In the beginning there will be increased pulse rate, but with the advent of raised intracranial pressure the pulse rate will be gradually slowed down. Headache, irritability, drowsiness and tendency to vomiting are the usual features of this condition. CSF will show increased number of cells and high protein content.

Chronic state will be evident by fall in temperature and pulse rate, but appearance of a few particular physical signs. These physical signs will depend on the location of the abscess. In cerebellum—nystagmus, ataxia, incoordination and decreased tone will be evident on the affected side. In temporal lobe—upper motor neuron type of paralysis of the affected side, and in frontal lobe—contralateral facial weakness may be seen. Pallor, cachexia, intermittent headache are the general features accompanied with this condition. If the abscess continues to be enlarged any excess intracranial space will be utilized and gradually the clinical features of increased intracranial pressure will be evident.

Examinations of the ear and sinuses are very essential as intracranial infection often originates from infected condition of these regions.

Algorithmic Approach to Patient with Intracranial Space-occupying Lesions

Patient presents with headache, seizures, or neurological deficit

↓

Is there a history of trauma?
- Yes → Consider **chronic subdural hematoma, post-traumatic abscess**
- No → Consider **primary or secondary tumors, vascular lesions**

↓

Assess symptoms of raised intracranial pressure (ICP)
- Present (headache, vomiting, papilledema, bradycardia, altered consciousness)?
  – Yes → Perform **fundoscopy, CT/MRI brain**
  – No → Consider **localizing symptoms for focal lesion**

↓

Assess neurological deficits and seizures
- Focal deficits (hemiparesis, cranial nerve palsies)? → Suggests **mass effect from tumor or abscess**
- Seizures (first-time in adult)? → Suspect **space-occupying lesion**

↓

Is there a mass effect on imaging (CT/MRI)?
- Yes → Proceed with **biopsy or neurosurgical referral**
- No → Consider **infective, inflammatory, or vascular causes**

↓

Perform special investigations
- CSF analysis (lumbar puncture) – avoid if papilledema
- EEG (for seizure activity in suspected tumor)
- PET scan (for metastatic workup, if primary tumor suspected)

↓

Determine need for surgery, radiotherapy, or chemotherapy
- Surgical resection? → If resectable tumor or abscess
- Radiotherapy and chemotherapy? → If glioblastoma, metastatic tumor
- Medical management? → If benign tumor, infection, or nonoperable condition

↓

Admit and monitor for neurological deterioration
- Monitor for worsening GCS, seizures, or new-onset symptoms
- Repeat imaging in progressive cases

Examination of Spinal Injuries

CHAPTER 18

HISTORY

The type of spinal injury depends on the severity of the violence. Sudden jolt as may occur in car or bus accident or at the time of lifting weight from bent position may cause injury to the spinal ligaments. Fractures and fracture-dislocation usually result from severe violence, e.g., fall from a height or fall of a heavy weight on the back. Diving is shallow water may cause dislocation of the cervical vertebrae. Pure dislocation is not seen in thoracic or lumbar region. Car accident following a sudden break when the seat-belt is fastened may cause injury to the lumbar vertebrae. This is commonly known as 'seat-belt injury'. In civil life most injuries are due to indirect violence and the most common site of lesion is about C6. The second most frequent site is in the region of L1. The thoracic region is seldom involved. If there is paralysis, enquire into the time and mode of its onset. Immediate paralysis is due to compression or crushing of the spinal cord in fracture-dislocation. Paraplegia which has occurred late and is gradually extending upwards may be due to traumatic intraspinal hemorrhage. Hemorrhage may occur within the cord itself (hematomyelia) or in the extramedullary region (hematorrachis). In the latter condition the blood will escape either into the extradural space or into the cerebrospinal fluid. The patient must be asked whether there is any sense of constriction around the trunk (girdle pain). If present, note its level.

History in spinal injuries

Aspect	Clinical significance	Patient-friendly questions
Mechanism of injury	Helps differentiate **fracture, dislocation, ligament injury**	"How did the injury happen? Were you in a car accident, fall, or direct impact?"
Immediate vs delayed symptoms	**Immediate paralysis** → Spinal cord injury; **Delayed** → hemorrhage or edema	"Did you feel weakness or numbness immediately after the injury, or did it develop later?"
Pain characteristics	**Localized pain** → Fracture; **Radiating pain** → Nerve root compression	"Do you have pain in your back or does it radiate to your arms or legs?"
Loss of sensation	Suggests **spinal cord or nerve root injury**	"Do you have numbness or tingling anywhere?"
Weakness or paralysis	Indicates **spinal cord or peripheral nerve involvement**	"Can you move your arms and legs normally?"

Contd...

Contd...

Aspect	Clinical significance	Patient-friendly questions
Bowel and bladder dysfunction	**Urinary retention → Cauda equina syndrome**	"Are you having trouble urinating or controlling your bowels?"
Previous spinal problems	**History of disc disease or Osteoporosis → Higher risk of injury**	"Have you had any previous back or neck issues?"

■ EXAMINATION FOR SPINAL CORD INJURIES

This should be carried out before examination of the spinal column since in presence of cord lesion, patient should be disturbed as little as possible.

A. UPPER LIMBS

1. **Attitude (Figs. 18.1A and B):** According to the level of fracture-dislocation of the cervical region, the upper extremities assume a characteristic attitude. If they lie immobile against the trunk and complete- ly paralyzed the level of *injury is at the 5th cervical segment*, because any severe lesion above this level will cause paralysis of the phrenic nerve and will lead to immediate death. When the *lesion is at the 6th cervical segment* the patient lies helplessly on the back with the arm abducted and externally rotated and the forearm flexed and supinated. The attitude is caused by irritation of the 5th cervical segment which supplies supraspinatus and deltoid to cause abduction of the shoulder; infraspinatus and teres minor to cause lateral rotation of the shoulder; biceps causes flexion and supination of forearm. In *lesion of the 7th cervical segment* the arm is partially abducted and internally rotated with the forearm flexed and pronated—possibly due to irritation of the 6th cervical segment which supplies teres major, anterior fibers of deltoid and subscapularis to cause internal rotation of shoulder; biceps and mainly brachioradialis to cause midprone flexion of elbow. In case of *lesion of the 8th cervical and 1st dorsal segments*

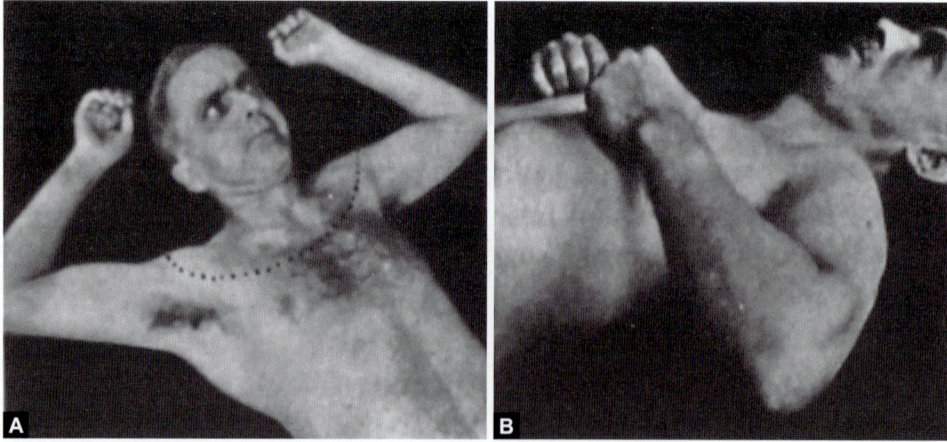

Figs. 18.1A and B: Show the attitudes in lesions at the 6th and 7th cervical segments caused by irritation of the 5th and 6th segments respectively. The dotted line in the A represents the upper limit of the sensory loss obtained in both the lesions.

there will be paralysis of the intrinsic muscles of the hand and will lead to a deformity known as 'main-en-griffe'. Any *lesion below the 1st dorsal segment* will not cause any impairment of the movement of the upper extremities upto the finger tips.

2. **Sensation:** Sensation of various parts of the upper limb is tested by pin prick, a wisp of cotton, a test tube with cold or hot water or with reverse of a tuning fork. Loss of sensation will be according to the level of cord lesion. There is a zone of hyperaesthesia between the normal and anesthetic skin.

3. **Muscle power:** This is tested of various muscles against resistance. According to the level of cord lesion, various muscles of the upper limb will lose power.

B. LOWER LIMBS

1. **Attitude:** The whole of the lower limb will lie helplessly paralyzed when the level of the spinal cord injury is at or above 10th thoracic vertebra. When the injury is below the 1st lumbar vertebra only the cauda equina will be injured and the lower limb below the knee will be affected and will lie flaccid paralyzed.

2. **Muscle power:** If the patient walks about, it may be assumed that there is no injury to the cord. In the supine position the patient is asked to move his ankles and toes against resistance. The patient is also asked to raise the legs one after the other. By this one can assess the muscle power of the lower limb muscles. Similarly, the patient is asked to move the upper limb against resistance.

3. **Sensation:** This is tested by pin prick, a wisp of cotton or a test tube with hot or cold water. Loss of sensation will be according to the level of cord lesion or injury to the cauda equina. Run the point of a pin from anesthetic to the normal area and note if there is a zone of hyperesthesia intervening. In cauda equina lesion, the sacral roots may be involved producing anesthesia in the back of the legs and a saddle area of the perineum with urinary retention.

4. **Reflexes:** Initially, all the reflexes may be lost during the stage of spinal shock. Gradually, the reflexes reappear according to the level of the lesion. The time laps between disappearance and reappearance of the reflexes depends on the severity of the cord lesion. In severe cases it may take as long as 3 weeks for the return of reflexes. If the reflexes fail to return by this time complete transverse section of the cord may be suspected. The bladder center is situated at the lumbar enlargement representing the 2nd to the 4th sacral segments. This center is concerned in supplying the detrusor muscle of the bladder and injury to this level of cord will lead to paralysis of the detrusor muscle resulting in overflow incontinence. The patient however retains the nerve supply of the abdominal muscles which may be contracted voluntarily at a time interval to evacuate the bladder. This process may be assisted by suprapubic compression with the help of the patient's both hands. In case of lesion of the spinal cord above the lumbar enlargement, after an initial phase of retention due to spinal shock, the bladder reflexes reappear and become uninhibited by the superior control resulting in an automatic bladder, i.e., the bladder evacuates by itself as soon as the intravesical pressure rises to a certain extent. The patient has to wear a receptacle in these cases.

Note the nature of the **respiration**. It is abdominal in lesion above T_2 due to paralysis of the intercostal muscles.

Look for the **distended bladder, incontinence of urine** and **priapism** (persistent erection of the penis).

In long standing cases one may expect presence of **trophic ulcer**—bed sores over the pressure points.

EXAMINATION OF THE SPINAL COLUMN

When the patient is brought in with paralysis, utmost care has to be exerted during the examination of the spinal column. If the patient is rotated, the unstable fracture may increase damage to the spinal cord. Even without paralysis these cases should be handled with extreme care. The patient may be lifted by an assistant just sufficiently to permit the surgeon's hand to be introduced under the site of the lesion. The patient may be examined in a better way if he is very carefully turned by at least two, preferably by three persons on to one side.

Only in cases when the surgeon is absolutely confident that the patient does not suffer from any unstable injury to the spinal column that the patient may be examined in standing or sitting posture.

A. Inspection

At first the skin of the back is inspected for presence of any abrasion or bruising to indicate the probable level of injury. One should also look for a swelling, which may indicate a hematoma or a prominent spinous process due to fracture-dislocation.

B. Palpation

First of all the spinal column is palpated by running a finger along the spinous processes and transverse processes. *Holdswath test* is performed by running a finger along the spinous processes. Abnormal gap in the line of the spinous processes indicates tear in the interspinous ligament which indicates unstable fracture. Abnormal prominence of a spinous process indicates fracture-dislocation of the spine, the most prominent spinous process is the one below the displaced vertebra. But in compression fracture the most prominent spine is the one above the crushed vertebra. Swelling in this region usually indicates a hematoma which will elicit fluctuation.

Pressure is exerted along the line of the spinous processes of the vertebrae with the thumb of the clinician **(Fig. 18.2)**. In case of sprain of the spinal column, there will be localized tenderness at the site of the ligamentous injury. If the muscle fibers are torn similar tender spot can be elicited. In fracture of the vertebra, however minor, will produce tenderness when pressure is exerted on the corresponding spinous process.

Active testing for abnormal mobility is **contraindicated** in suspected spinal injuries, as it may **worsen spinal cord damage**. Instead, priority should be given to **immediate immobilization and radiographic assessment** to confirm spinal stability.

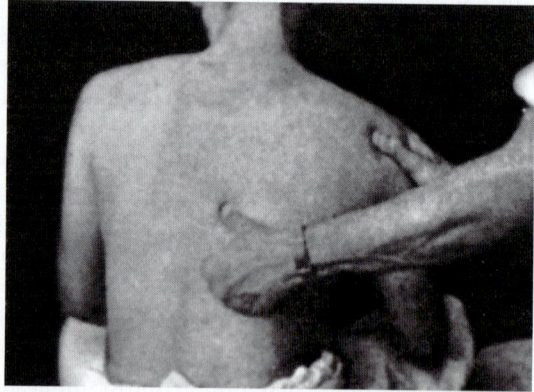

Fig. 18.2: Shows how to examine for tenderness of the corresponding spinous process in injury to the vertebral column.

Percussion—gently with fingertip over the spinous processes will elicit tenderness if there is fracture of the spinal column.

Movements of the spinal column are *not* tested at this stage until and unless the clinician is sure that the patient is not having any fracture of the spinal column which may cause injury to the spinal cord due to such movement.

Rectal examination will help in detecting fracture of the coccyx.

GENERAL EXAMINATION

A **thorough secondary survey** should be performed to assess for associated injuries, particularly **abdominal trauma**, which is a leading cause of mortality in spinal injury patients and often requires urgent surgery. **Head trauma** must also be carefully evaluated, given the high co-occurrence of spinal and cranial injuries in falls and road traffic accidents. A careful watch must be made all throughout the scalp along with palpation to exclude such injury. Next comes the **thoracic injury**. Transverse pressure towards the midline from both sides of the thoracic cage will elicit tenderness if there is any fracture of the rib of sternum. To exclude sternal fracture the clinician should press along the sternum from above downwards for its whole extent, which is often missed. **Injury to the pelvis** is excluded by a transverse pressure on both the iliac crests with both hands towards the midline (*see* **Fig. 13.27**). Fracture of the ilium will show tenderness. Lastly one should exclude any **injury to the limb** which may be associated with such type of injury.

SPECIAL INVESTIGATIONS

X-RAY EXAMINATION

Two views anteroposterior and lateral must always be taken and compare the depths of the vertebrae. A **slight reduction in vertebral body height** on a lateral X-ray may be the only sign of a wedge or compression fracture, making it easily missed. **Unlike Pott's disease, compression fractures do not cause narrowing of the adjacent intervertebral disc spaces**. It may be emphasized here that there will be no narrowing of the intervertebral space (**Fig. 18.3**) (cf. Pott's disease, *see* **Fig. 19.28** page 347). In case of fracture-dislocation the line of the posterior surfaces of the bodies of the vertebrae is noted. If any vertebra has encroached on the spinal canal that vertebra is supposed to be fracture-dislocated. A fracture of the transverse process of the vertebra is best seen in the anteroposterior view.

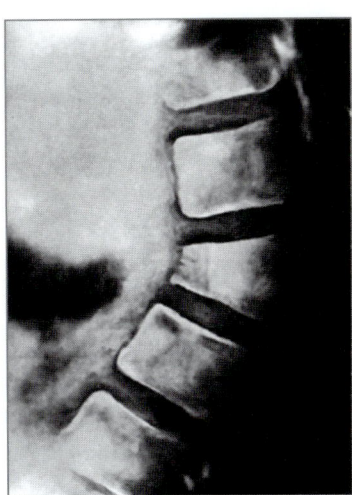

Fig. 18.3: Wedge or compression fracture following flexion injury. Note that there is no narrowing of the intervertebral space above and below the affected vertebra.

DIAGNOSIS

FRACTURES OF THE SPINE

As fracture of the spine is often associated with damage to the spinal cord, the fracture of the spine is best classified into *stable* and *unstable* fractures. **STABLE** fractures are those which are not associated with cord damage and movement of the spine is safe. Whereas **UNSTABLE** fractures are either associated with cord damage or if not, movement of the spine can damage the spinal cord. Various types of spine fractures are shown in **Figures 18.4A to D**.

Stability does not depend on the fracture itself only, but on the integrity of the ligaments, particularly the posterior ligament complex, being formed by the supraspinous, interspinous ligaments, the capsules of the facet joints and possibly the ligamentum flavum.

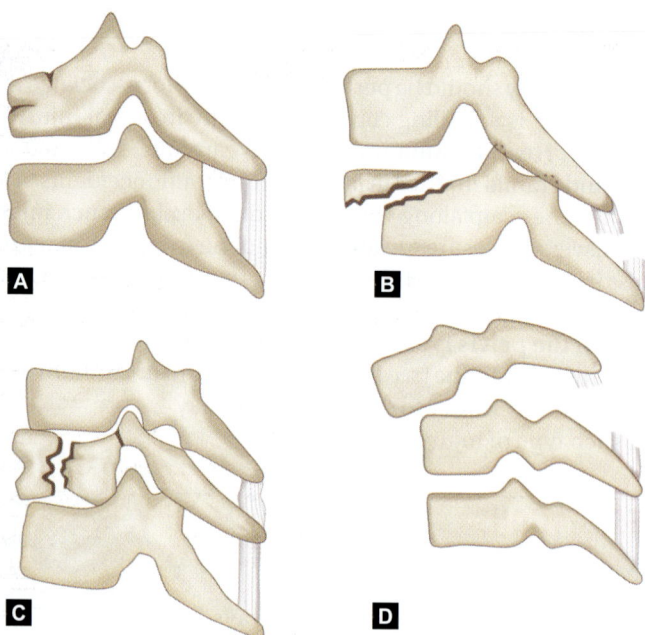

Figs. 18.4A to D: Diagrammatic representation of various types of fractures of the spine.
(A) Crush fracture; (B) Fracture-dislocation; (C) Burst fracture; (D) Dislocation without fracture.

Burst fracture: Here the compression force acts on the straight position of the spine. The body of the vertebra fractures vertically. This is a stable injury.

Backward hinge (extension injury): In the cervical region it may fracture atlas or axis, anterior ligaments may tear. This is also stable injury. In the lumbar region it may result in fractured lamina. Young toddler, who falls on his buttock, may sustain such an injury and may be the starting point of spondylolisthesis.

Forward hinge (flexion injury)—is common in lumbar vertebrae. The posterior ligaments will remain intact but the body of the vertebra crumples. This is stable. These injuries are rare in the neck as the chin touches the sternum before any fracture occurs.

Shearing force—causes instability. Rotation causes ligamentous damage. Usually rotation is associated with flexion. A slice of bone may be sheared off the top of one vertebra and the posterior facet is fractured.

Fractures of the spinous processes, transverse processes and laminae are grouped under the nomenclature of *'incomplete fractures'*. These are mostly due to direct violence. Spinous processes are most liable to fracture in the dorsal region, and Shoveller's fracture of the 7th cervical spine is really a stress fracture. Transverse processes are most prone to be fractured in the lumbar region as they are longer and rather unprotected.

DISLOCATION OF THE SPINE

A dislocation without fracture occurs mostly in the cervical region. The oblique and vertical directions of the articular processes in the thoracic and lumbar regions, respectively, will not allow dislocation without a fracture. Barring dislocation following hanging, which occurs between the atlas and axis, dislocation of the cervical spine usually occurs between the 4th and 5th or 5th and 6th, caused by acute flexion resulting from fall on the head. In unilateral cases, the head is deviated to the opposite side with severe pain referred along the corresponding nerve root which is nipped in the intervertebral foramen. In the lumbar spine a comparable mechanism occurs in the so called 'seat-belt fracture', where following a car accident the body is thrown forward against the seat belt. The posterior ligaments are torn but there may be no fracture. The spine however is angulated and the upper facet may leap-frog over the lower.

INJURY TO THE CORD

Typically four types of injury to the cord may be seen:

1. **Cord concussion (shock):** The disturbance is one of function without any demonstrable and anatomical lesion. Motor paralysis (flaccid), sensory loss and visceral paralysis—all occur below the level of the injury to the cord. Recovery begins within 6 hours and it is always complete.
2. **Complete contusion of the cord:** This condition is produced by nipping of the cord between the lamina of the displaced vertebra above and the edge of the fractured vertebra below. It causes transverse contusion, above and below of which there will be minute petechial hemorrhage. Immediately after injury there will be a stage of spinal shock. After this period, the cord below the transection recovers from the shock and acts as an independent structure. The plantar reflex becomes extensor, the anal and bladder reflexes return. The tendon reflexes will be exaggerated with presence of the clonus. Flexor spasms may develop and sensation never returns. There will be retention of urine and the bladder becomes 'automatic'.
3. **Root transection:** It occurs due to injury of the nerve roots. There will be motor paralysis, sensory loss and visceral paralysis along the distribution of the damaged roots. Root transection differs from cord transection in two ways: (i) Residual motor paralysis is always flaccid in nature and (ii) Regeneration is theoretically possible (being peripheral nervous system). Cauda equina injury comes under this category.
4. **Traumatic intraspinal hemorrhage:** Hemorrhage may occur either within the cord itself (hematomyelia) or in the extramedullary region (hematorrachis). In the latter condition blood escapes either into the extradural space or into the cerebrospinal fluid. Intradural hemorrhage leads to paralysis without causing prior spinal irritation. But in extramedullary hemorrhage there will be spinal irritation, hyperesthesia, pain etc., which will precede paraplegia due to progressive compression of the cord from below upwards.

Algorithmic Approach to Patient with Spinal Injuries

Patient presents with back or neck pain after trauma

↓

Is the patient conscious?
- Yes → Proceed with **neurological deficit assessment and history-taking**
- No → **Immediate airway and spine stabilization**

↓

Is there a history of high-energy trauma?
- Yes → Assume **unstable spinal injury until proven otherwise**
- No → Consider **soft tissue injury or stable fracture**

↓

Assess for neurological deficits (motor, sensory, reflexes)
- Complete spinal cord injury → No sensation or movement below lesion
- Incomplete spinal cord injury → Variable weakness and sensory loss

↓

Is there bowel/bladder dysfunction?
- Yes → Consider **cauda equina syndrome or high spinal cord injury**
- No → Monitor for progressive neurological deterioration

↓

Perform imaging based on stability and symptoms
- X-ray/CT → Best for fractures, dislocations
- MRI → Best for cord compression, hemorrhage, ligament injury

↓

Determine management based on stability
- Stable fracture → Conservative management (brace, physiotherapy)
- Unstable fracture → Surgical fixation and spinal decompression

↓

Admit and monitor for neurological deterioration
- Frequent GCS and motor sensory assessments
- Prepare for rehabilitation and long-term management if needed

Examination of Spinal Abnormalities

CHAPTER 19

HISTORY

1. **Age:** Spina bifida is seen in newborn babies. Spina bifida occulta may present late till adolescent or adult stage. It may be revealed accidentally later in life during X-ray examination for some other reason. Pott's disease is more often seen among children. Disc prolapse is seen commonly in middle aged persons. Idiopathic spondylolisthesis is commonly seen in individuals of 4th and 5th decades of life. Ankylosing spondylitis is a disease of young adult affecting usually individuals between the ages of 15 and 35 years. Majority of the primary carcinomas of the vertebral column occur in children and young adults, whereas secondary deposits in the vertebral column are common in aged people above 40 years of age.
2. **Sex:** Ankylosing spondylitis, prolapsed intervertebral disc and osteoarthritis are common in males. Psychogenic backache, osteomalacia and ligamentous strain are more common in females.
3. **Trauma:** An enquiry must be made whether trauma initiated the presenting complaints or it aggravates these. Very often the patient complains that while raising a weight from the floor he suddenly experienced a strain or catch or bursting pain in the spine. This history itself is very suggestive of lumbar disc prolapse.
4. **Pain:** This is in fact the most common symptom of spinal column abnormalities. An enquiry must be made about onset, exact site, its nature, any radiation or presence of any referred pain. Dull and continuous pain is a feature of inflammatory lesion of the spine which will be aggravated by movement. A sudden sharp pain may be complained of in case of prolapse of the intervertebral disc during lifting weight in the stooping position. In majority of pathological lesions of the spine movement aggravates the pain.
   a. *Site:* While taking history, ask the patient to point out from where actually the backache started—in the cervical region, or in the dorsal region, in the lumbodorsal region or in the lumbar region, in the lumbosacral region or in the sacral region.
   b. *Mode of onset:* Whether the pain started immediately after trauma or lifting weight or during strenuous exercises as seen in prolapsed intervertebral disc or whether the pain appears late only after the pathology is well established, e.g., tuberculosis of the spine.
   c. *Nature of pain:* Pain is sharp stabbing or of shooting in nature in case of prolapse of the intervertebral disc. It is of continuous and throbbing type in case of acute osteomyelitis. Pain is usually intermittent and dull, which gets worse after exercises in case of spondylolisthesis. Pain comes on suddenly and is very severe while the patient bends back in case of fibrositis or lumbago. Pain is usually mild in nature but is aggravated by movement of the spine in case of secondary carcinoma of the spine. It must be remembered that such pain is increased with the increase in intradural pressure, e.g., coughing, sneezing or defecation. Pain is of dull ache character in Pott's disease (spinal tuberculosis). In thoracolumbar tuberculous disease one may

experience 'girdle pain'. Pain increases at night, which is known as 'night cry'. Pain of ankylosing spondylitis is usually intermittent and is mainly experienced on getting up in the morning. This is often accompanied with stiffness of the spine.

d. **Radiation:** In majority of pathological conditions of the spinal column pain usually radiates along the course of the spinal nerves. A careful history must be taken about the precise nature of such radiation. In case of prolapsed intervertebral disc pain radiates along the root of the nerve affected. In case of spondylolisthesis sciatic pain along one or both lower limbs is sometimes complained of. In case of extramedullary tumors, e.g., neurofibromas affecting posterior nerve roots, pain radiates along the nerve roots. In caries (tuberculosis) of the cervical spine pain is often referred over the occiput and to the arms.

Pain radiation follows **nerve root involvement**:
- **Cervical tuberculosis** → Pain radiates to occiput and arms.
- **Thoracic tuberculosis** → Pain follows **intercostal nerve** distribution.
- **Lumbar tuberculosis** → Pain radiates to **hip and legs** (mimicking sciatica).

In thoracolumbar caries one may experience 'girdle pain' or epigastric pain. In ankylosing spondylitis pain is sometimes complained of along the distribution of the sciatic nerve (sciatica), but the peculiarity is that it alternates from one side to the other.

e. *Aggravating factors:* As mentioned above in majority of pathological lesions of the spine, movement aggravates the pain. In case of secondary carcinoma of the vertebral body, increase in intradural pressure, e.g., coughing, sneezing or defecation will cause increase in pain. In the initial stage of tuberculosis of spine the pain is of dull ache character, which gets worse during standing or jolting. In spondylolisthesis pain is usually intermittent and of dull ache nature which gets worse after exercise.

f. *Relieving factors:* In majority of spinal column pathologies pain is usually relieved by rest.

5. **Deformity:** In a number of cases of spinal pathologies patients present with deformity of the spine. A swelling is seen in meningocele. In spina bifida occulta there may be a dimple or a tuft of hair or dilated vessels or fibrofatty tumor or a naevolipoma over the bony deficiency in the lumbosacral region. Scoliosis or kyphosis or lordosis is often noticed in pathologies of spine. These are discussed later in this chapter in the section of 'Differential Diagnosis'. A typical deformity is also seen in case of spondylolisthesis in which the sacrum becomes unduly prominent with deep transverse furrows seen on both sides of the trunk between the ribs and iliac crests (*see* **Figs. 19.4A and B**).

6. **Stiffness of the back:** This is occasionally complained of alongwith pain and definitely the latter symptom predominates. Only in ankylosing spondylitis stiffness of back is a prominent symptom, though this is sometimes complained of in cases of tuberculosis of the spine.

7. **Other symptoms:** Enquiry must be made if there is any complaint of the abdomen or gynecological problem or genitourinary problem or vascular disorders. These conditions may give rise to low back pain.

8. **Family history:** Tuberculosis of the spine and ankylosing spondylitis sometime run in families. Even prolapsed intervertebral disc has been seen to involve more than one member in a family. So family history is important.

History in spinal abnormalities

Aspect	Clinical significance	Patient-friendly questions
Age	Helps diagnose **age-related spinal conditions**	"How old are you?"
Onset of pain	Acute → Trauma/disc prolapse, chronic → Degenerative/infective	"Did the pain start suddenly or gradually?"

Contd...

Aspect	Clinical significance	Patient-friendly questions
Radiation of pain	Follows nerve root compression patterns	"Does the pain travel down your legs or arms?"
Stiffness	Prominent in ankylosing spondylitis	"Do you feel stiff in the morning?"
Night pain	Red flag for tumors, infections	"Does the pain wake you up at night?"

GENERAL SURVEY

The victims of tuberculosis of the spine are usually from low social class with malnutrition, anemia and sometimes cachexia. In case of secondary carcinoma of the spine, patients often give history of quick loss of weight in near past. Spondylolisthesis is often seen among over weight individuals. In ankylosing spondylitis malaise, fatigue and loss of weight are often complained of.

Fever or rise of temperature is mainly come across in inflammatory conditions of the spine. Rise in night temperature is noticed in tuberculosis of the spine.

LOCAL EXAMINATION

A. INSPECTION

For proper inspection exposure of the entire posterior aspect of the patient from head to foot is required, even the shoes are removed to avoid the effect of high heel. The arms should hang by the side.

1. **Attitude and deformity:** In caries of the cervical spine the child often supports his head with both the hands under the chin and twists his whole body in order to look sideways. Later on the position of the head becomes similar to that in torticollis. In tuberculosis of the dorsolumbar region there will be a prominent gibbus and the spinal column becomes kyphosed **(Figs. 19.1A and B)**. Its level must be determined.

The back of the patient is carefully observed. Starting from above note: (i) Position of the head, whether bent or twisted to one side; (ii) the level of the shoulders; (iii) the position of the scapulae, whether one is elevated or displaced forward, backward, laterally or medially; (iv) the lateral margins of the body from axilla to the crest of the ilium—whether the affected

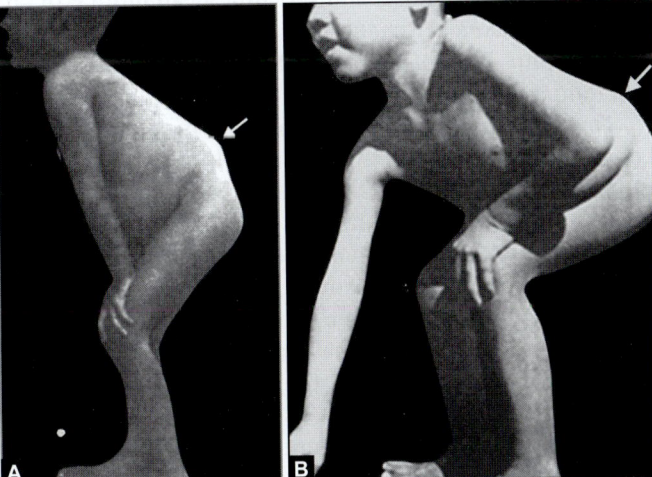

Figs. 19.1A and B: (A) The attitude in caries on the dorsolumbar region. The arrow shows the gibbus; (B) The boy with caries of the dorsolumbar region is picking up a coin from the floor by bending the knees.

side is flatter or more curved than the other; (v) the relative prominence of the iliac crest, e.g., spondylolisthesis; (vi) the curvature of the spine, whether there is kyphosis **(Fig. 19.2)**, i.e., forward bending; lordosis, i.e., backward bending; or scoliosis, i.e., side-bending with rotational deformity. In each case the level of deformity is always estimated **(Fig. 19.3)**.

In case of *scoliosis,* ascertain the side of primary curve. To determine, the spinous processes are marked out with a skin pencil. It should be remembered that the bodies of the vertebrae are rotated towards the convexity of the curve and the spinous processes are rotated towards the concavity. Differentiation should immediately be made between mobile scoliosis (transient) and fixed scoliosis (structural). In case of scoliosis if the patient is asked to lean forward, postural scoliosis will disappear whereas structural scoliosis will be more prominent. In case of compensatory scoliosis, mostly due to short lower limb the patient is asked to sit down and this scoliosis disappears.

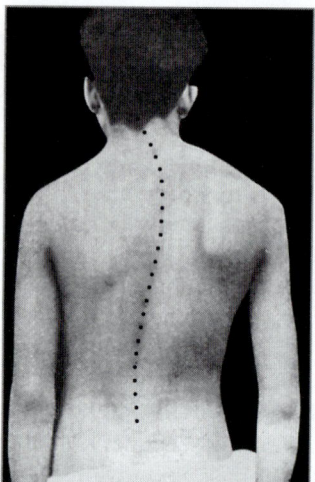

Fig. 19.2: Scoliosis with convexity to the right side. The spinous processes are marked with dots. Note that the scapula of the right side is elevated.

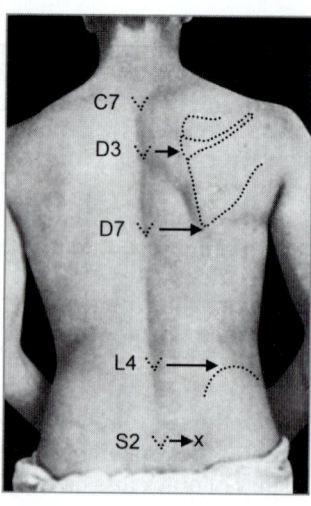

Fig. 19.3: Shows the landmarks which help to ascertain the various levels of the spine.

In case of *kyphosis* the type of deformity must be noted—whether of the "knuckle" type, i.e., one spinous process becomes prominent indicating collapse of one vertebra as occurs in tuberculosis; or "angular" resulting from collapse of two or three vertebral bodies as occurs in late cases of tuberculosis and secondary carcinoma; or "round" where several vertebrae are affected as occurs in Scheuermann's disease and in senile kyphosis. It must be remembered that in kyphosis age of the patient is very important in determining the underlying disease (*see* differential diagnosis).

Lordosis is mostly compensatory and may be due to flexion deformity of the hip, bilateral congenital dislocation of the hip or rarely due to kyphosis of the dorsal region.

In *spondylolisthesis,* a transverse furrow is seen encircling the body between the costal margin and the iliac crest with diminution of this space. The upper angle of the sacrum forms a distinct prominence with a depression just above it **(Figs. 19.4A and B)**.

Now the front of the patient is carefully observed. In scoliosis, the chest diagonally opposite to posterior convexity is more prominent. In advanced kyphosis, the sternum also becomes convex anteriorly to compensate for the diminished vertebral measurement of the thorax. The ribs are crowded together. The anterior superior iliac spines are noted whether they are in same level or not.

2. **Gait:** As soon as the patient enters the clinic one can come to a diagnosis by just looking at the gait. In caries of the spine the patient walks with short step and often on the toes to avoid jerking on the spine. In case of sciatica the patient accounts the typical gait. In case of sacroiliac arthritis the patient may limp and if this condition is bilateral a 'waddling gait' may be seen.

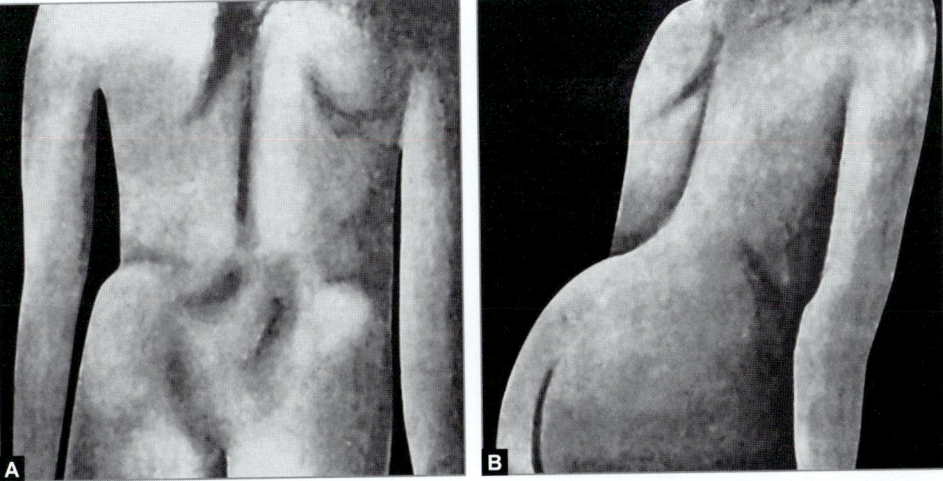

Figs. 19.4A and B: Spondylolisthesis—showing a transverse furrow just above the iliac crest. Note that the upper edge of the sacrum is prominent.

3. **Swelling:** In spina bifida **(Fig. 19.5)**, a meningocele may be present in the sacral or in the occipital region. If this is detected one should look for talipes (*see* **Fig. 21.1**) which may be associated with it. In spina bifida occulta, there may be a swelling, a tuft of hair, dilated vessels, a fibrofatty tumor or even a dimple to show the point of attachment of membrana reuniens to the skin. Congenital sacrococcygeal teratoma is occasionally seen in the sacrococcygeal region. In Pott's disease abscess may be seen in various places—paravertebral abscess, psoas abscess, behind the sternomastoid muscle, abscess on the lateral chest wall following the lateral cutaneous nerve, at the Petit's triangle, abscess in the buttock, etc.

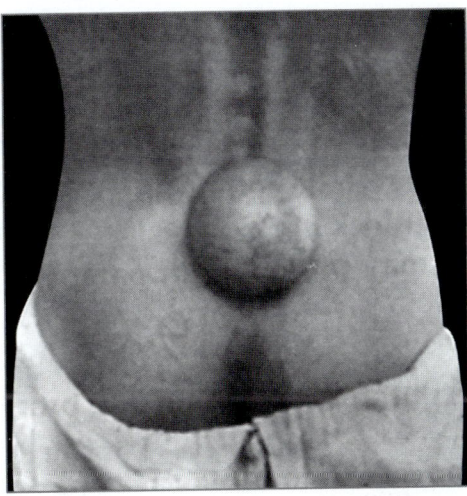

Fig. 19.5: A lipoma in spina bifida occulta.

4. **Paraplegia:** In caries of the thoracic region the patient may present with paraplegia which is quite obvious on inspection.

B. PALPATION

This is carried out in the standing and prone positions:

Tenderness: A thumb may be pressed along the spinous processes from above downwards along its whole extent. Note the level of maximum tenderness. Tenderness may be elicited by pressing upon the side of the spinous process in an attempt to rotate the vertebra **(Fig. 19.6)**. This can also be elicited by applying gentle blows on either side of the spine **(Fig. 19.7)**. Tenderness can also be elicited by percussing on the spinous processes with a finger **(Fig. 19.8)**. An exquisitely tender area may indicate torn muscle fiber or ligamentous tear. It must be remembered that at times the patient may flinch with pain as soon as the skin is being touched. In such cases pinch up the skin to differentiate whether the pain is in the skin or in the spine. In hysterical

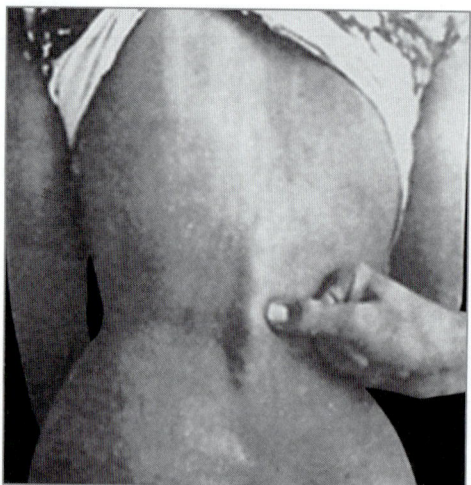

Fig. 19.6: An attempt is being made to rotate the vertebra by pressing on the side of the spinous process. This will elicit tenderness in pathologies of the spinal column.

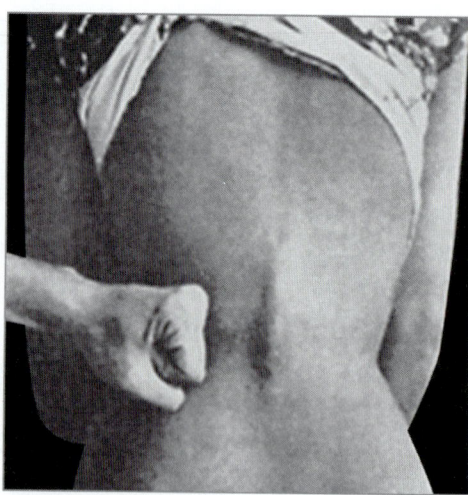

Fig. 19.7: Gentle blows are made on either side of the spine to elicit tenderness.

spine there is always cutaneous hypersensitivity. It is not advisable to perform the *anvil test* **(Fig. 19.9)** always to elicit tenderness in the spine. In this test sudden jerk is applied over the head or the patient is asked to jump down from a chair. However this test should be reserved just to exclude any tenderness in the spine.

1. **Swelling:** Swellings are of two types in relation with spinal pathology: (i) Cold abscess **(Figs. 19.10 to 19.13)** arising from the spinal column and may be seen in different places, e.g., behind sternomastoid muscle (in cervical caries), in the mediastinum, in the lateral thoracic wall (in thoracic caries), psoas abscess, lumbar abscess, abscess in the buttock and pelvic abscess

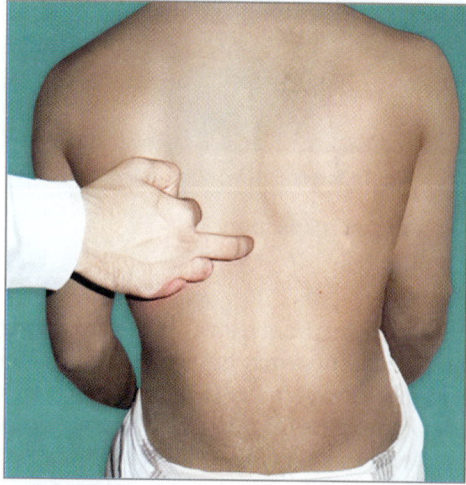

Fig. 19.8: Method of eliciting tenderness by percussing on the spinous processes with a finger in case of pathology of the vertebrae.

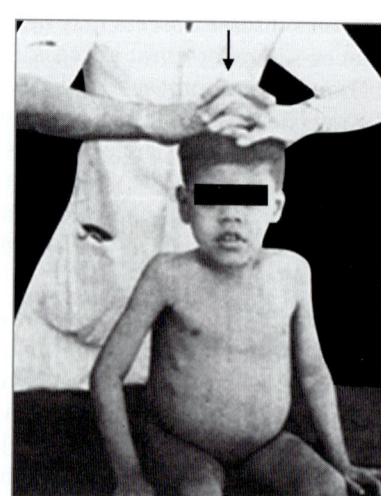

Fig. 19.9: Anvil test. See the text.

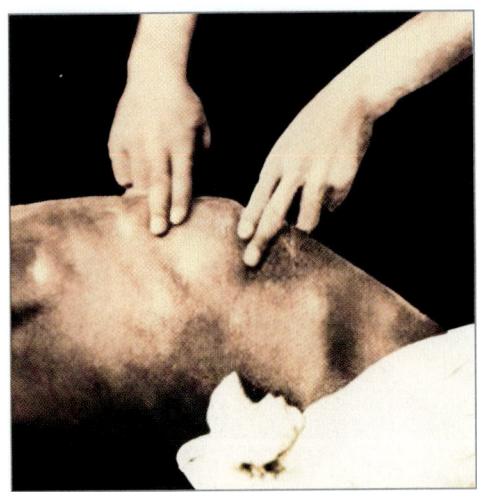

Fig. 19.10: Cold abscess at the lateral thoracic wall in Pott's disease.

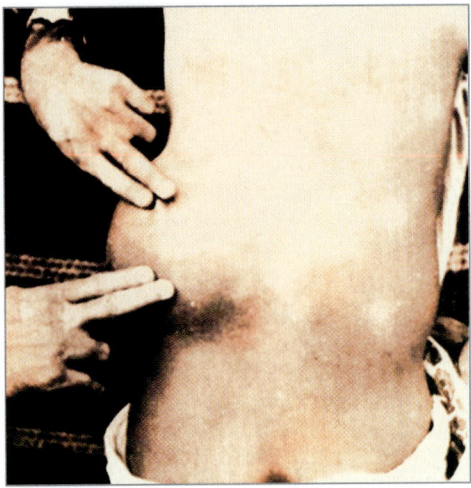

Fig. 19.11: Cold abscess at the lower lumbar triangle (Petit's triangle) in Pott's disease. Fluctuation test is being performed.

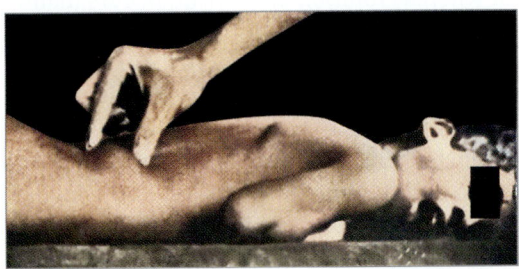

Fig. 19.12: A lumbar cold abscess—feeling for an impulse on coughing (which is more marked in a lumbar hernia).

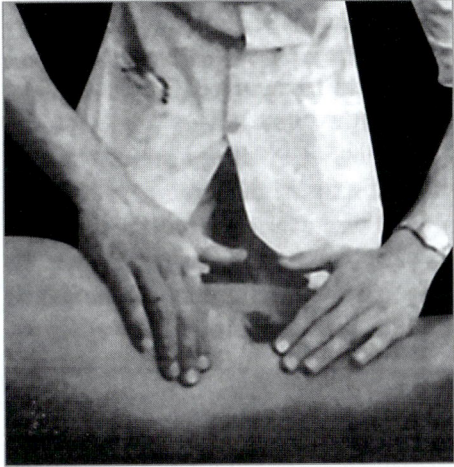

Fig. 19.13: Iliac cold abscess extending into the thigh under the inguinal ligament. This is being determined by eliciting cross fluctuation.

(in lumbar caries). (ii) Meningocele—in case of spina bifida, mostly in the lumbosacral or occipital region **(Fig. 19.14)**.

In both these cases an *impulse on coughing* may be elicited. In case of children the meningocele may be pressed with one hand keeping the other hand on the anterior fontanelle to feel for the impulse **(Fig. 19.15)**.

2. **Wasting and rigidity** of the erector spinae muscle must be felt for.

C. **PERCUSSION** over the spine is sometimes performed to elicit tenderness in addition to the method already described.

D. **MOVEMENTS** of the spine are flexion, extension, lateral flexion and rotations. Normally, *flexion* of the spine occurs mostly in the lumbar region and is possible to the extent of obliteration of the normal convexity. *Extension* is free in the lumbar and lumbodorsal regions. *Lateral flexion* is not possible without rotation of the vertebrae. This movement is permitted chiefly in the dorsal region. Rotations occur more often in the dorsal and cervical regions. *Nodding movement* of

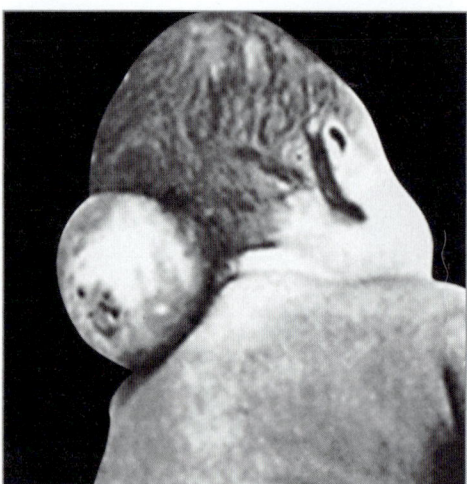

Fig. 19.14: Occipital meningocele.

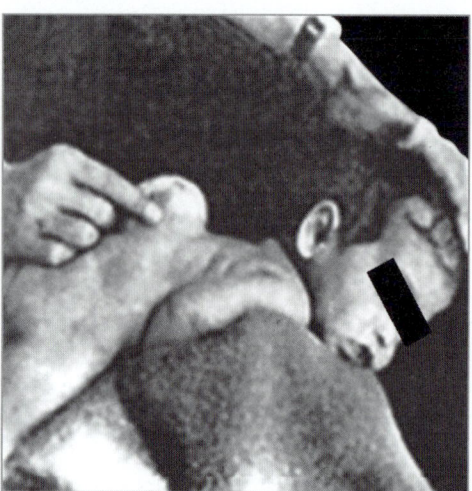

Fig. 19.15: Feeling for an impulse at the anterior fontanelle while the meningocele is being compressed.

the head takes place at the atlanto-occipital joint whereas *rotation of the head* occurs mainly at the atlantoaxial joint.

Cervical spine movements must be examined **cautiously**, especially in suspected **atlantoaxial instability**, as **excessive force may cause fatal spinal cord injury**. Passive testing should be **avoided** unless **radiological clearance is obtained**.

Mobility of the **costovertebral** joints is judged from the range of chest expansion. The normal difference of the chest girth between full expiration and full inspiration is about 2½ inches. This may be affected in conditions which may lead to rigidity of these joints, e.g., ankylosing spondylitis.

Movements of **dorsal and lumbar spine**: **RIGIDITY OF THE SPINE** is a constant feature of ankylosing spondylitis and Pott's disease. In the early stage it is due to reflex muscular spasm—a natural attempt to immobilize the painful part. Later on fibrous or bony ankylosis is the cause of rigidity. Presence of rigidity is determined by testing the different movements of the spine as follows:

(i) *Flexion*: In an adult, flexion is tested by asking him to lean forward keeping the knees straight. The clinician places his hands over the spine to note the movements of the spinous processes. It must be noted how much of the movement occurs at the spine and how much by hip flexion. It may be possible to touch the toes by excessive flexion of the hips while the spine remains stiff.

In case of children, they may not act accordingly so it is better to ask them to pick up an object from the floor. When the spine is rigid the child will stoop bending his knees and hips keeping the spine straight. While raising the body he puts his hands successively on the legs, knees and thighs as if he is climbing up his own legs.

(ii) *Extension*: The adult patient may be asked to lean backwards, i.e., to look up at the ceiling. Note the range of extension movement. This movement mainly occurs in the lumbar region and will not be affected until this region of the spine is involved **(Fig. 19.16)**.

In case of children, the patient is laid on his face. The clinician lifts up his legs in an attempt to bend the lumbar spine whilst the other hand fixes the dorsal spine. If the lumbar spine is affected it cannot be bent but will be lifted as one piece **(Fig. 19.17)**.

(iii) *Lateral flexion:* Adults are asked to bend sideways while standing, i.e., to slide each hand down the thigh and leg whilst the clinician holds firmly his pelvis from his back **(Fig. 19.18)**. In children these movements are demonstrated by lifting up the legs as in testing extension and then by carrying the legs first to one side and then to the other in order to bend the spine sideways. The other hand of the clinician is placed on the thoracic spine to detect the movement of the spine **(Fig. 19.19)**.

(iv) *Rotations* **(Figs. 19.20 and 19.21)**: The patient is always asked to sit down so as to fix his pelvis. He is then instructed to rotate the trunk to the right and to the left. Passively these movements can be performed by moving the shoulders.

E. **MEASUREMENT:** The lengths of the lower limbs must be measured to exclude shortening of any limb as the cause of scoliosis.

F. **STRAIGHT-LEG RAISING TEST (FIG. 19.22):** The patient lies supine on the examining table. First exclude that there is no compensatory lordosis by insinuating a hand beneath the lumbar spine. The patient is now asked to raise one lower limb keeping knee straight. He should continue to raise the leg till he experiences pain as evidenced by watching his face. The angle at which the pain was experienced is recorded. To be sure the test is repeated and as the

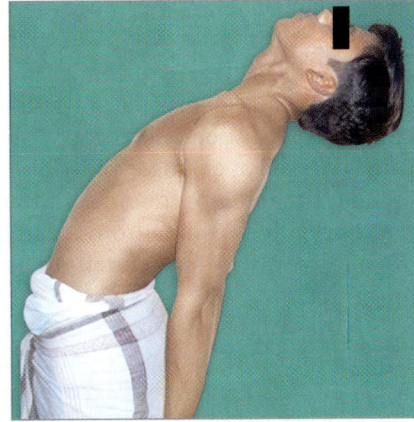

Fig. 19.16: Method of extension of spine in case of an adult.

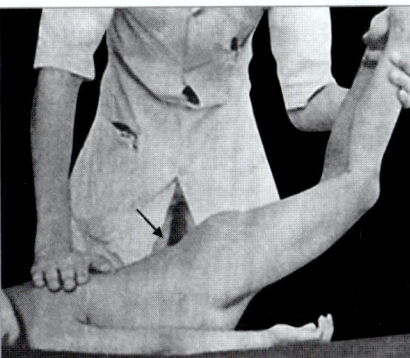

Fig. 19.17: Testing the extension of the spine. In a child the spine can normally be bent to about 60°.

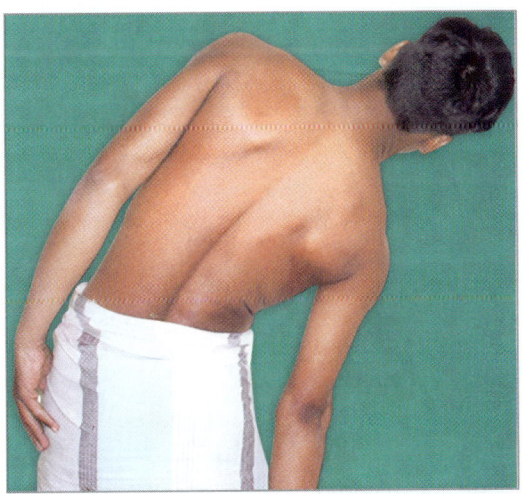

Fig. 19.18: Method of lateral flexion in case of an adult.

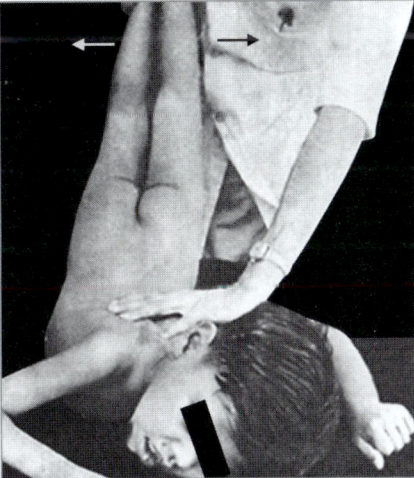

Fig. 19.19: Testing lateral flexion of the spine. In a child this is possible to the extent of 30° to 40° from the median line.

angle is approached additional care is exercised to note when the pain started. If the pain is evoked under 40° it suggests impingement of the protruding intervertebral disc on a nerve root. If the pain is evoked at an angle above 40° it indicates tension on nerve root that is abnormally sensitive from a cause not necessarily an intervertebral disc protrusion.

At the angle when the patient experiences first twinge of pain, *the ankle is passively dorsiflexed* **(Fig. 19.23)**. This causes aggravation of the pain due to additional traction to the sciatic nerve *(LASSEGUE'S SIGN)*. It suggests irritation of one or more nerve roots either by disc protrusion or from some other space occupying lesion. This second part of the test is important to differentiate sciatica from diseases of the sacroiliac joint. In the latter condition straight leg raising test will be positive but there will be no aggravation of pain during passive dorsiflexion of the ankle.

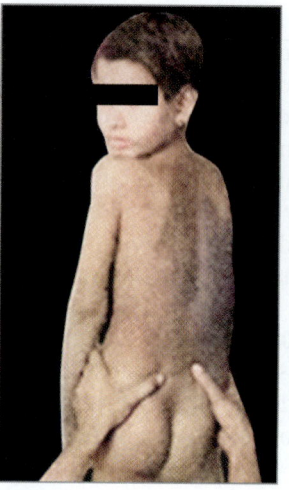

Fig. 19.20: Testing rotations of the spine. Note that the pelvis is being steadied by the clinician. The patient may be seated to fix the pelvis.

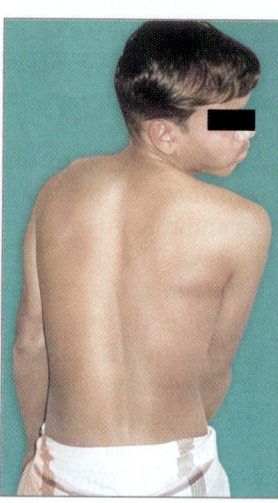

Fig. 19.21: Rotation of spine in case of adult. Note that the patient is sitting on a stool to fix his pelvis.

G. **FEMORAL NERVE STRETCH TEST:** Very rarely a patient with lumbar disc prolapse may complain of pain in front of the thigh. This indicate that probably the protruding disc is L2-3 which is irritating the femoral nerve. The patient is asked to lie on his abdomen and flex the knee of the affected side. If this maneuver reproduces the same pain the patient complained of, it is confirmatory that the L2-3 lumbar disc is protruded to cause stretching of the femoral nerve root.

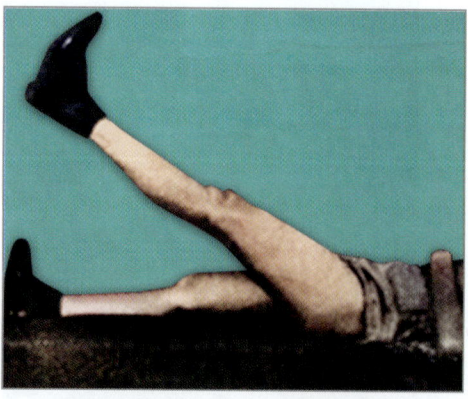

Fig. 19.22: Active straight-leg raising test. See the text.

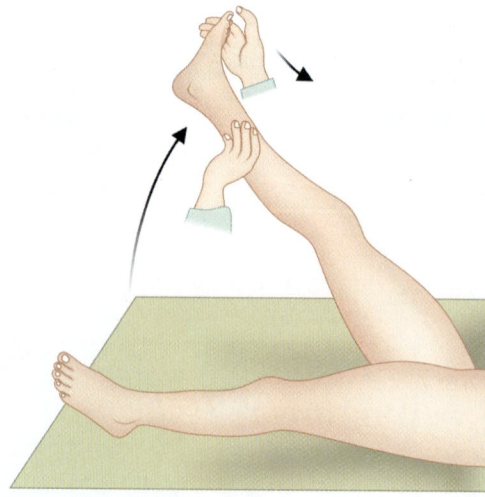

Fig. 19.23: Passive straight-leg raising test. This is important to differentiate the sacroiliac lesion from sciatica.

H. **NAFFZIGER'S TEST:** Pressure on the jugular vein if increases pain in prolapsed intervertebral disc, this test becomes positive.

I. **LHERMITTE'S SIGN (FIG. 19.24):** This sign detects protrusion of cervical intervertebral disc or an extradural spinal tumor irritating the spinal duramater. The patient sits on an examining table. Now the head of the patient is bent down passively (flexing the cervical spine) and simultaneously the lower limbs are lifted (flexing the hip joints) keeping the knees straight. This will cause sharp pain radiating down the spine and to both the extremities.

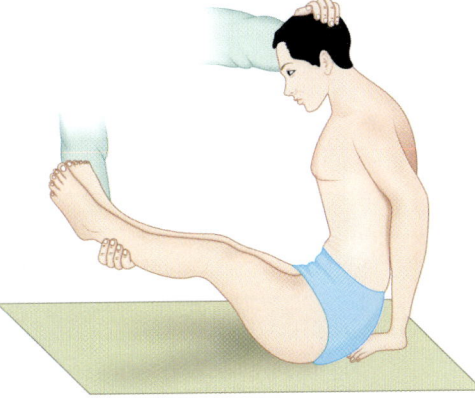

Fig. 19.24: Lhermitte's sign. Neck and hip are simultaneously flexed keeping the knees in full extension. Sharp pain is experienced down the spine into the upper or lower extremity due to irritation of the spinal dura either by tumor or by protruded intervertebral disc.

SACROILIAC JOINT

This joint deserves special mention as it requires different techniques of examination to elicit any pathology therein.

A. INSPECTION

The patient is stripped and examined in standing, sitting and recumbent positions. The position of the sacroiliac joint is determined by presence of a dimple situated just medial to the posterior superior iliac spine.

In standing position the patient is asked to point out the site of pain and the direction in which it radiates. In recumbent position it should be noted whether the hip and knee joints are slightly flexed or not.

B. PALPATION

Tenderness is elicited by placing the thumb over the dimple and exerting pressure while the patient is asked to bend forward. It may also be elicited by compressing the two iliac crests together. A search for presence of a cold abscess should be made over the buttock, iliac fossa and pelvis (by rectal examination).

C. MOVEMENTS

Any movement which throws strain upon this joint will cause pain. Forward bending in standing position becomes painful but in sitting position it will be painless as the pelvis becomes fixed (cf. prolapsed intervertebral disc, in which pain is also felt in sitting position). Rotatory movements are also painful (cf. prolapsed intervertebral disc, in which rotation is painless). There are certain tests to demonstrate movements of these joints.

1. **GENSLEN'S TEST (FIG. 19.25):** The hip and knee joints of the affected side are flexed to fix the pelvis and the hip joint of the unaffected side is hyperextended over the edge of the examining table. This will exert a rotational strain on the sacroiliac joint and will cause sharp pain.

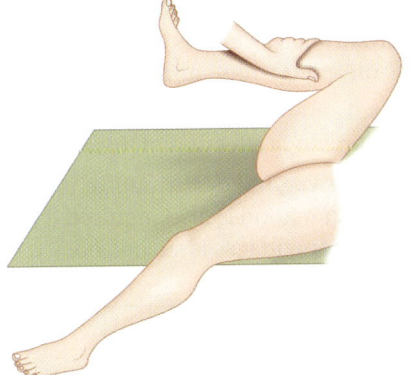

Fig. 19.25: Genslen's test. See the text.

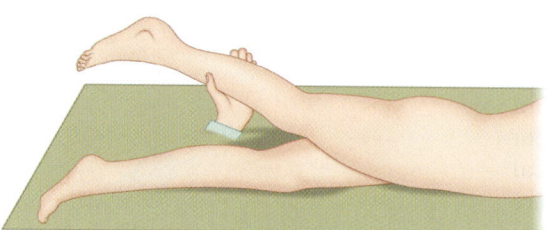

Fig. 19.26: Gillie's test. See the text.

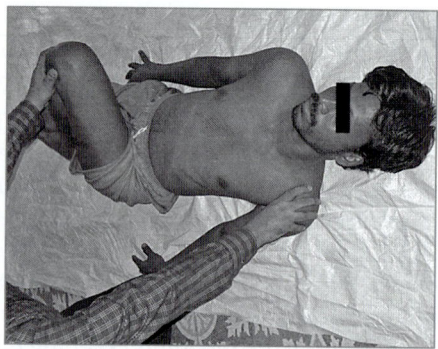

Fig. 19.27: Pump-handle test. See the text. Note the placing of the two hands of the clinician.

2. **GILLIE'S TEST (FIG. 19.26):** The patient lies prone on the bed. The pelvis of the patient is kept steadied by clinician's hand on the normal sacroiliac joint. The thigh of the affected side is hyperextended passively with the other hand of the clinician. A sharp pain is felt by the patient when the concerned sacroiliac joint is diseased.

3. **PUMP-HANDLE TEST (FIG. 19.27):** This test is performed with the patient supine on the examining table. First the normal side is examined. The patient is steadied on the table by grasping the shoulder of the side to be tested. The leg of that side is held with the other hand just below the knee. The knee and hip of that side are flexed and brought up towards the shoulder of the opposite side. In case of normal sacroiliac joint no pain is felt. But when this test is performed on the affected side a severe pain is complained of in the affected sacroiliac joint.

Straight-leg raising test: The patient is asked to lift the thigh up with the knee extended as shown in **Figure 19.23**. This will cause pain at the pathological sacroiliac joint due to the rotational strain imposed on this joint.

Passive straight-leg raising test: This test can differentiate sacroiliac lesion from sciatica. The patient is asked to lie completely relaxed. There should be no compensatory lordosis. The ankle is held with one hand and the leg is gradually raised. Normally the leg can be raised to about 90°. Note the angle at which pain is felt. Next the foot is passively dorsiflexed. In case of sciatica, pain will be aggravated by this maneuver. It should be noted that in sacroiliac lesion pain starts with the maneuver and continues to be worsen as the leg is being passively elevated. There is hardly a definite angle in which pain appears (cf. prolapsed intervertebral disc, in which pain appears at a certain angle, which is below 40° when it indicates impingement of a protruding intervertebral disc on a nerve root; and if it is above 40° it indicates tension on a nerve root from any cause).

Measurement: Girth of the lower limb may give some indication of wasting which is so evident in tuberculous affection of this joint.

Rectal or vaginal examination is sometimes required to exclude presence of pelvic abscess. This examination is also required if pathological condition of the prostate, seminal vesicles or uterine appendages is suspected.

GENERAL EXAMINATION

1. **Look for neurological signs** especially in the affection of the thoracic region where the spinal canal is very narrow. Different sensations, muscle powers and reflexes are tested to know

if there is any evidence of cord compression. Pott's paraplegia is not unusual in tuberculosis of the spine.
2. **Cold abscess** must be sought in cases of tuberculosis of the spine. It must be looked for in suboccipital region, posterior triangle of the neck, in the paravertebral region, the lateral aspect of the chest, the loin the Petit's triangle, the iliac fossa, the groin (psoas abscess), the pelvis and the ischiorectal region *Rectal examination* is very much essential to exclude pelvic extension of this abscess.
3. **The chest** should be carefully examined to exclude any previous operation as may be the cause of scoliosis.
4. **The primaries** should be looked for when secondary carcinoma of the spine is suspected. The lungs, the thyroid, prostate, breasts, kidneys should be the intervertebral space with hazy outline of the adjoining vertebral surfaces seems to be the early manifestation. Later on one may find paravertebral abscess and even psoas abscess. Wedging and gross destruction of the adjoining vertebrae are late features. In *compression fracture* the vertebrae may be wedged but the intervertebral space remains normal. In *secondary carcinoma,* examined to detect any primary lesion there.

SPECIAL INVESTIGATIONS

X-RAY EXAMINATION: This is by far the most important special investigation and most of the cases are diagnosed by this. Both anteroposterior and lateral views should be taken. In *tuberculosis of the spine* diminution of osteolytic changes are evident in the bodies of the vertebrae **(Figs. 19.28 and 19.29)**. Here also the intervertebral space remains unchanged. Osteosclerotic change may be seen in prostatic carcinoma. In *Scheuermann's disease* the vertebral epiphysis may be irregular, dense, similar to the osteochondritic changes. In *Paget's disease* coarse trabeculation with cystic changes may be seen. In *senile osteoporosis* the vertebrae are less dense than normal. In *osteoarthritis* characteristic

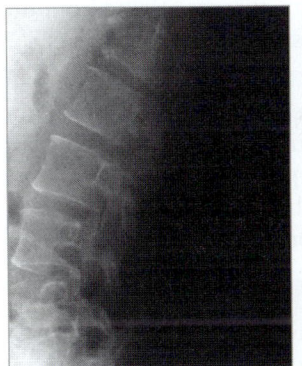
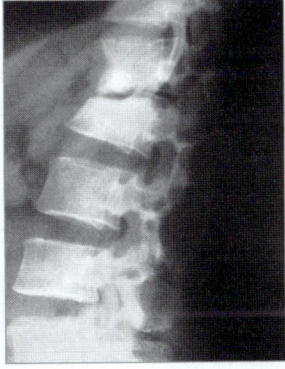

Fig. 19.28: Pott's disease showing diminution of the intervertebral space and destruction of the opposing surfaces of the vertebrae.

Fig. 19.29: Skiagram of a case of caries spine. Note the diminution of the intervertebral space shown by arrow.

peripheral lipping when present, leaves no doubt about the diagnosis. *Spina bifida* will be obvious when a gap in the laminae is seen in X-ray. In *prolapsed intervertebral disc* the affected intervertebral space becomes narrowed. In *spondylolisthesis* **(Figs. 19.30A and B)** the lateral view is very important in which the 5th lumbar vertebra with the upper articular process slides forward over the sacrum and its lower articular process. This is due to the developmental defect of the pedicle of the 5th lumbar vertebra. In *tuberculous affection of the sacroiliac joint,* the joint line becomes blurred with osteolysis of the neighboring bones. In *ankylosing spondylitis* X-ray will reveal irregular marginal sclerosis with indistinct joint outline **(Fig. 19.31)**.

BONE SCAN: *See* page 180.

MYELOGRAPHY: Light lipiodol is introduced through the lumbar puncture needle or heavy lipiodol is injected by cisterna puncture into the subarachnoid space. X-ray picture is taken to find out if there is any filling defect by a protruding disc or any space occupying lesion in the subarachnoid space.

EPIDUROGRAPHY (FIGS. 19.32A AND B): Injection of water soluble contrast medium is often preferred due to the risk of possible long-term sequel of oily contrast medium. The most commonly used medium is urografin (sodium diatrizoate) 60%.

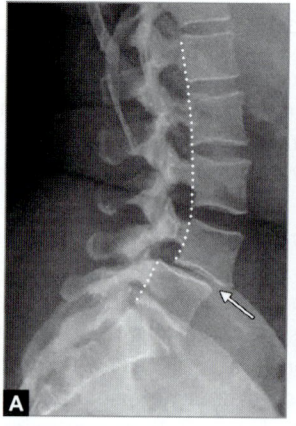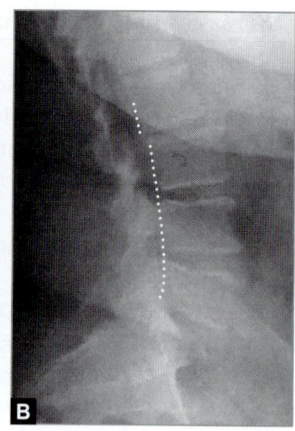

Figs. 19.30A and B: Skiagram of spondylolisthesis. (A) The structural defect in the pars interarticularis can be seen. (B) There is forward displacement of the fifth lumbar over first sacral vertebra (congenital spondylolisthesis).

Anteroposterior film will show central filling defect, peripheral filling defect or interruption of the nerve root out line. Lateral X-rays will reveal the filling defect from disc intrusion. Epidurography is found useful in the investigation of prolapsed intervertebral disc, epidural and periradicular lesions, spina bifida occulta, tumors arising from the intradural, vertebral and paravertebral tissues, spondylolisthesis, subdural hematoma, etc.

DISCOGRAPHY (FIG. 19.33): Indications of lumbar discography are: (i) clinically protruded intervertebral disc but a negative myelogram, (ii) uncertain clinical evidence of prolapse of a specific disc and (iii) when pain recurs following surgery as defects in myelogram may then be due to adhesions and postoperative distortion of the theca. The main complication of discography is infection which of course can be minimized by strictly aseptic technique. The other potential complication is prolapse of the punctured disc. Its incidence can also be reduced

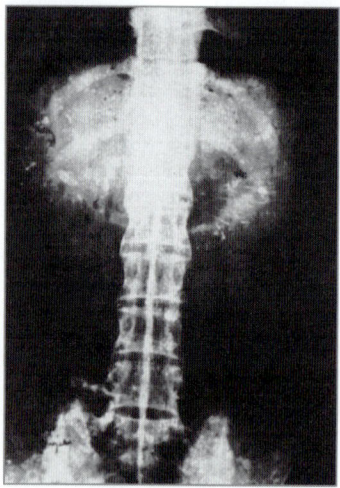

Fig. 19.31: A straight X-ray of ankylosing spondylitis (late stage).

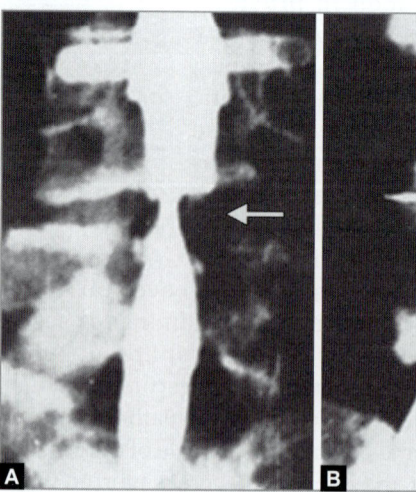

Figs. 19.32A and B: Anteroposterior and lateral views with radio-opaque dye showing filling defect at the level between L4 and L5 shown by arrows due to lumbar disc protrusion.

by using a very fine needle. It is usual to inject the lower three or sometimes four discs with water-soluble contrast medium after confirming that the needles appear to be in about the center of the nucleus pulposus on lateral radiographs. Injection of a normal disc frequently causes some backache. Radiographs are then made in lateral and posteroanterior projections. A normal nucleus is well-circumscribed and is confined by annulus fibrosus. In degenerated discs the nucleus is usually narrowed and may bulge the annulus. A disc prolapse fills beyond the confines of the intervertebral space and if the annulus is torn the contrast may extravasate. Accentuation of symptoms, which may quickly recede again makes discography an unpleasant procedure even with adequate premedication. But it is preferred to negative surgical exploration.

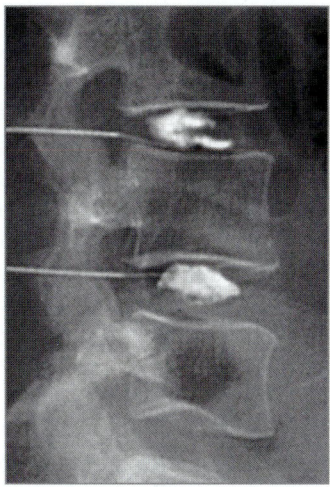

Fig. 19.33: A normal discography.

ILIAC AND INFERIOR VENACAVOGRAPHY: The venogram is simple, performed by percutaneous catheterization of the femoral vein with simultaneous injection of suitable contrast medium on both sides. The patient is kept mobile to discourage thrombus formation. This investigation reveals a retroperitoneal mass which may cause backache.

LYMPHOGRAPHY: Malignant lesions causing referred pain are usually sufficiently advanced to show obvious abnormalities in lymphogram. With this investigation one can confirm their positions and may give a good indication of their nature.

MRI: This has revolutionized the investigation of these cases as soft tissue abnormalities can be detected by this method, e.g., disc prolapse, spinal cord tumor, spinal column tumor are all detected in early stages. MRI with contrast medium (*see* page 44) is particularly helpful to detect spinal cord tumor **(Fig. 3.44)**.

DIFFERENTIAL DIAGNOSIS

■ CONGENITAL ANOMALIES

Spina bifida: This condition develops due to failure of fusion of the posterior part of the spine resulting in a defect through which the membranes and even the spinal cord may herniate. Usually it affects one vertebra most commonly in the lumbosacral region and less often in the cervico-occipital region. The different types of spina bifida are as follows:

1. *Spina bifida occulta* is due to failure of the neural arches to unite posteriorly, but no protrusion of the cord or membrane is noticed. Almost always this condition is seen in the lumbosacral region and it is suspected by presence of a cicatricial thickening or a dimple or a tuft of hair or dilated vessels or a fibrofatty tumor or a naevolipoma over the bony deficiency. A fibrous band, the membrena reuniens, connects the skin to the spinal theca. As soon as the child grows older the theca is pulled down by membrana reuniens and symptoms like backache, enuresis, foot drop, weakness of the lower limbs and even paralysis may appear. A few cases may remain symptomless and are only diagnosed when X-ray is taken for some other reason.
2. *Meningocele:* When meninges protrude through the defect in the spine this condition develops. It contains only cerebrospinal fluid.

3. *Meningomyelocele:* In this condition in addition to protrusion of the membrane, normally developed spinal cord and cauda equina lie within the sac and may be adherent to the posterior aspect of the sac. This condition is quite common in living children and is differentiated from the previous condition by presence of dark shadows of the cord or nerves on transillumination.
4. *Syringomyelocele:* In this condition the central canal of the spinal cord becomes dilated and the cord lies within the sac and becomes adherent to the posterior part of the sac.
5. *Myelocele:* This is probably the most common type of spina bifida but is incompatible with life. The central canal of the spinal cord opens out on the surface and discharges cerebrospinal fluid continuously. Paralytic deformities of foot and incontinence of urine and feces are almost always accompanied with these conditions.

DEFORMITIES OF THE SPINE

SCOLIOSIS

Scoliosis is a **lateral deviation of the spine**, often accompanied by **vertebral rotation**. While **transient scoliosis** can occur after **trauma or infections (e.g., tuberculosis)**, **structural scoliosis** is a progressive deformity requiring differentiation from congenital, neuromuscular, and idiopathic causes. Lateral curvature of scoliosis is almost always associated with the rotation of the spine. Mainly two types of scoliosis are noticed in surgical practice—mobile scoliosis (transient) and structural scoliosis (permanent).

MOBILE SCOLIOSIS is transient that means it is never transformed into fixed scoliosis and in this type the vertebrae are not rotated. In this group three types are noticed—(i) *Postural scoliosis,* particularly seen in adolescent girls and the curve is mild and convex to the left. The main diagnostic feature is that when the patient bends forward, the spine straightens completely (cf. structural scoliosis in which the curve becomes excessive on bending forward). (ii) *Compensatory scoliosis* is seen in patients with unilateral short legs, ocular disorders, torticollis, etc. The diagnostic feature in case of short leg is that the curve disappears when the patient sits. (iii) *Sciatic-scoliosis* is usually accompanied by sciatica with prolapsed lumbar disc. The clinical features signify the underlying cause.

STRUCTURAL SCOLIOSIS is always associated with rotation of the vertebrae. The bodies rotate towards convexity of the curve and the spinous processes towards the concavity. Once the deformity develops, it is liable to be increased due to greater pressure on the epiphyses on the concave side which retards growth. The curvature ceases to be increased when the growth of the patient stops completely. An index to spinal maturity is the complete appearance of the iliac apophyses in X-ray (Risser's sign). In this type of scoliosis three curves are found. The middle one is primary and the compensatory curves lie above and below the primary curvature. The different causes of fixed scoliosis are as follows:

(i) *Idiopathic* is most common. In this condition the primary curve is always thoracic and mental defect is a common accompaniment of this condition. This type is recognized by eliminating any identifiable cause. (ii) *Congenital* type is always associated with some form of radiologically demonstrable anomaly such as hemivertebrae, fused vertebrae, absent ribs or fused ribs, absent discs, etc. Some obvious congenital abnormality may be found on the surface, e.g., naevi, angioma, excess of hair, a dimple or a pad of fat. This type of scoliosis is usually mild. A careful neurological examination should always be carried out as spina bifida or other neurological deficits may be present along with this condition. (iii) *Paralytic* scoliosis is due to paralysis from poliomyelitis, cerebral palsy, muscular dystrophy, etc. Unbalanced paralysis affecting intercostal and lateral abdominal muscles is the cause of this scoliosis. (iv) About l/3rd of the patients suffering from *multiple neurofibromatosis* develop scoliosis.

Generally the patients with scoliosis complain of the deformity only. A few of them may present with backache in whom lumbar curves or combined curves may pass unnoticed. In all cases of scoliosis one must not forget to examine the heart and lungs as congenital heart disease may be associated with this condition and an increasing thoracic scoliosis may lead to gradual respiratory embarrassment.

KYPHOSIS

Excessive posterior convexity of the thoracic spine is defined as kyphosis. The different causes of kyphosis worth mentioning are: (i) *Postural* kyphosis is usually associated with such defects as flat foot, is seen in girls approaching puberty, women after child birth or with obesity. (ii) *Compensatory* kyphosis is seen in lumbar lordosis, congenital dislocation of hip or fixed flexion deformity of the hip. (iii) *Scheuermann's disease*—is nothing but osteochondritis affecting the epiphyseal plates of the vertebrae. The victims are usually teen-agers and the usual complaint is the backache. Thoracic 6th to 10th vertebrae are usually involved and become wedge shaped, narrower in front. The epiphyseal plates appear fragmented especially anteriorly. They may contain small translucent areas (Schmorl's nodes). (iv) *Ankylosing spondylitis* is an autoimmune disease with a definite genetic background. Prostatitis probably plays a part. The underlying pathology is that the intervertebral discs are first replaced by vascular connective tissue and then undergo ossification affecting the periphery of the annulus fibrosus and the intervertebral ligaments. The disease often starts around the sacroiliac joint in the form of osteitis. Pain and stiffness of the lumbar spine and buttocks are the main presenting symptoms. Occasionally, the pain may mimic that of sciatica, but in contradistinction to the disc prolapse the pain alternates its side. The onset is insidious and only noticed during getting up of the bed. Malaise, fatigue, loss of weight are the general symptoms which the patient may complain of. The victims are usually men between the ages of 15 to 35 years. They are undernourished and in half of the cases the process stops before significant deformity has occurred. In the other half of the cases the process continues for many years with phases of activity and it does not stop till the entire spine and the several large joints have stiffened. The general attitude of the patient is to stand with kyphosis and the knees are bent to maintain balance. The sarco-iliac joints may be painful particularly so when the two iliac crests are pressed inwards from both the sides. It must be noted that small joints are always exempted. Anemia and raised sedimentation rate are the abnormalities found in routine blood examination. X-ray shows blurred and irregular joint lines with surrounding sclerosis, joint spaces are gradually diminished and may be obliterated. The vertebral bodies lose their normal anterior concavity and look square. Calcification of the intervertebral ligaments and well defined borders with sclerosis complete the classical picture of a 'bamboo' spine. (v) *Senile kyphosis* is the kyphosis seen in old people. Degeneration of intervertebral discs produce increasing stoop characteristic of the aged. The disc spaces become narrowed and the vertebrae slightly wedged. There is hardly any pain unless osteoarthritis affects the intervertebral joints. Kyphosis may also be seen in cases of widespread osteoporosis, Paget's disease and secondary malignant deposits affecting the vertebrae. (vi) Kyphosis may also follow a fracture of the vertebra, *tuberculosis* or *Calve's disease* which is a rare condition and is the sequel to an eosinophilic granuloma affecting one vertebra (the disc space remains normal).

LORDOSIS

This is an increased anterior curvature of lumbar spine. It may be postural as compensatory to fixed flexion deformity or congenital dislocation of the hip. Tuberculosis of the hip and malunited

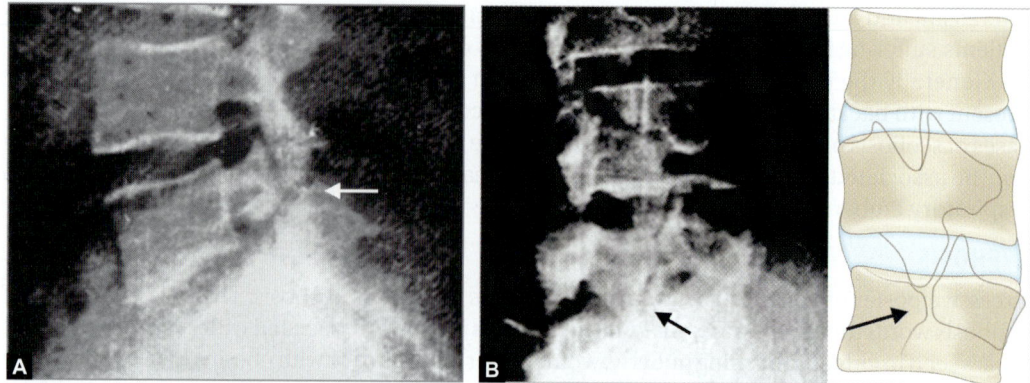

Figs. 19.34A and B: (A) The lateral view is shown. It is a typical case of moderate spondylolisthesis of L5 and S1 is being shown with an obvious bony defect in the interarticularis zone. (B) Spondylolisthesis is better diagnosed however in oblique view. An outline of a 'Scot's terrier' can easily be seen in this view with the neck formed by the pars interarticularis. When there is a break, as shown by arrow, the terrier is decapitated and the lesion in the pars is seen.

fracture of the femur may lead to this condition. The deformity may also develop to correct the center of gravity of the body as required in last trimester of the pregnancy, large uterine fibroid or a big fatty abdomen.

SPONDYLOLISTHESIS (FIGS. 19.34A AND B)

This means forward shift of the spine. The shift nearly always takes place between L4 and L5 or between L5 and S1. The pathology lies either in the lamina which may be in two pieces or unduly elongated or in the facets which are poorly developed. The *congenital* variety is by far the commoner and constitutes no less than 75% of the cases. *Degenerative* variety constitutes about 20% of cases and is due to the degenerative changes in the facet joints as also the discs, which permit the forward shift despite intact lamina. *Traumatic* variety constitutes about 5% of cases and may follow either a single major injury or repeated minor injuries. In the congenital variety there is developmental defect of the pedicle of the 5th lumbar vertebra. This part which is called 'Pars interarticular' is divided in two parts being connected by fibrous tissue which is shown as a gap in X-ray. The lower articular processes remain with the sacrum in situ whilst the upper articular processes along with the spinal column above move forward. The main complaint is the backache which becomes more obvious after exercise or strain. The pain may radiate down to the legs and there may be weakness of the lower extremities. This is due to the pressure on the cauda equina and the emerging nerve roots. Disc prolapse is liable to occur. This condition may affect any age but degenerative variety is obviously rare before the age of 40 years. On examination the trunk appears shorter, the buttocks look flat, the upper angle of the sacrum forms a distinct prominence on the back with depression just above it. The most important finding on inspection is a transverse furrow encircling the body between the ribs and the iliac crests. On palpation a definite prominence at the upper angle of the sacrum will be obvious when the clinician runs his fingers down along the spinous processes. X-ray shows the upper border of the 5th lumbar vertebra is too low in anteroposterior view, whereas lateral view demonstrates clearly the forward shift of the spinal column, a gap in the lamina, elongated lamina or defective facets if they are present. To demonstrate the gap in the lamina which may not be so obvious in lateral view, oblique views may be required.

INFLAMMATORY CONDITIONS

TUBERCULOSIS OF THE SPINE (POTT'S DISEASE)

This is the most important disease that affects the spine in this country. It attacks children and adolescents more commonly than the adults. In prodromal stage, the patient gets tired, there are loss of weight and evening rise of temperature. Pain is usually the main complaint. It is slight in the beginning and dull ache in character. It becomes worse on walking or jolting. The pain may be localized or referred due to involvement of the nerve-roots. Rigidity is the next complaint. It restricts all movements. Deformity in the form of a hump or angular kyphos leading to hunchback is not uncommon. On palpation one can detect localized tenderness if pressed on the particular spine. Slight angular deformity also becomes obvious in palpation. The two common complications are *cold abscess formation* and *paraplegia*. Fluctuation test will be positive with the formation of the abscess. Movements become diminished in all directions. This becomes obvious in the involvement of the lumbar spine than that of the thoracic spine. Attempt to movement will provoke muscular spasm. "Coin test" gives a good indication as to the limitation of the flexion movement of the spine.

X-ray findings are important in which the adjacent bodies will show destruction with diminution of the intervertebral space (cf. secondary deposit in the spine will cause destruction of the bodies with intact intervertebral disc). Anteroposterior view may show the soft tissue shadow of paravertebral abscess. The legs must always be examined for presence of neurological deficits.

A summary of the clinical features according to the region affected is as follows:

(i) **CERVICAL:**
(a) Besides localized pain, it may be referred to the back of the head or arm depending on the nerve-root affected by pressure.
(b) Attitude—the head being supported by the patient's hand.
(c) Rigidity of the neck.
(d) Deformity in the form of torticollis.
(e) Abscess—in the retropharyngeal space (causing dysphagia and dyspnea), in the posterior triangle of the neck whence it may travel down towards the mediastinum or along the brachial nerve to the axilla or in the suboccipital region.

(ii) **THORACIC:**
(a) Pain may be localized or referred to the chest, abdomen or sometimes girdle pain.
(b) Rigidity is not so obvious in tuberculosis of this region of the spine.
(c) Deformity in the form of kyphosis and gibbus.
(d) Abscess formation in the paravertebral region and it may burrow following the cutaneous branches of the intercostal vessels and nerves to the anterior and lateral thoracic region. From the posterior mediastinum it may gravitate down beneath medial or lateral arcuate ligament to become psoas or lumbar abscess respectively. The psoas abscess comes out through the medial aspect of the upper part of the thigh; whereas the lumbar abscess becomes superficial in the Petit's triangle, formed by the iliac crest and the adjacent borders of the latissimus dorsi and the external oblique muscles.
(e) *Nervous manifestations* are most frequently noticed in the affection of this region. *Paraplegia is quite common due to the fact that the spinal canal is narrowest in the region.*

(iii) **LUMBAR:**
(a) Pain is mostly localized in this region but may be referred to the lateral aspect of the thigh.
(b) Limitation of movements is mostly noticed in this region.
(c) Deformity is minimum.
(d) Abscess formation is not uncommon mainly in the form of iliopsoas abscess which may burrow into the thigh under the inguinal ligament or into the pelvis and perineum where a fistula forms on bursting or it may travel to the buttock from the pelvis passing through the sciatic foramen.
(e) Nervous symptoms are rare as the spinal canal is spacious.

Pott's paraplegia is due to compression of the spinal cord more frequently by soft inflammatory material (the abscess, a caseous mass and granulation tissue) or less frequently by solid material (a bony sequestrum, sequestrated disc or the ridge of the bone at the kyphos). Occasionally fibrous tissue is the compressing agent.

ACUTE OSTEOMYELITIS OF THE SPINE

This condition is very rare. It is characterized by sudden onset of fever and severe local pain. There is hardly any collapse of the affected vertebrae owing to early recumbency by the patient, rapid new bone formation and paravertebral calcification. In late cases there will be pyogenic abscess and not a cold abscess. The condition culminates in bony ankylosis and not fibrous ankylosis (cf. tuberculosis of the spine). The prognosis is dismal as there always remains the chance for the infection to spread and involve the meninges.

◼ DISORDERS OF INTERVERTEBRAL DISCS

In this group the most important condition is the disc prolapse. Only other condition which deserves mention is protrusion of the disc into the vertebral bodies causing Schmorl's node. This is seen in Scheuermann's disease.

LUMBAR DISC PROLAPSE (FIGS. 19.35 AND 19.36)

The various factors which may cause this condition are: (i) *Injury:* A lifting strain with the back bent may tear the posterior longitudinal ligament causing the tense disc to bulge backwards. The annulus fibrosus may also be torn and the nucleus pulposus may bulge out. If the tear does not heal properly further prolapse is likely to take place with trivial strain. (ii) *Increased tension* within the nucleus pulposus is sometimes seen in some physical illnesses and emotional stress. Extra fluid is absorbed, the nucleus swells and may even burst through the annulus. (iii) *Degeneration* is probably most common cause in which the fluid content of the disc decreases with changes in the character of the collagen

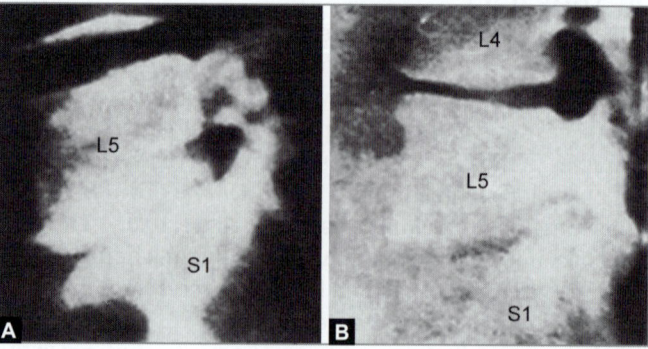

Figs. 19.35A and B: Note considerable diminution of the intervertebral space between L5 and S1. (A) Due to lumbar disc prolapse. (B) Can see the normal intervertebral space.

fibers so that the disc loses elasticity and may liable to bulge with body weight.

Prolapsed disc may press on the duramater causing backache or on the nerve roots causing backache or sciatica or both. The prolapse of a disc occurs nearly always just above or below the 5th lumbar vertebra (i.e., between L4 and L5 or L5 and S1). As edema subsides the prolapsed disc may shrink or slip back into place. Sometimes it may not be absorbed and becomes adherent to root sheaths. Long-standing prolapse may disturb the mechanism of the intervertebral joints.

The first attack is often sudden in onset and occurs while lifting weight from bent position. The patient complains of excruciating backache and sciatica may or may not follow soon after. The symptoms subside in a few days or weeks. Sciatica is at first located in the buttock but it soon spreads to the thigh, leg along the posterior aspect even up to the toes. Subsequent attacks are also sudden in onset but may follow trivial injury such as coughing, etc. *On examination,* the patient is found to stand with a characteristic attitude—lumbar scoliosis with convexity to the affected side, kyphosis and slight flexion of the hips and knees. Local deep tenderness is elicited on or slightly lateral to the affected spine. Pressure on the jugular vein often induces pain over the lesion (Naffziger's test). Flexion and extension of the spine are greatly restricted. Lateral flexion on the side of the lesion is also very painful, but rotation may be free and painless. Knee jerk may be diminished (in case of lesion between L3 and L4), but tendo Achillis jerk is almost always absent. Extension of the great toe against resistance will show weakness of the extensor hallucis longus. This indicates nervous involvement.

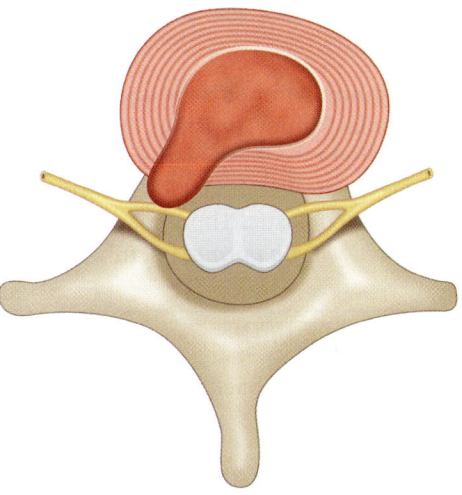

Fig. 19.36: Diagrammatic representation of lumbar disc prolapse in which the prolapsed disc is pressing on a spinal nerve root on the left side.

After first attack there may not be any X-ray changes. But after many months or years with subsequent attacks there will be narrowing of the intervertebral space with lipping of the vertebral bodies, i.e., secondary osteoarthritic changes develop. Myelography is helpful in diagnosing this condition. Recently discography is often done to delineate the protrusion of the disc. Epidurography is also helpful so far as the diagnosis of this condition is concerned. MRI is probably the best method of investigation at the present (*see* **Fig. 30.6** of the author's 'A Concise Textbook of Surgery').

LUMBAR SPONDYLOSIS

This is a degenerative condition which involves not only the disc space but also the interarticular joints. The discs degenerate and lose the normal elasticity. There will be lipping of the vertebral bodies. Osteophytes will be seen around the interarticular joints. Sometimes the disc material may extrude with a pressure of the body and press on the duramater leading to backache. Osteophytes and protruded disc may also press on the nerve roots causing sciatica. Patients are invariably over 40 years of age. There will be tenderness of the affected vertebrae. All lumbar movements are limited and painful. Neurological examination may elicit some deficit in the lower extremities. X-ray will show diminution of the intervertebral space. The interarticular joints are narrowed and irregular. There will be lipping at the corners of the vertebral bodies and presence of osteophytes around the interarticular joints.

TUMORS OF THE SPINAL COLUMN

Most common tumor is the **secondary carcinoma**, the primary being in the breast, bronchus, suprarenal, kidney, prostate, thyroid, etc. The main features are severe local pain with collapse of the vertebral column with or without symptoms of cord compression. X-ray shows osteolytic changes in the vertebral bodies, barring in case of secondaries from the prostate when the lesion will be osteoblastic. There may be collapse or wedging of the vertebra, *but the intervertebral space will remain normal* (cf. tuberculosis of the vertebra).

LOW BACK PAIN

The causes of low back pain can be classified in the following way:

A. **In the back**

(i) **CONGENITAL**

(a) Spina bifida; (b) Spondylolisthesis; (c) Hemivertebra (when one of the two centers of ossification for the vertebral body fails to develop); (d) Split vertebra (when there is a definite gap between the two centers of ossification); (e) Abnormality in the articular processes (articular facets of the 5th lumbar vertebra may take the form like that of articular processes of the thoracic vertebra); (f) Besides lack of fusion between the two halves of the neural arch which produces the condition of spina bifida, the lamina may fail to fuse with the body of vertebra; (g) Sacralization of the transverse process of the 5th lumbar vertebra.

(ii) **TRAUMATIC**

(a) Lumbosacral strain

(b) Injuries to the intervertebral joints, ligaments and muscles. These injuries are produced by external violence which may overstretch the spinal column. The pain is sudden and although increased by certain movements, it is a constant excruciating pain during the acute stage which is only partly relieved by rest. It is sometimes difficult to find out the exact sign of the lesion. In case of muscle strain the common site being the origin of the sacrospinalis from the back of sacrum or the origin of the gluteus maximus from the posterior superior iliac spine. The underlying pathology is simply the rupture of some fibers with consequent exudation and swelling. Novocaine injection abolishes the local pain. In ligamentous injury the pain is deep-seated and can be elicited both by pressure with the finger or by movement of the spine.

(c) Spondylolisthesis: Many orthopedic surgeons are of the opinion that trauma plays a significant role so far as the etiology of this condition is concerned. Minor repeated trauma may lead to this condition which may be incriminated as a congenital lesion.

(d) Compression fracture

(e) Vertebral process fracture (transverse or spinous processes)

(f) Ruptured disc

(iii) **FUNCTIONAL DEFECTS**

(a) Anteroposterior imbalance (pregnancy, pot belly, fixed flexion deformity of the hip joints etc.)

(b) Lateral imbalance (scoliosis, leg length discrepancy, etc.)

(iv) **INFLAMMATORY**

(a) Pyogenic osteomyelitis

(b) Tuberculosis

(c) Rheumatoid arthritis

(d) Brucellosis
(e) Ankylosing spondylitis
(f) Myositis
(g) Fibrositis
(v) **DEGENERATIVE**
(a) Osteoarthritis (spondylosis)
(b) Senile osteoporosis
(c) Degenerative disc disease
(vi) **NEOPLASTIC**
(a) Primary tumors, e.g., multiple myeloma, eosinophilic granuloma, hemangioma, osteoid osteoma
(b) Metastatic tumors from breast, bronchus, kidney, suprarenal, prostate, thyroid, gastrointestinal tract.

B. **Other than the back**
(i) **ABDOMINAL DISORDERS**, e.g., pancreatitis (very important), cholecystitis, biliary calculus, peptic ulcer, hiatus hernia, etc.
(ii) **PELVIC DISORDERS**, e.g., inflammatory condition of the ovaries and tubes, any intrapelvic tumor, etc.
(iii) **GENITOURINARY CAUSES**, e.g., renal infection, renal or ureteric calculus, prostatitis, prostatic carcinoma, seminal vesiculitis etc.
(iv) **VASCULAR DISORDERS**, e.g., ischemic pain from occlusion of the aorta or iliac arteries and aneurysmal dilatation of the aorta may cause backache.

LUMBOSACRAL STRAIN

This condition develops from mechanical stress and strain which the lumbosacral region renders itself. It is the site of great shearing strain and it is the junction between the mobile and the fixed part of the spinal column. It occurs in both acute and chronic forms. The acute form may be due to sudden blow forcing the joint into positions beyond the normal range of movement. The spinal muscles yield when they are off guard and thus the ligaments sustain the full force of injury. The chronic form is usually insidious in onset but may follow an acute strain which may or may not be recognized. It occurs mostly in individuals with poor musculature and an increase in the normal lumbar lordosis (usually a woman with a pendulous abdomen). Gradually, the attacks become more and more frequent and the pain may become constant as the age advances. Sciatic pain may be present if there is root pressure.

FIBROSITIS (LUMBAGO)

Fibrositis causing backache often reveals one or more tender nodules lying superficially in the erector spinae or its attachments. In the lumbar region it is called lumbago. This tender nodules may be found in the buttocks. The etiology is not very clearly known. It may be rheumatic fibrositis or local muscular spasm due to nerve root irritation. The pain comes on suddenly when the patient bends his back and it is very severe. Recurrences are common and the condition may become chronic. If neurological signs are present, it is probable that a disc has been protruded.

MALINGERER'S LOW BACK PAIN

In this condition though the patient constantly complains of low back pain, yet no organic cause can be found out. Patient is mostly psychic with depression and anxiety states. Two tests can be performed to detect such cases—(i) AIRD'S TEST: The patient is first asked to flex forward to touch his toes in standing position keeping the knees straight. He usually fails and complains of pain. He is now asked to sit down on an examining table and advised to touch his toes by flexing the spine. This he is often able to do as there is no organic lesion of the spinal column. (ii) MAGNUSON'S TEST: The patient is asked to point the most painful area of the spine and this is pointed out with a skin pencil. Now the patient's attention is diverted by examining his throat, eyes, rectum, abdomen, etc., and then asked to point again the most painful spot on his back. He shows a different spot as he has forgotten by that time which spot did he show earlier, as there is no organic lesion.

SACROILIAC STRAIN

When there is definite pain on one sacroiliac joint, but no definite cause can be detected the condition is called 'sacroiliac strain'. Though the tests for the sacroiliac joint are positive, yet the X-ray and other investigations are all negative.

SACROILIAC ARTHRITIS

This is quite rare. It may be a complication of Reiter's disease. This joint is almost always involved in ankylosing spondylitis. A few patients with ulcerative colitis suffer from this disease. Leading symptom is painful stiffness of the back as first thing in the morning. There may also be pain of band-like distribution across the sacrum and buttocks. Patient may limp, and if the condition is bilateral 'Waddling gait' may be seen.

TUBERCULOSIS OF THE SACROILIAC JOINT

This is a rare disease. When in a patient with persistent low back pain no cause could be found out one must keep in mind this condition. It is a condition which usually affects young adults. Pain is often of central low back or groin pain or sciatica. Only in half the cases pain is localized to the joint. At the time of cold abscess formation pain is severe. Patient also complains of night pain. When pus erodes the ligamentous coverings of the joint, pus comes superficial and presents as fluctuating swelling. In 70% of cases the abscess appears over the joint and in the rest the abscess tracks down either to the groin or to the iliac fossa or in the femoral triangle.

Chapter 19: Examination of Spinal Abnormalities

Algorithmic Approach to Patient with Spinal Abnormalities

Patient presents with back pain or spinal deformity

↓

Assess history for underlying cause (trauma, infection, degenerative, neoplastic)

↓

Recent trauma?
- Yes → Consider **fracture, ligament injury, or disc prolapse**
- No → Proceed to **chronic pain assessment.**

↓

Pain worse at night?
- Yes → Consider **tumor (metastases, multiple myeloma) or spinal tuberculosis**
- No → Evaluate **mechanical vs Inflammatory pain**

↓

Morning stiffness lasting >30 min?
- Yes → Consider **inflammatory conditions (e.g., ankylosing spondylitis)**
- No → Likely **mechanical back pain (spondylosis, postural strain)**

↓

Perform neurological examination and assess deformity
- Assess for weakness, sensory loss, reflex changes
- Check for spinal curvatures (scoliosis, kyphosis, lordosis)

↓

Are neurological deficits present?
- Yes → Urgent **MRI or CT scan** to assess for **cord compression or nerve root impingement**
- No → Consider **conservative management (physiotherapy, pain management, lifestyle modifications)**

↓

Determine need for surgery vs conservative care
- **Surgical intervention?** → If spinal cord compression, severe deformity, or unstable fracture
- **Conservative management?** → If mild to moderate mechanical back pain

CHAPTER 20

Examination of the Hand

HISTORY

A careful history should be elicited as to what is the complaint and how is he suffering from it. The onset is very important. Whether it follows injury, a sequel of abrasion or a prick or of insidious onset.

History in hand diseases

Aspect	Clinical significance	Patient-friendly questions
Onset of symptoms	Acute → Trauma, infection; gradual → Degenerative, neurological	"When did your symptoms start? Was it sudden or gradual?"
Mechanism of injury	Helps determine **fractures, ligament tears, nerve injuries**	"Did you injure your hand? Was there a fall, crush, or cut?"
Pain characteristics	Sharp pain → Fracture, nerve injury; throbbing → Infection	"Is the pain sharp, burning, or throbbing? Does it spread?"
Pain aggravating factors	Movement-related → Joint/Tendon injury; worse at night → Carpal tunnel syndrome	"What makes the pain worse? Activity, rest, or nighttime?"
Numbness or tingling	Median nerve → Thumb, index, middle fingers; ulnar nerve → Ring and little finger	"Do you feel numbness or tingling in any fingers?"
Weakness in hand	Intrinsic hand muscle weakness → Ulnar nerve; grip weakness → Carpal tunnel, radial nerve palsy	"Have you noticed any weakness when gripping objects?"
Joint stiffness	Morning stiffness (>30 min) → Rheumatoid arthritis; postactivity stiffness → Osteoarthritis	"Is your hand stiff in the morning? Does it improve with movement?"
Swelling or redness	Localized swelling → Trauma or infection; diffuse swelling → Autoimmune arthritis	"Has your hand been swollen or red? Does it feel warm?"
Finger locking or clicking	Trigger finger (tendon thickening)	"Do your fingers get stuck or click when bending?"

Contd...

Contd...

Aspect	Clinical significance	Patient-friendly questions
Previous hand surgeries or injuries	Recurrent trauma → Chronic nerve compression or post-surgical scarring	"Have you had any hand injuries or surgeries in the past?"
Occupation and repetitive hand use	Frequent hand use → Carpal tunnel, tendinitis	"Do you perform repetitive hand movements at work or hobbies?"
History of systemic diseases	Diabetes → Increased risk of neuropathy and infections; autoimmune diseases → Rheumatoid arthritis, psoriasis	"Do you have diabetes, arthritis, or any long-term illness?"
Recent infections or fever	Hand infections (felon, paronychia, tenosynovitis)	"Have you had any recent cuts, wounds, or infections on your hand?"

LOCAL EXAMINATION

A. INSPECTION
Careful inspection is crucial for diagnosing hand conditions:
- **Mallet finger** → Flexed DIP joint due to **extensor tendon rupture**.
- **Trigger finger** → Painful **finger locking on flexion** due to thickened tendon sheath.
- **Claw hand** → Hyperextension of MCP, flexion of IP joints due to **ulnar nerve palsy**.
- **Volkmann's ischemic contracture** → Fixed **wrist flexion with clawing of fingers** from ischemia.
- **Dupuytren's Contracture** → Progressive **flexion of the ring/little finger due to palmar fascia thickening**.

Deformity is so characteristic of Dupuytren's contracture that nothing more could be asked from the patient. *Swelling* may be *localized* as in localized abscess (e.g., paronychia, subcuticular abscess, terminal pulp-space abscess, web-space abscess) or other local swellings as may be found anywhere in the body. *Diffuse* swelling and redness of lymphangitis, cellulitis and erysipelas are also not uncommon. *Always compare with the normal hand side by side.* Wasting of thenar or hypothenar eminence or interossei between the metacarpals can be best diagnosed by such comparison. Similarly ischemic atrophy is also diagnosed in this way.

B. PALPATION
Hand is carefully palpated to note if there is any change *of temperature* (warm or cold). In case of inflammatory lesions, e.g., cellulitis, erysipelas, abscess, arthritis, etc., there will be rise of temperature; whereas in case of ischemic lesion (cervical rib syndrome, thoracic outlet syndrome, scalenus anticus syndrome, Raynaud's disease, etc.) the hand will be cold. If there is any localized *swelling*, e.g., implantation dermoid of finger, ganglion or compound ganglion such swelling should be examined according to the plans set out in Chapter 3 'Examination of a lump or a swelling'. In case of trigger-finger thickening of the fibrous sheath of the flexor tendon can be palpated. Similarly subcutaneous nodules may be palpated in Dupuytren's contracture. Hand is also carefully palpated to detect any point of *tenderness*. This is significant to diagnose both spreading and localized infections (see below) of the hand.

Feel **both pulses** (radial and ulnar) at the wrist. Sometimes the digital arteries can be felt on either side of the base of the fingers. A rough indication of the arterial flow to the fingers can be obtained by watching the rate of feeling of the vessels beneath the nail after emptying them by pressing down on the tip of the nail.

There are certain conditions which may involve the **nerves** which supply the muscles and the skin of the hand. These nerves are mainly the median nerve, the ulnar nerve and the radial nerve. These nerves may be involved singularly or plurally in various medical conditions and surgical conditions, e.g., thoracic outlet syndrome, cervical rib syndrome, leprosy, Carpal-Tunnel syndrome (median nerve), elbow tunnel syndrome (ulnar nerve) and in various fractures and dislocations of the arm and forearm.

SENSATION: Carefully palpate the hand to locate loss of sensation or paresthesia. A few terms should be remembered in this regard—(i) paresthesia means altered sensations felt in the form of pins and needles, tingling and numbness, etc. (ii) Hyparesthesia means the skin has become hypersensitive to normal stimuli. (iii) Hypoesthesia means decreased feeling of sensation. (iv) Anesthesia means total loss of sensation of the affected part.

Assess nerve function to localize the lesion:
- **Median nerve** (Carpal tunnel syndrome) → Numbness in **thumb, index, middle fingers**, positive **tinel's and phalen's test**.
- **Ulnar nerve** (Cubital tunnel syndrome) → Numbness in **ring and little finger**, weak finger adduction (Froment's sign).
- **Radial nerve** (Wrist drop) → Loss of **wrist and finger extension**, sensation loss over **dorsal hand**.

With a fine pin, a wisp of cotton and a test-tube of warm and cold water one can test the various sensations of the hand and fingers to note which nerve has been affected. In **Figure. 9.21** the sensory distribution of these 3 nerves in the hand has been shown. One should also know the dermatomes of the hand means the sensory distribution of the spinal segment—the medial part of the hand, the whole of the little finger and a portion of the medial aspect of the ring finger are supplied by the segment C8. The lateral part of the hand, the whole of the thumb and a portion of the lateral aspect of the index finger are supplied by the segment C6. The middle portion of the hand, the whole of the middle finger, the major portion of the lateral aspect of the ring finger and the major portion of the medial aspect of the index finger are supplied by the segment C7 **(Figs. 9.23A and B)**.

MOTOR SUPPLY: The muscles that control the movement of the hand are either *intrinsic* (short muscles lying within the hand) or *extrinsic* (the long flexors and extensors of the fingers which take origins in the forearm). It is necessary to examine all the motor functions of the 3 principal nerves to know the level at which the nerve is damaged. This has been elaborately described in the chapter of 'Examination of the peripheral nerve'. In this chapter we shall only discuss the motor deficits of the hand which may occur due to affection of the individual nerve. In case of *median nerve* palsy there will be: (i) inability to abduct the thumb, (ii) inability of opposition of the thumb, (iii) inability of flexion of the terminal interphalangeal joints of the thumb and index finger, and (iv) wasting of the thenar eminence. In case of *ulnar nerve* palsy there will be (i) inability to flex the ring and the little fingers, (ii) inability of adduction and abduction of fingers and (iii) wasting of hypothenar eminence and hollows between the metacarpals. In case of *radial nerve* palsy there will be: (i) inability to extend the wrist (wrist drop), (ii) inability to extend the metacarpophalangeal joints of all the fingers and (iii) inability to extend interphalangeal joint of the thumb.

C. MOVEMENTS

Both active and passive movements of all the important joints of the hand should be performed to know of various affection of the joints. The following joints are important in the hand:

(i) **WRIST JOINT:** The movements of the wrist joint or the radiocarpal joint occur in association with the movement of the midcarpal joints. The active movements of these joints are flexion, extension, adduction (ulnar deviation), abduction (radial deviation) and circumduction. When the wrist is *flexed* both the radiocarpal and midcarpal joints are implicated, though the range of movement is greater at the latter joint. In *extension*, the reverse is the case and most of the movement takes place at the radiocarpal joint. The range of adduction is considerably more than that of abduction may be due to shortness of the styloid process of the ulna. In *adduction*, most of the movement occurs at the radiocarpal joint. In *abduction*, the movement takes place almost entirely at the midcarpal joints. *Circumduction* of the hand results from the movements of flexion, adduction, extension and abduction carried out in that order or in the reverse order.

(ii) **CARPOMETACARPAL JOINT** of the thumb permits flexion, extension, adduction, abduction and opposition.

(iii) **METACARPOPHALANGEAL JOINTS** of the fingers permit flexion, extension, adduction and abduction.

(iv) **INTERPHALANGEAL JOINTS** of the fingers permit only flexion and extension.

Inability of active movement of a joint may be due to involvement of motor nerve supplying the muscles concerned with the movement or due to injury to the tendons of the muscles concerned with the movement. Passive movement of the joint and both active and passive movements of joint will be interfered with in cases of intra-articular pathologies or extra-articular pathologies, e.g., sprain of the ligaments, ligamentous adhesions, adhesions of the tendons, etc.

INFECTION OF THE FINGERS AND HAND

Hand infections are classified as follows:
- **Spreading infections** → Lymphangitis, cellulitis, erysipelas.
- **Localized infections** → Paronychia, pulp space infection (felon), web space abscess.
- **Tendon sheath infections** → Suppurative tenosynovitis (kanavel's signs).
- **Deep space infections** → Thenar, midpalmar, ulnar bursitis.

SPREADING INFECTIONS

Lymphangitis: The organisms gain entrance through a minute abrasion which is often forgotten by the patient. Soon the hand becomes swollen with severe constitutional disturbances like high fever. Hand becomes painful, red, warm and tender. Considerable edema is the characteristic feature. In fair-skinned person red streaks may be noticed along the lymph vessels. The regional lymph nodes become enlarged and tender. For the lateral half of the hand the axillary nodes become first involved whereas in the affection of the medial half of the hand, the supratrochlear group of lymph nodes will be enlarged.

Cellulitis: *See* page 51.

LOCALIZED INFECTIONS

Intracutaneous abscess: This can also be designated as septic blister. This is often seen on the palmar surface of the digits and the webs. Pus collects within the layers of the skin to elevate the epidermis from the dermis. Sometimes an intracutaneous abscess may communicate with subcutaneous abscess through a small hole and this is called a *Collar-stud abscess.* So during evacuation of pus care must be taken to lay open the deep abscess also.

Paronychia: The inflammation commences beneath the eponychium. Suppuration usually follows which may burrow beneath the base of the nail. The infection is subcuticular since it is situated entirely within the dermis in which the nail is developed. The infection arises from careless nail paring or from manicurist's unsterile instrument. The diagnosis is obvious on inspection which shows redness and swelling of the nail fold. Excruciating pain on touch is the characteristic feature.

Chronic paronychia: This condition affects women more often than men and those who do much washing. The onset is insidious (the condition has already existed for months). It seldom follows acute paronychia. On inspection the eponychium is glazed and faintly pink (cf. acute paronychia, where it is angry red). The nail may become cross-ridged and pigmented (cf. acute paronychia in which the nail remains absolutely normal but there may be subungual extension of pus). This condition may be multiple (cf. acute paronychia which is almost always a single lesion).

Apical space infection: This is a tiny abscess at the tip of the finger just under the nail. Though this condition is exquisitely painful, there is comparatively little swelling. Sometimes this condition is associated with redness extending along one or both the lateral nail folds and to add to fallacy this may be prolonged even into the eponychium. Paronychia is excluded by finding out the area of greatest tenderness which is always just above the distal edge of nail in case of apical space infection. In advanced untreated cases there is likelihood of osteomyelitis of the end of the distal phalanx with possible sequestration and prolonged sinus formation.

SUBCUTANEOUS INFECTIONS

PULP SPACE INFECTION (FELON)

The term denotes a subcutaneous infection of the terminal segment of a digit. This condition is quite common as the pulp of the finger is subjected to pricks and abrasions. The terminal pulp space of the finger is subdivided into 15–20 compartments by fibrous septa stretching between the periosteum of the phalanx and the skin **(Fig. 20.1)**. These compartments are limited proximally by a transverse septum of deep fascia, which is attached to the base of the distal phalanx at the level of the epiphyseal line. This arrangement has an important bearing on localization and spread of pulp infections. The strong proximal boundary of the fascial compartment acts as an effective barrier to infection spreading proximally up the finger. This leads to increase in tension within the closed compartments which may affect the blood supply of the distal 4/5th of the distal phalanx leading to necrosis of that part of the bone.

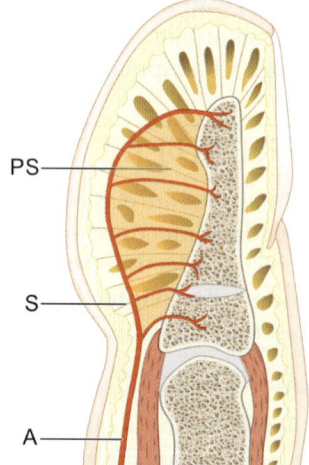

Fig. 20.1: Shows the pulp space (PS), which is a closed space bounded proximally by a fibrous septum (S) at the level of the epiphyseal line of the terminal phalanx. The space is traversed by fibrous strands from the skin to the periosteum and carry blood vessels to the bone. In pulp space infection (Felon) the tension in this closed space becomes increased. The blood vessels are occluded causing necrosis to the distal four-fifths of the terminal phalanx. The proximal one-fifth (the epiphysis) gets the supply from a twig from below the septum and hence not affected by this affection and remains viable althroughout.

This condition starts with pain which increases in intensity very fast and swelling. Soon the pain becomes severe and throbbing in nature. Swelling is maximum at the center where abscess develops. This condition should be recognized as early as possible and the pus should be drained before the disease has involved the bone. When following drainage of the space, the wound continues to discharge with sprouting granulation tissue at the mouth of the sinus, it is quite certain that necrosis of the terminal phalanx has occurred. X-ray will confirm the diagnosis.

Complications: (i) Osteomyelitis of the terminal phalanx. (ii) Pyogenic arthritis of the distal interphalangeal joint. (iii) Spread of infection to the flexor-tendon sheath, probably due to the fact that the incision has been wrongly extended proximally to the sheath.

INFECTION OF THE MIDDLE AND PROXIMAL VOLAR SPACES

This condition is less common than the preceding one. The pus becomes localized above and below by flexion creases. There is tender induration of the affected space. The finger is held in semiflexion position. In case of proximal volar space infection, the web space is frequently involved. Middle volar space infection is sometimes difficult to differentiate from suppurative tenosynovitis, the only differentiating feature being relatively pain-free movement of the fingers in case of the former.

Complications: The infection in these spaces tend to spread to the (i) web space, (ii) interphalangeal joint and (iii) tendon sheath.

WEB SPACE INFECTION

There is only loose fat in the web space. Infection of the proximal volar space or the web space gives rise to considerable swelling with separation of the adjacent fingers. The swelling also spreads to the dorsum of the hand. Maximum tenderness is found on the palmar aspect of the web and on the adjacent bases of the fingers. In untreated cases the pus tends to point under the thinner skin on the dorsal aspect. Gradually, the adjacent webs may be involved.

■ SUPPURATIVE TENOSYNOVITIS (INTRATHECAL WHITLOW)

This is an infection of the flexor tendon sheath **(Fig. 20.2)**. The infection is mainly a direct one from a prick of a needle, a thorn or a dorsal fin of a fish. The prick is obviously through the skin overlying the tendon sheath, mostly through a digital flexion crease as at this part the skin surface is remarkably nearer to the sheath. Sometimes this condition may develop from injudicious incision for drainage of the distal pulp space or from spread of infection from the middle and proximal volar spaces. The whole sheath is rapidly involved. The patient feels throbbing pain in the affected digit, the finger becomes red and swollen and the patient's temperature rises. Infection of the thumb or little finger spreads up to the palm to involve the radial or ulnar bursa respectively. The cardinal features of this condition are: (i) Uniform swelling of the whole finger except the terminal segment where there is no tendon sheath. (ii) Typically, the finger is held in flexed position. This is an early sign. (iii) Tenderness over the anatomical disposition of the sheath. To determine the area of tenderness the end of a match stick serves the purpose admirably. Accurate localization of tenderness is not possible with the examiner's finger tip which covers too wide an area. Usually the tenderness is most marked at the proximal ends of the sheaths in case of the index, middle and ring fingers. In case of ulnar bursa, a point of maximum tenderness is obtained over the part of the bursa lying between the two transverse palmar creases—*Kanavel's sign*. (iv) The patient is asked to move the fingers. Slight movement of the metacarpophalangeal joint by contraction of the lumbrical and interosseous muscles may be possible but movement of the interphalangeal joint is completely restricted, (v) Any attempt to straighten the finger actively or passively causes exquisite pain.

Complications: (i) Necrosis of the tendon and adhesion of the tendon with the sheath result in permanent stiffness of the finger in flexed position. (ii) Spread of infection from one tendon sheath to another is not impossible since the ulnar and radial bursae inter-communicate in 80% of cases and occasionally the tendon sheath of the index or the middle or the ring finger communicates with the ulnar bursa.

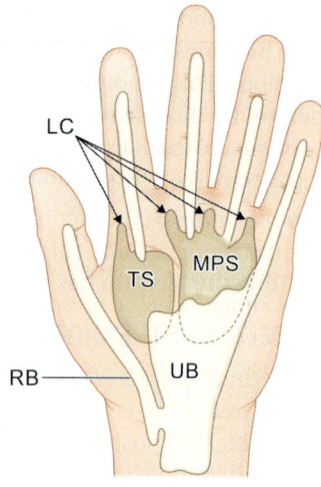

INFECTION OF THE ULNAR BURSA

This is probably the most serious of all infections in the hand. The infection may result from a direct spread from tenosynovitis of the 5th finger. The clinical features of this condition are: Flexion of mainly the little finger and other fingers if the sheaths of their tendons communicate with the ulnar bursa, but if the sheath has already ruptured this finding may not be possible. The features are—fullness of the palm **(Fig. 20.3)**; maximum tenderness towards the ulnar side between the two palmar creases (Kanavel's point) **(Fig. 20.4)** and edematous swelling of the dorsum of the hand.

Fig. 20.2: Shows anatomical disposition of the tendon sheaths and fascial spaces. (UB: ulnar bursa; RB: radial bursa; TS: thenar space; MPS: middle palmar space; LC: lumbrical canals)

INFECTION OF THE RADIAL BURSA

In fact true synovitis of the flexor pollicis longus always brings about this condition. This is evident by the fact that swelling of the thumb is seen to extend into the thenar eminence. The thumb is held flexed. Swelling may be seen just proximal to the flexor retinaculum on the lateral side.

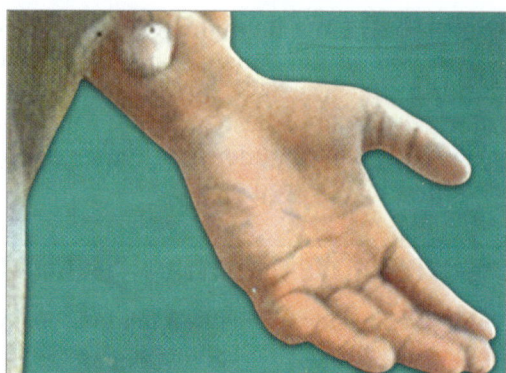

Fig. 20.3: Infection of the ulnar bursa. See how the hypothenar eminence, the little and the ring fingers are swollen and red.

■ INFECTIONS OF THE FASCIAL SPACES

There are a few cellular spaces in the hand as shown in **Figure 20.5**. In the dorsum, where the importance of these cellular spaces is very much insignificant, there are only two spaces—(i) Subcutaneous (superficial to the aponeurosis extending between the extensor tendons) and (ii) Subaponeurotic (deep to the extensor expansion). In the palm, there are (i) Subaponeurotic space (just deep to the palmar fascia but superficial to the flexor tendon sheath). The space deep to the flexor tendon sheaths is the main cellular space which may becomes infected and is divided into two compartments—(ii) Thenar space (which lies deep to the thenar muscles and superficial to the adductor pollicis) and (iii) Middle palmar space (which is situated deep to the flexor tendons and superficial to the medial three metacarpals and the intervening interossei). These two compartments are separated by a septum which is attached to the 3rd metacarpal bone posteriorly and to the flexor tendon sheath anteriorly between the tendons for the index finger and the middle finger. The septum is obliquely placed. These two spaces are continuous proximally with the Parona's space, which lies in front of the pronator quadratus and behind the flexor tendons.

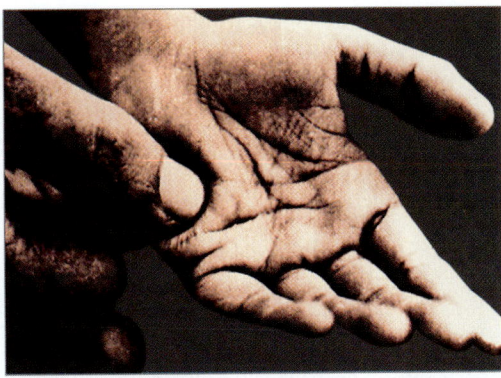

Fig. 20.4: Shows how to examine for Kanavel's sign. See the text.

INFECTION OF THE SUBAPONEUROTIC SPACE

This may follow pricks. The palm looks swollen and tender. The pus often tracks through a point in the palmar fascia to be superficial, forming a Collar-stud abscess.

INFECTION OF THE THENAR SPACE

The characteristic feature is the "ballooning" of thenar eminence **(Figs. 20.6A and B)**. The thumb is held abducted and flexed. The web space between the thumb and the index finger is swollen. This condition should be differentiated from tenosynovitis of the flexor pollicis longus. This can be done by passive extension of the thumb, which is very painful and not allowed in case of the latter.

INFECTION OF THE MIDDLE PALMAR SPACE

There may not be much swelling of the palm, but obliteration of the normal hollow of the palm is noticed. This is due to the fact that the pus is situated beneath the thick, strong and resistant

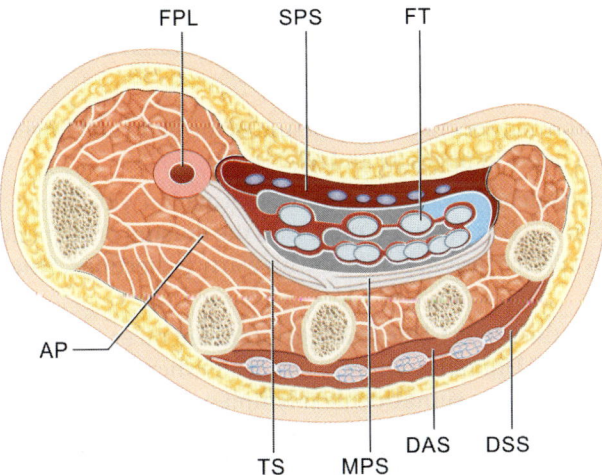

Fig. 20.5: Cross section of the palm showing: FPL: tendon of flexor pollicis longus in radial bursa; SPS: superficial palmar space; FT: flexor tendons to all fingers (except the thumb) in ulnar bursa; AP: adductor pollicis; TS: thenar space; MPS: middle palmar space; DAS: dorsal subaponeurotic space; DSS: dorsal subcutaneous space.

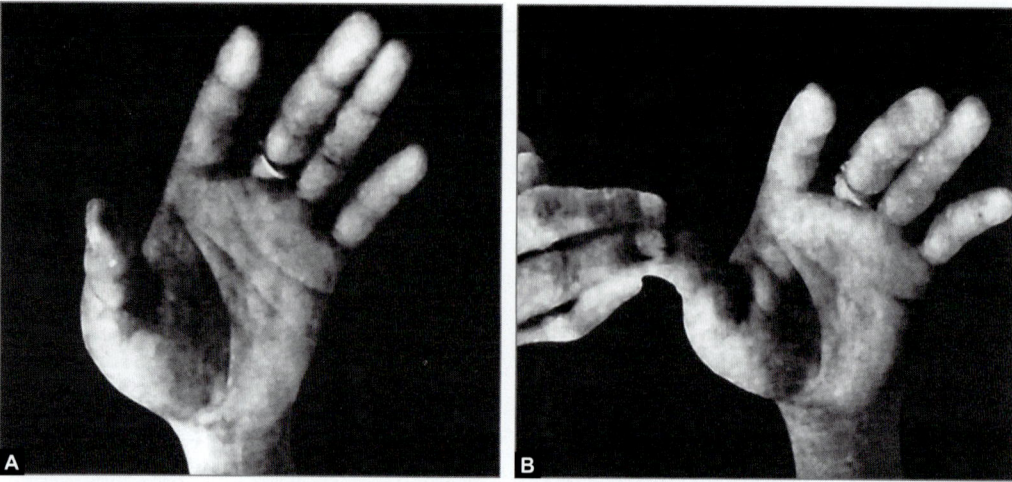

Figs. 20.6A and B: Showing swollen thenar eminence in thenar space infection. Note that passive extension of the thumb is possible and not painful. This excludes infection of the radial bursa.

palmar fascia. Fluctuation is difficult to elicit. The fingers are held in flexion. But their movement and passive extension are not so painful as in the case of tenosynovitis.

It must be remembered that in all infections of the palm there will be considerable swelling on the dorsum. This is because the lymphatics from the palm pass over to the dorsal aspect of the hand and also due to the fact that the skin and subcutaneous tissue on the dorsum are more loose and elastic.

INFECTION OF THE PARONA'S SPACE

Besides proximal extension of the infection from middle palmar and thenar spaces, this space may be infected in suppurative tenosynovitis. Deep-seated abscess may develop. Fluctuation is difficult to elicit. But brawny induration that pits on pressure suggests abscess formation.

OTHER INFECTIONS OF THE HAND

Carbuncle and **furuncle** may occur on the dorsum of the hand and finger. The clinical picture has been described in detail in pages 52 and 53.

Verruca necrogenica (Butcher's wart) is caused by inoculation with *Mycobacterium tuberculosis* through an abrasion in the skin. It is seen mostly on the dorsum of the hand. It begins as bluish red patch, later on its surface becomes raised with warty projections. Small pustules surround this warty mass.

Hunterian chancre of the finger: This painless indurated ulcer, which is more often seen on the index finger, is a typical Hunterian chancre found anywhere in the body. The regional lymph node is enlarged, which may be supratrochlear lymph node or axillary lymph node.

Dactylitis: This term denotes infection of the phalanges or metacarpals. Two types are commonly seen—tuberculous dactylitis and syphilitic dactylitis. In tuberculous dactylitis, the affected bone becomes enlarged, spindle-shaped and painful. There is a great tendency to soften, ulcerate or involve the neighboring joint. X-ray shows osteolytic changes. In syphilitic dactylitis, there

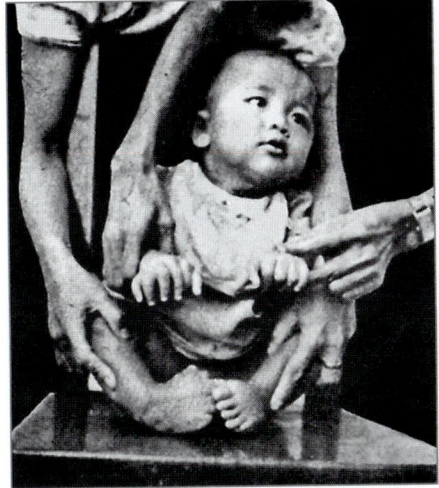

Fig. 20.7: Polydactylism.

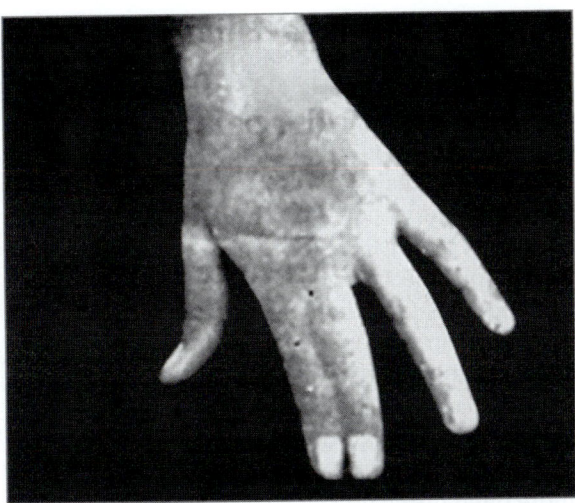

Fig. 20.8: Syndactylism.

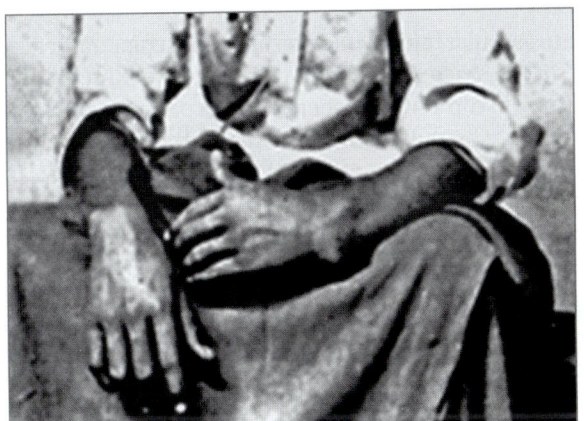

Fig. 20.9: Madelung's deformity of the left hand.

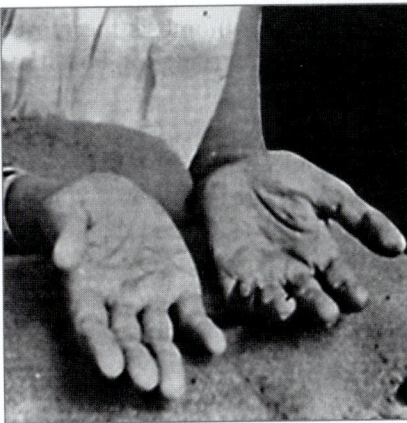

Fig. 20.10: Showing Dupuytren's contracture affecting left hand. See the difference with the normal right hand. The little and the ring fingers are affected by contracture. The thickened nodule is shown by an arrow.

is also a swelling but it is painless. X-ray will show sclerosis of bone. Other syphilitic stigmas will confirm the diagnosis.

OTHER LESIONS OF THE HAND

A. **CONGENITAL DEFORMITIES** include: *Polydactylism*, i.e., supernumerary fingers (**Fig. 20.7**); *Ectrodactylism*, i.e., absence of digits; *Syndactylism*, i.e., webbing of the fingers (**Fig. 20.8**); *Macrodactylism*, i.e., overgrowth of fingers; *congenital contracture of the little finger*; *Madelung's deformity*, i.e., congenital subluxation of the lower end of the ulna (**Fig. 20.9**).

B. **ACQUIRED DEFORMITIES**

Dupuytren's contracture—is an affection of the palmar aponeurosis which is thickened and contracted (**Fig. 20.10**). Usually, the ring finger is affected and this condition is more commonly seen in men. Usually, a nodule is palpated in the subcutaneous tissue of the palm. Thickened palmar aponeurosis is also felt in certain cases. First the proximal phalanx and then the middle phalanx are flexed but the terminal phalanx remains unaffected since the palmar aponeurosis does not extend to that phalanx (cf. *congenital contracture of the little finger* in which the first phalanx is hyperextended and the 2nd and 3rd phalanges are flexed). The finger can neither be straightened actively nor passively even on flexing the wrist (cf. Volkmann's ischemic contracture). Its incidence is curiously more in epileptic and cirrhotic individuals. Those, who work with vibratory machines, are more often the victims. It has got an unknown relationship with Paronie's disease of penis and Pellegrini Stieda's disease.

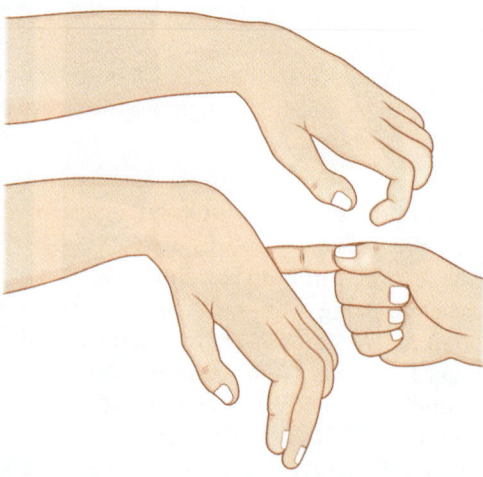

Fig. 20.11: Volkmann's ischemic contracture. Fingers can be extended to some extent if the wrist is passively flexed.

Volkmann's ischemic contracture—is due to vascular injury which result in muscular infarction and subsequent contracture **(Fig. 20.11)**. *In the stage* of *ischemia* the signs like *p*ain, *p*allor, *p*uffiness (edema), *p*ulselessness and *p*aralysis (five 'p's) will be seen. Pain on passive extension of the fingers is probably the first sign to appear. The radial pulse is constantly absent and the skin temperature of the affected hand will definitely be lower than its healthy counterpart. *In the stage of contracture* the fingers become flexed but they can be, at least partially, extended when the wrist is flexed (cf. Dupuytren's contracture in which the affected finger can never be extended).

Congenital contracture of the little finger—is commonly seen during early childhood. It is frequently bilateral. In many ways it mimics Dupuytren's contracture, but absence of thickening of the palmar fascia is the pathognomonic feature of this condition. Moreover the ring finger is rarely involved. The pathology is the contracture of the soft tissues.

Burns contracture can be diagnosed easily by the history itself.

Mallet finger is a typical deformity in which there is persistent flexion of the terminal phalanx. This is due to rupture of the extensor tendon either at its insertion or due to an avulsion fracture of the base of the terminal phalanx.

Trigger finger is a condition in which the extension of the affected finger becomes difficult and unequal, so that the patient's initial effort does not produce any extension and later on the finger is extended suddenly with a click. This action is more or less like a trigger of a pistol and hence the nomenclature. The middle-aged women are frequently the victims and the most commonly affected finger is the middle or the ring finger. A palpable nodular thickening may develop in the long flexor tendon opposite the head of the metacarpal or there may be a constriction in the tendon sheath which is responsible for this condition. In children this condition may occasionally be seen and the thumb is the most affected finger and is often called 'Snapping Thumb'. An orange-pip like swelling can be felt over the head of the 1st metacarpal bone. Extension is brought about with a click.

Attrition rupture of the extensor pollicis longus is also a condition most commonly seen in middle-aged women. This is usually due to rheumatoid arthritis or occasionally may complicate a Colles' fracture. While working with the thumb suddenly the patient experiences a snap and the thumb falls adducted helplessly and the patient fails to extend the terminal interphalangeal joint of the thumb.

Rheumatoid arthritis of the hand: The metacarpophalangeal joints are most commonly affected, the proximal interphalangeal joints are next to be involved. In the beginning, there will be hypertrophy of the synovial membrane of the joints *(Pannus)*. Gradually, the overlying skin becomes shiny and atrophic. The affected joints are swollen and become fusiform in shape. Muscle wasting is quite significant. Deformity is the most prominent feature in late cases—(i) *Ulnar drift* is common at the metacarpophalangeal joint as the normal line of the pull of the finger tendon is slightly towards the ulnar side, synovial swelling tends to push the extensor tendon medially and in the normal resting posture gravity favors ulnar deviation; (ii) *Swan-neck deformity,* i.e., hyperextension at the proximal interphalangeal joint and flexion at the distal interphalangeal joint, is due to forward subluxation at the proximal interphalangeal joint or attrition rupture of the sublimis tendon or impediment of action of flexor sublimis tendon by synovial swelling; (iii) *Boutonniere deformity,* i.e., flexion of the proximal interphalangeal joint and hyperextension at the distal, occurs when the middle slip of the extensor tendon undergoes attrition rupture; (iv) *Dropped fingers* is a late feature following rupture of extensor tendons usually at the level of the wrist.

Heberden's nodes: These are small long swellings about the size of small peas which are seen at the terminal interphalangeal joints of all fingers except the thumb. It is felt as definite bony ridge across the palmar and dorsal surfaces of the affected joints. These nodes are due to osteoarthrosis, though these do not herald osteoarthrosis of other joints. Women near menopause are usually involved, though males are also rarely involved due to repeated trauma to the finger in games like cricket or baseball and the lesion is almost always solitary in males. Pain is conspicuous by its absence in this lesion.

Barber's pilonidal sinus: Barbers may have interdigital pilonidal sinus at the web space often between the middle and ring fingers of the right hand. Clipped hairs usually have beveled tips like those of hypodermic needles which may penetrate the skin of the web space which does not have hair follicles. The lesion looks like a black dot at the dorsum of the affected cleft. When palpated with the thumb and index finger, a nodule is palpated. This lesion is liable to be inflamed. In 80% of cases the lesion is multiple. In female hair dressers such lesion may be seen in interdigital clefts between the toes in those who are accustomed not to use stockings particularly in hot climate.

C. SWELLINGS OF THE HAND: (i) Implantation dermoid is caused by prick by different pointed objects such as needle, bone of a fish, etc. The epithelium of the skin is driven in and causes such condition. A soft cystic swelling is found mostly in the finger and occasionally in the hand which is neither attached to the skin nor to the deeper structures. Fluctuation can be elicited.

(ii) Ganglion: This is commonly seen on the dorsum of the wrist or even on its volar aspect. This has been discussed in page 169.

(iii) Glomus tumor: This is a red or violet color small tumor mostly seen beneath the nail. Considering its size it is an exquisitely tender tumor. The tumor is derived from a glomus body—an arteriovenous anastomosis incorporating nerve tissue. This is believed to help in regulating body temperature. A peculiar characteristic feature is that the tenderness is reduced considerably by applying a sphygmomanometer cuff and inflating it above the systolic blood pressure.

(iv) Compound palmar ganglion (Fig. 20.12): Probably this condition is still a feature of tuberculous tenosynovitis of the ulnar bursa in this country, but in western countries it is mostly associated with rheumatoid arthritis. The main feature is an hour-glass shaped swelling bulging above and below the flexor retinaculum. Cross fluctuation can be elicited from the swelling above and below the flexor retinaculum. With careful palpation one can feel movements of the melon-seed bodies within the bursa.

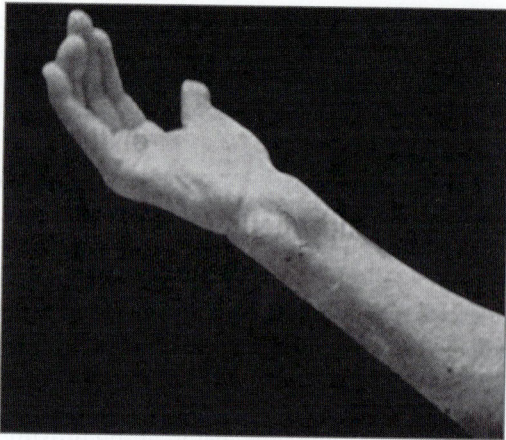

Fig. 20.12: Compound palmar ganglion. Note the swelling above and below the flexor retinaculum.

Algorithmic Approach to Patient with Hand Conditions

Patient presents with hand pain, numbness, weakness, or deformity

↓

Is there a history of trauma?
- Yes → Consider **fracture, dislocation, ligament injury, or tendon rupture**
- No → Assess **for neurological or systemic causes**

↓

Is there numbness or tingling?
- Yes → Perform **nerve examination (median, ulnar, radial nerves)**
- No → Assess for **structural deformities or joint pathology**

↓

Does the patient have swelling or warmth?
- Yes → Consider **infection (cellulitis, abscess, tenosynovitis, septic arthritis)**
- No → Evaluate for **degenerative (osteoarthritis) or autoimmune (rheumatoid arthritis) causes**

↓

Perform motor testing to identify nerve deficits
- **Thumb opposition weakness** → **Median nerve involvement (carpal tunnel syndrome)**
- **Finger abduction weakness** → **Ulnar nerve involvement (cubital tunnel syndrome)**
- **Wrist drop** → **Radial nerve involvement (nerve palsy)**

↓

Perform imaging to confirm diagnosis
- **X-ray** → For **fractures, dislocations, bony deformities**
- **MRI** → For **soft tissue injury, nerve compression**
- **Nerve conduction study** → For **peripheral neuropathy**

↓

Determine need for surgery vs conservative management
- **Surgical intervention?** → If **tendon rupture, severe nerve compression, unstable fracture**
- **Conservative management?** → If **mild to moderate carpal tunnel syndrome, arthritis, or trigger finger**

CHAPTER 21

Examination of the Foot

■ HISTORY

Patients with foot conditions usually present with **pain, deformity, or functional impairment**. A structured history should include:
- **Pain location:** Heel, midfoot, forefoot, toes.
- **Onset and duration:** Sudden (trauma, infection) vs gradual (degenerative, congenital).
- **Precipitating factors:** Walking, standing, footwear.
- **Radiation of pain:** Suggestive of nerve involvement (Morton's neuroma, radiculopathy).
- **Associated deformities:** Progressive vs static conditions.

This is so typical at times that this history itself can give the diagnosis. Pain at the neck of the 2nd metatarsal bone after a long walking is probably due to march fracture (stress fracture). When a young girl complains of pain at the head of the 2nd metatarsal bone whose onset is rather insidious, the condition is probably one of Freiberg's disease. Pain between the heads of the 3rd and 4th metatarsals radiating to the adjacent sides of the toes indicates Morton's metatarsalgia. Plantar fasciitis gives rise to pain on the ball of the heel particularly on walking.

In case of ***deformity***, one should carefully note the type of deformity, its duration and whether it is associated with any other deformity in the body.

History in foot diseases

Aspect	Clinical significance	Patient-friendly questions
Age	Helps diagnose **age-related spinal conditions**	"How old are you?"
Onset of pain	Acute → Trauma/Disc prolapse, Chronic → Degenerative/Infective	"Did the pain start suddenly or gradually?"
Radiation of pain	Follows nerve root compression patterns	"Does the pain travel down your legs or arms?"
Stiffness	Prominent in ankylosing spondylitis	"Do you feel stiff in the morning?"
Night pain	Red flag for tumors, infections	"Does the pain wake you up at night?"

■ PHYSICAL EXAMINATION

A. INSPECTION

The patient is asked to stand evenly on both feet and observe if there is any deformity. Foot examination should include:

- **Weight-bearing and nonweight-bearing inspection:** Identify postural abnormalities.
- **Arch assessment:** Pes planus (flat foot) vs Pes cavus (high arch).
- **Toe deformities:** Hallux valgus, hammer toe, curly toes.
- **Skin changes:** Corns, callosities, ulcers (diabetic foot, neuropathy).
- **Gait analysis:** Antalgic gait (pain-related), equinus gait (contracture-related).

In talipes equinovarus the forefoot is adducted and points downwards. In pes planus, the longitudinal arch is flattened so that the navicular region may be seen bulging. In pes cavus the longitudinal arch is higher than normal. In talipes calcaneovalgus the forefoot looks upwards and abducted. There may be swelling, ulcer or sinus in the foot, which is examined in the usual way as described in the respective chapters.

B. PALPATION

When the main complaint is pain, the point of maximum tenderness must be noted carefully. Tenderness beneath the heel may be due to plantar fasciitis or a bony spur underneath the calcaneal tuberosity. Localized tenderness over the back of the calcaneal tuberosity, particularly in boys of about 10 years of age, is usually due to Sever's disease (apophysitis of the calcaneus); this may also be due to bursitis just above the insertion of the tendo Achillis. Tenderness at the neck of the 2nd metatarsal bone after a long march is due to march fracture. Tenderness between the heads of the 3rd and 4th metatarsal bones is due to Morton's metatarsalgia.

C. MOVEMENTS

At the ankle joint (talocrural joint) the active movements are dorsiflexion and plantar flexion. In *dorsiflexion* the angle between the front of the leg and the dorsum of the foot is diminished. In *plantar flexion* this angle is increased, the heel is raised and the toes point downwards. A considerable range of rotatory movement is permitted at both talocalcanean (subtalar) joint and talocalcaneonavicular joint. The calcaneus and the navicular carrying the foot with them can be moved medially on the talus and this movement results in elevation of the medial border and corresponding depression of the lateral border of the foot so that the plantar aspect of the foot faces medially and this is called *inversion* of foot. The greater part of this movement occurs at the above-mentioned two joints. The axis of this rotation movement runs from back of the calcaneus, through sinus tarsi to emerge at the superior and medial aspect of the neck of the talus. The obliquity of this axis accounts for the adduction and slight flexion of the foot that accompany inversion. The opposite movement of this is known as *eversion,* the range of which is much more limited due to tension of the tibialis anterior and tibialis posterior and the strong deltoid (medial) ligament of the ankle joint.

Both active and passive movements of these should be carefully measured to know the excessive limitation of a particular movement. Since flexion and extension take place at the talocrural (ankle) joint, the passive movements of these can be tested by holding with one hand the lower end of the leg and with the other hand the proximal part of the foot so as to include the talus within the hand and both flexion and extension passive movements are tested. In case of *inversion* and *eversion*, the passive movements are tested by holding the very lower end of the leg with one hand to fix the talus and then with other hand hold the heel of the foot and then twist the foot medially and laterally. *Adduction and abduction* movements mainly take place in the midtarsal joints and ranges of passive movements are tested by holding the heel with the lower part of the leg with one hand and the forefoot with the other hand and then by adducting and abducting the forefoot one can assess the ranges of passive movements.

D. NEUROLOGICAL EXAMINATIONS

Neurological examination is critical in foot disorders, as deformities may be linked to systemic neurological conditions:
- **Sensation testing:** Light touch, pinprick, vibration (diabetic neuropathy, peripheral nerve lesions).
- **Motor function:** Weak dorsiflexion (common peroneal nerve injury), weak toe flexion (Tibial nerve injury).
- **Reflex testing:** Absent ankle jerk (S1 lesion, neuropathy).
- **Spinal screening:** Talipes equinovarus (spina bifida), foot drop (L5 radiculopathy).

Deformity of foot is sometimes due to abnormality affecting spinal column. Talipes equinovarus is often an accompaniment of spina bifida **(Fig. 21.1)**.

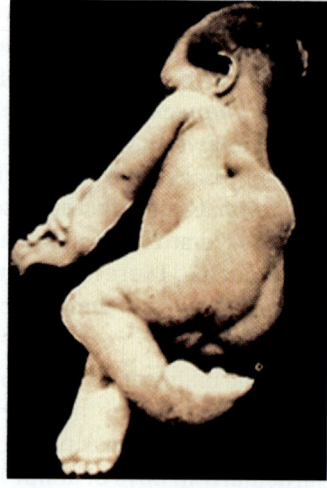

Fig. 21.1: Talipes equinovarus as an accompaniment of spina bifida.

E. EXAMINATIONS OF THE KNEE, HIP AND SPINE

As has been mentioned earlier that the spinal column must be examined thoroughly to exclude any abnormality there in cases of deformities of the foot. Genu valgus is sometimes associated with pes planus. Limb rotation is also seen to be associated with pes planus. Coxa vara may be associated with some form of deformity of the foot.

SPECIAL INVESTIGATIONS

X-ray examination is quite helpful in the diagnosis of different deformities of the foot as well as to know a few pathologies involving the foot.

DIAGNOSIS

DEFORMITIES of the foot and toes **(Figs. 21.2A to C)** are as follows:

Talipes: The different types are: (i) *Talipes equinus*—the patient walks on toes. (ii) *Talipes calcaneus*—the patient walks on the heel. (iii) *Talipes varus*—the patient walks on the outer border of the foot (i.e., the sole of the foot looks medially). (iv) *Talipes valgus*—the patient walks on the medial border of the foot (i.e., opposite of talipes varus). (v) *Talipes equinovarus* and *talipes calcaneovalgus* are two common combinations and mixture of two different deformities stated above. Talipes equinovarus is the more common.

Common foot deformities:
- **Talipes equinovarus (clubfoot)** → Forefoot adduction, hindfoot varus, ankle equinus.
- **Pes planus (flat foot)** → Loss of longitudinal arch, medial bulging.
- **Pes cavus (high arch foot)** → Excessive arch, clawing of toes.

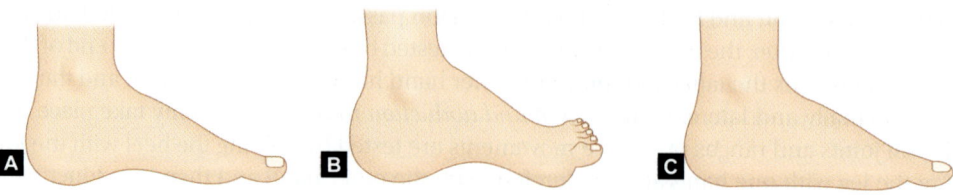

Figs. 21.2A to C: Deformities of the arch of the foot: (A) Normal foot; (B) Claw-foot; (C) Flat foot.

- **Hallux valgus (bunion)** → Lateral deviation of great toe, metatarsal prominence.
- **Hammer toe** → Hyperextension of MTP joint, flexion at PIP joint.
- **Claw toe** → Flexion of PIP & DIP joints, overpowered intrinsic muscles.

1. **Talipes equinovarus or club foot:** It is a combination of three elements—equinus, varus (i.e., inversion) and adduction. The talus points downwards (equinus), the calcaneum faces inwards (varus) and the forefoot is adducted. The *congenital* variety is by far the commoner. This type is recognized by the following points: (i) Present from birth. (ii) usually bilateral, and (iii) presence of a transverse crease across the sole of the medial side. Later on when the child has walked, callosities and bursae develop on the outer border. The *acquired* type is usually unilateral and shows trophic changes in the skin which may be cold and blue. There may be infantile paralysis (the muscles are flaccid and wasted) or spastic upper motor neuron type of paralysis.

2. **Pes planus or flat foot**—is flattening of the longitudinal arch of the foot. Flat foot may be of anatomical or physiological type. *Anatomically*, it may be due to: (1) External rotation of tibia; (2) Genu valgum; (3) Equinus position of the foot or (4) Varus position of the forefoot. *Physiologically* they are of: (1) Congenital variety with vertical talus (boat shaped foot); (2) Infantile flat foot—before the child learns to walk; (3) Middle aged flat foot in case of flabby obese individual; (4) Postural flat foot with weak intrinsic muscles of the foot, with or without other postural defect like kyphosis, etc.; (5) Temporary flat foot following long standing chronic illness when the patient first stands on his feet, the feet become flat and the patient complains of 'foot strain', i.e., strain of the inferior calcaneonavicular ligament.

    Spasmodic flat foot is absolutely a separate entity due to spasm of peroneal muscles. This is found mostly in 12–16 years old boys. Often it is due to tarsal coalition, i.e., presence of abnormal bony or cartilaginous bar extending from calcaneus to talus or navicular bone. Probably, the spasm is due to faulty movement of the subtaloid and midtarsal joints.

    The diagnosis is made by looking at the medial side of the foot. Instead of the normal concavity, there is flattening or even convexity with prominence of the tarsal navicular. Examine the shoes the patient is wearing. The sole and the heel are worn away more on the inner side and the inner side of the shoe often bulges medially and downwards. There are often two physical signs, viz. limitation of movements of the tarsal joints and localized tenderness over the 'spring' ligament (inferior calcaneonavicular ligament).

3. **Pes cavus or claw foot:** The deformity consists of a high-arched foot with dorsiflexion or even dorsal subluxation of the metatarsophalangeal joints and plantar flexion of interphalangeal joints. The intrinsic muscles of the foot, in this condition, become weak and are overpowered by the long toe muscles. This weakness may be due to neurological disease, myopathy, vascular lesion or idiopathic (probably the commonest). Idiopathic pes cavus is first noticed at the age of 8–10 years in an otherwise fit child.

4. **Talipes calcaneovalgus:** This deformity is quite uncommon and it is important to exclude congenital dislocation of the hip in this condition.

5. **Hallux valgus (Fig. 21.3):** The great toe is abducted at the metatarsophalangeal joint. The inner portion of the head of the first metatarsal bone forms a marked prominence. An adventitious bursa which is liable to inflammation, suppuration and sinus formation may develop. The condition is usually bilateral. The other toes are crowded together and the 2nd toe may be a hammer toe. Metatarsus primus varus is the basic deformity which may be congenital or acquired. In the acquired variety

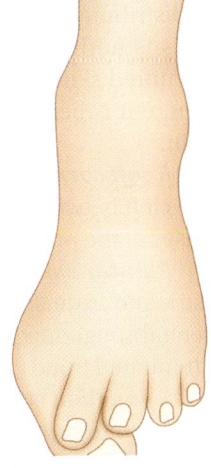

Fig. 21.3: Hallux valgus.

generally the middle-aged obese person with splayed forefoot may lead to varus deformity of the first metatarsal bone. Shoe, at times, is incriminated for this deformity, as short and pointed shoe may lead to this condition.

6. **Hallux rigidus:** This means stiff great toe with painful limitation of dorsiflexion with fixity in the position of slight plantar flexion. This can also be a congenital or acquired deformity. In case of acquired deformity three causes have been found out which may lead to this deformity: (i) The hallux is longer than the 2nd toe so that it may be stubbed repeatedly against the toe cap of the shoe; (ii) Splitting osteochondritis of the head of the first metatarsal bone and (iii) Sesamoid chondromalacia is another possible precursor. The chief complaint is pain on walking especially on rough grounds and slopes. This condition is often bilateral. Adult males are mainly affected but adolescents of either sex are not completely exempt from this condition.

7. **Hammer toe:** The 2nd toe on one or both the feet is commonly affected. Hallux valgus is often associated with this condition. The metatarsophalangeal joint is hyperextended and the proximal toe joint is fixed flexed. A corn or a bursa is often present on the dorsum of the first interphalangeal joint.

8. **Curly toes:** The metatarsophalangeal joints are hyperextended and the toe joints are flexed. Several toes are generally affected. The condition is often bilateral and may be associated with pes cavus deformity. A positive family history is often elicited. Painful callosities may develop on the dorsum of the toes.

9. **Rare congenital deformities:** There may be supernumerary toes, *absence of toes* (Fig. 21.4), *bifid foot,* overlapping 5th toe, etc. These are often associated with congenital deformities of the fingers.

SWELLINGS: *Corns* and *callosities* occur at the sites of intermittent pressure. A corn consists of a conical wedge of highly compressed keratotic epithelial cells. This occurs over a very limited area and impinges on the nerve endings. This gives rise to pain. A callosity on the other hand is distributed over a comparatively large area. This is nothing but a greatly thickened and cornified skin which ceases at the periphery where it is being continued with the normal skin.

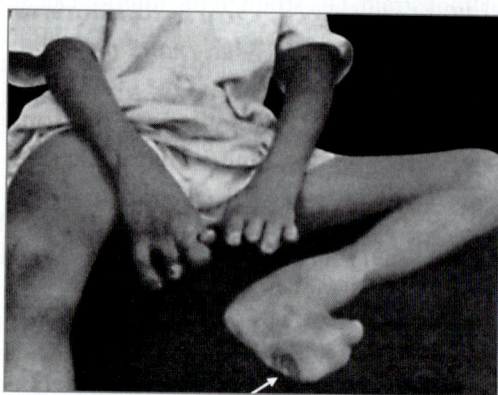

Fig. 21.4: Congenital absence of toes of left foot with congenital constriction of the lower leg resulting in a trophic ulcer (shown by arrow). Note also congenital deformities of the fingers.

A *soft corn* occurs where the skin is macerated between the toes. This is commonly seen in the cleft between the 4th and 5th toes where the soft skin is subjected to pressure between the bases of the proximal phalanges.

Plantar wart is commonly seen on the weight-bearing portion of the sole. These warts are dark and exquisitely tender. These differentiate this condition from corn or callosity. When seen through magnifying glass, one may find red or black spots which are hemorrhages from attenuated fronds of the submerged papillomas.

A *ganglion* is more or less similar to that found in the hand and wrist.

A *bursa* superficial to the tendo Achillis may be enlarged due to inflammation.

Swelling of the ankle joint may be due to *effusion* in the joint.

Other causes of swellings of the foot are the *tumors* affecting the foot. Of the tumors most common is malignant melanoma followed by squamous cell carcinoma. **Malignant melanoma** occurs mainly on the medial aspect of the sole where the skin is relatively soft. The swelling is asymptomatic in the beginning. Pigmentation and ulceration are the usual features. Regional lymph nodes are always enlarged and occasionally the liver may be involved by metastasis. **Squamous cell carcinoma** on the other hand affects the weight-bearing areas of the forefoot where the skin is relatively hard **(Fig. 21.5)**. Due to pressure of the weight the tendons and bones are soon infiltrated and the tumors become fixed to the deeper structures.

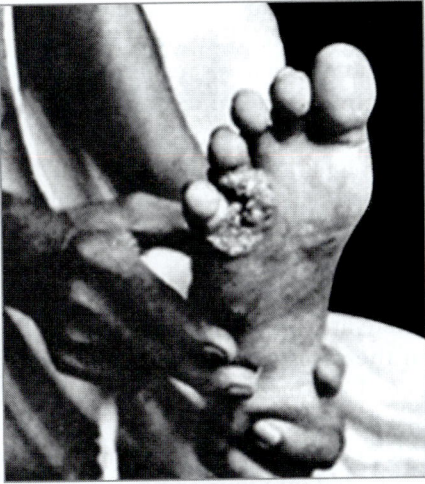

Fig. 21.5: Squamous cell carcinoma affecting the fore-foot.

ULCERS: Ulcers of the foot are more often seen in tropical countries and are caused by various infective agents. Of these **tuberculosis** is by far the most common. Besides these infective ulcers, one may come across **perforating ulcers (Fig. 21.6)** in denervated sole. These are mainly situated on the weight-bearing zones, such as ball of the great or little toe or heel. These ulcers are usually surrounded by indurated skin and the ulcers tend to perforate right up to the bone justifying its nomenclature. Ulcers may develop from *ingrowing toe-nail* and *subungual exostosis* due to repeated friction of the skin against the nail or the bony exostosis. The surface becomes granulating.

Madura foot is a tropical disease caused by mycotic infection. This condition commonly affects persons who move about barefooted and in the great majority of cases infection is introduced by prick of a thorn. Firm, painless and pale nodules develop on the foot. They increase in size and gradually vesicles appear on the surface of the nodule. Each vesicle bursts and a sinus develops which discharges purulent mucoid fluid containing the characteristic tiny granules. Lymphadenitis is conspicuous by its absence. Gradually the nodules infiltrate the underlying structures such as muscle, bone, etc. Tendons and nerve tissues are resistant to invasion. Blood borne dissemination is also absent. Lymphadenitis may occur from secondary infection. This condition mimics actinomycosis.

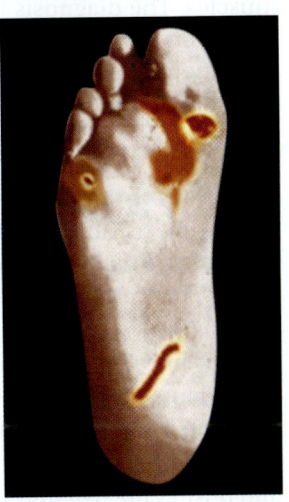

Fig. 21.6: Perforating ulcer.

The other rare cause of ulcer in the foot is **Kaposi's sarcoma**. This is commonly seen in the Jews, Italian and Eastern Europeans. Males in the middle of their lives are more susceptible to this condition. Multiple, painless, plum-colored nodules particularly affecting the lower extremities are the characteristic features of this condition. The last but not the least is the *malignant melanoma* in the list of causes of ulcer of the foot.

INFECTIONS OF THE FOOT (Figs. 21.7A and B): By this we mean pyogenic infection of the foot and in many respects this is similar to that of the hand. In the sole, there are the *superficial* *plantar space* and *deep plantar space* lying superficial and deep to the plantar aponeurosis respectively.

Infection of the superficial fascial space is mainly seen in: (i) the sole of the foot (in those who walk bare-footed), (ii) the web space, (iii) interdigital subcutaneous space and (iv) the heel space.

Infection of the deep fascial space: There are three deep fascial spaces in the sole—medial, central and lateral. The medial and lateral spaces are less important and are rarely infected. The central plantar space is divided into four compartments between the five layers of the muscles. The diagnosis is made by the history of a penetrating injury, pain, tenderness and swelling. The swelling becomes more prominent on the dorsum even if the pus is situated under the sole.

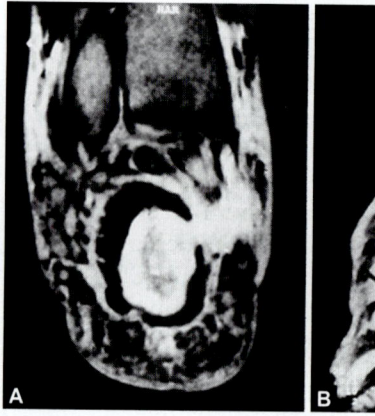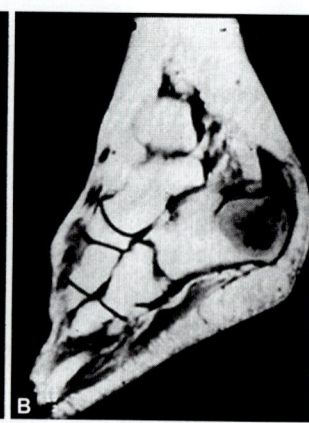

Figs. 21.7A and B: MRI showing tuberculous cavity of the calcaneum with a track through which cold abscess is burrowing superficially and if allowed to burst a sinus will form. Note how MRI is helpful in locating the track so that proper surgery can be performed to excise the track and the tuberculous cavity.

■ DEFORMITIES AND LESIONS AROUND NAILS

1. **Ingrowing toe-nail:** This occurs due to excessive lateral growth of the nail into the nail-fold may be due to trimming of the corners of the nail. The sharp lateral edge of the nail digs into and lacerates the nail-fold. Infection starts here and recurrent attacks of painful acute and subacute paronychia continue. Gradually, the resulting granulation tissue may protrude. Usually, the great toe is involved.

2. **Onychogryphosis (Ram's horn nail):** This is a condition in which usually nail of the great toe becomes thickened, crooked and over-grown. The cause is oft repeated trauma or fungus infection. Usual victims are bedridden old people.

3. **Subungual exostosis:** It is an exostosis growing from the dorsal aspect of the distal phalanx and pushes the nail upwards which becomes discolored. At this stage this condition becomes painful and results in deformity of the displaced nail which gradually splits and becomes a source of infection with severe pain. Ultimately the nail breaks away and the exostosis reaches the surface only covered with a mass of granulation tissue.

4. **Onychomycosis:** This condition, which is a fungus affection of the nail of the great toe, mimics the early stage of the previous condition. It is a rare entity in which the nail becomes brittle, discolored and split longitudinally at several places.

5. **Subungual malignant melanoma:** A malignant melanoma sometimes grows as a pigmented nodule beneath a nail or nail groove. In a matter of months the nail is lifted up and eventually lost due to quick proliferation of the growth. Ultimately the growth ulcerates and becomes secondarily infected. Though it retains its characteristic brown-black color, occasionally it may be colorless *(amelanotic melanoma)*.

6. **Glomus tumor**—may occur below the tip of a toe nail as finger and is discussed in detail in pages 51 and 371.

PAIN IN THE FOOT

Pain in the foot can be classified according to the region affected.

A. **Pain in the heel:** This can be subdivided into (a) *pain within the heel,* e.g., fracture or disease of the calcaneum (osteomyelitis or tumor or Paget's disease) and arthritis of the subtaloid joint; *(b) Pain behind the heel,* e.g., tendo Achillis bursitis, retrocalcaneum bursitis, apophysitis of the calcaneum (Sever's disease) and rupture and paratendinitis of the tendo Achillis; and (c) *Pain beneath the heel,* e.g., infracalcaneum bursitis and plantar fasciitis (Policeman's heel).

Calcanean spur: This is usually revealed in X-ray and is a bony projection forwards from undersurface of the calcaneal tuberosity. It is nothing but ossification of the plantar fascia at its calcaneal end. This has very little significance so far as the pain in the heel is concerned. That means if a patient complains of pain in the heel and on X-ray one can find the presence of calcanean spur, the clinician cannot infer that the calcanean spur is the cause of pain. Very often inflammation of the soft tissue or a bursa beneath the spur gives rise to pain.

B. **Pain in the midfoot:** A *strain on the inferior calcaneonavicular ligament* (spring ligament) occurs when the foot flattens rapidly due to weakness of the short muscles of the sole or after a prolonged confinement in the bed. *Kohler's disease* (osteochondritis of the navicular bone) is another cause of the pain in the midfoot. The usual victim is the child under 5 years of age. Painful limp and tenderness over the navicular bone are the diagnostic considerations, the navicular bone becomes dense with altered shape. An *"overbone"* connecting the dorsal surfaces of the medial cuneiform and the base of the 1st metatarsal bone gives rise to pain in the midfoot. A tender and bony lump just proximal to the base of the 1st metatarsal bone is the diagnostic feature of this condition.

C. **Pain in the forefoot or metatarsalgia:** (a) DISORDERS OF THE FOOT may give rise to pain in the forefoot, e.g., splay foot associated with hallux valgus, curly toes, a claw-foot with claw toes, etc. (b) DISORDERS OF INDIVIDUAL TOES, e.g., hallux valgus, hallux rigidus, ingrowing toe-nail, hammer, toe, etc. (c) SPECIAL VARIETIES OF METATARSALGIA: This includes (i) *Freiberg's disease:* This is nothing but crushing type of osteochondritis affecting the head of the 2nd or 3rd metatarsal bone. It is generally seen in young adults and girls predominate. A bony lump or irregularity is palpable which is tender and the affected joint becomes irritable. X-ray shows dense and the flattened epiphysis, increase in joint space and a thick neck (similar to what is seen in Perthes' disease).
(ii) *Morton's metatarsalgia:* This is a fibroneuroma affecting usually the 3rd digital nerve just before its division into two branches. Middle-aged women are more often affected. Sharp intermittent pain shoots into the affected toes. Sensation may be diminished in the adjacent toes. Localized tenderness can be elicited over the neuroma. Relief is obtained by taking the shoe off and squeezing or massaging the forefoot.
(iii) *March or stress fracture:* This usually affects the 2nd or 3rd metatarsal bone. It occurs in young adults after unaccustomed long walking. Swelling and tenderness may be felt on the dorsum of the affected metatarsal bone. X-ray appearance is at first normal but later on one may find a fusiform callus around a fine transverse fracture in about 2–3 weeks time.

Algorithmic Approach to Patient with Foot Conditions

Patient presents with foot pain, deformity, or swelling
↓

Is there a history of trauma?
- **Yes** → Consider **fracture, ligament injury, stress fracture**
- **No** → Assess for **neurological, inflammatory, or mechanical causes**

↓

Pain localized to heel, midfoot, or forefoot?
- **Heel pain** → Consider **plantar fasciitis, achilles tendinitis, calcaneal spur**
- **Midfoot pain** → Consider **spring ligament strain, kohler's disease**
- **Forefoot pain** → Consider **morton's neuroma, freiberg's disease, metatarsalgia**

↓

Is there a visible deformity?
- **Yes** → Assess for **flat foot (pes planus), clubfoot (talipes equinovarus), hallux valgus, pes cavus**
- **No** → Evaluate for **neuropathy, arthritis, or overuse injury**

↓

Perform neurological exam
- Test sensation (light touch, vibration, pinprick) → Peripheral neuropathy, radiculopathy
- Test reflexes (ankle jerk, babinski sign) → Spinal cord involvement
- Assess motor strength (toe flexion, ankle dorsiflexion) → Nerve compression, myopathy

↓

Imaging (X-ray, MRI, CT) based on clinical findings
- **X-ray** → For **fractures, deformities, joint space changes (arthritis)**
- **MRI** → For **soft tissue injury, nerve compression, infection**
- **CT scan** → For **complex bony abnormalities (tarsal coalition, tumors)**

↓

Determine need for surgery vs conservative management
- **Surgical intervention?** → If **severe deformity, progressive nerve compression, unstable fracture**
- **Conservative management?** → If **mild to moderate arthritis, plantar fasciitis, nonprogressive deformities**

Examination of the Head and Face

CHAPTER 22

The clinical examination of swellings and ulcers on the head and face is carried out as discussed in the general chapters. Here differential diagnosis of various lesions of the head and face are discussed below:

DIFFERENTIAL DIAGNOSIS

A. CONGENITAL LESIONS: *Hydrocephalus* is a condition of excess of cerebrospinal fluid in the cranium, commonly due to failure of development of the arachnoid villi through which absorption takes place. There is often a huge enlargement of the head with widening of the anterior fontanelle which normally becomes obliterated between 15th and 18th months. The eyes are bulging and looking downwards **(Fig. 22.1)**. *Meningocele* (protrusion of the meninges), *encephalocele* (protrusion of the brain) or *meningoencephalocele* (protrusion of the meninges as well as the brain) are sometimes met with at the root of the nose, the occipital region or anterior fontanelle **(Figs. 22.2 and 22.3A)**. They are diagnosed by their typical situation (in the midline), impulse on coughing **(Fig. 22.3B)** (crying in case of children) and translucency. *Dermoid cysts* occur in the line of ectodermal fusion. They are commonly met with just above the outer canthus of the eye, behind the ear (postauricular dermoid cyst) and in the midline. Clinically they are cystic, free from the skin but are often fixed to the underlying skull in which a saucer-shaped depression with a peripheral ridge may be felt. *Cleft (hare) lip*

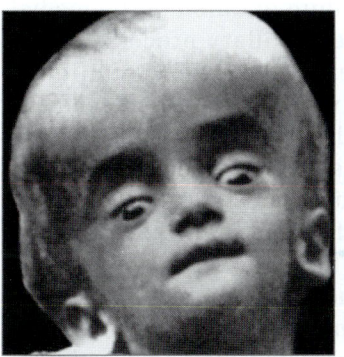

Fig. 22.1: Hydrocephalus.

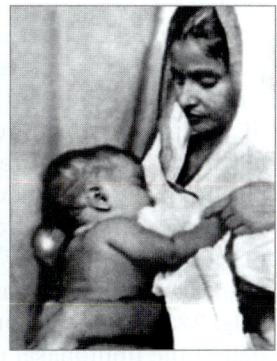

Fig. 22.2: Meningocele at the occiput.

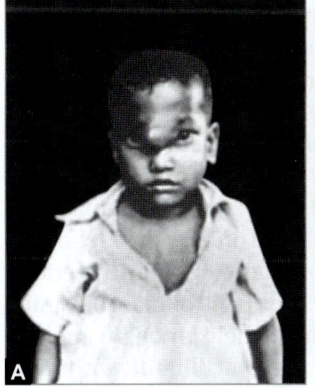

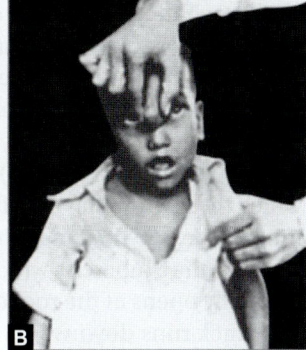

Figs. 22.3A and B: (A) Meningocele at the root of the nose. (B) An impulse on coughing is felt.

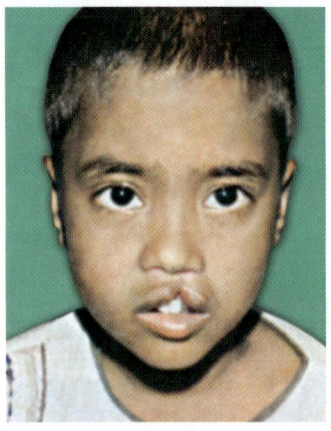
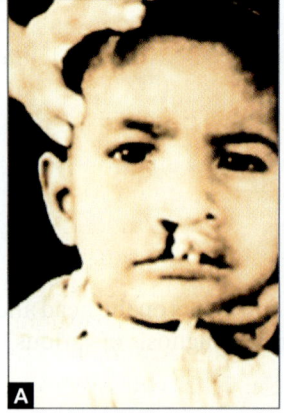
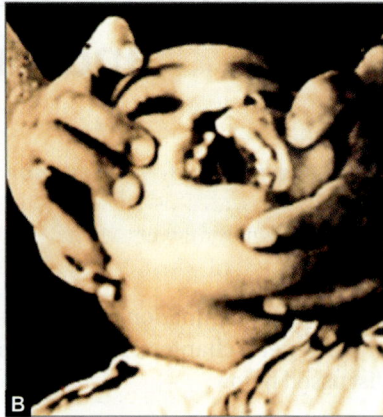

Fig. 22.4: A typical case of unilateral hare lip.

Figs. 22.5A and B: Unilateral cleft lip with cleft palate.

(Fig. 22.4) is due to failure of union of the medial nasal process with the maxillary process. It may be unilateral or bilateral. The latter condition is frequently associated with forward displacement of the premaxilla and cleft palate. *Cleft palate* (Figs. 22.5A and B) results from failure of the two palatine plates of the maxillary processes to fuse together and with the premaxilla developed from the frontonasal process. Note whether the nasal septum is hanging free or is attached to one side of the cleft. *Bifid nose* (Fig. 22.6) is a developmental curiosity in which one half of the frontonasal process remains isolated from the rest. If the lateral nasal process fails to unite with maxillary process, a fissure known as *facial cleft* will be evident extending from the upper lip to the inner canthus of the eye along the side of the nose. *Macrostoma* (Fig. 22.7), or abnormally large size of the mouth, results from imperfect union of the maxillary process with the mandibular arch. *Macrocheilia* or hypertrophy of the lip is usually congenital but may be due to lymphangiectasis. *Mandibular cleft* (Fig. 22.8) is a very rare abnormality in which the mandibular arch fails to unite with its fellow in the midline. *Preauricular sinus* develops from imperfect fusion of the 6 tubercles which form the pinna. This sinus generally opens at the root of the helix or on the tragus. The track runs downwards and ends blindly. At times the mouth of the sinus becomes closed, a cyst develops and becomes infected. Later on it may burst and an ulcer develops. This ulcer refuses to heal as infection is maintained within the sinus. *Congenital short frenum of the upper lip* may be seen with a wide gap between the

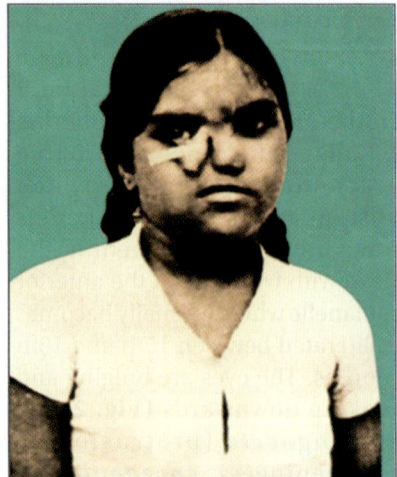

Fig. 22.6: Bifid nose.

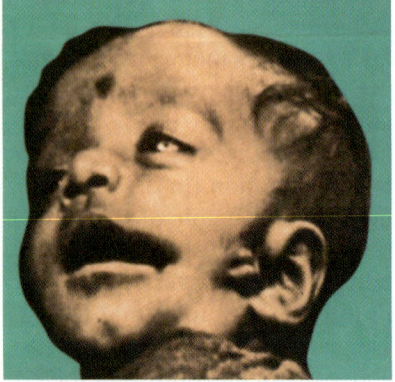

Fig. 22.7: Macrostoma. Note the nodules in front of the pinna—another developmental anomaly.

permanent incisor teeth. *Congenital fistulae of the lower lip* are rarely found as two blind pits one on either side of the midline. These are wide-open mucus secreting glands which are found in certain quadrupeds.

Figures 22.9 A and B shows the development of the face.

TRAUMATIC LESIONS: Hematoma and fracture are the two main traumatic causes of swellings in this region. Details of fractures which may occur in skull bone have been mentioned in the chapter of 'Head Injury'. Fractures of facial bones are not quite common and do not come in the domain of such book. **Hematoma of the scalp** quite commonly occurs in head injury. Such hematoma usually occurs in either in the second connective tissue layer of the scalp or in the 4th layer which consists of loose areolar tissue of the scalp. While bleeding in the second layer of the scalp above the galea aponeurotica is a localized hematoma, hemorrhage in the 4th layer of the scalp below the galea aponeurotica (subaponeurotic) spreads considerably and is limited posteriorly by the attachment of the aponeurotic layer with the occipital region of the skull, laterally by the zygomatic arch, but anteriorly this aponeurosis has no bony attachment so blood may track into the root of the nose and the eyelids. **Cephal hematoma** (subpericranial hematoma) occurs due to accumulation of blood beneath the pericranium. It is commonly seen in the parietal region often following forceps delivery. It may also occur along with fracture of the skull. It forms a localized swelling being limited to the affected bone bounded by its suture lines. The swelling is soft and fluctuant but is not translucent. The swelling gradually disappears over a period of weeks or months.

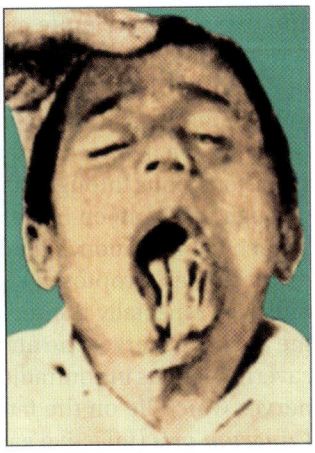

Fig. 22.8: Mandibular cleft.

INFLAMMATORY LESIONS: *Pott's puffy tumor* is nothing but localized pitting edema of the scalp over the cranial bone which has been affected with osteomyelitis. Acute localized pain, localized tenderness and swelling over the affected bone are the clinical features of this condition. Extradural abscess may develop in the deeper aspect. *Boils, carbuncles, cellulitis*

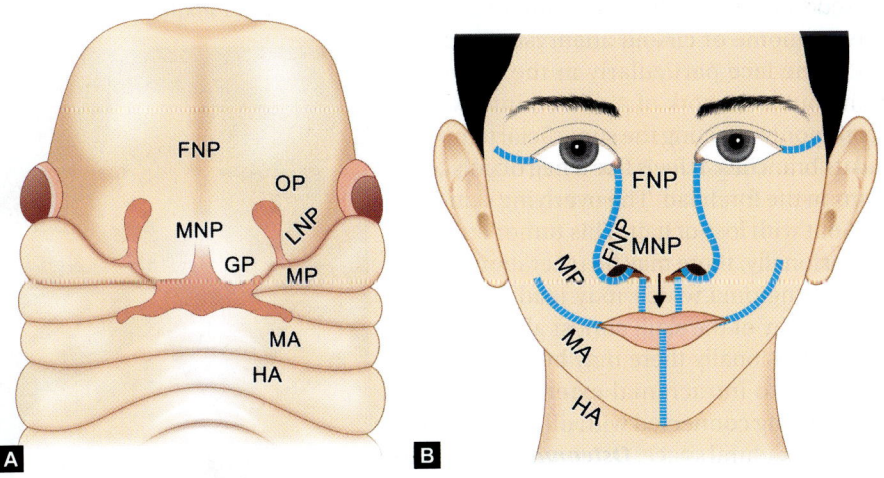

Figs. 22.9A and B: Show the development of the face. FNP: frontonasal process; MNP: medial nasal process; LNP: lateral nasal process; OP: olfactory pit; GP: globular process; MP: maxillary process; MA: mandibular arch; HA: hyoid arch; D: dermoid cyst at the commonest site.

and *erysipelas* are quite common in the head and face. The serious complication of such infections is the cavernous sinus thrombosis. The infection spreads (i) along the angular vein to the ophthalmic vein—a tributary of the cavernous sinus or (ii) along the deep facial vein which communicates with the cavernous sinus through the pterygoid plexus of veins passing through the foramen ovale and foramen lacerum. Diagnosis of such complication is made by noting severe constitutional disturbances, proptosis, squint and paralysis of the ocular muscles, especially the rectus lateralis which is supplied by the abducent nerve. The nerve is situated in the interior of the cavernous sinus in contradistinction to the 3rd and 4th cranial nerves which lie on the lateral wall of the cavernous sinus. **Cancrum oris** (infective gangrenous stomatitis) **(Fig. 22.10)** occurs more often in debilitated children after long-continued typhoid fever or kala-azar.

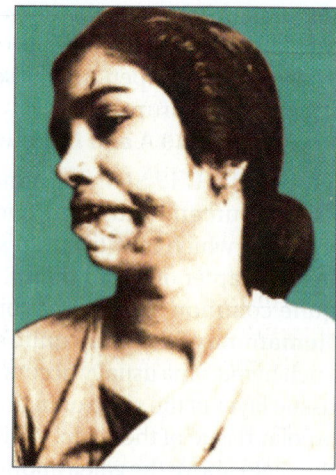

Fig. 22.10: Cancrum oris.

ULCERS: *Lupus vulgaris* (cutaneous tuberculosis) is a chronic ulcer found in the face in tropical countries. *Rodent ulcer* is commonly found in the face particularly above the line joining the angle of the mouth to the tragus of the ear. *Actinomycosis* rarely affects the lower jaw and may cause multiple sinuses of the face with surrounding induration discharging pus with sulfur granules. Lymph nodes are usually not involved. In the lip, most common cause of ulcer is *carcinoma of the lip. Extragenital chancre or mucous patches or condylomas* (manifestations of syphilis) may be seen in the lip.

TUMORS and CYSTS: Benign and malignant tumors originate from the skin, subcutaneous tissue or bone.

Benign tumors, e.g., papilloma, lipoma (subcutaneous and subpericranial), hemangioma, cirsoid aneurysm, neurofibroma, osteoma and osteoclastoma may be seen. *Hemangioma* **(Fig. 22.11)** is quite common in the face. Capillary hemangiomas are more common which are discussed in Chapter 3 'Examination of a Lump or a Swelling'. Plexiform hemangioma or arterial hemangioma or cirsoid aneurysm is almost only seen in the face particularly in the forehead. It is nothing but a network of a dilated interwoven arteries commonly affecting the superficial temporal artery and its branches. It feels like a bag of pulsating earthworms in the forehead. The overlying skin may be thinned out with loss of hair. This tumor enlarges slowly. Occasionally, there may be ulceration of skin over this hemangioma which may lead to serious hemorrhage. X-ray of the skull almost always shows erosion and occasionally there may be perforations in the skull due to intracranial extension of such hemangioma being connected with dilated tortuous vessels in the extradural space. *Osteoma* particularly sessile type (compact osteoma or ivory exostosis) is a tumor commonly seen affecting the outer table of the skull. The frontal, parietal and occipital bones are

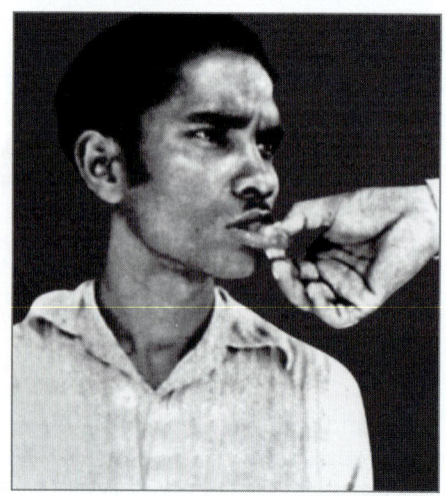

Fig. 22.11: Hemangioma of the lip.

often involved. Very occasionally this tumor may originate from the inner surface of the skull when it may give rise to focal epilepsy. This osteoma is known for its stony hard consistency. The adolescents or young adults are the common victims and the presenting symptom is the hard painless lump.

Among **malignant tumors** squamous cell carcinoma **(Figs. 22.12A and B)**, malignant melanoma, osteosarcoma and secondary carcinoma in the skull may occur. Ectopic salivary tumor may be rarely

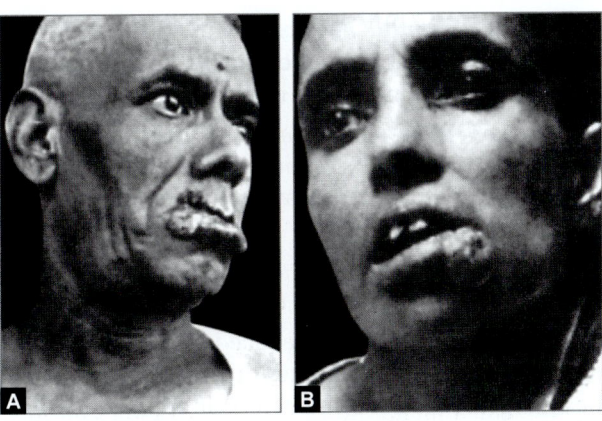

Figs. 22.12A and B: (A and B) Squamous cell carcinoma of the lip. (A) Note the 'kiss lesion' affecting the upper lip as well.

seen particularly in the lip of a young adult male. A tumor arising from the skin or subcutaneous tissue can be moved freely over the bone. Skin can be moved freely over the tumor which is arising from subcutaneous tissue or bone. *Cylindroma* (turban tumor) occurs very occasionally in the scalp involving whole of it and that is why it is also known as 'Turban tumor'. It forms a red, lobulated swelling, which grows slowly. It is considered to be a type of basal cell carcinoma, though a few pathologists are of the opinion that it is an endothelioma. But it is definitely a locally malignant tumor. It is almost always associated with alopecia of the area affected. *Secondary carcinoma* is not uncommon tumor of the skull. Though skull is not a very common site of bone involvement of secondary carcinoma, yet of the tumors of the skull secondary carcinoma is one of the common tumors. It is usually caused by blood borne metastasis and it commences in the diploe. It presents as solitary or multiple swellings of the skull. The consistency varies from stony hard to very soft depending on its vascularity. Soft and very vascular metastases often show pulsation presenting as pulsatile swelling.

Paget's disease of the skull: Though it is not a tumor or cyst but this malformation syndrome of bone often affects the skull. This condition almost always affects the skull and the skull enlarges so that the patient often requires a bigger hat after certain time interval. This disease usually affects old individuals above 40 years and males are more often affected. Pain is often an important symptom. The thickened cranial bones are sometimes quite vascular so as to produce systolic bruit on auscultation.

Among the **cysts,** *sebaceous cysts* occur quite frequently in the scalp and face. They may suppurate and ulcerate to give rise to *Cock's peculiar tumor* (this looks like a squamous cell carcinoma). *Mucous cysts* are often found on the mucous surface of the lip and cheek (these are recognized by their blue color and translucency). *Dermoid cysts* are discussed earlier.

SOME CHARACTERISTIC FACIES: In a few surgical conditions the face of the patient assumes a characteristic appearance. These are discussed below:

The Hippocratic facies: This characteristic facial appearance is almost pathognomonic of advanced diffuse peritonitis. The eyes are sunken, but bright, the nose is pinched. The forehead is cold and clammy. There are crust on the lips. The tongue is dry and shriveled. It is in fact due to dehydration rather than peritonitis that the appearance of sharp nose, hollow eyes and collapsed temples are produced. But when this facial appearance is combined with thready pulse and a grossly distended abdomen, the condition is nothing but an advanced case of diffuse peritonitis.

The facies of hepatic cirrhosis: The eyes are sunken and there is variable degree of icterus present in the watery conjunctivae. There is also presence of spider naevi and all these indicate a moderately advanced case of hepatic cirrhosis.

The adenoid facies: A high arched palate, narrow dental arch and protruding incisor teeth are the characteristic features found in a patient with enlarged adenoids. However this concept has been challenged nowadays and these features are not considered to be pathognomonic of enlarged adenoids.

The moonface of Cushing's syndrome: The face becomes round shaped like a full moon and often the lips are pursed in a case of Cushing's syndrome.

The facies of cretinism: The face is pale, puffy and wrinkled. The skin is dry and cold. The tongue is protruded. The anterior fontanelle remains open. The thyroid gland may or may not be enlarged. This is the characteristic appearance of a case of cretinism.

Carcinoid facies: This occurs when a carcinoid tumor metastasizes in the liver and excess of serotonin is secreted. This condition produces characteristic facial flushing, which is known as carcinoid facies.

Differential diagnosis of head and face

Condition	Facial features
Hippocratic facies (peritonitis)	Sunken eyes, pinched nose, dry tongue
Cushing's syndrome (moon face)	Rounded face, red cheeks, excessive hair
Myxedema (hypothyroidism)	Puffy face, coarse skin, dry hair
Cretinism (congenital hypothyroidism)	Protruding tongue, flat nasal bridge, thick lips
Carcinoid syndrome	Flushing, telangiectasia, sweating

Algorithmic Approach to Patient with Head and Face Lesions

Patient presents with swelling, ulcer, or deformity on head/face

↓

Is the lesion congenital?
- **Yes** → Consider **hydrocephalus, meningocele, cleft lip, dermoid cyst**
- **No** → Assess for **traumatic, inflammatory, or neoplastic causes**

↓

Recent trauma?
- **Yes** → Consider **hematoma, fracture, soft tissue injury**
- **No** → Assess for **infection or tumor**

↓

Is there fever or redness?
- **Yes** → Consider **cellulitis, cavernous sinus thrombosis, abscess**
- **No** → Evaluate **for tumors (benign vs malignant)**

↓

Is the mass soft and mobile?
- **Yes** → Consider **lipoma, sebaceous cyst, benign tumor**
- **No** → Consider **malignant tumor (SCC, melanoma, osteosarcoma)**

↓

Perform imaging (X-ray, MRI, CT) based on findings
- **X-ray** → For **bony abnormalities (fractures, osteoma)**
- **MRI** → For **soft tissue masses, neural lesions**
- **CT scan** → For **complex facial fractures, skull base tumors**

↓

Determine need for surgery vs conservative management
- **Surgical intervention?** → If **large tumors, progressive neurological deficits, or infected lesions**
- **Conservative management?** → If **small cysts, lipomas, or stable lesions**

Examination of the Jaws and Temporomandibular Joint

CHAPTER 23

HISTORY TAKING

History in examination of Jaws and TMJ

Aspect	Clinical significance	Patient-friendly questions
Onset of swelling	Acute → Abscess, trauma; chronic → Tumor, cyst	"When did you first notice the swelling?"
Pain characteristics	Dull → Abscess, tumor; sharp → Fracture	"Is the pain sharp, dull, or throbbing?"
Nerve symptoms	Trigeminal nerve involvement → Numbness, neuralgia	"Do you feel tingling or numbness in your jaw?"
Clicking/locking jaw	TMJ dysfunction, disc displacement	"Do you hear a clicking sound when chewing?"

THE UPPER JAW

Maxilla, which constitutes the upper jaw has got **five surfaces**. These surfaces are examined systematically **(Figs. 23.1A to D)**.

1. *Anterolateral surface (superficial surface):* It is most obviously available for examination. The condition of the skin is noted. The upper lip is everted to expose a portion of this surface. When a swelling is present, examine it with a finger.

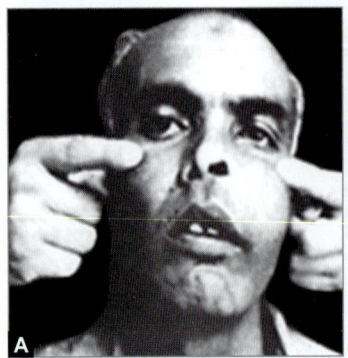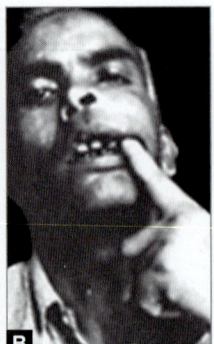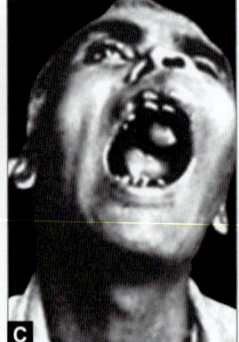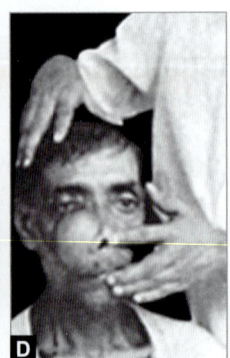

Figs. 23.1A to D: Examining the orbital, superficial, palatine and nasal surfaces of the maxilla. In (D) the patient has been asked to breathe through the naris of the affected side while his other naris and mouth are kept closed. Any obstruction present is thus demonstrated.

2. ***Superior surface (orbital surface):*** This surface constitutes the floor of the orbit. The inferior orbital margins of both sides are palpated and note any difference in sharpness and level. If this surface is bulged upwards, it causes proptosis and diplopia. One may have a glance at each profile of the patient in order to consider relative protuberance of the eyeball.
3. ***Inferior surface (palatine surface):*** The patient is asked to open his mouth. Note if there is a swelling. It is examined in the usual manner. The nasopharynx is also examined. The teeth are examined. If there is any missing tooth, careful examination may reveal an odontome.
4. ***Medial surface (nasal surface):*** This forms the lateral wall of the nostril. The patient is asked to blow through his nose occluding the nares one at a time. If the nostril on the affected side is not blocked, it is obvious that the medial wall of the maxilla is not bulging to any great extent. This surface can only be seen with the help of a nasal speculum. The patient should be asked if any discharge is coming out through the nostril of the affected side. Whether the discharge is purulent or sanguineous? Constant overflow of tears from the eye (epiphora) indicates obstruction of the nasolacrimal duct.
5. ***Posterior surface:*** The surface forms the anterior boundary of the pterygopalatine fossa and is absolutely beyond our reach. Only extension of the growth from this surface may firstly be felt in the infratemporal region. So this region must be palpated before completion of the palpation of the surfaces of the maxilla.

While examining these surfaces, if any **swelling** or **ulcer** is discovered, examine it in the usual way. When there is a growth arising from the mucoperiosteum, i.e., **epulis**, note whether it is sessile or pedunculated, soft or firm, bleeds easily during palpation or not.

If there is any tenderness in the maxillary antrum without any distension of its wall, it may suggest empyema of the antrum. This of course may be associated with unilateral purulent nasal discharge. This is confirmed by anterior rhinoscopy, posture test, transillumination, X-ray and aspiration of the antrum through the inferior meatus.

The **teeth** should be count. Dental cyst is frequently associated with caries tooth. Dentigerous cyst is invariably associated with unerupted permanent tooth.

The **cervical lymph nodes** must always be examined, particularly the submandibular group. Any inflammatory lesion or carcinoma will lead to enlargement of the regional lymph nodes. But sarcoma of the upper jaw does not lead to enlargement of the regional lymph node.

The 2nd division (maxillary division) of the 5th cranial nerve **(trigeminal nerve)** is always tested for its integrity. This nerve and its branches are likely to be involved when the growth extends backwards and upwards.

THE LOWER JAW

When there is a history of trauma look for evidence of **fracture of the mandible**.
Mandibular fracture assessment includes:
- **Common sites:** Canine region (weakest point), condylar process, symphysis.
- **Signs:**
    - Malalignment of teeth → Suggests displaced fracture.
    - Loss of mandibular contour → High suspicion of fracture.
    - Crepitus and tenderness → Confirms bony discontinuity.
- **Bimanual palpation:** One finger intraorally, one externally to detect discontinuity.
- **Skiagraphy (X-ray/CT):** Essential for definitive diagnosis.

When the patient tries to support the fragments with his hands, speech is impossible and when the saliva is blood-stained (as the fracture of the mandible is nearly always *compound* into the mouth), one may suspect the case is one of fracture of the mandible. The intimately adherent mucoperiosteum always gives way in case of fracture of the mandible to make the fracture compound. Majority of the fractures of the mandible occur in the horizontal portion (at the region of the canine tooth as the bone is weak due to deep canine socket). Contour of the alveolus is carefully noted as also alignment of the teeth. Loss of continuity of the lower border and crepitus leave no doubt about the diagnosis. When the fracture occurs above the angle of the mandible the diagnosis may not be made with certainty. But swelling at the site of fracture, localized tenderness and skiagraphy help to make the diagnosis.

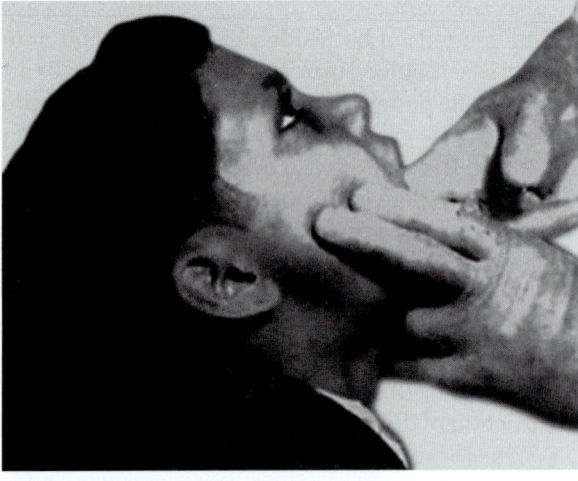

Fig. 23.2: Bimanual palpation of the lower jaw.

The body, the angle and the inferior part of the ramus are accessible to the palpating fingers. Examination can be done both from without and from within the mouth. *Bimanual palpation* (**Fig. 23.2**), i.e., one finger inside the mouth and fingers of the other hand applied externally can palpate comparatively inaccessible portion of the mandible. In case of **swelling** enquire particularly its duration. A long history of a slow growing large tumor would suggest adamantinoma. The swelling is examined in the usual way, noting its position, size, shape, consistency (whether uniform or variable), pulsation, egg-shell crackling, mobility, etc.

Examine the **lymph nodes** of the neck particularly the submandibular lymph nodes.

THE TEMPOROMANDIBULAR JOINT

The patient is asked to open and close his mouth. Normally, one can open the jaw to the extent of 2–5 cm distance between the upper and lower incisor teeth. Place the fingers over the joint just below and in front of the tragus to appreciate the movements of the condyle and to feel if there is any crepitus (as in osteoarthritis) or clicking (as in a loose meniscus). One may auscultate with a stethoscope placed over the joint to know more about crepitus and click.

TMJ Examination:
- **Range of motion:** Normal opening **(3–5 cm)**, lateral movements **(1 cm each side)**.
- **Palpation:** Place fingers over the joint (in front of tragus) to detect crepitus or clicking.
- **Clinical signs:**
    - **Clicking or Popping** → Suggests TMJ dysfunction (displaced articular disc).
    - **Crepitus** → Indicative of **osteoarthritis**.
    - **Restricted opening (Trismus)** → Seen in **tetanus, pericoronitis, TMJ ankylosis**.

- **Confirmatory tests:**
  - **MRI:** Best for soft tissue involvement (disc displacement).
  - **CT scan:** Best for **bony deformities or ankylosis**.

Ankylosis of the mandibular joint is evident by restriction in opening the mouth. False ankylosis may be seen in osteoarthritis or fibrosis resulting from virulent infections like cancrum oris.

The patient sometimes cannot open his mouth because of muscular spasm which is known as *trismus*. Severe trismus may complicate any inflammatory process or painful condition in the neighborhood of the joint. Erupting 3rd molar tooth (wisdom tooth), a dental abscess or parotitis may cause trismus. Trismus is also seen in tetanus with a characteristic facies—risus sardonicus (painful smiling appearance).

Displaced articular cartilage of the temporomandibular joint may lead to clicking jaw. This condition occurs more in females and in the first instance the patient hears snap in the ear and subsequently almost every time she opens her mouth, a click can be heard. Locking of the jaw occurs suddenly when the patient opens her mouth during yawning and fails to close the mouth. This is accompanied by pain which radiates to the pinna.

Dislocation of the temporomandibular joint can be either bilateral or unilateral. In case of bilateral dislocation, the mouth is open and fixed, a prognathous deformity may be evident. In case of unilateral dislocation, the partially opened jaw is deviated to the opposite side. A small hollow can be felt just behind the dislocated condyle. In a suspected case, a little finger is inserted into the external ear with the pulp directed forwards. The movement of the condyle will not be felt on the dislocated side when the mouth opens and closes.

SWELLINGS OF THE JAW

Classification of jaw swellings:
- **Mucoperiosteal swellings:**
  - **Granulomatous epulis** → Carious tooth association.
  - **Fibrous epulis** → Slow-growing, firm, arises from periodontal membrane.
  - **Myelomatous epulis** → Soft, lobulated, purplish, associated with osteoclastoma.
- **Odontogenic tumors:**
  - **Dental cyst** → Associated with carious tooth, expansile.
  - **Dentigerous cyst** → Surrounds unerupted tooth, common in molars.
- **Osseous tumors:**
  - **Osteoclastoma** → Locally aggressive, soap-bubble appearance on X-ray.
  - **Adamantinoma** → Honeycomb appearance, slow-growing but malignant potential.
- **Inflammatory conditions:**
  - **Alveolar abscess** → Dull pain, gum swelling, risk of Ludwig's angina.
  - **Osteomyelitis** → Bone infection, tenderness, and nonhealing ulcers.

DIFFERENTIAL DIAGNOSIS

Epulis means 'upon the gum'. There are several types: ***Granulomatous*** (or false) type is a mass of granulation around carious tooth. ***Fibrous epulis*** is most common and is a slow-growing firm growth **(Fig. 23.3)**. It arises from the periodontal membrane. It is red, firm, sessile or pedunculated lesion. Although it is benign yet it has a tendency to recur after operation, if its root is not thoroughly excised. ***Sarcomatous epulis*** is differentiated from the fibrous type by its more rapid growth, softer feel and bleeding more readily. It is bluish-red in color and of varying consistency. ***Myelomatous epulis*** or periosteal osteoclastoma produces a sessile swelling, soft, lobulated purplish in color. Egg-shell crackling may be palpated, regional lymph nodes are not enlarged and in X-ray typical soap-bubble appearance is produced. It may undergo malignant change—malignant myelomatous epulis, which is characterized by bleeding on touching and ulcer formation. ***Carcinomatous epulis***—an undesirable term given to epithelioma—is not uncommon in the gum. It is an infiltrating lesion around the tooth or its socket which may invade the bone, ulcerate or fungate. There is always lymph node enlargement.

Odontomes: In the development of the tooth, downward extension of epithelium takes place which later forms the enamel organ. A cluster of this epithelium persists as '**epithelial debris'** from which the epithelial odontomes are formed, e.g., dental cyst, dentigerous cyst **(Fig. 23.4)** and adamantinoma.

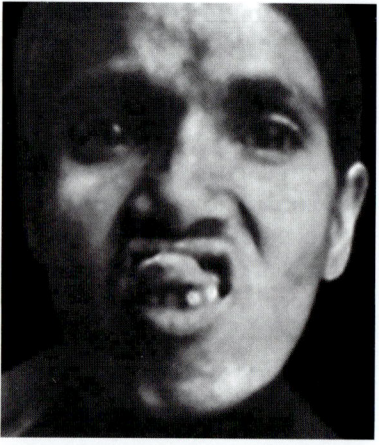

Fig. 23.3: Fibrous epulis from the mucoperiosteum of the upper jaw.

Dental cyst (radicular or periapical cyst): This condition occurs in association *with a carious tooth* and develops at the apex of the tooth with necrotic pulp. Once the cyst develops, it enlarges slowly by resorption of adjacent bone and expansion of the jaw. It usually affects the upper jaw, where it tends to enlarge to fill the maxillary sinus. In case of lower jaw, if untreated, it involves greater part of the body of the mandible even including the ramus. There may be 'egg-shell crackling' when the bone is thinned out or it may even elicit fluctuation when the bone is completely destroyed. The fluid within the cyst is clear and may contain cholesterol crystals. X-ray is helpful in diagnosis.

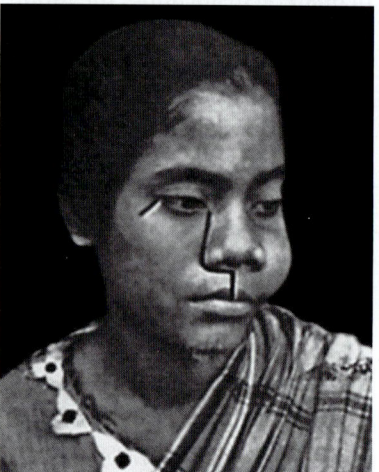

Dentigerous cyst (follicular odontome): It is associated *with unerupted permanent tooth.* This develops from

Fig. 23.4: Dentigerous cyst. Skiagram of this patient showed two unerupted teeth.

enamel epithelium from the surface of the crown of an unerupted tooth with accumulation of fluid inside it. This cyst also enlarges like the dental cyst. The unerupted tooth is displaced deeper by the cyst thus preventing its eruption. The crown of the tooth protrudes into the cyst cavity and the cyst lining is attached around the neck of the tooth. The upper or lower third molar tooth is usually affected. The cyst contains viscid fluid and unerupted tooth. It may also produce egg-shell crackling on palpation. Condition is confirmed by X-ray.

Adamantinoma (multilocular cystic disease or ameloblastoma): It gives rise to a multilocular cystic swelling commonly occurring in the lower jaw **(Figs. 23.5A and B)**. Differentiation from osteoclastoma is really difficult even by skiagraphy as both these conditions cause expansion of bone with trabeculae in the interior. But it more looks like a honey-comb. Adamantinoma is a more slow-growing tumor but locally malignant. Usual victims are between 20 to 30 years of age. Almost always the mandible is affected and the tumor expands at the cost of the outer table.

Solitary bone cyst: This resembles solitary bone cyst of long bone. It usually involves the premolar or molar region of the mandible. In the beginning, the bone cavity is round and oval, but it gradually bulges outwards in a lobulated fashion. Histological examination reveals bone resorption and certain amounts of bone deposition at the periphery. Complication like hemorrhage inside the cyst is quite common from the thin-walled vessels in the wall.

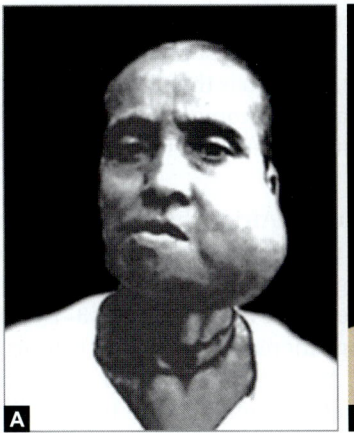 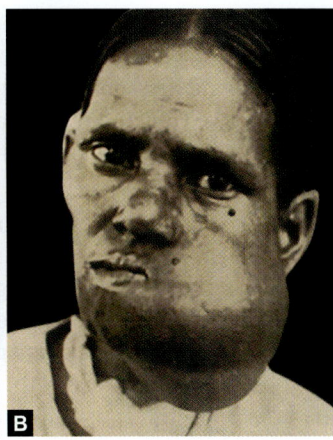

Figs. 23.5A and B: (A) Adamantinoma of the lower jaw; (B) Adamantinoma of the lower jaw affecting the left mandible.

That is why in aspiration the fluid looks yellow containing high bilirubin level. Unlike fluid from other jaw cyst, it will clot.

Giant-cell granuloma: This lesion usually occurs centrally in the jaw either in the mandible or in the axilla. It presents as a lobulated tumor.

It often erodes through the cortex and is covered by a thin layer of subperiosteal new bone. The roots of adjacent teeth are misplaced. It should not be confused with a giant-cell epulis. Histologically, it bears resemblance with osteoclastoma of long bone, but it is quite benign. It contains a stroma of connective tissue, scanty collagen, thin-walled blood vessels and numerous osteoclasts-like giant-cells. Histiocytes may be present scattered throughout the lesion. So histologically it resembles giant-cell epulis and brown tumor of hyperparathyroidism. It is differentiated from osteoclastoma of the jaw by histology.

Tumors of the upper jaw: Besides the benign tumors, e.g., ivory osteoma and osteoclastoma, the upper jaw may be affected with malignant growths—osteosarcoma and carcinoma arising from columnar epithelium lining the maxillary antrum or from squamous epithelium overlying the hard palate. Their *clinical features* vary according to the direction in which the tumor spreads. If the roof of the antrum is invaded, there will be proptosis and diplopia; if the anterolateral wall is involved, there will be obvious swelling of the face; if the medial wall is affected, there will be nasal obstruction, epistaxis and epiphora; if the floor is invaded, there will be bulging of the hard palate. In the early stage, it is extremely difficult to distinguish a sarcoma from a carcinoma arising from the lining membrane of the maxillary antrum. A diagnosis of carcinoma is suggested when the tumor burrows through one of its walls and ulcerates or when the submandibular lymph nodes are involved.

Tumors of the lower jaw: Benign tumors are mainly of three types: (i) Fibro-osseous group: The mandible being mainly a membranous bone this type of tumor may obviously occur in this bone. If it is localized it is called monostotic fibrous dysplasia and if it is diffuse it is called polyostotic fibrous dysplasia. According to the portion of the fibrous tissue and bone this tumor may be either soft or hard. (ii) Paget's disease may be part of the generalized Paget's disease or confined mainly to the jaws. Old person complains of pain and swelling of the affected bone. X-ray shows the typical appearance of Paget's disease. (iii) Giant-cell tumor or osteoclastoma: This lesion occurs between the ages of 10 and 25 years, though this tumor in other sites appears between 25 to 40 years of age. Females are more often affected. The usual complaint is painless swelling. X-ray is characteristic of osteoclastoma anywhere in the body.

Malignant neoplasm is rare, more so is the primary variety. The mandible however may be involved by an advancing primary carcinoma of the tongue or the floor of the mouth. Neoplastic involvement may also occur from the secondarily involved facial lymph nodes lying by the sides of the facial artery.

Burkitt's tumor: In many parts of Africa this is the most common neoplasm in children of first decade. It is a type of multifocal lymphoma whose etiology is not very clear. Viral origin has been strongly suggested. Age distribution has been very characteristic in the sense that majority of the patients are in the range of 3–7 years of age. Involvement becomes progressively diminished as age increases. Maxillary tumors generally present in relation to the molar and premolar teeth. As the tumor develops the alveolus expands on both sides and the affected teeth loose their attachments to the bone. Subsequently, the tumor develops around the teeth with an external swelling which appears under the cheek distorting the face. Mandibular tumors develop in the same way with marked distortion of the face though without significant ulceration and often with surprisingly little evidence of pain. Multiple jaw lesions with involvement of several jaw quadrants are one of the characteristic features. When two jaw quadrants are involved it is nearly always the maxilla and the mandible of the same side. Radiological features of this tumor in the jaws are disappearance of the lamina dura round the affected teeth. Subsequently multiple small areas of bone dissolution appear and eventually coalesce forming larger areas of bone destruction. So the bone involvement is essentially osteolytic. Abdominal tumors are the second most frequent mode of presentation. Retroperitoneal mass, liver enlargement or ovarian tumors may be seen. The adrenal and pancreatic involvements are also common. Enlargement of mesenteric lymph nodes can give rise to an epigastric mass. Splenic involvement is not very significant. Lesion involving the spinal nerves is the 3rd most common mode of presentation. Radiographs frequently show paravertebral mass in the lower dorsal or upper lumbar region. Intracranial lesions in the form of cranial nerve palsies may be seen in this condition. This tumor may affect the salivary gland, the thyroid, the breast, the bones and lymph nodes.

Alveolar abscess: This condition mainly affects children and early adults. In children abscesses may occur in either jaw while in case of early adults this abscess develops mainly in the lower jaw. The disease starts as acute pulpitis which gradually affects the osseous tissue through the root of the tooth, localized osteitis and later on abscess develops. These abscesses tend to bulge towards the external surface, barring the one in relation to the upper lateral incisor and in relation to an impacted wisdom tooth. In both these conditions abscesses show a natural tendency to bulge on the medial aspect, so that in case of the former, a swelling becomes evident on the palate and in case of the latter, the abscess may burst through the medial wall to cause the dangerous Ludwig's angina. Alveolar abscess if not treated properly by antibiotic therapy and drainage, osteomyelitis of the jaw may be expected.

The patient complains of dull and constant aching. Later on swelling of the cheek becomes evident with redness and edema of the gum. Excruciating pain is the characteristic feature and the regional lymph nodes are almost always enlarged. X-ray may show rarefaction around the root of the affected tooth in late cases (no less than 10 days).

COMPLICATIONS OF ALVEOLAR ABSCESS: Infection from lower teeth may spread lingually to cause cellulitis of the sublingual space. Apical abscesses of the 2nd and 3rd molars may perforate the lingual plate below the mylohyoid muscle to spread into the submandibular space. Bilateral sublingual and submandibular space infections constitute *Ludwig's angina*. Backward spread from here around the sublingual vessels results in edema of the epiglottis and respiratory obstruction. From molars there may be posterior spread to the pterygoid space between the pterygoid muscles and the medial side of the ramus. From here infection spreads to the cavernous sinus by way of emissary vein. Abscess from upper canine tooth may travel up to the medial corner of the eye and may cause thrombophlebitis of the angular vein and cavernous sinus thrombosis. Alveolar abscess of the apex of the upper lateral incisor is closer to the palatal surface than the labial cortex and thus causes a palatal abscess. Pus from lower third molar may travel back beneath the masseter as a submasseteric abscess. Pus from the lower incisors may erode the bone below the origin of the mentalis muscle. Gradually, the abscess reaches the surface between the two muscles and drains via a sinus in the midline of the chin, known as *Median mental sinus*.

Osteomyelitis of the jaw: Three types of osteomyelitis are come across in jaws:
(i) *Acute osteomyelitis* is occasionally seen in infants as a complication of acute fevers like measles or scarlet fever. Either the upper or the lower jaw may be affected. Swelling, redness and puffiness are the features. In case of maxilla pressure may cause pus to come from the nostril. X-ray is not much helpful.
(ii) *Subacute osteomyelitis* is the most common of the three varieties. Adults are mainly affected. Epical dental infection or alveolar abscess or fractured jaw or injudicious extraction of tooth with poor general condition is the main cause of this condition. Endarteritis of the artery supplying the mandible will cause obstruction to the blood supply leading to bone necrosis. The maxilla is rarely affected due to the fact that series of vertical arteries anastomose and maintain the blood supply to the bone.

Pain, swelling, tenderness and irregularity of the bone are usual features of this condition. Increased tension in the dental canal compresses the inferior dental nerve causing numbness of the chin in the distribution of the mental nerve. X-ray may show bone necrosis in very late cases (no less than 3 weeks time).
(iii) *Chronic osteomyelitis* also affects the mandible more often than maxilla. This condition usually follows apical dental infection or alveolar abscess or fractures. Patient seeks advice many months after the original disease. X-ray will show local osteitis, localized abscess (similar to Brodie's abscess) or formation of sequestrum.

Chronic osteomyelitis may also follow radiation or chemical necrosis due to phosphorus poisoning. Tuberculous, syphilitic and actinomycotic necrosis may also be found.

Median mental sinus is a form of chronic osteomyelitis, which is produced by an apical abscess on one or more of the lower incisors. The cortical plate is penetrated and the abscess accumulates deep to the mentalis muscles. The pus ultimately escapes to the surface only in the midline through a sinus in a center of the chin.

Actinomycosis: Faciocervical actinomycosis is the most common actinomycosis occurs in the human body. The lower jaw is usually involved adjacent to a carious tooth. The gum becomes indurated. Nodules gradually appear which soften. The overlying skin becomes indurated and bluish in color which gradually softens in patches. Ultimately abscesses burst through the skin and multiple sinuses form. Swelling, brawny induration, irregularity of the bone with multiple sinuses are the features of this condition. The multiple sinuses discharge sulfur granules which is pathognomonic. X-ray appearance is usually normal.

Micrognathism: Occasionally, the mandible may be excessively small, when it is called 'Micrognathism'. There may be respiratory obstruction in case of neonates with micrognathism, as this deformity results in backward displacement of the tongue. Oral cavity is also small. Special airway plates should be used to prevent airway obstruction, which is much better than sewing of the tip of the tongue to the lower lip. Nowadays monoblock orthodontic appliance has been devised to correct this small mandible.

Mandibular prognathism: When the mandible is larger than average and protrudes, it is called mandibular prognathism. Occasionally, the maxilla may be hypoplastic producing a relative mandibular prognathism.

Algorithmic Approach to Patient with Jaw and TMJ Disorders

Patient presents with jaw pain, swelling, or clicking TMJ

↓

Is there a history of trauma?
- Yes → Consider **fracture, hematoma, dislocation**
- No → Assess for **inflammatory, neoplastic, or TMJ causes**

↓

Is there a localized swelling
- Yes → Consider **abscess, dental cyst, odontogenic tumor**
- No → Assess for **TMJ dysfunction or neuropathy**

↓

Is there clicking or locking of the TMJ?
- Yes → Consider **TMJ dysfunction (disc displacement, osteoarthritis)**
- No → Evaluate for **nerve involvement (trigeminal neuralgia, tumor)**

↓

Perform imaging based on clinical findings
- X-ray → For **fractures, bony lesions, TMJ degeneration**
- MRI → For **soft tissue abnormalities (disc displacement, neural involvement)**
- CT scan → For **complex mandibular fractures or tumors**

↓

Determine need for surgery vs conservative management
- Surgical intervention? → If **fracture, large tumor, TMJ ankylosis**
- Conservative management? → If **mild TMJ dysfunction, small cysts, nonprogressive lesions**

Examination of the Palate, Cheek, Tongue and Floor of the Mouth

CHAPTER 24

HISTORY

1. **Age and sex:** Cleft lip and cleft palate are seen since birth. Stomatitis may occur at any age. Mucous retention cyst also occurs at any age. Carcinoma of lip and carcinoma of tongue occur more often in males above 50 years of age.
2. **Occupation:** Carcinoma of lip is commonly seen in men involved in outdoor activities and that is why it is often called 'countryman's lip'.
3. **Residence:** White Caucasians residing in Australia are the major sufferers of lip cancer. Negroes are less susceptible to this disease.
4. **Swelling or ulcer:** The lesions of the lip, cheek, tongue and floor of the mouth usually present as a swelling or an ulcer. Enquire about the onset, duration and progress of the lesion. While a *mucous retention cyst* usually occurs on the inner side of the lip or cheek and grows very slowly and presents for quite a long time; a *cancer of the lip* may present as a swelling or ulcer, gives a relatively short history though it is a slow-growing cancer and a *cancer of the tongue* gives an even shorter history.
5. **Pain:** This is an important symptom of these lesions. A careful history must be taken about its site, radiation or referred pain. Stomatitis is a painful condition particularly aphthous stomatitis. Similarly dental ulcer is very painful, but tuberculous ulcer is less painful. Pain is conspicuous by its absence in leukoplakia, mucous retention cyst and early stage of carcinoma of lip or tongue. If an old patient presents with ulcer of his tongue, but without pain, is an ominous sign. But it must be remembered that in late cases pain appears even in carcinoma of tongue. Site of pain is important, e.g., pain is complained of at the side of the tongue in case of dental ulcer. In certain late cases of carcinoma of tongue pain is referred to the ear of the affected side as lingual nerve and auriculotemporal nerve supplying the anterior surface of the external ear are both the branches of the mandibular nerve.
6. **Certain specific complaints:** Excessive salivation is a very common specific complaint of carcinoma of tongue. If an old patient is seen in surgical outdoor holding handkerchief in his mouth, he is most probably suffering from carcinoma of tongue. Inability to protrude the tongue is a symptom of tongue-tie and late cases of carcinoma of tongue with invasion to the floor of the mouth. Difficulty in speech is the main complaint of cleft lip and cleft palate and carcinoma of tongue. Deviation of tip of the tongue when protruded towards the side of the lesion is a sign of carcinoma of tongue. Alteration of voice may be the first symptom in carcinoma of posterior 1/3 of the tongue which may remain unnoticed for quite sometime.
7. **Personal history:** Enquiry must be made whether the patient smokes a lot or in the habit of drinking alcohol or taking spicy food. These may cause leukoplakia which is a premalignant condition. Similarly habit of taking betel nut and *supari* or *'khaini'* is quite common among the sufferers of carcinoma of the cheek.

Chapter 24: Examination of the Palate, Cheek, Tongue and Floor of the Mouth

History in examination of oral cavity

Aspect	Clinical significance	Patient-friendly questions
Onset of symptoms	Acute → Trauma, infection; chronic → Tumor, leukoplakia	"When did you first notice the ulcer/swelling?"
Pain	Painful → Aphthous, dental ulcer, infection; painless → Carcinoma, leukoplakia	"Does it hurt when you eat or talk?"
Ulcer duration	Short duration → Stomatitis; long duration → Neoplasm, syphilis	"Has the ulcer been present for weeks or months?"
Nerve involvement	Referred ear pain → Carcinoma of tongue	"Do you feel any pain in your ear?"

PHYSICAL EXAMINATION

A. INSPECTION

Inspection of inside of the mouth should be carried out preferably in daylight or in good light and you should always use a spatula.
Add after this:
Oral cavity examination steps should include:
- **Use good lighting:** Preferably daylight or a focused light source.
- **Inspect with a spatula:** Retract lips, cheeks, and tongue systematically.
- **Examine lips:** Look for clefts, pigmentation (Peutz-Jegher's syndrome), and neoplastic changes.
- **Assess the tongue:** Check for leukoplakia, glossitis, ulcers, or macroglossia.
- **Palate and floor of mouth:** Identify clefts, perforations (syphilitic gumma), ranula, or dermoid cysts.
- **Buccal mucosa and gums:** Check for leukoplakia, mucous cysts, or Vincent's stomatitis.
- **Cervical lymph nodes:** Palpate for submental, submandibular, and deep cervical involvement.

To inspect the *lips* properly not only the outer surfaces of the lips are examined, but also the lips are retracted to see the mucosal surface of the lips. Similarly, the *cheeks* are retracted outwards to see the buccal mucosal surface of the cheek as also the buccal side of the gum. To see the inside of the gum and floor of the mouth, the tongue is pushed away to one side or the other. For inspection of the tongue, the mouth is fully opened and the tongue is protruded to see the anterior 2/3rd of the tongue. To see the lateral aspect of its posterior third the tongue is pushed to one side or the other with a spatula. To see the fauces, tonsils and the beginning of the pharynx, one should depress the tongue with a spatula.

1. **Lips:** Cleft lip is obvious in inspection. ***Cleft lip*** may be complete when there is total failure of fusion and then the cleft extends up to the corresponding nostril. In case of incomplete cleft lip the cleft does not extend up to the nostril. There may be bilateral complete cleft lip in which there is also a cleft palate and a protuberant premaxilla. A ***facial cleft*** is a cleft between the maxilla and the side of the nose. ***Pigmentation of the lips*** and buccal mucous membrane is sometimes seen in Addison's disease. Small bluish-black spots on the lips and on the buccal and palatal mucous membrane are seen in Peutz-Jegher's syndrome. This syndrome is a familial disease which is inherited by autosomal dominant gene and the main pathology lies in the small bowel in the form of adenomatous polyp which may cause intussusception or intestinal colic,

but rarely undergo malignant change. **Chancre of the lip** presents as a painless ulcer with dull red color. **Cracked lips** are indolent cracks in the midline of the lower lip as a result of exposure to cold weather. These may occur more often in the angles of the mouths. **Ectopic salivary neoplasms** are usually seen in the upper lip as slow growing lobulated tumors. **Carcinoma of the lip** is seen in old individual which presents as erosion in the early stage—as red granular appearance with whitish flecks followed by yellowish crusting in the middle of the erosion. Gradually, the center becomes ulcerated and the margin becomes everted. The skin over the tumor becomes red and vascular. **Macrocheilia** means thickening of the lip which often involves the upper lip.

2. **Tongue:** Ask the patient to open the mouth and note: (a) The *volume* of the tongue; massive tongue *(macroglossia)* is commonly due to lymphangioma **(Fig. 24.1)**, hemangioma **(Fig. 24.2)**, neurofibroma and muscular macroglossia commonly seen in Cretins. (b) Its *color*—the white color of leukoplakia (chronic superficial glossitis), the 'red glazed tongue' when the leukoplakia plaques are desquamated, the blue color of venous hemangioma and black hairy tongue due to hyperkeratosis of the mucous membrane in heavy smokers or caused by a fungus called *Aspergillus niger* are very characteristic. (c) Any *crack or fissure*; note the direction of the fissures. Congenital fissures are mainly transverse whereas syphilitic fissures are usually longitudinal. (d) *Swelling* and (e) An *ulcer* if any.

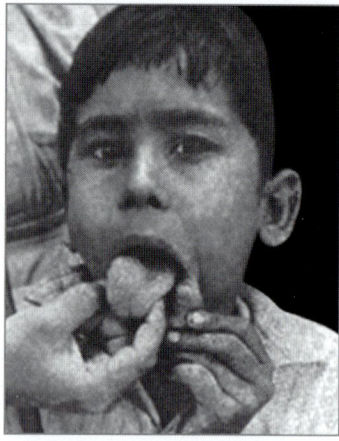

Fig. 24.1: Lymphangioma of the right half of the tongue.

If there is a swelling or an ulcer, note its site, size, shape, color, surface, margin, etc., as discussed in chapters 3 and 4 respectively. Note also whether it has extended to the floor of the mouth, to the jaw or tonsil. The site of the ulcer is usually characteristic, e.g., the dental ulcer occurs on the side of the tongue where they come in contact with sharp teeth or dentures, tuberculous ulcers on the tip and sides, gummatous ulcer on the dorsum and carcinomatous ulcers occur usually on the margin of the tongue (on the dorsum where superimposed on chronic superficial glossitis).

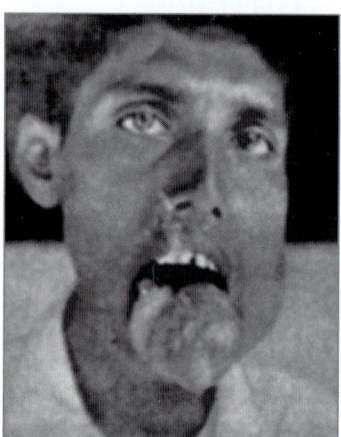

Fig. 24.2: Hemangioma of the left half of the tongue.

Very rarely one can discover an angioma-like swelling in the region of the foramen cecum—this is **lingual thyroid (Fig. 24.3)**. This may be the only thyroid gland the patient possesses and therefore should not be removed.

Lastly, the **mobility of the tongue** is tested. Ask the patient to put the tongue out and move it sideways. Inability to put the tongue out completely is due to ankyloglossia. If the tongue deviates to one side during the protrusion, it indicates impairment of nerve supply to that half of the tongue. This may be noticed in advanced carcinoma **(Fig. 24.4)** of the tongue which has damaged the nerve supply of the consequent side. If a child with impaired speech fails to protrude the tongue, it is possibly due to tongue-tie; look for the short frenum linguae.

3. **Palate:** Is there a congenital cleft, perforation, ulceration or a swelling? In case of a **congenital cleft (Fig. 24.5)**, note the extent of the cleft (involving only the uvula, only the soft palate or part

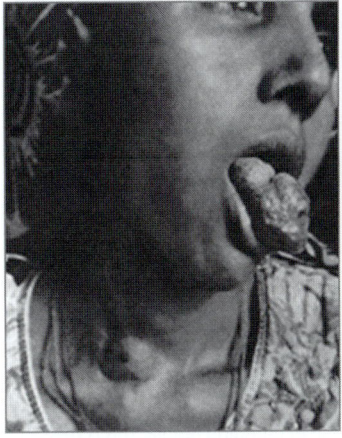 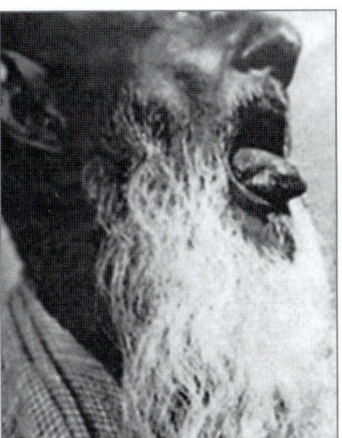 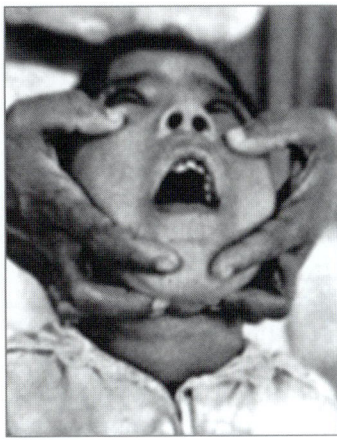

Fig. 24.3: Lingual thyroid with a branchial fistula in front of the lower part of the sternomastoid.

Fig. 24.4: Carcinoma at the right border of the tongue.

Fig. 24.5: Congenital cleft of the palate.

or whole of the hard palate) and also whether the nasal septum is hanging free or is attached to one side of the cleft. **Perforation** of the hard palate is usually caused by gumma (syphilitic affection) **(Fig. 24.6)**. The student must be careful to note if there is any scar of operation around or such history, as sometimes a hole may persist after an operation for closure of a congenital cleft. An *ulcer* or a *swelling* is examined in the usual way **(Fig. 24.7)**.

4. **Gums:** In order to examine the gums each lip must be everted fully. A spatula and a torch will be essential to visualize more posterior portions of the gums. Healthy gums are bright pink in color. The earliest sign of **pyorrhea alveolaris** is a deep red line along the free edge of the gum. **Vincent's stomatitis** is an inflammatory condition of the gingivae. There is ulceration of the gingival margin and formation of a pseudomembrane. This condition is often associated with very bad smell. **Cancrum oris** starts with a painful purple-red indurated papule found on the alveolar margin in the region of the molar or premolar teeth. Later on an ulcer forms which rapidly exposes the underlying bone and extends to the cheek and lip. This is also associated

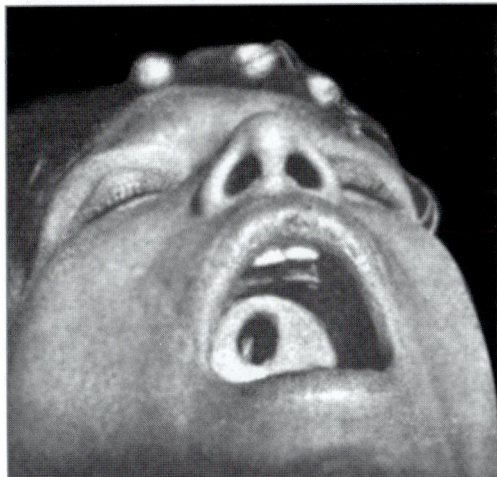 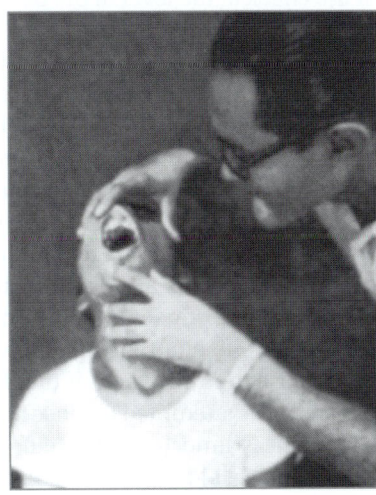

Fig. 24.6: Gummatous perforation of the hard palate.

Fig. 24.7: Swelling at the hard palate.

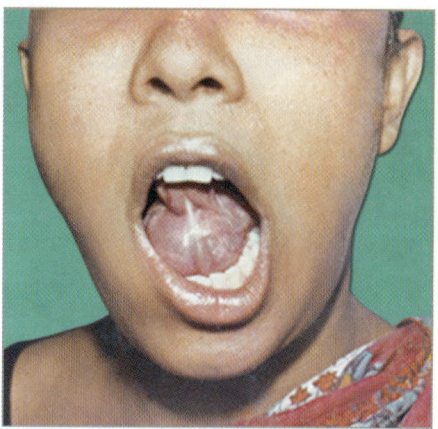

Fig. 24.8: A typical ranula at the floor of the mouth. Note its bluish color.

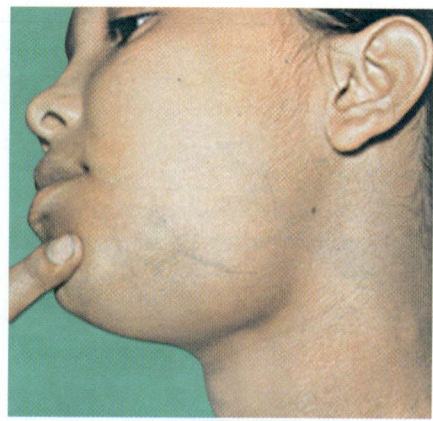

Fig. 24.9: A case of plunging ranula. This is the same case as shown in Fig. 24.8. Note how the swelling is so obvious in the submandibular triangle.

with foul smell. Swollen gum is sometimes a feature of dental abscess. A blue line may be seen in case of patients who work with lead.

5. **Floor of the mouth:** Ask the patient to open his mouth and to keep the tip of his tongue upwards to touch the palate. This will expose the floor of the mouth. When a swelling is present, note amongst other features, its color and position. A *ranula* appears as a unilateral bluish translucent cyst over which Wharton's duct can often be seen **(Fig. 24.8)**. A *sublingual dermoid* is opaque, lies exactly in the midline and may extend into the submental region. A deep or plunging ranula **(Fig. 24.9)** may have a cervical prolongation into the submandibular region.

6. **Cheek:** Examine the inside of the cheek for aphthous ulcer, leukoplakia, mucous cyst, lipoma, mixed salivary tumor, papilloma or carcinoma **(Fig. 24.10)**. Pigmented patches may be seen in Addison's disease and in Peutz-Jegher's syndrome. Of the above list, *mucous cyst* deserves special mention. Such cyst may develop anywhere on the inner side of the lips and the cheek, though more common on the inner side of the lower lip and on the buccal mucous membrane of the cheek at the level of the bite of the teeth.

B. **PALPATION**

1. **Lip:** Any lesion of the lip should be carefully palpated. While benign neoplasms are firm and lobulated, that the tongue should be relaxed and at rest within the mouth. If it is kept protruded, the contracted muscles may carcinoma of the lip is hard in consistency. Hunterian chancre is rubbery hard, whereas carcinoma of lip is stony hard. When carcinoma of lip is an ulcer hold the base of the ulcer with index finger and thumb which is always hard. With one hand the lip is now fixed and with the other hand the lesion of the lip is held by two fingers and is attempted to move against the lip. The carcinoma is almost always fixed. Mucous retention cyst **(Fig. 24.11)** is often seen on the inner surface of the lip (mostly in the lower lip). Fluctuation and

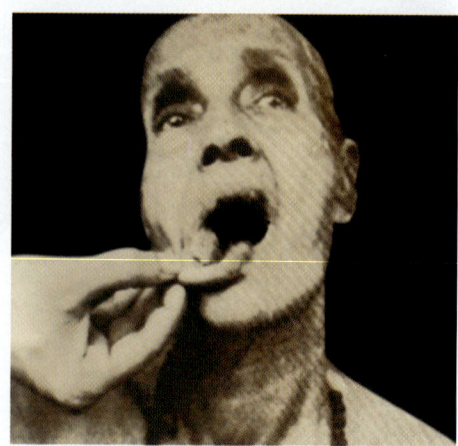

Fig. 24.10: Carcinoma of the cheek.

transillumination test are positive when the cysts are large. But these tests are not easy to perform in the lip. For fluctuation test one should follow the technique for small swelling as mentioned in chapter 3 (page 26). Regional lymph nodes are always felt in the submental and submandibular region **(Figs. 24.12 and 24.13)**.

2. **Tongue:** While palpating for *induration* **(Fig. 24.14)** of the base of an ulcer, it is desirable give a false impression to induration and lead to error in diagnosis **(Fig. 24.15)**. Induration is an important clinical sign of epithelioma. It may be present in gummatous ulcer but is absent in tuberculous ulcer. Note whether the *ulcers bleed readily during palpation*. This usually occurs in a malignant ulcer. Palpate carefully for a sharp tooth or tooth plate against an ulcer in the tongue.

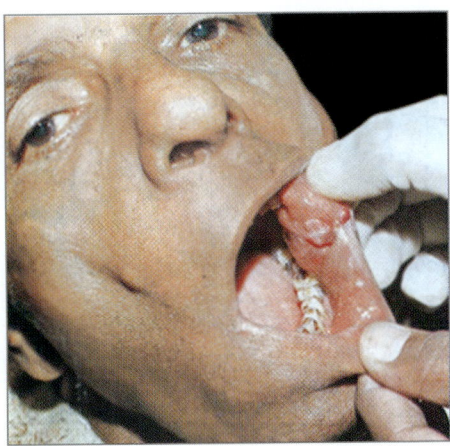

Fig. 24.11: Mucous retention cyst at the inner surface of the cheek.

Palpate the back of the tongue for any ulcer or swelling. The patient sits on a stool. The examiner stands on his right. The head is first fixed by holding it firmly against him with the left hand; the index finger of this hand is pushed in between the upper and lower jaws over the cheek to prevent closing of the mouth and biting the examiner's finger. The right index finger is then passed behind the soft palate. The back of the tongue and the pharynx are explored.

3. **Palate:** A tender fluctuating swelling close to the alveolar process is an alveolar abscess. A soft swelling in the middle of the hard palate is usually a gumma. An ulcer or a swelling is examined in the usual way. Mixed tumor of ectopic salivary gland may be felt in the palate.

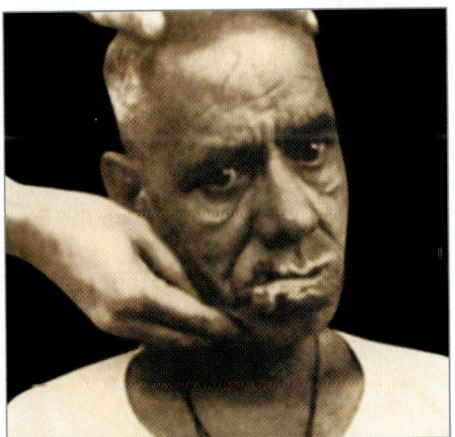

Fig. 24.12: Method of palpation for enlarged submandibular lymph nodes in a case of carcinoma of the lip. Note that the carcinoma originally affected the lower lip and now 'kiss lesion' is seen in the upper lip. Carefully note the method of palpation of submandibular lymph nodes. The head is bent to the side being palpated with one hand to relax the platysma and the muscles of that side of the neck for better palpation with the other hand.

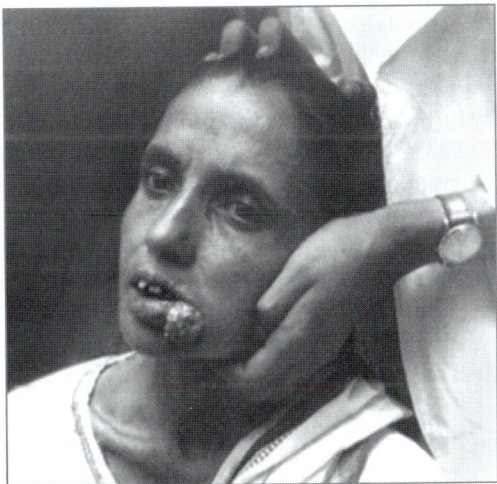

Fig. 24.13: Another case of carcinoma of the lip where the submandibular lymph nodes are being palpated for enlargement. Note the method of palpation.

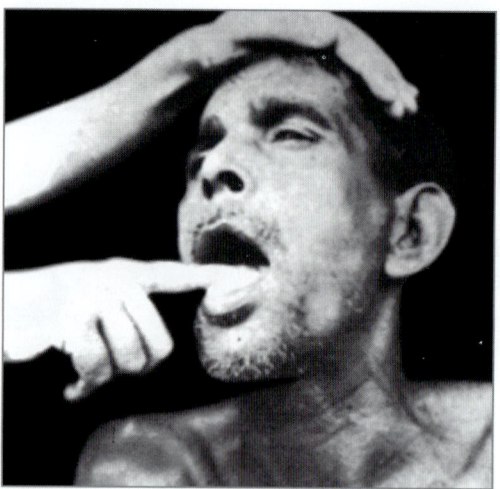
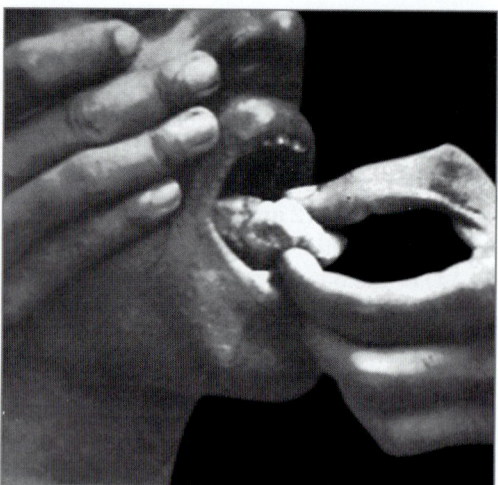

Fig. 24.14: The correct method of palpation of the tongue for induration (which is a characteristic feature of carcinoma of the tongue). The tongue must lie at rest within the mouth.

Fig. 24.15: The wrong method of palpation for induration of the base of an ulcer. If the tongue is kept protruded, the contracted muscles may give an impression of induration.

4. **Gums:** As age advances the gums recede and the teeth appear longer. The gums may bleed on palpation, which become swollen, spongy and tender in *scurvy*. Gums may bleed in uremia but they may not be as spongy as in scurvy. *Epulis* is a swelling of the alveolar margin of the gum. The margin, consistency, surface, mobility should be noted to come to a definite diagnosis of the type of epulis. These have been discussed in details in Chapter 23.

5. **Floor of the mouth:** A ranula is a fluctuating swelling with positive translucency **(Fig. 24.16)**. To know its extent, bimanual palpation of the floor of the mouth on one side and submandibular triangle on the other hand is necessary. Sublingual dermoid is not a translucent swelling but it is a tense fluctuant swelling on the midline. Carcinoma of the floor of the mouth may be revealed by its indurated base and probable fixation to the underlying structures.

6. **Cheek:** Mucous cyst has a smooth surface and is movable over the deeper structures. Fluctuation can be elicited by pressing on the top of the cyst while the sides are palpated by other two fingers. Papilloma is a solid tumor with irregular surface and mobile on the deeper structures. Carcinoma is fixed and indurated.

Examine the cervical lymph nodes (*see* 'Examination of the neck'), particularly the **(Fig. 24.17)**: (i) submental, (ii) submandibular, (iii) jugulodigastric and (iv) jugulo-omohyoid groups. The lymph nodes of both sides must be examined even if the lesion is unilateral as the lymph vessels decussate.

GENERAL EXAMINATION

1. If the ulcer of the tongue seems to be tuberculous, look for the primary focus in the lungs.
2. In *gummatous ulcer*, look for syphilitic lesions in other parts of the body. Since an epithelioma may develop on a syphilitic base, a positive WR will not exclude a carcinoma.

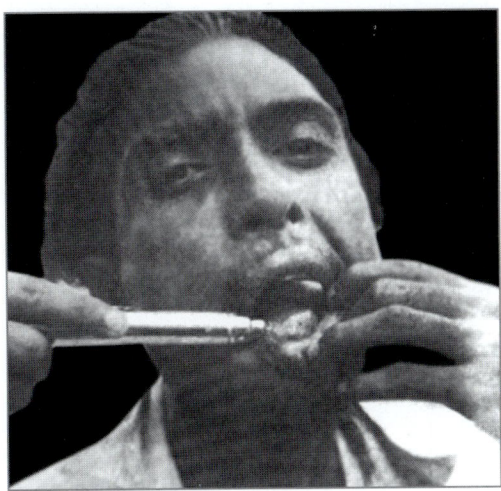

Fig. 24.16: A ranula is being tested for translucency.

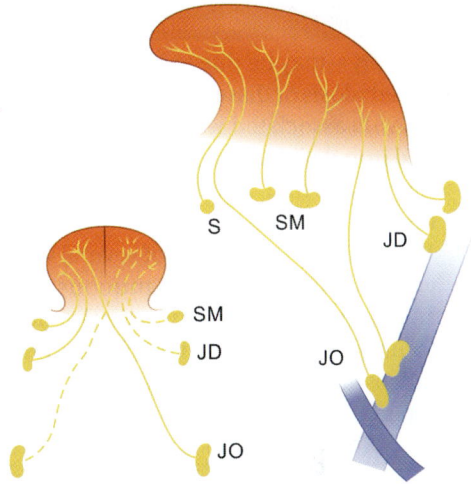

Fig. 24.17: Lymph drainage of the tongue. From the tip—to the submental (S) and jugulo-omohyoid (JO); from the margin—to the submandibular (SM) and upper deep cervical group; from the back—to the jugulodigastric (JD) and (JO). (B) Decussation of lymph vessels.

DIFFERENTIAL DIAGNOSIS

MUCOUS RETENTION CYST

This cyst usually develops due to obstruction of the duct of a small mucous secreting gland. So this cyst may occur anywhere on the inner surface of the lips, cheek and the mouth where these mucous secreting glands are present. It is most common on the lower lip and in the buccal mucous membrane of the cheek at the level of the bite of the teeth. The cyst may occur at any age. The main complaint is a lump on the inner side of the lip or cheek, which is *not* painful, but grows slowly and interferes with eating and may get bitten. The color of such cyst varies according to the state of the overlying epithelium. If the epithelium is healthy the cyst is pale-pink with gray glairy appearance of the mucus inside the cyst. If the epithelium is damaged it looks white, scarred and obscure the color of the mucus inside the cyst. This cyst is usually spherical with smooth surface and consistency varies from soft to hard according to the tension of fluid inside the cyst. Fluctuation and transillumination tests are positive when the cysts are large enough. This cyst is neither fixed to the overlying mucous membrane, nor fixed to the deeper structures, e.g., underlying muscles—orbicularis oris or buccinator. The regional lymph nodes are not enlarged.

STOMATITIS

This is a general term to describe inflammation of any kind of the lining membrane of the mouth. There are various *causes* of stomatitis which can be broadly classified into two groups—general causes and local causes.

General causes	Local causes
1. *Debility*—may be due to lack of nutrition, tuberculosis or disseminated carcinoma. 2. *Anemia* associated with vitamin B$_{12}$, folic acid and iron deficiency which make the mucous membrane thin, atrophic with loss of papillae of the dorsum of the tongue. 3. *Vitamin deficiency*: Lack of several varieties of vitamin B may lead to red mucous membrane and angular cheilitis. Vitamin C deficiency (scurvy) causes ulceration of gums and buccal mucosa due to interference in collagen synthesis. Vitamin B and C deficiency are also come across in sprue, celiac disease, pellagra and kwashiorkor.	1. Poorly fitting denture, sharp tooth and excessive smoking. 2. Infections with Vincent's angina, *Candida albicans*, monilia or herpes virus. 3. *Trauma*—mechanical, chemical, thermal or X-rays. 4. Foot and mouth disease.
4. *Blood diseases*, e.g., leukopenia, agranulocytosis, aplastic anemia and hypogammaglobulinemia and severe anemia are the conditions which reduce ability of the oral mucosa to deal with various infections and thus lead to stomatitis. 5. *Drugs*: Certain drugs, e.g., adrenal cortical steroid, phenobarbitone, phenytoin, lead, mercury, bismuth or sulfur poisoning. Excessive ingestion of iodides may also lead to stomatitis or sore mouth and excessive salivation. 6. An autoimmune mechanism is often believed to be at the root of forming stomatitis. 7. Secondary syphilis.	

Infecting organisms of this disease can be classified into two groups—(i) Facultative pathogens, that means the pathogens which are normal oral commensals, but take advantage of any weakness in the defense mechanism of the oral mucosa to produce localized or generalized infection of the mouth. These are streptococci, staphylococci and occasionally Vincent's organism. (ii) True pathogens, which are real pathogens and produce specific infections. *The followings are the different varieties of stomatitis*:

❖ **Catarrhal stomatitis:** The whole of the mucous membrane of the mouth becomes edematous and red. This usually occurs in association with acute upper respiratory tract infection and acute specific fever.

❖ **Aphthous stomatitis:** In this condition the inside of the mouth is covered with small painful vesicles with hyperemic base. The vesicles break and ulcers form which are round or oval in shape, with yellow base and red erythematous margin. These ulcers are exquisitely painful and are usually associated with generalized debilitating diseases. These ulcers are seen on the inside of the cheek, lips, soft palate and floor of the mouth. These usually heal within 10–14 days. These are more frequently seen in women than in men.

❖ **Monilial stomatitis (thrush):** This condition occurs due to oral infection with a fungus— *Candida albicans*. This is more commonly seen in children and in people with debilitating disease and also as a complication of a long continued antibiotic therapy. This may accompany the onset of AIDS. Small red patches appear on the buccal mucosa and tongue, which gradually turn white. This white color is due to a layer of edematous desquamating epithelium which is heavily contaminated with the fungus. This is also a very painful condition with excessive salivation.

❖ *Ulcerative stomatitis (Vincent's angina):* This condition is caused by **Borrelia vincentii** and **Bacillus fusiformis**. *Borrelia vincentii* is a mobile spirochaete whereas fusiformis fusiformis is a rod shaped organism with pointed ends. Both of these are anerobic and Gram negative. In this condition the gums are swollen, inflamed and painful with numerous small ulcers that are covered with yellow slough. These ulcers bleed easily and patients often complain of spontaneous gingival hemorrhage with fetor oris. This condition is mainly seen in adolescents and young adults. Patients are often unwell in particularly acute cases with fever and loss of appetite. The cervical lymph nodes are often enlarged and tender.

❖ *Gangrenous stomatitis (cancrum oris):* It is a severe form of stomatitis affecting the young and poorly nourished children. Malnutrition is the main predisposing cause and sometimes a complication of measles and leukemia. It begins as an area of edema and induration on the gums which becomes necrotic. The area of necrosis spreads on to the inside of the cheek, the lips and then through to the skin surface, producing a large area of full-thickness tissue loss. This is an extremely painful condition and the patient is very ill with anorexia, malaise and pyrexia.

❖ *Angular stomatitis (angular cheilosis):* In this condition there are moist, infected reddish-brown fissures at the angles of the mouth. The saliva usually leaks at the corners of the mouth and the moist skin becomes infected by Candida and staphylococci. It may occur in children who rub or lick the corners of their mouths, when it is called 'Perleche'. This condition may also occur in middle-aged and elderly using dentures.

Occasionally, small radiating cracks in the corners of the mouth may develop in patients with congenital syphilis, the condition is known as 'Rhagades'.

HUNTERIAN CHANCRE OF THE LIP

The features of primary chancre of the lip are similar to those of one on the genitalia. Initially, there is an elevated, pink macule. This grows slowly into hemispherical papule. Up to this stage the condition is painless. Gradually, the mucosal covering breaks down and a superficial ulcer forms which is often covered with a thick crust. The base of this ulcer is rubbery hard. This ulcer is slightly painful. The regional lymph nodes in the neck become enlarged and slightly tender. This ulcer is highly contagious. Ultimately the ulcer heals leaving a fine permanent superficial scar.

THE MUCOUS PATCH OF SYPHILIS

In the secondary stage of syphilis mucous patches are seen on the inside of the lips, cheeks and on the pillers of the fauces. These are grayish white in color due to edema and desquamation of the epithelium. When this gray patch of dead epithelium separates, the underlying mucosa is seen raw and bleeding. These mucous patches are also highly contagious. The patient with these mucous patches often complain of sore throat.

SNAIL TRACK ULCER

These ulcers form due to coalescence of a number of small mucous patches. So these ulcers are also seen on the inside of the lips, cheeks and mainly on the pillers of the fauces. These look like linear ulcers which are covered with white boggy epithelium and thus these are called 'snail track' ulcers.

BENIGN NEOPLASMS OF THE LIP

These are quite rare in the lip. Only when benign neoplasms develop in minor salivary glands such tumors are seen. Usually the upper lip is affected. Firm, slow growing, lobulated and mobile tumors are seen which are nothing but pleomorphic adenomas of the ectopic salivary glands. In extreme rare cases malignancy may develop in these ectopic salivary glands.

CARCINOMA OF THE LIP

Usually, males over 50 years of age become the victims of this disease. It usually occurs in individuals who are involved in outdoor occupations and that is why this condition is sometimes called 'Countryman's lip'. White Caucasians residing in Australia are often affected. Exposure to sunlight, especially the ultraviolet part, seems to be an important etiological factor. Leukoplakia of the lip, recurrent trauma from pipes and cigarettes are other etiological factors. The lower lip is involved in more than 90% of cases. Upper lip is affected in only 5% of cases and 1% for each corner of the lip. Initially patient complains of blistering, thickening or white patches on the lips which are persisting. Gradually, a nodule appears, the center of which becomes ulcerated and the margin becomes everted. Such ulcer fails to heal. As the ulcer grows it gradually invades into deeper structures, it often bleeds and may produce offensive discharge. It must be remembered that this condition is *painless*. The regional lymph nodes are almost always enlarged and the patients often show lumps under their chins.

TONGUE-TIE

It is a developmental anomaly, in which the frenum of the tongue is short and thicker. This frenum holds the tip of the tongue close to the lower central incisors. So the patient fails to protrude the tongue. Such attempt will cause eversion of the lateral margin of the tongue and heaping up of the midportion of the dorsum. It usually does not cause any other disability.

LEUKOPLAKIA (CHRONIC SUPERFICIAL GLOSSITIS)

In this condition normal surface of the dorsum of the tongue is lost and white color of thickened patches of epithelium which have lost their papillae cover the dorsal surface of the tongue. The lesion starts as thin and wrinkled white patches which gradually coalesce to form creamy-white thick surface. Later on this surface becomes dried and cracked. If the superficial epithelium is shed over a considerable area a 'red glazed tongue' may develop. In early cases if one is suspicious about this condition one may press a glass slide on the surface of the tongue which makes the thickened epithelium more obvious. While palpating, one must be careful to palpate the whole of the tongue to exclude any induration anywhere to suggest the malignant change which might occur.

Though syphilis was by far the commonest cause previously, yet carcinoma is gradually taking over this place. The other predisposing causes are smoking, spirit, sepsis and spices. So, students should remember of five 'S' as the predisposing factors of this condition. No less than 30% of cases of carcinoma of the mouth is being preceded by leukoplakia.

Five stages are recognizable in this condition:
Stage I: Mild thickening of the surface with hypertrophy of the papillae and hyperkeratosis.
Stage II: Stage of leukoplakia—the tongue is covered with smooth paint.
Stage III: The surface becomes irregular like dried paint.
Stage IV: Warty projections appear with cracks and fissures (precancerous stage).

Stage V: Desquamation of the abnormal mucosa leading to 'red glazed tongue'. This condition may gradually lead to carcinoma.

MACROGLOSSIA

This means chronic painless enlargement of the tongue. The causes are lymphangioma, hemangioma (which may be associated with congenital arteriovenous fistula), plexiform neurofibroma, muscular macroglossia (is often a feature of cretinism) and amyloid infiltration.

MANIFESTATIONS OF SYPHILIS IN THE TONGUE

Primary syphilis: Extragenital chancre may occur in the tongue with enlargement of the regional lymph nodes (submandibular and submental lymph nodes).

Secondary syphilis: Multiple shallow ulcers may be found on the under surface and sides of the tongue. Mucous patches may be seen on the dorsum of the tongue as well as in the fauces. Hutchinson's Wart (a condyloma) may be seen on the middle of the dorsum of the tongue.

Tertiary syphilis: Gumma of the tongue always occupies the midline position on the dorsum.

BLACK HAIRY TONGUE

This is due to hyperkeratosis of the mucous membrane caused by a fungus, *Aspergillus niger*. Generally heavy smokers are the victims.

MEDIAN RHOMBOID GLOSSITIS

A reddish color may be seen in the midline just in front of the circumvallate papillae. This is probably due to inadequate covering of the tuberculum impar in the formation of the anterior part of the tongue. This condition is often mistaken for syphilitic wart or epithelioma of the tongue.

CONGENITAL FISSURING OF THE TONGUE

Usually there is a deep median furrow from which transverse furrows originate on both sides. This condition usually reveals itself at the age of 3 years.

SYPHILITIC FURROWING OF THE TONGUE

In contradistinction to the congenital fissures, the syphilitic fissures are generally longitudinal in direction and the intervening epithelium is either hyperkeratotic or desquamated.

ULCERS OF THE TONGUE

Various types of ulcers may be found in the tongue. Of these the important ulcers are described below:

Aphthous (dyspeptic) ulcer—is a small painful ulcer seen on the tip, undersurface and sides of the tongue in its anterior part. The ulcer is small, superficial, with white floor, yellowish border and surrounded by a hyperemic zone. This condition is quite painful and usually starts in early adult life. These ulcers tend to recur and show a familial predisposition. Women suffer from this condition more often than men.

Dental ulcer—is caused by mechanical irritation either by a jagged tooth or denture. These ulcers occur at the periphery or on the undersurface of the tongue at the sides. This ulcer is elongated, often presents a slough at its base and surrounded by a zone of erythema and induration. This ulcer is quite painful.

Syphilitic ulcer—has been discussed above under the heading of 'Manifestations of syphilis in the tongue'.

Tuberculous ulcer—is shallow, often multiple and greyish yellow with slightly red undermining margin. These ulcers are also seen at the margin, tip or dorsum. This ulcer when occurs in the anterior 2/3rd of the tongue becomes very painful. Tuberculosis of the lungs or larynx is frequently associated with.

Postpertussis ulcer occurs only in children with whooping cough. It is usually seen at the frenum linguae.

Chronic nonspecific ulcer usually occurs in the anterior 2/3rd of the tongue. No etiological factor can be found out. It is moderately indurated and not very painful.

Carcinomatous ulcer is painless to start with and only becomes painful in late cases. Pain may be referred to the ear. The ulcer has a raised and everted edge with indurated base. Lymph node involvement is also quite early.

CARCINOMA OF THE TONGUE (FIG. 24.18)

It is highly important to know the *precancerous conditions* which are (i) chronic superficial glossitis, (ii) smoking pipes and cigars, (iii) syphilis, (iv) sessile papilloma and (v) Plummer vinson syndrome.

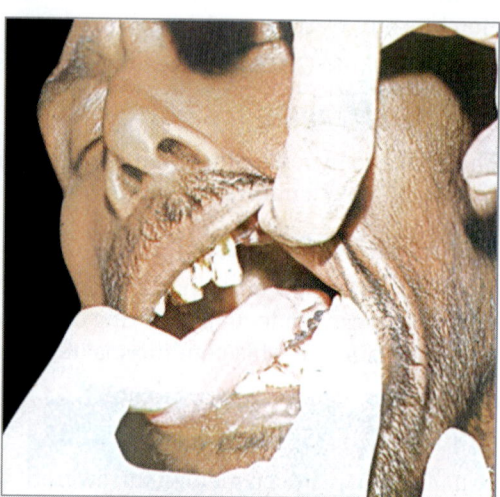

Fig. 24.18: Carcinoma at the left border of the tongue.

CLINICAL TYPES: (i) fungating or warty type; (ii) ulcerating or excavating type; (iii) fissure or cracked type following chronic superficial glossitis; (iv) nodular type and (v) 'frozen' type, when the tongue is transformed into an indurated mass. Of these, the first 3 types are common.

CLINICAL FEATURES: Carcinoma of the tongue should be diagnosed whenever an elderly man (sometimes a woman) presents a fungating growth or an ulcer having raised and everted margin with indurated base at the lateral border of the anterior 2/3rd of the tongue. There is little pain in the tongue; in late cases one may complain of pain and it may be referred to the ear since irritation of the lingual nerve is referred to the auriculotemporal nerve. *Profuse salivation* is common and an elderly man sitting in the surgical outpatient department with handkerchief continuously pressed at the mouth to soak saliva, is probably suffering from this condition. This is partly due to irritation of the nerves of taste and partly due to difficulty in swallowing due to *ankyloglossia*, that means the patient cannot protrude the tongue out of the mouth. This indicates that the carcinomatous process has infiltrated the lingual musculature and even the floor of the mouth. Besides these, in late cases there will be difficulty in speech, *dysphagia*, i.e., difficulty in swallowing and *faetor* (offensive smell).

Growth at the posterior third of the tongue often escapes the notice and in these cases *alteration of the voice* and *dysphagia* are the important symptoms. Diagnosis is made by palpating the growth which has been described in the section of "palpation" and by laryngoscopy.

SPREAD occurs (i) *locally* into the floor of the mouth and mandible when the growth is situated on the anterior 2/3rd of the tongue; and on the sides into the tonsil, fauces, epiglottic vallecula and soft palate when occurring on the posterior 3rd of the tongue. (ii) *Lymphatic spread* takes place into the submental, submandibular, jugulo-digastric and jugulo-omohyoid groups of lymph nodes of the same side as well as of the opposite side. Lymph node enlargement becomes more conspicuous in carcinoma of posterior 3rd of the tongue where growth is relatively out of sight. (iii) *Blood spread* is exceptional and only seen in cases of growth situated in the extreme posterior part of the tongue.

DEATH results from (i) inhalation bronchopneumonia due to aspiration, (ii) cancerous cachexia and starvation, (iii) hemorrhage from the primary growth and also from carotid artery when eroded by metastatic lymph nodes and (iv) asphyxia due to pressure on the air passages by metastatic lymph nodes or edema of the glottis.

RANULA

It is a translucent cystic swelling with bluish tinge situated on one side of the frenum linguae. It is almost always unilateral. Often the submandibular duct can be seen traversing the dome of this swelling. A big ranula may fill the floor of the whole mouth.

Deep or plunging ranula: When a ranula extends into the neck so that it can be palpable in the submandibular triangle, it is called a 'deep or plunging ranula'. Bimanual palpation will reveal cross fluctuation between the floor of the mouth and its cervical extension. This type of ranula probably derives from the cervical sinus.

SUBLINGUAL DERMOID

This is a congenital condition, but unfortunately is not seen before 10 years and majority of the patients when enter the surgical clinic are in their 20s. Thus ranula which is an acquired condition, becomes the most important condition in differential diagnosis. Though median variety is more common yet lateral sublingual dermoids are not unseen. While the median variety develops from inclusion of ectoderm between the two halves of the developing mandible, the lateral variety develops from the 2nd branchial cleft. It is an opaque and nontranslucent swelling in the floor of the mouth when situated above the mylohyoid. When situated below the mylohyoid, a cystic swelling develops either just below the chin, giving rise to a double chin or in the sub-mandibular region giving rise to a cystic swelling there. It is filled with sebaceous material and unlike other dermoid cysts does not contain hair.

Algorithmic Approach to Patient with Oral Cavity Disorders

Patient presents with oral ulcer, swelling, or pain
↓

Is the lesion congenital?
- **Yes** → Consider **cleft palate, lingual thyroid, macroglossia**
- **No** → Assess for **inflammatory, neoplastic, or infectious causes**

↓

Is there a localized ulcer?
- **Yes** → Consider **aphthous ulcer, syphilitic ulcer, carcinoma**
- **No** → Evaluate for **leukoplakia, glossitis, or stomatitis**

↓

Is the ulcer painful?
- **Yes** → Consider **aphthous ulcer, vincent's angina, tuberculous ulcer**
- **No** → Consider **carcinoma, leukoplakia, syphilitic ulcer**

↓

Perform imaging based on clinical findings
- **Biopsy** → For **suspected malignant or chronic ulcers**
- **X-ray** → For **bony involvement (osteomyelitis, jaw tumors)**
- **MRI** → For **soft tissue assessment (carcinoma, deep infections)**
- **CT scan** → For **complex oral cavity tumors or structural anomalies**

↓

Determine need for surgery vs conservative management
- **Surgical intervention?** → If **carcinoma, large cysts, advanced infections**
- **Conservative management?** → If **minor ulcers, leukoplakia, stomatitis**

Examination of the Salivary Glands

CHAPTER 25

THE PAROTID GLAND

History in examination of salivary glands

Aspect	Clinical significance	Patient-friendly questions
Onset of symptoms	Acute → Infection, abscess; chronic → Tumor, autoimmune	"How long have you had this swelling?"
Pain	Painful → Sialadenitis, abscess; Painless → Tumor	"Does the swelling hurt?"
Meal-related swelling	Sialolithiasis → Swelling increases at mealtime	"Does your swelling increase when you eat?"
Facial weakness	Malignant tumors involving facial nerve	"Have you noticed difficulty moving your face?"
Dry mouth, dry eyes	Sjogren's syndrome	"Do you have dry eyes or mouth?"

A. HISTORY

1. **Swelling:** Careful history must be taken as 'How did the swelling start?' 'Where exactly was the swelling first noticed?' 'How long is the swelling present?' 'Has the swelling enlarged uniformly throughout the period?' or 'Has it suddenly enlarged very recently?' So, the onset of the swelling, exact site of the swelling, duration of the swelling and growth of the swelling are noted. In dehydrated patient with poor oral hygiene if he complains of sudden increase in size of both the parotid glands with considerable pain, the case is probably one of acute parotitis. If there is brawny edematous swelling of the parotid region with pain, this is probably a case of parotid abscess. When there is generalized enlargement of all major salivary glands including lacrimal glands, it is called Mikulicz's syndrome. If this is associated with dry eyes and generalized arthritis the condition is called Sjogren's syndrome. A slow-growing tumor having duration for years or months of the parotid gland is the pleomorphic adenoma. When such a tumor suddenly starts growing rapidly and becomes painful, it is highly suggestive of malignant transformation of this adenoma (mixed parotid tumor). Site is important as adenolymphoma, which is also a slow-growing painless tumor, arises in the lower part of the parotid gland at the level of the lower border of the mandible slightly lower than the usual site of pleomorphic adenoma. 'Does the swelling increase in size, becomes tense and painful during meals?' This is characteristic of obstruction of the parotid duct with stone.

2. **Pain:** Acute parotitis is a painful condition. It must be remembered that mumps is the most common cause of bilateral parotitis (*see* **Fig. 25.12**). Throbbing pain is the characteristic feature of parotid abscess. Excruciating pain, slight swelling and redness in the region of the parotid gland are characteristic features of parotid abscess. In case of obstruction of the parotid duct

with a stone or stricture patient will complain of colicky pain during meals when the swelling of the parotid gland will also be increased.

3. **Watery discharge** from a sinus in the region of the parotid gland or its duct particularly during meals is significant for a parotid fistula.

B. **INSPECTION and PALPATION**

1. **Swelling:** The students must keep in mind the position of the parotid gland, which is below, behind and slightly in front of the lobule of the ear **(Figs. 25.1A and B)**. A swelling of the parotid gland thus obliterates the normal hollow just below the lobule of the ear. This position of the parotid gland is very important as many of the lymph node swellings are often mistaken for parotid gland tumor and vice versa. While examining the swelling its extent, size, shape, consistency, etc., should be noted as in any other swelling. Whether the swelling is fixed to the masseter muscle or not is examined by asking the patient to clinch his teeth and the mobility of the swelling is tested over the contracted masseter muscle **(Figs. 25.2A and B)**.

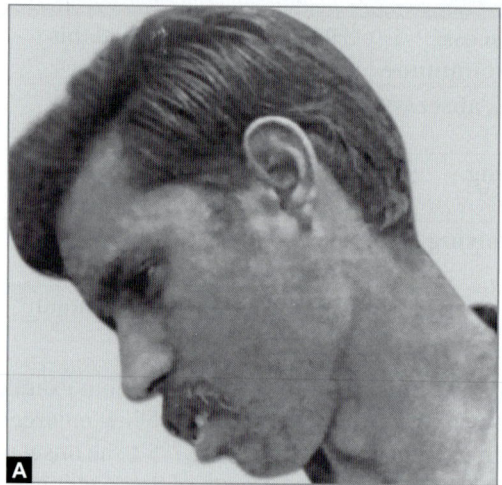
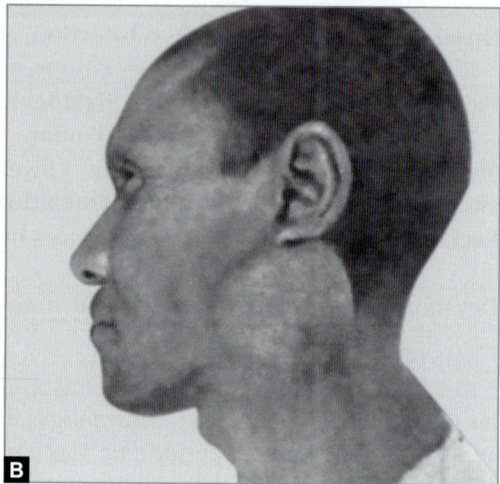

Figs. 25.1A and B: Note the typical site of the mixed parotid tumor.

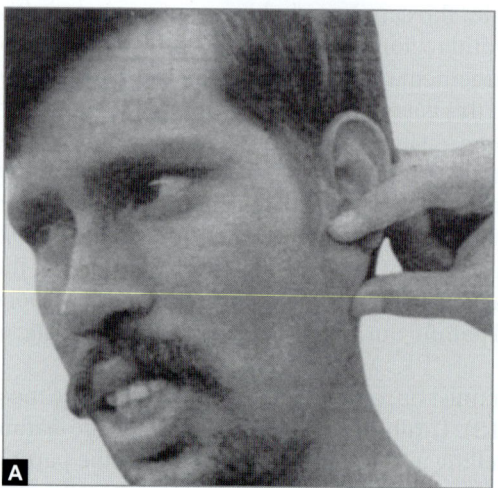
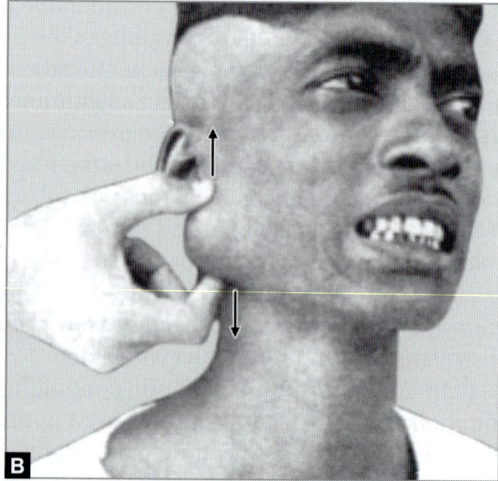

Figs. 25.2A and B: Testing for mobility over the contracted masseter. The patient is asked to clinch his teeth to make the masseter contracted.

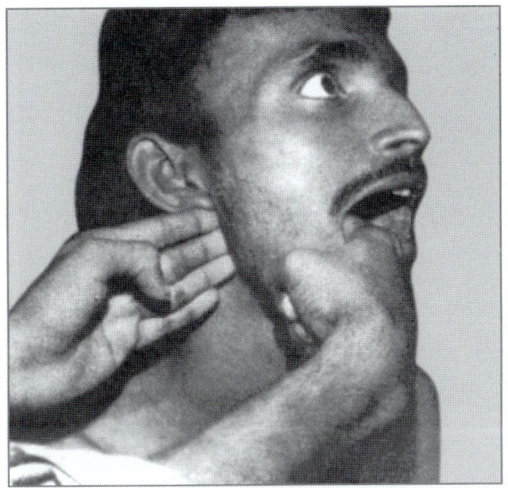

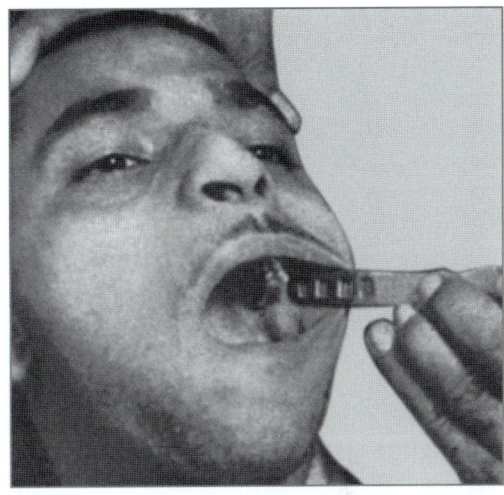

Fig. 25.3: Method of palpation of the deep lobe of the parotid gland. See the text.

Fig. 25.4: Method of palpation of the deep lobe of the parotid gland. See the text.

Enlargement of the deep lobe of the parotid gland, though occasionally seen is not very easy to diagnose. The examinations detailed above are all for the superficial lobe. A bimanual examination with one finger of one hand inside the mouth just in front of tonsil and behind the 3rd molar tooth and one finger of the other hand externally behind the ramus of the mandible is necessary for palpation of the deep lobe **(Fig. 25.3)**.

2. **Skin over the parotid gland:** Careful inspection and palpation must be made for the skin over the parotid gland. In case of parotid abscess the skin becomes brawny oedematous with pitting on pressure. It must be remembered that fluctuation is a very late feature of a parotid abscess as there is strong parotid fascia overlying the parotid gland. So, the findings of the skin mentioned above should be considered as conclusive evidence for the diagnosis. The skin will also be warm and extremely tender. One should also look for any scar or fistula in this region. When parotid malignancy is suspected careful examination must be made to exclude if there is infiltration of the skin by the tumor.

3. **Duct:** The parotid (Stensen's) duct starts just deep to the anterior border of the gland and runs superficial to the masseter muscle, then it curves inwards to open on the buccal surface of the cheek opposite the crown of the upper second molar tooth. For its proper inspection, one has to retract the cheek with spatula **(Fig. 25.4)**. If one suspects the case to be one of suppurative parotitis, gentle pressure over the gland will cause purulent saliva to come out of the orifice of the duct. Similar pressure may find blood to come out in case of malignant growth of the gland. While the duct rounds over the masseter muscle one can feel the duct by rolling the finger over the taut masseter muscle. The terminal part of the duct is best palpated bidigitally between the index finger inside the mouth and the thumb over the cheek **(Fig. 25.5)**.

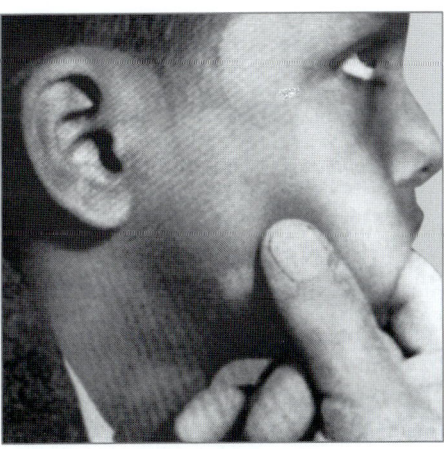

Fig. 25.5: Bidigital palpation of the terminal part of the parotid duct.

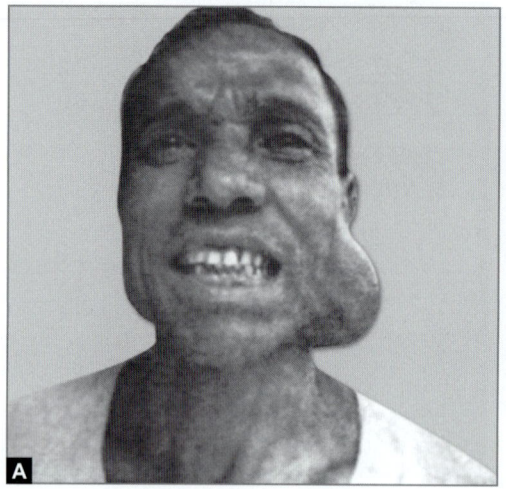
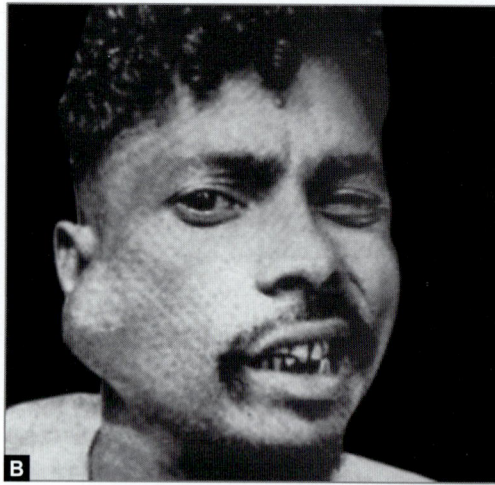

Figs. 25.6A and B: Examination is being performed to test the integrity of the facial nerve. (A) No paralysis of the facial nerve whereas in (B) There is definite paralysis of the facial nerve.

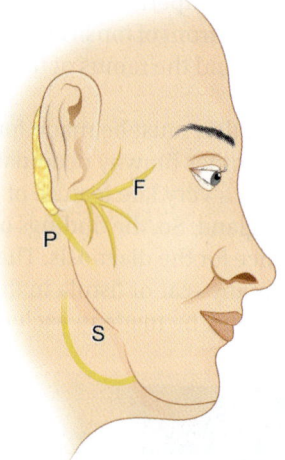

Fig. 25.7: A diagrammatic representation of the position of the facial nerve (F), the parotid gland (P) and the submandibular gland (S).

4. **Fistula:** If there is a parotid fistula, note its position: whether in relation to the gland or the duct (masseteric or premasseteric).

Examine the facial nerve as discussed in page 317.

The facial nerve is not involved in a benign tumor of the parotid gland, but is involved in a malignant growth **(Figs. 25.6A and B)**. The relationship of facial nerve to parotid gland and submandibular gland is shown in **Figure 25.7**.

Lymph nodes: Lymph nodes of the neck must be examined as a routine. The preauricular, the parotid and the submandibular groups of lymph nodes are mostly involved.

Movements of the jaw may become restricted if the growth is malignant and has involved the periarticular tissue of temporomandibular joint.

Sialography: A watery solution of lipiodol (neohydriol) is injected into the orifice of Stensen's duct and a skiagram is taken. Any obstruction of the duct by a calculus or dilatation of the ducts and acini (sialectasis) may be demonstrated. In parotid fistula, it helps to locate the site of lesion—whether in the main duct or in a ductule.

SUBMANDIBULAR SALIVARY GLAND

HISTORY: Appearance of a swelling in the submandibular region with colicky pain at the time of meals is diagnostic of stone in the submandibular duct. This swelling is tense and painful **(Fig. 25.8)**. *Otherwise, swelling in this region is more often due to lymph node enlargement rather than salivary gland tumors.*

LOCAL EXAMINATION

INSPECTION: If the patient gives the history which is very much suggestive of a stone in the submandibular salivary duct, the patient may be asked to suck a little lemon or lime juice. The swelling will at once appear. In *Mikulicz's disease* submandibular salivary glands along with the parotid glands and lacrimal glands may be enlarged **(Fig. 25.9)**. Otherwise, majority of the swellings in this region are due to enlarged lymph nodes. But a careful palpation must be performed to come to the definite diagnosis rather than biased by assumptions.

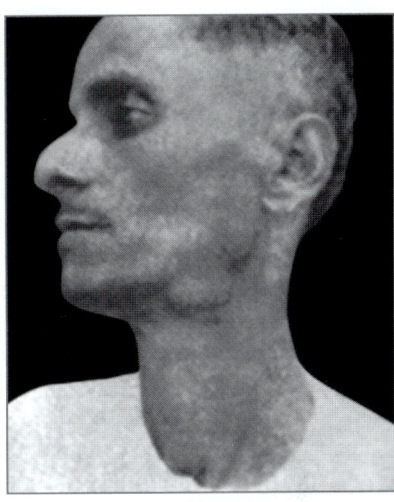

Fig. 25.8: A swelling of the submandibular salivary gland. The patient states that the swelling gets tense and tender during meals—stone in the salivary gland.

Inspection of the orifices of the submandibular (Wharton's) ducts **(Fig. 25.10)** is made by means of a torch on the floor of the mouth. The orifices are situated on either side of the frenulum linguae. It is noted whether each orifice looks inflamed or swollen due to impaction of a stone in the duct. Occasionally, a stone may be impacted in the ampulla just deep to the orifice and can be seen if inspected carefully. If the salivary gland is infected, slight pressure on the gland will extrude pus through the respective orifice. If a stone is impacted in one duct, saliva will be seen coming out with normal flow from the other orifice while the orifice concerned remains dry. This may be tested by putting two dry swabs one on each orifice and some lemon juice is given on the dorsum of the tongue. A minute later the patient is asked to move the tongue up and the two swabs are taken out. The swab on the orifice of the duct where the stone is impacted will remain dry.

PALPATION: Palpation must be done very carefully as lymph node swellings are quite common in this region. Nodular swelling either discrete or matted is suggestive of lymph node

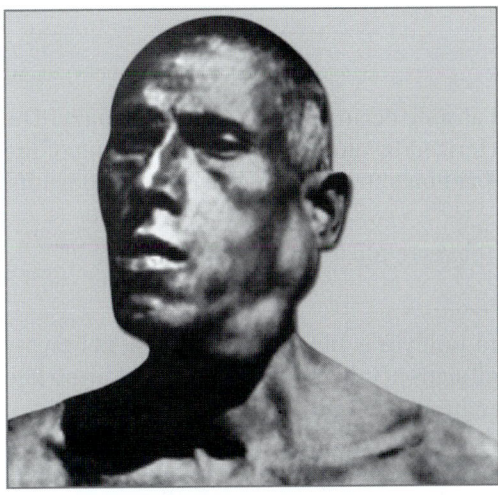

Fig. 25.9: Mikulicz's disease.

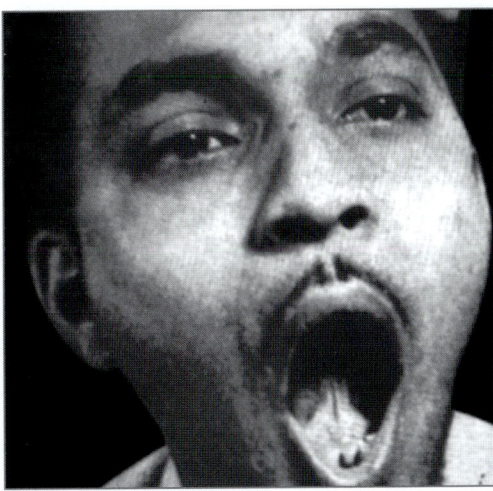

Fig. 25.10: Examining the orifice of the Wharton's duct.

enlargement. In case of submandibular salivary gland enlargement, it is one swelling and not a few nodular swellings. Submandibular salivary gland is best palpated *bimanually* **(Fig. 25.11)**. The patient is asked to open his mouth. One finger of one hand is placed on the floor of the mouth medial to the alveolus and lateral to the tongue and is pressed on the floor of the mouth as far back as possible. The fingers of the other hand, in the exterior, are placed just medial to the inferior margin of the mandible. These fingers are pushed upwards. This helps to palpate both the superficial and deep lobes of the salivary gland. Presence of a calculus is also appreciated by this bimanual examination. *This examination also differentiates an enlarged salivary gland from enlarged submandibular lymph nodes.* The finger inside the mouth can

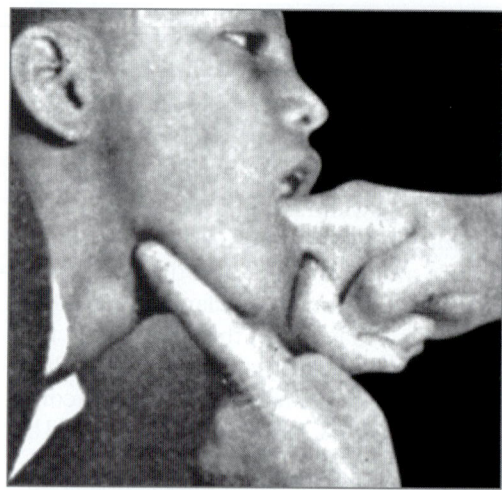

Fig. 25.11: Shows bimanual palpation of the submandibular salivary gland.

feel the deep part of the salivary gland but not the lymph nodes as the former is situated above the mylohyoid muscle and the latter below the muscle. To exclude impaction of stone in the duct, the whole duct must be palpated bimanually.

So far as the lymph node swellings are concerned the students must remember that the swelling may be due to primary or secondary involvements of lymph nodes. For the latter case one must examine thoroughly the inside of the mouth including the upper lip, the lower lip, the cheeks, the tongue and the floor of the mouth.

X-ray: In case of stone in the salivary gland or duct this special investigation is very helpful, as majority of the stones here are radio-opaque.

DIFFERENTIAL DIAGNOSIS

■ THE PAROTID GLAND

CONGENITAL SIALECTASIS

It is a condition of dilatation of the ductules and alveoli, occurring in one gland usually. The symptoms commence in infancy and are characterized by attacks of painful swelling of the parotid gland, often accompanied by fever. Some patients show an allergy to certain foodstuffs. Diagnosis is established by sialography.

Calculus is rarely formed in the parotid gland as the secretion is watery.

ACUTE SUPPURATIVE PAROTITIS

Infection reaches the gland from the mouth and rarely it is blood-borne. There is brawny edematous swelling over the parotid region with all signs of inflammation. Fluctuation is a late feature owing to the presence of strong fascia over the gland.

THE AURICULOTEMPORAL (FREY'S) SYNDROME

This condition follows injury to the auriculo-temporal nerve while incising for the suppurative parotitis. At the time of meals, the parotid region and the cheek in front of it become red, hot

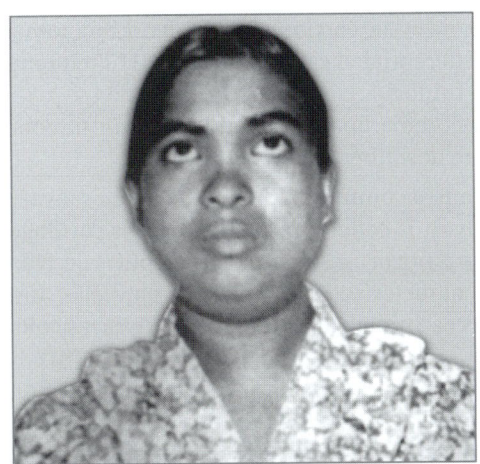

Fig. 25.12: Acute parotitis due to mumps.

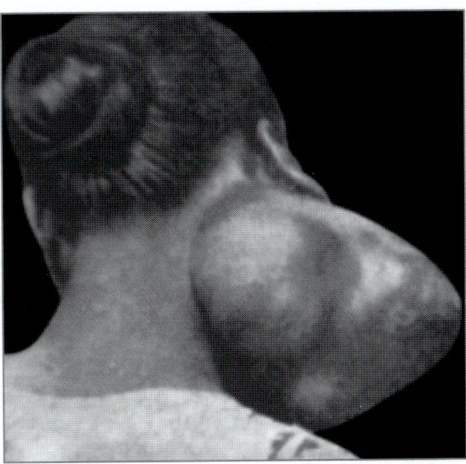

Fig. 25.13: A huge parotid tumor. For the last month it is growing rapidly.

and painful; very soon beads of perspiration appear on this area. Cutaneous hyperesthesia is also present over this area and becomes evident to the patient while shaving.

ACUTE PAROTITIS

Due to mumps, is a nonsuppurative condition. It may be unilateral to start with but becomes bilateral within a few days. It is associated with constitutional disturbances and other manifestations of mumps **(Fig. 25.12)**.

SUBACUTE AND CHRONIC PAROTITIS

This affection may be unilateral or bilateral. Patient complains of recurrent swelling of the parotid gland. The swelling is particularly seen during meals. The gland feels firmer, slightly tender and rubbery. Diagnosis is confirmed if purulent saliva or watery saliva can be ejected from the opening of the duct while gentle pressure is exerted over the gland.

PAROTID TUMORS (FIG. 25.13)

Approximately 90% of the neoplasms of the salivary glands occur in the parotid glands, 10% in the submandibular glands and very rarely in the sublingual and ectopic salivary glands. Approximately 3/4th of the epithelial lesions in the parotid are clearly benign; the remaining 1/4th is composed of definite carcinomas alongwith the mucoepidermoid and acinic cell tumors which are generally considered to be cancers of variable aggressiveness. But in submandibular gland majority of the tumors are malignant. The most common cancers in the salivary glands are in descending order of frequency—mucoepidermoid tumors, adenoid cystic carcinoma, adenocarcinoma, epidermoid carcinoma, undifferentiated carcinomas and carcinomas arising in pleomorphic adenomas (malignant mixed tumors).

After considering the general points, as have been mentioned in the previous paragraph, we now consider classification of the tumors of the salivary glands. They are classified as follows:

A. Epithelial tumors: Benign—(1) Pleomorphic adenoma (mixed tumor), (2) Papillary cystadenoma lymphomatosum (adenolymphoma or Warthin's tumor) and (3) oxyphil adenoma (oncocytoma).

Malignant: (1) Mucoepidermoid carcinoma, (2) Adenoid cystic carcinoma, (3) Adenocarcinoma, (4) Epidermoid (squamous cell) carcinoma, (5) Undifferentiated carcinoma and (6) Carcinoma arising in pleomorphic adenoma (malignant mixed tumor).

B. **Connective tissue tumors**: *Benign*—hemangioma, fibroma, lipoma, etc. and *malignant* tumors.

C. **Metastatic tumors**: Only the common tumors are described below:

Pleomorphic adenoma (mixed tumor): This is the most common tumor of the major salivary glands and its marked feature is histologic diversity. It is called 'mixed' as there is cartilage besides epithelial cells. It is believed that the cartilage is not of mesodermal origin but is derived from mucin secreted from the epithelial cells. It is characterized principally by epithelial and myoepithelial components distributed in varied patterns through an abundant matrix of mucoid, myxoid or chondroid supporting tissue.

Diagnosis is made by the presence of a lobulated and painless swelling over the parotid region being present for many months or years. It is neither adherent to the skin nor to the masseter muscle. The tumor is generally firm but variable consistency is the diagnostic feature. The facial nerve remains free. Sometimes it is difficult to enucleate completely despite encapsulation. Adding to the difficulty, the capsule may at points be thinned and somewhat deficient to define surgically. At such places of capsular deficiency, small pseudopods of tumor may protrude and left behind after enucleation. Thus, recurrences following resection are reported to occur from 5 to 50% of cases with a higher incidence in tumors of the minor salivary glands. These recurrences may not become apparent until one to two decades later.

Though rare yet malignant transformation of this tumor may occur in approximately 3% to 5% of cases. This *malignant transformation* is suggested when the tumor: (a) becomes painful, (b) starts growing rapidly, (c) feels stony hard and (d) gets fixed to the masseter and mandible deeply or to the skin superficially and (e) involves the facial nerve—an important feature. (f) The cervical lymph nodes are enlarged and (g) movements of the jaw may be restricted.

Papillary cystadenoma lymphomatosum (Warthin's tumor): This represents about 5–15% of parotid tumors and *almost always occurs in the lower portion of the parotid* overlying the angle of the mandible. Infrequently these tumors occur bilaterally or in other salivary glands. It is the only salivary neoplasm that occurs preponderantly in males above 40 years. This tumor presents as a slow-growing painless swelling over the angle of the jaw. The overlying skin looks normal. The surface of the swelling is smooth and well defined and the margin is distinct. Consistency is soft, often fluctuate, but not translucent. The regional lymph nodes are *not* enlarged. This tumor was previously considered to be teratoid or branchiogenic in origin. But today it is believed that the tumor is essentially epithelial in origin and that the lymphoid component represents reactive element perhaps of immunologic origin, comparable to that seen in Hashimoto's thyroiditis or Sjogren's syndrome.

This tumor is composed of cystic or glandular spaces lined by columnar epithelium within an abundant lymphoid tissue, harboring germinal centers. The cells are eosinophilic. Though this tumor may be firm, yet it may be soft and frequently cystic. Irregular papillary processes of tall columnar epithelium project into the cystic spaces.

This tumor is more often seen in white races and not seen in Negroes. These are encapsulated lesions and do not undergo malignant transformation. However, they are susceptible to infection and may sometimes be converted into abscesses.

Carcinoma of the parotid gland (adenocarcinoma, epidermoid and undifferentiated carcinoma): The patients are usually over 50 years of age. Males and females are equally affected. The main complaint is a rapidly enlarging swelling in the parotid region which was painless to start with, but becomes painful at later stage particularly during movements of the jaw. The pain may radiate to the ear and over the side of the face. On examination there is often infiltration of the tumor to the overlying skin, when the skin becomes tethered and reddish blue. It also becomes hyperemic. But the tumor is not tender (cf. acute parotitis when the swelling is extremely tender). The surface is irregular and the margin is often indistinct. Consistency is firm to hard. The swelling is fixed to deeper structures and gradually restricts the jaw movements. The facial nerve is often infiltrated by the tumor which becomes irritable initially with muscle spasm and ultimately leads to facial paralysis. The cervical lymph nodes are always enlarged and hard. General examination must be made to exclude disseminated blood-borne metastases.

Oxyphil adenoma: When Warthin's tumor becomes devoid of lymphoid element and is composed entirely of epithelium it is called an oxyphil adenoma.

Mucoepidermoid tumor: This accounts for 6–8% of all neoplasms in the major salivary glands. This occurs more frequently in parotid rather than submandibular glands. This tumor has variable level of aggressiveness and sometimes subdivided into high, intermediate and low variants. The majority are slow-growing cancers which can be successfully treated by adequate radial excision. On cross section they may be solid, cystic or semicystic. The fluid within the cyst is clear, mucous or thick turbid secretion. Histologically, there are cords or sheets of squamous, mucous or intermediate cells. The cells range from well differentiated cells with small regular nuclei to less differentiated cells with hyperchromatism and mitotic figures in the nuclei. These tumors yield to about 85% 5-years' survival rate.

Adenoid cystic carcinoma (cylindroma): These are poorly encapsulated infiltrating tumors to which the name 'Cylindroma' is commonly applied. Approximately 10% of the malignant tumors of the salivary gland are of this type. Though this tumor arises more frequently in the parotid glands yet in the submandibular and ectopic salivary glands this represents a higher proportion of all tumors (20%). The tumor cells are small, darkly stained with relatively little cytoplasm and are arranged about the stromal elements in a pseudoglandular (adenoid) pattern. They display a wide range of patterns—either tubular or cribriform or solid. The stroma in most of these tumors is moderately cellular fibrous tissue but is strikingly hyalinized.

This tumor is slow-growing and may be mistaken as a mixed tumor. But local recurrence and continuous growths involving the surrounding structures soon reveal itself. Local pain is prominent and sometimes an early symptom. The tendency of this tumor to invade the perineural lymphatics accounts for the high frequency of facial nerve paralysis. Five-year cure rate has been quoted as less than 25%.

THE SUBMANDIBULAR SALIVARY GLAND

CALCULUS

This is more common in the submandibular than in the parotid gland, as the secretion is more watery in the latter gland. It has the same composition as that of the tartar formed upon the teeth, viz., calcium and magnesium phosphates. It may occur within the gland or its duct. The pathognomonic feature of the salivary calculus is the swelling of the gland during meals, often preceded by salivary colic. When this history is forthcoming, the patient should be given some lemon juice and the swelling can be reproduced. At the same time examination of the orifice of the affected duct shows little or no ejection of saliva. The stone, if it is situated in the duct, can be easily palpated bidigitally. Radiograph is often helpful in confirming the diagnosis. Ultrasound

(**Fig. 25.14**) is nowadays more often used as this noninvasive technique is more competent to detect stone in the submandibular salivary gland or duct.

THE TUMORS OF THE SUBMANDIBULAR SALIVARY GLANDS

Tumors in this gland are uncommon in comparison to the parotid tumors. Enlargement of this gland is more due to calculus rather than a tumor. Of the tumors seen in this gland, the *mixed* tumor is the commonest. Mixed tumor presents as a slow growing tumor of moderate size. The swelling is hard but not stony hard. One must exclude lymph nodes swelling in this region before coming to this diagnosis.

Carcinoma of the submandibular gland is extremely rare.

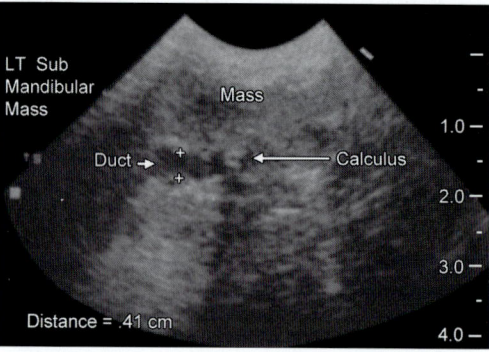

Fig. 25.14: Ultrasonography showing calculus in the submandibular salivary duct with enlarged submandibular salivary gland noted as 'mass'.

THE SUBLINGUAL AND ECTOPIC SALIVARY GLANDS

MUCOUS CYST (RETENTION CYST)

This is the result of cystic degeneration of the sublingual salivary gland or of glands of Blandin and Nuhn that are situated in the floor of the mouth or under-surface of the tongue.

TUMORS

Tumors of the minor salivary glands, mostly mixed tumors, are encountered frequently in the palate. The upper lip is second in frequency. But these are also encountered in the nasopharynx, larynx, bronchi and nasal sinuses. Adenoid cystic carcinomas also occur in the bronchi, trachea, pharynx, paranasal sinuses and lacrimal glands.

MIKULICZ'S DISEASE (SYNDROME)

This disease is characterized by: (i) symmetrical and usually progressive enlargement of all the salivary glands—both parotids, both submandibulars, both sublinguals and frequently the accessory salivary glands. (ii) Enlargement of the lacrimal glands. This causes a bulge below and outer ends of the eyelids, thus narrowing the palpebral fissures. (iii) Dry mouth. The enlargement of the lacrimal and salivary glands is due to replacement of the glandular tissue by lymphocytes. Usually, the disease occurs in persons between 20 and 40 years of age. In the beginning one salivary gland or often the lacrimal gland is attacked and the disease may be localized in that gland for quite a long time before involving the others. Mikulicz disease is probably due to an autoimmune process in the glands and is often looked upon as a clinical variant of Sjogren's syndrome. The diagnosis is established only by histological examination.

SJOGREN'S SYNDROME

This syndrome is characterized by all the features of Mikulicz's syndrome *plus:* (i) dry eyes (keratoconjunctivitis sicca) and (ii) generalized arthritis (rheumatoid). Enlargement of the salivary glands is often not so gross as seen in Mikulicz's disease. Recently other connective tissue diseases such as systemic lupus erythematosus or scleroderma has been seen to be associated with it. In this condition the salivary and lacrimal glands are also infiltrated with lymphocytes and the acini are progressively destroyed. The epithelium of the ducts becomes hyperplastic and may form casts within the lumen blocking smaller ducts. Thus blocking of the ducts, strictures, proximal duct dilatations and ascending infection may complicate the syndrome. This condition is also considered to be an autoimmune disease as autoantibodies and hypergammaglobulinemia are usually detected. $^{99}Tc^m$ Technetium scan may be performed to know the function of the gland.

Algorithmic Approach to Patient with Salivary Glands Disorders

Patient presents with swelling or pain in salivary gland

↓

Is the swelling acute or chronic?
- **Acute** → Consider **infection (mumps, parotitis, abscess)**
- **Chronic** → Assess **for obstruction, tumor, or autoimmune disease**

↓

Does swelling increase during meals?
- **Yes** → Consider **sialolithiasis (salivary duct stone)**
- **No** → Assess for **tumors or chronic inflammation**

↓

Is the swelling painful?
- **Yes** → Likely **infection, abscess, or sialolithiasis**
- **No** → Likely **benign tumor or autoimmune condition (Sjogren's syndrome, Mikulicz's disease)**

↓

Is facial nerve involved?
- **Yes** → High suspicion for **malignancy (adenoid cystic carcinoma, SCC, mucoepidermoid carcinoma)**
- **No** → Likely **benign lesion (pleomorphic adenoma, Warthin's tumor)**

↓

Perform imaging based on clinical findings
- **Ultrasound** → First-line for **salivary gland swellings, stones, tumors**
- **Sialography** → For **ductal obstruction and chronic sialadenitis**
- **CT/MRI** → For **deep tumors, suspected malignancy, facial nerve involvement**

↓

Determine need for surgery vs conservative management
- **Surgical intervention?** → If **obstructing sialolithiasis, tumor, or malignant lesion**
- **Conservative management?** → If **minor infections, small nonprogressive cysts, autoimmune disorders**

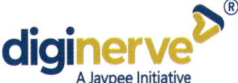

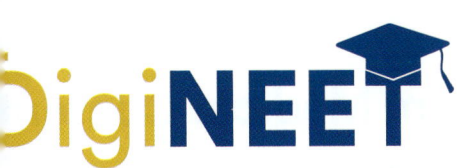

plify your undergraduate studies and NEET PG preparation
this comprehensive program covering all 19 subjects.
fted by India's top faculty, it includes video lectures, printed
es, OSCEs, a QBank, test series, and the innovative Dr. Wise
Chatbot.

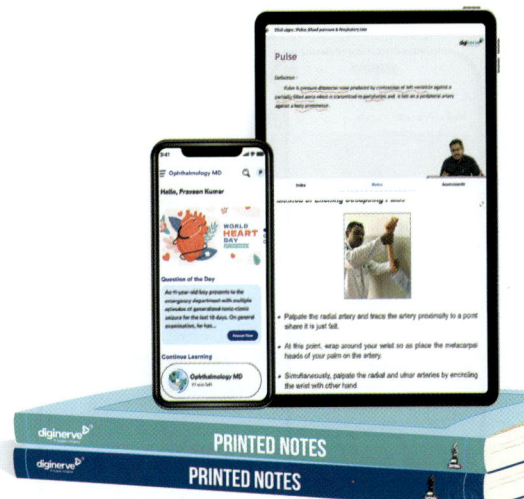

Course Features

1400+ hrs Video Lectures

1500+ Topics in Notes

15000+ Questions in QBank

1800+ GEMS

450+ OSCEs

Test Series

Dr. Wise AI Chatbot

Drug Chart

Regular Webinars by Esteemed Faculty

Access Anytime, Anywhere

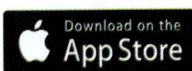
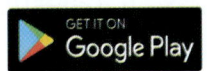

📞 +91-8800-418-418   ✉ marketing@diginerve.com

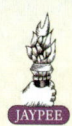 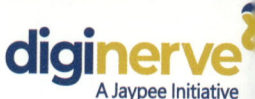

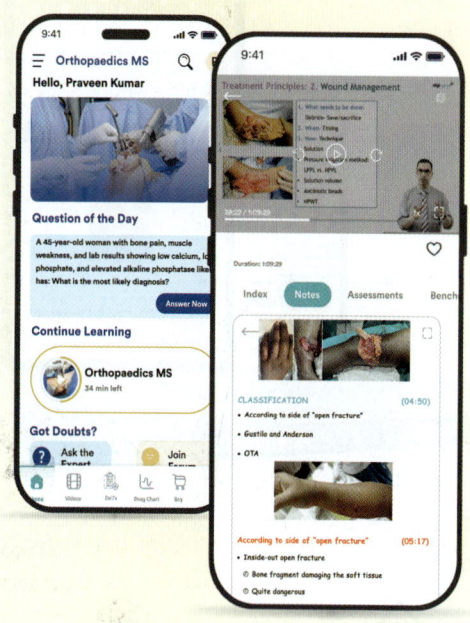

Premium Medical Content Anytime, Anywhere

Trusted by 150K+ Users

20+ Courses **3600+** Hrs of Video Content **790** Mentors

A host of features for UnderGrads, PostGrads and Professionals

Available on

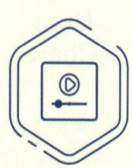 Video Lectures
 Notes
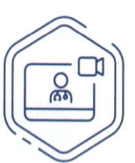 OSCEs

 Drug Chart
 Question Bank
 Dr. Wise AI Chatbot

+91-8800-418-418   marketing@diginerve.com

Examination of the Neck (Excluding the Thyroid Gland)

CHAPTER 26

HISTORY

The most common cause of swelling in the neck is enlarged lymph nodes.

a. **Age** is useful so far as conditions in the neck are concerned. Sternomastoid 'tumor' occurs in the newborn baby and there is often a history of difficult labor. Both branchial cyst and branchial fistula **(Fig. 26.1)**, though congenital, are more often seen in early adult life. Cystic hygroma is met with in infancy or in early childhood. Inflammatory swellings may occur at any age but commonly seen in early adults. Carcinomatous swelling is more common in the old.

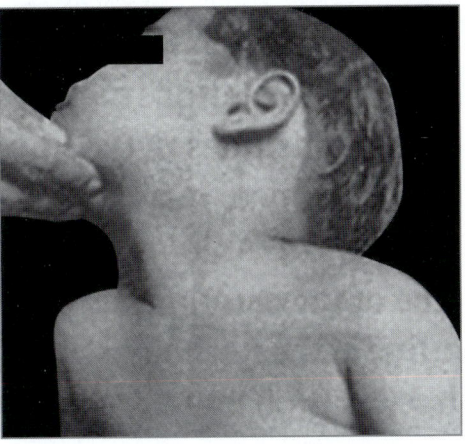

Fig. 26.1: Branchial fistula is shown. Note the typical site.

b. **Swelling:** Swelling is a very common symptom of the lesions of the neck. A careful history to know the *mode of onset* and *duration* is very essential. Swellings with long history are generally benign. Tuberculous lymphadenopathy and cold abscess also give history of more than a month. Quickly-grown swellings within a short span of time are mostly malignant tumors. But swelling due to acute lymphadenitis is also of short duration.

c. **Pain:** It is always an important symptom and question must be asked 'whether the swelling is *painful or not?*' Inflammatory swellings are always painful. This distinguishes acute lymphadenitis from a malignant growth as the former is extremely painful whereas the latter is painless unless in late stages when there may be nerve involvement. A swelling in the submandibular triangle particularly seen during meals with pain is due to calculous obstruction of the duct of the submandibular salivary gland.

History in examination of neck

Aspect	Clinical significance	Patient-friendly questions
Onset of swelling	Acute → Infection, abscess; Chronic → Tumor, cyst	"How long have you noticed the swelling?"
Pain	Painful → Lymphadenitis, abscess; Painless → Tumor, cyst	"Does the swelling hurt?"
Swallowing and tongue protrusion	Moves with swallowing → Thyroglossal cyst	"Does the swelling move when you swallow?"

LOCAL EXAMINATION

A. INSPECTION

For proper inspection of the neck, it has to be exposed up to the level of the nipples. The students often forget of the supraclavicular fossa. Enlargement of the left supraclavicular lymph nodes is an important sign so far as the cancer of breast and cancer of many abdominal organs are concerned.

1. **Swelling:** As in other places, whenever there is a swelling, note its *number, situation, size, shape, surface*, etc. Multiple swellings indicate the diagnosis of enlarged lymph nodes. The SITUATION is very important as it often indicates the diagnosis by itself. The **branchial cyst*** is situated in the upper part of the neck with its posterior half lying under cover of the upper 3rd of the sternomastoid muscle **(Fig. 26.2)**. In the submandibular triangle, besides lymph nodes, there may be enlarged **submandibular salivary gland and deep or plunging ranula (Fig. 26.3)**. A **dermoid cyst** occurs in the midline of the neck, either in the most upper part giving rise to double chin or in the most lower part in the space of Burns. **Cystic hygroma (Fig. 26.4)** is commonly seen in the posterior triangle of the neck in its lower part. Sometimes in the lower part of the posterior triangle one may look for the prominence of a **cervical rib**. An *aneurysm* is likely to be seen in the line of the carotid artery. An oval swelling along the line of the sternomastoid muscle in a newly-born baby is probably a **sternomastoid 'tumor'**. A **carotid body tumor** lies under the anterior margin of the sternomastoid at the level of bifurcation of the common carotid artery, i.e., at the level of the upper border of the thyroid cartilage. At last the *swellings that occur over the known sites of the lymph nodes should be considered to have arisen from them* unless some outstanding clinical findings prove their origin to be otherwise. Different regions of swelling in neck is shown in **Figure 26.5**.

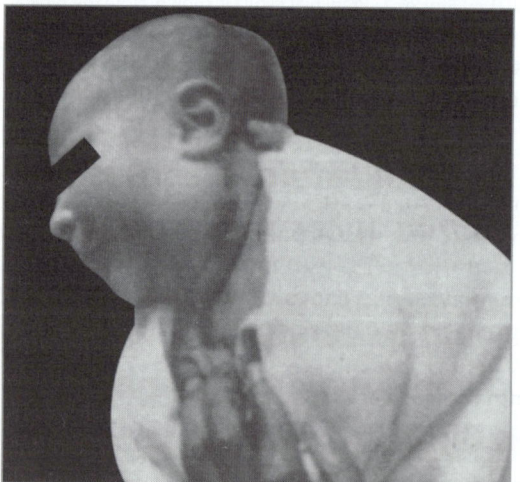

Fig. 26.2: Branchial cyst in its typical position.

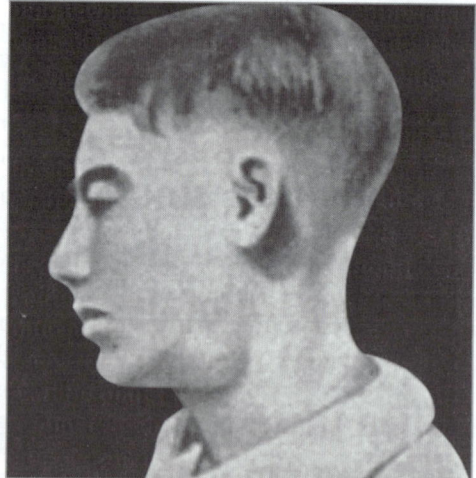

Fig. 26.3: Deep or plunging ranula in the submandibular triangle.

---

* Branchial cyst develops from the buried ectodermal pouch formed under the 2nd branchial arch which overlaps the 3rd and the 4th and fuses with the 5th. A branchial fistula is formed if this pouch communicates with the exterior due to failure of fusion. So, structures developed from the 2nd branchial arch lie superficial to this fistula whereas structures developed from the 3rd and 4th branchial arches lie deep to this fistula.

The patient is asked to swallow and note whether the swelling moves on deglutition or not. The swellings which are adherent to the larynx and trachea move upwards on swallowing, e.g., thyroid swelling, thyroglossal cyst and subhyoid bursitis. Tuberculous and malignant lymph nodes when they become fixed to the larynx or trachea will also move on deglutition.

2. **Skin:** A sinus, fistula, ulcer or scar should be noted during inspection of the skin of the neck. *Tuberculous sinus or ulcer* arising from bursting of caseous lymph nodes is not uncommon in the neck. Undermining edge is typical of this ulcer. Puckering scar may also be found on the skin after healing of these ulcers or sinuses. *Sinus due to osteomyelitis of the mandible* is usually single and lies a little below the jaw, whereas multiple sinuses over an indurated mass at the upper part of the neck would suggest *actinomycosis*. Sulfur granules in the pus is very much confirmatory of actinomycosis. A *branchial fistula* is seen just in front of the lower 3rd of the anterior border of the sternomastoid muscle. *Gummatous* ulcer rarely occurs in the sternomastoid muscle. For *thyroglossal fistula* see the next chapter.

When there is a swelling, the condition of the skin over the swelling should be carefully noted. Redness and edema are features of inflammation. Presence of subcutaneous dilated veins indicate lymphosarcoma. Skin may be infiltrated by the *malignant growth* **(Fig. 26.6)** and the skin is stuck down to the growth causing a fold of skin to stand out above it. This is a characteristic feature of secondary carcinoma of lymph nodes.

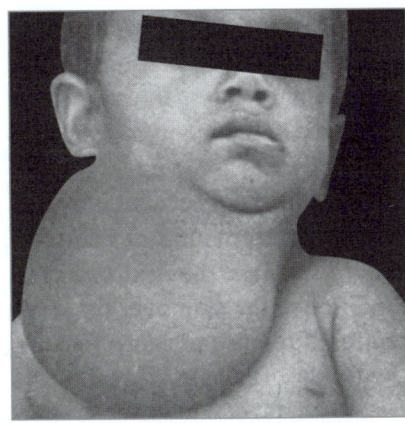

Fig. 26.4: Cystic hygroma.

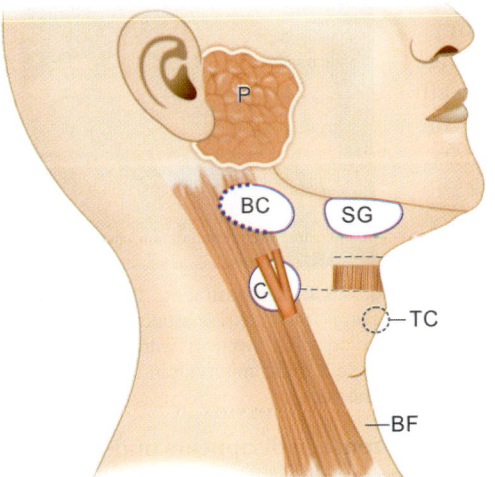

Fig. 26.5: Showing the situation of different swellings of the neck. (P: parotid gland; SG: submandibular salivary gland; BC: branchial cyst, posterior part is covered by the sternomastoid muscle; C: carotid body tumor situated behind the bifurcation of the common carotid artery; TC: thyroglossal cyst; BF: indicates the position of branchial fistula)

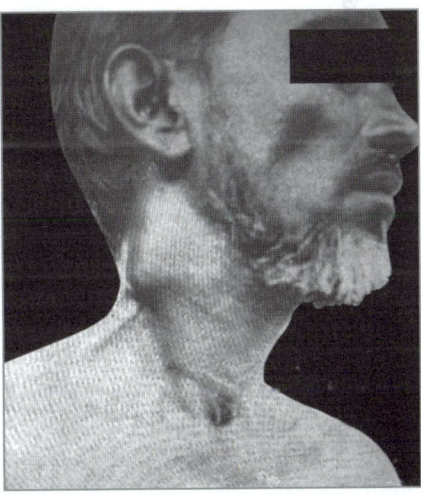

Fig. 26.6: Secondary carcinoma of the lymph nodes. Observe the fold of skin below the swelling. This is due to infiltration of the skin and platysma by the carcinomatous growth.

One should also inspect for presence of visible and dilated cutaneous veins. These are sometimes present around malignant tumors especially the lymphosarcoma.

3. The *face* and *upper part of chest* are also noticed to see if there is any venous engorgement due to pressure of cervical lymphadenopathy over the jugular vein. There may be torticollis in case of acute cervical lymphadenitis or tuberculous lymphadenitis or in case of sternomastoid tumor. Enlarged lymph nodes may also press on the nearby nerves to cause wasting of the muscles.

B. PALPATION

The swellings of the neck are best palpated from behind. The patient sits on a stool and the examiner stands behind the patient. Natural tendency of the patient is to extend his neck while the clinician starts palpating the neck. This obscures the swelling. So, the patient's neck is passively flexed with one hand on his head and the other hand is used for palpating the swelling **(Fig. 26.7)**. The head is also flexed passively towards the side of the swelling for proper palpation. This is to relax the muscles and fasciae of the neck.

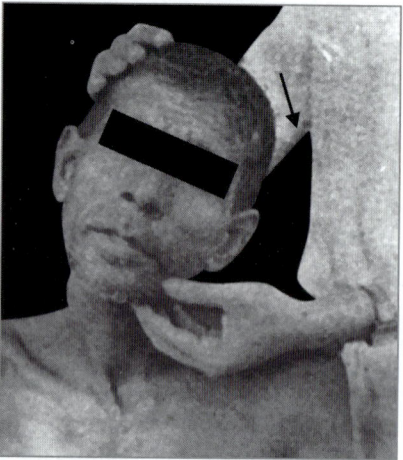

Fig. 26.7: Method of palpating a swelling in the submandibular triangle. Note that the head is passively flexed towards the side of the swelling to relax the muscles and fasciae of the neck.

1. **Swelling:** Examine the swelling systematically noting its situation, size, shape, surface, margin, consistency, reducibility, impulse on coughing, translucency, mobility, pulsation (expansile or transmitted), etc., as discussed in Chapter 3. Mobility should be tested in all directions. A carotid body tumor or an aneurysm can be moved across but not along the line of the carotid artery.

Determine the *relation of the swelling with the sternomastoid muscle* **(Fig. 26.8)**. To test one side place your hand on the side of the patient's chin *opposite* to the side of the lesion and tell him to nod the head to that side against the resistance of your hand. To test both sides simultaneously, put your hand under the point of the chin and ask him to press down against resistance when both sternomastoids are put into action. If the swelling lies deep to the muscle which is a common occurrence, it disappears under the taut muscle either completely or partially depending on the size of the swelling; the mobility of the swelling becomes very much restricted at the same time. If the swelling is situated superficial to the muscle, it will be more prominent and movable over the contracted muscle.

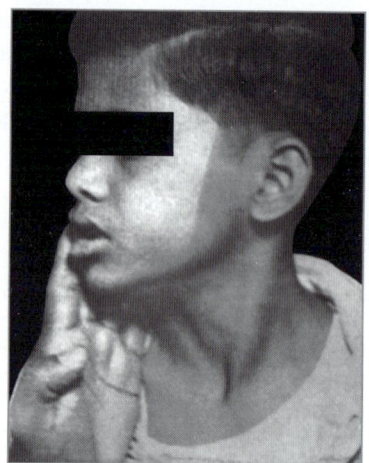

Fig. 26.8: Demonstrating the method of making the sternomastoid muscle taut. Relation of a swelling with sternomastoid muscle is quite important in the examination of the neck.

Whether the swelling has *involved the neighboring structures* such as the larynx, trachea, esophagus, blood vessels, nerves, etc., should also be determined. A malignant growth lying just below the angle of the jaw may involve the hypoglossal nerve and lead to paralysis of the same half of the tongue. The patient is asked to put his tongue out. In case of paralysis, the tongue

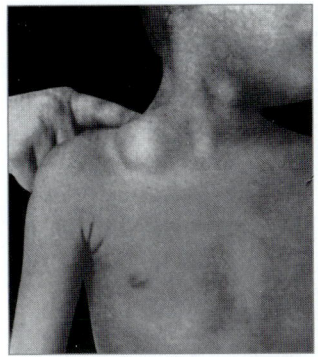
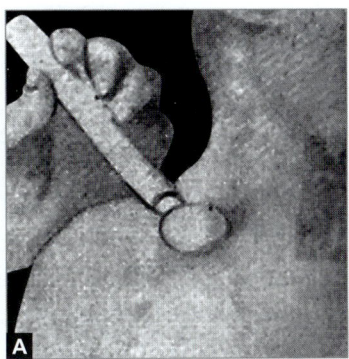
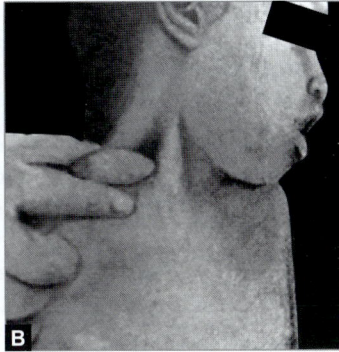

Fig. 26.9: A cystic hygroma in the posterior triangle of the neck.

Figs. 26.10A and B: Testing for an impulse on coughing and translucency in a case of cystic hygroma shown in Figure 26.8.

will deviate towards the side of lesion. *Involvement of the skin* with the growth should also be examined. This is done by pinching the overlying skin off the tumor or by gliding the overlying skin over the tumor. Skin is often involved in case of malignant lymphatic growths and in case of certain benign conditions, e.g., acute lymphadenitis or tuberculous lymphadenitis with cold abscess just on the verge of bursting to the exterior.

One should carefully note whether the swelling is *pulsatile* or not. In case of pulsatile swellings one should differentiate between transmitted pulsation and expansile pulsation. In case of aneurysm of the carotid artery there will be expansile pulsation, whereas a tumor in front of the carotid artery will give rise to transmitted pulsation, e.g., carotid body tumor or malignant lymph node enlargement around the carotid artery. Cystic hygroma **(Figs. 26.9 and 26.10)** is a brilliantly translucent swelling, whereas branchial cyst or cold abscess are not translucent, so *transillumination test* is also important in case of a swelling of the neck. Any cystic swelling of the neck will elicit *fluctuation test* positive, e.g., cystic hygroma, branchial cyst, thyroglossal cyst, dermoid cyst, subhyoid bursal cyst, cold abscess and pharyngeal pouch.

2. **Lymph nodes:** In case of palpation of the cervical lymph nodes one should follow the same technique as used for palpation of swelling in the neck **(Fig. 26.11)**. A system should be maintained to palpate all the groups of lymph nodes in the neck. It may be started from below with supraclavicular group, then moving upwards palpating the lymph nodes in the posterior triangle, jugulo omohyoid group, jugulodigastric, submandibular, submental, preauricular and occipital groups. (a) In case of enlargement of lymph node one should examine the *drainage area* for inflammatory or neoplastic focus. (b) *Other groups of lymph nodes* lying in other parts of the body should also be examined in case of enlargement of cervical lymph nodes. These groups include the axillary, the inguinal and abdominal groups. The causes of generalized

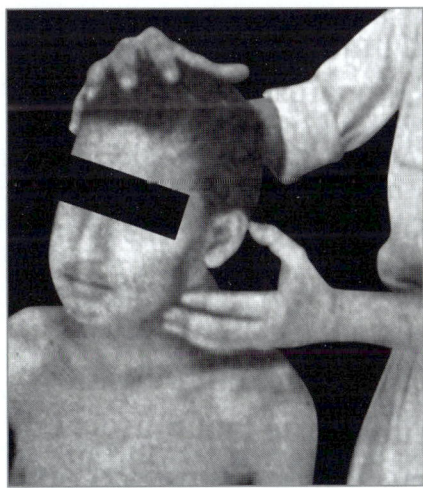

Fig. 26.11: Shows the method of palpation for enlargement of lymph nodes by the side of internal jugular vein. Note that the head is passively flexed towards the side of examination to relax the muscles and fasciae of the neck.

enlargement of lymph nodes are discussed in chapter 8. (c) The *spleen* and the *liver* should be examined in case of Hodgkin's disease and (d) the *lungs* for tuberculosis.

Examination of the drainage area: If the *submental group* is involved examine the chin, central part of the lip, gingiva, floor of the mouth and tip of the tongue. If the *submandibular group* is affected, one should examine the palate, the tongue, floor of the mouth, the lower lip, cheek, gingiva, nose and antrum. Involvement of the *jugular chain* should draw one's attention to the tongue, mouth, pharynx, larynx, upper esophagus and thyroid. The *tonsillar node* which lies below the angle of the mandible at the junction of the facial vein and the internal jugular vein may be enlarged in case of inflammatory or neoplastic lesion of the tonsil

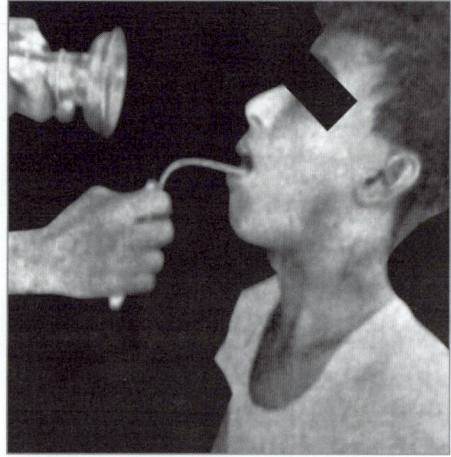

Fig. 26.12: Examining the inside of the mouth as well as the tonsils in case of enlarged lymph nodes at the angle of mandible.

(Fig. 26.12). If the *supraclavicular (Virchow's) nodes* are enlarged (Troisier's sign), one should examine not only the arm, breast and chest (bronchus) but also the abdomen right down to the testis.

Percussion: This is not very important examination, yet a rare disease—laryngocele may be revealed by the tympanic note which is connected with the larynx through a narrow neck. The swelling becomes more apparent when the patient blows his nose.

Auscultation: A bruit may be heard over an aneurysm or carotid body tumor.

Movements: A patient with cold abscess of the posterior triangle of the neck may not be able to move his neck due to tuberculous affection of the cervical vertebrae. All movements of the neck will be restricted. Care must be taken to minimize forceful movements of the neck as sudden death is on record following examination of movements of the neck in this condition from dislocation of the atlantoaxial joint (the dens pressing on the medulla).

Special investigations will be carried out along the lines discussed in Chapter 3 and 8. The fluid *aspirated* from a branchial cyst often contains cholesterol crystals. X-ray is helpful in the diagnosis of the caries of the cervical spine and cervical rib. A radio-opaque fluid (uropac) may be injected into a branchial fistula to determine its extent. A complete fistula will extend up to the supratonsillar fossa. Barium swallow (a little amount) or urografin pushed through a Ryle's tube will diagnose pharyngeal pouch in skiagraphy. In case of secondary malignant lymph nodes: (a) **Laryngoscopy** if laryngeal carcinoma is suspected, (b) **bronchoscopy**, if bronchial carcinoma is suspected, (c) **X-ray chest** and **mediastinoscopy** if mediastinal growth or lung cancer is suspected, (d) **Esophagoscopy** and **barium swallow** in esophageal cancer and (e) **mammography** in case of breast cancer may be performed to come to a definite diagnosis. Above all excision biopsy of the affected lymph nodes is of immense value.

DIFFERENTIAL DIAGNOSIS OF SWELLINGS OF THE NECK

For differential diagnosis, swellings of the neck can be divided into: (a) midline swellings and (b) lateral swellings according to their site of origin.

Midline swellings of the neck from above downwards are: Ludwig's angina, enlarged submental lymph nodes, sublingual dermoid and lipoma in the submental region; thyroglossal cyst and subhyoid bursitis; goiter of the thyroid isthmus and pyramidal lobe, enlarged lymph nodes and lipoma in the suprasternal space of Burns, retrosternal goiter and thymic swelling. A dermoid cyst may occur anywhere in the midline.

Lateral swellings according to their sites may be divided into the following regions: (i) *SUBMANDIBULAR TRIANGLE*: Besides the lymph nodes and enlarged submandibular salivary gland, there may be deep or plunging ranula and extension of growth from the jaw. (ii) In the *CAROTID TRIANGLE* aneurysm of the carotid artery, carotid body tumor, branchial cyst and branchiogenic carcinoma may be met with. Thyroid swellings will be deep to the sternomastoid, a sternomastoid tumor may develop in a newborn baby. (iii) In the *POSTERIOR TRIANGLE*— besides enlarged supraclavicular lymph nodes, there may be cystic hygroma, pharyngeal pouch, subclavian aneurysm, aberrant thyroid, cervical rib, lipoma (Dercum's disease), etc.

For clinical diagnosis the swellings of the neck may also be divided into acute and chronic swellings. **Acute swellings** are cellulitis including Ludwig's angina, boil, carbuncle and acute lymphadenitis. **Chronic swellings** may be further subdivided into: (a) *Cystic*—branchial cyst, thyroglossal cyst, dermoid cyst, cystic hygroma, sebaceous cyst, cystic adenoma of the thyroid gland, cold abscess etc., (b) *Solid* swellings are swellings arising from thyroid, branchiogenic carcinoma, sternomastoid tumor, etc. (c) *Pulsatile* swellings are aneurysm of the carotid or subclavian artery, carotid body tumor, lymph node swellings lying in close proximity to the carotid artery to elicit transmitted pulsation and a few primary toxic goiter.

Brief descriptions of the important swellings of the neck are described below:

LYMPH NODE SWELLINGS

No doubt lymph node swellings occupy the most important position so far as the swellings of the neck are concerned. Of the lymph node swellings, tuberculous lymph nodes, carcinomatous lymph nodes (secondary) and various types of lymphoma comprise major components in this group.

Tuberculous lymph nodes: In Indian subcontinent, this is probably the most common cause of lymph node swelling in the cervical region **(Fig. 26.13)**. The pathology passes through various stages and has been discussed in detail in Chapter 8. The first stage is solid enlargement which goes by the name of lymphadenitis. Subsequently periadenitis develops and the glands become matted. Later on the whole matted mass liquifies and "cold abscess" develops deep to the deep cervical fascia. Fluctuation can be elicited with difficulty at this stage due to the presence of tough fascia superficial to the abscess. In a very late stage the deep cervical fascia gives way forming a "collar stud" abscess. At this stage fluctuation can be elicited more easily. In the last stage, the skin over the swelling becomes inflamed and the abscess finds its way out through a sinus which refuses to heal.

Carcinomatous lymph nodes (secondary): Usually, the patients are elderly above 50 years of age. The only exception is papillary carcinoma of the thyroid, which

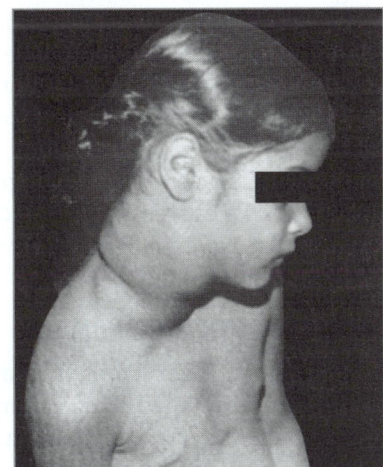

Fig. 26.13: A typical case of cervical lymph node enlargement due to tuberculosis.

occurs and metastasizes at young age. Men are usually more often affected than women. The swelling is always painless and grows relatively fast. New lumps may appear by the side. On examination there is no rise of temperature and the swelling is not tender. The surface is usually nodular and the consistency is hard (often stony hard). The swelling may be fixed to the skin and to the deeper structures at later stage, so the swellings become immobile at this stage. Majority of these swellings lie deep to the anterior edge of the sternomastoid muscle. Rarely such swelling may be pulsatile when it lies just in front of the carotid artery. The students must remember that the greater cornu of the hyoid bone may be mistaken for carcinomatous lymph nodes. The patient may be asked to swallow, in which case the bone will move up but not the lymph nodes. Whenever a secondary carcinomatous lymph node is detected, a careful search should be made for the primary focus in the mouth, tongue, nasopharynx, larynx, thyroid, external auditory meatus, lungs and in case of left supraclavicular lymph nodes, the abdomen and testis.

Lymphoma: In this group the common members are Hodgkin's disease, lymphosarcoma and reticulosarcoma. Detail description of these tumors are laid down in Chapter 8.

CELLULITIS

Cellulitis in the neck is the most serious form of its kind. The inflammatory exudates are held tightly under tension by the unyielding deep cervical fascia. So, the diagnosis becomes late. The neck becomes stiff and very painful with swelling in the submental region. This inflammatory exudate tends to track down towards the mediastinum. *Ludwig's angina* is the most serious form of cellulitis which affects the floor of the mouth and submental region. It produces a diffuse swelling beneath the jaw with redness and edema at that region. Besides fatal septicemia, edema glottis is the most dangerous and final complication of this condition.

BRANCHIAL CYST

Though congenital, it does not appear before adolescence and early adult life. The most common way of presentation is the (painless) cystic swelling of the upper part of the neck half in front and half deep to the sternomastoid muscle. The cyst is usually ovoid in shape with its long axis running forwards and downwards. Majority of branchial cysts are between 5 and 10 cm wide. Its surface is smooth and the margin is distinct. The consistency depends on the tension of fluid inside the cyst. When lax it feels soft and when tense it is hard. Fluctuation test is positive. Transillumination test is usually negative. The content of the cyst is thick and white and contains desquamated epithelial cells. The fluid may be golden yellow-containing fat globules and cholesterol crystals. This cyst cannot be compressed or reduced. The local deep cervical lymph nodes are usually not enlarged. If these are palpable you should reconsider the diagnosis in favor of cold abscess or so. The cyst may become inflamed and confuses the clinician to be misdiagnosed as an inflammatory swelling. The diagnosis is confirmed by finding cholesterol crystals in the aspirate.

BRANCHIOGENIC CARCINOMA

This condition is very rare and diagnosis is made mainly by exclusion. Whenever a swelling in the neck is deemed to be carcinomatous, possibility of secondary carcinomatous lymph nodes should be considered and a thorough search should be made for the primary focus. If the primary source is not available, one may think in the line of branchiogenic carcinoma. It is a tumor arising from the remnants of branchial cleft.

CYSTIC HYGROMA

It is a type of congenital lymphangioma and the common victims are infants and children. The swelling is soft cystic and brilliantly translucent as it contains clear fluid. As it is a multilocular swelling fluid of one locule can be *compressed* into the other. It generally positions itself at the root of the neck and may extend its pseudopods deep into the muscles or down to the mediastinum and pectoral region. Mediastinal extension may be suspected if it shows impulse on coughing. The swelling is a multilocular one but occasionally it may be unilocular where the term 'hydrocele of the neck' is used. It may be inflamed as a result of nasopharyngeal infection to cause some confusion to the diagnosis. There is no lymph node enlargement unless infected. Occasionally, it may occur in other places like axilla, mediastinum and very rarely in the groin.

BRANCHIAL FISTULA

It is diagnosed by the typical site of the external orifice of this fistula which is situated in the lower 3rd of the neck near the anterior border of the sternomastoid. Occasionally, it may be bilateral. This fistula represents a persistent 2nd branchial cleft. This fistula is a congenital one and must not be confused with an acquired sinus which may result from incision of an inflamed branchial cyst. In this case the sinus will be situated in the upper 3rd of the neck. This fistula often becomes the seat of recurrent attacks of inflammation. The fistula often discharges mucus, the amount of which varies. This fistula is frequently a sinus that is an incomplete one. When complete the internal orifice of the fistula is situated on the anterior aspect of the posterior pillar of the fauces.

PHARYNGEAL POUCH

It is a pulsion diverticulum of the pharynx through the gap between the lower horizontal fibers and upper oblique fibers of the inferior constrictor muscle. The victims of this condition are usually, but not necessarily, the middle-aged or old men. The main complaint is regurgitation of undigested food long time after meal. It may be during turning from one side to the other at night, when the patient wakes up by a bout of coughing or during swallowing of the next meal. At this stage abscess of the lung may result from aspiration from the pouch. In the last stage gurgling noise in the neck may be heard when the patient swallows. The pouch may form a visible swelling in the posterior triangle of the neck particularly when the patient drinks. Increasing dysphagia is probably the last symptom which compels the patient to visit a surgeon. Radiology with a very thin emulsion of barium particularly in semilateral view is diagnostic.

LARYNGOCELE

This is an air-containing diverticulum from herniation of the mucous membrane through the thyrohyoid membrane at the point where it is pierced by the superior laryngeal vessels. It is a resonant swelling and appears prominently when the patient blows his noses. It is probably commoner in trumpet-blowers, glass-blowers and those with chronic cough.

STERNOMASTOID 'TUMOR'

It is a swelling in the middle third of the sternomastoid muscle which results from birth injury. It is seen in newborn babies. It is a circumscribed firm mass within the muscle. This swelling usually subsides spontaneously but the abnormal segment of muscle becomes fibrotic and contracted which may, later on, lead to torticollis. The tumor is fusiform with its long axis along the line of sternomastoid muscle. Its surface is smooth. Its anterior and posterior margins are distinct whereas upper and lower margins are indistinct and continuous with normal muscle. At first the lump is firm, gradually becomes hard and then begins to shrink.

CAROTID BODY TUMOR

This tumor is located at the bifurcation of the common carotid artery. It forms a slowly growing painless hard ovoid lobulated swelling, which is movable laterally but not vertically. Transmitted pulsation is often seen. A few patients complain of attacks of faintness on pressure over the lump—carotid body syncope. It is a very slowly growing tumor and remains localized for years. Regional metastasis occurs in 1/5th of the cases and distant metastasis is almost unknown.

Cervical rib: See page 105.

TORTICOLLIS

Torticollis or wryneck is a deformity in which the head is bent to one side whilst the chin points to the other side **(Figs. 26.14A and B)**. In long-standing cases, there may be atrophy of the face on the affected side. The measurement from the outer canthus of the eye to the angle of the mouth is smaller, the eyebrow is less arched, the nose is somewhat flattened and the cheek is less full than on the sound side. These phenomena are probably due to imperfect vascular supply resulting from the restricted mobility. The

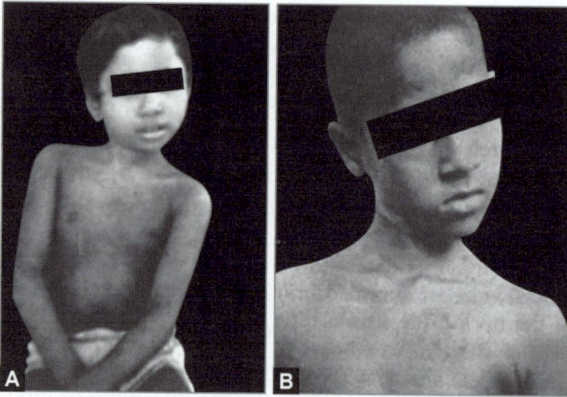

Figs. 26.14A and B: Cases of torticollis..

different varieties of wryneck are: (a) *Congenital*: The diagnosis is made by a history of difficult labor, followed by the appearance of a sternomastoid 'tumor'. The affected muscle feels firm and rigid. (b) *Traumatic*—fracture dislocation of the cervical spine. (c) *Rheumatic*—sudden appearance of wryneck after an exposure to cold or draught is suggestive. (d) *Inflammatory*—e.g., from inflamed cervical lymph nodes. (e) *Spasmodic*—when the sternomastoid of the affected side and the posterior cervical muscles of the opposite side are found in a state of spasm. (f) *Compensatory*—e.g., from scoliosis, defect in sight (ocular torticollis). (g) *From Pott's disease* of the cervical spine. (h) *From contracture*—e.g., after burns, ulcers, etc.

Chapter 26: Examination of the Neck (Excluding the Thyroid Gland) 437

Algorithmic Approach to Patient with Neck Swelling

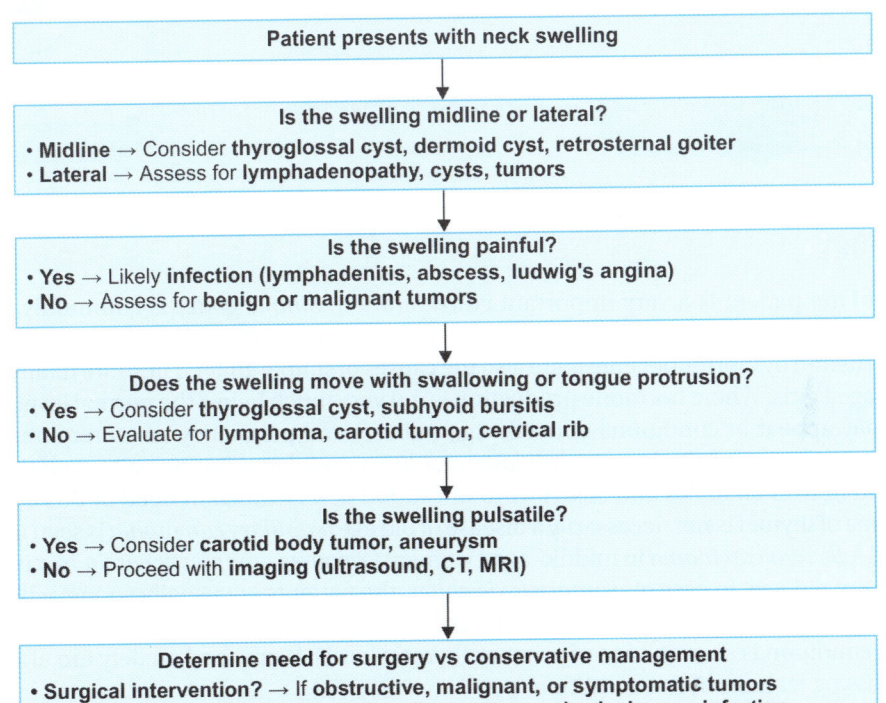

Examination of the Thyroid Gland

CHAPTER 27

HISTORY

1. **Age** of the patient is a very important consideration. *Simple goiter* is commonly seen in girls approaching puberty. In endemic areas deficient iodide is the cause of the simple goiter. Goitrogens and dyshormonogenesis are also the causes of simple goiter. These are mainly found in teen-aged girls. Where hormone production is not very much below the normal level, simple goiter may appear in conditions of need, e.g., puberty and pregnancy when requirement of hormone is augmented. Both *multinodular* and *solitary nodular goiters* as well as *colloid goiters* are found in women of 20s and 30s. A word of caution is very much in need in this context—carcinoma of thyroid is not necessarily a disease of old age. *Papillary carcinoma* is seen in young girls and *follicular carcinoma* in middle-aged women. Of course, *anaplastic carcinoma* is mainly a disease of old age. In case of *primary toxic goiter*, the patients are usually young, whereas in *Hashimoto's disease* the victims are usually middle-aged women. Patients with unbalanced psychic condition is seen in case of primary thyrotoxicosis. Worry and anxiety are always the embarrassing features of this condition.

2. **Sex:** Majority of thyroid disorders are seen in females. All types of simple goiters are far more common in the female than in the male. Thyrotoxicosis is eight times commoner in females than in males. Even thyroid carcinomas are more often seen in females in the ratio of 3:1.

3. **Occupation:** Though occupation has hardly any relation with thyroid disorders, yet thyrotoxicosis may appear in individuals working under stress and strain. The patients with primary toxic goiter may be psychic.

4. **Residence:** Except endemic goiter due to iodine deficiency, no other thyroid disorder has any peculiar geographical distribution. Certain areas are particularly known to have low iodine content in the water and food. Residents of these areas often suffer from iodine deficiency endemic simple goiter. These areas are near rocky mountains, e.g., Himalayas, the Vindyas, the Satpuda ranges which form the goiter belts in India. Such goiter is also probably more common in Southern India than in Northern India. In Great Britain such areas are in the Mendips, Derbyshire, Yorkshire, etc. Endemic goiter is also found in low land areas where the soil lacks iodides or the water supply comes from far away mountain ranges, e.g., Great Lakes of North America. In the mountains of Bulgaria arises the river Struma, which flows into the Aegean Sea. Along its banks and those of its tributaries endemic goiter has been prevalent. Calcium is also goitrogenic and areas producing chalk or lime stone are also goitrogenic areas, e.g., Southern Ireland and Derbyshire.

5. **Swelling:** In case of thyroid swellings history about the *onset, duration, rate of growth* and whether *associated with pain* should be noted. In case of any thyroid swelling it should be asked 'how does the patient sleep at night?' 'Does she spend sleepless nights?' In primary thyrotoxicosis patients often complain of sleepless nights. Whether the patient is very worried,

stressed or strained. These are also features of thyrotoxicosis. Palpitation and ectopic beats and even congestive cardiac failure (CCF) may be noticed in cases of secondary thyrotoxicosis. These symptoms may develop in already existing thyroid swelling cases for years. In secondary thyrotoxicosis the brunt of the attack falls more on the cardiovascular system, whereas in primary thyrotoxicosis the brunt of attack falls more on the nervous system. Sudden increase in size with pain in a goiter indicates hemorrhage inside it. A thyroglossal cyst may be present since birth. The rate of growth of the swelling is quite important. While simple goiter grows very slowly or may remain of same size for quite sometime, multinodular goiter or solitary nodular goiter or colloid goiter increases in size though extremely slowly for year. These goiters may also increase in size little faster than before. A special feature of papillary and follicular carcinoma of the thyroid is their slow growth. They may exist as a lump in the neck for many year before metastasizing. Anaplastic carcinoma however is a fast-growing swelling.

6. **Pain:** The goiter is usually a painless condition. Inflammatory conditions of thyroid gland are painful. Malignant diseases of the thyroid gland are painless to start with, but become painful in late stages. In Hashimoto's disease there is discomfort in the neck. Anaplastic carcinoma is more known to infiltrate the surrounding structures and the nerves to cause pain.

7. **Pressure effects:** Enlarged thyroid may press on the trachea to cause *dyspnea* or may press on the esophagus to cause *dysphagia* or press on the recurrent laryngeal nerve to cause *hoarseness of the voice*. It must be remembered that thyroid swellings can rarely obstruct the esophagus as it is a muscular tube and can be easily stretched or pushed aside. As in the first stage of deglutition the thyroid gland moves up, so an enlarged thyroid gland makes swallowing uncomfortable but usually this is not true dysphagia. An enlarged thyroid may compress on the trachea or deviate it to one side or the other to cause difficulty in breathing. This symptom is often worse when the neck is flexed forwards or laterally. When air rushes through a narrowed trachea, a whistling sound is produced which is called *stridor*. Hoarseness is usually due to paralysis of one recurrent laryngeal nerve and anaplastic carcinoma infiltrating the nerve is often the cause.

8. **Symptoms of primary thyrotoxicosis:** It is quite important to know the symptoms of primary thyrotoxicosis as often in these cases there is not much enlargement of the thyroid gland and only these symptoms will indicate the presence of this disease. The most significant symptom is *loss of weight* inspite of good appetite. *Preference for cold* and intolerance to heat and *excessive sweating* are the next symptoms. Nervous excitability, irritability, insomnia, tremor of hands and weakness of muscles are the symptoms of involvement of nervous system which are the main features of primary thyrotoxicosis. Cardiovascular symptoms are not so pronounce as seen in secondary thyrotoxicosis, but even then palpitation, tachycardia (rise in sleeping pulse) and dyspnea on exertion are symptoms of this disease. Exophthalmos is often associated with this condition. The patient may complain of *staring* or *protruding eyes* and difficulty in closing her eye lids. Double vision or diplopia may be caused by muscles weakness (ophthalmoplegia). Edema or swelling of the conjunctiva (chemosis) is seen in very late cases of exophthalmos alongwith persistent primary thyrotoxicosis. Ultimately the patient may get pain in the eye if the cornea ulcerates. Some women may have a change in menstruation, usually amenorrhea.

9. **Symptoms of secondary thyrotoxicosis:** When a longstanding solitary nodular goiter or multinodular goiter or colloid goiter shows manifestations of thyrotoxicosis the condition is called *secondary thyrotoxicosis*. As mentioned above the brunt of the attack falls more on the cardiovascular system than on the nervous system. Palpitations, ectopic beats, cardiac arrhythmias, dyspnea on exertion and chest pain are the usual symptoms. Even congestive cardiac failure may appear at late stage with swelling of ankles. Nervous symptoms and eye symptoms may be mild or absent.

10. **Symptoms of myxedema (hypothyroidism):** Increase of weight is often complained of inspite of poor appetite. Fat accumulates particularly at the back of the neck and shoulders. Intolerance of cold weather and preference for warm climate is noticed. There is minimal swelling of thyroid. The skin may be dry. There may be puffiness of the face with pouting lips and dull expression. Loss of hair is a characteristic feature and 2/3rds of the eyebrows may fall off. Muscle fatigue and lethargy are important symptoms with failing memory and mild hoarseness due to edema of vocal cords. Constipation and oligomenorrhea are sometimes complained of.

11. **Past history:** Enquiry must be made about the course of treatment the patient had and its effect on the swelling. In case of thyroglossal fistula there may be a previous history of an abscess (an inflamed thyroglossal cyst) which was incised or burst spontaneously. The patient should also be asked if she was taking any drugs, e.g., PAS or sulfonylurea or any antithyroid drugs as these are goitrogenic.

12. **Personal history:** Dietary habit is important as vegetables of the brassica family (cabbage, kale and rape) are goitrogens. Persons who are in the habit of taking a kind of sea fish which has particularly low iodine content, may present with goiter.

13. **Family history:** It is often seen that goiters occur in more than one member in a family while endemic goiters may affect more members in the same family. Similarly enzyme deficiency within the thyroid gland which are concerned in the synthesis of thyroid hormones are also seen to run in families. Primary thyrotoxicosis has been seen in more than one member of the same family. Thyroid cancers are seen to involve more than one member of the same family.

History in patients with thyroid disorders

Aspect	Clinical significance	Patient-friendly questions
Onset and duration	Acute → Thyroiditis, hemorrhage; Chronic → Goiter, malignancy	"When did you first notice the swelling?"
Progression	Slow-growing → Benign (multinodular goiter, colloid goiter); Rapid growth → Malignancy, hemorrhage	"Has the swelling grown rapidly over weeks or months?"
Pain	Painful → Thyroiditis, hemorrhagic cyst; Painless → Benign/malignant tumor, goiter	"Do you feel any pain in your neck?"
Change in size during infection/stress	Increase with infection → subacute thyroiditis	"Has the swelling worsened during illness?"
Symptoms of hyperthyroidism	Increased metabolic activity due to excessive thyroid hormone	"Do you feel overly energetic, hot, or have frequent bowel movements?"
Symptoms of hypothyroidism	Reduced metabolic activity due to low thyroid hormone	"Do you feel sluggish, cold, or constipated?"
Presence of hoarseness or voice changes	Indicates recurrent laryngeal nerve involvement (thyroid malignancy, goiter compression)	"Have you noticed any recent changes in your voice?"

Contd...

Contd...

Aspect	Clinical significance	Patient-friendly questions
Dysphagia or difficulty breathing	Compression of esophagus or trachea (retrosternal goiter, thyroid malignancy, large nodules)	"Do you feel difficulty swallowing or breathing?"
Neck pain or radiation to ear/jaw	Suggests thyroiditis, malignancy with local spread	"Do you have pain that radiates to your ears or jaw?"
Weight changes	Weight loss → Hyperthyroidism, malignancy; weight Gain → Hypothyroidism	"Have you lost or gained weight unintentionally?"
Palpitations, sweating, heat intolerance	Seen in hyperthyroidism (graves' disease, toxic goiter)	"Do you experience a racing heart or excessive sweating?"
Cold intolerance, fatigue, hair loss	Suggestive of hypothyroidism (hashimoto's, myxedema)	"Do you feel tired, cold, or have thinning hair?"
Eye symptoms (protrusion, dryness, double vision)	Exophthalmos (graves' disease), orbital compression (malignancy)	"Have your eyes become more prominent or irritated?"
Past history of radiation exposure	High risk for papillary or follicular thyroid cancer	"Have you ever received radiation therapy to your head or neck?"
Family history of thyroid disease	Increased risk for autoimmune thyroiditis, medullary thyroid carcinoma (MEN syndrome)	"Does anyone in your family have thyroid disease or cancer?"

A. PHYSICAL EXAMINATION

GENERAL SURVEY

1. **Build and state of nutrition:** In thyrotoxicosis the patient is usually thin and underweight. The patient sweats a lot with wasting of muscles and in hypothyroidism the patient is obese and overweight. In case of carcinoma of thyroid there will be signs of anemia and cachexia.
2. **Facies:** In thyrotoxicosis one can see the facial expression of excitement, tension, nervousness or agitation with or without variable degree of exophthalmos. In hypothyroidism one can see puffy face without any expression (mask-like face).
3. **Mental state and intelligence:** Hypothyroid patients are naturally dull with low intelligence. This is more obvious in cretins.
4. Not only the **pulse rate** becomes rapid, but it becomes irregular in thyrotoxicosis. Irregularity is more of a feature of secondary thyrotoxicosis. Particularly *sleeping pulse rate* is a very useful index to determine the degree of thyrotoxicosis. In case of mild thyrotoxicosis, it should be below 90, whereas in case of moderate or severe thyrotoxicosis it should be between 90 to 110 and above 110 respectively. In hypothyroidism the pulse becomes slow (bradycardia).

5. **Skin:** The *skin* is moist particularly the hands in case of primary thyrotoxicosis. The clinician while feeling for the pulse should take the opportunity to touch the hand as well. Hot and moist palm to come across in primary thyrotoxicosis. Skin is dry and inelastic in myxedema.

B. LOCAL EXAMINATION

Examination of the thyroid swelling should be made as discussed in Chapter 3 under 'Examination of a swelling', besides these examinations peculiar to the thyroid gland will be described below:

A. INSPECTION

Normal thyroid gland is not obvious on inspection. It can be seen only when the thyroid gland is swollen. In case of obese and short-necked individual inspection of the thyroid gland becomes more difficult. To render inspection easier one can follow *Pizzillo's method* **(Figs. 27.1A and B)** in which the hands are placed behind the head and the patient is asked to push her head backwards against her clasped hands on the occiput. The thyroid swelling may be uniform involving the whole of the thyroid gland (physiological goiter, colloid goiter **(Fig. 27.2)**, Hashimoto's disease, etc.) or isolated nodules of different sizes may be seen in the thyroid region

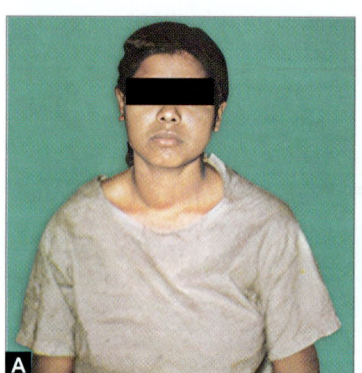
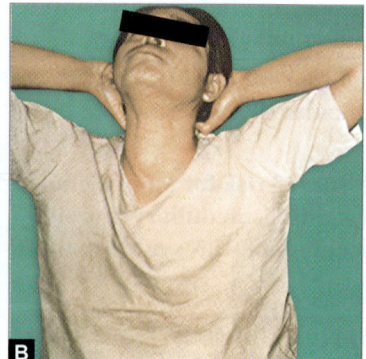
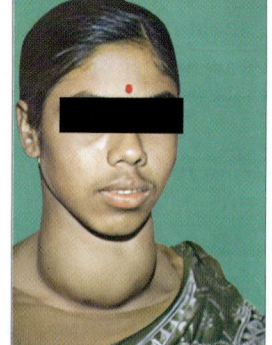

Figs. 27.1A and B: Shows how Pizzillo's method improve inspection of a goiter. (A) shows inspection in normal position and (B) shows Pizzillo's technique.

Fig. 27.2: A typical case of colloid goiter.

(Figs. 27.3 and 27.4) (nodular goiter). Rarely, a swelling on the lateral side of the neck is not due to enlargement of an aberrant thyroid gland but is caused by metastasis in lymph nodes from hidden carcinoma of the thyroid gland.

Ask the patient to swallow and watch for the most important physical sign—*a* **thyroid swelling moves upwards on deglutition.** This is due to the fact that the thyroid gland is fixed to the larynx. *Other swellings which may move on deglutition* are thyroglossal cysts, subhyoid bursitis and prelaryngeal or pretracheal lymph

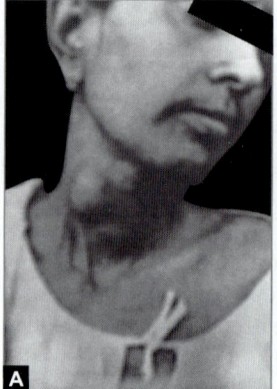
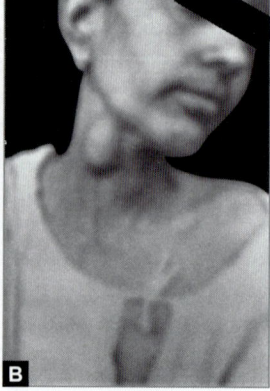

Figs. 27.3A and B: Nodular goiter. Note how the swelling moves up during swallowing in the second picture.

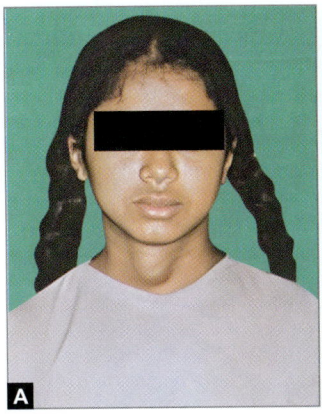
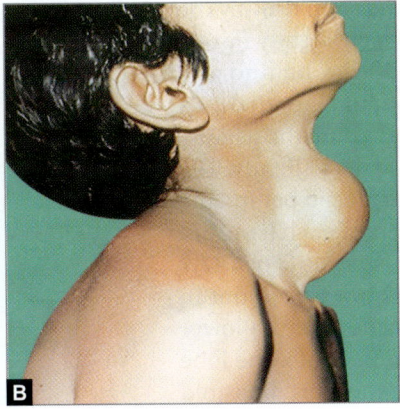
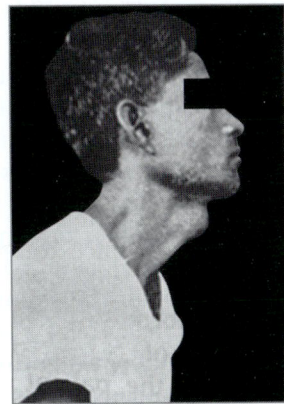

Figs. 27.4A and B: (A) A typical case of solitary nodule of the thyroid; (B) A large solitary nodular goiter in a woman of 40 years of age.

Fig. 27.5: The typical position of a thyroglossal cyst.

nodes fixed to the larynx or trachea. Such movement of the thyroid becomes greatly limited when it is fixed by inflammation or malignant infiltration.

In *retrosternal goiter*, pressure on the great veins at the thoracic inlet gives rise to dilatation of the subcutaneous veins over the upper anterior part of the thorax. When these are present, ask the patient to swallow and determine, on inspection, the lower border of the swelling as it moves up on deglutition. This is not possible in case of retrosternal goiter. The patient should be asked to raise both the arms over his head until they touch the ears. This position is maintained for a while. Congestion of face and distress become evident in case of retrosternal goiter due to obstruction of the great veins at the thoracic inlet.

A *thyroglossal cyst* **(Fig. 27.5)** also moves upwards on deglutition. But the pathognomonic feature is that it moves upwards with protrusion of the tongue since the thyroglossal duct extends downwards from the foramen caecum of the tongue to the isthmus of thyroid gland **(Figs. 27.6A and B)**.

Thyroglossal fistula is seen near the midline a little below the hyoid bone. The opening of the fistula is indrawn and overlaid by a crescentic fold of skin.

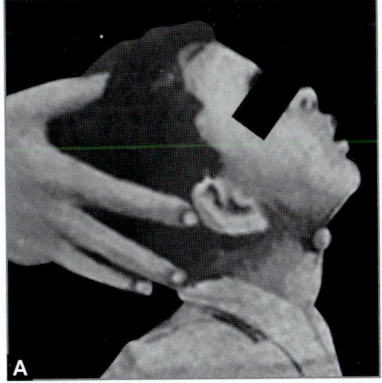
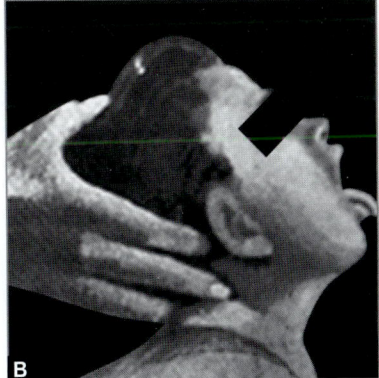

Figs. 27.6A and B: Show that the thyroglossal cyst moves up with protrusion of the tongue.

PALPATION: The thyroid gland should always be palpated with the patient's neck slightly flexed. The gland may be palpated from behind and from the front. The patient should be sitted on a stool and the clinician stands behind the patient. The patient is asked to flex the neck slightly. The thumbs of both the hands are placed behind the neck and the other four fingers of each hand are placed on each lobe and the isthmus **(Figs. 27.7 and 27.8)**. Palpation should be carried out in their entirety. Careful assessment of the lower margin. Additional information about one lobe may be obtained by relaxing the sternomastoid muscle of that side by flexing and rotating the face to the same side.

To get more information about a particular nodule of the thyroid gland one may ask the patient to extend the neck. This only makes the nodule more prominent for better the margins of the thyroid gland is important, particularly palpation.

Fig. 27.7: Shows how to get below the thyroid swelling to exclude presence of retrosternal prolongation. The patient is asked to swallow. The thyroid swelling moves up. Clinician now puts his fingers at the lower margin of the thyroid to be sure that there is no further downward extension of the thyroid tissue.

Palpation of each lobe is best carried out by Lahey's method **(Figs. 27.9 and 27.10)**. In this case the examiner stands *in front* of the patient. To palpate the left lobe properly, the thyroid gland is pushed to the left from the right side by the left hand of the examiner. This makes the left lobe more prominent so that the examiner can palpate it thoroughly with his right hand.

During palpation the patient should be asked to swallow in order to settle the diagnosis of the thyroid swelling. Slight enlargement of the thyroid gland or presence of nodules in its substance can be appreciated by simply placing the thumb on the thyroid gland while the patient swallows. (Crile's method).

During palpation the following points should be noted:

(i) **Whether the whole thyroid gland is enlarged?** If so, note its surface—whether it is smooth (primary thyrotoxicosis or colloid goiter) or bosselated (multinodular goiter) and

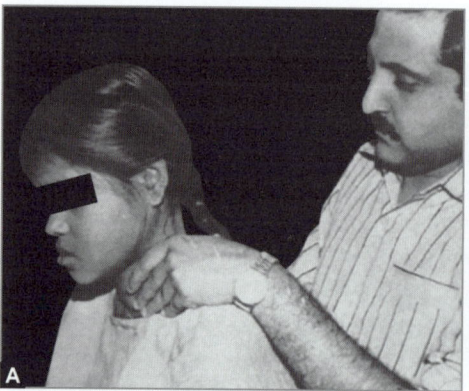
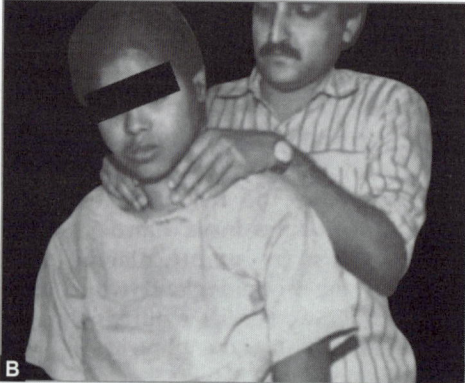

Figs. 27.8A and B: Show the method of palpation of the thyroid gland from behind. Note how the thumbs are placed on the occiput to flex the neck in the lateral view (A), and how the four fingers are placed on the lobes of the thyroid for better palpation in the anteroposterior view (B).

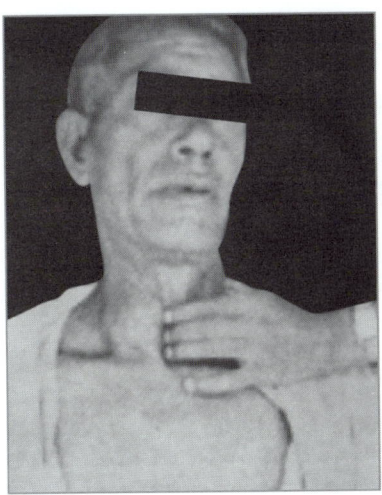

Fig. 27.9: Shows the Lahey's method of palpation of each lobe of the thyroid gland. The right lobe is pushed to the right by the examiner to make the lobe prominent for better palpation.

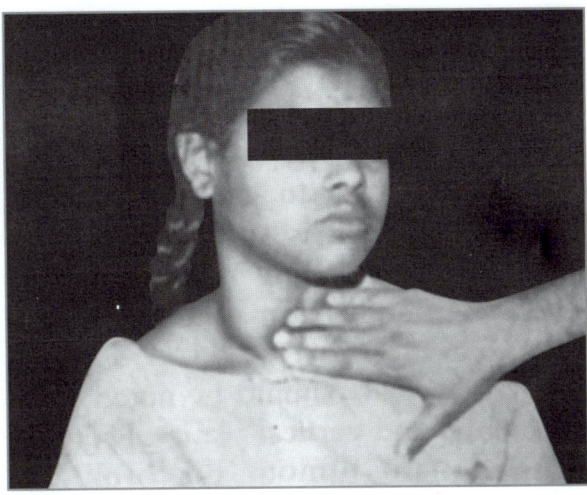

Fig. 27.10: Lahey's method for palpation of the right lobe of the thyroid gland. In this case the right lobe is pushed to the right by the right hand of the clinician to make it more prominent, so that he can palpate with his left hand easily.

its consistency whether uniform or variable. It may be firm in case of primary thyrotoxicosis, Hashimoto's disease, etc., it is slightly softer in colloid goiter and hard in Riedel's thyroiditis or carcinoma in which the consistency may be variable in places.

(ii) **When a swelling is localized,** note its position, size, shape, extent and its consistency. It must be remembered that a cystic swelling in the thyroid gland often feels firm due to great tension within the cyst which is surrounded by relatively soft surrounding tissue of the gland. A calcified cyst may even feel hard.

(iii) The **mobility** should be noted in both horizontal and vertical planes. Fixity means malignant tumor or chronic thyroiditis.

(iv) **To get below the thyroid gland** is an important test to discard the possibility of retrosternal extension. Clinician's index finger is placed on the lower border of the thyroid gland. The patient is asked to swallow, the thyroid gland will move up and the lower border is palpated carefully for any extension downwards **(Fig. 27.11)**.

(v) **Pressure effect** from the thyroid swelling should be carefully looked for. Pressure may be on the *trachea* **(Fig. 27.12)** or *larynx*, which may lead to stridor (inspiratory noise of inrushing air through narrowed trachea) and later on dyspnea. Pressure may be on the *esophagus* which may lead to dysphagia. Pressure may be on the *recurrent laryngeal nerve*, which may lead to hoarseness of voice. Pressure may be on even the *carotid sheath* **(Fig. 27.13)**. If pressure on trachea is suspected, slight push on the lateral lobes will produce stridor **(Kocher's test)**. This test, if positive, indicates an obstructed trachea.

Kocher's test: Gentle compression on lateral lobes may produce stridor. This is due to narrow trachea. This test is particularly positive in multinodular goiters and carcinoma infiltrating into trachea which produce narrowed trachea. The position of the larynx and trachea should also be noted. This may be assessed by placing stethoscope on the suspected zone. Passage of air will indicate the position of the trachea. Simple palpation by an experienced hand will indicate the position of the trachea. Finally, X-ray may be advised to know the exact position of the trachea.

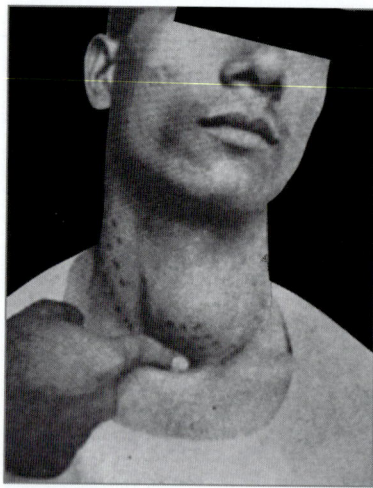

Fig. 27.11: Shows how to get below the thyroid gland. The patient is asked to swallow. The thyroid gland will move up and the lower border is palpated carefully to exclude any extension downwards.

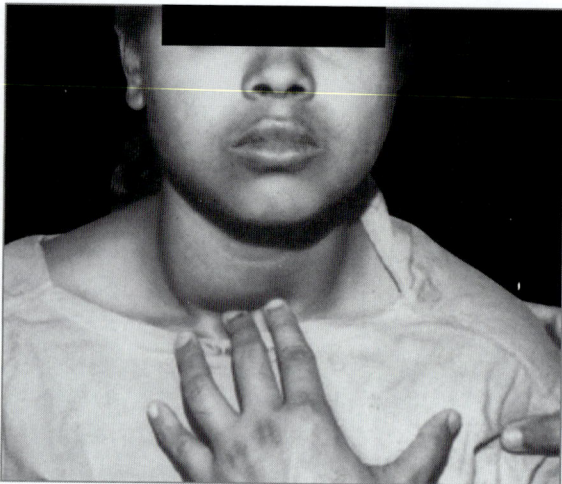

Fig. 27.12: Shows how to palpate the trachea to ascertain its position or any pressure effect being exerted on it due to thyroid enlargement.

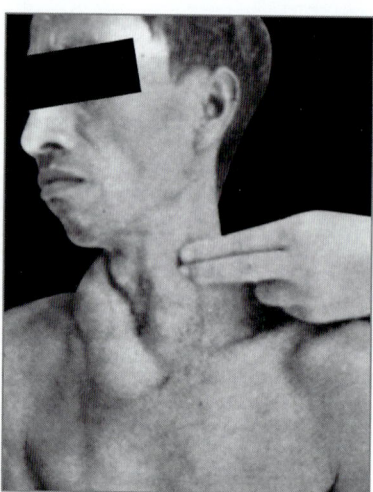

Fig. 27.13: Shows how to feel for carotid pulsation. A malignant thyroid may engulf the carotid sheath so that no pulsation can be felt.

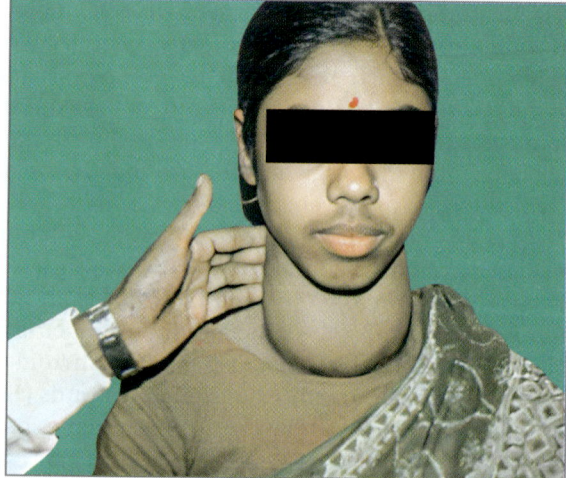

Fig. 27.14: Shows how to feel for the carotid pulsation in case of thyroid enlargement. In certain pathological conditions of the thyroid the pulse may be obliterated. See the text.

Narrowing of the trachea, i.e., 'Scabbard' trachea becomes quite obvious in skiagram. The carotid sheath may be pushed backward by a benign swelling of the thyroid gland where the pulsation of the carotid artery may be felt **(Fig. 27.14)**. A malignant thyroid may engulf the carotid sheath completely and pulsation of the artery cannot be felt. Sympathetic trunk may also be affected by thyroid swelling. This will lead to Horner's syndrome, i.e., slight sinking of the eyeball into the orbit (enophthalmos), slight drooping of the upper eyelid (pseudoptosis), contraction of the pupil (miosis) and absence of sweating of the affected side of the face (anhidrosis). Obstruction

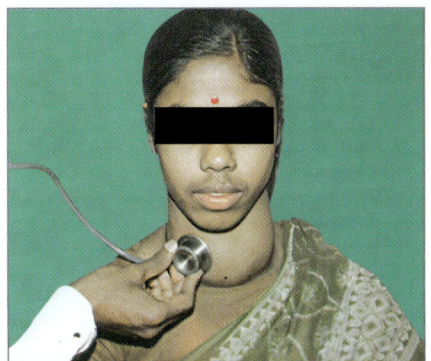
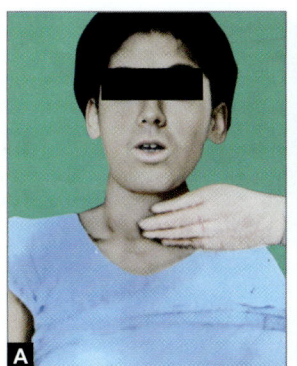
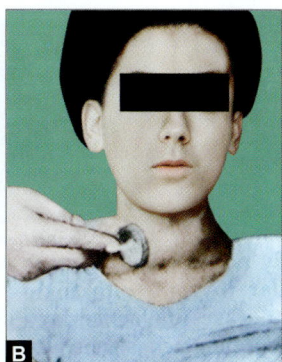

Fig. 27.15: Auscultation of the thyroid to exclude presence of bruit there.

Figs. 27.16A and B: Feeling and auscultating the thyroid for thrill and bruit in a case of slightly exophthalmic goiter.

to the major veins in the thorax causes **engorgement of neck veins** are not uncommon. This sign becomes obvious when the patients are asked to raise the hands above the head and the arms touch the ears. This is known as **Pemberton's sign**.

(vi) Whether there is any *toxic manifestation* or not. Primary toxic thyroid is generally not enlarged whereas an enlarged thyroid or nodular thyroid with toxic manifestation is generally a case of secondary thyrotoxicosis. In this case the brunt of attack is generally borne by the cardiovascular system whereas in primary thyrotoxicosis it is the nervous system which is mainly affected.

(vii) Whether there is any evidence of myxedema or not.

(viii) Whether the swelling is a malignant one or a benign one.

(ix) Is there any pulsation or thrill in the thyroid?

(x) **Palpation of cervical lymph nodes:** This is extremely important particularly in malignancy of thyroid. Occasionally only cervical lymph nodes may be palpable, while the thyroid gland remains impalpable. Papillary carcinoma of thyroid is notorious for early lymphatic metastasis when the primary tumor remains quite small. Such enlargement was called 'aberrant thyroid' previously, which is nothing but metastatic enlarged lymph nodes.

Percussion: This is employed over the manubrium sterni to exclude the presence of a retrosternal goiter. This is more of theoretical importance rather than practical.

Auscultation: In primary toxic goiter a systolic bruit **(Figs. 27.15 and 27.16)** may be heard over the goiter due to increased vascularity.

Measurement of the circumference of the neck at the most prominent part of the swelling may be taken at intervals. This will determine whether the swelling is increasing or decreasing in size.

GENERAL EXAMINATION

In general examination one should look for (i) primary toxic manifestations in case of goiters affecting the young, (ii) secondary toxic manifestations in nodular goiter and (iii) metastasis in case of malignant thyroid diseases.

(i) **Primary toxic manifestations:** One should look for five cardinal signs **(Fig. 27.17)**:

1. *Eye signs:* There are four important changes that may occur in the eyes in thyrotoxicosis **(Figs. 27.18A to C)**. Each one may be unilateral or bilateral:

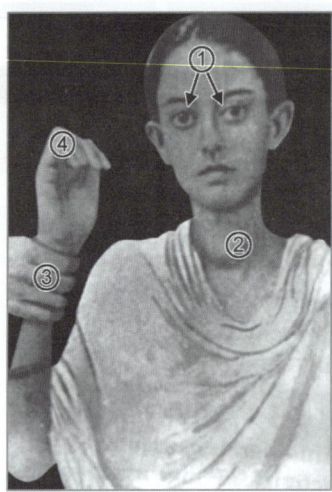

Fig. 27.17: The four cardinal signs of primary toxic goiter are shown by numbers. 1. Exophthalmos; 2. thyroid swelling with or without thrill; 3. tachycardia and 4. tremor.

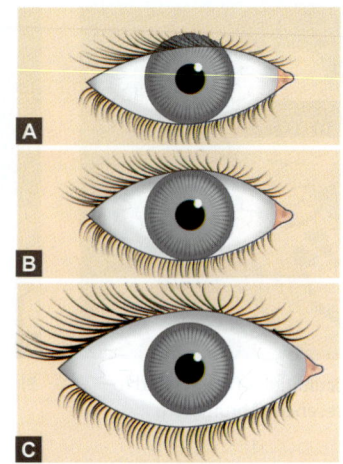

Figs. 27.18A to C: (A) Normal eye. (B) Lid retraction of the upper eyelid, whereas lower lid is normal. This is not exophthalmos. (C) Exophthalmos, where both lids are moved away showing sclera both below and above the iris.

(i) **Lid retraction:** This sign is caused by over- activity of the involuntary (smooth muscle) part of the levator palpebrae superioris muscle. When the upper eyelid is higher than normal and the lower eyelid is in its normal position this condition is called lid retraction. 'Lid lag' is a different term. This means the upper eyelid cannot keep pace with the eyeball when it looks down following an examiner's finger moving downwards from above. Both lid retraction and lid lag are not exophthalmos.

(ii) **Exophthalmos (Fig. 27.19A and B):** When eyeball is pushed forwards due to increase in fat or edema or cellular infiltration in the retro-orbital space the eyelids are retracted and sclera becomes visible below the lower edge of the iris first followed by above the upper edge of the iris. Now the following tests or signs are:

(a) *Von Graefe's sign*: The upper eyelid lags behind the eyeball as the patient is asked to look downwards.

(b) *Joffroy's sign*: Absence of wrinkling on the forehead when the patient looks upwards with the face inclined downwards.

(c) *Stellwag's sign*: This is staring look and infrequent blinking of eyes with widening of palpebral fissure. This is due to toxic contraction of striated fibres of levator palpebrae superioris.

(d) *Moebius' sign*: This means inability or failure to converge the eyeballs.

(e) *Dalrymple's sign*: This means the upper sclera is visible due to retraction of upper eyelid.

(iii) **Ophthalmoplegia:** There may be weakness of the ocular muscles due to edema and cellular infiltration of these muscles. Most often the superior and lateral rectus and inferior oblique muscles are affected. Paralysis of these muscles prevents the patient looking upwards and outwards.

(iv) **Chemosis:** This is edema of the conjunctiva. The conjunctiva becomes edematous, thickened and crinkled. Chemosis is caused by obstruction of the venous and lymphatic drainage of the conjunctiva by the increased retro-orbital pressure.

2. ***Tachycardia*** or increased pulse rate without rise of temperature is constantly present in primary toxic goiter. Sleeping pulse rate is more confirmatory in thyrotoxicosis. Regularity of the pulse may be disturbed and a rapid irregular pulse should arouse suspicion of auricular fibrillation **(Fig. 27.20)**.

3. ***Tremor*** of the hands (a fine tremor) **(Figs. 27.21 to 27.23)** is almost always present in a primary thyrotoxic case. Ask the patient to straight out the arms in front and spread the fingers. Fine tremor will be exhibited at the fingers. The patient is also asked to put out the tongue straight **(Fig. 27.21B)** and to keep it in this position for at least 1/2 a minute. Fibrillary twitching will be observed. In severe cases the tongue and fingers may tremble.

4. ***Moist skin*** particularly of the hands and feet are quite common in primary thyrotoxic cases. It should be a routine practice to feel the hands just after feeling the pulse at the wrist. The palms are hot and moist and the patients cannot tolerate hot weather, on the contrary tolerance to cold is increased.

5. ***Thyroid bruit*** is also quite characteristic in Graves' disease (primary thyrotoxic goiter). This is due to increased vascularity of the gland **(Fig. 27.15)**. But this sign is a relatively late sign and mostly heard on the lateral lobes near their superior poles.

(ii) **Secondary thyrotoxicosis** may complicate multinodular goiter or adenoma of the thyroid. The cardiovascular system is mainly affected. Auricular fibrillation is quite common. The heart may be enlarged. Signs of cardiac failure such as edema of the ankles, orthopnea, dyspnea while walking up the stairs may be observed. *Exophthalmos* and *tremor* are *usually absent*. Patients in this group are generally elderly.

(iii) **Search for metastasis:** When the thyroid swelling appears to be stony hard, irregular and fixed losing its mobility even during deglutition a careful search should be made to know about

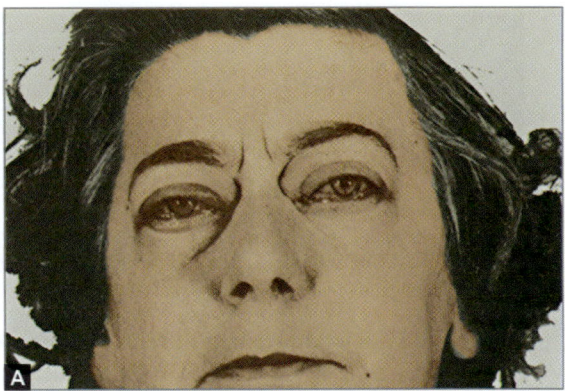
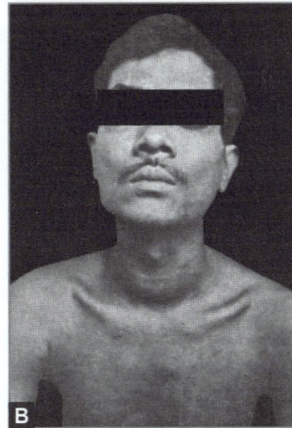

Figs. 27.19A and B: (A) Progressive (malignant) exophthalmos which developed over a period of 3 months following radioiodine therapy for thyrotoxicosis. Extensive chemosis and periorbital edema obscures the degree of exophthalmos; (B) A typical exophthalmic goiter.

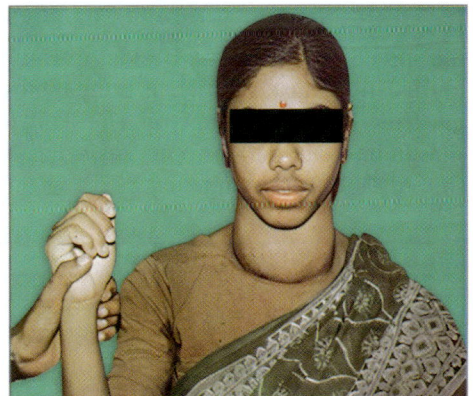

Fig. 27.20: Shows how to feel for the pulse of a thyroid patient. In primary toxic goiter the pulse rate will be fast. Secondary toxic goiter also manifests through it. Pulse may be irregular in the latter case. See the text.

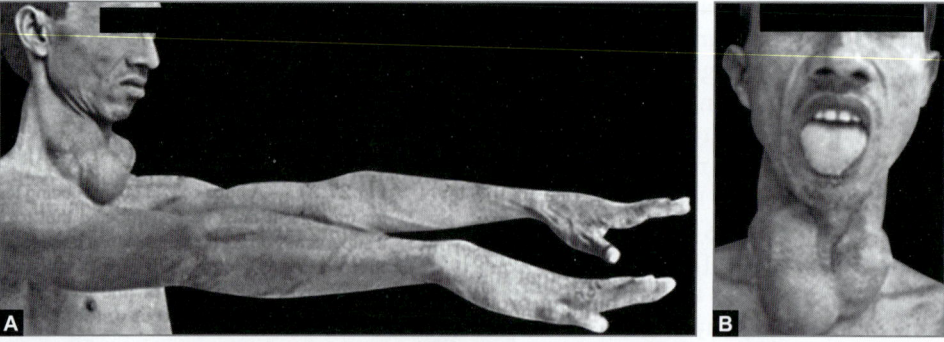

Figs. 27.21A and B: Tremor is a sign of primary thyrotoxicosis. It is mainly looked for in two sites—(A) fingers of an outstretched arm and (B) the protruded tongue.

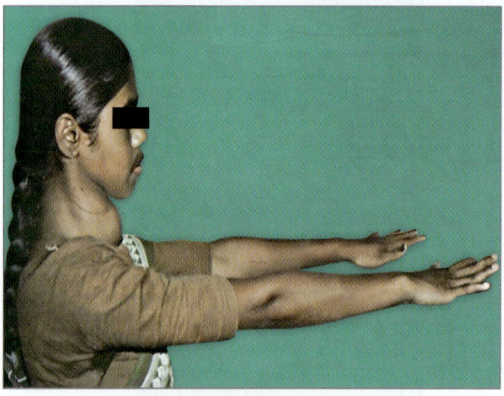

Fig. 27.22: Shows how to look for tremor in the extended fingers. This is a manifestation of primary toxic goiter and not of the secondary toxic goiter.

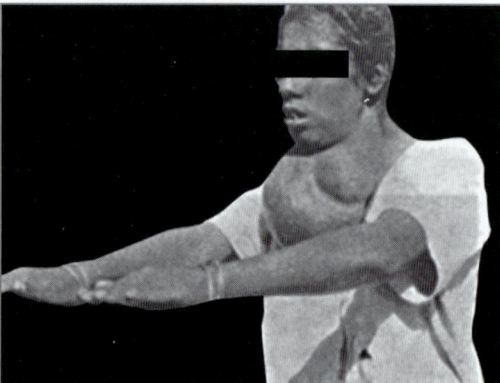

Fig. 27.23: A huge colloid goiter is being tested for tremors. It must be remembered that toxicity if supervenes on such a goiter, it will be secondary thyrotoxicosis. Manifestations of secondary thyrotoxicosis are mainly on the cardiovascular system and not on the nervous system. So tremors are usually not seen in these cases.

the spread of the disease. Besides examining the cervical lymph nodes, one should also look for distant metastasis such as bony metastasis which is quite common in thyroid carcinoma particularly the follicular type. The skull, the spine, the ends of the long bones, the pelvis, etc., should be examined for metastasis. Lastly metastasis in the lungs, which is not uncommon, should also be excluded.

SPECIAL INVESTIGATIONS

THYROID FUNCTION TESTS

The most important investigation of thyroid function is meticulous clinical assessment of the patient. But clinical diagnosis has to be confirmed by investigations to know exactly the hormonal status of the thyroid and also its relation with the anterior pituitary and hypothalamus. The following tests are useful to detect the function of the thyroid gland.

A. **Invitro tests:**
1. **SERUM PROTEIN BOUND IODINE (PBI):** In euthyroid condition, the range is 3.5–8 µg per 100 mL. It is cheap and can be easily assessed, but it lacks specificity in that it measures nonhormonal forms of iodine in the blood. False positive results are found in pregnancy, persons taking iodides in various forms particularly the contrast media, expectorants containing potassium iodide and in those taking oral contraceptives. False negative results are found in persons taking salicylates, androgens, hydantion-like drugs and in nephrotic syndrome.
2. **SERUM THYROXIN (T4):** Thyroxin is transported in the plasma mainly in the bound form with the thyroxin binding globulin (TBG) and by thyroxin binding prealbumin. Only a small amount circulates in the blood in the free form. Measurement is more difficult and can be measured only by competitive protein binding or radioimmunoassay method. The normal range varies from 3.0–7.5 µg per 100 mL.
3. **TOTAL SERUM TRI-IODOTHYRONINE (T3):** The estimation is very difficult and is only possible by radioimmunoassay method. This test is more effective in the sense that some cases of hyperthyroidism are due to excessive production of T3 without any accompanying rise in the level of serum T4.
4. **T3 RESIN UPTAKE:** The patient's serum is incubated with radioactive T3 so that the latter becomes fixed to any thyroid-binding protein not carrying T3 or T4. The amount so fixed can be measured and thus the number of binding sites in the serum which are unoccupied can be measured. Naturally in hyperthyroidism the number of free binding sites is low and in hypothyroidism this number is high. The secondary binder, where the unutilized radioactive T3 become fixed, was a resin previously and later on Thyopac or Sephadex was used. The fraction of labelled T3 taken up by the resin can be compared with that of a standard serum and this test goes by the name of "resin uptake ratio". The normal range being .91–1.21 µg. While using the Thyopac method one may take 100% as the mean normal value for free binding sites. In this case 85% or less will suggest hyperthyroidism as in this case the number of free sites will be less and a figure of 120% or more will suggest hypothyroidism as the number of free sites is high in this case.
5. **FREE THYROXIN INDEX (FTI):** This is calculated from the formula that FTI is equal to serum T4 (or PBI) × T3 uptake percent. The normal range is from 3.5 to 8. It correlates closely with the level of free T4 in serum and thus accurately reflects the thyroid status of an individual. This can be considered as the best single test available at present.
6. **SERUM THYROID STIMULATING HORMONE (TSH):** The serum concentration of TSH is measured by immunoassay. The normal level is about 1 µu/mL. It is raised in primary hypothyroidism and almost undetectable in hyperthyroidism. This test is more of help in the diagnosis of hypothyroidism rather than hyperthyroidism. It is also of value to measure TSH level following radioiodine therapy and subtotal thyroidectomy.
7. **TEST OF HYPOTHALAMIC-PITUITARY AXIS:** When thyrotrophin-releasing hormone (TRH) is given I.V. in a dose of 200 µg to a normal individual, the level of TSH in the serum rises from a basal level of about 1 µu/mL to a mean pick concentration of about 10 µu/mL at 20 minutes and returned to normal by 120 minutes. In hypothyroidism there is an exaggerated rise of an already elevated TSH level but in hyperthyroidism there is no response of a depressed TSH level. Its importance remains to certain extent in the diagnosis of T3 thyrotoxicosis if it is not possible to measure the circulating level of T3. Many drugs interfere with the result, e.g., T4, antithyroid drugs, corticosteroids, estrogens and levodopa. These modify the TSH response to

TRH. Probably its main indications remain in cases of mild hyperthyroidism when diagnosis is in doubt, in hypopituitarism and in ophthalmic Graves' disease.

B. **In vivo tests:** These tests hardly help in the diagnosis of hypothyroidism. These are mainly used in the diagnosis of thyrotoxicosis and in the assessment of functional activity of thyroid nodules by scanning. The radioisotopes are mainly used and ^{99m}Tc (Technetium) is gradually replacing iodine isotopes because of the low energy and short half-life of the former. The radiation dose to the thyroid is about 1/10000 time that of ^{132}I. Moreover Technetium is concentrated in the thyroid gland in the same way as iodine but is not bound to tyrosine. Therefore, it gives a more accurate measure of the iodine trap.

1. **UPTAKE TESTS:** The rate at which the thyroid gland traps iodine reflects the rate of secretion of the thyroid hormone. In hyperthyroidism both the proportion of the tracer dose taken up and the rate at which this takes place are increased. The best time to measure the isotope uptake is between 10–120 minutes after administration. At this stage there is no additional discharge of radioactivity from the gland. The tracer dose of ^{131}I is 5 microcuries. The uptake is first measured and then the radioisotope passes back into the serum being incorporated into the T3 and T4 molecules and can be measured as protein bound ^{131}I. ^{132}I may also be used as a diagnostic tracer but only for thyrotoxicosis as it has a short life (2.3 hours as opposed to 8 days of ^{131}I). One point must be remembered that in case of hyperplastic nontoxic goiter of iodine deficiency will show an increase uptake and lead to an erroneous diagnosis of toxic goiter. This test cannot be performed immediately after contrast medium X-rays such as IV pyelography, cholecystogram, etc. The contrast medium is excreted in about 2 weeks time after IV pyelography and more than a month after cholecystogram and even years after bronchography and myelography.

This test should not be performed in children or during pregnancy because of whole body radiation. But isotopes with shorter half-life, e.g., ^{132}I or ^{99m}Tc may be used.

2. **T3 SUPPRESSION TEST (WERNER):** This test differentiates thyrotoxicosis from other causes of raised uptakes, e.g., iodine deficiency and the autonomous thyroid nodules. This test is dangerous in elderly patients and those with heart failure as there always remains a potential risk of inducing transient hyperthyroidism.

The initial uptake is measured. 40 μg of tri-iodothyronin is given 8 hourly by mouth for 5 days, after which the uptake is repeated. T3 is used because of its more rapid effect and its shorter half-life. Considerable suppression in thyroid uptake is noted in the range of 50–80% by this amount of exogenous hormone. Slight suppression in the range of 10–20% is noted in thyrotoxicosis. The TRH test gives similar information and has replaced the T3 suppression test in centers where a radioimmunoassay of serum TSH is available. In patients who are on antithyroid drug treatment for thyrotoxicosis, this test may be used as an indicator of remission of the disease. A return to normal suppressibility in treated patients usually indicates remission.

3. **THYROID SCAN:** Scanning with a tracer dose will show which part of the gland is functioning or which part is not functioning (hot or cold). Both ^{131}I and ^{99m}Tc can be used. ^{131}I scan can be obtained at 24 hours whereas ^{99m}Tc scan is obtained at about 1/2 hour. It is not useful to scan all enlarged glands, but it is helpful to scan the thyroid when (i) a solitary nodule is palpated, (ii) in case of suspected retrosternal goiter or (iii) ectopic thyroid tissue. *A single non-functioning thyroid nodule is an indication for surgery*. Only histological examination can reveal whether it is a carcinoma or one of other causes of nonfunctioning nodules such as a cyst, colloid-filled adenoma or a focal area of autoimmune thyroiditis. If a nodule is autonomous most of the isotopes will accumulate in the nodule and the rest of the gland will show little activity. But if

the nodules are functioning but not autonomous, both the nodules and the rest of the gland will take up the isotopes.

Metastasis can be demonstrated by scanning the whole body of the patient but there should be no functional thyroid tissue as the thyroid cancer cannot compete with the normal thyroid tissue in the uptake of iodine.

C. **Miscellaneous tests:** These comprise the **BMR**, serum cholesterol, serum creatine, measurement of tendon reflexes, ECG, etc. Of these **BMR** and measurement of tendon reflexes may help in the diagnosis of hypothyroidism. Other tests are of little value.

Radiography: This is helpful to diagnose the position of the trachea—whether displaced or narrowed. Straight X-ray is also helpful in diagnosing retrosternal goiter. In case of malignant thyroid, the bones (especially the skull) if suspected to be secondarily involved should be X-rayed for evidence of metastasis.

X-ray after barium swallow may indicate whether there is any pressure effect on the esophagus or not.

Selective angiography can also differentiate between a functioning and nonfunctioning thyroid nodule. Moreover it may indicate presence of retrosternal goiter.

Bone scan may be done to exclude early bony metastasis.

Fine needle aspiration cytology (FNAC): This is an excellent, simple and quick test for thyroid cysts which can be performed as outpatient method. Thyroid conditions which may be diagnosed by this technique are—thyroiditis, colloid nodule (quite common), benign tumors like follicular adenoma, follicular carcinoma, papillary carcinoma, anaplastic carcinoma, medullary carcinoma and lymphoma.

Ultrasound: It has a value to differentiate between solid and cystic swellings. It also demonstrates impalpable nodules. But its value to diagnose malignancy is limited.

CT and MRI: These newer methods have not yet proved themselves very helpful in detecting day-to-day thyroid disorders. These are still in the experimental stage.

DIFFERENTIAL DIAGNOSIS OF THYROID SWELLINGS

A thyroid swelling is recognized by its position, its shape and by the fact that it moves upwards during deglutition.

GOITER

The term "goiter" denotes here any enlargement of thyroid gland irrespective of its pathology.
Differential diagnosis of thyroid swellings include:
- **Nontoxic goiter:**
  - **Colloid goiter** → Slow-growing, soft, nontender.
  - **Multinodular goiter** → Irregular, asymmetrical, may compress trachea.
- **Toxic goiter (Thyrotoxicosis):**
  - **Graves' disease** → Diffuse goiter, exophthalmos, pretibial myxedema.
  - **Toxic multinodular goiter** → Hyperthyroid symptoms in a nodular gland.
- **Thyroid malignancies:**
  - **Papillary carcinoma** → Slow-growing, lymphatic spread, young females.
  - **Follicular carcinoma** → Hematogenous spread, middle-aged females.

- **Anaplastic carcinoma** → Rapid growth, fixed, poor prognosis.
- **Medullary carcinoma** → Associated with MEN syndrome, calcitonin marker.
• Thyroiditis:
  - **Hashimoto's thyroiditis** → Autoimmune, firm, associated with hypothyroidism.
  - **De Quervain's thyroiditis** → Painful, viral etiology, transient thyrotoxicosis.
• Other conditions:
  - **Thyroglossal cyst** → Moves with tongue protrusion.
  - **Riedel's thyroiditis** → Hard, fibrotic, mimics anaplastic carcinoma.

DIFFUSE PARENCHYMATOUS (HYPERPLASTIC) GOITER

It occurs especially in endemic area affecting the children and adolescents between the ages of 5 and 20. There is uniform enlargement of the thyroid gland and it feels comparatively soft. This is due to increased TSH stimulation in response to low level of circulating thyroid hormones. (i) Iodine deficiency, (ii) goitrogenic substances like turnips, brassica family of vegetables (e.g., cabbage, kale, rape etc.), soyabean, antithyroid drugs, para-amino salicylates, etc., and (iii) genetic factors with deficiency of some enzymes of thyroid concerned with production of hormones, are the factors responsible for the development of this type of goiter. At the time of puberty when the metabolic demands are high and in pregnancy when there is too much stress, this goiter may develop *physiologically*. This goiter usually subsides by itself (natural involution) or with iodine therapy. But it may lead to colloid goiter when TSH stimulation ceases and the follicles become inactive and filled with colloid. Fluctuating TSH levels may lead to areas of active and inactive lobules (nodular goiter).

COLLOID GOITER (FIG. 27.24)

The patients usually present between the ages of 20 and 30 years, i.e., after physiological hyperplasia should have subsided. The whole gland becomes enlarged, soft and elastic. There is no other trouble. Pressure effects, e.g., dyspnea, venous engorgement and discomfort during swallowing are rare unless the swelling is enormous.

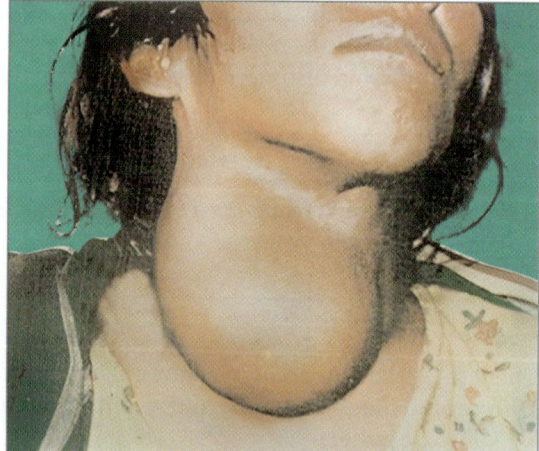

Fig. 27.24: A huge colloid goiter.

NODULAR GOITER

There may be a single nodule—*solitary nodular goiter* (syn. adenoma) or a number of nodules—*multinodular goiter* (syn. adenoparenchymatous).

MULTINODULAR GOITER: Cut surface of multinodular goiter reveals nodules with hemorrhagic and necrotic areas separated by normal tissue which contains normal active follicles. In endemic areas this goiter appears early between 20 and 30 years, whereas in sporadic areas it appears late between 30 and 40 years. This goiter is found six times commoner in females than males. It presents as slowly enlarging painless lump in the neck. Sudden enlargement with pain is complained of when there is hemorrhage into the inactive nodules. Pressure symptoms, e.g., dyspnea, engorged neck veins, discomfort during swallowing, stridor, etc., are complained of when the swelling becomes quite large. Secondary thyrotoxicosis occurs in approximately 25% of cases. In long standing multinodular goiters most of the nodules gradually become inactive and myxedema may ensue by the time she reaches 60 or 70 years of age. *On examination*, the gland assumes asymmetrical shape and its surface becomes smooth and nodular. Consistency of the nodules vary from soft to hard (nodules which are tense with hemorrhage).

SOLITARY NODULAR GOITER: It must be remembered that approximately half of the patients who present with solitary nodules actually have multinodular goiters. A solitary nodule may be present anywhere in the thyroid gland, though its common site being the junction of the isthmus and one lateral lobe. In general, in case of nodular goiters the patient seeks medical advice for disfigurement, dyspnea (from pressure on the trachea) or toxic symptoms (see secondary toxic goiter).

Complications such as hemorrhage, calcification, secondary thyrotoxicosis and carcinoma may develop especially in the nodular type. Sudden hemorrhage into the goiter may cause dyspnea, demanding immediate tracheostomy.

PRIMARY TOXIC GOITER (GRAVES' DISEASE OR EXOPHTHALMIC GOITER)

Primary toxic goiters are said to be due to increased long acting thyroid stimulating (LATS) in the form of IgG (a form of gammaglobulin) in the serum. This humoral agent is supposed to be derived from lymphocytes. This occurs in a previously healthy gland (cf. secondary toxic goiter). Commonly seen in young women. A history of overwork, worry and severe mental strain is often obtained. The disease is characterized by five features: (1) exophthalmos; (2) some enlargement of the thyroid gland; (3) loss of weight inspite of good appetite; (4) tachycardia and (5) tremor **(Fig. 27.25)**. In addition to these, there may be thirst and disturbed menstrual function. The basal metabolic rate is increased to even 100%. Thyroid gland is enlarged, firm or soft, a bruit may be present mostly near the upper pole.

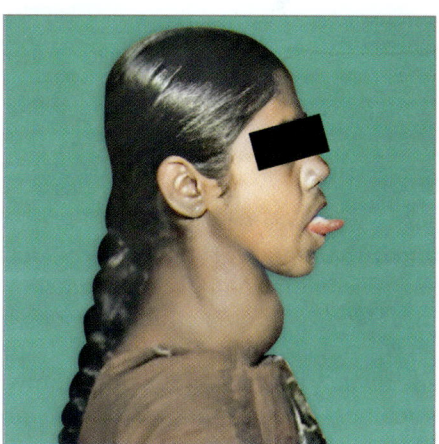

Fig. 27.25: Shows how to examine for tremor in a protruded tongue, which is a manifestation of primary toxic goiter (and not of secondary toxic goiter). See the text.

SECONDARY TOXIC GOITER

Toxicity is superimposed on a previously diseased gland more commonly a nodular goiter. It must be remembered that the brunt of attack falls on the cardiovascular system. There may be no exophthalmos, no tremor and no tachycardia but the pulse becomes irregular in rate and rhythm. The patient complains of precordial pain and exhaustion, later on auricular fibrillation and heart failure may set in.

RETROSTERNAL GOITER

It may be *substernal*, wholly *intrathoracic* or *plunging*, i.e., intrathoracic but is forced into the neck while coughing. The patient becomes dyspneic on lying on one side only—right or left. The most diagnostic feature is the presence of engorged veins over the upper part of the chest. X-ray pictures will show soft tissue shadow in the superior mediastinum or calcification. Compression or deviation of trachea may be seen. I^{131} scan can locate the gland. Arteriography also helps in the diagnosis.

TUMORS

Benign tumors are rare and can be either papillary adenoma or follicular adenoma. They present as solitary nodules.

Malignant tumors may be primary or secondary. Primary malignant tumors can be either (1) Carcinoma or (2) Medullary carcinoma or (3) Malignant lymphoma. Carcinoma is again classified as follows:

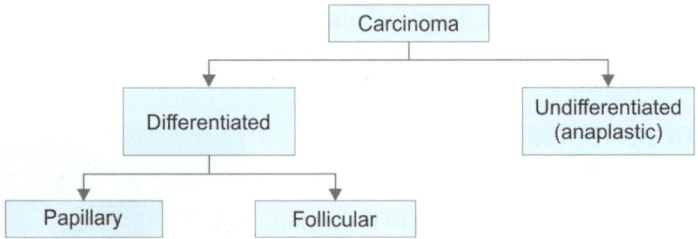

CARCINOMA

There are three types: (i) *Papilliferous* (in the young), (ii) *Follicular* (in the middle-aged) and (iii) *Anaplastic* (in the elderly). It is more common in goitrous districts. The diagnosis is suggested by the hard feel and indistinct outline of the thyroid swelling. It gradually infiltrates into the neighboring structures such as the trachea, esophagus, recurrent laryngeal nerve, infrahyoid muscles etc., causing dyspnea, dysphagia and hoarseness of voice. The carotid sheath may be surrounded by the growth so that its pulsation cannot be felt at the back of the swelling. Metastasis in bone may be the first symptom with pathological fracture or pulsating bone tumor.

Papillary carcinoma: Females are affected 3-4 times more than males. Common presenting symptom is relatively slow growing painless lump in the neck for more than a year. The lump is hard and not tender. This spreads by lymphatic channel in the early phase, so enlargement of regional lymph nodes is early. Multiple foci may be seen in the same thyroid due to lymphatic spread. These carcinomas are TSH dependent, so responds to thyroxin very well.

Follicular carcinoma: Females are more often affected. Presenting symptoms are similar to those of papillary carcinoma, but the age of the patient is more and there may be pain in the bones due to metastasis. These often metastasize through blood to bones or lungs in the first instance. 50% remains noninvasive. These respond to radio-iodine more than the former.

Anaplastic: Females are again more often affected. There may be aching pain alongwith the lump. The lump is slightly tender, hard, irregular and the margins are diffused due to infiltration. Dyspnea, pain in the ear, hoarseness of voice are the complaints due to infiltration of surrounding structures. Thyroid may not move up during deglutition due to fixity to the surrounding structures. Though lymph nodes are almost always enlarged and hard, yet such enlargement may be obscured by the primary mass. General malaise and weight loss are common features. *Duration of symptoms is much less* (months) than the preceding varieties of carcinoma. These metastasize through lymphatics, bloodstream and local infiltration. These are extremely lethal.

MEDULLARY CARCINOMA

These tumors derive from the parafollicular (C) cells, which are derivatives of ultimobranchial body (5th arch). Patients are between 50–70 years. When these affect the younger group, a familial incidence is often found. The common presentation is firm, smooth and distinct lump in the neck, indistinguishable from any other form of thyroid solitary nodule. *Diarrhea* is an important symptom which is complained of by at least 1/3 of the patients. These patients may also have pheochromocytoma, parathyroid tumor, neuromas of the skin or mucous membrane etc. Lymph node metastasis is found in half the patients and blood-borne metastasis is not very rare. High serum calcitonin is seen which is secreted by the tumor cells. Patients often complain of diarrhea due to high 5HT or prostaglandin.

MALIGNANT LYMPHOMA

This presents as a rapidly enlarging firm, painless mass in older woman. Symptoms caused by compression of the trachea and esophagus are common. So clinical presentation is almost similar to anaplastic carcinoma. It represents only 5% of thyroid malignancy and it is related to Hashimoto's thyroiditis and may develop from pre-existing thyroiditis. It is a radiosensitive tumor. This tumor is very difficult to differentiate from anaplastic carcinoma without biopsy.

OTHERS

Secondary growths—are rare and may be involved from local infiltration from adjacent organs or from blood borne metastasis from kidney, lung, breast, colon or melanoma of any site.
Acute suppurative thyroiditis is quite uncommon. Almost invariably it follows an acute upper respiratory tract infection.

AUTOIMMUNE THYROIDITIS (HASHIMOTO'S DISEASE)

This is the most common form of chronic thyroiditis. Four autoantigens have been detected—thyroglobulin, thyroid cell microsomes, nuclear component and nonthyroglobulin colloid. Of these antimicrosomal and antithyroglobulin antibodies can be measured in the patient's serum. There is some evidence of genetic predisposition. The thyroid is symmetrically enlarged, soft, rubbery and firm in consistency in 80% of cases. The enlargement may be asymmetric, lobulated and even nodular in rest of the cases. Though the disease is focal in the beginning yet it extends to involve one or both lobes and the isthmus. Majority of patients are women of an average age of 50 years. The most frequent complaints are enlargement of the neck with slight pain and tenderness in that region. Coughing is a common symptom. Shortness of breath, increasing fatigue and increase in weight are more related to hypothyroid state. There may be transient hyperthyroidism, but hypothyroidism is inevitable. There may be pressure symptoms on the esophagus and trachea. Increased incidence of other autoimmune diseases, e.g., rheumatoid arthritis, disseminated lupus, hemolytic anemia, purpura, myasthenia gravis and pernicious anemia may be found in these patients or in their families. There may be associated other endocrine organ failure syndrome, e.g., Addison's disease, diabetes mellitus and ovarian or testicular insufficiency. In special investigation one may find low T4, T3 and FTI values. Diagnosis is confirmed by demonstrating high titres of thyroid antibodies in the serum. Biopsy may be indicated in case of asymmetric and nodular goiters to rule out carcinoma.

GRANULOMATOUS (SUBACUTE OR DE QUERVAIN'S) THYROIDITIS

Etiology is controversial yet viral origin has been advocated and it is not an autoimmune disease. Majority of the patients are females around 40 years of age. Firm and irregular enlargement of the thyroid with adhesion to surrounding tissues is quite common. But these adhesions are separable. Fever, malaise and pain in the neck often accompany. In 10% of cases the onset is acute, the goiter is painful and tender and there may be symptoms of hyperthyroidism. White blood cells count is usually normal but ESR is almost always raised and ^{131}I uptake is usually low. Needle biopsy is quite helpful in diagnosis as enlargement of the follicles with infiltration by large mononuclear cells, lymphocytes, neutrophils and foreign body type of giant cells containing many nuclei can be detected easily.

RIEDEL'S (STRUMA) THYROIDITIS

It is a rare chronic inflammatory process involving one or both lobes of the thyroid even extending to the surrounding tissues. The gland is firmly attached to the trachea and surrounding tissues. When it is unilateral it is indistinguishable clinically from carcinoma. Women around 50 years are usually affected. Slight enlargement of the gland with difficulty in swallowing and hoarseness are usual symptoms. In the beginning serum PBI and radio-iodine uptake are normal. But in late cases these are lowered. Some patients may have circulating thyroid autoantibodies but in lower titers than in patients with Hashimoto's disease.

THYROGLOSSAL CYST (FIG. 27.26)

Though this cyst can appear at any time of life, yet it is commonly seen in early childhood (cf. branchial cyst). The thyroglossal cyst is mainly diagnosed by its characteristic position. It being a cyst of the thyroglossal tract, it is mainly a midline structure. The most common position is the *subhyoid* (just below the hyoid bone) and next common is the *suprahyoid* (just above the hyoid bone) position. The cyst is essentially midline in position in these two places. In case of suprahyoid position one must carefully differentiate this cyst from the sublingual dermoid cyst. Thyroglossal cyst may be seen *at the level of the thyroid cartilage*, when it is slightly shifted to the left and must be differentiated from cervical lymph node enlargement. The least common position is *at the level of the cricoid cartilage* when it may mimic an adenoma of the isthmus of the thyroid.

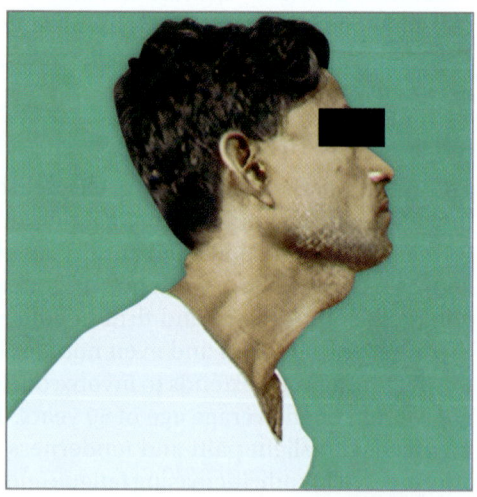

Fig. 27.26: A typical case of thyroglossal cyst.

The cyst is usually too small or the content is too tense to exhibit definite fluctuation. That the swelling moves up during swallowing and *that it moves upwards when the tongue is protruded* are the two pathognomonic features of this condition. One thing must be remembered that this cyst is very much liable to be infected.

THYROGLOSSAL FISTULA

This condition is usually an acquired one either from bursting or incision of an inflamed thyroglossal cyst or from local removal of the thyroglossal cyst leaving behind the thyroglossal tract. It is also a midline fistula **(Figs. 27.27 and 27.28)**.

HYPERPARATHYROIDISM

It must be remembered that parathyroid disease presents as a disturbed endocrine function and never as a swelling in the neck.

Primary hyperparathyroidism is due to increased secretion of parathyroid hormone which mobilizes calcium from bone, increases calcium uptake and causes phosphate loss from renal tubules resulting in hypercalcemia. Such overactivity of the parathyroid usually result from an adenoma (90% of cases), or due to hyperplasia (9%) or rarely due to carcinoma (1%). Patients may present with symptoms of hypercalcemia or the case may remain asymptomatic only to be revealed on routine serum analysis. Recurrent renal calculus is the most common presenting feature. There are certain gastrointestinal symptoms—features of peptic ulceration due to hypercalcemia-induced gastrin secretion. There may be acute or chronic pancreatitis. Bone manifestation is more common histologically and is not often clinically evident. Radiological appearances resembling rickets may occur in

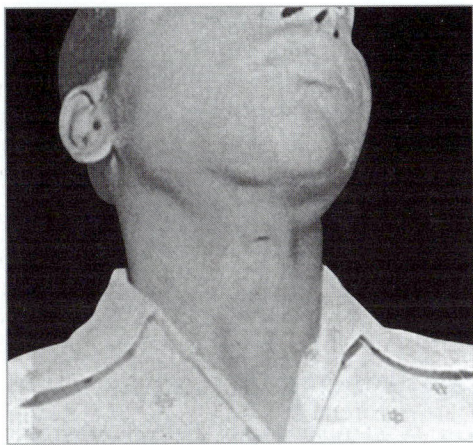

Fig. 27.27: Shows thyroglossal fistula in the suprahyoid position, which is not very common.

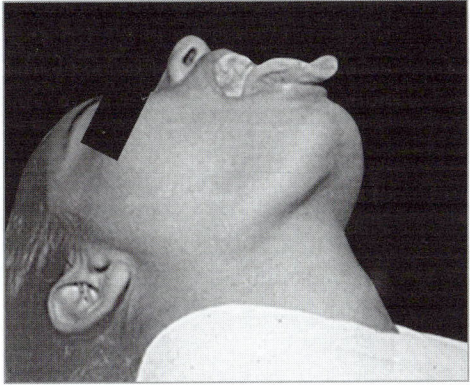

Fig. 27.28: Note how a thyroglossal fistula moves up when the tongue is protruded.

children from resorption of metaphyseal bones. Osteitis fibrosa cystica (brown tumor) arises from a process of subperiosteal bone resorption with patchy fibrous replacement. Mental disturbances with psychosis, dementia and behavioral changes are often noticed. Calcification may occur in other tissues such as cartilage resulting in pseudogout, in the cornea there may be a band—keratopathy. Other features of hypercalcemia include myopathy and hypertension.

This condition must be differentiated from sarcoidosis, milk-alkali syndrome, disseminated malignancy and excessive vitamin D ingestion, all of which cause hypercalcemia.

It must be remembered that hyperparathyroidism may be a feature of *multiple endocrine neoplasia syndrome* (MEN). In MEN type I there are parathyroid tumor, islet tumors of the pancreas producing gastrin to cause Zollinger-Ellison syndrome, medullary carcinoma of the thyroid and pituitary chromaffin adenomas-producing prolactin or giving rise to acromegaly.

In MEN type IIa there is parathyroid hyperplasia, together with medullary carcinoma of thyroid and pheochromocytoma. In MEN type IIb in addition there are features of neurological complications with the presence of neuromas of the lips and eyelids and ganglioneuromatosis together with even megacolon.

Secondary hyperparathyroidism is a reactive hyperplasia of the parathyroid glands in response to chronic calcium-losing conditions, chronic renal failure or malabsorption. There is unlikely of any clinical manifestation.

Tertiary hyperparathyroidism results from overactivity of the parathyroids associated with chronic calcium loss which may become autonomous later on. It may occur after renal transplantation.

It is rather impossible to palpate an enlarged parathyroid gland be it a case of hypertrophy or adenoma. But a systemic palpation should always be made to discover enlarged parathyroid gland. One thing must be remembered that even in presence of hyperparathyroidism if one finds a swelling at the posterior aspect of a thyroid lobe, very often it is a thyroid adenoma rather than parathyroid adenoma.

PARATHYROID TETANY

This is mainly a complication of thyroidectomy and reveals itself within first 5 days after operation. Early complaints are tingling and numbness of the lips, nose and the extremities. Later on painful cramps of the hands, feet and ultimately all the muscle of the body may occur. Strong adduction of the thumbs is a common feature of this condition and this when coupled with strong extension of the feet, constitutes the "carpopedal spasm". Lastly, the muscles of respiratory system may be affected which results in severe dyspnea. Blurring of vision due to spasm of intraocular muscles is not uncommon. The two common signs associated with this condition are: (i) *Chvostek-Weiss sign* in which a gentle tap on the facial nerve as it emerges in front of the external auditory meatus will invite a brisk muscular twitch of the same side of the face. (ii) *Trousseau's sign* in which a sphygmomanometer cuff is placed around the arm and the pressure is raised to 200 mm Hg. Within 5 minutes typical contractions of the hand can be seen, i.e., the fingers are extended but the metacarpophalangeal joints are slightly flexed and the thumb is strongly adducted—the so called 'Obstetrician's hand'.

Algorithmic Approach to Patient with Thyroid Swelling

Patient presents with thyroid swelling

↓

Is the swelling diffuse or nodular?
- **Diffuse** → Consider **goiter, thyroiditis, graves' disease**
- **Nodular** → Assess for **solitary vs multinodular swelling**

↓

Is the patient hyperthyroid or hypothyroid?
- **Hyperthyroid symptoms** → Suspect **graves' disease, toxic nodular goiter**
- **Hypothyroid symptoms** → Consider **hashimoto's thyroiditis, myxedema**

↓

Is the nodule solitary or multiple?
- **Solitary** → **Assess risk of malignancy (FNAC, ultrasound, TFTs)**
- **Multiple** → Likely **benign multinodular goiter**

↓

Are there compressive symptoms? (dyspnea, dysphagia, hoarseness)
- **Yes** → Consider **malignancy, retrosternal goiter, large goiter**
- **No** → Likely **benign process**

↓

Is the nodule hard, fixed, or associated with lymphadenopathy?
- **Yes** → High suspicion for **thyroid malignancy (papillary, follicular, anaplastic, medullary)**
- **No** → Consider **benign adenoma, colloid goiter**

↓

Perform thyroid function tests (TFTs)
- **Is TSH suppressed?**
  – **Yes** → Hyperthyroid workup (T3, T4, radioiodine uptake scan)
  – **No** → hypothyroid workup (anti-TPO antibodies, TSH levels)

↓

Perform imaging (ultrasound, FNAC, CT if retrosternal involvement suspected)
- **Ultrasound features suggestive of malignancy:** Hypoechoic, irregular margins, microcalcifications, increased vascularity
- **FNAC indications:** Suspicious solid nodules >1 cm, nodules with high-risk features, rapidly growing nodules

↓

High suspicion for malignancy?
- **Yes** → FNAC, surgical referral
- **No** → Follow-up and conservative management

Examination of Injuries of the Chest

CHAPTER 28

HISTORY

A careful history must be taken about the nature of violence. In civil practice road accidents and stab wounds are the main forms of chest injuries. Crush injuries are the severe forms of chest injuries in which apart from contusion of the chest wall and rib fractures there may be stove-in-chest, flail chest, lung contusion or laceration, aortic rupture, etc. The patient must always be asked whether he has coughed up any blood or not. This indicates injury to the lung.

Examination in chest injuries

Aspect	Clinical significance	Patient-friendly questions
Mechanism of injury	Blunt → Rib fracture, flail chest, hemothorax; Penetrating → Pneumothorax, tamponade	"How did the injury happen?"
Respiratory symptoms	Dyspnea → Pneumothorax, flail chest, tamponade	"Are you feeling breathless?"
Chest pain	Localized → Rib fracture; sharp, radiating → Myocardial contusion	"Where exactly do you feel pain?"
Coughing blood	Hemoptysis → Lung contusion, pulmonary laceration	"Have you coughed up any blood?"

PHYSICAL EXAMINATION

General Survey: The patient must be stripped properly and immediate careful observation must be made althroughout the body. Chest injuries are often associated with injuries of the abdomen which are more serious and may demand immediate surgical intervention, head injury and injuries of the limb. Note whether the patient is lying quiet (shock) or is restless and gasping (internal hemorrhage). Is the patient cyanosed or dyspneic? In traumatic asphyxia, which may complicate compression injuries of the thorax, petechial hemorrhages due to extravasation of blood from compressed venules may be seen in the face, conjunctivae and neck.

LOCAL EXAMINATION

A. INSPECTION

For proper inspection of the chest the patient should be stripped to the waist.

1. **Skin:** Any bruise or ecchymosis should be noted. These may indicate as to the nature of injury. If there is a wound assess whether it has penetrated the pleura or not. In a penetrating injury, air and blood will pass in and out of the wound with a loud sucking noise. This may be associated with pneumohemothorax and surgical emphysema. If the opening is quite large, the patient will be in great distress. Under such circumstances, a detailed examination should be deferred and *the wound should be immediately occluded by a pad of sterile gauze and strappings*. This avoids harmful effects of open pneumothorax and mediastinal flutter. Subsequently, the patient should be taken into the operation theater and the wound should be excised and closed.
2. **Respiration:** Note the *character* of breathing (hyperpnea, shallow breathing or dyspnea) and the *type* (abdominal or thoracic). The patient is asked to take a deep breath in. In fracture of the ribs the patient experiences an excruciating pain whose site he can point out.

    Note if there is any *paradoxical respiration,* i.e., collapse of the chest wall during inspiration and expansion during expiration. This is mainly seen in multiple rib fractures particularly when ribs are fractured at two places (at the anterior and posterior angles). This may lead to *flail chest,* i.e., a flaccid unstable chest wall which is sucked in by negative pressure within the pleural cavity during inspiration and pushed out in expiration by air coming from the good lung to the lung of the affected side **(Figs. 28.1A and B)**.
3. **Swelling:** This is not very frequently seen, neither very significant so far as injuries of the chest are concerned. Mostly a swelling is a hematoma. *Surgical emphysema* does not give rise to a localized swelling but may produce a diffuse swelling or a puffy appearance. The students must remember that surgical emphysema resulting from chest injury may not be localized to the chest wall but may spread to the neck, face, abdomen and even to the scrotum.
4. If the patient coughs out **sputum,** the students must make a careful look at it. A blood-stained sputum indicates nothing but injury to the lung or to the upper respiratory tract and mouth.

B. PALPATION
1. **Palpation of the ribs:** When injury is severe causing multiple fractures of the ribs, a careful assessment must be made as to which ribs are affected and the sites of fractures. More difficult is the case of simple crack fracture of a single rib when the patient may not attend the doctor

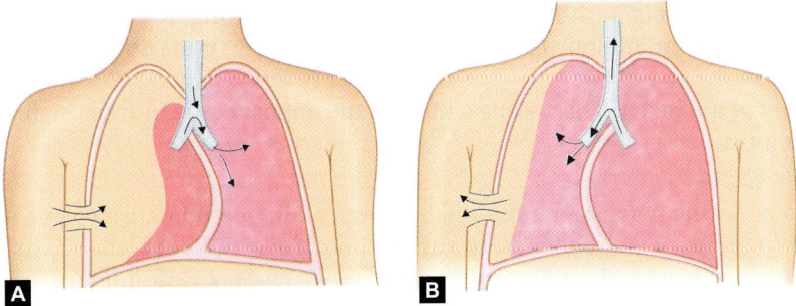

Figs. 28.1A and B: The mechanism of mediastinal flutter and paradoxical respiration. When the opening of the chest wall is large the lung of the affected side shrinks during inspiration as the air rushes into the pleural cavity through open wound pushing the mediastinum towards the healthy side pressing upon the unaffected lung whose aeration is also impaired. (B) During expiration, the mediastinum is pushed towards the affected side with air pushing from the good lung to the affected lung. The side-to-side movement of the mediastinum is known as 'mediastinal flutter' and since the heart and the great vessels are implicated it leads to shock with rapid pulse. During inspiration the affected lung collapses and during expiration it expands, i.e., reversal of the normal process. This is referred to as 'paradoxical respiration'. It is more evident from outside in a case of 'flail chest' when the two ends of the ribs are fractured.

immediately after the injury but will report only when the pain persists even after a few days of injury. If the patient can locate the exact site of pain the clinician should run his finger along the concerned rib to find out local bony tenderness, bony irregularity and crepitus. This indicates fracture of the rib. When the patient cannot indicate the exact site of pain the clinician must try to discover the site of fracture by "*compression test*".

Compression test (**Fig. 28.2**): The patient stands with both hands on the head. The clinician places the base of one hand on the sternum and the other hand on the spine. The thoracic cage is now *compressed anteroposteriorly*. If any rib is fractured this maneuver causes pain at the site of fracture.

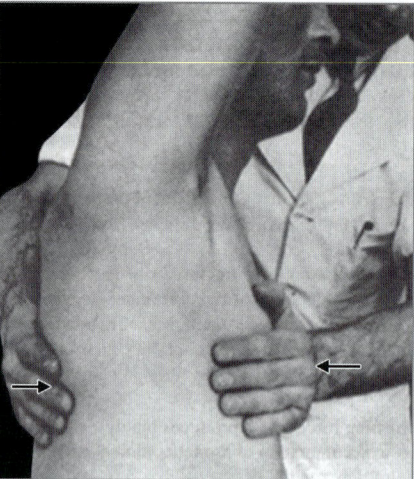

Fig. 28.2: Compression test. The patient stands with both hands on the head. The clinician places his one hand on the sternum and the other hand on the spine. The thoracic cage is now compressed anteroposteriorly. If any rib is fractured this maneuver causes pain at the site of fracture.

2. **Palpation of the sternum:** Fracture of the sternum is often missed by the students. It should form a part of the routine examination to run the finger along the anterior surface of the sternum. A crack fracture will thus be diagnosed. Displaced fracture is easier to diagnose as consequent deformity will attract the attention immediately. In majority of cases the upper fragment overrides the lower. *Whenever a fracture of sternum is detected, the spine must be examined for evidence of fracture, since these two conditions coexist quite frequently.*

3. **Swelling:** If there is a diffuse swelling, put your hand on the swelling. The typical crepitant feel of *surgical emphysema* once experienced is never forgotten. In fracture of the ribs, the surgical emphysema appears first at the site of the fracture, whereas in the *mediastinal emphysema* due to rupture of the bronchus or esophagus the surgical emphysema starts in the neck and rapidly spreads to the face, chest and abdomen.

Usual findings of a swelling should be noted. Besides these one should feel for impulse on coughing. This is present in subcutaneous herniation of the lung.

4. **Vocal fremitus:** Diminution of absence of the vocal fremitus is the finding in pneumothorax and hemothorax.

5. **Apex beat of the heart:** This will be shifted to the opposite side in cases of pneumothorax and hemothorax.

C. PERCUSSION

In pneumothorax the percussion note will be resonant. In hemothorax it will be dull. In right sided pneumothorax, it may obliterate the upper limit of liver dullness, whereas on the left side it may obliterate the normal cardiac dullness. In case of hemopericardium the area of cardiac dullness is increased.

D. AUSCULTATION

1. *Crepitus* may be heard when the bell of the stethoscope is placed exactly over the site of the rib fracture. This may be confused with surgical emphysema.
2. *Lungs:* In cases of pneumothorax and hemothorax the breath sounds and vocal resonance will be diminished or absent.
3. *Heart:* 'Silent heart' is pathognomonic of hemopericardium.

SPECIAL INVESTIGATIONS

1. **X-ray examination:** Importance of this investigation cannot be emphasized too hard. Fractures of the ribs with or without displacement are clearly seen. Pneumothorax and amount of air inside the pleural cavity can be diagnosed. The outer margin of the lung is also clearly delineated in X-ray. In hemopneumothorax the horizontal level of blood in the pleural cavity is easily seen in X-ray **(Fig. 28.3)**. Skiagraphy will also diagnose rupture of diaphragm and esophagus as also hemopericardium. Aortography is helpful when injury to major artery is suspected.

2. **Estimation of blood gases:** Regular estimation of arterial oxygen and carbon dioxide partial pressure will give a clue to the amount of respiratory insufficiency particularly in cases of paradoxical respiration.

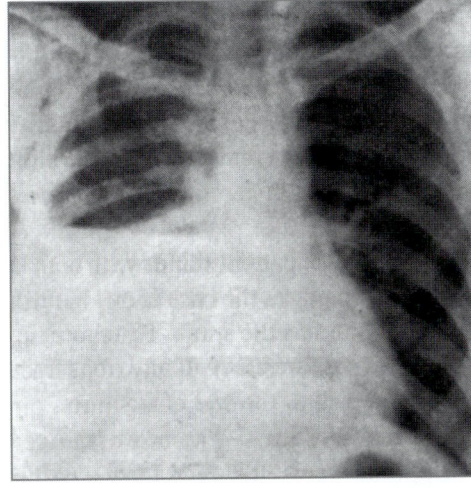

Fig. 28.3: Hemopneumothorax showing the horizontal level of blood in the right pleural cavity.

3. **Aspiration:** This test is better avoided for diagnostic purpose only, as there remains a chance of empyema to develop from secondary infection. In case of hemothorax blood can be aspirated out. This can be done after several days or weeks as the blood does not tend to coagulate due to constant movement of the lungs. Pleural shock must be avoided by properly infiltrating the parietal pleura with local anesthetic.

DIFFERENTIAL DIAGNOSIS

Fracture of the rib: The main complaint of the patient is pain while taking a deep breath in. Nothing more can be elicited from inspection except presence of slight bruising. On palpation, local bony irregularity, tenderness and crepitus are the findings of fractured rib. The compression test becomes positive. The clinician should run his finger along each rib in the region of injury to reveal local bony tenderness. The students must not forget to look for signs of other concomitant injury such as lung, liver (on the right side) and spleen (on the left side). Surgical emphysema denotes injury to the lung. Skiagraphy though confirmatory yet may miss a hair-line crack fracture.

Stove-in-chest: This condition develops from an extensive localized crushing force which produces multiple rib fractures. This results in depression of the chest wall in that region. Relative immobility leads to accumulation of bronchopulmonary secretions. This condition, if associated with depressed fractured clavicle, becomes a serious condition.

Flail-chest: This condition also develops from crushing injury. Multiple ribs fracture anteriorly at the costochondral junction and posteriorly near the angle of the ribs. This results in a fragment of the chest wall which becomes unstable having no bony connections. This part moves in during inspiration and moves out during expiration resulting in paradoxical movement of the chest wall. This condition very badly affects aeration of the lung and progressive accumulation of carbon dioxide. It may so happen that a number of ribs or costal cartilages on either side of sternum a little away from it may be fractured and then it becomes a flail sternum. It must be remembered that with quiet respiration paradoxical movement may not be apparent, but if the patient coughs or takes deep breathing paradoxical movement becomes obvious. Immediate surgical intervention in the form of tracheostomy and positive pressure respiration should be called for. If slight paradoxical movement still persists the ribs should be exposed and the ends joined by stainless-steel wire or nails.

Surgical emphysema: This means air in the subcutaneous tissue. The mechanism is injury to the lung through which air is forced into the chest wall. *This may not be associated with pneumothorax*, the rent in the lung being sealed off. This should not be confused with mediastinal emphysema which is a sequel of rupture of the bronchus or esophagus. In this condition emphysema is first noticed in the neck and it rapidly spreads to the face, chest wall, abdominal wall and even to the scrotum. The tension may rise sufficiently to cause embarrassment to the heart and great veins.

Traumatic pneumothorax: Air in the pleural cavity is called "pneumothorax". In majority cases of trauma blood is associated with air in the pleural cavity and then it is called hemo-pneumothorax. Air may reach the pleural cavity through a small rent in the lung which may subsequently be closed (*closed pneumothorax*). Air may enter the pleural cavity through a wound in the chest wall (*open pneumothorax*). Sometimes the leak in the lung through which air comes out becomes valvular, i.e., air enters the pleural cavity from the lung during inspiration but cannot leave the pleural cavity during expiration as the leak in the lung becomes closed. That means with each inspiration more air is drawn into the pleural cavity causing collapse of the injured lung. This condition is called *tension pneumothorax*. The mediastinum deviates to the healthy side. The onset of this emergency is suggested by increasing dyspnea and cyanosis. The trachea with the mediastinum shifts to the opposite side. Immediate aspiration of the air through the second intercostal space anteriorly is a life-saving procedure.

Pneumothorax, as a whole, is easily recognized by varying degrees of dyspnea, pain, shock, cyanosis etc. Hyperresonance, absence of breath sounds and shifting of the trachea and apex beat towards the opposite side are the findings of this condition.

Traumatic hemothorax: This means accumulation of blood in the pleural cavity. This results from contusion of the lung or injury to the parietal vessels. The diagnosis is made by dullness on percussion, weak breath sounds, impaired vocal resonance, etc. Hemothorax may be complicated by infection.

Contusion and laceration of the lung: Contusion generally results in areas of consolidation and usually resolves spontaneously whereas laceration permits leakage of blood and air into the pleural cavity. Minor lacerations also heal spontaneously but severe degrees of lacerations require exploration by thoracotomy.

Injury to the lung is clearly evidenced by *hemoptysis*. In every case of thoracic injury, the patient must be questioned whether he has coughed up any blood or not. Even a small quantity of frothy blood if coughed up is an indication of injury to the lung. *Surgical emphysema* is another strong evidence of lung injury. It must be remembered that besides the common surgical emphysema which is seen on the chest wall, *injury to the lung may result in mediastinal emphysema*. If the visceral pleura remains intact, air comes out through the traumatic rupture of the pulmonary tissue and accumulates to the hilum of the lung, from there to the mediastinum and neck.

Traumatic asphyxia occurs in crushing injury of the chest. Blood from the heart being driven into the veins of the head and neck and upper part of the chest causing extravasation of blood into the conjunctivae and skin of those regions.

Injury to the heart and **hemopericardium (cardiac tamponade):** When the heart is injured by penetrating wound blood accumulates in the pericardium. This compresses the heart and the circulation fails considerably. The three classical signs are: (i) "silent heart", i.e., diminution of cardiac sounds; (ii) increased area of cardiac dullness; and (iii) steady fall of arterial pressure with gradual rise of venous pressure. Immediate aspiration of the pericardium through the left costoxiphoid angle should be carried out as a life-saving measure.

Rupture of the thoracic aorta—is rare and fatal. Patients only come to the hospital when mediastinal pleura or adventitia holds the pulsating hematoma. Widening of the superior mediastinum with tracheal shifting in straight X-ray will give a clue, which will be confirmed by aortography.

Tear of the bronchus—is rare and may occur in severe chest injury. A continuing massive leakage of air indicates a torn bronchus which may develop into a severe mediastinal emphysema culminating in surgical emphysema which may extend into the scrotum. Bronchoscopy will finally diagnose this condition.

Rupture esophagus: This condition is very rare after injury to the chest, though perforation of esophagus does develop through inexpert use of esophagoscope or a gastroscope. Great pain and dyspnea give indication towards the diagnosis. X-ray will reveal air in the mediastinum, the pleural cavity and in the neck. Radiograph may be taken after swallowing a small quantity of lipiodol to diagnose this condition. Urgent operation under antibiotic cover is the main solution to this problem.

Rupture of the thoracic duct—is also and will cause chylothorax. Aspiration of chyle during pleural-tapping will confirm the diagnosis. If the patient is asked to ingest cream containing confectioner's green, this will mark the tear on thoracotomy.

Injury to the diaphragm and diaphragmatic hernia: Rupture of diaphragm is often associated with thoracic injury and this may lead to diaphragmatic hernia. Increasing dyspnea after injury, which cannot be explained otherwise, straight X-ray showing abnormal gas shadow within the thorax and barium swallow examination will reveal coils of intestine inside the thoracic cavity.

Injury to the subdiaphragmatic organs: An account of thoracic injury cannot be made complete without mentioning about injury to the abdominal organs. This is important as this injury requires more attention than injury to the chest proper. This is fatal and demands immediate surgical intervention. The liver, the spleen, the kidney, stomach, colon are the organs which may be involved in injury and is discussed in the Chapter on "Examination of abdominal injuries".

Algorithmic Approach to Patient with Chest Trauma

Patient presents with chest trauma

↓

Is the trauma blunt or penetrating?
- Blunt → Consider **rib fractures, pulmonary contusion, pneumothorax, hemothorax**
- Penetrating → High risk **of pneumothorax, hemothorax, cardiac injury**

↓

Is the patient in respiratory distress?
- Yes → Assess for **flail chest, tension pneumothorax, hemothorax**
- No → Proceed with **systematic examination**

↓

Is there tracheal deviation or jugular venous distension?
- Yes → High suspicion for **tension pneumothorax or cardiac tamponade**
- No → Proceed with **chest palpation and percussion**

↓

Percussion findings: Hyperresonant or dull?
- Hyperresonant → **Pneumothorax suspected**
- Dull → Consider **hemothorax or cardiac tamponade**

↓

Is there paradoxical chest wall movement?
- Yes → **Flail chest likely**
- No → Proceed with **chest auscultation**

↓

Breath sounds absent or muffled?
- Absent → Suggests **pneumothorax or hemothorax**
- Muffled → Highly suggestive of **cardiac tamponade**

↓

Emergency interventions
- Immediate needle decompression → If **tension pneumothorax suspected**
- Chest tube insertion → If **hemothorax or pneumothorax confirmed**
- Pericardiocentesis → If **cardiac tamponade suspected (Beck's triad: Hypotension, JVD, muffled heart sounds)**

↓

Further imaging for definitive diagnosis
- Chest X-ray → Identify rib fractures, pneumothorax, hemothorax, cardiac enlargement
- FAST ultrasound → Rapid detection of pericardial effusion and pleural fluid
- CT chest → Evaluate pulmonary contusions, mediastinal injuries, aortic trauma

Examination of Diseases of the Chest

CHAPTER 29

This chapter is mainly on physician's interest and elaborately described in the books of medicine. Here, only conditions of surgical importance will be discussed.

HISTORY

A careful history must be elicited. Whether the patient is in early postoperative period or not? How did the disease start—spontaneously, after an attack of acute lobar pneumonia (e.g., acute empyema) or following inhalation of a foreign body (e.g., lung abscess). Sudden acute pain in the chest to collapse after 7–10 days of operation may indicate pulmonary embolism. The appearance of dyspnea, cyanosis and fall of blood pressure on the second postoperative day suggests pulmonary atelectasis. Inquiry must be made about fever, pain in the chest, cough, sputum, haemoptysis, etc.

1. **Pain:** This is the most common symptom of diseases of the chest. Pleural conditions like pleurisy, empyema, pneumothorax and haemothorax all give rise to chest pain. Lung conditions like lung abscess, bronchiectasis, infarction, embolism, atelectasis and late cases of bronchogenic carcinoma give rise to this symptom. Pain is intermittent and throbbing in lung abscess. Radiation of pain along an intercostal space is typical of intercostal neuralgia. In acute empyema pleural pain is quite significant. About half of the patients with carcinoma of lung complain of chest pain when first seen by a doctor. It is often described as 'heaviness'. Constant pain indicates poor prognosis. Shoulder pain radiating to the corresponding arm is a feature of Pancoast (apical) tumor.

2. **Fever:** This is a common symptom of empyema, lung abscess, bronchiectasis, etc. Inquiries about its onset, nature, duration and timings.

3. **Dyspnea**—is also a very common symptom of almost all pleural and pulmonary diseases. Inquiries about its onset, type, whether continuous or only on exertion.

4. **Cough**—with or without sputum (dry) is a characteristic symptom of a few diseases of the lung. It is quite common in lung abscess and bronchiectasis. In bronchiectasis, the cough is chronic and productive with purulent expectoration, whereas in lung abscess cough is productive with foul-smelling sputum. In carcinoma of the lung this is the most common manifestation and it may or may not be productive. This is a rare complaint of pleural diseases.

5. **Hemoptysis:** This is a very significant symptom of a few lung disorders. Whereas tuberculosis is the most common cause of hemoptysis in India, yet a few surgical conditions also manifest with this symptom. It is seen in bronchiectasis. It is an alarming symptom of lung carcinoma and occurs in approximately 1/3 of cases. Occasionally hemoptysis may be massive in this condition constituting a surgical emergency.

6. **Loss of weight:** It is complained of in lung abscess, but it is significantly present in carcinoma of the lung. In tuberculosis, also it is seen, but basically it is a medical disease and very occasionally it may need surgery.

7. **Sinus formation:** Patients may present with this. Sinus formation may occur from empyema necessitatis. It is also a characteristic feature of actinomycosis of the lung in which the patient presents with multiple sinuses in the chest wall with induration and bluish skin around.

8. **Past history:** This is important particularly in tuberculosis, empyema and spontaneous pneumothorax. In a case of swelling of the chest wall or in a case who presents with hemoptysis and fever past history of tuberculosis suggests the possibility of a cold abscess of flaring up of the old infection. Past history of pneumonia suggests the postpneumonic empyema which is the most common cause of empyema. A recent past history of persistent cough treated by medicine and now the patient presents with cough, dyspnea, hemoptysis and weight loss should arouse suspicion of carcinoma of the lung.

9. **Personal history:** Excessive smoking for quite sometime is still considered to be the most common etiological factor of carcinoma of the lung.

History in chest diseases

Aspect	Clinical significance	Patient-friendly questions
Cough type	Dry → Pneumonia, TB; Productive → Bronchiectasis, lung abscess	"Is your cough dry or with mucus?"
Hemoptysis	Mild → TB, Bronchiectasis; Massive → Carcinoma, lung abscess	"Have you noticed blood in your sputum?"
Weight loss	Suggests malignancy, TB, lung abscess	"Have you lost weight recently?"

PHYSICAL EXAMINATION

General appearance: Presence of cyanosis, anemia, clubbing should be noted. Whether the patient is dyspneic or not? Emaciation is a feature very often seen in malignant diseases. The patient must be asked whether he is losing weight very fast or not.

LOCAL EXAMINATION

A. INSPECTION

1. **Contour of the chest:** Look at the chest as a whole, whether there is any abnormal prominence or retraction. If present, ask whether it was present previously or appeared after the beginning of the present illness. If there is undue prominence of the ribs anteriorly on one side, exclude scoliosis before considering an intrathoracic disease.

Funnel chest (pectus excavatum): There is posterior concavity of the body of the sternum from above downwards deepest above its junction with the xiphoid. The lower costal cartilages dip posteriorly to meet the depressed sternum. So there is concavity from above downwards, antero-posteriorly and side-to-side of the chest giving rise to the appearance of a funnel. It predisposes repeated respiratory infection and cardiovascular disturbances.

Pigeon chest (chicken breast or pectus carinatum): This is also a congenital deformity with occasional association with congenital heart disease. It is also a sequel to chronic respiratory disease in childhood. In this the sternum appears prominently bowed forward along with the costal cartilages, often accompanied by endowing of the ribs to form symmetrical horizontal grooves (Harrison's sulci).

Barrel shaped chest: It commonly occurs in obstructive emphysema of the lungs. Anteroposterior diameter of the chest is greater than the transverse diameter. There are prominent sternal angle and wide subcostal angle.

Flat chest: Here, the transverse diameter is more than the anteroposterior diameter.

Thoracic kyphoscoliosis: This may have profound effects on pulmonary function, as the chest deformity reduces the ventilatory capacity of the lungs.

Rachitic chest: This occurs in rickets. There are bead-like prominences at the costochondral junction known as 'Rickety rosary'.

2. **Respiratory movements:** Note the rate, character and type of breathing. It is always advisable to compare both the sides. Sluggish movement on one side of the chest may be due to pleural effusion, consolidation, collapse, etc.

3. **Apex beat of the heart:** It is better palpated than inspected. Collection of effusion, blood or air in one pleural cavity will push the apex beat to the opposite side, whereas in massive collapse the apex beat will be shifted to the same side.

4. Any **swelling** or a **sinus** must be carefully looked at and examined. They are always very significant in surgical conditions. The methods of examination have been discussed thoroughly in Chapters 3 and 5 respectively.

5. **Neck veins** may be engorged due to congestive cardiac failure or secondary to long-standing lung disorders.

B. PALPATION

1. **Respiratory movements:** The clinician places his hands on the chest—each hand on each side of the chest. They are so placed that the tips of the two thumbs come in contact with each other in the center. The patient is now asked to take a deep breath in and out. See how each thumb moves away from the midline with each inspiration. Deficient movement or immobility of one thumb indicates pleural effusion, consolidation, collapse, etc., of that side.

2. **Apex beat of the heart:** Place the palm of the hand on the apex beat of the heart. One can easily assess whether it is shifted medially or laterally.

3. **Position of trachea** should be examined to know if this is shifted to one side or the other.

4. **Feel for vocal fremitus:** It is much **diminished** in pleural effusion or pneumothorax, whereas it is increased in consolidation of the lung.

5. **Swelling:** Test for its consistency, mobility, compressibility, reducibility, fluctuation, impulse on coughing, etc. Bony hard swelling arising from a rib is a *tumor*. Soft, fluctuating swelling mainly on the anterior axillary line or parasternal line is a *cold abscess*. Presence of impulse on coughing means empyema necessitatis (**Figs. 29.1 and 29.2**). Reduction is often complete in *empyema necessitatis*. A cold abscess arising from caries of

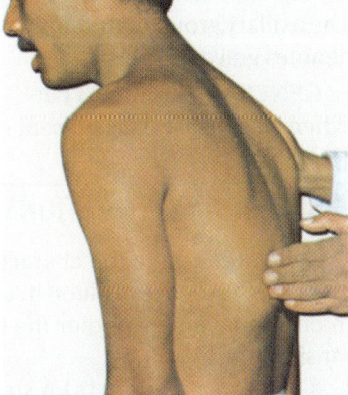

Fig.29.1: Lipoma affecting lower part of the left chest which clinically simulates empyema necessitatis. It is being excluded by looking for impulse on coughing which is positive in case of the latter but not in case of a lipoma.

the rib is compressible. Ascertain the mobility of the swelling over the chest wall and note whether the swelling is free or fixed to the chest wall. Fixed swellings are those arising from the ribs or may grow from within the thorax, e.g., parietal carcinoma of the lungs, endothelioma of the pleura, etc. If the swelling is pulsatile, note whether it is an expansile or transmitted pulsation. An expansile pulsating swelling is probably an *aneurysm*.

6. **Sinus:** Single sinus is mostly due to bursting of a long-standing *cold abscess*. Palpate the neighboring ribs for tenderness, irregularity, thickening, etc., to denote the origin of this condition. Multiple sinuses with marked induration may be due to *actinomycosis of the lung*. If they extrude sulfur granules diagnosis is confirmed.

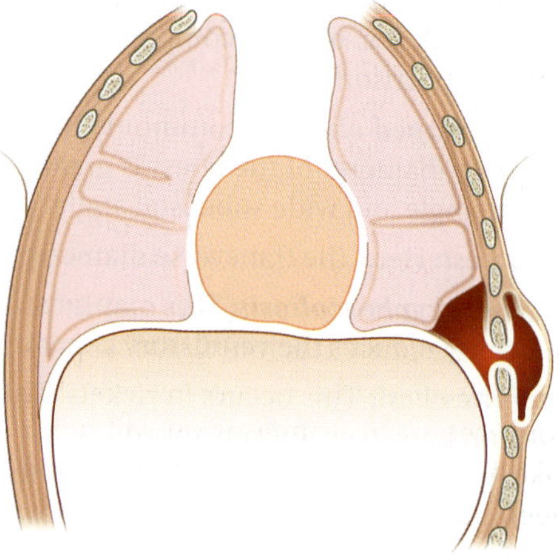

Fig. 29.2: Diagram of empyema necessitatis showing encapsulated pleural empyema, a narrow opening between the ribs through which the empyema has burrowed externally presenting a collection of pus in the subcutaneous tissues giving rise to a fluctuating swelling.

C. PERCUSSION

A dull note over a normally resonant area indicates thickened pleura, pleural effusion, consolidation of the lung or a tumor. Increased resonance suggests pneumothorax or emphysema of the lung. Define the area of cardiac dullness. In pleural effusion the heart may be displaced to the other side.

D. AUSCULTATION

Character of the breath sounds should be noted. *Diminished* breath sounds will be heard in pleural effusion, pneumothorax, hemothorax, etc., whereas *increased* breath sound will be heard in consolidation. Note the nature of vocal resonance.

E. EXAMINATION OF LYMPH NODES

The axillary group or the supraclavicular group may be involved in carcinoma of the lung. This denotes grave prognosis.

F. GENERAL EXAMINATION

When a cold abscess is present on the chest wall examine the spine for Pott's disease.

SPECIAL INVESTIGATIONS

1. **Aspiration:** Note the character of the fluid after aspiration. This often gives a clue to the diagnosis. Presence of blood in unknown cases of pleural effusion indicates malignant disease. In empyema note whether the fluid is turbid or thick pus. It should be sent for culture and sensitivity tests.

2. **X-ray examination:** (a) A straight film is of great value in detecting a bony lesion, pleural effusion, air or blood in the pleural cavity, aneurysm, bronchial carcinoma, mediastinal tumor, etc. In case of bronchial carcinoma it may show a hilar or peripheral shadow and features of obstructive emphysema, atelectasis or consolidation as secondary changes. (b) In chronic empyema with a sinus, *injection of lipiodol followed by skiagraphy* will show the position and extent of the empyema cavity. In bronchopleural fistula, if a few crystals of Sudan III are added

to the injected lipiodol, the sputum is colored pink. (c) *Bronchography* is done by injecting a radio-opaque substance, e.g., neohydriol, into the bronchial tree through the trachea. The 'rat-tail' deformity of the main bronchus is pathognomonic of carcinoma of the bronchus. Diagnosis of bronchiectasis can also be made with certainty by this method. (d) *Tomography* is very helpful in studying a cavity inside a dense shadow which is not clearly visualized in an ordinary film. Skiagram is taken while the tube is moving in one direction and the film in the opposite direction, so that all the objects above and below the cavity throw blurred shadows but the cavity stands out clearly. This will also help in demonstrating enlarged mediastinal nodes and lung cancer. (e) *Skiagraphy after barium swallow* may show deviation of the oesophagus in the case of mediastinal deposits.

3. **Bronchoscopy:** This is an important investigation so far as bronchogenic carcinoma is concerned. This examination will reveal the lesion which is centrally placed. It also helps to take a biopsy from the tumor under vision. Bronchoscopy gives useful information regarding operability of the tumor. Widening of the carina, involvement of the main bronchus within 1.5 cm from the carina, compression of the trachea and paralysis of the vocal cord are the features of nonoperability. This examination, of course, fails to reveal any lesion in the segmental division of the upper bronchus and the peripheral lesions. Cytology study can be performed by bronchial washing and brushing through bronchoscopy. Even biopsy specimen may be taken through bronchoscopy.

4. **Laryngoscopy:** A left-sided paralysis suggests a tumor under the arch of the aorta whereas a right-sided paralysis indicates an apical tumor spreading below the subclavian artery.

5. **Mediastinoscopy:** Through a small incision just above the sternum the instrument is introduced to know involvement of the mediastinal structures particularly the lymph nodes.

6. **Cytological examination:** In carcinoma of the lung, the sputum or the aspirated material from the pleura can be examined histologically for malignant cells by papanicolaou's technique.

7. **Scalene node biopsy**—is done as a routine in certain centers. Involvement excludes the possibility of radical operation.

8. **C.T. scan** is extremely helpful in detection of pulmonary metastasis. It can detect small pulmonary nodules, identifies enlarged mediastinal nodes. It is used to stage carcinoma of lung.

9. **Screening of diaphragm** will give a clue whether the phrenic nerve has been involved or not.

10. **Liver, brain** and **bone scanning** should be done if these organs are suspected to be involved.

11. **Lung function test** is very important and always done before operation.

12. **Exploratory thoracotomy** should be performed if an early diagnosis and radical extirpation are desired.

DIFFERENTIAL DIAGNOSIS

SOLID SWELLINGS OF THE THORACIC WALL

These are the usual *tumors of the skin, subcutaneous tissue* and *bone*. Tumors of the rib and nerve deserve special mention. Other group of swelling is *costochondritis* be it tubercular or nonspecific.

Rib tumors may be primary or secondary. Primary rib tumor may be a chondroma, osteoma, osteoclastoma, chondrosarcoma, osteosarcoma, etc. Secondary carcinoma of rib may be seen in cancer of the breast, bronchus, suprarenal, prostate, kidney, etc. In case of benign tumors swelling and deformity are the main symptoms. In case of malignant tumors pain and tenderness are often come across, which become more obvious in case of secondary growths.

Two types of *tumors of the nerve* may be seen in the thorax. Neurofibroma arising from the intercostal nerves and ganglioneuroma from the sympathetic chain. The former appears close to the neck of the rib while the latter lies more medially close to the vertebral bodies. These tumors are detected by straight X-ray as they tend to erode the adjacent ribs and the vertebrae. Some may extend through the intervertebral foramina into the neural canal. Here, they may press upon the spinal cord to cause paraplegia.

Costochondritis is nothing but a swelling at the junction of a rib and the costal cartilage. Pain is quite prominent which attracts attention towards the swelling. This swelling must not be confused with the breast swelling as the whole of the breast can be moved over the swelling.

CYSTIC SWELLINGS OF THE THORACIC WALL

By far the most important in this group is the cold abscess. Empyema necessitatis and hernia of the lung are rare entities.

Cold abscess mainly originates from the tuberculous lymphadenitis of the posterior mediastinal group of lymph nodes in front of the necks of the ribs or the internal mammary group or from the Pott's disease affecting the vertebrae. Only rarely perinephric abscess may burrow superficially to give rise to an abscess in the posterior aspect. Cold abscess in the chest wall is usually seen along the anterior axillary line and the parasternal line. This is because of the fact that the abscess follows the lateral and the anterior cutaneous branches of the intercostal nerves to become superficial.

Empyema necessitatis means pus of the empyema burrows to the chest wall and becomes superficial either in the lateral or anterior aspect (*See* **Fig. 29.2**). This is mostly seen between 3rd and 6th intercostal spaces. This condition is diagnosed by presence of impulse on coughing and reducibility.

Hernia of the lung is very rare and seen usually at the root of the neck behind the clavicle.
It is a tympanitic cystic swelling which can be reduced completely.

SINUS OF THE CHEST WALL

Three types of sinuses may be seen—1. chronic empyema sinus; 2. sinus following cold abscess and 3. actinomycotic sinus. The last named sinus is extremely rare.

1. *Chronic empyema sinus* only develops when the empyema cavity was drained but (a) drainage was ineffective or (b) presence of foreign body within the empyema cavity or (c) there is some underlying lung pathology.

2. *Cold abscess sinus* develops from an inadvertent attempt to drain a cold abscess or a long-standing cold abscess ultimately burrows superficially and drains itself forming a sinus.

3. *Actinomycotic sinus* is usually multiple. Surrounding induration, dusky hue and linear puckering of the skin are the characteristic features of this condition. It must be remembered that most often it is secondary to actinomycosis elsewhere.

EMPYEMA

It is a collection of pus in the pleural cavity. It may be an acute or chronic empyema.

Acute empyema: In this condition there is profound toxemia and shock with pleural pain. Collection of pleural fluid is the diagnostic point, which should be confirmed by needle aspiration. Chest X-ray will confirm the diagnosis.

Chronic empyema: This is a localized empyema walled off by a thick wall. It results from mismanagement of an acute empyema or due to underlying pathology in the lung, e.g., bronchiectasis, lung tumor, etc. The symptoms are usually vague like ill health, febrile bouts, malaise, etc. Chronic empyema may develop due to delay in drainage of acute empyema. A chronic empyema ultimately may discharge outside continuously or intermittently through a sinus in the chest wall. Persistence of chronic empyema may result from either bronchopleural fistula or tuberculosis of the lung or the bronchiectasis or lung abscess or foreign body or rib sequestrum. Diagnosis is established by finding pus with an exploring needle and chest X-ray. If iodized oil is injected into the empyema and subsequent radiographs are taken, the cavity will be outlined.

LUNG ABSCESS

It is a localized area of suppuration and cavitation in the lung. It usually occurs as a result of aspiration of a bit of septic debris from the oropharynx (with gingivodental disease or oral sepsis) into the lung. Such aspiration may occur during periods of unconsciousness from general anesthesia, alcoholism, cerebral vascular accident, epilepsy or immersion. Direct route of the infected aspirated embolus in supine position is through the right main bronchus to the superior division of the right lower lobe or posterior segment of the right upper lobe. So these two segments are the common sites of primary lung abscesses. The organisms responsible for this disease are alpha- and beta-hemolytic streptococci, staphylococci, nonhemolytic streptococci, E. Coli and anaerobic bacteria. *Common presentations* are cough, foul- smelling sputum, fever, chest pain, weight loss and night sweats. *Chest X-ray* (thoracic roentgenogram) is not always diagnostic particularly in early stages. In erect posture or lateral decubitus position air fluid level is diagnostic. *CT Scan* is more helpful in delineating the abscess.

BRONCHIECTASIS

This means dilatation of bronchi. Bronchial obstruction, and dilatation and infection beyond the obstruction are the reasons. Bronchial obstruction may result from a foreign body, plug of tenacious mucopurulent material, tumor and extra bronchial occlusion by lymph nodes. Mucopurulent material fills the bronchi beyond the obstruction with subsequent infection of the bronchial wall with destruction of its muscle and elastic tissue. It is a disease of young people before 20 years of age. As bronchi of children are small, obstruction occurs easily. Cough with purulent expectoration, hemoptysis and recurrent localized pneumonitis are the main clinical manifestations. Bronchoscopy and bronchography are helpful to diagnose this condition.

CARCINOMA OF THE LUNG

Carcinoma originates from the primary or secondary bronchus or peripherally from small bronchi. There is no pathognomonic symptom, but a patient complaining of vague symptoms with heavy smoking habit should be suspected of this condition. The patient may complain of cough, hemoptysis, dyspnea, pain in the chest, loss of weight and appetite and wheezing. Finger clubbing is a frequent sign. Any of the above symptoms appearing in a middle-aged person should demand further investigation. In majority of cases the disease starts with influenza-like symptoms. Only a minority of cases start with haemoptysis. Symptoms often simulate those of chronic bronchitis and the clinician wastes valuable time in treating the condition as one of chronic bronchitis. Atelectasis or emphysema may be presented with as these are the obstructive features of a carcinoma of the bronchus. Pleural effusion may be present which may be sanguineous.

Patient may present first with secondary deposits. Deposits in the bone may lead to aching and even pathological fracture. Enlarged stony hard lymph nodes may be seen in the neck and axilla. Recurrent laryngeal nerve paralysis in the absence of thyroid cancer should arouse suspicion of this condition. Pancoast's tumor commences from the apex of the lung and is a type of peripheral tumor. It produces a syndrome known as "Pancoast's syndrome". This comprises Horner's syndrome (ptosis, miosis, enophthalmos and anhidrosis) due to pressure on the sympathetic chain, distension of the veins of the face, neck and thorax due to pressure on the superior vena cava and shooting pain down the arm due to pressure on the nerve trunks of brachial plexus. Later on paralysis of the lower brachial plexus develops.

IMPORTANT POSTOPERATIVE CHEST COMPLICATIONS

1. **Aspiration pneumonia:** Sometimes following general anesthesia, unconsciousness or semiconscious patient vomits and inhales the vomitus. A surgeon may be called to a dyspneic patient recovering from general anesthesia. Smell of vomitus from the mouth and presence of some of it on the pillow may clinch the diagnosis. Open the mouth, draw forward the tongue and insert a finger far back into the laryngopharynx to look out a piece of food or denture. A bronchoscope may be used if this method fails to remove anything in the trachea or main bronchus to save the patient.

2. **Atelectasis (collapse) of the lung:** This is the most frequent postoperative pulmonary complication. This is essentially blockage of some part of the bronchial tree with inspissated mucus plug. In 80% of cases atelectasis occurs in the right lung and within 1–2 days following operation. Infection often occurs in the uninflated portion of the lung. Three varieties are usually seen:

a. *Lobular or segmental atelectasis*: Basal part is usually affected. There is little or no constitutional disturbance. The most important early sign is presence of sonorous rhonchi over the base. Cough and pyrexia are only seen when infection supervenes. If untreated this condition is followed by bronchopneumonia and is called 'postoperative pneumonia'.

b. *Lobar atelectasis*: This is characterized by rise of temperature, dyspnea and chest pain. On examination, there is limited movement of respiration on the affected side.

c. *Massive atelectasis (collapse)*: This occurs when a plug of mucus obstructs the main bronchus, commonly the left one. There is absolutely no respiratory movement of the affected side. Trachea is displaced to the side of lesion. The apex beat is shifted to the side of lesion. The sternal head of the sternomastoid muscle of the affected side becomes more tense than its fellow as this is an accessory muscle of respiration. This is known as 'Sternomastoid sign'. Cyanosis of the nail beds is almost always seen.

3. **Pulmonary embolism:** This condition is a contributing factor in the deaths of even a large number of patients than previously. Mortality from this complication following surgical procedures is about 0.11%. More importantly, the clinical diagnosis was frequently not made or even considered. To the contrary it should be remembered that the clinical findings alone are insufficient to establish a diagnosis of pulmonary embolism. These findings resemble those of other serious cardio-respiratory diseases. Therefore before starting medical or surgical treatment

for pulmonary embolism, an objective diagnosis should be established either by perfusion lung scan or by pulmonary arteriography.

Dyspnea, chest pain, hemoptysis and hypotension are often present. Physical examination may reveal presence of tachycardia, accentuation of the second pulmonary sound and dilatation of the cervical veins. Hypoxia and peripheral cyanosis may be present particularly in severe pulmonary embolism.

The electrocardiographic changes are not specific but should be borne in mind. Enlargement of P waves, ST segment depression and/or T wave inversion especially in leads III, AVF, V_1, V_4 and V_5 may be noticed. The most common abnormality is ST segment depression probably due to accompanying myocardial ischemia.

Chest X-ray may show diminished pulmonary vascular markings, though this finding should not be relied upon for diagnosis, as it returns to normal within 24 hours.

Elevated serum lactic dehydrogenase (LDH activity), increased serum bilirubin concentration and normal serum glutamic oxaloacetic transaminase (SGOT) are often the findings of this condition.

Radioisotope scanning of the lungs is a reliable method for diagnosis of pulmonary embolism. Macroaggregated particles of human serum albumin tagged with ^{131}I (10 to 100 micra) are injected intravenously. These particles lodge in the pulmonary arterioles and capillary bed and a scan delineates the distribution of pulmonary arterial blood flow to the various parts of the lungs.

Pulmonary arteriography is also a reliable test. The filling defects in the large pulmonary arteries are diagnostic.

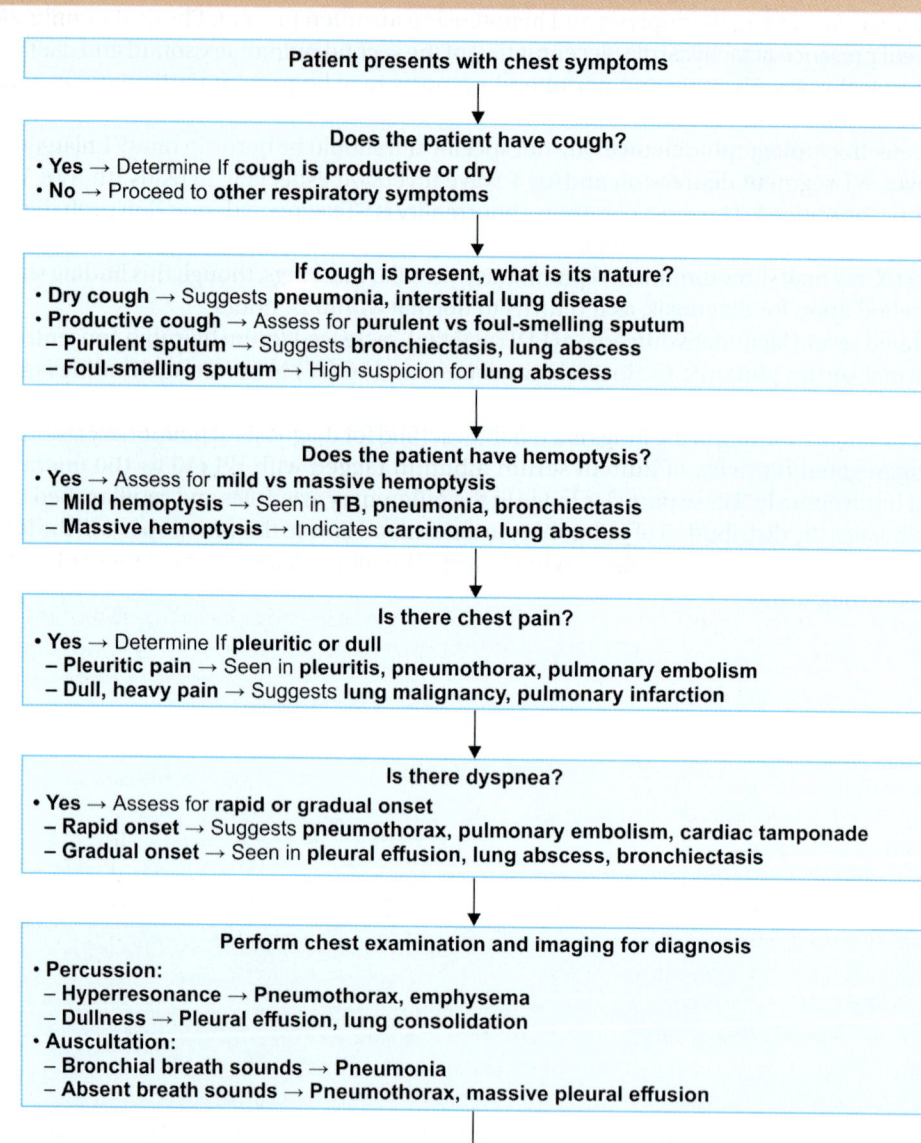

Examination of the Breast

CHAPTER 30

HISTORY

Majority of women who come to the surgical outpatient department complain of either pain or lump in the breast or discharge from the nipple. History is taken in the usual manner as mentioned in the Chapter 1. Here only specific points are discussed.

1. **Age:** Fibroadenoma usually occurs in females below 35 years of age. Fibroadenosis may occur at any age, though more common in the middle age. Intramammary breast abscess is most commonly seen in young lactating women and is often referred to as 'mastitis of lactation'. *Carcinoma of the breast* occurs usually in women above 40 years of age, though rarely it may occur earlier, so age should not be the criterion to exclude the diagnosis of breast carcinoma.

2. **Residence:** Carcinoma of breast and fibroadenosis (mammary dysplasia) are more common in the western world with high incidence in England and Wales. Breast carcinoma is rare in Japan.

3. **Social status:** Carcinoma of breast and fibroadenosis are more seen in the 'developed' world. There may be a link between diets rich in saturated fatty acids and breast carcinoma (in fact majority of breast diseases). Both these diseases are common in nulliparous women and who have refused the intended purpose of the breasts, i.e., breastfeeding. These diseases are less common in 'underdeveloped' world where women give birth to multiple children.

4. **Lump:** The most common mode of presentation of diseases of the breast is 'lump'. Enquiry must be made about its *mode of onset, duration* and *rate of growth*. A lump may develop in the breast following trauma which is either a hematoma or fat necrosis. Trauma may simply attract attention of the patient towards a pre-existing lump. A lump with a long history and slow-growth is a benign condition—either fibroadenosis (mammary dysplasia) or fibroadenoma. A lump with a short history and fast growth is probably a carcinoma, though atrophic scirrhous carcinoma is a slow growing tumor. The average duration between the patient finding the lump and reporting it to a surgeon is about 6 weeks in case of carcinoma of the breast.

5. **Pain:** The student must remember that carcinoma of the breast is a painless condition. A lump which is painless and accidentally felt during washing may be a breast carcinoma and the clinician must be more particular in examining this case rather than ignoring it. Pain is the main complaint of acute mastitis. The pain is of throbbing nature when pus has formed. Pain is also a common complaint in case of fibroadenosis (mammary dysplasia) which becomes aggravated during menstruation. This type of cyclical breast pain is more common in young women with fibroadenosis. In case of fibroadenosis affecting women after menopause there is also localized breast pain which may be due to periductal mastitis or there may be referred pain from musculoskeletal disorders. The students must remember that all neoplasms of the breast—either benign or malignant including carcinoma are painless to start with.

In case of relatively long-standing carcinoma of the breast enquiry must be made regarding pain at the back, hip or shoulder. Patients may ignore their presence considering them to be due to rheumatism and not having any relation with the 'lump of the breast'. Such pain may be due to bony metastasis of the carcinoma of the breast.

6. **Discharge from nipple:** This may be the only complaint which has brought the patient to a surgeon. Fresh blood or altered blood may be discharged in case of duct papilloma or carcinoma. Pus may be discharged in case of mammary abscess. Milk may be discharged during lactation or galactocele or from mammary fistula due to chronic subareolar abscess. Serous or greenish discharge is seen in case of fibroadenosis (mammary dysplasia) and mammary duct ectasia.

7. **Retraction of nipple** may be rarely a complaint which may bring the patient to a surgeon. Retraction for quite a long time or since puberty may be developmental. Recent retraction is of importance and is usually due to underlying carcinoma of the breast.

8. **Loss of weight** is often complained of in case of carcinoma of breast or tuberculosis of breast or chest wall tuberculosis leading to retromammary abscess.

9. **Past history:** Recurrence of abscess is sometimes seen in congenital retraction of nipple. Tuberculosis of breast may recur. Fibroadenosis (mammary dysplasia) may give rise to symptoms after a good gap. So that if asked carefully the patient may confess that similar problems she had a few years back which disappeared with some sort of treatment. Above all it must be remembered that carcinoma may recur in the opposite breast.

10. **Personal history:** Marital status of the patient must be enquired into. Fibroadenosis and carcinoma of breast are more common in unmarried or nulliparous women. Menstrual history must be taken so that relation of pain with menstruation may be assessed. Lactational history should also be taken. Suppurative mastitis particularly occurs in women during first lactational period.

11. **Family history:** Majority of the breast diseases including carcinoma often recur in a family. If especially asked for it may be revealed that the patient's mother or grandmother or sister also suffered from the similar disease.

History in patients with breast diseases

Aspect	Clinical significance	Patient-friendly questions
Age of onset	Young (<30 years) → Likely **fibroadenoma, fibrocystic disease**. Middle-aged (30–50 years) → Consider **fibrocystic disease, intraductal papilloma**. Elderly (>50 years) → High suspicion for **breast carcinoma**	"How old were you when you first noticed the lump?"
Nature of the lump	**Painless, slow-growing, mobile lump** → Suggests **fibroadenoma**. **Tender lump with cyclical pain** → Suggests **fibrocystic disease**. **Rapidly growing, fixed lump with skin dimpling**→ Consider **carcinoma**	"Is the lump painful? Does it move when you press it? Has it changed in size?"

Contd...

Contd...

Aspect	Clinical significance	Patient-friendly questions
Pain in the breast	**Throbbing pain with redness** → Likely **mastitis or abscess**. **Dull, aching pain aggravated by menstruation** → Suggests **fibrocystic disease** **Painless lump initially, later with deep-seated pain**→ Suggests **carcinoma**	"Do you experience pain in your breast? Is it linked to your menstrual cycle?"
Nipple changes and discharge	**Bloody discharge** → Suggests **duct papilloma or carcinoma** **Purulent discharge** → Indicates **breast abscess** **Greenish or serous discharge** → Seen in **fibrocystic disease, duct ectasia**	"Have you noticed any discharge from your nipple? What color is it?"
Family history of breast cancer	**Mother, sister, grandmother with breast carcinoma**→ Increased risk	"Does anyone in your family have breast cancer?"
Previous breast lumps or surgeries	**History of prior lump excision** → May suggest **recurrence or malignancy**	"Have you had any previous breast lumps or surgeries?"

PHYSICAL EXAMINATION

LOCAL EXAMINATION

The patient must be stripped to the waist to expose completely both the breasts before inspection is commenced. There must be adequate privacy so that the patient can be relaxed. The examining area must be well lighted so that subtle changes in the skin can be identified. The examination of breast is performed mainly with the patient in *sitting posture*. This gives more information regarding the level of the nipples **(Fig. 30.1)**, a lump and palpation of the axillary lymph nodes. Examination may also be performed in *semirecumbent* (45°) *position*. This position is a good compromise between lying flat which makes the breasts flatten out and fall sideways, and sitting upright which makes the breasts pendulous and bulky. Examination can also be performed in the *recumbent position* so as to palpate the breasts lump against the chest for more information. If in doubt one can examine the patient in *bending forward position* which gives information regarding retraction of the nipple. Always compare both the breasts in inspection.

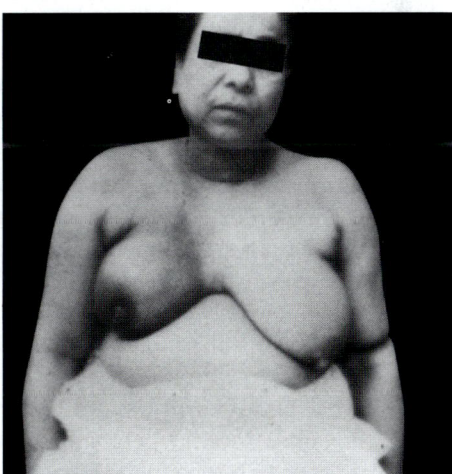

Fig. 30.1: Compare the level of the nipples. The nipple of the right breast is raised.

A. INSPECTION

This is carried out: (i) with the arms by the side of the body, (ii) with the arms raised straight above her head when the lump or dimple may be more marked, (iii) with the hands on her hips pressing and relaxing as the surgeon commands when abnormal movement of the nipple or exaggeration of skin dimples may be evident and lastly (iv) with the patient bending forwards from the waist so that the breasts fall away from the body. Any failure of one nipple to fall away from the chest indicates abnormal fibrosis behind the nipple. Inspection of the whole breast should be done systematically.

1. **Breasts:** Both the breasts are inspected in their entirety and the following points are noted—(i) *Position*—whether displaced in any direction. (ii) *Size* and *shape*—whether larger or smaller than its fellow **(Fig. 30.2)**. Sometimes males breast becomes enlarged—the condition is known as gynecomastia. (iii) *Any puckering or dimpling*? In scirrhous carcinoma the breast may be shrunken and drawn in towards the growth. Dimpling of the skin may be made prominent by lifting the breast gently upwards **(Fig. 30.3)**. In presence of a **swelling** or an **ulcer** determine its position (in relation to four quadrants of the breast), *size, shape* and *surface*.

2. **Skin over the breast:** (i) *Color* and *texture*: In acute mastitis the skin becomes red, warm and edematous. Similar picture may be seen very rarely in acute mastitis carcinomatosa (acute lactational carcinoma). (ii) *Engorged veins*: Presence of engorged veins is commonly seen in large soft fibroadenoma (cystosarcoma phyllodes) and in rapidly growing sarcoma. Engorged veins may also be seen when there is presence of acute lactational mastitis with huge breast abscess. (iii) *Dimple, retraction* or *puckering* is often noticed in scirrhous carcinoma of the breast **(Figs. 30.4 and 30.5)**. (iv) *Peau d' orange* is a classical sign in case of carcinoma of the breast **(Fig. 30.6)**. This is due to blockage of subcuticular lymphatics with edema of the skin which deepens the mouths of the sweat glands and hair follicles giving rise to the typical 'orange peel' appearance. (v) *Nodules* may be observed in the breast which are often metastatic. (vi) *Ulceration* and *fungation*: There may be ulceration in any part of the skin of the breast which are examined according to Chapter 4. Fungation of the skin is a late feature of advanced carcinoma of the breast due to infiltration of the skin by the growth **(Fig. 30.7)**. Fungation may also occur in case of large soft

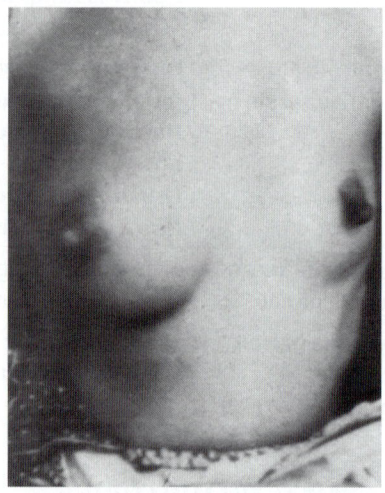

Fig. 30.2: Note congenital asymmetrical breasts. The left breast is abnormally small.

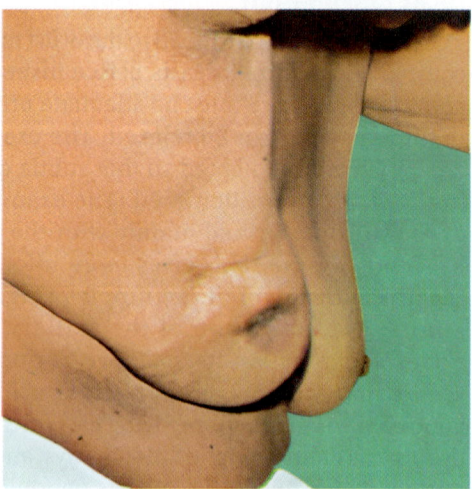

Fig. 30.3: Shows how retraction of nipple due to carcinoma (right side) can be so well detected in bending forward position.

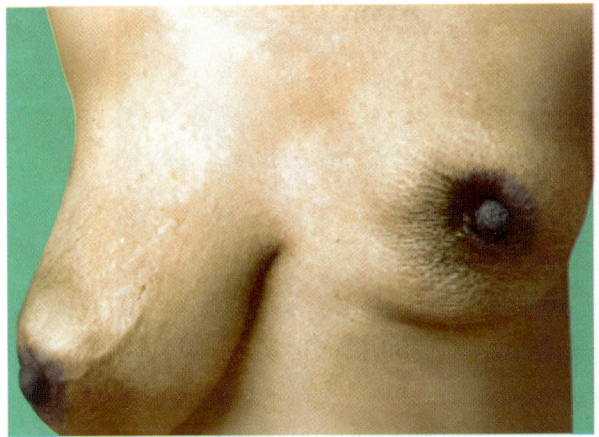

Fig. 30.4: Showing considerable retraction of the left nipple due to carcinoma.

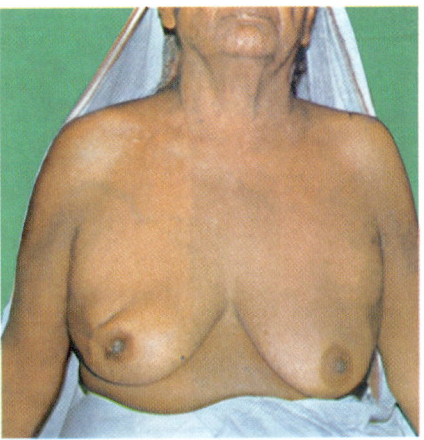

Fig. 30.5: Note how the nipple is retracted towards the carcinomatous lump on the right side. This is even obvious in sitting posture.

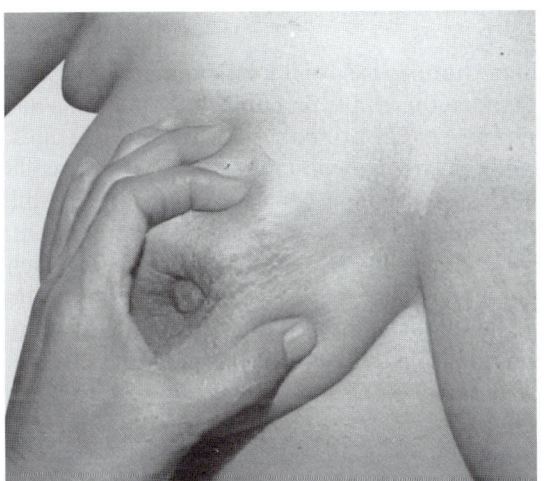

Fig. 30.6: A fine demonstration of peau d' orange.

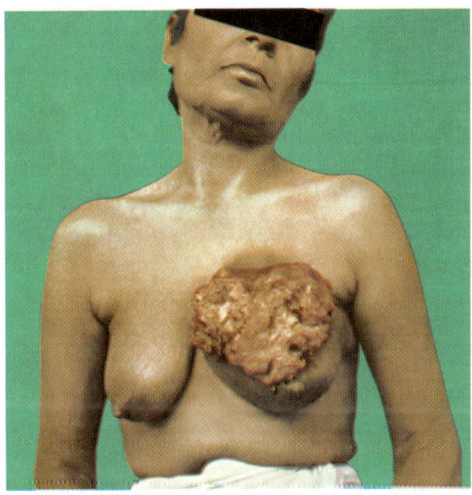

Fig. 30.7: An advanced carcinoma showing fungation and excavation.

fibroadenoma or in a rapidly-growing sarcoma due to the fact that the skin becomes atrophied at the site of maximum pressure over the huge swelling and ultimately gives way so that the growth fungates out. But in this case the skin is not infiltrated. This can be demonstrated by means of a probe which can be passed underneath the skin margin in this case, but this is not possible in case of a fungating carcinoma where the skin is infiltrated.

3. **Nipple:** (i) *Presence*: Are both nipples present and symmetrical or one is retracted or destroyed. (ii) *Its position*: Compare the level of the nipples on both sides **(Fig. 30.8)**. Vertical distance from the clavicle and horizontal distance from the midline should be considered. In carcinoma, nipple of the affected side is drawn up towards the lump. It should be remembered that inflammatory fibrosis may cause similar elevation of the nipple. This elevation of the nipple will be more marked if the patient is asked to raise both the hands above the head

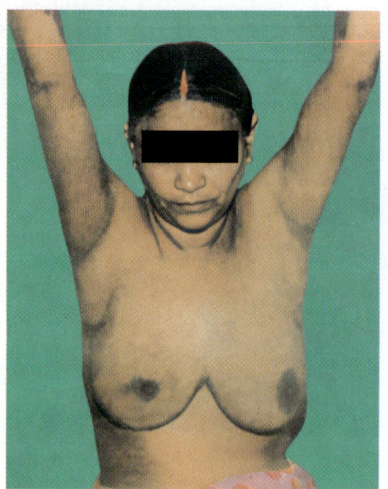
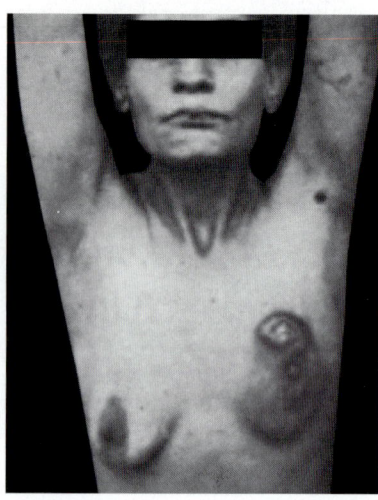

Fig. 30.8: Best method to demonstrate the levels of the nipples. Note slight elevated level on the right side affected by carcinoma.

Fig. 30.9: Note how retraction of the nipple can be made more prominent by raising both hands above the head.

(Fig. 30.9). Nipple may be displaced away from the lump in case of fibroadenoma. Nipple may be destroyed when Paget's disease has almost eroded the nipple or a fungated carcinoma has destroyed the nipple. (iii) *Number*: Accessory nipples may be present besides the normal ones. These are usually found anywhere along the milk line (ridge) which extends from the axilla to the groin. Such accessory nipple has also been seen on the inner aspect of the thigh. Milk may discharge through these nipples also during lactation. (iv) *Size* and *shape*: Is it prominent, flattened or retracted? Prominence of the nipple may be due to an underlying swelling such as a cyst. Slight retraction may be seen since puberty. Recent retraction of the nipple with the onset of the present illness is very much significant. Most often it is due to carcinoma of the breast and occasionally due to chronic inflammation **(Figs. 30.10 to 30.12)**. In Paget's disease, the nipple is completely destroyed, a red and flat ulcer being present in its place. (v) *Surface*: Look for cracks, fissures or eczema. (vi) *Discharge* if any: Note the character (see above). Is the discharge coming from the nipple or from its immediate neighborhood (mammary fistula)?

4. **Areola:** The normal areola is slightly corrugated and contains a few small nodules—Montgomery's glands. These glands become larger during pregnancy when these are known as Montgomery's tubercles. (i) *Color*: The skin of areola of young girl is pale pink, but it becomes slightly darker in adult life. It becomes brown during pregnancy. (ii) *Size*: It becomes larger in case of a huge swelling of soft fibroadenoma or sarcoma. Diminution of the size of the areola is sometimes noticed in scirrhous carcinoma. (iii) *Surface* and *texture*: Look for crack, fissure, ulcer, eczema, swelling or discharge. In Paget's disease, the areola becomes bright red in the early stage and is destroyed leaving a red weeping ulcer later on. It is useful to remember that eczema is usually a bilateral affection, whereas Paget's disease is purely unilateral. As mentioned earlier glands of Montgomery may become hypertrophied during pregnancy and lactation to produce small swellings here. This is not a pathological condition. Occasionally Montgomery's gland may be enlarged forming a retention cyst similar to a sebaceous cyst. Such cyst may become infected.

5. **Arm and thorax:** After completing inspection of the breast a quick look at the arm of the affected side and the thoracic wall may be well informatory. *'Cancer en cuirasse,'* i.e., multiple

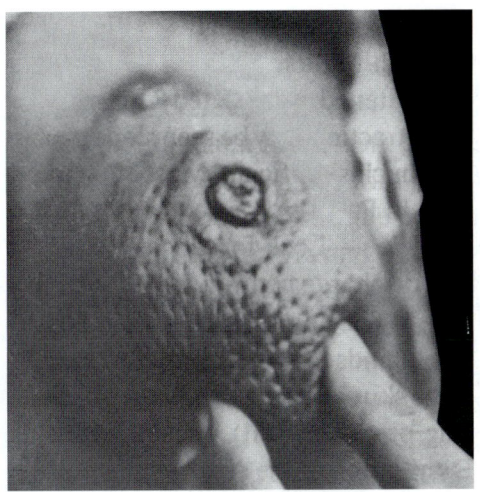

Fig. 30.10: Note retraction of the left nipple due to presence of carcinoma at the upper and outer quadrant shown by an arrow. One can detect a swelling there.

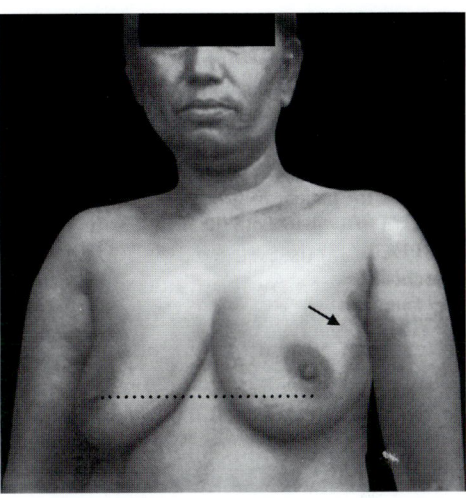

Fig. 30.11: A fine demonstration of 'peau d' orange'.

cancerous nodules and thicken infiltrated skin like a coat of armour may be seen in the arm and the thoracic wall. *Brawny edema* of the arm may be due to extensive neoplastic infiltration of the axillary lymph nodes. It is mainly due to lymphatic blockage. Edematous arm may also be seen after radical mastectomy. It is also a feature of lymphatic obstruction, but infection may play a contributory role.

6. **Axilla and supraclavicular fossa:** These regions should particularly be inspected for any swelling due to enlarged lymph nodes. The students must make a habit of inspecting these regions, so that he should never ignore these regions. Subsequently he has to palpate these regions.

7. **The patient is asked to raise her arms above her head.** This is the last part of inspection and should not be missed. The change in the shape of the breast caused by lifting the arms often reveals lumps, puckering and distortion, not visible when the arms are by the sides. This action also reveals the lower surfaces of the breasts. If the submammary fold is still not visible, lift up the breast and inspect it. This may reveal a swelling which was missed so long, as also skin nodules (metastatic) or presence of any skin disease. In this position the clinician should inspect the axillae properly for swelling, skin puckering and ulceration. The shoulder movements are also noticed which may be affected by lymph node enlargement in the axilla.

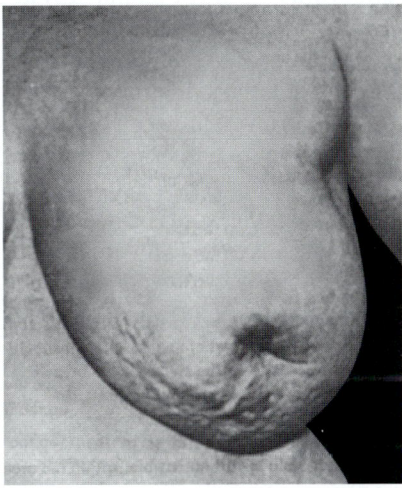

Fig. 30.12: Retraction of nipple with peau d' orange is clearly seen in a case of carcinoma of the left breast.

B. **PALPATION**

Palpation should be made initially in sitting position, in semirecumbent (45°) position and later on in recumbent position. It is advantageous to put a small pillow under the scapula on the side to be examined, so that the breast concerned rests evenly on the chest wall and does not fall to the side of the body. Sometimes it is necessary to put her arm above her head during palpation.

It is advisable to **palpate the normal breast first.** The texture of the breast varies from woman to woman. In some it is soft and smooth when it is quite difficult to distinguish the glandular tissue from the subcutaneous tissue; whereas in others it is firm lobulated with nodularity. Palpation should be made with **palmar surface of the fingers (Fig. 30.13)** with the hand flat and not with the 'flat of the hand' as this means with the palm of the hand which is not correct. Palpation should also be made between the pulps of the fingers and the thumb to know more about a swelling. The normal breast gives a firm lobulated impression with nodularity. **Now the affected side is palpated** in a similar fashion keeping in mind the findings of the normal side and comparing them with those of the affected side. The **four quadrants** should be palpated systematically. Also feel the *axillary tail.* Do not miss to palpate just *behind the nipple.*

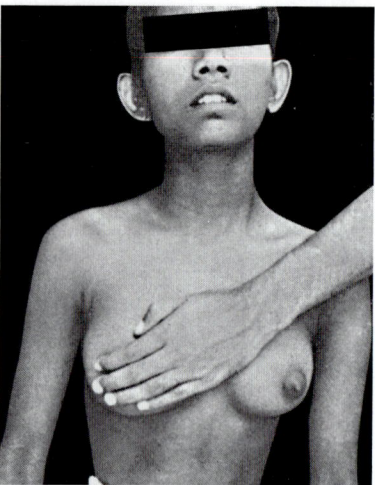

Fig. 30.13: Palpating the breast with the palmar surface of the fingers with the hand flat. Remember breast carcinoma is best felt with this method and with the flat of the hand.

There may be a small lump here and no other abnormality in the whole of the breast. This will be missed if the students do not make habit of this examination as a routine. While palpating this region an eye must be kept on the nipple—whether any discharge is being expressed out of the nipple or not. In case of duct papilloma or duct carcinoma blood will come out.

If any lump is detected in this examination, it should be felt by the palmar surfaces of the fingers with the hand flat. Remember, breast cancer is best felt by the hand flat, which being less sensitive fails to feel any other lump than carcinoma (e.g., fibroadenosis, fibroadenoma, etc.).

If a lump is detected the following points should be noted:
1. **Local temperature and tenderness:** Local temperature is best felt by the back of the fingers. A warm and tender swelling is generally inflammatory in origin, but one should keep in mind acute mastitis carcinomatosa which may present the similar features.
2. **Situation** (in which quadrant): Carcinoma can occur anywhere in the breast including the axillary tail (a prolongation of breast tissue into the axilla), but is commonly found in the upper and outer quadrant. Fibroadenosis also occurs more often in the upper and outer quadrant and in the axillary tail. Fibroadenoma is more commonly seen in the lower half than in the upper half though it may occur in any part of the breast.
3. **Number:** Though majority of the breast lesions are solitary, yet fibroadenosis is known for its multiplicity. Multiple lumps are felt. Even the opposite breast may be affected.
4. **Size and shape:** Whether globular (fibroadenoma) or uneven (carcinoma).
5. **Surface:** Smooth surface is a feature of benign condition, whereas an uneven surface is a significant feature of carcinoma.
6. **Margin:** In case of fibroadenosis the margin is ill-defined. In case of fibroadenoma (a firm tumor within the soft tissue) and more so in carcinoma (stony hard tumor within the soft surrounding) the margin is well defined. In fibroadenoma the margin is regular and tends to slip off the palpating fingers, whereas in carcinoma the margin is very much irregular and does not tend to slip away from the palpating fingers as it is fixed to the breast tissue.

7. **Consistency:** Consistency of the lump must be assessed properly—whether cystic, firm, hard or stony hard. In case of soft cystic swelling test for fluctuation. A firm, sotty or diffuse India-rubber feel is characteristic of fibroadenosis. A fibroadenoma is a firm encapsulated tumor, whereas carcinoma is stony hard in consistency. In case of sarcoma consistency may vary from place to place.

8. **Fluctuation:** A cystic swelling should be tested for fluctuation **(Fig. 30.14)**. The clinician stands behind the patient, who sits on a stool. His two hands should go above the patient's shoulder. With one hand he holds the cyst and with index finger of the other hand gentle tap is made on the center of the cyst. Besides a cyst the fluctuation test will be positive in chronic abscess (it may not be tender) and lipoma. A very tense cyst may not show fluctuation test positive.

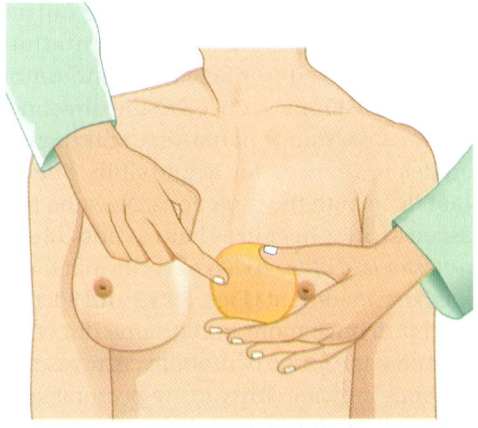

Fig. 30.14: Shows the method to elicit fluctuation in a case of a breast lump. The examination is carried out from behind. With one hand using two fingers the lump is held by the sides (watching fingers) and kept fixed, whereas with index finger of the other hand (displacing finger) the center of the lump is pressed to displace fluid within the lump.

9. **Transillumination test:** This can only be effectively carried out in a dark room. The torch is placed on the undersurface of the breast so that the light is directed through the breast tissue to the examiner. Fat is translucent but a solid tumor is opaque.

10. **Fixity to the skin:** This can be tested in the following ways: (i) An attempt to move the tumor side to side or up and down will make the appearance of dimpling or tethering of the skin; (ii) the skin is made to slide over the tumor which is not possible; (iii) the skin over the tumor is pinched up, this is also not possible if the tumor is fixed to the skin. When a wide area of the skin over the tumor is attempted to pinch up, peau d' orange will become prominent. Hard nodules may be felt in the skin in late stage of breast cancer as part of cancer-en-cuirase.

Two terms must be understood in this respect—*'Tethered'* to the skin and *'fixed'* to the skin. (i) The term *'tethered'* to the skin means that the malignant disease has spread to the fine fibrous septae that pass from the glandular tissue of the breast to the skin. These are called Astley Cooper's ligament. Infiltration of these strands makes them shorter and inelastic and thus pull the skin inwards resulting in puckering of the skin. The lump at this stage can still be moved independently of the skin for some distance after which this may cause puckering of the skin. So tethering of the lump to the skin can be tested by moving the lump side to side and watching if the skin dimples at the extremes of movement. (ii) *'Fixity'* means that there is direct and continuous infiltration of the skin by the tumor and the tumor cannot be moved independent of the skin and the overlying skin cannot be pinched up.

It must be remembered that any tumor lying immediately deep to the nipple will be fixed to the nipple be it benign or malignant as the main mammary ducts may have traveled through the growth and so the nipple becomes fixed.

11. **Fixity to the breast tissue:** This is demonstrated by holding the breast tissue with one hand and gently moving the tumor with other hand. A fibroadenoma is not fixed to the breast tissue and can be easily moved within the breast substance. That is why it is called a 'Breast mouse'. A carcinoma on the other hand is fixed to the breast substance and cannot be moved within it. Fibrous strands can be felt radiating from the mass into the breast substance.

12. **Fixity to the underlying fascia and muscles** (pectoralis major and serratus anterior): The patient is asked to place her hand on her hip lightly. The lump is moved in the direction of the fibers of pectoralis major first and then at right angles to them as far as possible. The lump is mobile in both the directions. Now the patient is asked to press her hip as hard as possible. *Feel the anterior fold of the axilla* to verify that the muscle has been made taut (**Figs. 30.15 and 30.16**). Move the lump once more in the same directions and compare the range of mobility. Any restriction in mobility indicates fixity to the pectoral fascia and pectoralis major. There will be total restriction of mobility along the line of the muscle fibers if it is fixed to it but slight movement along the right angle of the fibers may be possible.

A swelling occupying the outer and lower quadrant of the breast will lie on serratus anterior, to which it may be fixed. This is ascertained by asking the patient to push against a wall with the outstretched hand of the affected side while the mobility of the swelling is tested. The swelling, if fixed to serratus anterior, will move very little.

13. **Fixity to the chest wall:** If the tumor is fixed irrespective of contraction of any muscle, it is fixed to the chest wall.

14. **Palpation of the nipple:** It is very important to palpate the nipple and the breast tissue just deep to the nipple. Tumor just deep to the nipple is usually fixed to the nipple. The underlying lump is moved and see if this movement causes or increases nipple retraction. Gentle pressing of such tumor may express discharge from the nipple. Note its color and nature. Note whether it appears from one or many ducts. When the discharge is visible, try to decide its nature—whether blood, serum, pus or milk. Take the bacteriological swab for culture. The source of such discharge must be found out by gently pressing on each segment of the breast and areola. If the nipple is *retracted*, press gently from both sides deep to the nipple. This will evert it if the retraction is congenital or spontaneous. If it is due to carcinoma the nipple cannot be everted like this.

If there is any **ulcer**, examine it as discussed in Chapter 4.

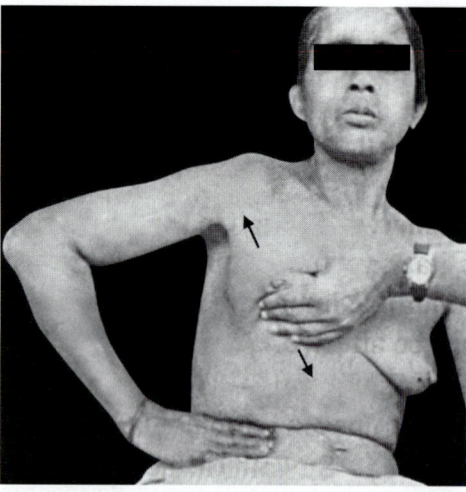

Fig. 30.15: Testing a lump in the breast for fixity to the pectoralis major by moving the lump in the direction of its fibers while the muscle is made taut by asking the patient to press her hip as hard as she can.

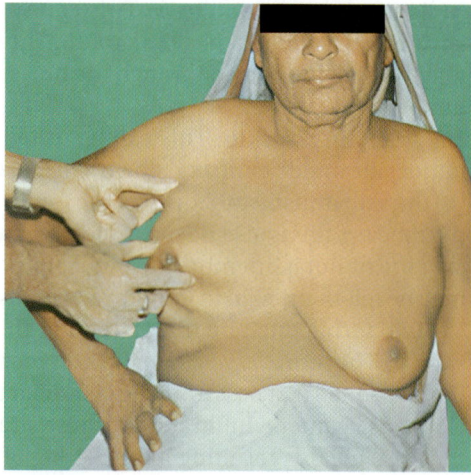

Fig. 30.16: See how to examine for fixity of the breast lump with the pectoralis muscle or pectoral fascia.

EXAMINATION OF LYMPH NODES

This examination is very important. On the finding of this examination the staging of the breast cancer can be judged as also the prognosis. This examination is carried out in sitting position. The muscles and fasciae around the axilla should be relaxed. If this cannot be properly achieved this examination can be done in lying down position.

A. **Palpation of the axillary group of lymph nodes**

1. **PECTORAL GROUP:** This group is situated just behind the anterior axillary fold. The patient's arm is elevated and using the right hand for the left side the fingers are insinuated behind the pectoralis major. The arm is now lowered and made rest on the clinician's forearm **(Fig. 30.17)**. This will relax the pectoralis minor. With the pulps of the fingers try to palpate the lymph nodes. The palm should look forward. The thumb of the same hand is used to push the pectoralis major backwards from the front **(Fig. 30.18)**. This facilitates palpation.

2. **BRACHIAL GROUP:** This group lies on the lateral wall of the axilla in relation to the axillary vein. To palpate this group left hand is used for the left side. The group is felt with the palm directed laterally against the upper end of the humerus (*see* **Fig. 30.22**).

3. **SUBSCAPULAR GROUP:** This lies on the posterior axillary fold and is best examined from behind. Standing behind the patient the examiner palpates the anterointernal surface of the posterior fold while with the other hand the patient's arm is semilifted. Now the nodes are palpated lying on this surface with the palm of the examining hand looking backwards **(Fig. 30.19A)**.

Figure 30.20 shows the lymphatic drainage and blood spread in case of carcinoma breast.

Method of examination for various groups of lymph nodes involvement in carcinoma of the breast (Figs. 30.21 to 30.25). See the text.

4. **CENTRAL GROUP:** This group of the left side is examined with the right hand. At first the patient's arm is slightly abducted and pass the extended fingers right up to the apex of the axilla directing the palm towards the lateral thoracic wall. The patient's arm is now brought to the side of her body and the forearm rests comfortably on the clinician's forearm. The other hand of the clinician is now placed on the opposite shoulder to steady the patient. Palpation is carried out by sliding the fingers against the chest wall when the lymph nodes can be felt to slip out from the fingers **(Fig. 30.24)**.

5. **APICAL GROUP:** Examination is carried out in the same manner as the previous one, but the fingers are pushed further up. If the lymph nodes are very much enlarged they may push themselves through the clavipectoral fascia to be felt through the pectoralis major just below the clavicle.

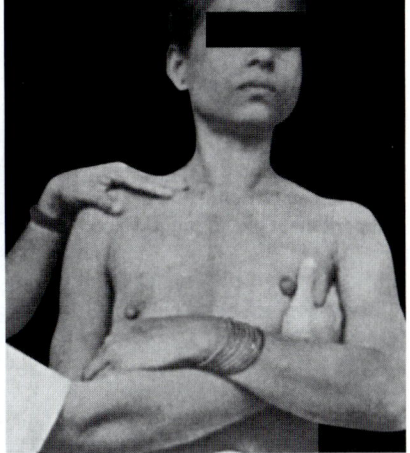

Fig. 30.17: Show the position of the arm while examining the lymph nodes of the axilla. Note that the arm is adducted and allowed to rest comfortably on the clinician's forearm.

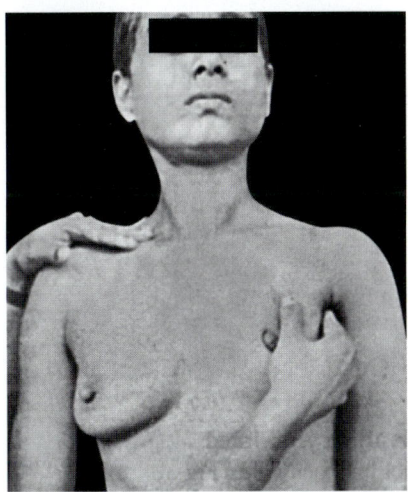

Fig. 30.18: Method of palpation of the pectoral group of lymph nodes.

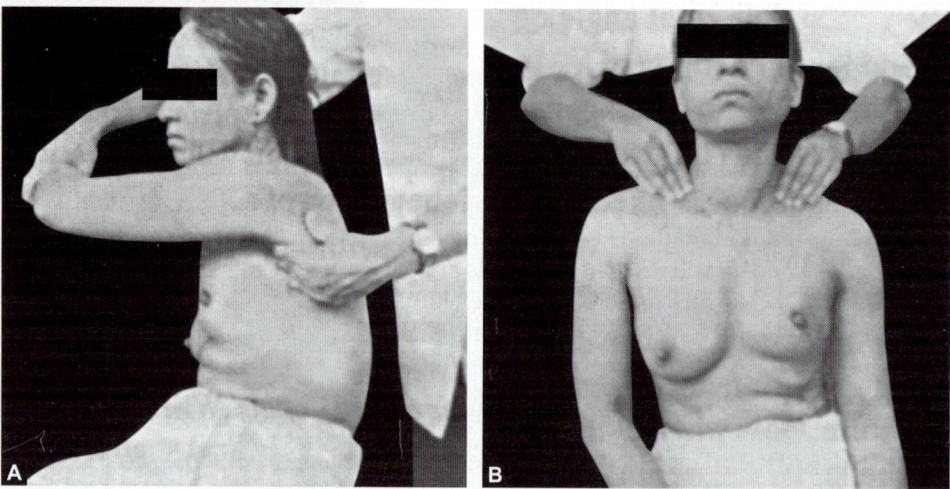

Figs. 30.19A and B: Method of palpation of the subscapular and supraclavicular group of lymph nodes.

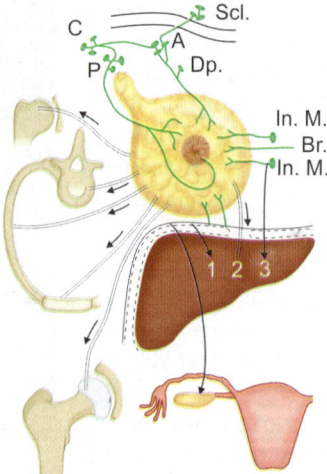

Fig. 30.20: Diagrammatic representation of lymphatic drainage (single line) and blood spread (double line) in carcinoma of the breast. Lymphatic drainage from the subareolar plexus of Sappey and outer quadrant of the breast takes place first to the pectoral (P), then central (C) and lastly to the apical (A) group of axillary lymph nodes. The other two groups of the axillary nodes, viz. the subscapular and lateral group may be involved in a retrograde way. From the apical group the supraclavicular group may be affected. On the left side the supraclavicular group is affected by retrograde permeation. The upper quadrant of the breast drains partly to the deltopectoral node but mainly to the apical group. From the inner quadrant the lymph spread occurs to the internal mammary group (In. M) and to the other breast (Br). From the lower and inner parts of the breast the lymph vessels form a plexus over the rectus sheath and pierce the costal margin to communicate with the subperitoneal lymph plexus. From this place, cancer cells may drop by gravity into the pelvis (transcoelomic implantation) and may cause metastases in the ovary (Krukenberg's tumor). It may be noted that the liver may be involved in two ways—subperitoneal plexus and by blood spread.

Blood spread—occurs in addition to the liver, to the bones, especially to the sternum, ribs, spine and upper ends of the humerus and femur. Lungs may be affected.

B. Palpation of cervical lymph nodes

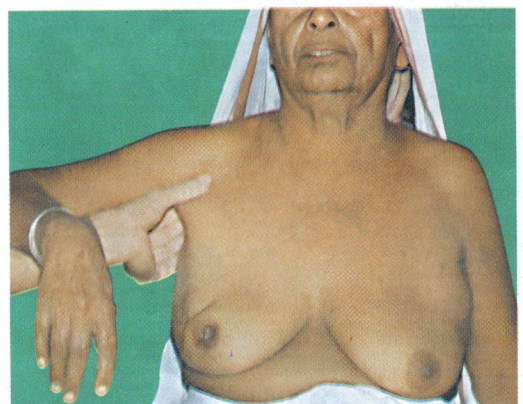

Fig. 30.21: Pectoral group.

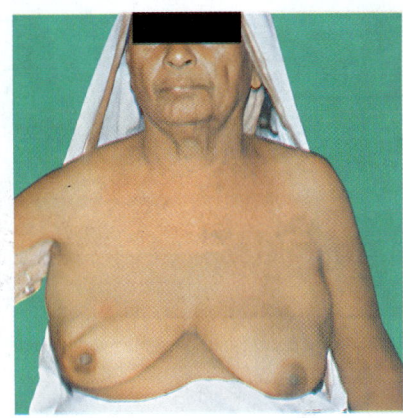

Fig. 30.22: Brachial group.

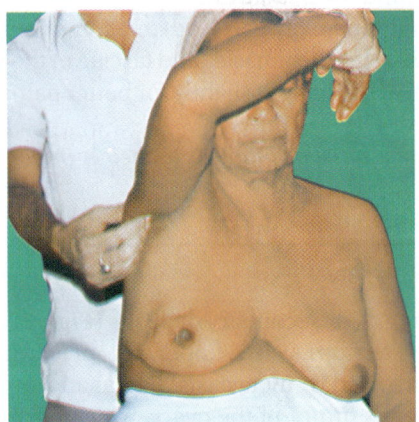

Fig. 30.23: Subscapular group.

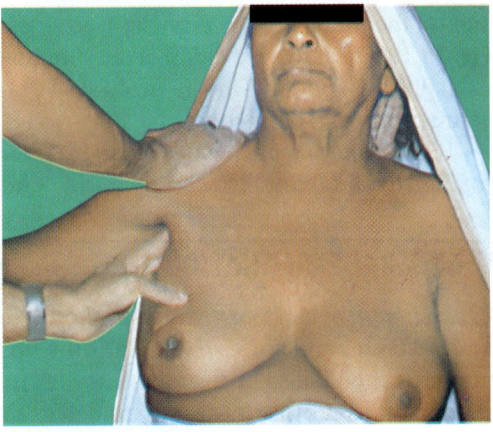

Fig. 30.24: Central group.

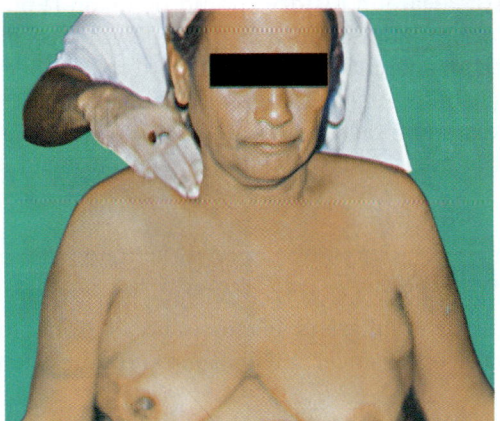

Fig. 30.25: Supraclavicular group (both sides should be palpated).

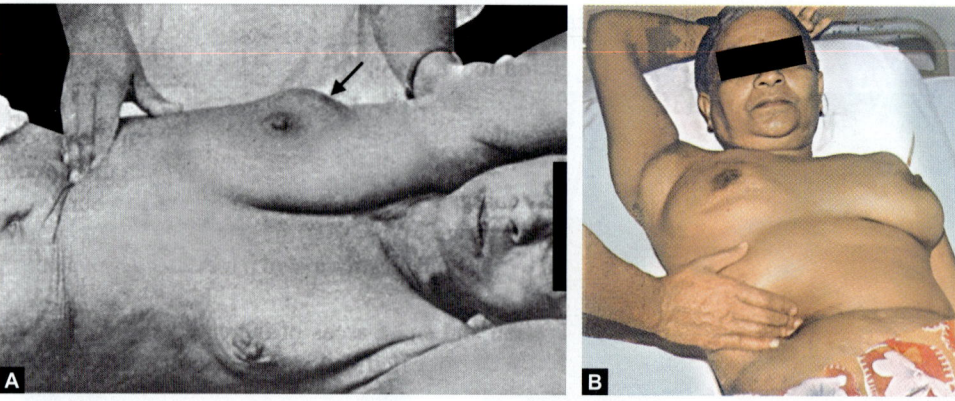

Figs. 30.26A and B: (A) Examining the liver in a case of carcinoma of the right breast; (B) The best method of palpation of liver in case of carcinoma of the breast.

One must always examine the *supraclavicular group* to conclude the examination of the lymph nodes. To examine this group the clinician stands behind the patient and dips the fingers down behind the middle of the clavicle. Two sides are simultaneously palpated and compared (*see* **Fig. 30.19B**). Passive elevation of the shoulders would relax the muscles and fasciae of the neck to facilitate palpation. One must always flex the neck of the patient slightly for better palpation of this group of lymph nodes.

While palpating the lymph nodes careful assessment must be made as to their number, size, consistency, mobility, etc., as discussed in Chapter 8.

GENERAL EXAMINATION

In *carcinoma of the breast*, the **liver** should be examined for secondary deposits **(Figs. 30.26A and B)**. **Lungs** and **bones** particularly the ribs, spine, sternum, pelvis, upper ends of femur and humerus should also be examined as they may be involved by metastasis. **Rectal** and **vaginal** examinations are also necessary to detect Krukenberg's tumor of the ovary, which occurs by transcoelomic implantation or lymphatic permeation.

In *gynecomazia* firstly a careful history should be taken **(Fig. 30.27)**. Patients having stilbestrol as treatment of prostatic cancer may present with this condition **(Fig. 30.28)**. The testis should be examined for anorchism, cryptorchism, teratoma or chorionepithelioma. Liver should be examined for cirrhosis. Associated leprosy may cause enlargement of breast in males. Certain drugs like digitalis, spironolactone, isoniazide may initiate enlargement of breast. Of course, certain amount of breast enlargement in male is noticed during puberty, which is considered normal.

SPECIAL INVESTIGATIONS

These are mainly used firstly to differentiate cancer breast from other benign lesions of the breast, secondly to detect an early cancer and finally to know the extent of the cancer, its spread and staging.

1. **Aspiration:** This is performed in case of cystic lumps of the breast which were preliminarily thought to be benign. But if the aspirated fluid is blood-stained, if the mass does not completely

condition. Moreover this lump will be quite soft at the center while a carcinoma is harder at the center. Aspiration is the final court of appeal in doubtful cases.

MAMMARY FISTULA

This is a chronic discharging fistula. The usual sufferers are women of 3rd decade. It occurs unilaterally or bilaterally. The fistula communicates with one of the major ducts. This condition may be a frequent complication of long-standing retraction of the nipple and infection being restricted to a single obstructed duct. The abscess ruptures and subsides only to repeat the cycle till it forms the mammary fistula. This condition may also result from periductal mastitis, which has affected all the major ducts.

MAMMARY DUCT ECTASIA (PLASMA CELL MASTITIS)

This is generalized dilatation of the major duct system of the breast with retrograde dilatation of the lobular ducts. The lining epithelium is atrophic and the ducts are filled with secretion. This secretion is made up of amorphous debris and lipoid-containing macrophages. The fluid within the ducts which causes the nipple discharge, varies and may be colored green, brown, viscous or even white. Due to leakage of lipoid through the thin duct wall, there is periductal mastitis, the cellular element of which is predominantly plasma cells. The associated periductal fibrosis often leads to nipple retraction. This inflammatory process regresses within a few days, but recurs again with more severe form. UItimately, an abscess develops at the edge of the areola.

Patients are usually in 40–55 years age group. Younger women with congenitally inverted nipples may be affected with this condition early. The disease may remain asymptomatic, but a persistent nipple discharge or a lump in the breast in the para-areolar region is the usual complaint. The problem is that if the abscess is drained, it leads to a fistula into the affected duct, which is known as *mammary duct fistula*. In chronic cases the characteristic appearance is a mammary duct fistula, with inverted nipple and distortion of the areola. Sometimes a chronic abscess may be formed which presents as a tender mass with skin fixity, nipple retraction and enlarged axillary lymph nodes—almost simulating a carcinoma. Diagnosis is established by needle biopsy.

BENIGN BREAST DISEASE

It is a very common condition occurring in women between the ages of 20 and 40 years. It is mostly seen in them who have denied its intended function, e.g., spinsters, childless married women or multiparous women who have not suckled their children. The incidence strictly falls after menopause, in contrast to malignant breast disease. Various names were given over the past few years, e.g., fibroadenosis, chronic mastitis, fibrocystic disease, cystic hyperplasia, benign mammary dysplasia, cystic mastopathy, etc. None of these nomenclatures is now acceptable. These actually described the histological features of breast biopsies of this disease, such as fibrosis, epithelial hyperplasia, adenosis, microcyst formation and lymphocytic infiltration. These changes are quite nonspecific and have been noticed even in breasts without any complaint. These aberrations are believed to be caused by very minor hormonal imbalances during the multiple menstrual cycles of the reproductive period.

The best nomenclature which is now accepted for this condition is:

ABERRATIONS OF NORMAL DEVELOPMENT AND INVOLUTION (ANDI). The etiology is poorly understood but it seems to involve the action of cyclical circulating hormone levels on breast tissue. This is influenced by cyclical changes in the hormonal environment, oral contraceptives, hormone replacement therapy and probably some factors such as diet and smoking.

Microscopic changes include adenosis, cyst formation, papillomatosis, epithelial hyperplasia, fibrosis and lymphatic infiltration.

The most common **MANIFESTATIONS** of **ANDI** are cyclical **pain** and nodularity. When pain is a dominant symptom, it needs to be assessed apart from nodularity. Such pain can be divided into cyclical (premenstrual) and noncyclical (irregular or continuous) mastalgia. Cyclical mastalgia is often related with **ANDI**. But noncyclical mastalgia is usually not associated with **ANDI**, but may be associated with musculoskeletal origin of the chest wall or may be associated with inflammatory episodes caused by duct ectasia or periductal mastitis. It must be remembered that a persistent, localized pain or discomfort may be a symptom of cancer.

Nodularity or **lump** in the breast is a very common symptom. It may be associated with certain amount of pain (mastalgia), which has been described in the previous paragraph. Though lump is present for sometime, yet it is often the pain which draws the patient's attention towards the lump. These nodules are often in the upper and outer quadrant of the breast and it must be remembered that lump in this region is noticed earlier than lump in the center and inner half of the breast. The lumps usually become larger and more tender premenstrually. Though it is difficult for the patient to judge whether the lump is progressively becoming larger or not, yet if the patient suggests that the lump *fluctuates in size* is typical of this condition and it almost excludes the diagnosis of carcinoma. Lumps can be single or multiple and characteristically sudden in onset. Lumps are often cysts, as changes in the secretory activity of breast tissue commonly give rise to such a cyst. Cysts may be single or multiple and vary from barely palpable to very large size. The cysts are usually smooth, round and of variable consistence. Fluctuation of the cyst can be elicited if the lump is relatively superficial and is often best elicited from behind **(Fig. 30.13)**. It must be remembered that very tense cyst is often hard and not fluctuant.

One must consider during examination whether the nodularity is focal or diffuse. When it is focal, one must take it seriously. *Diffuse nodularity* is often bilateral and found mainly in the upper and outer quadrant. If the patient is seen first in premenstrual period, it is useful to examine her again in the first half of the cycle.

Focal nodularity should be examined very carefully to exclude malignant condition. One must differentiate between a benign lump and a cyst. It is advisable to apply further diagnostic tests to obtain a definite diagnosis. One of the easiest method is fine-needle aspiration. The aspirate should be sent for cytological examination to exclude presence of malignant cells. Following successful aspiration, there should not be residual mass and the breast should be re-examined several weeks later to ensure that it has not reaccumulated.

A benign lump or a cyst from this condition is neither fixed nor tethered to the skin or the underlying muscle and is usually moderately mobile within the breast. The axillary nodes are usually not enlarged. It must be remembered that the other breast may be affected with the similar condition.

Patient usually complains of pain in one breast, which becomes worse just before menstruation. Pain is also felt after over-using the arm. There may be greenish or serous discharge through the nipple. On examination, simultaneous palpation of both the breasts in standing posture from behind may reveal nodular breasts on both sides. They may be slightly tender. The nodules are better felt by the fingers and thumb, *but cannot be felt by the palmar surfaces of the fingers.* The nodules are firm and rubbery in texture without any fixation with the skin or pectoralis fascia. These are more often felt in the upper and outer quadrant. Cysts may or may not be palpable. Axillary lymph nodes may occasionally be slightly enlarged and tender.

Cysts and swellings simulating cysts arise from various conditions: (i) Cystic hyperplasia of fibroadenosis; (ii) Chronic abscess; (iii) Hematoma; (iv) Galactocele; (v) Hydatid cyst; (vi) Lymph cyst; (vii) Serocystic disease of Brodie; (viii) Colloid degeneration of carcinoma; (ix) Papillary cystadenoma, etc.

Solitary cyst of the breast is diagnosed by the fluctuation test. The swelling is held with one hand and with the other hand the center of the swelling is pressed. This displaces the fluid towards periphery to displace the fingers which are used to hold the swelling. The solitary cyst presents as the blue-domed cyst of Bloodgood. Aspiration of the cyst is diagnostic. (i) If the aspirate is not blood-stained, (ii) if there is no residual lump after aspiration, (iii) if the cyst does not refill and (iv) if the cytological examination of the aspirated fluid does not show evidence of malignant cells, *the cyst is considered to be not malignant.*

TUMORS OF THE BREAST

BENIGN TUMORS

1. **Fibroadenoma:** Two histological varieties of fibroadenoma are seen—(a) *Pericanalicular* fibroadenoma which consists of fibrous tissue surrounding a few small tubular glands. This type of fibroadenoma is smaller in size and hard. (b) *Intracanalicular* fibroadenoma contains more glands which become stretched into elongated spidery shapes and become indented by fibrous tissue. This type of fibroadenoma is larger in size and comparatively soft.

The pericanalicular fibroadenoma (hard) occurs in young girls between 15 and 30 years, whereas the intracanalicular (soft) variety is seen in middle-aged women between 35 and 50 years. The main symptom is *a painless lump* in the breast. It is a slow growing tumor and remains more or less same size for quite a long time. This may occur anywhere within the breast substance, though more often seen in the lower half than in the upper half.

On examination, the swelling is not tender and without any rise in temperature. It is smooth, firm and possesses a well-defined margin. This tumor is not fixed to the skin or deeper structure. It is a highly mobile tumor without any tethering inside the breast substance. That is why it is often called a "breast mouse" or a "floating tumor". There is *no enlargement of the axillary lymph nodes.* Sometimes a soft fibroadenoma undergoes cystic degeneration leading to cystadenoma which is ultimately transformed into cystosarcoma phyllodes.

Cystosarcoma Phyllodes (serocystic disease of Brodie): This is a real giant fibroadenoma, seen in women of over 40 years of age. Main complaint is huge swelling, though occasionally the patients may complain of serous discharge through the nipple. This is not a malignant condition. The tumor does not infiltrate the skin though the overlying skin becomes thin and tense. The subcutaneous veins become prominent. This tumor is not fixed to deeper structures. The axillary lymph nodes become rarely enlarged only secondary to infections.

2. **Duct papilloma:** This tumor occurs in one of the major ducts. Occasionally two or more ducts of the same breast may be affected. Majority of the patients are above 30 years of age. *Bloody discharge* from the nipple is the main symptom. Generally it is bright red blood and less often dark blood. A cystic swelling may sometimes be felt just deep or lateral to the areola. If this swelling be pressed bloody discharge will come out from the affected duct. This should be considered as premalignant condition and the axillary lymph nodes are only enlarged when the growth has become malignant.

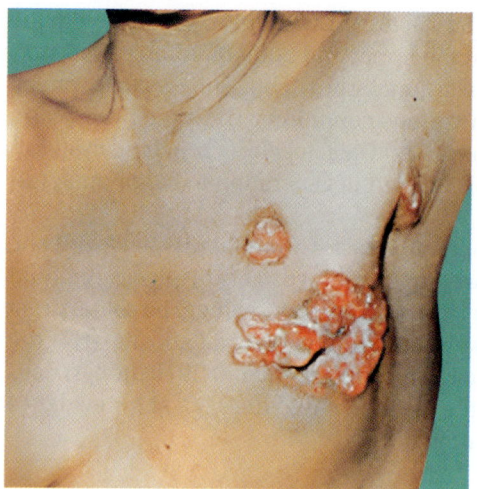

Fig. 30.35: Fungated carcinoma. Note the everted edge.

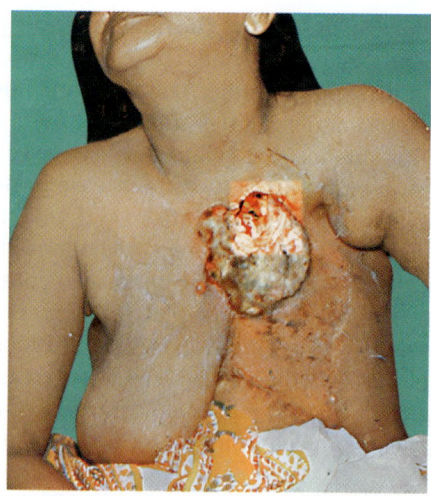

Fig. 30.36: Fungated recurrence after mastectomy.

Other benign tumors like neurofibroma, lipoma, papillary cystadenoma, etc., are rarely found in the breast.

MALIGNANT TUMORS are: atrophic scirrhous carcinoma—the least malignant, scirrhous carcinoma—the commonest type, encephaloid (medullary) carcinoma, comedocarcinoma, colloid carcinoma and mastitis carcinomatosa—the most malignant, duct carcinoma, Paget's disease of the nipple and sarcoma.

1. **Carcinoma (scirrhous) (Figs. 30.35 to 30.37):** Since there is great hope of curing this disease only when it is still localized to the breast tissue, *a diagnosis of carcinoma should be made in the early stage. A lump, as discovered by palpation with the flat of the hand, is painless, stony hard and irregular in surface and outline, is a carcinoma.* Carcinoma should not be excluded if the patient is young or the lump is free from the skin or deeper structure or if the lymph nodes are not involved. Involvement of lymph nodes determines the prognosis of the case. There may be dimpling, retraction or puckering of the skin (resulting from invasion of the ligaments of Cooper followed by contraction), retraction of the nipple (due to extension of the growth along the lactiferous ducts with subsequent fibrosis) or *peau d' orange* (i.e., edema with pitting; edema being due to obstruction of the lymphatics by cancer cells and pitting being due to fixation of the hair follicles and sebaceous glands to the subcutaneous tissue). Late features include adhesion to the deep fascia, pectoral muscle and chest wall, presence of distant subcutaneous nodules, fungation, brawny induration of the arm, *cancer en cuirasse* and distant metastases in the liver, lungs, bones (by blood) and ovary (by transcoelomic implantation).

Clinical stages: **Stage I**—The growth is limited to the breast. There may be a small area of adherence to the skin. **Stage II**—In addition to the growth in the breast, the axillary lymph nodes

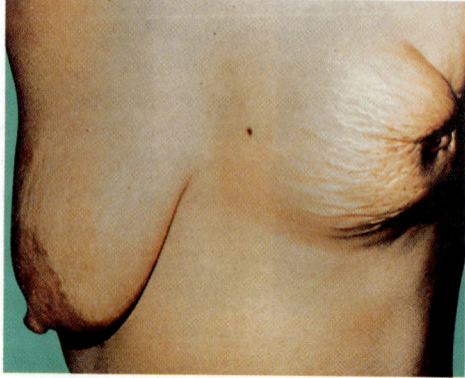

Fig. 30.37: Demonstration of extreme retraction of nipple due to carcinoma on the left side.

are involved but they are still mobile. There may be just tethering of the growth to the pectoral muscle. **Stage III**—The growth is fixed to the pectoral muscle or the skin involvement is larger than the tumor. **Stage IV**—The growth is fixed to the chest wall; axillary nodes are no longer mobile; supraclavicular nodes are affected; and there is metastasis in the opposite breast, skin away from the tumor, liver, lungs, bones or other distant organs such as the ovary.

International Classification and TNM Classification: This is advocated by International Union against cancer. T denotes the characteristic of the tumor, N—the characteristic of the lymph nodes (particularly the axillary group) and M—the presence or absence of metastasis.

T1—means the size of the tumor is same as or less than 2 cm diameter. No fixation or nipple retraction. T2—more than 2 cm but less than 5 cm diameter. No pectoral fixation but skin may be tethered. T3—more than 5 cm but less than 10 cm diameter. There may be pectoral fixation. Skin infiltrated or ulcerated. T4—more than 10 cm diameter. Chest wall fixation. Skin involved, but not beyond breast. N0—No palpable lymph nodes. N1—Axillary lymph nodes are palpable and mobile. N2—Axillary nodes are palpable and fixed. N3—Supraclavicular nodes are involved. M0—No Metastasis. M1—Metastases are present including involvement of the skin beyond the breast and contralateral nodes. This TNM classification can be applied in clinical staging:— Stage I—T1, T2 and N0, Stage II—T1, T2 and N1; Stage III—T3, T4 and M0; Stage IV—T4, N3 and M1.

Prognosis: In assessing prognosis in a case of carcinoma of the breast, the following points should be taken into consideration: (1) **Age**: The younger the patient, the worse becomes the prognosis. Prognosis is better when the growth occurs within 5 years of menopause. (2) Sex: Carcinoma of the male breast carries a bad prognosis owing to early fixation to the chest wall. (3) **Site:** Growths occurring at the inner and lower quadrant convey a bad prognosis owing to early metastasis into the mediastinum and abdomen. (4) **Nature of the growth**: The prognosis is the worst with the mastitis carcinomatosa whereas it is much better with the atrophic scirrhous as the spread is limited by extensive fibrosis. Contradictory to the common belief the prognosis is better with medullary carcinoma than with scirrhous. (5) **Metastasis:** It must be remembered that there is 75% chance of cure if the carcinoma is operated upon before the involvement of lymph nodes; whereas the percentage comes down to 25 as soon as the axillary nodes are invaded—so the importance of diagnosing carcinoma before the involvement of lymph nodes cannot be too strongly impressed. Involvement of distant lymph nodes, lung, liver, bones, etc., makes the case hopeless.

2. **Atrophic scirrhous:** The patient is very old and the tumor grows slowly for years. Due to excessive fibrosis, the spread and metastasis are limited.

3. **Comedocarcinoma:** Tumors arising in peripheral ducts confine within the ducts and the proliferation of cells leads to central plug of necrotic neoplastic cells. These extrude from the cut surface of the growth.

4. **Colloid carcinoma**—is cystic and occurs in older patients. Microscopically, the cells lie in pool of extracellular mucin. Prognosis is better than scirrhous carcinoma.

Encephaloid type occurs in young women. The tumor grows rapidly to give rise to a soft swelling which becomes adherent to the surrounding structures. There may be no retraction of the nipple. The lymph nodes are soon involved. This type of cancer has a high degree of lymphocytic infiltration, a factor which in itself is associated with a favorable prognosis.

5. **Acute lactation carcinoma or mastitis carcinomatosa or inflammatory carcinoma** is extremely malignant. It occurs during pregnancy or lactation. This often produces obstruction of subepithelial lymphatics and veins resulting in redness and edema. This gives a false

impression of inflammation. It has been mistaken for acute mastitis and incised to let out pus. Differentiation is made by the facts that pain and tenderness are comparatively slight and there may be fever but no rigor.

6. **Duct carcinoma:** The symptoms are very much similar to those of duct papilloma. On examination a *solid swelling* may be felt at the region just beneath or around the areola. The axillary lymph nodes are enlarged. Diagnosis is mainly established by mammography and finally by biopsy.

7. **Paget's disease:** This is a malignant condition characterized by gradual destruction of the nipple and *development of a carcinoma within the breast* usually close to the nipple. At first the nipple and areola become red and covered with scales. Subsequently, the scales are detached and the nipple is destroyed. Ultimately, the nipple disappears completely, leaving a flat bright red weeping surface. In the early stage this condition very much resembles eczema of the nipple. The differentiating features are: (i) Eczema is often bilateral, whereas Paget's disease is unilateral; (ii) Eczema is often seen during lactation, whereas Paget's disease is seen at menopause; (iii) Eczema itches, but Paget's disease does not itch; (iv) Vesicles are formed in eczema whereas vesicles are not found in Paget's disease; (v) In eczema the nipple remains intact, but in Paget's disease the nipple may be destroyed; (vi) In eczema no lump can be felt deep to the nipple, whereas in Paget's disease one may feel a lump deep to the nipple.

8. **Carcinoma of the male breast**—is a more serious condition than that in the female since it affects the chest wall more readily, owing to much less amount of tissue between the carcinoma and the chest wall. It has all the characteristic features of carcinoma with a great tendency to fungate quite early **(Fig. 30.38)**.

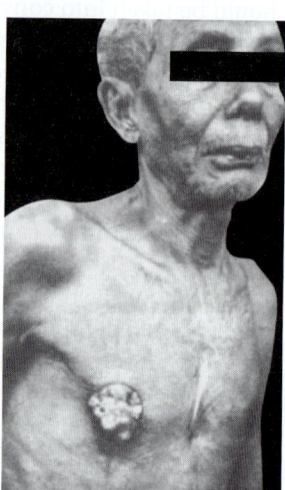

Fig. 30.38: Carcinoma in a male breast showing fungation.

9. **Sarcoma:** Sarcomatous changes in a soft fibroadenoma account for more than half the cases of sarcoma of the breast. A history of swelling, which is present for months or years and has recently enlarged rapidly, is frequently obtained. On examination, a large prominent swelling with dilated subcutaneous veins and without retraction of the nipple is observed. It is of inequal consistency, parts of it being hard, parts soft and parts fluctuating, due to cystic degeneration or hemorrhage. Only in the late stages does the skin become adherent (without being infiltrated) or fungation occurs. Lymph nodes are not involved until very late.

Gynecomastia: Increase in the ductal and connective tissue element of the male breast is called gynecomastia. Though this condition may occur commonly at puberty idiopathically, yet one or other cause may be found out. It may occur in liver failure, in Klinefelter's syndrome, in leprosy, in chorioncarcinoma and Sertoli cell tumors of the testis, in bronchial carcinoma (ectopic hormonal production), in adrenal or pituitary diseases, after stilboestrol therapy for prostatic carcinoma and after ingestion of certain drugs like digitalis, isoniazide, spironolactone, certain tranquilizers, steroid and a few other diuretics. The common idiopathic variety found at puberty among school boys is a firm disc of breast tissue beneath the areola and is called the 'hard' type. It may be slightly tender and is called 'true gynecomastia'. But the variety which develops following estrogen therapy is of soft consistency and is called 'soft' type of 'mammaplasia'.

Chapter 30: Examination of the Breast

Algorithmic Approach to Patient with Breast Lump

Patient presents with a breast lump

↓

Is the lump painful?
- Yes → Consider **breast abscess, mastitis, or fibrocystic disease**
- No → Evaluate for **benign or malignant etiology**

↓

Is the lump mobile or fixed?
- **Mobile lump** → Likely **benign (fibroadenoma, cyst)**
- **Fixed lump** → High suspicion for **carcinoma**

↓

Is there associated nipple discharge?
- Yes → Determine **type of discharge**
  - **Bloody discharge** → Consider **duct papilloma or carcinoma**
  - **Purulent discharge** → Suggests **breast abscess**
  - **Serous/greenish discharge** → Seen in **duct ectasia, fibrocystic disease**

↓

Is there skin or nipple retraction?
- Yes → Suggests **carcinoma**
- No → Proceed with further assessment

↓

Perform imaging (mammography, ultrasound) for further evaluation
- **Cystic lesion** → Likely benign
- **Irregular solid mass** → High suspicion for malignancy

↓

Perform FNAC or biopsy for definitive diagnosis
- **Benign lesion** → Conservative management
- **Malignant lesion** → Requires surgical and oncological treatment

↓

Manage based on specific diagnosis (medical vs surgical)
- **Medical treatment** → Antibiotics, hormonal therapy for fibrocystic disease
- **Surgical intervention** → Excision for fibroadenoma, mastectomy for carcinoma

Examination of a Case of Dysphagia

CHAPTER 31

HISTORY

1. **Age:** Carcinoma of the esophagus is a disease of old age (50–70 years). To the contrary in infancy the common causes of dysphagia are esophageal atresia, dysphagia lusoria and congenital cardiospasm. In children dysphagia may be caused by impaction of a foreign body, paralysis of the soft palate (due to diphtheria) and acute retropharyngeal abscess. In young girls hysterical spasm may be seen. In middle age the common causes of dysphagia are benign stricture (may occur at any age of adult life), achalasia (30–40 years) and Paterson-Kelly (Plummer-Vinson) syndrome.
2. **Sex:** Paterson-Kelly syndrome (sideropenic dysphagia) occurs almost exclusively in females nearing menopause (over 40 years of age). Achalasia occurs in both sexes, though women may dominate. Carcinoma of esophagus mainly affects men.
3. **Mode of onset and progress:** A sudden onset may suggest foreign body obstruction or acute esophagitis. A comparatively short history of difficulty in swallowing (a few months duration) in the elderly suggests carcinoma of esophagus. A slow onset with a long history obtained in benign stricture, achalasia, pharyngeal pouch, etc. Progressively worsening dysphagia is typical of carcinoma and stricture. In case of spastic lesions, (Paterson-Kelly syndrome and Schatzki's rings) there may be periods of remission. Difficulty in swallowing first with solids and subsequently with liquids points to mechanical obstruction. This is mainly seen in carcinoma of the esophagus. Difficulty in swallowing first with liquids and subsequently with solids is typical of achalasia (cardiospasm). In the latter condition the weight of the solid helps in overcoming the spasm.
4. **Regurgitation:** This is often seen in achalasia, but may be seen in sliding hiatus hernia with stooping or straining. Pharyngeal pouch may cause regurgitation. In this case, a lump in the neck may be visible, which may be emptied with pressure.
5. **Pain:** Typical pain along with dysphagia is only complained of in reflux esophagitis or in corrosive stricture. But the majority of patients with dysphagia will complain of some sort of discomfort at the site of obstruction. This type of pain is mainly felt just beneath the sternum. According to the site of obstruction, this is felt either behind the upper part of the sternum or behind its lower part.
6. **Vomitus:** If present, should be examined noting the amount, reaction (it is generally not acid in causes other than reflux esophagitis), odor and presence of blood (carcinoma or esophageal reflux or very rarely in achalasia). When the esophagus has been marked by dilatation, the patient may complain of vomiting of foul-smelling stagnated intraesophageal contents of 2–3 days old. Postprandial vomiting is also complained of in paraesophageal hernia. This condition may cause hematemesis.
7. **Coughing**—is not a common symptom in these cases. Persistent coughing is only come across due to irritation by a mediastinal mass. Coughing occurring immediately after feeds indicates

tracheoesophageal fistula. Coughing, which occurs sometime after ingestion of meals may be due to regurgitation of food in case of cardiospasm or pharyngeal pouch.

8. **Loss of weight:** This is quite appreciable and is common in achalasia and malignant lesion of the esophagus.

Past history: A history of radiation, instrumentation or swallowing of corrosive such as concentrated acid or alkali may be obtained in simple stricture of esophagus. Past history of vagotomy indicates periesophagitis to be the cause of dysphagia. Similarly previous history of hiatus hernia repair indicates excessive tightness of the repair to be the cause of dysphagia. Diphtheria may result in dysphagia. Symptoms of other bowel diseases may indicate a rare entity—Crohn's disease of esophagus.

History in examination of case of dysphagia

Aspect	Clinical significance	Patient-friendly questions
Onset and progression	Acute → Foreign body, stroke; Progressive → Cancer, achalasia	"When did you first notice difficulty swallowing?"
Type of dysphagia	Liquids first → Achalasia, Neuromuscular; Solids first → Obstruction	"Do you struggle more with solids or liquids?"
Associated symptoms	Weight loss → Cancer; Regurgitation → Achalasia	"Have you lost weight unintentionally?"

■ PHYSICAL EXAMINATION

General survey: Emaciation is usual in a case of dysphagia but is much more prominent in case of achalasia and malignant diseases. Anemia is very much evident in Paterson-Kelly syndrome and carcinoma of esophagus and in reflux esophagitis. Radial pulses will be inequal on two sides in case of aneurysm of the aorta. Concave and spoon-shaped nail is peculiar of Paterson-Kelly syndrome. The tongue is also smooth, pale and devoid of papillae in Paterson-Kelly syndrome.

1. **Examination of the mouth and pharynx:** Tonsils and fauces should be examined for any lesion. Test the mobility of the soft palate to determine if it is paralyzed or not. The posterior wall of the pharynx is examined to exclude retropharyngeal abscess.

2. **Examination of the neck:** An obvious swelling like enlarged thyroid or lymph nodes may press upon the pharynx or esophagus to cause dysphagia. A soft swelling which appear during meals just above the left clavicle is the third stage of pharyngeal pouch. Pressure over such swelling will cause regurgitation of food into the mouth. 'Tracheal tugging' is a sign of aneurysm of the arch of the aorta. The clinician stands behind the patient and holds the cricoid cartilage with a little upward traction. The downward tug can be felt with each throb of the aorta. It must be remembered that if no relevant sign can be elicited on examination of the neck one must palpate the left supraclavicular fossa to exclude presence of enlarged lymph nodes which may be the only sign in case of carcinoma of the esophagus.

3. **The chest:** This should be examined routinely but in majority of cases there will be hardly any abnormality in a case of dysphagia. One may get pleural effusion in a late case of esophageal carcinoma. Aspiration pneumonitis, which may cause lung abscess, bronchiectasis, hemoptysis may be seen in achalasia. In this condition when the esophagus is hugely dilated dyspnea may be complained of with displacement of adjacent structures. On careful examination one may detect intrathoracic hernial sac in case of paraesophageal hernia.

4. **The abdomen:** Barring an abnormal mass due to infiltration of esophageal carcinoma to the upper end of the stomach and enlarged liver due to metastasis in carcinoma of the cardia, there will be hardly any abnormality in a case of dysphagia.

5. **The spine:** If Pott's disease is suspected to cause dysphagia due to its cold abscess pressing on the pharynx or esophagus one should examine the cervical region of the spine.

SPECIAL INVESTIGATIONS

1. **Laryngoscopy:** This should be better performed by ENT specialist.
2. **Esophagoscopy:** This is an important investigation so far as a case of dysphagia is concerned. In case of *achalasia of the esophagus* as soon as the instrument has passed the cricoid cartilage it appears to enter a cave partially filled with dirty water. When the fluid is aspirated the cardiac orifice can only be located with difficulty due to its contracted condition. In case of *benign stricture* this investigation not only helps in the diagnosis but also can be used to dilate the stricture with an esophageal bougie. In *carcinoma of esophagus* it is not only diagnostic but also gives an indication about the histology of the cancer by taking biopsy specimen through esophagoscopy. Cytologic examination may be performed from brushing to establish the diagnosis. In *reflux esophagitis* this investigation shows inflammation of the mucosa of the lower end of the esophagus.
3. **Chest X-ray:** Chest X-ray may show an air-fluid level in the mediastinum behind the heart which is diagnostic of paraesophageal hernia. However, barium swallow radiography confirms the diagnosis. In achalasia with a moderately dilated esophagus if a lateral chest X-ray is taken a typical air-fluid level may be seen in the posterior mediastinum which along with the typical symptoms is diagnostic of achalasia. Conditions like Pott's disease and aneurysm of the aorta (calcification of the wall) can be diagnosed by straight X-ray.
4. **Radiography with barium meal:** This is by far the most important investigation in dysphagia. More or less all the conditions which may give rise to dysphagia will be diagnosed by this investigation. If a **pharyngeal pouch** (Fig. 31.1) is suspected a thin emulsion of barium should be used for barium swallow. This will show that the barium first feels the pharyngeal pouch, and then overflows from the top. In **stricture** the meal is first arrested in the dilated esophagus immediately above the constriction and gradually trickles down through the stricture. The stenosed portion is usually smooth and does not produce any soft tissue shadow as may be obtained in carcinoma. In case of **carcinoma** the dilatation of the esophagus above the tumor is less marked. Moreover, the constricted part is extremely irregular (the filling defect which is often called 'Rat-tail' deformity) and a 'shouldering' may be seen at the proximal end of the filling defect. A soft tissue shadow of the tumor can be obtained. In **achalasia** the radiographic appearance varies according to the extent of the disease. In early stage there is only mild dilatation of the esophagus, whereas in late stage there is massive dilatation and tortuosity of the esophagus. Retained intraesophageal contents are typically seen. The hallmark of achalasia on barium swallow examination is the distal 'bird-beak' taper of the esophagogastric junction at the distal

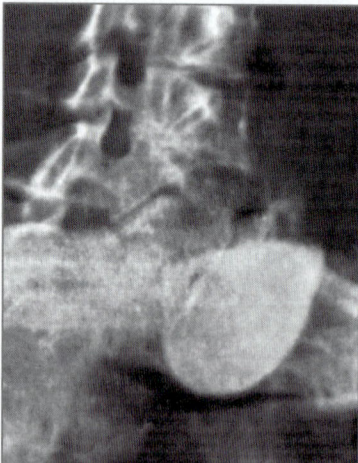

Fig. 31.1: The typical barium meal X-ray of a pharyngeal pouch.

end of the dilated esophagus. No benign esophageal tumors produce characteristic features in barium swallow examination. In case of **leiomyoma** there is a smooth filling defect. In case of **polyps** there is also characteristic filling defect detected in this examination. Barium swallow esophagogram is quite helpful in diagnosing both type I and type II **hiatus hernia**. In type I the gastroesophageal junction is above the level of the diaphragm, whereas in type II one can see the barium filled part of stomach in the thorax. In **gastroesophageal reflux** during the course of barium swallow examination reflux can be demonstrated. To demonstrate such reflux one can even use 'water-sipping' test accompanied by abdominal compression. Swallowing of water will cause relaxation of the distal esophagus.

5. **Manometric examination:** This examination is helpful to diagnose a case of achalasia by showing the failure of the lower esophageal sphincter (LES) to relax reflexly with swallowing and lack of progressive peristalsis throughout the length of the esophagus. In *diffuse esophageal spasm* this is the main test to diagnose this condition. This study shows multiphasic, repetitive and high-amplitude contractions that occur after swallowing in the smooth muscles of the esophagus. This study is also helpful in diagnosis of *scleroderma*. In case of *gastroesophageal reflux*, pH recording in the esophagus 5 cm above the distal esophageal high-pressure zone shows decline in pH to less than 4, which is a clear evidence of gastroesophageal reflux.

6. **Exfoliative cytology:** To examine the esophageal lavage for malignant cells is a good investigation to discover esophageal carcinoma in quite early stage when radiology is negative. This is more efficiently done through esophagoscope.

7. **Ultrasound and CT scan:** The value of these investigations is not much in finding out the cause of dysphagia. These investigations however may find out abnormal masses in the mediastinum and aortic aneurysm which may press on the esophagus to cause dysphagia.

CAUSES OF DYSPHAGIA

1. **In the mouth:** Tonsillitis, quinsy (peritonsillar abscess), certain varieties of stomatitis, carcinoma of the tongue and paralysis of the soft palate (due to diphtheria in children and bulbar paralysis in adults).
2. **In the pharynx**
i. *In the lumen:* Impaction of a foreign body (e.g., coin, tooth and denture).
ii. *In the wall:* Acute pharyngitis, malignant growth, hysterical spasm, Paterson-Kelly syndrome.
iii. *Outside the wall:* Retropharyngeal abscess, enlarged cervical lymph node, malignant thyroid, etc.
3. **In the esophagus**
i. *In the lumen*—impaction of foreign body.
ii. *In the wall*—(a) Atresia of esophagus; (b) Benign stricture—may be due to reflux esophagitis, swallowed corrosives, tuberculosis, scleroderma, radiotherapy, etc.; (c) Spasm—Paterson-Kelly syndrome, achalasia, webs and rings, diffuse esophageal spasm, etc.; (d) Diverticulum; (e) Neoplasms—mainly malignant; (f) Nervous disorders—bulbar paralysis, postvagotomy; (g) Miscellaneous—Crohn's disease, etc.
iii. *Outside the wall*—malignant or any large thyroid swelling, retrosternal goiter, pharyngeal diverticulum, aneurysm of the aorta, mediastinal growth, dysphagia lusoria, periesophagitis after vagotomy, hiatus hernia particularly paraesophageal (type II) and tight esophageal hiatus repair.

DIFFERENTIAL DIAGNOSIS

ATRESIA OF ESOPHAGUS WITH DISTAL TRACHEOESOPHAGEAL FISTULA

This is the most common form of esophageal atresia occurring in about 90% of patients. The proximal esophagus ends as a blind tube and the distal esophagus is joined to the lower part of the trachea with a tracheoesophageal fistula. During fetal life this condition may be recognized by presence of hydramnios, but this may not be present. The most important clinical presentation is that the infant has an abundance of saliva which may bubble out from the mouth. 'Spitting up' or frank vomiting during feeding is a characteristic sign. Aspiration, choking, cyanosis and respiratory distress are often noticed. The abdomen may be progressively distended. Attempts to push a nasogastric tube will be stopped at the upper mediastinum. When the tip of this tube is radio-opaque, straight X-ray in situ can diagnose this condition. Straight X-ray also reveals intestinal gas which indicates communication of distal trachea with distal esophagus. The greatest risk of this condition is that there is a great possibility of aspiration of gastric juice, which is highly injurious to the lungs.

PATERSON-KELLY SYNDROME (PLUMMER-VINSON SYNDROME)

This syndrome was first described by Paterson and Kelly in 1919 and subsequently more elaborately described by Plummer and Vinson in 1921. The patient is nearly always a middle-aged woman who presents with difficulty in swallowing. Glossitis, anemia and dysphagia form the important triad of this disease. The tongue becomes devoid of papillae, smooth and pale. The lips and corners of the mouth are often cracked. Hypochromic anemia is almost always present. The nails become brittle and spoon shaped (Koilonychia). Dysphagia is due to spasm of the circular muscle fibers at the extreme upper portion of the esophagus. There may be formation of webs. The mucous membrane is hyperkeratotic at places and desquamated at others. This lesion is considered to be precancerous.

PHARYNGEAL POUCH

It is also called Zenker's diverticulum occurring at the upper end of the esophagus protruding posteriorly through a gap between two parts of the inferior constrictor muscle—i.e., oblique thyropharyngeal part and transverse cricopharyngeal part. It may be considered as a Pulsion diverticulum—herniation of the esophageal mucosa and submucosa through the weakened area. This diverticulum mainly affects subjects over 50 years of age and more frequently men than women. Regurgitation of undigested food at an unpredictable time or after turning from one side to the other is often the main complaint in the beginning. Sometimes the patients may wake up from sleep with a feeling of suffocation followed by a severe cough. When the pouch enlarges it tends to compress the esophagus which leads to dysphagia. When the patient drinks the pouch can be seen to be enlarging with gurgling noise in the neck. X-ray with a very thin barium emulsion should be performed as thick mixture refuses to be washed out from the pouch following examination.

Traction diverticula may be occasionally seen in the middle portion of the esophagus near tracheal bifurcation. These result from pull of scar tissue from an adjacent inflammatory process, usually tuberculous lymph nodes. These diverticula are often symptomless.

BENIGN STRICTURE (FIG. 31.2)

The causes of benign stricture have been set out above. Past history must carefully be taken to find out the cause. Difficulty is more with solids than with liquids. X-ray with barium meal will show a long tortuous stricture with some dilatation of the proximal esophagus and without any shouldering at the proximal end of the stricture.

ACHALASIA OR CARDIOSPASM (FIG. 31.3)

This represents failure of the lower esophageal sphincter to relax with deglutition. The number of ganglion cells in the myenteric plexus seems to be diminished. Usually, women around 40 years of age are affected. Regurgitation of food even several hours after meal is the main complaint. Dysphagia is more with liquids and less so with solid (weight of the food helps). Complications like pneumonia, bronchiectasis and lung abscess may take place. X-ray with barium meal will reveal enormous dilatation with smooth termination (smooth pencil-shaped 'bird-beak') and lack of fundal gas in the stomach. Esophageal varix is shown in **Figure 31.4**.

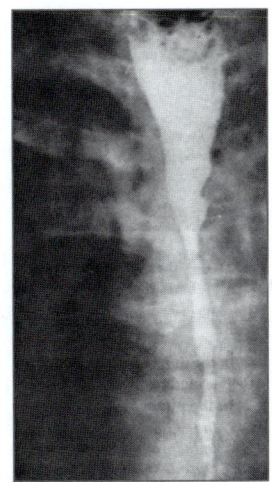

Fig. 31.2: Barium meal X-ray of benign stricture of the esophagus. Note the long irregular narrowing with slight dilatation of the esophagus above the stricture. There is no 'shouldering'.

DIFFUSE ESOPHAGEAL SPASM

The etiology of this condition is not known and the patients usually complain of chest pain and dysphagia due to repetitive and high-amplitude esophageal contractions. Some sort of emotional stress and anxiety are often associated with along chest pain and dysphagia. There is also regurgitation of food, though many patients experience regurgitation of intraesophageal saliva during esophageal colic. Ingestion of cold liquids and food aggravate the condition. Irritable bowel syndrome, pylorospasm, peptic ulcer disease, gallstone and pancreatitis may stimulate diffuse esophageal spasm. Esophageal manometry has been considered the ultimate test in the diagnosis of this condition.

SCLERODERMA

Esophageal motor disturbances occur in scleroderma or systemic sclerosis. This is due to fibrous replacement of esophageal smooth muscle and then the distal esophagus loses its tone and normal response to swallowing and gastroesophageal reflux occurs. In distal 2/3rds or 3/4ths of the esophagus normal peristalsis gives way to weak nonpropulsive contractions.

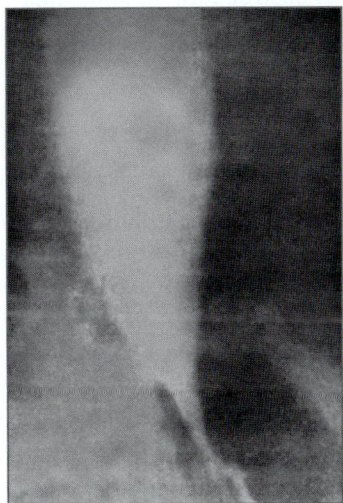

Fig. 31.3: Barium meal X-ray of a case of cardiospasm. Note the huge dilatation of the esophagus above the smooth narrowing of the lower end of the esophagus.

DIVERTICULA OF ESOPHAGUS

Esophageal diverticula are epithelial-lined mucosal pouches that protrude from the esophageal lumen. All of them are acquired and occur mainly in adults. These commonly occur at 3 separate sites—I. At its most upper part at the pharyngo-esophageal junction and is known as *pharyngo-esophageal diverticulum* or *pharyngeal pouch* which has been discussed above. II. *Parabronchial* or midesophageal near the bifurcation of the trachea and III. *Epiphrenic* or supradiaphragmatic which arises from the distal esophagus.

PARABRONCHIAL or MIDESOPHAGEAL DIVERTICULUM: This is a traction diverticulum which comes out from the midesophagus and is in fact a true diverticulum. This occurs in association with tuberculosis or histoplasmosis of the subcarinal and parabronchial lymph nodes to which this diverticulum becomes adherent. This condition rarely causes symptom and is discovered accidentally on barium esophagogram.

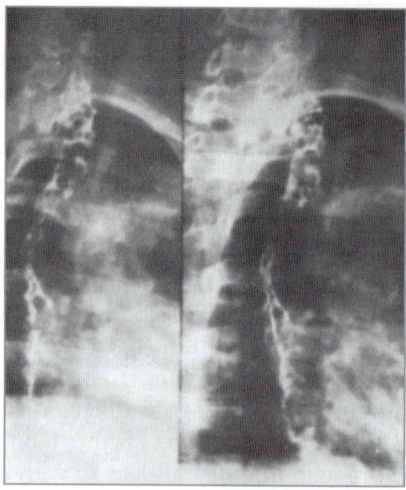

Fig. 31.4: Barium meal X-ray of a case of esophageal varix.

EPIPHRENIC DIVERTICULUM: Occurs within the distal 4 inches of the esophagus and is a pulsion diverticulum same as pharyngeal pouch. This is due to esophageal motor dysfunction of the distal esophagus leading to mechanical distal obstruction. An abnormal elevation of intraluminal pressure occurs and this blows out the mucosa and submucosa of the esophagus through its muscles. Many patients may remain asymptomatic though dysphagia, regurgitation and retrosternal pain are the main symptoms. This condition is diagnosed by barium esophagogram, though esophageal manometry should be performed to identify the exact motor disturbance.

WEBS AND RINGS

Membranous or partially fibrous structures extending across the lumen of the esophagus and thus constricting the esophagus partially are called webs or rings. In Paterson-Kelly syndrome this type of web is seen in the upper esophagus. A lower esophageal ring (Schatzki's ring) has been found with increasing frequency in patients with hiatus hernia. It is generally located at the esophagogastric junction and has squamous epithelium on one side, gastric mucosa on the other side and fibrous tissues in the center. Dysphagia to solid food occurs when the diameter of the lumen is under 13 mm. Careful X-ray examination with contrast will define the level of the web or ring.

CARCINOMA OF ESOPHAGUS (FIGS. 31.5 AND 31.6)

It should be suspected when a man above 40 years complains of heaviness or oppression behind the sternum at the time of meals. Pain is conspicuous by its absence. Indeed, the main complaint is dysphagia, which is steadily progressive. Due to sloughing of a portion of the growth dysphagia may be eased out temporarily. Difficulty is first felt with solid and then with liquid. Unfortunately the patient fails to report in the early stage and majority of them come to the surgical clinic when they are feeling difficulty in swallowing semisolids. By this time 3/4 of the circumference has been involved. Pseudovomiting, i.e., regurgitation of food is often seen. Regurgitated material is usually alkaline mixed with saliva and streaked with blood from malignant growth. Anorexia is another symptom but more often seen in growths at the lower end of the esophagus. Barium meal X-ray is confirmatory (*see* 'radiography with barium meal' under 'special investigations'), but too much stress should not be given on negative results. By esophagoscopy one will be able to see the growth and to take biopsy from it. Exfoliative cytology from esophageal lavage may clinch the diagnosis very early even when radiology has not been positive. In late stages pressure on recurrent laryngeal nerve may cause hoarseness of voice or erosion of bronchus may lead to broncho-esophageal fistula. Erosion of aorta, though very rare, is a fatal complication.

PARAESOPHAGEAL HIATUS HERNIA

In this condition the esophagus remains in its normal position, but a peritoneal hernia occurs alongside the esophagus through the esophageal hiatus. Usually a part of stomach herniates. This condition may remain symptomless. If symptoms occur these are usually fullness after meals, early satiety and postprandial vomiting. Dysphagia is another important symptom. Gastroesophageal reflux, which is a very common occurrence in sliding or axial or type I hiatus hernia, does not take place in this condition.

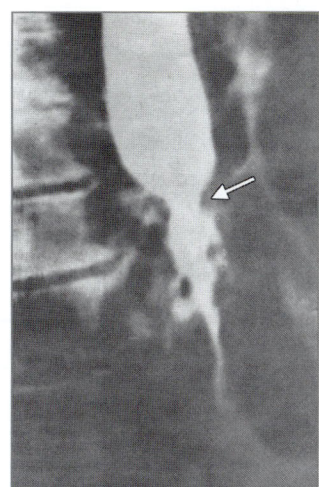

Fig. 31.5: Barium meal X-ray of a case of carcinoma of the esophagus. There is virtually no dilatation of the esophagus above the growth. The constricted part is very much irregular—'rat-tail' deformity of the lower end of the esophagus. Shouldering is shown by an arrow.

DYSPHAGIA LUSORIA

During development of the aortic arch if the proximal portion of the right fourth arch disappears instead of the distal portion, the right subclavian artery will arise as the last branch of the aortic arch and then it courses behind the esophagus (or in rare instances in front of the esophagus between the esophagus and the trachea or in front of the trachea) to supply the right arm. Due to its courses it presses on the esophagus to cause dysphagia which is known as 'dysphagial lusoria' and it was first recognized by Bayford in 1974.

GASTROESOPHAGEAL REFLUX

Slight amount of regurgitation of gastric contents into the esophagus after a large meal is not uncommon. It is only when reflux occurs with increased frequency and at times

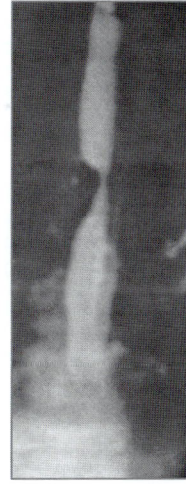

Fig. 31.6: Barium meal X-ray of malignant growth of the esophagus in its middle third. The filling defect is usually more irregular than is shown in this case.

when the stomach is not distended that pathologic gastroesophageal reflux is considered. The symptoms of this reflux are heartburn and regurgitation aggravated by postural change. These are associated with dysphagia, substernal chest pain, sensation of something sticking in the throat and bleeding. Reflux of gastric contents irritates the esophagus causing secondary muscle spasm along with inflammation of the mucosa leading to fibrosis and stricture.

A Manual on Clinical Surgery

Algorithmic Approach to a Patient with Dysphagia

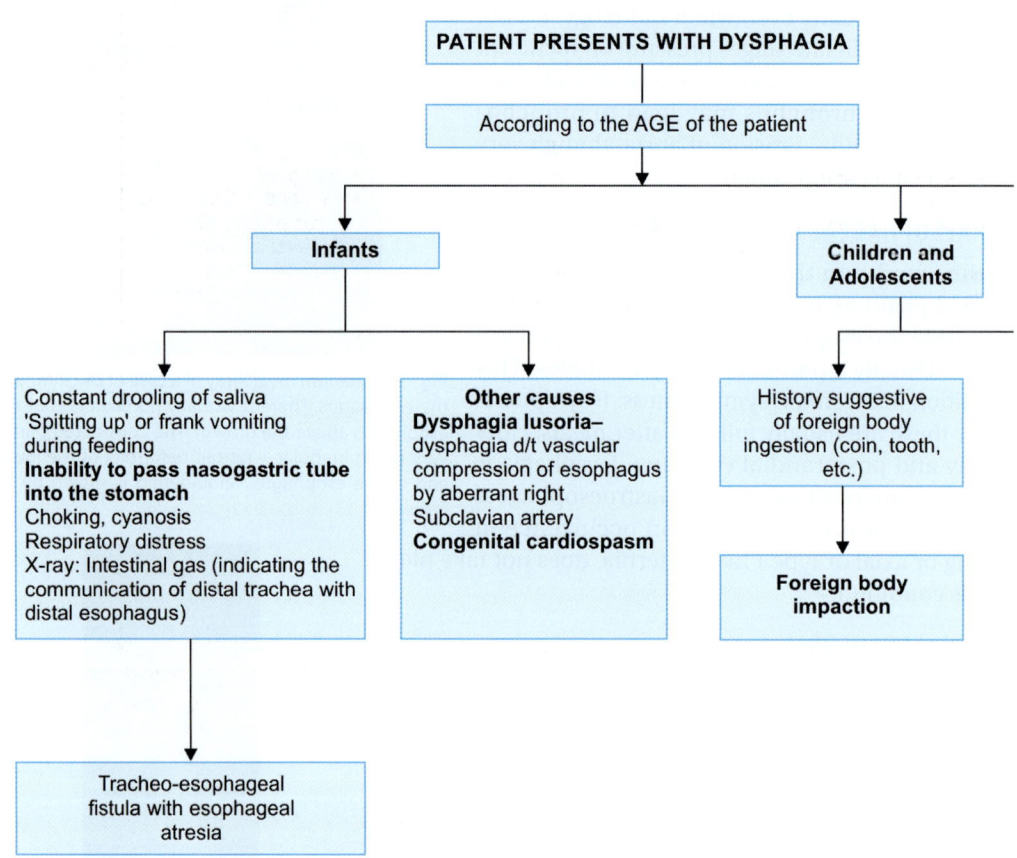

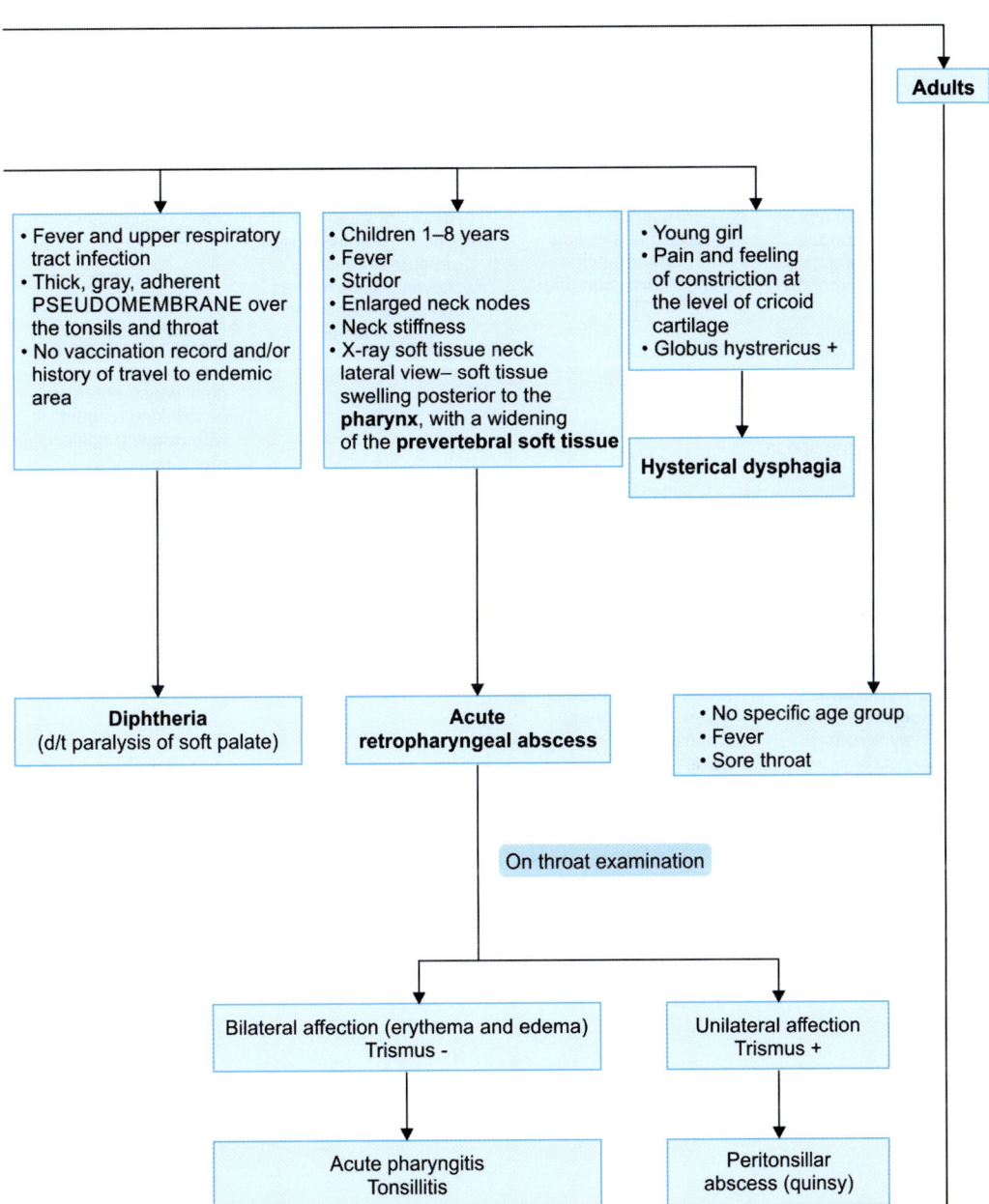

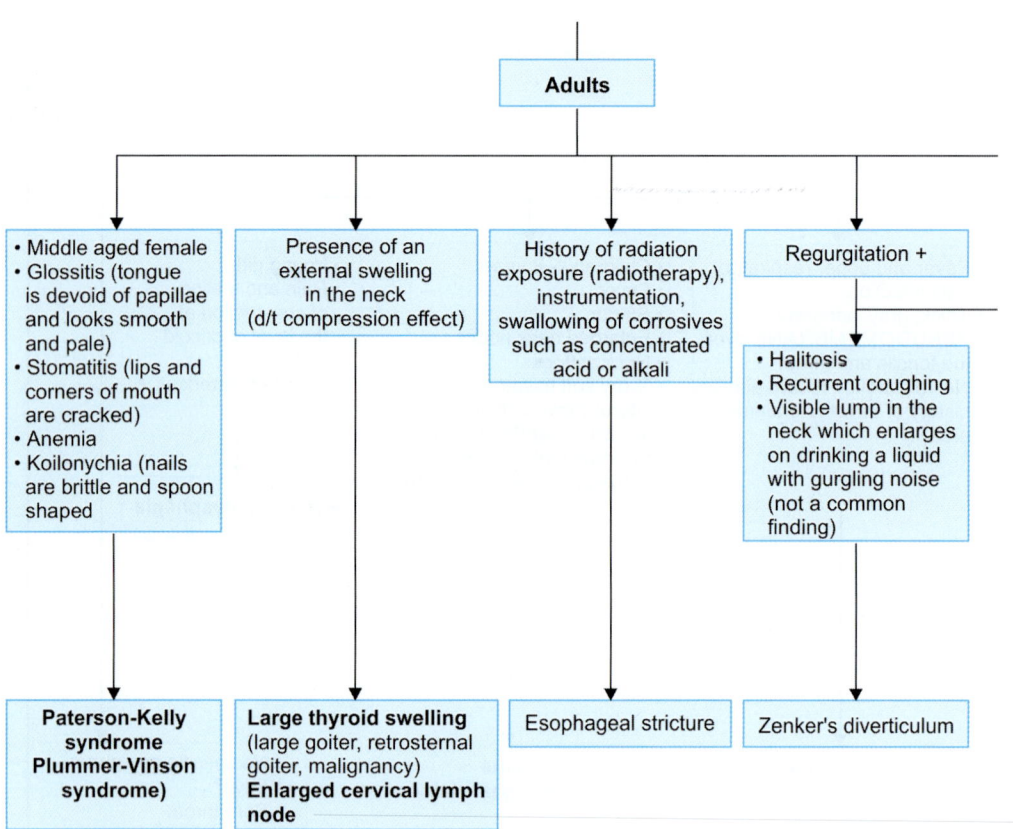

Chapter 31: Examination of a Case of Dysphagia

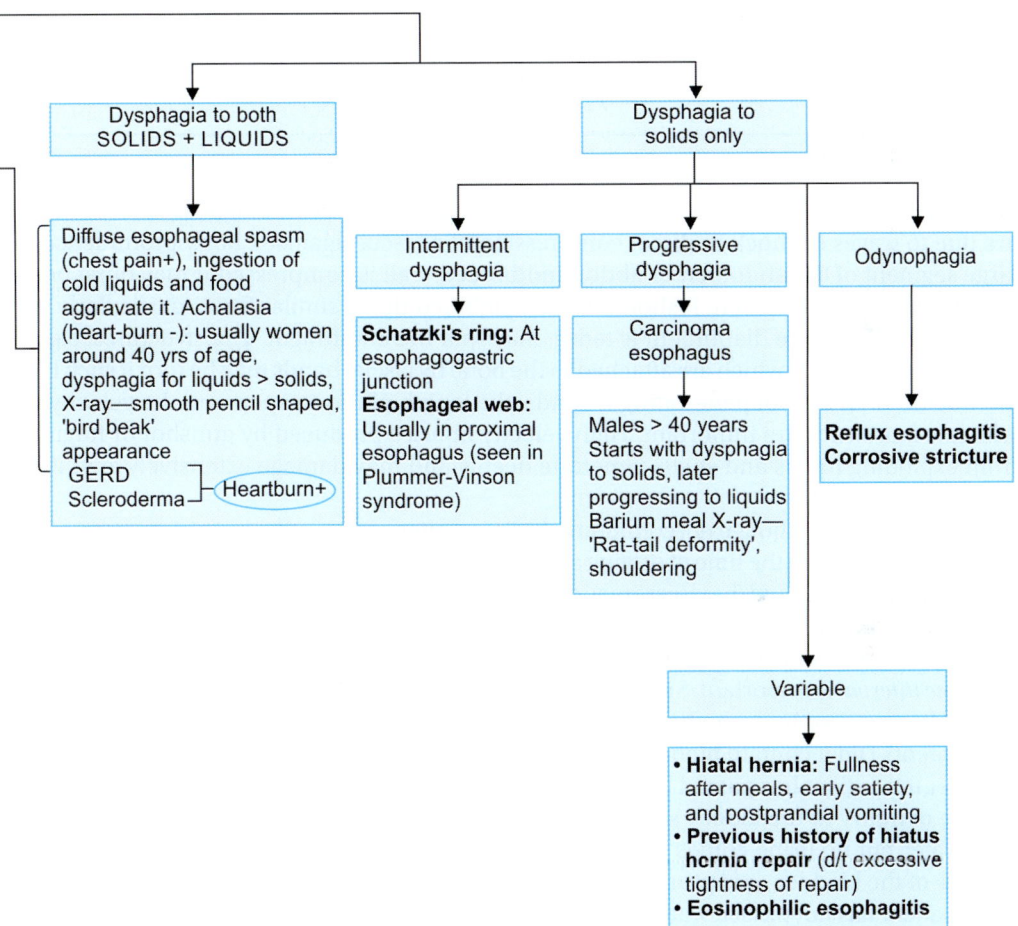

CHAPTER 32

Examination of Abdominal Injuries

HISTORY

Mechanism of injury should be enquired into. It may give a clue to the diagnosis. Closed injuries are due to waves of shock or direct compression of a viscus against a bony prominence. If a large segment of the abdomen or abdominothoracic wall is compressed it may burst or split organs like liver and spleen. It should be remembered that a similar force, particularly if the breath is held and the diaphragm is tense, may split the diaphragm. The structures, e.g., the bladder, urethra, etc., which are attached to the bone by fascial bands may be torn if such bones are fractured. In case of penetrating wounds, the length of the weapon and the velocity with which it was struck are important. High velocity injuries produced by gunshot or fragments from exploding mines and shells penetrate deeply and may damage extensively anything in or around their paths.

Seat-belt injuries, though not common in India, yet often seen in other countries where wearing a seat-belt is a must at the time of driving a car. The harness may impinge heavily on the points of contact with the trunk and the viscera may continue to move when the abdominal wall has suddenly been decelerated. The combination of these two factors may result in contusion of the abdominal contents, detachment of the gut from its mesentery and less commonly rupture of solid viscera.

Time interval is important. Similarly exact spot where the blow was struck is also important. It must be enquired into whether the patient has vomited following injury. If he has, what was the content? Did it contain blood? In suspected injury to the kidney and pelvic bones enquire whether the patient has passed urine or not. If the patient has passed blood mixed with urine, chance of injury to the kidney should be kept in mind. If the patient shows intense desire to pass water but no urine comes out, instead a few drops of blood comes out, extraperitoneal rupture of the bladder or rupture of the membranous urethra is the most probable diagnosis. If the patient has not passed water and has no intention to do so, possibility of intra-peritoneal rupture of bladder should be kept in mind.

Comprehensive history-taking for abdominal trauma should include:
- **Mechanism of injury:**
  - **Blunt trauma** → Motor vehicle accidents, falls, blows to the abdomen, crush injuries.
  - **Penetrating trauma** → Stab wounds, gunshot injuries, impalement.
- **Nature of impact:**
  - **Seatbelt injury** → Mesenteric tear, bowel perforation, vertebral column compression.
  - **Direct blow to epigastrium** → Pancreatic injury.
  - **Blow to the flank** → Renal or splenic trauma.
- **Symptoms indicating severity:**
  - **Abdominal distension** → Hemoperitoneum, bowel obstruction.
  - **Vomiting (bloody or bile-stained)** → Hollow viscus perforation.

- Hematuria → Possible **renal or bladder rupture**.
- Inability to pass urine → **Bladder or urethral trauma**.
- **Signs of shock:**
  - **Hypotension, tachycardia, pale skin** → Internal bleeding (liver, spleen, major vessels).
  - **Cold, clammy extremities** → Late-stage hemorrhagic shock.

History in abdominal injuries

Aspect	Clinical significance	Patient-friendly questions
Mechanism of injury	Blunt → Solid organ rupture; Penetrating → Bowel perforation	"How did you get injured?"
Abdominal pain	Generalized → Peritonitis; Localized → Organ injury	"Where exactly do you feel pain?"
Vomiting and nausea	Bloody vomit → Stomach perforation; Bilious → Bowel injury	"Have you vomited? Did you notice blood?"

PHYSICAL EXAMINATION

GENERAL SURVEY

The patient is quiet in peritonitis but restless in intraperitoneal hemorrhage. Note the pulse, respiration and temperature. Signs of hypovolemia out of proportion of external injury, if blood in the chest can be excluded, is an almost cardinal indication for opening the abdomen. Note the appearance. The patient becomes pale in internal hemorrhage. Tachycardia and tachypnoea are noticed in internal hemorrhage. Subnormal temperature and low blood pressure are features of shock.

LOCAL EXAMINATION

A. *INSPECTION*:

1. **Skin over the abdomen:** This is carefully inspected. Particularly in unconscious patient this is the only sign of site of injury. If the patient is conscious and indicates the site of pain with one finger—'*Pointing sign*', it becomes rather easier to come to a diagnosis. Bruise, laceration or perforating wound is the external sign of injury which one may locate on careful inspection and injury to internal organ may be at the depth of this external wound. There may be 'pattern' bruising (an imprint of clothing or seatbelt) on the abdominal skin that indicates crushing force which may have ruptured the bowel against the vertebral column – known as 'London's sign'.
2. **Respiratory movements:** These should be carefully observed. There will be absence of abdominal movements in respiration due to peritonitis from perforation or due to internal hemorrhage.
3. **Contour:** One should carefully look whether there is generalized distension of the abdomen (*meteorism*) or localized distension of the abdomen. Generalized distension of the abdomen occurs in internal hemorrhage or in late case of peritonitis. Localized distension may be due to localized internal hemorrhage or localized peritonitis due to adhesion of the neighboring structures and 'policeman-like' action of the greater omentum.
4. **Umbilicus** may be bulged due to distension of the abdomen caused by internal hemorrhage, late cases of peritonitis, intraperitoneal rupture of the urinary bladder and paralytic ileus.

B. **PALPATION**:
1. **Tenderness and rebound tenderness:** Localized tenderness is felt on the injured organ. If it be hollow viscus peritonitis will ensue. When adhesion of the surrounding viscera and greater omentum succeed in keeping the peritonitis localized, there will be *localized tenderness*. When peritonitis becomes generalized, there will be *generalized tenderness*. Similarly, if the viscus is a solid one injury will cause internal bleeding. When the internal bleeding is localized there will be localized tenderness and when the internal bleeding is generalized, there will be generalized tenderness.

Rebound tenderness can only be elicited when the parietal peritoneum is inflamed or irritated due to internal hemorrhage. Clinician's hand is gently placed on the abdomen and gradually pressure is applied with that hand. Now suddenly the hand is taken off the abdomen and the patient winces in pain. This occurs due to the fact that the irritated parietal peritoneum suddenly moves up along with the abdominal musculature on withdrawal of the examiner's hand.

2. **Muscle guarding and rigidity:** Muscle guarding is an excellent sign of irritation of the parietal peritoneum due to peritonitis, presence of internal bleeding or presence of contents of hollow viscus in the peritoneal cavity. The abdominal muscles in the vicinity of the irritant parietal peritoneum go into involuntary spasm, leading to *muscle guard*. Generalized muscle guard occurs when there is generalized peritonitis or when internal bleeding has spread all over the peritoneal cavity.

Voluntary muscular rigidity means rigidity of the abdominal musculature brought about by the patient himself due to fear of being hurt during examination and also indicates abdominal injury underneath but no parietal peritonitis.

3. **Swelling:** Carefully palpate the whole abdomen gently to find out any lump or swelling. Such swelling may be present due to subcapsular hematoma of the spleen or liver, or distended bladder in rupture of posterior urethra. In case of injury to the kidney there may be fullness of the loin. There may be bruise with hematoma affecting lumbar region which should arouse suspicion of renal injury. Similarly bruising with hematoma affecting lower ribs should arouse suspicion of liver or splenic injury according to the side of injury. In case of rupture of anterior urethra there will be perineal swelling or swelling due to extravasation of urine.

4. **Fluid thrill** will be present when there is free fluid in the peritoneal cavity.

C. **PERCUSSION:**
1. Obliteration of liver dullness indicates perforation of a hollow viscus.
2. **Shifting dullness** test becomes positive when there is free fluid inside the peritoneal cavity. This may occur from internal hemorrhage without localization, in late case of generalized peritonitis, ascites, etc.
3. **Percuss the suprapubic region** to know if the urinary bladder is distended or not.

D. *AUSCULTATION*

Auscultation of the abdomen is very important as absence of bowel sound means peritonitis from injury to hollow viscus, internal hemorrhage and retroperitoneal hemorrhage. Normal bowel sound almost excludes any serious injury to the abdominal viscera. But this examination should be repeated as it takes sometimes for disappearance of bowel sound after injury to the viscera. Auscultation of the chest may indicate presence of bowel sound in case of rupture of the diaphragm.

GENERAL EXAMINATION

Respiratory, cardiovascular, nervous, muscular system and bones should be examined properly to exclude any injury there.

The spine and pelvis (compression test) must be examined properly to exclude any injury here. Abdominal injury is often associated with these injuries. Patients often complain of abdominal pain in case of injury to the intercostal nerves (T7–T12).

Head, face and neck should be thoroughly examined.

Rectal and vaginal examinations should always be performed. Fluid in the rectouterine or rectovesical pouch indicates free fluid in the peritoneal cavity, intraperitoneal rupture of urinary bladder and intraperitoneal hemorrhage. This examination also reveals pelvic visceral injury.

Genital examination: The external urethral meatus is examined and blood drop there indicates injury to the anterior urethra. Perineum should also be examined.

Repeated examinations: It cannot be emphasized too strongly that repeated examinations are highly important to come to a diagnosis in these cases. In many cases you will find that no definite clue can be received in the first examination, but characteristic signs appear later to clinch the diagnosis.

SPECIAL INVESTIGATIONS

1. **Blood** is examined for Hb, PCV, serum amylase level, grouping and cross-matching.
2. **Urine** for routine examination and hamaturia (microscopic or macroscopic).
3. **X-ray chest** to exclude thoracic injury and presence of abdominal viscus in case of rupture of diaphragm.
4. **Straight X-ray of the abdomen** particularly in sitting position may reveal gas under the diaphragm—a definite sign of rupture of a hollow viscus. Along this one can also assess injury to the chest, lumbar spine and the pelvis. Loss of psoas shadow may be helpful in the diagnosis of retroperitoneal effusion of blood. Even in case of intraperitoneal hemorrhage one can find a bigger blur gap between the air-fluid intestinal loops.
5. **Contrast radiography:** (a) **Angiography** is a more vigorous undertaking. Individual circulations are outlined by selective catheterization in case of hepatic, splenic, renal and superior mesenteric arteries. The signs of bleeding are stretching of vessels around an area of swelling and escape of contrast medium into the hematoma space. (b) IVU in renal injury. (c) **Gastrografin** test for stomach or duodenum injury.
6. **Endoscopy:** (a) Gastroduodenoscopy may be performed in case of suspected injury to the stomach or duodenum.
(b) Proctoscopy, sigmoidoscopy and colonoscopy should be performed in case of suspected injury to the anal canal, rectum and colon respectively.
(c) Cystoscopy is of high value in diagnosis of urinary bladder injury.
7. **Scanning** may be applicable in case of liver, spleen and kidney injuries. This investigation is definitely helpful in both positive and negative results. Particularly in delayed rupture of the spleen, the diagnosis is established much before and operation can be undertaken earlier which would otherwise have been postponed until actual rupture has taken place.
8. **Diagnostic aspiration of peritoneal fluid** (Peritoneocentesis): A four-quadrant peritoneal tap with No. 19 gauge needle is said to be a reliable test. First of all this test should only be ventured by those who are very much experienced in doing this test and secondly a negative result does

not exclude intra-abdominal injury. Fluid should be sent for physical, chemical, microscopic and bacteriological examinations.

9. **Peritoneal lavage:** It is indicated when the previous test has failed to produce any information. In this technique 250 ml saline solution is introduced in the peritoneal cavity. After a few minutes this fluid is aspirated out and examined thoroughly to come to a diagnosis.

DIFFERENTIAL DIAGNOSIS

Abdominal injuries can be broadly classified into two groups—1. Closed (blunt or crush) injury and 2. Open (penetrating or stab) injury.

1. **Closed injury** is caused by compression force such as fall from a height, blow by fist or by blunt instruments, e.g., 'lathi'. Crush injuries may occur in run-over accidents or fall of heavy objects on the abdomen. Seatbelt injury is also included in this group in which during driving a car sudden break will cause the trunk and viscera to move forward with the abdominal wall and become decelerated against the seatbelt and compressed against the spinal column behind. This causes even rupture of solid viscera and/or hollow viscera (e.g., small and large intestine). There may be even detachment of the gut from the mesentery and contusion of the abdominal contents.

2. **Open injury** is usually caused by a sharp cutting instrument, e.g., knife or razor or by penetrating injury, e.g., bullet or missile. In this type of injury the peritoneal cavity is exposed outside and peritonitis is almost inevitable. The intra-abdominal organ which may be injured by such injury depends on the site of this penetrating wound. As for example stab injury to the right upper quadrant of the abdomen may injure the liver.

The main concern of abdominal injury is injury to the viscera inside the abdomen. This often causes internal hemorrhage and/or peritonitis from injury to the hollow viscus. Internal hemorrhage produces certain general signs which are common for injury to any viscus inside the abdomen. But the local signs depend on injury to the concerned viscus.

In case of internal hemorrhage, increasing pallor, restlessness, small thready pulse, deep and sighing respiration (air-hunger), subnormal temperature and collapse are the **general signs**. The **local signs** are discussed below.

LIVER

In case of injury to the lower part of the chest on the right side one may suspect of ruptured liver. Liver injury may occur as a result of a penetrating wound by stabbing or bullet injury. Right lobe is more commonly injured (5 : 1) than the left lobe as it is less mobile and large. Patient complains of pain in the right upper quadrant of the abdomen. Occasionally when the central part of liver is ruptured bleeding occurs into the large radicles of the biliary tree so that liquid blood is carried along the bile passages into the duodenum and there is hematemesis. Examine for tenderness and rigidity in the right hypochondriac region. Look for increased area of liver dullness, shifting dullness and silent abdomen. Scanning with radioactive isotopes like colloidal gold or ^{99}Technetium may detect injury to the liver. Straight X-ray may show increased haziness around the liver region and the diaphragm becomes immobile. Fracture of lower ribs or transverse processes of first two lumbar vertebrae may become evident. Selective angiography may be diagnostic.

SPLEEN

Injury to spleen is usually caused by closed (blunt) left upper abdominal injury and only occasionally it may be caused by penetrating injury to the left lower costal region. This is more common in tropical countries where spleen is diseased by malaria. Rupture of spleen manifests itself in one of the three following types—1. The patient succumbs rapidly; 2. There are immediate signs of rupture (common group); 3. Delayed type:

1. ***The patient succumbs rapidly:*** This occurs due to tearing of the splenic vessels and complete avulsion of the spleen from its pedicle. This leads to catastrophic internal hemorrhage and becomes fatal within a few minutes.

2. ***Immediate signs of rupture:*** This is the most common group seen in surgical practice. There are signs of initial shock when it may not be possible to state precisely which organ has been damaged. Gradually this initial shock is recovered and the signs of intra-abdominal bleeding caused by ruptured spleen will become evident. The general signs have already been discussed in the beginning of 'differential diagnosis'. After moderate intra-abdominal hemorrhage, adequate clotting occurs to control the hemorrhage temporarily. Thus, when the patient is first seen the general signs may not be that alarming, but the local signs become more important to come to a diagnosis.

Local Signs: (a) There are tenderness and muscle guard over the left upper abdomen. (b) Abdominal distension (meteorism) gradually appears about 3 to 4 hours after the accident. It is due to paralytic ileus. **(c) *Kehr's sign:*** Pain is referred to the left shoulder due to irritation of the left half of the diaphragm by splenic blood. There may be hyperesthesia in the area of left shoulder. This sign may be demonstrated by elevating the foot of the bed for 15 minutes, by which time blood will accumulate below the left cupula of the diaphragm. (d) Presence of shifting dullness in the flanks is fairly common. ***Ballance's sign***—persistent dullness on the left side of the abdomen due to early coagulation of splenic blood. Even at this stage shifting dullness is present on the right side. (e) Rectal examination may reveal tenderness and sometimes a soft swelling due to presence of blood or clot in the rectovesical pouch. (f) ***Saegesser's splenic point*** is the point in the lower part of the posterior triangle of neck between the left sternomastoid and the scalenus medius muscles above the clavicle. Application of pressure on this point will give rise to exquisite pain. Among the *investigations* (g) *straight X-ray of the abdomen* is important so far as the diagnosis of rupture of spleen is concerned. A well-outlined spleen is a reliable negative sign. The positive radiological signs are : (i) Obliteration of splenic outline. (ii) Obliteration of left psoas shadow. (iii) Elevation of the left side of the diaphragm. (iv) Fracture of one or more ribs on the left side. (v) Indentation of the gastric fundal gas shadow from the left. (vi) Presence of free fluid between gas-filled intestinal coils. (vii) Downward displacement of the splenic flexure. (h) *Ultrasound* examination of the spleen is the investigation of choice when there is difficulty in diagnosis. The spleen may be visualized with a surrounding hematoma which suggests rupture. (i) Four-quadrant *peritoneal aspiration* may reveal frank blood but the source is not evident by this investigation.

3. ***Delayed type:*** In this type, following the accident, there is a period of comparative freedom of symptoms for a few days (15 days or more). After which the patient is often readmitted with well-marked signs of internal hemorrhage. The causes of this delayed hemorrhage are—(i) the coagulum which was sealing the rent suddenly gives way (a type of reactionary hemorrhage). (ii) Infection may lyse the coagulum to cause such hemorrhage (a type of secondary hemorrhage). (iii) The greater omentum which performs as a policeman to shut off the rent in the spleen gives way. (iv) A subcapsular hematoma bursts later on to cause this hemorrhage. Scanning of the spleen and angiography are helpful in diagnosing subcapsular hematoma with no sign of intraperitoneal hemorrhage.

MESENTERY

Both closed and open injury can result in mesenteric laceration. An expanding hematoma which compresses the arterial arcades may threaten the viability of a segment of intestine. So after injury to the abdomen when tenderness and rigidity persist and the patient's condition gradually deteriorates in spite of a good resuscitative treatment one should immediately consider of opening the abdomen.

THE DUODENUM

The *intraperitoneal rupture* gives rise to the similar clinical picture as perforation of peptic ulcer. *Retroperitoneal ruptures* are more difficult to detect. Symptoms develop a few hours or even a day after the injury. Severe pain in the epigastrium, in the back, associated with intractable vomiting, is the most important symptom. Generalized appearance of sepsis and systemic upset become apparent. On examination, epigastric and flank tenderness can be elicited. The abdomen may be slightly distended and on auscultation there will be diminished peristaltic sound. A straight X-ray not infrequently shows the presence of small bubbles of air in the region of right kidney and sometimes the margin of the right psoas muscle may be outlined by gas shadow. X-ray after a thin barium suspension swallow may show the retroperitoneal leak.

SMALL INTESTINE

Rupture of small intestine may also occur from blunt injury or penetrating injury of the abdomen. In case of penetrating injury the symptoms and signs are more or less like perforation of peptic ulcer. In case of blunt injury the symptoms and signs may not appear early and this delay is due to appearance of traumatic necrosis involving the parts of the injured intestine. The fixed parts of the small intestine are more vulnerable to blunt injury particularly when the blow impinges these parts against the vertebral column. It is the first two feet of jejunum and last two feet of terminal ileum which are most vulnerable to closed traumatic rupture. Early diagnosis is highly important. The time interval between the perforation and development of peritonitis depends on the size of the rupture, whether the perforation occurs into the free peritoneal cavity and on the character of the intestinal contents. *Pointing test* is an important sign in rupture intestine. The patient is asked to point which is the most painful area or where the pain started. This often indicates the site of perforation. *London sign* indicates pattern of bruising of the skin (i.e. an imprint of clothing or a seat-belt is noted on the skin) with the type of crushing force applied to the abdomen against the vertebral column. *Local tenderness* is highly important as it often indicates the site of rupture. Rebound tenderness means peritonitis has set in due to rupture of small intestine.

LARGE INTESTINE

Rupture of large intestine may be intraperitoneal or extraperitoneal. Rupture of ascending and descending colon may be intra- or extraperitoneal, whereas rupture of transverse and sigmoid colon is often intraperitoneal. Intraperitoneal rupture will lead to severe peritonitis as the contents of the large gut are highly infective. The condition is lethal. Radiography can be helpful mainly in that a large pneumoperitoneum suggests escape from the predominantly gas containing large bowel. Extraperitoneal injury will lead to spreading cellulitis and surgical emphysema in the loins. Gas gangrene may supervene. Very occasionally rupture of large intestine may be delayed. The colon is bruised by the trauma. Necrosis sets in slowly involving the thin colonic wall which takes sometime and suddenly the gangrenous portion perforates.

THE KIDNEY

Renal injuries can be classified into slight, severe and critical. Slight injuries comprise those where the parenchyma is damaged without rupture of the capsule or extension of the laceration into the renal pelvis or calyx. This also includes a contusion of the cortex of the kidney without tear of the capsule and this produces a subcapsular hematoma. This condition does not produce hematuria but slight tenderness at the renal angle can be elicited. *Severe injuries* are those where the capsule is broken, renal pelvis or calyx is distorted. This produces hematuria or a mass in the loin from a perirenal hematoma. There may be clot colic. There may be leakage of urine in the retroperitoneal tissue. Perinephric hematoma is suspected when there is flattening of the normal curvature of the loin. In many cases of renal injuries there will be generalized abdominal distension (Meteorism) which is caused by retroperitoneal hematoma pressing on the splanchnic nerves. One must continue to examine the urine for hematuria both macroscopic and microscopic. If hamaturia gradually ceases, it is a good sign but the patient should be kept at rest for a few days more as such cessation of hematuria may be due to occlusion of the ureter by blood clot. A *critical injury* is such when the kidney is shattered or there is a tear in the renal artery or one of its branches. The patient rarely survives after this type of injury. *Delayed rupture* is very rare, though is occasionally seen in renal injury. A patient who after injury did not reveal any sign of kidney injury suddenly suffers from profuse hamaturia usually between 3rd and 5th days of accidents. This usually occurs due to some movement which dislodges the clot into the renal pelvis. So rest in bed is extremely important even when minimum injury to kidney is suspected.

X-ray will show obliteration of the renal and pass shadows. I.V.P. is important not only to diagnose the condition, but also to know that the other kidney is functioning alright. Scintiscan is also important to know the portion of the kidney affected.

URINARY BLADDER

This may be injured intraperitoneally or extraperitoneally. The rupture is extraperitoneal in 90% of cases. Intraperitoneal rupture can only occur when someone is drunk so that his abdominal musculature remains relaxed during the blow and the bladder is full. Symptoms of ruptured bladder are usually masked due to multiple injuries and shock. A question must be asked 'Has the patient passed urine since the accident?'

Extraperitoneal rupture: It is usually associated with fractured pelvis. This is ascertained by 'compression test' by compressing the pelvis laterally inwards or by distraction test by distracting the pelvis. Fracture is indicated by pain. Extravasation occurs into the prevesical space **(Figs. 32.1A and B)**. After a few hours there will be increasing tenderness over the lower abdomen and the pulse rate will rise. These factors in association with failure to pass urine and no evidence of bladder distension will confirm the diagnosis. This condition is often confused with rupture of membranous part of the urethra. This is differentiated by rectal examination in which the prostate may not be palpable as it is displaced upwards in rupture of membranous part of urethra (Vermooten's sign) and some amount of blood will definitely leak from the urethral meatus in the latter condition.

Intraperitoneal rupture: In this condition the physical findings are those of peritonitis. Patient complains of agonizing pain and is often accompanied by severe shock. There will be varying degrees of abdominal rigidity and a few hours later abdomen becomes obviously distended. Though the patient has not passed urine he does not show any intention whatsoever to do so.

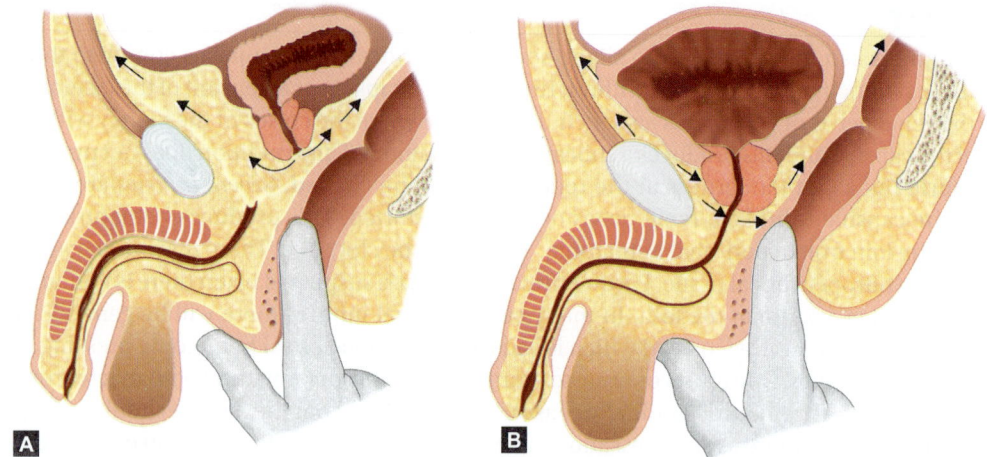

Figs. 32.1A and B: Show deep extravasation of urine by dotted areas; (A) Deep extravasation is due to rupture of membranous part of the urethra which usually tears the puboprostatic ligaments and thus the prostate is displaced posterosuperiorly and has gone beyond the reach of the finger in rectal examination; (B) Deep extravasation of urine is due to extraperitoneal rupture or perforation of the bladder, in which the prostate is in its normal position and can be well felt by rectal examination.

There is no dullness just above the pubis as the bladder is not distended. But tenderness will be present in the hypogastrium. Shifting dullness is usually present. Rectal examination reveals a bulged rectovesical pouch.

To confirm the diagnosis, a straight X-ray in the erect position will show ground glass appearance in the lower abdomen due to presence of urine. Descending cystography will confirm the diagnosis. In case of intraperitoneal rupture retrograde cystography is very helpful and may show the site of rupture. But retrograde cystography may be performed in extraperitoneal rupture when a diagnosis of rupture of urethra has definitely been ruled out. But the last-mentioned investigation does provide a serious risk of introducing infection, hence better be avoided.

Chapter 32: Examination of Abdominal Injuries

Algorithmic Approach to a Patient with Abdominal Injury

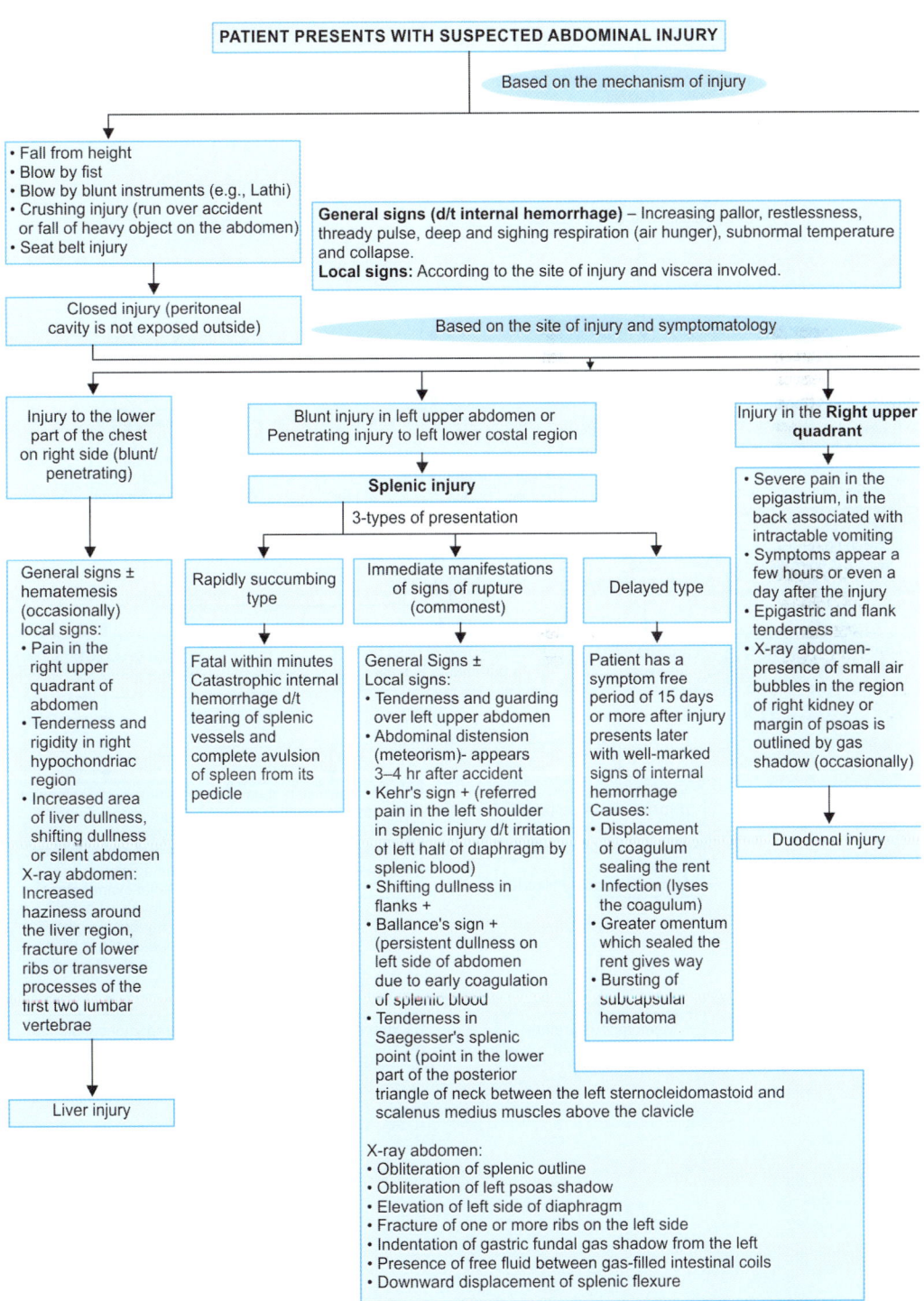

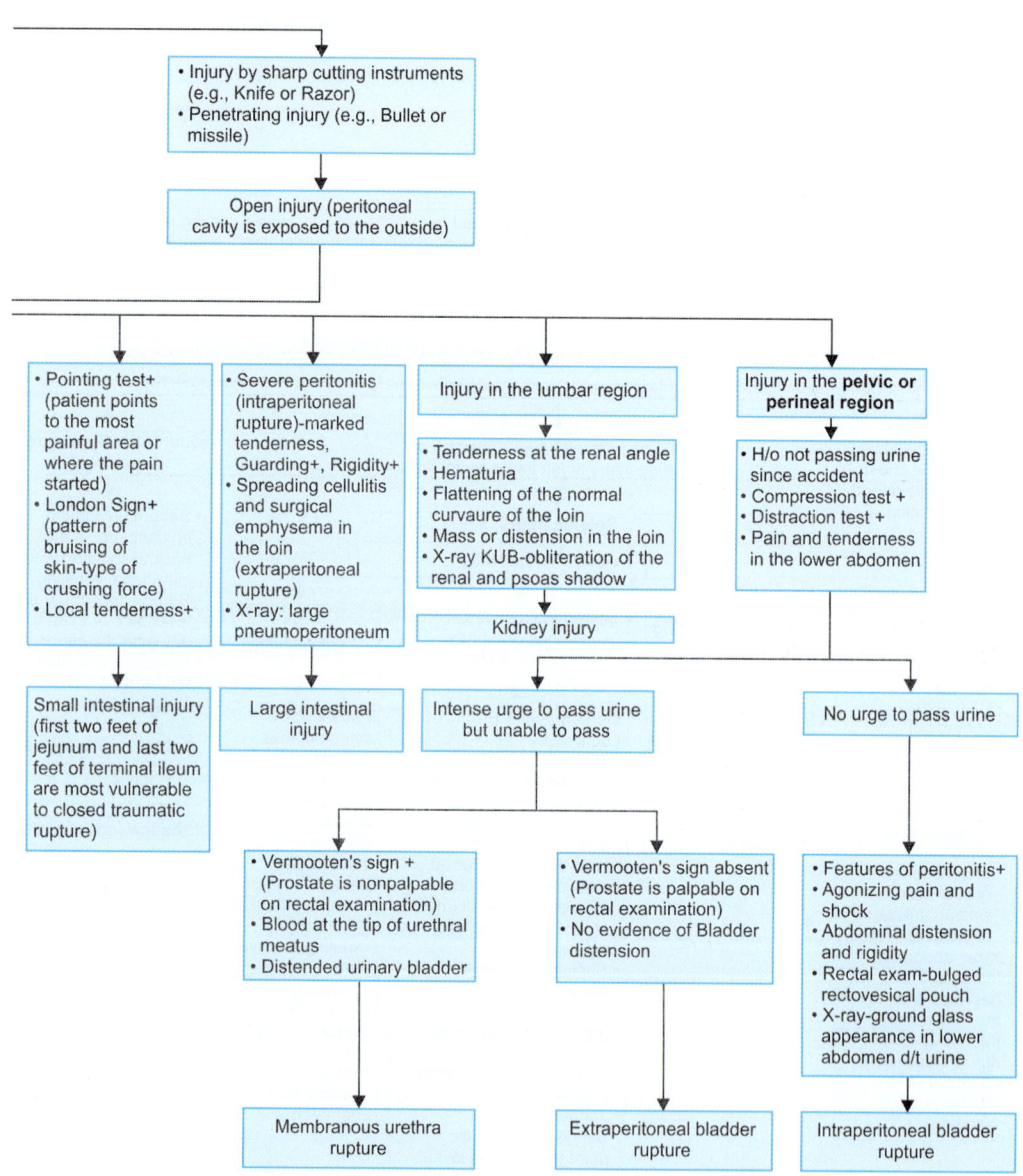

Examination of an Acute Abdomen

CHAPTER 33

'Acute abdomen' means the patient complains of an acute attack of abdominal pain that may occur suddenly or gradually over a period of several hours and presents a symptom complex which suggests a disease that possibly threatens life and demands an immediate or urgent diagnosis for early treatment. A careful history should be taken indicating the symptoms of the patient and a careful examination to find out the physical signs and their interpretations which are of high significance to come to a diagnosis in these cases. It goes without saying that how important it is to make the diagnosis as early as possible in these conditions. Delay will definitely worsen the condition of the patient and may lead to fatal outcome.

HISTORY

1. **Age:** A few acute abdominal conditions are peculiarly seen at a definite age group. In **NEWBORNS**, intestinal obstructions due to intestinal atresia and stenosis, meconium ileus, meconium peritonitis, imperforate anus and annular pancreas are commonly seen. In **INFANTS**, midgut volvulus, intussusception and Meckel's diverticulitis are common. In **CHILDREN**, appendicitis, nonspecific mesenteric lymphadenitis, primary pneumococcal or streptococcal peritonitis and round worm intestinal obstruction are commonly come across. In **YOUNG ADULTS** appendicitis and Meckel's diverticulitis are common. In **ADULTS** perforation of peptic ulcer, acute cholecystitis and acute pancreatitis are more common. In **ELDERLY** sigmoid volvulus, intestinal obstruction from malignant growth, diverticulitis and mesenteric occlusive disease are commonly seen.

2. **Sex:** Ruptured ectopic gestation, twisted ovarian cyst, acute salpingitis are obviously the diseases of women. But a few acute abdominal conditions are peculiarly more often seen in females than males. These are acute cholecystitis, acute appendicitis, primary peritonitis, etc. Whereas perforation of peptic ulcer, pancreatitis, volvulus, intussusception, etc., are more common in men.

3. **Occupation:** Painters may have recurrent abdominal colic due to lead poisoning, similarly workers in arsenic industries may suffer from similar disease.

4. **Residence:** Peptic perforation is more common in northern India and in southern India due to their habit of taking very spicy food. Acute cholecystitis is more common in Eastern India and Southern India. Amoebic typhlitis is only seen in tropical countries. Pancreatitis is more common in western countries, due to their habit of consuming alcohol. Appendicitis is also more common in Western countries may be due to their habit of taking low residue diet.

5. **Social status:** Appendicitis is more common in high income group probably they tend to take more protein as the main dish and ignore vegetables. Peptic perforation is more common in low income group as they tend to ignore peptic ulcer disease at the early stage.

History in acute abdomen

Aspect	Clinical significance	Patient-friendly questions
Onset and progression	Sudden → Perforation, rupture; Gradual → Inflammatory conditions	"When did your pain start? Has it gotten worse over time?"
Character of pain	Colicky → Obstruction; burning → Peritonitis	"Is your pain constant or does it come and go?"
Radiation of pain	RUQ to back → Cholecystitis; flank to groin → Renal colic	"Does the pain spread anywhere else?"

■ CHIEF COMPLAINTS

1. **Pain**

a. *Time of onset:* The pain of acute appendicitis starts in the early morning, whereas sudden pain due to perforation of a peptic ulcer usually takes place in the afternoon after the lunch break but the patient is often brought to the hospital at night.

b. *Mode of onset:* This is sudden in perforation, colic, torsion, volvulus, etc. In acute intestinal obstruction the pain may not be severe at the onset but gradually increases in intensity. In acute appendicitis the pain becomes boring in the beginning and suddenly becomes acute in case of obstructive appendicitis which often wakes up the patient in the early morning. 'Acute abdomen' is sometimes precipitated by administration of purgatives (e.g., acute appendicitis), by straining (e.g., perforation) or by jolting (ureteric colic).

c. *How long is the history of present complaint of pain?* Similar type of pain with varying intensity appearing on and off for the last few years is the feature of appendicitis, cholecystitis, etc. In peptic ulcer a periodicity is noted before perforation.

d. *Site of pain:* It usually coincides with the position of the affected organ. The patient is asked to indicate the site of pain with tip of one finger (pointing test) **(Fig. 33.1)**. If the pain is diffuse the patient will obviously use his whole hand instead of one finger to locate its site. If the pain is at the flank—renal origin is considered. When it is below the right costal margin—liver or gallbladder disease is suspected. If it is in the epigastric region, peptic ulcer perforation, acute pancreatitis, etc., are considered.

e. *Shifting of pain:* This is characteristically seen in acute appendicitis. The pain is initially felt around the umbilicus, but later on shifts to the right iliac fossa with the onset of parietal peritonitis.

f. *Radiation of pain:* In spreading peritonitis the pain is first complained of at the region of the affected organ but it soon spreads all over the abdomen. In case of peptic perforation the pain is at first felt at the right hypochondriac region, but soon it is radiated towards the right iliac fossa as the gastric contents gravitate down the right paracolic gutter. At this time this condition mimics acute appendicitis. When the

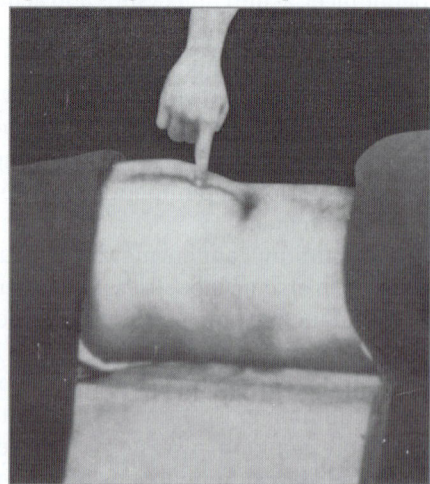

Fig. 33.1: The patient is always asked to show the site of pain with one finger. This figure shows the typical site of pain in a case of peptic ulcer.

patient complains of a radiating pain towards the left iliac fossa while he is suffering from acute appendicitis, the condition is one of spreading peritonitis.

g. *Referred pain (Fig. 33.2):* The pain is said to be referred when it is felt at some other regions having the same segmental innervation as the site of the lesion. In lesions of the stomach, duodenum and jejunum (T.5–8) the pain is felt in the epigastrium; in affections of the ileum and appendix (T.9–10) around the umbilicus, whereas in case of colon (T.11–12, L1–2) in the hypogastrium. The diaphragm is supplied by the phrenic nerve (C.3–5 of which the main supply comes from the fourth). The cutaneous nerves from the same segments are concerned in supplying the skin over the shoulder as also the upper part of the front of the chest through the supraclavicular nerves (C.3–4). Any irritation on the undersurface of the diaphragm either by gastric contents or blood or bile (after operation on the biliary tract) or inflammatory exudate may give rise to referred pain to the corresponding shoulder. In suspected cases the foot-end of the bed may be raised by about 18 inches to allow the exudates to gravitate down towards the undersurface of the diaphragm which will obviously initiate pain on the corresponding shoulder. In renal colic, pain is referred from the loin to the groin, testis and inner side of the thigh, i.e., the distribution of the genitofemoral nerve (L.1–2). The same segments supply the ureter also. In biliary colic the pain radiates from the right hypochondrium to inferior angle of the right scapula since the gallbladder is supplied by the 7th–9th thoracic segments. In passing, it must be emphasized that the segmental nerve supply as has been referred to in this section is the sympathetic supply of the viscus. Of course the same viscus also receives the parasympathetic supply mostly from the vagus (the sole exception being the hindgut and the bladder which receive the sacral sympathetic supply).

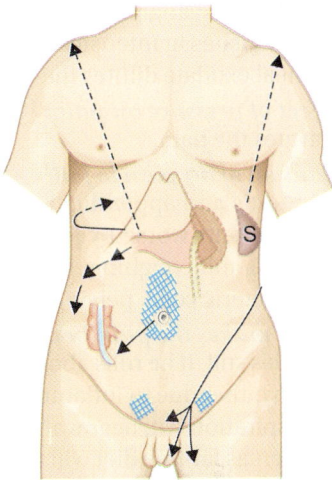

Fig. 33.2: A diagrammatic representation of various types of pain seen in acute abdomen. In perforation of peptic ulcer pain is frequently referred to the right shoulder and migrates along the right paracolic gutter towards the right iliac fossa. Pain originating in the gallbladder may radiate to the back just below the inferior angle of the scapula and even to the right shoulder. Splenic (S) pain is referred to the left shoulder (Kehr's sign). In appendicitis the pain occurs primarily at the umbilical or epigastric region and shifts subsequently to the right iliac fossa. Renal colic is referred to from the loin to the groin, testis and inner side of the thigh. Bilateral pain and tenderness over the hypogastrium (shown by criss-cross) characterize acute salpingitis.

Similarly irritation of the parietal pleura may occur in pleurisy, hemothorax or pneumothorax may initiate referred pain to the abdominal wall as may mimic acute abdominal conditions.

h. *Character of pain:* (i) *Colicky pain:* It is a sharp intermittent griping pain which comes on suddenly and disappears suddenly. It indicates obstruction to a hollow organ—either bowel obstruction (intestinal colic) or obstruction of the common bile duct with a stone (biliary colic) or obstruction of the renal pelvis or ureter with a stone (renal or ureteric colic). (ii) *Constant burning pain* is a feature of peritonitis and often seen in perforated peptic ulcer. (iii) *Severe agonizing pain* is very much characteristic of acute pancreatitis or of torsion. (iv) *Throbbing pain* is suggestive of inflammation, e.g., hepatitis or cholecystitis.

Change in character of the pain is sometimes noticed. Colicky pain of acute intestinal obstruction may change into constant burning type which indicates strangulation. Diminution of pain is not always a happy symptom. In acute appendicitis it may indicate perforation of an obstructive gangrenous appendix. In 2nd stage (stage of irritation) of peptic perforation, pain diminishes in intensity although the disease is continuing. This is due to the fact that the peritoneal exudate dilutes the irritant gastric content.

i. **Effect of pressure on pain:** In colics pressure gives relief but in inflammatory conditions it aggravates the pain.

j. **Relation of the pain to jolting, walking, respiration and micturition:** In amoebic hepatitis, cholecystitis and appendicitis the pain aggravates during walking and jolting. Ureteric colic sometimes gets worse by jolting. In diaphragmatic pleurisy pain is aggravated during deep inspiration and coughing. Pain during the act of micturition or 'strangury' is frequently met with in ureteric colic, pelvic appendicitis or even pelvic abscess.

k. **What makes the pain better or worse?** In case of peritonitis, pain is slightly relieved if the patient lies still. If he rolls about the pain becomes worse. In case of pain due to diaphragmatic irritation either due to inflammatory exudate or due to blood from injury to the liver or spleen deep inspiration will aggravate the pain. In case of cholecystitis fatty foods will aggravate the pain whereas fat-free diet will give some relief. In case of peptic ulcer alkalis will make the pain better whereas alcohol, spicy food or drugs like aspirin will aggravate the pain. In case of hiatus hernia and reflux esophagitis, stooping will make the pain worse.

l. **How is the pain relieved?** Vomiting sometimes relieves the pain in peptic ulcer. In colics vomiting temporarily relieves the pain which reappears immediately. In acute pancreatitis the pain is relieved to a certain extent by sitting up from the recumbent position. Application of local pressure relieves colicky pain (biliary ureteric or intestinal).

2. **Vomiting:**

a. **Character of the act:** The vomiting may be projectile i.e., involuntary forceful ejection of a large quantity of vomitus in high intestinal obstruction, toxic enteritis, etc. In case of peptic ulcer perforation or general peritonitis the vomiting is quiet regurgitation of mouthfuls.

b. **Vomitus:** In intestinal obstruction at first the stomach contents, next the duodenal contents (bilious) and lastly the intestinal contents (feculent) are voided. True fecal vomiting is not common. It is also seen in gastrocolic fistula. In case of biliary colic the vomiting is usually bilious. In case of peptic ulcer the vomitus is nothing but gastric contents. In late cases of peritonitis the vomitus becomes dark brown, feculent being mixed with altered blood. This type of vomitus is also seen in uremia.

c. **Frequency and quantity:** Vomiting is constant, frequent and profuse in acute intestinal obstruction and acute pancreatitis. In peptic ulcer vomiting is periodical. *In perforation of a peptic ulcer vomiting is not a diagnostic feature.* It may be once or twice during the first stage, it is more or less absent in the second stage and may reappear in the last stage with the characteristic vomitus of diffuse peritonitis. Similarly in acute appendicitis it may or may not be present. But nausea is more often complained of. Both nausea and vomiting are the characteristic complaints in pre- or post-ileal appendicitis.

d. **Its relationship with pain:** Pain precedes vomiting in acute appendicitis, acute pancreatitis, peptic ulcer, biliary and renal colics. In high intestinal obstruction, vomiting appears almost simultaneously with the pain. In obstruction of the lower end of the ileum vomiting may not occur in the beginning but follows after a few hours; in large bowel obstruction vomiting is absent or is a late feature. Vomiting relieves pain in case of peptic ulcer but in colics it relieves pain temporarily so that it reappears immediately.

3. **Bowel habit:** Absolute constipation i.e., arrest of both feces and flatus is the usual accompaniment of intestinal obstruction and peritonitis. A history of one motion in the

beginning of intestinal obstruction is not unusual. In acute appendicitis history of constipation is often received. In pelvic appendicitis or pelvic abscess, irritation of the rectum may lead to 'Tenesmus', i.e., ineffectual straining at stool with passage of mucus and blood. In children features of intestinal obstruction accompanied by passage of mucus and blood per annum is suggestive of acute intussusception. In mesenteric thrombosis, blood and putrid stool may be noticed. Diarrhea occurs in acute ulcerative colitis, regional ileitis and acute enteritis.

4. **Micturition:** 'Strangury', i.e., painful and frequent attempts at micturition passing only a small quantity each time is often come across in case of stone impacted in the lower end of the ureter and stone in the bladder. In inflammatory conditions in the neighborhood of the bladder and ureter, such as retrocecal appendicitis, pelvic appendicitis and pelvic peritonitis, they may give rise to the same condition. Even retrocecal appendicitis lying in very close proximity to the ureter, may lead to hematuria which may mislead the clinician.

Personal history: In women the *menstrual history* is very important and should never be missed. A history of missed period is often present in rupture of ectopic gestation. If a patient presents with symptoms very much similar to acute appendicitis in the middle of her menstrual period one should suspect ruptured follicular (lutein) cyst. Smoking and alcoholic habits should always be enquired into.

Past history:

a. In perforation of peptic ulcer previous history of ulcer pain may be elicited, even there may be history of hematemesis and melaena.
b. In suspected cases of acute appendicitis, biliary and renal colics, history of previous attacks may be presented which the patient may consider to bear no relation with the present illness.
c. In intestinal obstruction one may get a history of previous abdominal operation.
d. In acute cholecystitis there may be a past history of biliary colic, high rise of temperature and jaundice.

■ PHYSICAL EXAMINATION

GENERAL SURVEY

1. **Appearance:** In 'acute abdomen' the patient usually presents a peculiar facial expression—*'abdominal facies',* which helps the clinician to discriminate an abdominal from an extra-abdominal case. In terminal stage of peritonitis, the typical *'facies Hippocratic'* can be observed. An anxious look, bright eyes, pinched face and cold sweat on the surface are the features of this type of facies, which once seen will never be forgotten. The *facies of dehydration* is also typical and consists of sunken eyes, drawn cheeks and dry tongue. The peculiar lividity or *blueness (cyanosis) of the face* is a feature which is characteristic, though not often found, in acute hemorrhagic pancreatitis. Extreme pallor and gasping respiration in a woman of child bearing age should arouse suspicion of ruptured tubal gestation.
2. **Attitude:** In *colic* the patient is either tossing on the bed, doubled up or rolls in agony seeking in vain a position of comfort. In *peritonitis* the patient remains quiet because movements will only increase the pain. Only in the last stage of peritonitis and postoperative peritonitis the patient becomes highly excitable which is evidenced by throwing of bed clothes, tossing of the head, grumbling, ineffective movements of the hands and feet, etc., nothing seems to give him comfort.
3. **Pulse:** In the early stage of many acute abdominal conditions, e.g., acute intestinal obstruction, acute hemorrhagic pancreatitis, perforation of peptic ulcer, the pulse remain normal

in rate, volume and tension. But it is said to be a good diagnostic guide in acute appendicitis. Sometimes the patient who cannot locate the abdominal pain properly, probably the pulse plays an important role, so far as the diagnosis of acute appendicitis is concerned. In internal hemorrhage pulse becomes immediately rapid. In peptic perforation the pulse may become normal in the early stage but with the spread of peritonitis the pulse begins to quicken and becomes small in volume. In acute intestinal obstruction though the pulse remains normal in the beginning but with the advent of dehydration the volume and tension fall and its rate increases with no tendency to return to normal.

4. **Respiration:** Barring internal hemorrhage and late cases of peritonitis, the respiration rate may seldom be high in acute abdominal conditions. If the temperature becomes high, the respiration rate will be proportionately increased. Increased rate with movements of alae nasi should direct one's attention to the thorax as the seat of the disease. Referred pain in the abdomen is quite common in lobar pneumonia, basal pleurisy, etc.

5. **Temperature:** In infective conditions the temperature will be raised. This rise of temperature varies from condition to condition. This may be quite high in case of acute appendicitis particularly in children, in acute cholecystitis it is raised to a moderate degree, whereas in acute pancreatitis or in acute diverticulitis the temperature may not be raised that much. But it must be remembered that rise of temperature is never an early sign, it occurs late in the disease, e.g., in acute appendicitis pain comes first followed by vomiting, and fever comes last of all (Murphy's syndrome).

6. **Tongue:** It is supposed to be an index of the state of the digestive system. Note whether it is dry or moist, coated or not. A dry tongue indicates dehydration. A dry and brown tongue signifies toxemia. Even in the early stage of appendicitis, it may be dry and thinly coated, as the patient might have vomited a good quantity.

7. **Anemia, cyanosis and jaundice:** Obvious pallor is seen in hemorrhagic conditions, e.g., ruptured ectopic gestation. Cyanosis is noticed in case of hemorrhagic acute pancreatitis. jaundice is often noticed after biliary colic and occasionally in acute pancreatitis.

EXAMINATION OF THE ABDOMEN

Examination in acute abdomen

Aspect	Clinical findings
General inspection	Facies hippocratica (sunken eyes, cold sweat) → Late-stage peritonitis Distended abdomen → Intestinal obstruction, ascites
Palpation	Localized tenderness → Suggests inflamed organ (**appendicitis, cholecystitis, diverticulitis**) Rebound tenderness and guarding → Indicates peritonitis (**perforation, ischemia**) Absent bowel sounds → Advanced peritonitis, paralytic ileus
Percussion	Shifting dullness → Free fluid in peritoneal cavity (**ruptured ectopic pregnancy, hemoperitoneum**) Liver dullness absent → Perforation with free gas under diaphragm
Auscultation	Hyperactive bowel sounds (borborygmi) → Early intestinal obstruction Silent abdomen → Advanced peritonitis or ileus

A. INSPECTION

The patient should lie flat on his back with legs extended. The whole abdomen from the nipples above down to the saphenous openings (thus the inguinal and femoral rings are exposed) must be exposed. Examination should be carried out in good light, preferably in day light.

1. **First inspect all the hernial orifices:** It is a good practice to start from the bottom. This should have been the last part of inspection. But if this examination be left for the last it may be missed and actual cause of acute abdomen may thus remain in the dark.
2. **Contour of the abdomen:** Distension of the abdomen in acute intestinal obstruction occurs gradually and may not be evident till sometime has elapsed. Distension is central in case of small bowel obstruction whereas it is peripheral in large bowel obstruction. In volvulus of the sigmoid colon and caecum distension almost immediately appears. In second stage of peptic perforation slight distension may be evident, on the contrary in biliary colic, acute cholecystitis, acute appendicitis and renal colic the contour of the abdomen remains normal.
3. **Respiratory movement:** Sluggish or no respiratory movement of the abdominal wall indicates wide spread irritation of the peritoneum as occurs in diffuse peritonitis (perforation of peptic ulcer) or hemorrhage into the peritoneal cavity (ruptured ectopic gestation). Similarly localized limitation of respiratory movement occurs in localized irritation of the peritoneum from inflammation of underlying organs, e.g., acute cholecystitis, appendicitis, etc.
4. **Peristaltic movements:** The characteristic 'ladder pattern' peristalsis may be found in small bowel obstruction. Watch for a while patiently to detect visible peristalsis.
5. **Look for a pulsating swelling:** In the case of leaking abdominal aneurysm the patient may come with acute pain in the abdomen.
6. **Skin:** Discoloration in the left flank (Grey Turner's sign) and bluish hue around the umbilicus (Cullen's sign) are occasionally seen in late cases of acute hemorrhagic pancreatitis with extensive destruction of the pancreas (*see* **Fig. 33.18**). Sometimes there may be redness and even blisters on the skin at the site of pain. This is an indication of hot application to the site of pain to get relief.

B. PALPATION

During palpation methods should be adopted same as those mentioned in chapter 34 of 'examination of chronic abdominal conditions'. Two points need special emphasis in this chapter. They are: (i) The volar surfaces of the fingers are employed for palpation. The forearm should be kept horizontal along the level of the abdomen so that the fingers are placed flat on the abdominal wall. They must not be held vertical to poke the abdominal wall. Rough palpation will lead to voluntary contraction of the abdominal muscles of the patient and this will definitely stand in the way of obtaining right information from palpation **(Figs. 33.3A and B)**. (ii) The clinician must keep his hands warm before palpation of the abdomen. This will gain confidence of the patient.

1. **Hyperesthesia:** Sometimes cutaneous hypersensitivity can be obtained due to the presence of inflamed abdominal organ underneath. This can be elicited by gently picking up a fold of skin and lifting it off the abdomen or by simply scratching the abdominal wall with finger. Presence of hyperesthesia in **Sherren's triangle** (this is formed by lines joining the umbilicus, right anterior superior iliac spine and symphysis pubis) is regarded as a good guide in the diagnosis of gangrenous appendicitis. If this hyperesthesia disappears during the process of illness it indicates bursting of the gangrenous appendix. An area of hyperesthesia between the 9th and 11th ribs posteriorly on the right side is known as **Boas's sign**—is suggestive of acute cholecystitis.
2. **Tenderness** is constant over an inflamed organ. Ask the patient to point out the site of pain (Pointing test). If this proves to be the site of maximum tenderness, it is certainly the site of

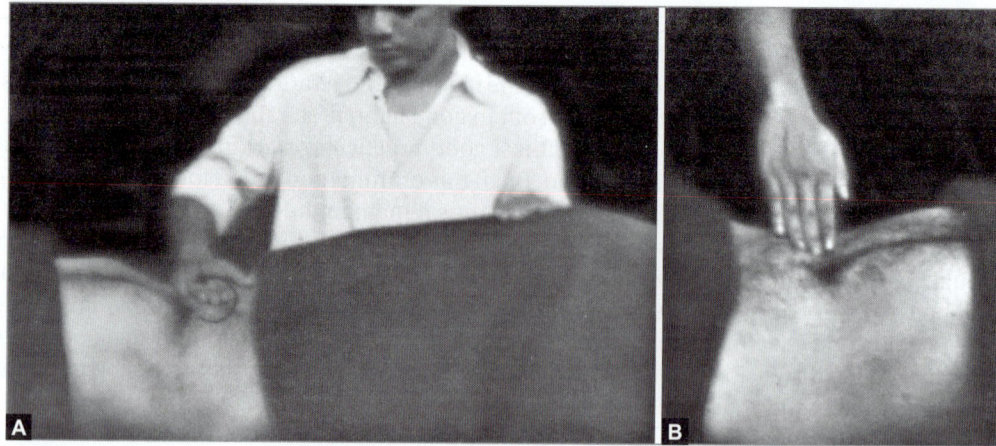

Figs. 33.3A and B: (A) During the palpation the volar surface of the fingers should be employed and moved gently as in 'pill rolling'. The forearm should be kept horizontal along the level of the abdomen; (B) The fingers are held vertical to poke the abdominal wall. *This is a wrong method of palpation.*

diseased viscus. In acute cholecystitis, tenderness is present just below the tip of the 9th costal cartilage on the lateral margin of the right rectus. In acute appendicitis, tenderness is present on the McBurney's point. This point is situated at the junction of the lateral 1/3 and medial 2/3 on the right spinoumbilical line joining the right anterior superior iliac spine and umbilicus. It is a good practice to ask the patient to show the tender area. If he is not definite about it, he may be asked to cough, when a sharp twinge of pain may be felt over the inflamed area. Note carefully the *degree* and *extent* of tenderness. These indicate severity of the disease. In doubtful cases one can percuss the abdomen. Presence of tenderness over the inflamed organ can be easily revealed by this technique.

The *bed-shaking test* (Bapat) can be applied whether early peritonitis is still on doubt. The foot-end of the bed is moved slightly and this will evoke pain at the position of inflamed organ.

Spread of tenderness, if present, should be noted. In acute appendicitis if there is tenderness also on the left iliac fossa, it indicates spreading peritonitis and demands immediate surgical intervention. Similarly in a case of peptic perforation tenderness may be elicited in the right iliac fossa as the gastric contents gravitate along the right paracolic gutter. Very often a case of peptic perforation has been diagnosed as acute appendicitis due to presence of right iliac fossa tenderness.

Appendicular tenderness can be best elicited in the left lateral position when the viscera shift to the left exposing the appendix to direct palpation. The abdominal wall also becomes relaxed in this position.

Differentiation from Thoracic disease (e.g., diaphragmatic pleurisy or basal pneumonia often refer pain to the abdomen) can be made by the fact that in these conditions the skin may become hyperesthetic but no definite tenderness can be elicited from deep palpation. Further if these cases complain of pain in the right iliac fossa and mimic appendicitis, pressure on the left iliac fossa will fail to elicit tenderness on the right iliac fossa (Rovsing's sign) which is typically present in appendicitis.

Rebound tenderness (Blumberg's sign or Release sign) **(Figs. 33.4A and B)**: This is mainly a sign of peritonitis due to presence of an inflamed organ underneath it. The suspected area is palpated. With each expiration the hand on the abdomen is gradually pressed down as the circumstances may allow. The hand is now withdrawn suddenly and completely. As a result of this abrupt removal the abdominal musculature springs back into its original place. The patient will immediately cry out or at least wince in pain. This is due to the fact that the parietal peritoneum which has already been inflamed due to the presence of underlying inflamed organ also springs back along with the abdominal muscles. This sudden movement of the inflamed peritoneum is very much painful. In presence of abdominal guarding due to generalized peritonitis this test may not be necessary. Presence of this sign in acute intestinal obstruction suggests strangulation of the gut. A few tests of eliciting tenderness are described below:

Rovsing's sign (Fig. 33.5): If the left iliac fossa is pressed, pain is appreciated on the right iliac fossa in the case of acute appendicitis. This is due to the fact that the coils of ileum shift slightly to the right and press on the inflamed appendix. This is a very important test to differentiate acute appendicitis from similar other abdominal conditions.

Cope's Psoas test (Fig. 33.6): A retrocecal appendix lies on the Psoas major muscle. Inflammation of this appendix will cause irritation of Psoas major muscle, which is concerned with flexion of the hip joint. When the right hip joint of the patient is hyperextended this muscle is stretched. This will initiate pain in case of retrocecal appendicitis. The patient is turned to the left and the right thigh is hyperextended.

The obturator test (Fig. 33.7): A pelvic appendix may lie on the obturator internus muscle. When this appendix becomes inflamed internal rotation of the hip joint will stretch the obturator internus and the patient will wince in pain.

Baldwing's test: A hand is placed over the flank of the patient. The patient is now asked to raise the right lower limb off the bed keeping the knee extended. The patient will immediately complain of pain in case of retrocecal appendicitis. Retrocecal appendix remains in close contact with the Psoas major muscle which becomes contracted during flexion of the hip joint.

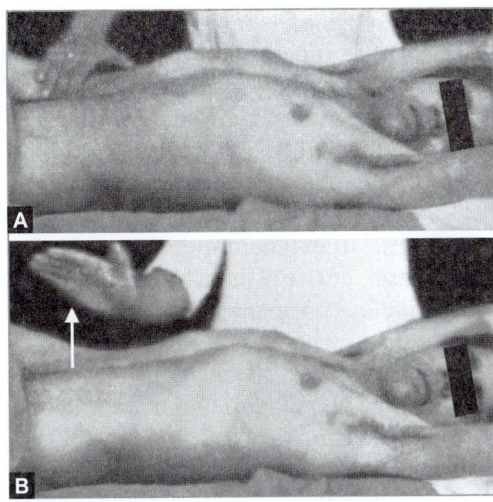

Figs. 33.4A and B: Showing how to elicit rebound tenderness; (B) The hand of the clinician has been suddenly lifted and the patient screams with pain.

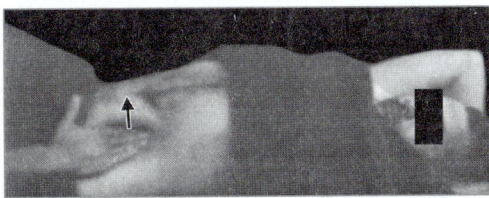

Fig. 33.5: Eliciting Rovsing's sign. The left iliac fossa is pressed and the pain is appreciated in the right iliac fossa in case of acute appendicitis.

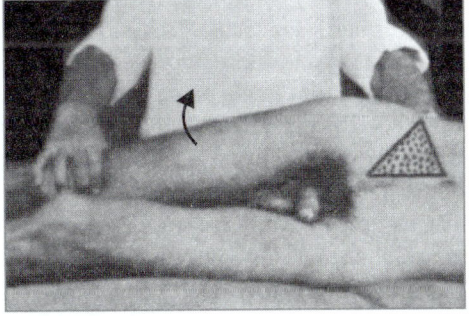

Fig. 33.6: Method of eliciting Cope's psoas test. The right thigh is being hyperextended which will initiate pain in a case of retrocecal appendicitis. Note the position of Sherren's triangle, indicated by dots.

In the passing it must be mentioned that in cases of retrocecal and pelvic appendicitis, tenderness and rigidity may not be that prominent on McBurney's point. Here lies the importance of the above-mentioned tests which become positive in retrocecal and pelvic appendicitis accordingly.

3. **Muscular rigidity (muscle guard):** Muscle guarding is an excellent indication of irritation of parietal peritonitis. This may be due to inflammation, presence of blood or contents of hollow organs within the peritoneal cavity. This is a part of the protective mechanism which is also seen in case of irritation of parietal pleura with restricted movement of the chest, irritation of the synovial membrane with restricted movement of the joint and irritation of the meninges in case of meningitis with rigidity of the neck.

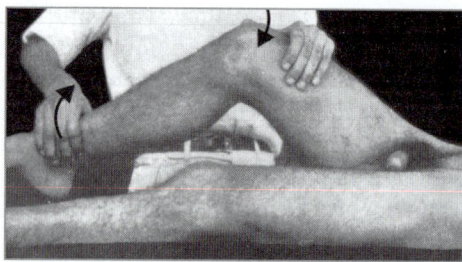

Fig. 33.7: Method of eliciting Cope's obturator test. The lower limb is being internally rotated which will stretch the obturator internus and will initiate pain in pelvic appendicitis.

It is of utmost importance to differentiate **voluntary** from **involuntary** muscular rigidity. While involuntary muscular rigidity or *muscle guard* indicates underlying parietal peritonitis and is one which the clinician is very much looking for, the *voluntary muscular rigidity* is simple rigidity of the abdominal musculature brought about by the patient himself due to fear of being hurt and resentment due to exposure of the abdomen.

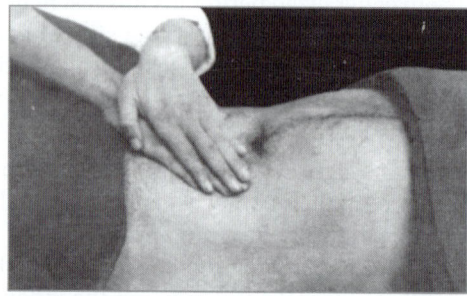

Fig. 33.8: Method of palpating the abdomen for muscle guard. The hand in contact with the abdomen feels for muscular rigidity whereas the hand over it applies pressure.

During palpation the hand must be placed flat on the abdomen using flexor surfaces of the fingers as the palpating media and must not try to poke the fingers deep into the abdomen. Gentle movement of the straight fingers will be able to find out presence or absence of involuntary muscle guard **(Fig. 33.8)**. This should be carried out all throughout the abdomen so as to detect localized muscle guard, if present. Another method of eliciting involuntary muscle guard is to use both hands during palpation one above the other. The hand in contact with the abdominal wall remains passive and wholly utilized to feel the condition of the abdominal musculature while the hand above is used to exert a slight and steady pressure to assist the hand below for better palpation. Patient's confidence must be gained by being gentle in your behavior. You may ask the patient to open his mouth and breathe deeply in and out. Unlike the involuntary muscle guard, the voluntary muscular rigidity will disappear during expiration and helps the clinician to palpate in a better way. The muscle guard usually corresponds to the area of tenderness.

Presence of a muscle guard over the upper half of the right rectus muscle in a patient who is seized with a sudden pain over the same region is strongly suggestive of perforation of a peptic ulcer and demands immediate surgical intervention. The Surgeon should not wait for board-like rigidity of the whole abdomen which is a late feature of this condition. In case of appendicitis the site of muscle guard varies according to the position of the appendix. In case of paracaecal appendix the rigidity will be present over the right iliac fossa, whereas in case of retrocecal appendicitis it will be present over the loin and in the pelvic type there may not be any rigidity of the anterior abdominal wall. Muscle guard will be conspicuous by its absence in case of all colics due to absence of irritation of the parietal peritoneum. Similarly acute intestinal obstruction without strangulation will not show any rigidity of the abdomen.

Differentiation of rigidity due to thoracic disease from that due to perforated peptic ulcer is made by asking the patient to take deep breath in and out with open mouth. During expiration the rigidity will be diminished in case of thoracic diseases whereas in case of peptic perforation it is always present.

4. **Distension:** In case of acute intestinal obstruction there will be central distension of the abdomen. The coils of intestine will be felt to harden and soften alternately. Generalized distension of the abdomen is a late feature of general peritonitis and the patient must not be allowed to reach that stage under any circumstances.
5. **Lump:** Appendicular lump may be felt in the right iliac fossa if the case is brought late to the surgeon. Carefully palpate the lump noting its position, size, shape, consistency and mobility. Appendicular abscess, cold abscess and interstitial hernia also produce lumps and should be differentiated. In intussusception, a sausage-shaped lump may be felt in the epigastrium or left lumbar region. It is usually associated with empty right iliac fossa (Sign-de-dance).
6. **Palpation of the hernial sites**—is very important. Quite a large number of cases of acute intestinal obstruction are due to strangulated hernias and can be very well managed by timely operation.

C. PERCUSSION

Light Percussion may be employed to elicit local tenderness.

1. **Shifting dullness (Fig. 33.9):** Presence of free fluid in the peritoneal cavity can be determined by eliciting shifting dullness. When the patient lies on his back the fluid gravitates down to the flanks and the intestine floats on the center of the abdomen which will therefore be resonant and the flanks dull. Percussion should be commenced from the center of the abdomen and is carried down to one flank. At the point where dullness starts the finger is kept in its position and the patient is asked to turn to the opposite side. That particular area is again percussed after waiting for a few minutes to allow the fluid to gravitate down. Now the note will be resonant to make the shifting dullness test positive.

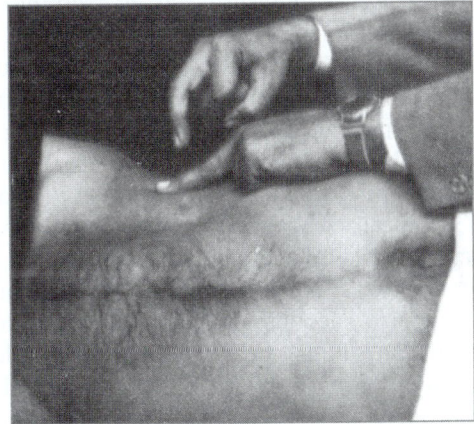

Fig. 33.9: Eliciting shifting dullness. The abdomen is percussed from the midline towards the flank. When the percussion becomes dull in the flank, the patient is turned to the opposite side. The figure shows that the flank is again percussed and the note becomes resonant.

There are many acute abdominal conditions of surgical importance in which free fluid can be accumulated in the peritoneal cavity. These are perforation of the peptic ulcer or typhoid ulcer, acute pancreatitis, ruptured ectopic gestation, etc.

Fallacy: Abnormal retention of enema may lead to distension of the intestine. In these cases shifting dullness test may be positive due to shifting of fluid inside the descending or ascending colon as the patient is rolled over. So the test becomes positive without the presence of free fluid inside the peritoneal cavity.

2. **Fluid thrill:** This test has been discussed in chapter 34 of 'Examination of Chronic Abdominal Conditions'. It also indicates presence of free fluid in the abdomen in large quantity.

3. **Obliteration of liver dullness:** Right midaxillary line is percussed from above downwards. The percussion note will be resonant in the upper part of the midaxillary line **(Fig. 33.10)**. At the upper border of the liver the resonant note is replaced by the dull note. If the liver dullness is replaced by a resonant note it indicates presence of *free gas* under the diaphragm as occurs in perforation of the gastrointestinal tract. It must be remembered that absence of this sign does not exclude perforation since this sign will only be present when there is sufficient leakage of air.

Fallacy: Considerable distension of the gut and emphysema of the lung may obliterate the area of normal liver dullness.

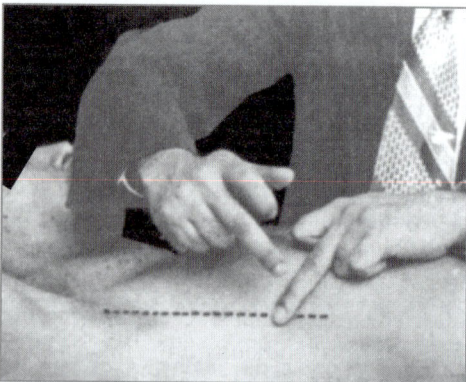

Fig. 33.10: Demonstrating the presence of resonance over the area of liver dullness by percussing along the right midaxillary line about 3 inches above the costal margin. Resonance here indicates gas under the diaphragm.

D. AUSCULTATION

This is a *very important part of examination* in acute abdominal conditions and should never be omitted **(Fig. 33.11)**. The student should be familiar with normal peristaltic sounds noting their character and frequency by studying them in healthy abdomen. The 'silent abdomen' is a pathognomonic feature of diffuse peritonitis. Even localized absence of peristaltic sound will be evident around acute inflammation of the organ concerned. To the contrary a 'noisy abdomen' is a feature of acute intestinal obstruction. Normal intestinal sound is heard as clicks and gurgles but in intestinal obstruction distinct metallic tinkles or borborygmi can be heard. In case of peritonitis or paralytic ileus when the intestinal sounds are absent peculiar respiratory and cardiac sounds may become audible.

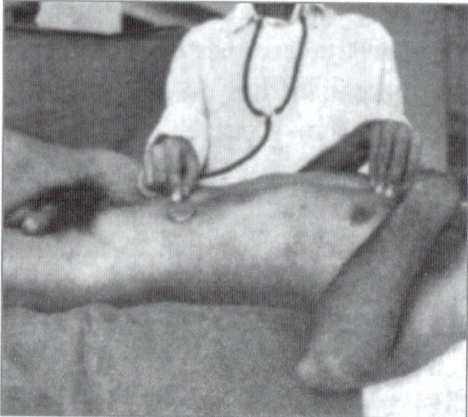

Fig. 33.11: Auscultation of the abdomen is of great value in differentiating peritonitis from intestinal obstruction. In peritonitis the abdomen is more or less silent—whereas in intestinal obstruction increased peristaltic sounds can be heard.

Measurement: Rate of distension in acute intestinal obstruction or paralytic ileus or postoperative peritonitis can be assessed through repeated measurements.

Rectal examination: No examination of an acute abdominal case is complete without the digital examination of the rectum. The right wall may be tender in pelvic type *appendicitis*, which may not show any tenderness or rigidity of the anterior abdominal wall. Tenderness is often elicited in the rectovesical pouch in *perforated peptic ulcer*. The bulging of the anterior wall of the rectum with tenderness is significant of a pelvic abscess. In *intussusception*, after the rectal examination has been finished one will find the gloved finger to be smeared with mucus and blood ('red-currant jelly') but there will be no fecal odor.

In majority of cases of acute abdomen there is ballooning of the rectum whose significance is yet to be found out.

Vaginal examination: Purulent discharge and tenderness in both fornices are suggestive of *acute salpingitis*. In case of *ruptured ectopic gestation*, the cervix feels softer and any movement of the cervix will initiate pain.

GENERAL EXAMINATION

When the abdominal findings are not sufficient to account for the symptoms the patient is complaining of, one should think of extra-abdominal causes and proceed to examine in the following way:

1. **Examine the chest and chest wall (Fig. 33.12):** Pain is often referred to the abdomen from the thorax in such conditions as diaphragmatic pleurisy, basal pneumonia, angina pectoris, myocardial infarction, etc. Pain may reflect from the upper and middle lobes of the right lung to the right hypochondrium and may wrongly lead to the diagnosis of acute cholecystitis. Similarly, referred pain from the right lobe to the right iliac fossa may lead to the false diagnosis of acute appendicitis. Abdominal distension if present, adds to confusion. Typical findings of pneumonia may be lacking but presence of fever, hurried respiration with lowered pulse/respiration ratio, working of the alae nasi and absence of vesicular breathing all lead to a probable diagnosis of lobar pneumonia.

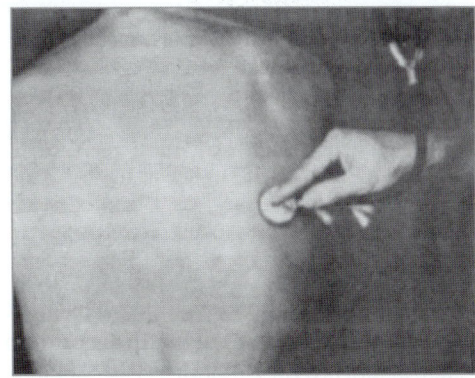

Fig. 33.12: The chest must be thoroughly examined in every case of acute abdomen. In diaphragmatic pleurisy and basal pneumonia pain is often referred to the abdomen.

In case of children, confusion is much more due to lack of good history. *Thoracic compression test* by compressing the lower part of the chest from side to side will bring about pain in presence of thoracic diseases but not with typical acute abdomen.

When pain radiates from the back along one or more spinal nerves of the lower thoracic segments to the midline anteriorly, one should think of herpes zoster as the probable condition. This often leads to confusion with acute cholecystitis, but skin hyperesthesia along the whole course of the affected nerve and absence of rebound tenderness may clinch the diagnosis.

2. **Examine the scrotum and spermatic cord for evidence of filariasis (Fig. 33.13):** This may lead to acute abdominal pain from retroperitoneal lymphangitis. Swelling, redness and tenderness of the groin due to filarial funiculitis supported by periodic fever should suggest this condition.

3. **Examine the spine for pott's disease (Fig. 33.14):** Compression of the spinal cord or more often the intercostal nerves by the granulation tissue of pott's disease may cause referred pain in the abdomen to mimic an acute abdomen.

4. **Examine the nervous system to exclude Tabes Dorsalis:** It may lead to gastric crisis consisting of pain in the abdomen and vomiting. A history of 'lightning pain' in the legs, Argyll-

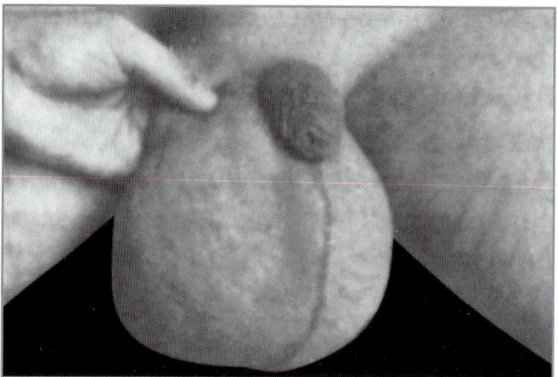

Fig. 33.13: The spermatic cord and scrotum should always be examined for evidence of filariasis in a case of acute abdomen. Cases are on record when the patient complains of acute pain in the abdomen when the pathology lies in the testis, e.g., pain complained in the right iliac fossa in case of torsion of the testis; abdominal pain sometimes in a child may be due to acute epididymitis.

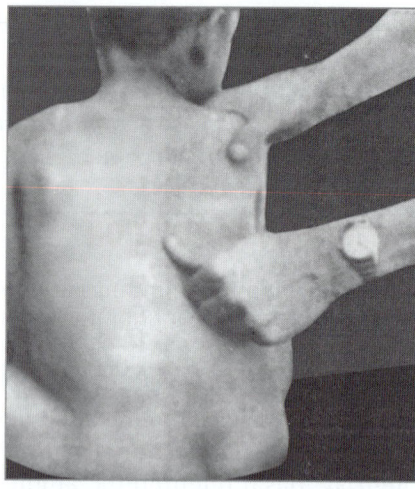

Fig. 33.14: Spine should be examined to exclude Pott's disease when the patient complains of abdominal pain.

Robertson pupil (i.e., pupil not reacting to light but retaining the accommodation reflex) and absence of ankle and knee jerks will settle the diagnosis.

There are a number of medical conditions which may mimic an acute abdomen. These are malaria, porphyria, diabetic crisis, Sickle-cell anemia, hemophilia, etc.

SPECIAL INVESTIGATIONS

1. **Blood:** (a) *Leukocytosis* indicates inflammatory condition. Its role in the diagnosis of acute appendicitis is considered very high. Besides this, it is almost always present in acute cholecystitis, acute pancreatitis, etc. Acute intestinal obstruction when complicated by strangulation may show presence of leukocytosis. (b) *Sugar* and *urea estimations* of the blood are important. Diabetic crisis may mimic an acute abdomen. Uremia may present itself with persistent vomiting accompanied by increasing distension of the abdomen to make this condition confused with acute intestinal obstruction. In pancreatitis, (c) the *serum amylase* estimation will be high. While the normal value is 80–150 Somogyi units, 400 units is considered to suggest presence of acute pancreatitis. The highest level (1,000–2,000 units) reaches within the first 24–48 hours, after which it may come down to normal. (d) The *serum calcium* level is lowered in acute pancreatitis as calcium is fixed in the formation of soap. It may take 5–8 days after the attack. The fall in the serum calcium level is a good index of the severity of acute pancreatitis. A level below 7 mg/100 mL is considered to be dangerous. (e) The *serum bilirubin* level is raised in acute pancreatitis. (f) The *plasma fibrinogen* is also raised at the end of first week and should return to normal within the 3rd week. It is of considerable prognostic value. (g) *Serum deoxyribonuclease, leucine amino-peptidase* (LAD) and *lecithinase A* may be raised and considered to be a definite diagnostic index so far as acute pancreatitis is concerned. (h) Increased *serum Methaemalbumin* indicates the presence of underlying hemorrhagic pancreatitis. Estimation of *C-reactive protein (CRP)* is important as high level in serum is considered to be diagnostic

of acute appendicitis. CRP is found to appear in sera of individual in response to various inflammatory conditions and tissue necrosis. This disappears when the inflammatory condition subsides. A venous blood sample is taken for estimation of CRP in plasma. CRP is estimated by extracting serum by centrifugation and determining the value by latex fixation test kit supplied by Ranbaxy India Ltd. When CRP value is more than 6 mg/L this is considered significant to be diagnostic of acute appendicitis.

2. **Blood pressure:** This becomes low in any hemorrhagic condition. In acute pancreatitis where shock is a prominent feature of the disease, the blood pressure will be lowered.

3. **Urine:** Routine urine examination should be a must in any case of acute abdomen. In acute appendicitis there may be presence of blood and pus cells in the urine due to approximation of inflamed appendix to the ureter. This does not indicate any disease of the urinary tract. Obviously in renal colic one may expect strick of hemorrhage in urine. *Estimation of urinary diastase* is an important laboratory test. In acute pancreatitis the diastase index may rise to 500 units or more from the normal 10 to 30 units. Glycosuria may be present in acute pancreatitis.

4. **X-ray examination:** Where there is facility, X-ray examination affords a distinct help in arriving at a diagnosis. In a straight X-ray multiple fluid levels and gas indicate *acute intestinal obstruction* (**Fig. 33.15**). Straight X-ray in sitting position when shows presence of gas under the diaphragm it indicates *perforation of the gastrointestinal tract*. In suspected gastroduodenal perforation 20–30 mL of air is injected into the stomach by means of Ryle's tube and a skiagram is taken in sitting position. Gas under the diaphragm confirms the diagnosis. Similarly, gastrografin may be used to mark the perforation.

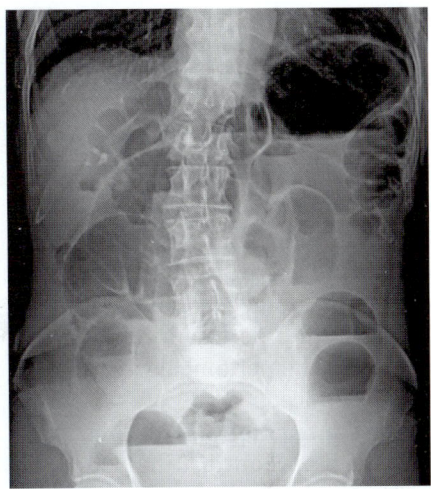

Fig. 33.15: Straight X-ray showing multiple fluid levels (shown by arrows) and gas in acute intestinal obstruction.

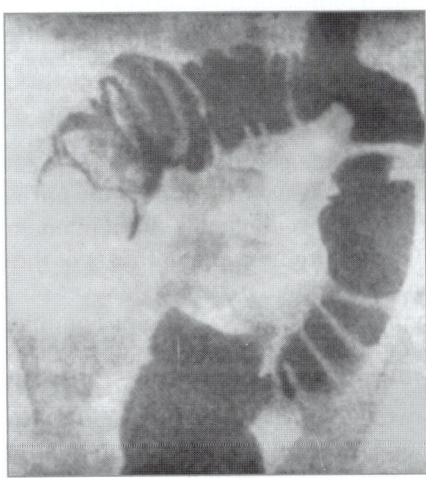

Fig. 33.16: Note the pincer-shaped ending of the barium enema—the pathognomonic feature of intussusception.

In *acute cholecystitis*, the bile ducts may be visualized by intravenous cholangiography with biligraffin but the gallbladder is not seen. If the gallbladder with the bile ducts is visualized it is not a case of cholecystitis. In *acute pancreatitis* gas in the duodenum and first coil of jejunum is sometimes seen. Stewart's sign i.e., gas filled hepatic and splenic flexures, no gas in the transverse colon is suggestive of this condition. Effacement of renal and psoas shadow and the film of fluid in between gas-filled ileal coils are additional evidences in favor of this condition. In case of *intussusception* screening and skiagraphy after a barium enema are of value in diagnosing the condition by showing pincer-shaped end of the barium enema (**Fig. 33.16**). It also helps in spontaneous reduction of the intussusception. In suspected *gallstone ileus*

(Fig. 33.17) the shadow of the stone near the termination of small intestine will clinch the diagnosis. To differentiate *renal colic* from appendicular colic, intravenous pyelography is very important. In *acute ulcerative colitis* a shadow of remarkable dilatation of the transverse colon—'toxic megacolon' may be seen. After perforation free air within the peritoneal cavity may be noticed.

5. **Barium enema examination:** This with air contrast may be helpful in detecting early stage of *acute ulcerative colitis*. Barium

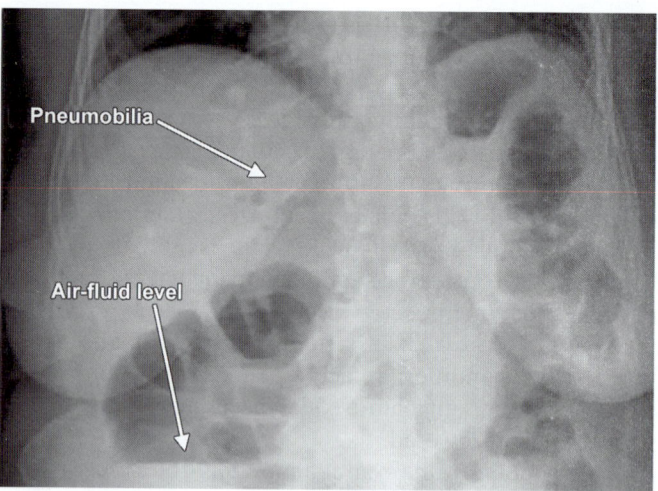

Fig. 33.17: Gallstone ileus—showing air in the biliary tree.

roentgenographic signs include loss of haustral markings and irregularities of the colon wall, which represent small ulceration. As the disease progresses pseudopolyps become prominent. When there are clinical signs of toxic megacolon, barium study is contraindicated. In *Crohn's disease* double-contrast barium study may reveal longitudinal and transverse mucosal ulcers or fissures may present as 'spicules'. The irregular network of intersecting ulcers combine with submucosal oedema to result in coarse nodularity or 'cobblestone' pattern. There may be filling defects due to hyperplastic lymph follicles. The hallmark of this disease is presence of 'skip lesions' with apparently normal intervening bowel which may measure a few inches to several feet in length. Barium enema examination of *diverticulitis* shows segmental spasm with serrations (saw-toothing) of the bowel. Mucosal oedema and narrowing of the lumen may be evident. It cannot be over-emphasized that barium enema examination is absolutely contraindicated in very acute conditions. This examination however may be performed when acute condition has subsided.

6. **Endoscopy:** Proctosigmoidoscopy is helpful in *acute ulcerative colitis* as the rectum is involved in 90–95%. The mucosa is usually erythematous and granular and bleeds easily. Superficial mucosal ulcers are seen. In *Crohn's disease* (regional ileitis) endoscopy reveals cobblestone appearance with deep linear ulceration. Colonoscopy will determine the extent of the disease in ulcerative colitis and in Crohn's disease 'skip lesions' become evident. In very *acute diverticulitis* sigmoidoscopy may be painful. The mucosa is inflamed and diverticula may be seen. But narrowing of the colon, spasm, fixation and angulation are more commonly seen.

7. **Enema:** Indiscriminate administration of enema in acute abdominal conditions must be *strongly condemned*. Nothing is more harmful than an enema given in a case of peritonitis. The only suitable subject for administration of an enema is one of the acute intestinal obstruction. In this condition the '*two enema*' *test* is of greater value. The first enema may show some result by evacuating the lower bowel. It is the result of the second enema given after an interval of 2 hours that leads to the diagnosis. In the presence of obstruction, the fluid of the second enema is either retained or rejected without any fecal matter. The patient is not relieved.

8. **Intravenous cholangiography permits visualization of the entire extrahepatic biliary tree:** Though this investigation was used earlier for acute cholecystitis as oral cholecystography is contraindicated, now it is losing ground in this condition.

9. **Ultrasonography:** This noninvasive imaging technique has become the routine investigation in acute cholecystitis. It demonstrates gallbladder calculi, bile duct calculi, dilatation of the gallbladder with stone and sludge, stone in the cystic duct, dilatation of biliary tree and even a tumor in the pancreas.

Ultrasonography is a significant tool in diagnosing appendicitis. The overall specificity and sensitivity was found to be 90% and 88% respectively, giving USG a high specificity and sensitivity value in diagnosing appendicitis. It also helps in diagnosing other causes of right lower quadrant pain.

10. **Radio-isotope scanning:** Cholescintigraphy with ^{131}I Rose Bengal or with a derivative of ^{99m}Technetium-iminodiacetic acid (technetium-IDA scan) has become more specific test than any other in acute cholecystitis. After intravenous injection this material is excreted by the liver into the biliary ductal system. This shows the extrahepatic biliary tree including gallbladder. In acute cholecystitis the gallbladder is not visualized as presumably the gallbladder outlet or the cystic duct is obstructed. It has an accuracy of almost 100%.

11. **Computed tomography (CT scan):** It provides almost similar informations as ultrasonography. It is probably useful for those in whom ultrasonography is difficult, e.g., in obese patients and in those having excessive bowel gas.

12. **Exploratory laparotomy:** On many occasions of acute abdomen the diagnosis is not established until a laparotomy is undertaken.

CAUSES OF 'ACUTE ABDOMEN'

A. INTRA-ABDOMINAL CAUSES

1. *Inflammation*—For example, acute appendicitis, acute cholecystitis, acute salpingitis, acute diverticulitis, acute regional ileitis, acute pneumococcal peritonitis, acute nonspecific mesenteric lymphadenitis, amoebic liver abscess.
2. *Perforation* of peptic ulcer, typhoid ulcer, diverticular disease, ulcerative colitis, etc.
3. *Acute intestinal obstruction:*
    a. *Mechanical:*
        i. In the lumen—Gallstone, round worms, faecolith, etc.
        ii. In the wall—Tubercular stricture, intussusception, growths, etc.
        iii. Outside the wall—Additional bands, volvulus, external and internal hernia, etc.
    b. *Toxic*—Paralytic ileus.
    c. *Neurogenic*—Hirschprung's disease.
    d. *Vascular*—Occlusion of mesenteric vessels by embolism or thrombosis.
4. *Hemorrhage*—For example, rupture of ectopic gestation, ruptured lutein cyst, spontaneous rupture of malarial spleen. Rupture or leaking aortic aneurysm, aortic dissecting aneurysm.
5. *Torsion of pedicle*—For example, twisted ovarian cyst, spleen, etc.
6. *Colics*—For example, (i) biliary, (ii) ureteric, (iii) appendicular and (iv) intestinal.

B. EXTRA-ABDOMINAL CAUSES

1. *Parietal conditions*—For example, superficial cellulitis of the abdominal wall, gas gangrene of the abdominal wall, abscess of the abdominal wall, rupture of rectus abdominis muscle and/or tearing of inferior epigastric artery.
2. *Thoracic conditions*—For example, diaphragmatic pleurisy, lobar pneumonia, spontaneous pneumothorax, pericarditis, angina pectoris, coronary thrombosis, etc.

3. *Retroperitoneal conditions*—For example, uremia, pyelitis, dietl's crisis, retroperitoneal lymphangitis and lymphadenitis, leaking aneurysm of the aorta, dissecting aneurysm of the aorta etc.

4. *Diseases of the spine, spinal cord and intercostal nerves*—For example, Pott's disease, acute osteomyelitis of lower dorsal or lumbar vertebrae, gastric crisis in Tabes Dorsalis, herpes zoster of lower intercostal nerves and intercostal neuralgia.

5. *General Diseases*—For example, malaria, typhoid fever, porphyria, diabetic crisis, sickle cell anemia, hemophilia, purpura, small pox, etc.

In children the following conditions are common :
a. Acute appendicitis;
b. Intussusception;
c. Intestinal obstruction by round worms, congenital band or by bands including Meckel's diverticula;
d. Acute nonspecific mesenteric lymphadenitis;
e. Meckel's diverticulitis;
f. Primary peritonitis.

In females the following conditions are common :
a. Ruptured ectopic gestation;
b. Ruptured lutein cyst;
c. Twisted ovarian cyst;
d. Acute salpingitis;
e. Tubo-ovarian abscess;
f. Torsion or degeneration of a uterine fibroid.

DIFFERENTIAL DIAGNOSIS

INFLAMMATION

ACUTE APPENDICITIS

The etiology of this very common condition is still not clearly known. However, diet (low residue diet), social status (high middle class and upper class), residence (European, American and Australian), familial susceptibility, obstruction of the lumen of the appendix with fecolith, foreign body, round worm or thread worm or a stricture and indiscriminate use of purgatives are all incriminated. Though no age is exempt, it is rare before the age of 2 years. It becomes increasingly common during childhood and adolescence and the maximum incidence is noticed between 20 and 30 years. Thereafter the incidence gradually drops. Clinically two varieties are seen—1. Nonobstructive type and 2. Obstructive type. *Nonobstructive* variety progresses slowly, whereas *obstructive* type progresses very fast, and gangrene and perforation are commonly seen in this type. A careful history must be taken. If the patient gets pain around the umbilicus or in the epigastrium in the beginning and later on this pain shifts to the right iliac fossa, he is undoubtedly suffering from an acute appendicitis. The initial pain is visceral and felt on the midline irrespective of the position of the appendix, since developmentally the midgut, from which appendix develops, is a median organ. The second pain is due to irritation of parietal peritoneum lying in close proximity to the appendix, therefore it depends on the position of the appendix. The pain is dull aching in character in nonobstructive type of appendicitis, whereas this is of colicky nature in obstructive appendicitis. Pain is followed by nausea and vomiting along with anorexia depending on the degree of distension of the appendix.

Fever is almost always associated with this condition. The sequence of symptoms, viz. *pain, vomiting* and *temperature*, is known as 'Murphy's syndrome'. So far as the bowel habit is concerned constipation is the usual accompaniment, but there may be diarrhea in case of acute pelvic appendicitis or with appendicular abscess.

Examination reveals presence of hyperesthesia in Sherren's triangle, tenderness at McBurney's point, muscle guard and rebound tenderness over the appendix. Positive Rovsing's sign is a definite diagnostic clue and should always be looked for. Within two or three days a tender and fixed lump develops at the site of the appendix, which is known as 'appendicular lump'. Sluggish peritoneal sound on the right iliac fossa is also evident in auscultation.

Should perforation take place, the outlook temporarily improves with disappearance of pain, but very soon the features of spreading peritonitis appears. Pain is complained of all over the abdomen, vomiting may become more marked, but more important is the pulse rate which gradually rises and the temperature becomes subnormal. Restricted movement of the abdominal wall, 'board-like' rigidity, spread of tenderness from the right iliac to the left iliac fossa and 'silent abdomen' on auscultation leave no doubt that the peritonitis is spreading. In estimating the degree of spread, the pulse rate is an important guide.

Variation of clinical features are observed according to the nature of the disease, the position of the appendix and the age of the patient.

Differentiation between catarrhal and obstructive appendicitis: In catarrhal appendicitis the onset is gradual, the pain is dull and aching, the patient carries on her usual duties but with discomfort in the abdomen, nausea, vomiting and even anorexia. In obstructive appendicitis the onset is sudden. The patient immediately goes back to her bed with severe colicky pain in the abdomen along with vomiting and rise of temperature.

Retrocecal appendicitis: When the organ is entirely retroperitoneal, there is hardly any tenderness and rigidity on the anterior abdomen. There may be some tenderness and rigidity in the right flank or more posteriorly. To elicit such tenderness the patient should be rolled to her left side. If the appendix lies in close relation to the right ureter, the patient may complain of hematuria and pain radiating from the loin to the groin. This confuses the clinician and the diagnosis of ureteric stone has often been wrongly made. The history of initial pain around the umbilicus, Rovsing's sign and Psoas test will guide the clinician to the diagnosis of appendicitis.

Pelvic appendicitis: Tenderness and rigidity may not be so prominent on the anterior abdominal wall as in normal. Moreover, the picture becomes more confusing due to the history of diarrhea and rise of temperature. Irritation of the bladder (strangury) and the rectum (passage of mucus per annum and tenesmus) are also very confusing. Even in this condition a careful history will elicit that pain started around the umbilicus. Presence of Rovsing's sign and obturator test will clinch the diagnosis. Rectal examination is often helpful as tenderness on the right side of the rectouterine pouch in females and rectovesical pouch in males will give definite clue to the diagnosis. A tender lump or cystic swelling in rectal examination is diagnostic of pelvic abscess.

Acute appendicitis in infancy and childhood: The constitutional disturbances are more in children. The temperature is often high along with the pulse rate, vomiting and diarrhea (instead of constipation) are the usual features. Elicitation of tenderness is not so easy as in case of adults. A good technique is to palpate the abdomen with the child's own hand. At the point of maximum tenderness the child will put its hand away. Appendicular lump is rarely seen due to short omentum and poor inflammatory response. For this, early perforation is the rule and the surgeon must diagnose the case very early and perform appendicectomy giving no chance to appendix to perforate by itself.

Acute appendicitis in the elderly: These patients with laxed abdominal wall hardly show any rigidity. Moreover, due to atherosclerosis of the appendicular artery chance of rapid gangrene and subsequent perforation becomes obvious. So distension of the abdomen in the second stage of peritonitis, with constipation and vomiting resemble the picture of intestinal obstruction. The clinician, may advice enema erroneously to make the patient's condition much worse.

Acute appendicitis in pregnancy: The enlarging uterus will cause an upward displacement of the caecum and thus confuse acute appendicitis with cholecystitis. Careful history with positive Rovsing's sign should help to make the diagnosis. Sometimes concealed accidental hemorrhage or necrobiosis of uterine fibroid may lead to similar pain as in acute appendicitis. With the patient in supine position, the most tender spot is marked with skin pencil. The patient is now turned to her left and is kept in this position for at least one minute. The most tender spot is again found out. If there is a shifting of tenderness, it indicates uterine pathology. Pyelitis and cystitis are also common during pregnancy. So, one should be careful to consider these conditions in the differential diagnosis.

ACUTE CHOLECYSTITIS

Fatty, fertile female of forty are the usual victims. A previous history of flatulent dyspepsia and belching and now with severe pain in the right hypochondriac region radiating to the inferior angle of the right scapula or to the top of the right shoulder are probable indications of a case of acute cholecystitis. Nausea, retching and vomiting, rise of temperature and an elevated pulse rate may be associated with this condition. Jaundice may be present in only 1/4 of the cases may be due to accompanying cholangitis or due to entry of the bile pigments into the circulation through the damaged gallbladder mucosa. Charcot's triad i.e., pain, jaundice and rigor (due to cholangitis and even septicemia) is very characteristic of this condition. Tenderness and rigidity can be easily elicited on the gallbladder point. Gallbladder is hardly palpable. If so, it is due to the organ being wrapped with greater omentum. Overlying rigidity stands in the way of better palpation. Very rarely an empyema of the gallbladder may become palpable if the clinician becomes very gentle **(Fig. 33.18)**. In *special investigations* blood examination is helpful as in 85% of cases there is elevation of W.B.C. count. In half the patients there is rise in serum bilirubin and in one-third of cases serum amylase will be

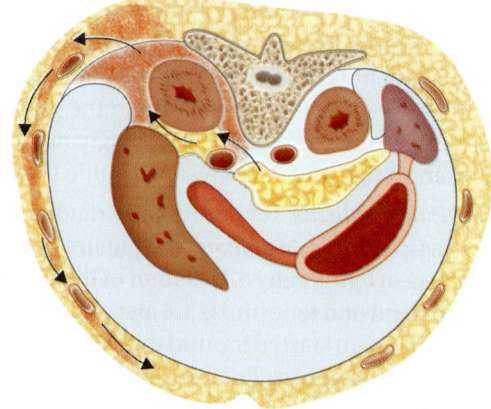

Fig. 33.18: Diagrammatic representation showing how hemorrhagic fluid from acute hemorrhagic pancreatitis tracks along the abdominal wall to cause discoloration of the loin (Gray-Turner's sign) and around the umbilicus (Cullen's sign).

increased. Oral cholecystography is contraindicated. Ultrasound and radioactive scanning are helpful in diagnosing this condition.

ACUTE PANCREATITIS

This condition is commonly seen over 30 years of age. Men slightly dominate over women. Pain which is felt over the epigastrium is excruciating and agonizing in nature. It is the first in severity considering all abdominal cases. It tends to pierce to the back or to the left loin, which becomes more severe when the patient lies down. So, the patient shows a tendency towards sitting on the bed leaning forward. The pain is *constant in nature* and not colicky. Vomiting is profuse, projectile and follows pain. Pulse rate is almost always quickened with the commencement of the disease. Shock and cyanosis are the two distinct features of this condition. Former is due to absorption of incompletely split products of protein and the latter to toxemia and anoxia caused by diminished excursion of the diaphragm resulting from the inflamed pancreas. Temperature is at first subnormal and does not rise over normal limit on the first day of the disease. While tenderness is very obvious just above the umbilicus, muscle guard is conspicuous by its absence. In acute pancreatitis the left costovertebral angle may be tender due to inflammation of the tail of the pancreas. In late cases muscular rigidity may be present to confuse this condition with peptic perforation. There may be some fullness of the epigastrium. Discoloration of the loin (Gray Turner's sign) and around the umbilicus (Cullen's sign) are late features of this disease **(Fig. 33.18)**. In *special investigations* estimation of serum amylase is the most widely used test. A serum level of more than 400 Somogyi units is suggestive whereas more than 1,000 Somogyi units is almost diagnostic. Urinary amylase will also be increased in this condition. Recently elevation in the serum and urinary lipase have been given importance but subject to limitations. Paracentesis fluid is analyzed and both amylase and lipase levels are raised. Straight X-ray findings have been discussed in the section of 'special investigations', but presence of 'sentinel loop'—a single dilated atonic loop of small bowel is a contributory evidence for diagnosis. In ultrasonography and CT scan one may detect an edematous pancreas **(Fig. 33.19)**. But the images are poor in the obese.

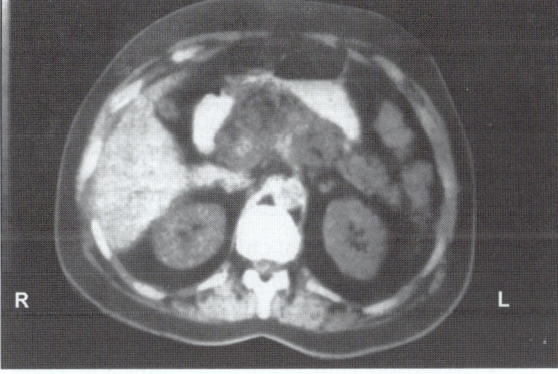

Fig. 33.19: CT scan of the abdomen showing edematous enlarged pancreas indicating acute pancreatitis.

ACUTE COLONIC DIVERTICULITIS

This condition mainly affects the pelvic colon. Typically the pain is complained of in the left iliac fossa. A tender, thick pelvic colon can be palpated in the left side of the abdomen. Perforation is not very common. More common is the localized peridiverticular abscess. In this condition the pus is confined, the mesocolon is greatly thickened and the bowel becomes swollen and edematous. Intestinal obstruction may result from thickened colon. Muscular rigidity is always present in this condition. Occasionally localized abscess may burst to the exterior (forming external fistula) or into any viscus viz. urinary bladder (forming internal fistula). Very rarely carcinoma may supervene. Sigmoidoscopy and barium X-ray are helpful in diagnosing this condition.

ACUTE REGIONAL ILEITIS

This condition in many respects resembles acute appendicitis. Pain in the right iliac fossa is common to both these conditions. But in this condition there may be a long previous history of intestinal colic (due to intestinal obstruction, which is a feature of this condition and never found in appendicitis) and diarrhea (it is again peculiar to this condition and never seen in appendicitis before the onset of the attack). A tender mass may be felt in the right iliac fossa and will be felt by pelvic examination. A patient when complains of pain in the right iliac fossa along with certain other complications like anal fissure, fistula or edematous skin tag, the diagnosis becomes certain. If an appendicular lump does not resolve by medical treatment, one should think of 4 conditions of which the first is Crohn's disease, the second is ileocecal tuberculosis, the third is actinomycosis and the last, though rare, is carcinoma. If after appendicectomy sinus complicates, one should think of the possibility of Crohn's disease.

ACUTE SALPINGITIS

Usually, the disease starts at the time of menstruation or during the first week after abortion or delivery. The pain of acute salpingitis is mainly felt on the sides of the hypogastrium or even in the iliac fossae. So, to differentiate from acute appendicitis, one should carefully take the menstrual history and ask "where did the pain start?" Normally in appendicitis the pain starts around the umbilicus and then shifts to the right iliac fossa, whereas in this condition the pain remains static at the iliac fossa. The temperature usually rises to 102°F or even more. Difficulty in micturition, e.g., scalding pain during micturition is a common accompaniment of this condition. Abdominal rigidity is not so pronounce as in appendicitis. Vaginal discharge is again a pathognomonic feature of this condition, it may be a recent onset or an exacerbation of a long-standing discharge. Vaginal examination will reveal a somewhat enlarged uterus when this condition has occurred following abortion or puerperium. The cervix may be softer but will cause tremendous pain if it is moved. Only when the acute stage is over, unilateral or bilateral swollen tubal mass may be discovered.

ACUTE NONSPECIFIC MESENTERIC LYMPHADENITIS

This is mainly a disease of children below six years of age. After 14 years it is better not to make this diagnosis. This condition mainly competes with acute appendicitis. The pain starts around umbilicus. The pain may be of colicky nature. Vomiting is usual and occurs in the beginning of the attack. The temperature may be raised just above normal. There is hardly any difference in pulse rate which is again a differentiating point against acute appendicitis. The patient indicates the site of pain a diffuse area above and medial to the position of appendix. The site of pain remains constant without showing any tendency to shift (cf. pain in appendicitis). On examination too much rigidity is never present. If one becomes gentle in palpation one may feel enlarged lymph nodes on deep palpation. Shifting tenderness (Klein's sign) is the pathognomonic feature of this condition. After locating the area of tenderness in the supine position, the patient is rolled to the left side and kept in this place for a few minutes. Tenderness moves to the left. This is a distinguishing feature from acute appendicitis, where tenderness is relatively fixed. Of course, the students should remember of Meckel's diverticulitis which shows similar type of shifting tenderness.

ACUTE ULCERATIVE COLITIS

Ulcerative colitis is mainly a chronic condition characterized by relapses and remissions. Only in 5% of cases it may present as an acute condition and deserves mention in this chapter. Incessant diarrhea containing blood, mucus and pus, high rise of temperature and a toxic state are the main features of this acute condition. When the whole or a substantial portion of the colon is involved the attack is likely to be more severe with some systemic upset. The depth of the ulcers are also an important feature in this respect. Deep ulceration extending up to the deep muscular layer will cause toxic colitis with severe systemic manifestations. Severe abdominal distension may occur from toxic megacolon. Depletion of protein with a low serum albumin and loss of body weight also accompany this condition. Erythema nodosum, pyoderma, arthritis, etc., are the complications of systemic involvement. It must be remembered that colitis in the elderly is much more dangerous than in young patients. Straight X-ray, endoscopy and rectal biopsy will clinch the diagnosis.

SUBDIAPHRAGMATIC (SUBPHRENIC) ABSCESS

This condition usually follows some intraperitoneal lesion, e.g., perforated peptic ulcer, abdominal trauma, acute appendicitis, operations on biliary tract and operations on the stomach. The patient usually runs temperature without any definite cause. Pulse rate and the rate of respiration also go up. Pain, if complained of, helps in the diagnosis. It is usually felt over the abscess in the hypochondriac region. Pain may be referred to the corresponding shoulder due to irritation of the diaphragm. On examination, careful palpation may elicit an area of tenderness over the abscess.

It must be confessed that there is hardly any definite diagnostic feature of this condition. Suspicion is the main help to the diagnosis. The popular aphorism that "signs of pus some where, signs of pus no where else, signs of pus there" is still to be remembered. Sluggish or no diaphragmatic movement in X-ray screening and elevation of the diaphragm on that side are diagnostic evidences.

AMOEBIC LIVER ABSCESS

It is not an uncommon condition to cause acute abdomen in tropical countries. Adult males are the usual sufferers. It is a complication of amoebic dysentery. The patient presents with acute pain in the right hypochondriac or epigastric region, which is increased by alcohol, walking, riding a vehicle and jarring. The patient often supports the upper right side of the abdomen with his hands when he expects jarring or vibration. Such pain is often associated with pyrexia, rigors and profuse sweating at night. On examination a swelling may be detected in the right hypochondriac or epigastric region which is extremely tender, moves with respiration and otherwise immobile. Aspiration reveals chocolate colored pus (anchovy-sauce). Radio-isotope liver scan, CT scan, sigmoidoscopy and Barium enema X-ray will reveal the diagnosis.

Complications are—Rupture of the abscess into (i) the peritoneal cavity (giving rise to acute peritonitis with board-like rigidity), (ii) the pleural cavity (empyema), (iii) into the lung (chocolate colored pus is expectorated) or (iv) into the intestine.

PERFORATION

PEPTIC PERFORATION

The clinical picture is described in three stages.
1. The first stage is known as *peritonism* i.e., irritation of the peritoneum. It is due to leakage of gastric juice into the peritoneal cavity (chemical peritonitis). This stage usually lasts for about six hours. Usually an adult male, who gives a previous history of peptic ulcer, is suddenly seized

with acute burning pain over the epigastrium. The pain may be referred to the tip of the right shoulder due to irritation of the under surface of the diaphragm. The pain may gradually gravitate down along the paracolic gutter to the right iliac fossa. At this stage one may misunderstand the pain to be due to acute appendicitis. The patient may or may not vomit. On examination there will be little change in the pulse, respiration and temperature. Tenderness and muscle guard are constantly present over the site of perforation i.e., upper half of the right rectus muscle. Great importance should be led on the diagnosis of this condition at this stage as chance of survival of the patient gradually declines with passage of time. Diagnosis in the first stage mainly rests on two features viz. onset of pain with a dramatic suddenness in a patient who has given a previous history of peptic ulcer and muscle guard over the upper half of the right rectus muscle. In the late phase of this stage pain may be felt on the right iliac fossa which adds confusion to this diagnosis.

2. The second stage is known as the *stage of reaction*. The irritant fluid becomes diluted with the peritoneal exudate. The intensity of the symptoms dwindles although the fire is still burning under the ashes. The patient feels comfortable and nothing is more deplorable than the attending doctor sharing the patient's comfort. Symptoms are no doubt relieved but the signs are there and should be looked for. Muscular rigidity continues to be present. The other two new features are obliteration of liver dullness and shifting dullness. Rectal examination may elicit tenderness in the rectovesical or rectouterine pouch. Straight X-ray in sitting position will show air under the diaphragm in 70% of cases.

3. The third or the final stage is the *stage of diffuse peritonitis* and it indicates that the patient has gone a step further towards the grave. The pinched and anxious face, sunken eyes and hollow cheeks—the so called facies hippocratic, with rising pulse rate which is low in volume and tension, persistent vomiting, 'board-like' rigidity of the abdomen, increasing distension of the abdomen all give hint to the diagnosis of this condition and imminent death.

PERFORATION OF A TYPHOID ULCER

This usually takes place in the 3rd or 4th week of the typhoid fever. Hemorrhage also occurs in this period. Sudden collapse, fast thready pulse and subnormal temperature indicate either perforation or hemorrhage. But a history of sudden pain, definite tenderness and rigidity (however slight it may be) will lead the diagnosis towards perforation. The liver dullness will be obliterated and shifting dullness test may be positive.

PERFORATION OF ULCERATIVE COLITIS

In only 4% of cases of ulcerative colitis perforation may complicate the fulminating type of the disease. It is usually preceded by toxic megacolon. Sudden pain of the abdomen with distension and shock should immediately rouse suspicion of this condition. Fecal contamination of peritoneum is more dangerous and should be operated on immediately.

PERFORATION OF DIVERTICULAR DISEASE OF COLON

Generalized peritonitis from perforation is extremely rare. More often a localized abscess results. If general peritonitis takes place mortality rate is very high and is not less than 50%.

ACUTE INTESTINAL OBSTRUCTION

The mortality rate from acute intestinal obstruction rises with each passing hour from the onset of the disease; so early diagnosis is imperative. The three main clinical manifestations of acute intestinal obstruction are—intestinal colic, vomiting and distension. The absolute constipation which was also considered to be one of the cardinal features should be excluded as it takes no less than 24 hours to develop this symptom.

1. *Intestinal colic:* When the obstruction lies in the jejunum or high in the ileum the colics appear in waves at intervals of 3–5 minutes. The pain lasts for about 30 seconds. This interval becomes longer in obstruction of the terminal ileum where it is about 8-10 minutes. The site of pain will give an indication as to the site of obstruction, e.g., small intestinal cramps are referred to the epigastrium or umbilical region whereas colonic cramps to the lower abdomen (hypogastrium).

2. *Vomiting:* This is a fairly constant symptom. The frequency of vomiting depends on the site of obstruction. In upper small bowel obstruction vomiting is much more frequent than obstruction in the terminal part of the small bowel. At first the vomitus is the gastric content i.e., ingested food particles and fluid, next it is the content of the duodenum, which is predominantly bile and lastly it is the content of the small intestine above the site of obstruction. Virtually it takes about 3-4 days in complete intestinal obstruction to vomit become feculant. This is a grave sign and should be diagnosed long before this.

3. *Distension:* It must be confessed that this may not be very early sign. But for an experienced clinician distension may be evident in the early stage and is considered to be a diagnostic feature.

4. *Absolute constipation:* It must be remembered that absence of history of recent constipation should under no circumstances exclude a diagnosis of intestinal obstruction. The patient might have moved his bowel in the morning. The symptoms started in the afternoon. For constipation to arrive as a significant sign one has to wait for another 24 hours. This only makes the diagnosis late in case one includes constipation to be one of the four major signs of this condition. Again absolute constipation appears later in the process as it means failure of passage of both feces and flatus. To add to more confusion intestinal obstruction may be accompanied by diarrhea. Mesenteric vascular occlusion, richter's hernia and a pelvic abscess associated with obstruction by adhesion—will produce diarrhea instead of constipation.

5. *Dehydration:* The higher is the obstruction more will be dehydration due to tremendous loss of water and electrolytes. To the contrary obstruction of the terminal ileum is associated with relatively small amount of loss of fluid and electrolytes as the secretions of the G.I. tract are reabsorbed. As a matter of fact dehydration appears late in obstruction of the terminal ileum but the distension becomes pronounce whereas in obstruction of the jejunum dehydration appears earlier but distension is much less.

On examination the patient looks anxious and restless. In the early stage pulse, respiration and temperature show no deviation from normal. Inspection rarely shows distension in the early stage, but a little fullness cannot be missed by an experienced clinician. *Distension* either central (small gut obstruction) or peripheral (large gut obstruction) or regional (volvulus of sigmoid colon or caecum) is a distinctive feature in acute intestinal obstruction. If the clinician becomes more patient and watchful he can discover *visible peristalsis* which is again diagnostic. Gentle flicking of the abdominal wall may initiate visible peristalsis. *It can't be over emphasized at this stage of inspection to inspect all the hernial sites, particularly inguinal, femoral and umbilical.* While umbilical hernia becomes obvious on inspection, inguinal and more often femoral herniae are missed if these sites are not looked for. On palpation muscle guard is conspicuous by its absence. If the hand is laid flat upon the abdomen the underlying coils of intestine may be felt to harden and soften alternately. During palpation one must be careful to discover a lump as may be found in intussusception, neoplasm of the small or large intestine or an intra-abdominal abscess.

Presence of muscle rigidity and rebound tenderness suggest internal strangulation.

Percussion is not much informative in the sense that it only reveals resonant note of gaseous distension of the bowel.

Auscultation is quite an important procedure, yet often missed. Presence of borborygmi which coincide with intestinal colic is very diagnostic. In a case of intestinal obstruction, "silent abdomen" suggests paralytic ileus. Localized absence of intestinal sounds means localized peritonitis or internal strangulation. **Rectal examination** is usually noninformative yet ballooning of the rectum is peculiarly noticed. Very occasionally one may detect pelvic abscess, a lump caused by intussusception or neoplasm of the small or large intestine.

Straight X-ray of the abdomen is very diagnostic. It shows gas-distended loops of the intestine and multiple fluid levels. *Gas-distended bowels* are seen earlier and for fluid levels to appear the fluid must be separated from the gas. Jejunum, ileum and colon may be seen distended with gas and will show characteristic appearances in X-ray. Jejunum is characterized by its valvulae conniventes which are placed at regular intervals giving rise to a concertina effect. Ileum is characterized by straight lines of its walls. Large intestine shows haustral folds, which leave indentations in the walls. While gas shadows can be seen even in the supine position, *fluid levels* are seen only in erect posture. The number of fluid levels is proportionate to the degree of obstruction and to its site. The number of fluid level is more, the nearer the obstruction is to the ileocecal valve. In paralytic ileus fluid level becomes more conspicuous and more numerous. In obstruction of the large intestine a gas-filled caecum becomes obvious in X-ray. In this context one should remember two fallacies—(i) in infants under the age of 2 years a few fluid levels in the small intestine are not abnormal. (ii) Two inconstant fluid levels may be seen in the duodenal cap and at the terminal ileum.

Having diagnosed that the case is one of acute intestinal obstruction, the clinician should proceed to detect (a) the site, (b) the nature and (c) the cause of the obstruction.

a. **THE SITE OF OBSTRUCTION:** In high intestinal obstruction vomiting is early and profuse. The vomitus consists of gastric fluid in the beginning and bile later on. Feculent vomiting is never seen. The patient becomes dehydrated very soon. The urine is scanty. Though distension is not a marked feature yet fullness of the epigastrium is often noticed. In this category acute dilatation of the stomach and pyloric stenosis may be included. In low small intestinal obstruction the onset is sudden. Pain is situated over the umbilical region. The vomiting is present but it is neither early and nor profuse. In the early stage the vomitus consists of gastric content later on bile and becomes feculent in the last stage. Distension is marked and is central, visible peristalsis in the form of "ladder pattern", is often noticed. In large gut obstruction the patient is usually elderly the onset is gradual (so it is often said to be chronic). Pain is not very prominent. If present, it is complained of in the hypogastrium. Vomiting is a very late feature and it may not be present altogether. Distension is more marked on the flanks. Careful palpation of the right iliac fossa may reveal the caecum to be distended and may harden under the examining finger. Rectal examination may reveal an annular growth.

b. **NATURE OF OBSTRUCTION:** Intestinal obstruction may be simple or strangulated and dynamic or paralytic. In *simple obstruction* there will be intestinal colic. Pulse, respiration, temperature and blood pressure remain unaffected. On palpation, muscle rigidity and rebound tenderness are conspicuous by their absence. *In strangulation* however, there is no complete remission of pain between colics. So colicky pain of simple obstruction is replaced by a continuous pain. Pulse becomes rapid, temperature may be elevated, there may be tachypnoea and blood pressure falls from the beginning. Presence of muscle rigidity and rebound tenderness immediately make the diagnosis. Two hours gastric suction if fail to relieve pain indicates internal strangulation. Though external strangulation is easier to diagnose by tense, tender and irreducible swelling without any impulse on coughing, yet internal strangulation is not so easy to diagnose and must be looked for.

Paralytic ileus—may occur in the early postoperative period after an abdominal operation or as a complication of diffuse peritonitis. It is differentiated from dynamic intestinal obstruction by the following points : (i) history of abdominal operation or features of peritonitis are present; (ii) gradual distension of the abdomen without visible peristalsis; (iii) absence of colicky pain; (iv) 'silent abdomen' in auscultation.

c. **CAUSE OF OBSTRUCTION:** In determining the cause of obstruction, age of the patient should be taken into consideration first. In the newborn, cause of obstruction is congenital malformation, e.g., congenital atresia of esophagus, congenital pyloric stenosis, meconium ileus, congenital atresia of the duodenum or ileum, Hirschsprung's disease, etc. In *infancy*, intussusception and obstruction due to warms. In *adolescence*, besides intussusception band or adhesion resulting from Meckel's diverticulum or local peritonitis due to appendicitis, tubercular peritonitis, tabes mesenterica, etc. In *adults*, obstruction by a band, volvulus or growth should be considered whereas in the old, carcinoma of the colon is the usual cause. A fatty woman of 40, with previous history of cholelithiasis, if presents with intestinal obstruction possibility of gallstone ileus should be considered. A strangulated hernia may occur at any age.

ACUTE INTUSSUSCEPTION

Usually, the patient is a lusty male baby between six to twelve months of age. The onset is usually sudden. The child screams in abdominal pain and draws his legs up. The attacks usually last for a few minutes and come back within fifteen minutes. In between the attacks the patient looks somewhat drawn. Facial pallor is an important sign which always associates with each attack. Vomiting is more often late to come—usually takes about 24 hours. Slight rise of temperature may be seen even during the first 24 hours. Absence of distension with severe colic in the abdomen and pallor should give the suggestion towards the diagnosis. Absolute constipation is rarely seen. In the early stage normal stools are passed frequently, later on blood and mucus are evacuated which is popularly known as "Red-currant Jelly".

On examination the abdomen is hardly distended. The main diagnostic feature is palpation of a lump which is curved, sausage shaped and in the line of the colon with its concavity towards the umbilicus. Should the lump harden under the examining fingers synchronously with the attacks of screaming, the diagnosis is established. The lump may not be felt when it is lying just under the right or the left costal margin. The examination must be gently conducted as contraction of the abdominal muscles may stand in the way of good palpation of the lump. A feeling of emptiness in the right iliac fossa is known as *signe-de-dance*. Too much stress should not be paid on this sign. When everything has been made ready for operation it is a good practice to search for the lump under general anesthesia. On *rectal examination* bloodstained mucus will be found on the examining finger. There is absolutely no fecal odour. If intussusception has travelled far enough, its apex may be felt per rectum and will be felt like cervix uteri. In very rare instance intussusception may project through the anus. This indicates that the patient possesses a long mesentery to render the small intestine unduly mobile. After six hours signs of dehydration will appear. After 24 hours the abdomen will start distending and vomiting becomes profuse. *X-ray is confirmatory:* Straight X-ray of the abdomen will reveal increased gas-shadows in the small intestine and absence of cecal gas-shadow. Barium enema X-ray, in presence of ileocolic intussusception, shows the typical pincer-like ending of the barium enema. Of course, in ileoileal intussusception barium enema X-ray will not be helpful if the ileocecal valve is competent.

VOLVULUS OF SIGMOID COLON

Usually middle aged or elderly males are sufferers. The onset is sudden with acute pain on the left side of the abdomen. Abdominal distension soon follows and in no other condition abdominal distension becomes so severe. Constipation is usually absolute but occasionally large quantities of flatus and feces may be voided due to untwist of the bowel. A straight X-ray is confirmatory, and it shows enormous distension of the sigmoid colon with gas.

VOLVULUS OF THE CAECUM

While volvulus of the sigmoid colon mainly affects middle aged and elderly, this condition is more common in young individuals between 20 and 30 years of age. This condition only occurs when the right half of the colon is laxed and mobile. Distension mainly prevails right lower abdomen which gradually involves the whole of the abdomen and picture becomes very much similar to low small bowel obstruction. Straight X-ray will show a large gas-filled caecum and later on loops of gas-filled ileum.

MECONIUM ILEUS

About 5–10% of infants born with fibrocystic disease of the pancreas will have small bowel obstruction due to abnormal inspissated meconium resulting from inadequate secretions of enzymes from the pancreas and intestinal mucosa. A family history is often noticed. The infant is born with intestinal obstruction. The typical radiograph shows distended loops of small intestine. There is scarcity or absence of fluid levels in the upright film. Air comes down the small intestine into the thick meconium causing a 'soap bubble' or 'ground glass' appearance.

VOLVULUS OF THE MID-GUT (VOLVULUS NEONATORUM)

Arrested rotation of the gut is responsible for this volvulus. Floating caecum together with whole of the small intestine rotates on a narrow stalk of mesentery. The child presents the symptoms of intestinal obstruction immediately after birth. The classical features and radiological findings are similar to any small bowel obstruction. Appearance of dehydration is very fast and treatment should be commenced as quickly as possible.

GALLSTONE ILEUS

Obese women within 40–50 years of age are usually the victims. Often the previous history of cholelithiasis can be obtained. The site of impact is about 2 ft. proximal to the ileocecal valve. This is the narrowest part of the small intestine. Symptoms are often illusive. Recurrent mild colics accompanied by vomiting is the usual presenting symptom. In majority of cases the obstruction is incomplete so there should be some result from enema. Abdominal distension is a late feature. Straight X-ray may reveal the stone to confirm the diagnosis, but even if it be not present, gas-distended loops of ileum should not be missed.

MESENTERIC VASCULAR OBSTRUCTION

This condition occurs in those who are known to be suffering from cardiac valvular diseases or atherosclerosis. Pronounced shock, colicky pain (which is quite severe), distension and frequent vomiting are the usual symptoms which may mimic acute appendicitis. Hematemesis and melaena occur in about a third of cases. On examination, localized rigidity and tenderness over the infarcted area can be elicited. The symptoms and signs just described are features of mesenteric arterial occlusion. Mesenteric venous occlusion shows different types of clinical features. An intra-abdominal obstruction or portal hypertension may predispose this condition.

INTESTINAL OBSTRUCTION DUE TO WORMS

Usually, children below 10 years of age in tropical countries are the victims. Aggregation of Ascaris Lumbricoides obstructs the lumen of the distal small bowel. On examination the child is very much undernourished. He may give history of vomiting a worm or of taking an anthelmintic. A swelling may be palpable in the right iliac fossa which pits on pressure. If this condition is suspected the stool is examined, blood is examined for eosinophilia. Straight X-ray may reveal the worm in a gas-filled loop of intestine. The only complication of significance is *perforation peritonitis* in which the worms penetrate the intestinal wall.

BOLUS OBSTRUCTION

This occurs when insufficiently masticated food obstructs the lumen of the distal small intestine (narrowest portion of the intestine is about 2 feet proximal to the ileocecal valve). This only occurs after partial gastrectomy as normally these foods are retained in the stomach till they are partially digested. Dried fruit, coconut, unmasticated orange pulp usually cause this type of intestinal obstruction by forming bolus.

HEMORRHAGE AND TORSION

RUPTURED ECTOPIC GESTATION

Sudden onset of acute pain over the hypogastrium with tremendous shock in a woman of child-bearing age, having a history of one or two missed periods is suggestive of this condition. Pain is often severe and mainly located in the hypogastrium with radiation backwards and downwards. Gradually the pain may involve whole of the abdomen and even to the tip of the shoulder due to irritation of the under surface of the diaphragm by sanguineous fluid (when hemorrhage is considerable and the foot of the bed is raised to combat shock). *On examination* there may be slight distension of the abdomen due to meteorism. Blue discoloration of the umbilical region, though very rare, is a distinguished sign of this condition. Palpation will reveal deep tenderness in the hypogastrium. Rigidity is not that pronounced as in inflammatory conditions. Rebound tenderness will be positive at an early stage. Shifting dullness will be positive when there is sufficient fluid blood in the peritoneal cavity. Vaginal examination is important and may be diagnostic. (i) That the cervix feels softer than normal; (ii) that all the fornices are tender (in acute appendicitis only the right fornix and in case of pelvic abscess the posterior fornix will be tender) and (iii) that gentle movement of the cervix will cause tremendous pain—give enough indications of the diagnosis of this condition. Later on, restlessness, air-hunger, increasing pallor and running thready pulse will leave no doubt about diagnosis.

RUPTURED LUTEIN (FOLLICULAR) CYST

If a young woman presents with lower abdominal pain in the middle of her menstrual period this condition should be suspected. When this problem affects the right side, it may mimic acute appendicitis. So, the history of the last menstrual period is very important and must always be asked. *That the pain commences in the right iliac fossa* and not that it started in the umbilical or epigastric region and then shifted to the right iliac fossa is very much suggestive of this condition. Last menstrual period is also important to exclude ruptured ectopic gestation. In exceptional cases intraperitoneal hemorrhage is considerable to make the shifting dullness test positive.

TWISTED OVARIAN CYST

If a woman be seized with colicky abdominal pain with vomiting at frequent intervals this condition should be thought of. If a lump is present, which is tense, tender and cystic with definite smooth margin moving in the lower abdomen—it is a twisted ovarian cyst. Overlying rigidity may mask the lump. If it be small enough to be situated entirely within the pelvis the lump will not be palpable abdominally. Vaginal examination in this case may be helpful. The history that the lump was present before will clinch the diagnosis.

RUPTURED OR LEAKING AORTIC ANEURYSM

When a patient, usually middle aged or elderly male, presents with severe upper abdominal or lower chest pain and marked shock, a few conditions should come in mind as probable diagnosis. These are perforated peptic ulcer, coronary thrombosis, acute pancreatitis and ruptured or leaking aortic aneurysm. The patient with this condition is often a known hypertensive patient, but when leakage starts the blood pressure falls catastrophically. He usually complains of severe upper or central abdominal pain radiating through to the back (cf. acute pancreatitis). On examination the patient is considerably anemic. The aneurysm may be palpable if leakage has not been much or not ruptured. If leakage has started there will be rigidity of the central abdomen more so a little to the left. A mass (blood clot) may be felt in the left iliac fossa resembling pericolic abscess in diverticulitis of sigmoid colon. Arterial pulses of the lower limbs are feeble or absent.

AORTIC DISSECTING ANEURYSM

Dissection usually starts in the aortic arch. Hypertension is often of high degree to cause this condition. Pain is excruciating, starts in the retrosternal region, radiates between the shoulders to the back and also spreads to the upper abdomen as dissection proceeds downwards. Signs of shock are apparent, but the blood pressure may be brought down to normal level in an otherwise highly hypertensive patient. Nothing very specific can be discovered on abdominal examination. There may be inequality of pulses of the superior and inferior extremities as the dissection progresses, ultimately there may be disappearance of pulses of one extremity or the other.

COLIC

The common features of colics are: (a) Sudden appearance of *griping pain* which stays for a period during which the patient almost tosses on the bed and then passes off as suddenly as it came. (b) Nausea, vomiting, belching, retching, etc. (c) Varying degree of collapse. (d) Absence of muscle guard (voluntary contraction of the abdominal wall may be mistaken for muscle guard).

BILIARY COLIC

Severe colicky pain over the right hypochondrium radiating to the inferior angle of the right scapula and right shoulder is a biliary colic. It is also called gallbladder (Gallstone) colic as it is caused by spasm of the gallbladder to force the stone down the cystic duct. Tenderness over the gallbladder region, jaundice may or may not be associated with depending on whether the stone is in the common bile duct or in the cystic duct. This pain is called a colic as it is intermittent, but the patient seldom describes it as a griping pain. The common bile duct has very little smooth muscle in its wall and this probably cannot be the source of a severe colicky pain.

URETERIC COLIC

Typically the patient is seized with sudden pain starting in the loin and radiating down to the testis, groin or inner side of the thigh (distribution of the genitofemoral nerve, L1 –2). The testis of the affected side may be drawn up. It is often accompanied by vomiting and profuse sweating. Tenderness can be elicited over the renal angle. Previous history of similar colic, passage of stone with urine and skiagraphy revealing the stone are confirmatory. Frequency of micturition and strangury may be present when the stone is impacted at the lower end of the ureter. Hematuria may be associated with. This colic occurs when a stone in the renal pelvis temporarily blocks the pelviureteric junction or enters the ureter to block it.

INTESTINAL COLIC

This occurs in small intestinal obstruction and also in toxic (catarrhal) enteritis. Catarrhal enteritis occurs due to improper food and must be distinguished from acute intestinal obstruction. History of improper diet, occurrence in other members of the same family having taken the same diet and presence of diarrhea will exclude organic obstruction. In **lead colic,** occupation of the patient as a painter, blue line on the gum and severe constipation are the distinguishing features.

APPENDICULAR COLIC

In obstructive appendicitis colicky pain in the right iliac fossa, vomiting and rise of temperature are the usual features. It is a far more serious condition than unobstructive appendicitis and demands immediate surgical interference due to greater possibility of gangrene and perforation of the appendix with resulting spreading peritonitis.

EXTRA-ABDOMINAL CAUSES

Rupture of Rectus abdominis muscle and/or tearing of the inferior epigastric artery: This may occur during a bout of coughing or in pregnancy or during anticoagulant therapy. An extremely tender lump is felt below the arcuate line and above the pubic bones, where the rectus ruptures. Such tender lump is often diagnosed wrongly as appendicitis when occurs on the right side. But this lump is more medially placed. Bruising of the overlying skin makes the diagnosis of tearing of inferior epigastric artery certain. If the patient is asked to lift both the legs keeping the knees straight the lump becomes more prominent and pain aggravates. Strangulated Spigelian hernia is difficult to differentiate from this condition, but absence of vomiting goes in favor of this condition.

Algorithmic Approach to a Patient with Acute Abdomen

Patient presents with abdominal trauma

↓

Is the trauma blunt or penetrating?
- **Blunt trauma** → Consider **solid organ injury (liver, spleen, kidney)** or hollow viscus injury (bowel, bladder, pancreas)
- **Penetrating trauma** → High risk of **bowel perforation, major vessel injury**

↓

Is the patient hemodynamically stable?
- **Stable** → Proceed with **physical examination and imaging**
- **Unstable** → Immediate **resuscitation and emergency surgery if needed**

↓

Does the patient have peritoneal signs? (rebound tenderness, guarding, rigidity)
- **Yes** → High suspicion for **hollow viscus injury or hemoperitoneum**
- **No** → Consider **retroperitoneal injury or minor trauma**

↓

Perform imaging and special tests
- **FAST ultrasound** → Detects free fluid (hemoperitoneum)
- **CT scan** → Identifies solid organ injury, bowel perforation, retroperitoneal hematoma
- **Diagnostic peritoneal lavage (DPL)** → For occult intra-abdominal bleeding

↓

Confirm diagnosis and initiate appropriate management
- **Nonoperative management** → For minor solid organ injuries (liver, spleen) if stable
- **Surgical intervention** → For major hemorrhage, bowel perforation, vascular injury

Examination of Chronic Abdominal Conditions

CHAPTER 34

HISTORY

In the diagnosis of chronic abdominal lesions, a careful history-taking is very essential as physical signs may be too meager.

Age and sex: Peptic ulcer is rare before 15 years of age. Incidence of duodenal ulcer is much more before the age of 35 years, whereas gastric ulcer occurs more frequently after 35 years. The ratio of duodenal to gastric ulcer varies from place to place and according to the age of the patient. In the western countries this ratio is about 4:1 below 35 years of age, while in India this ratio is 30:1. Carcinoma of stomach is a disease of old age. The majority of patients suffering from hiatus hernia are over 40 years of age. Hiatus hernia may occur in infants when the diagnosis becomes difficult. Diseases of gallbladder mainly affect women of fourth or fifth decade. Congenital pyloric stenosis is obviously a disease of new born babies who start their symptoms from the 2nd month of their lives. Chronic pancreatitis mainly affects individuals in their forties, fifties and sixties.

Peptic ulcer is mainly a disease of males. Carcinoma stomach is also commoner among males but gallbladder diseases and visceroptosis are met with in females more frequently than in males. Chronic appendicitis is more often seen among young girls. Chronic pancreatitis has no predilection towards sex. Congenital pyloric stenosis mainly affects first-born male babies. Women (female, fat, fertile fifty; cf. chronic cholecystitis) are clearly more often affected than men by hiatus hernia.

Occupation: Though a few professions have been incriminated as causing peptic ulcer, yet substantial evidences are lacking. These professions are bus conductors, clerks, civil servants, business executives, etc., who are habituated in drinking teas and coffees in odd times and indulged in excessive smoking. This of course is the statistics in India and may not tally with those of the Western countries.

Residence: The gallbladder disease is commoner in Eastern region of India, whereas peptic ulcer is more common in northern and southern parts of India due to the habit of taking excessive spicy foods.

History in chronic abdominal conditions

Aspect	Clinical significance	Patient-friendly questions
Age-based differential diagnosis	**Infants and children** → Intestinal malrotation, hirschsprung's disease, chronic appendicitis **Young adults (20–40 years)** → Peptic ulcer disease, inflammatory bowel disease (IBD), gallbladder disease	"What is your age group? Have you had any childhood digestive issues?"

Contd...

Contd...

Aspect	Clinical significance	Patient-friendly questions
	Middle-aged adults (40–60 years) → Chronic pancreatitis, gallstones, hiatus hernia, chronic cholecystitis **Elderly (>60 years)** → Colorectal cancer, chronic mesenteric ischemia, diverticular disease	
Symptoms and disease association	**Epigastric pain** → Peptic ulcer, gastritis, pancreatitis **RUQ pain** → Chronic cholecystitis, liver disease, gallbladder carcinoma **LUQ pain** → Chronic pancreatitis, splenic infarction **Periumbilical pain** → Small bowel obstruction, mesenteric ischemia **LLQ pain** → Diverticulosis, colorectal cancer, irritable bowel syndrome (IBS)	"Where exactly do you feel the pain? Does it spread anywhere?"
Relationship with food	**Gastric ulcer** → Pain occurs **immediately after meals** **Duodenal ulcer** → Pain occurs **2–3 hours after meals**, relieved by food **Gallbladder disease** → Pain after fatty meals **Chronic appendicitis** → Pain unrelated to food intake	"Do you notice the pain getting worse after eating? If yes, how soon after?"
Associated symptoms	**Flatulent dyspepsia** → Gallbladder disease, chronic pancreatitis **Nausea and vomiting** → Chronic appendicitis, pancreatitis, gastric carcinoma **Hematemesis and melena** → Peptic ulcer, esophageal varices, gastric carcinoma **Jaundice** → Biliary tract obstruction (stones, malignancy)	"Have you experienced nausea, vomiting, or noticed blood in your stool or vomit?"
Past medical and surgical history	**History of previous abdominal surgery** → adhesions, intestinal obstruction **Prior gastric ulcers** → Risk of malignancy or perforation **History of hepatitis** → Liver disease, cirrhosis	"Have you had any previous abdominal surgeries or conditions like ulcers or hepatitis?"

COMPLAINTS

1. **Pain:** This is the main symptom of majority of chronic abdominal conditions. Enquiry must be made mainly about the following points:

a. *Duration*: Ask the patient, 'how long is he suffering from pain?' When the duration is long, enquire if there is any *periodicity of attacks*. Note, how many attacks did he have, how long did each attack last and whether he was absolutely free from symptoms in the intervals. In peptic ulcer there is definite periodicity which lasts for several weeks and is followed by interval of freedom from pain for 2–6 months. The attacks are more evident in the spring and autumn. In appendicular dyspepsia and gallbladder disease this type of definite periodicity of attacks is not found, instead a mild pain continues even in the periods of remissions.

b. *Site*: In case of gastric ulcer pain is complained of in the midepigastrium or slightly to its left. In case of duodenal ulcer, the patient complains of pain on the transpyloric plane about one inch to the right of the midline (duodenal point). In cholecystitis pain is felt on the outer border of the right rectus muscle just below the costal margin. In case of chronic appendicitis, pain is felt in the right iliac fossa on the McBurney's point.

c. *Radiation*: When the pain radiates from the right hypochondrium to the right shoulder or to the inferior angle of the right scapula, it suggests gallbladder disease; from epigastrium penetrating through to the back—peptic ulcer penetrating into pancreas; from the left of the umbilicus to the left iliac fossa or to the back—gastrojejunal anastomotic ulcer; from the umbilicus to the right iliac fossa—appendicitis.

d. *Relationship with food*: In gastric ulcer food brings pain (*food-pain-relief*), whereas in duodenal ulcer food relieves pain (*food-relief-pain*). The time of appearance of pain in a peptic ulcer depends largely on the site of ulcer. In high gastric, pyloric and duodenal ulcer pain appears about 1/2 hour, 1½ hours and 2½ hours after the meals respectively. The time of appearance of pain is more or less constant in a particular case. So an enquiry should be made whether the patient gets pain when the stomach is empty, i.e., in the early hours of morning or in the afternoon (about 3–4 hours after having lunch); this is diagnostic of duodenal ulcer. If the pain starts immediately after taking food about ½ hour after meals the patient is probably suffering from gastric ulcer. If the pain is more or less constant aching between meals but is increased after intake of food one should suspect gastric carcinoma or complicated gastric ulcer, e.g., penetration into the pancreas or pyloric obstruction. That means a gastric ulcer patient, if loses his periodicity of pain one may suspect superimposition of carcinoma or penetration into the pancreas. In cholecystitis and appendicular dyspepsia pain has no relation with food, but it may so happen that a few cholecystitis patients may complain of pain after having fatty meals.

e. *Character*: Is the pain severe, griping or mild or burning in nature? A griping pain is often experienced in biliary colic which may be associated with cholecystitis. Pain may be severe in peptic ulcer. In appendicitis pain may be severe and even griping in nature (appendicular colic) with quite a few months of intervals between the attacks. In majority of cases of chronic appendicitis pain is mild aching in nature which gets worse on jolting and running.

f. *How relieved?* As has been mentioned earlier, in duodenal ulcer food relieves pain (hunger pain). Vomiting always relieves pain of peptic ulcer. The peptic ulcer pain is also relieved by taking alkalis.

2. **Flatulent dyspepsia:** This is often seen in diseases of gallbladder. The symptoms include a feeling of fullness after food, belching and heart-burn. Sometimes patients with esophageal hiatus hernia and chronic pancreatitis, may complain of flatulent dyspepsia. This may even be seen in certain cases of gastric ulcer. Heart-burn denotes hyperacidity.

3. **Nausea and vomiting:** Nausea is an early symptom of chronic appendicitis, pancreatitis and even gastric carcinoma. Nausea is also an early complaint of virus and serum hepatitis. If there is a history of vomiting, note:

a. *Character and amount*: 'Coffee ground' vomiting is seen in conditions where slow hemorrhage takes place in the stomach, e.g., carcinoma, gastric ulcer, etc. Bilious vomiting is often a feature of cholecystitis and intestinal obstruction. Too much acidic vomiting is a feature of duodenal ulcer. Projectile copious vomiting is often seen in pyloric stenosis complicating duodenal ulcer and in pancreatitis. In pyloric stenosis the vomitus often contains undigested food particles ingested even a day earlier.

b. *Frequency*: Vomiting is constant in pyloric obstruction and gastritis; it is frequent in gastric ulcer, appendicular dyspepsia, gallbladder disease and pancreatitis. It is usually absent in duodenal ulcer without obstruction.

c. *Relation to food*: Vomiting soon after the intake of food (within 2 hours) is usually seen in gastric ulcer. In pyloric stenosis it may occur at any time but usually takes place several hours after meal (more often in the evening). Vomiting from gallbladder diseases and pancreatitis (in which vomiting is a marked feature) has got no relation with food.

d. *Relief of pain*: Vomiting sometimes brings relief to pain. This is more often seen in case of gastric ulcer. Once the patient has learnt this fact he often resorts to it at the height of pain (induced vomiting) but vomiting affords little relief in pancreatitis, cholecystitis, carcinoma of the stomach and appendicitis.

4. **Hematemesis and melena:** Hematemesis means vomiting of blood and should be distinguished from hemoptysis which means coughing out of blood. Peptic ulcer hemorrhage is a likely complication of a posteriorly situated ulcer whereas perforation is more common in an ulcer lying anteriorly. Though the most common cause of hematemesis is a chronic peptic ulcer, yet acute peptic ulcer, multiple erosions, esophageal varices, carcinoma of the stomach, Mallory-Weiss syndrome, purpura, hemophilia, etc., are other causes of hematemesis. In a gastric ulcer the amount of vomited blood varies—it may be small or profuse depending on the size of the blood vessel involved. In profuse hemorrhage the color of the vomitus is bright red; whereas in slow and small bleeding the blood becomes partly digested and looks like 'coffee ground'.

Melena means passing of dark or tarry stool per annum. It occurs commonly in peptic ulcer, but may be seen in all cases which may have induced hematemesis. A history of fainting attack just before the melena may be obtained.

5. **Jaundice:** In surgical practice three groups of cases may present with jaundice—(1) Jaundice due to neoplasia; (2) Jaundice due to biliary tract calculus and (3) Jaundice from other causes.
1. *Neoplastic jaundice:* May be due to carcinoma of the head of the pancreas, carcinoma of the ampulla of Vater, carcinoma of the biliary tract including gallbladder, ca-liver and a further 4% of cases may be due to primary neoplastic disease elsewhere with metastatic involvement of the lymph nodes at the porta hepatis.
2. *Calculous jaundice:* Occurs consequent upon a stone or stones in the biliary duct system. Cholangitis from previous calculus may lead to jaundice and rise of temperature.
3. Among *other causes of jaundice:* Pancreatitis, pancreatic pseudocyst, cirrhosis of liver and virus hepatitis or serum hepatitis are important.

To ascertain yellow discoloration of sclera, skin, nail bed, under surface of the tongue, soft palate, etc., one should examine in day light. Jaundice is very liable to be overlooked in artificial light. Itching often accompanies jaundice, so presence of scratch marks on the chest or abdomen sometimes gives a clue to the diagnosis even if yellow discoloration is not that prominent. Itching is due to accumulation of bile salts in the blood. An enquiry must be made about the mode of onset, duration and its progressiveness (that means whether the jaundice is gradually deepening or intermittent). Is the jaundice associated with pain? Painful, intermittent jaundice is very much characteristic of stone in the common bile duct, whereas painless and progressively deepening jaundice is a feature of carcinoma of the head of the pancreas. In carcinoma of ampulla of Vater jaundice may be intermittent due to sloughing of tumor mass.

6. **Bowel habit:** Blood and/or mucus (slime) in the stool is suggestive of a colonic disease. Constipation is usually present in obstructive lesion of the stomach, gallbladder diseases, chronic appendicitis, etc. In case of carcinoma of colon a change of normal bowel habit is noticed such as increasing constipation or alternate diarrhea and constipation depending on the site of the lesion. The patient should be asked about the color and quantity of the stool whether black tarry [melena—which indicates hemorrhage in the upper gastrointestinal (GI) tract or ingestion of large doses of iron or bismuth]; or whitish or clay colored (indicates biliary obstruction either intra- or extrahepatic); or large, fatty and offensive (suggests chronic pancreatitis).

7. **Appetite:** Loss of appetite is an early feature of carcinoma affecting any part of the gastrointestinal tract. This is more prominent in gastric carcinoma. It must be remembered that appetite is never lost in a case of peptic ulcer. Only in case of gastric ulcer the patient becomes reluctant to take food more often due to immediate resumption of pain rather than anything else. In case of appendicitis the patient often rejects food because it initiates nausea and vomiting. Dislike for fatty foods characterizes gallbladder diseases (*qualitative dyspepsia*).

8. **Fever:** Evening rise of temperature is characteristic of tabes mesenterica as tuberculosis in any other parts of the body. Appendicitis and acute ulcerative colitis are always associated with varying degrees of temperature. Intermittent fever (Charcot's) occurring with rigor and jaundice is highly suggestive of a calculus in the common bile duct.

9. **Loss of weight:** In carcinoma particularly affecting GI tract there will be marked and progressive loss of weight. In pyloric obstruction and in cases with jaundice loss of weight is noticed. In case of gastric ulcer there may be slight loss of weight but in duodenal ulcer patient never loses weight on the contrary he may gain some weight.

Past history: This must be noted carefully. Whether the patient suffered from typhoid fever (in gallbladder disease), tuberculosis, syphilis, septic foci in the tonsil, throat or nose, jaundice, etc. This gives some clue to the present diagnosis. Drug history must be enquired into. Whether the patient was on any drug or not? This not only gives a clue to the diagnosis of the present condition (such as ingestion of aspirin in peptic ulcer) but also it has got importance from anesthesia point of view (the students are referred to the chapter on 'Anesthesia' in the treatise 'A Practical Guide to Operative Surgery' written by the author).

Whether the patient had undergone any operation or not? If so, the details of operation should be noted.

Personal history: The dietary habit of the patient must be noted. Majority of patients with peptic ulcer observe irregular dietary habit whereas patients with appendicitis or gallbladder diseases may maintain a regular dietary habit. The type of diet should be enquired into. Majority of the patients suffering from duodenal ulcer are accustomed to take spicy foods. Meat forms the major dish of patients with appendicitis as this is a disease of civilization.

Excessive smoking and worry have some bearing on the pathogenesis of peptic ulcer. Excessive alcohol consumption also worsens this condition. Cirrhosis of liver and portal hypertension are often accompaniments of excessive drinking of alcohol.

Family history: Some diseases often run in families—peptic ulcer, Crohn's disease, ulcerative colitis, diverticulitis, carcinoma affecting various parts of the GI tract, etc.

PHYSICAL EXAMINATION

A. GENERAL SURVEY

The general appearance of the patient should be noted—his build, emaciation, presence of anemia, jaundice, etc. Examine the teeth, fauces and tonsils. Look for signs of pyorrhea. Note the pulse, respiration and temperature.

B. ABDOMINAL EXAMINATION

INSPECTION: The patient should lie flat on his back with his legs extended. The whole of the abdomen from the level of the nipples above to the saphenous openings below should be completely exposed. It cannot be over emphasized how rewarding it is to spend sometime on inspection. Examination should be carried out in good light (preferably day light) looking first from the side then tangentially and finally from either end of the bed.

1. **Skin and subcutaneous tissue:** Firstly look carefully for any visible swelling. Then look for any erythema—this is due to hot-water bottle application and indicates the site of pain.

   If superficial veins are engorged, note (i) their positions—whether situated around the umbilicus (portal obstruction) or on the sides of the abdomen (obstruction of the inferior vena cava) and (ii) the direction of blood flow—whether away from the umbilicus (portal obstruction) or from below upwards (inferior vena cava obstruction). To determine the direction of blood flow two index fingers are placed close together on the vein. A portion of the vein is now emptied by milking it with one of the index fingers. The finger is now released. The rate at which the vein fills after releasing one finger should be noted. The process of emptying the vein is repeated and this time the other finger is taken off. The vein fills rapidly when the finger obstructing the flow of the blood is released. The scar, if any, should be noted. Whether it is linear scar (healing by first intention) or broad and irregular scar (indicating wound infection).

   Any hard subcutaneous nodules near the umbilicus, if present, are significant of an intra-abdominal carcinoma, especially that of the stomach.

2. **Umbilicus:** Umbilicus is normally placed almost in the middle of the line joining the tip of xiphoid process to the top of the symphysis pubis. The umbilicus is displaced upwards by a swelling arising from the pelvis or downwards by ascites (Tanyol's sign). The umbilicus may be everted (ascites) or tucked in (obesity). Any swelling on one side of the abdomen will push the umbilicus to the opposite side.

3. **Contour of the abdomen:** Normal abdomen is neither retracted nor distended. Generalized retraction is found in thin individual whilst symmetrical distension may be due to fat, fluid, flatus, feces or fetus. Distension due to obesity should be differentiated from distension due to intra-abdominal causes. In the former the umbilicus is deeply inverted whereas in the latter the umbilicus shows varying degree of eversion. In case of chronic intestinal obstruction there will be fullness of the right iliac fossa. The patient lies in the examination couch straight in such a way that an imaginary line through both the anterior superior iliac spines will be precisely at right angle to the long axis of the examining couch. Compare the left with the right iliac fossa. The fullness of the right fossa due to distended cecum is better seen than felt. In case of enlargement or distension of viscus of the upper abdomen there will be distension of the upper abdomen.

Similarly distension or tumor of the viscus of the lower abdomen will lead to distension of that region. In case of *visceroptosis* undue protuberance of the lower abdomen will be evident as soon as the patient stands.

4. **Movements:**
a. *Respiratory*: Localized limitation of respiratory excursion is indicative of subjacent inflammation.
b. *Peristaltic*: Peristalsis will be visible in pyloric stenosis and obstruction of the small and large intestines. In pyloric stenosis a rounded prominence will be seen travelling slowly from the left costal margin towards the right whereas peristalsis of the transverse colon will be seen in the reverse direction. Peristalsis of the small intestine is 'ladder pattern'. In suspected cases peristalsis can be induced by flicking the abdominal wall or by pouring a few drops of alcohol or ether on the abdomen.
c. *Pulsatile:* In thin persons epigastric pulsation may be seen. But a pulsatile swelling in the abdomen means either aortic aneurysm (expansile pulsation, see page 37) or a tumor in front of the abdominal aorta (transmitted pulsation).

5. **Swelling,** if present, should be examined as discussed in the next chapter under 'Examination Of An Abdominal Lump'.

PALPATION: During palpation patient's confidence must be gained. The patient should lie flat on his back comfortably with one pillow below his head. Ask the patient to lie relaxed and breathe slight deeply with mouth open. Under no circumstances he should be hurt. Otherwise abdominal muscles will go into spasm and important findings may be missed. (i) Routine palpation of the abdomen should be carried out with the flat of the hand using mainly the flexor surfaces of the fingers. The forearm should be in the horizontal plane so that the fingers lie flat on the abdomen. For this it is better for the clinician to seat on a chair or even to kneel upon the floor no matter how indignified this may appear. *The fingers must not be held vertical and poke the abdominal wall as shown in the* **Figure 33.3B**. The great enemy of efficient palpation is rigidity of the abdominal muscles. To avoid this (ii) the patient is asked to flex the hips and knees to release the abdominal muscles. A pillow may be placed under his knees to obviate the strain of keeping the legs flexed. (iii) The patient is advised to breathe quietly and deeply with his mouth open. (iv) In winter the hand of the clinician must be kept warm same as the patient's skin either by rubbing one hand against the other or by washing it with hot water. (v) It is a good practice to engage the patient in conversation while palpating so that his attention is taken off from clinician's palpation and the abdominal muscles become obviously relaxed. (vi) In obstinate cases some clinicians exert pressure on the lower end of the sternum with the base of the left palm (Nicholson's maneuver). This compels the patient to breathe abdominally as the movement of the thorax has been restricted. (vii) It is a routine practice to start palpation farthest from the site of the disease. For example, if the pain is located at the right iliac fossa, commence palpating the left hypochondrium and after palpating each quadrant in turn reach the affected area last of all. (viii) When the hand is over a particular region the mind should visualize the particular structures deep to the hand. (ix) While palpating the different regions of the abdomen keep an eye on the patient's face to know his reaction. He may wince at palpation of a region where he did not complain of pain and this may give a valuable clue to the diagnosis. (x) For *deep palpation* (Fig. 34.1) the whole of the volar surfaces of the fingers should be used and gradually tilted towards the abdomen. With each expiration more pressure is employed to feel deeper. It is a good practice to use both hands one above the other for deep palpation. While the upper hand puts more pressure, the lower

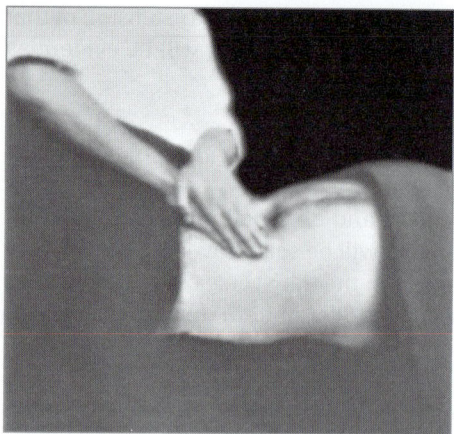

Fig. 34.1: Shows the method of deep palpation of the abdomen using both hands one above the other.

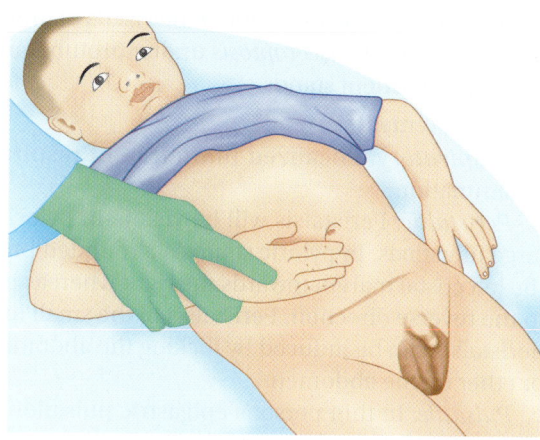

Fig. 34.2: It is often convenient to palpate a child's abdomen with its own hand. See the text.

hand remains passive to receive more information about the structures deep to this hand. (xi) *In case of children* who are not cooperative, their hands should be used for deep palpation **(Fig. 34.2)**. Child's one hand is placed on his abdomen and on that the examiner places his hand. Now all the quadrants are palpated like that. When a tender spot comes the child withdraws his own hand.

1. **Tender spot:** If the patient has complained of pain at the time of history-taking, ask him to point to its site so that you can begin palpation in a nontender area and move towards the tender spot **(Fig. 34.3)**. The area of tenderness should be detected by light palpation first. This should be done by gently resting the hand on the abdomen and pressing lightly. Move your hand systematically over all areas of the abdomen. If systematic light palpation over the whole abdomen elicits no pain, repeat the process pressing firmly and deeply to find out if there is deep tenderness. The area of tenderness can be drawn on the history sheet as a hatched area. The degree of tenderness must be assessed—whether it is mildly tender, moderately tender (which initiates slight tightening of the abdominal muscles) or severely tender (when the muscular rigidity becomes obvious).

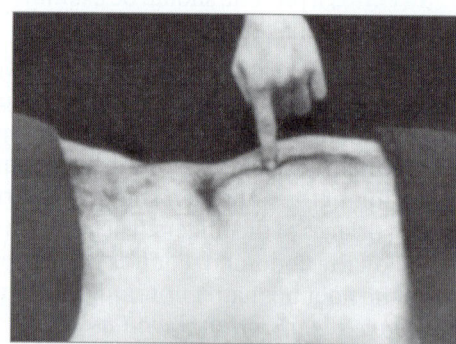

Fig. 34.3: The best method to locate the deep tender spot is with one finger.

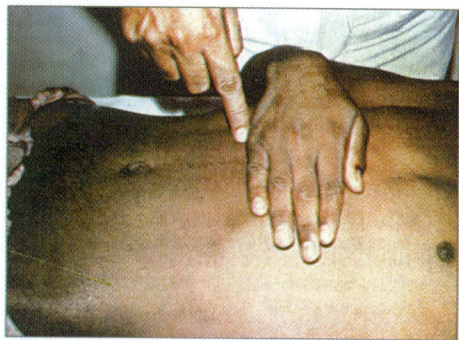

Fig. 34.4: Shows how to find out the transpyloric line (shown in figure by the index finger). On this line 1 inch to the right of the midline is the duodenal point.

In case of *gastric ulcer* tender spot is usually situated in the midepigastrium below the xiphoid process. In *duodenal ulcer* it is about 1½ inches to the right of the midline on the transpyloric plane **(Fig. 34.4)**. To elicit tenderness *in cholecystitis* one may place the right hand just below the right costal margin on the lateral border of the right rectus (the gallbladder point). Moderate pressure is exerted with the fingers to palpate the fundus of the gallbladder. The patient is now asked to take a deep breath in, the gallbladder descends and hurts the examining fingers. The patient will immediately wince with a 'catch' in the breath if the organ is inflamed. This is called Murphy's sign (Moynihan's method) **(Fig. 34.5)**. This examination can be performed with the patient sitting. The fingers are hooked under the right costal margin at the lateral border of the rectus and the patient is asked to take deep breaths in. The gallbladder descends further down and comes closure to the palpating fingers. Both sides should be similarly examined to note the difference. In cholecystitis the cartilage of the right 8th rib becomes tender (compare with the other side). This is a positive sign of cholecystitis. In case of *appendicitis* tenderness can be elicited on the McBurney's point, which is situated at the junction of the lateral 1/3 and medial 2/3 of the line joining the right anterior superior iliac spine and the umbilicus (spinoumbilical line).

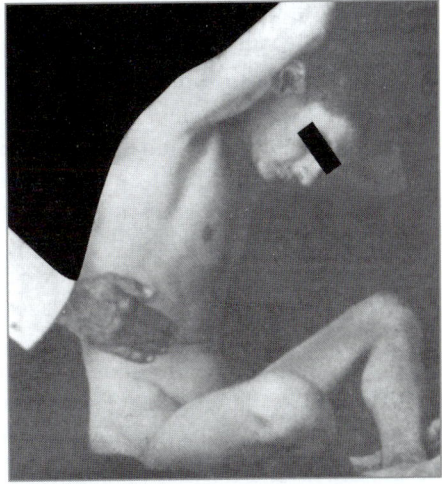

Fig. 34.5: Method of eliciting Murphy's sign. In Moynihan's method the patient lies down.

2. **Fluid thrill:** This is obtained when there is a large amount of fluid in the peritoneal cavity either free or encysted. This is obtained by a gentle tap applied to one flank of the abdomen while the thrill is felt with the other hand placed on the other flank of the abdomen **(Fig. 34.6)**. The patient's or an assistant's hand is placed vertically on the midline of the abdomen pressing deeply. This is intended

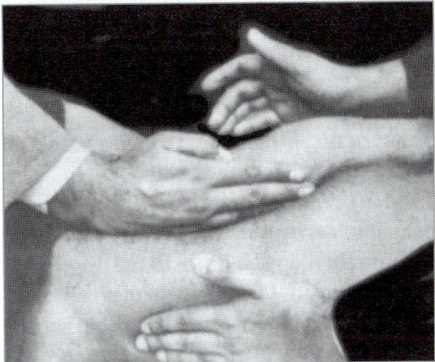

Fig. 34.6: Method of eliciting fluid thrill.

to cut off any transmitted wave through the subcutaneous fat which may travel along the abdominal wall to the other flank as also to increase the intra-abdominal fluid tension for better palpation of the fluid thrill. The fluid thrill is also obtained in case of encysted fluid such as a large *ovarian cyst which has touched both the abdominal flanks*. Differentiation between these two conditions can be done by shifting dullness test.

3. **Shifting dullness:** This is a valuable sign and even becomes positive when the quantity of fluid in the peritoneal cavity is comparatively small. The patient lies flat. Percussion is started from the midline and continued to any of the flanks till the percussion note becomes dull. The finger on the abdomen is kept as such and the patient is asked to turn to the opposite side. In this position wait for a minute or so in order to allow the fluid to gravitate down. That area is again percussed and it will be resonant now.

When there is much fluid in the abdomen palpation of different organs is carried out by 'dipping' the fingers. The quick action will displace the fluid and allows the organ to be felt. In the passing it may be mentioned that in surgical practice the common causes of ascites are portal hypertension, carcinomatosis peritonei and tuberculous peritonitis, but considering all cases including the medical conditions the most common cause is congestive cardiac failure in which there will be engorgement of the neck veins also.

4. **Palpation of the abdominal organs:**

A. **STOMACH:** Normally the stomach cannot be palpated. If there is any history suggesting pyloric stenosis, one should look for visible peristalsis. The sign of *splashing (succussion splash)* should be looked for in these cases. The hand is laid over the stomach. Short, sudden, jerky movements with fingers are made over the stomach area or the patient is shaken. A gurgle may be heard. In case of suspicion the patient may be asked to take fluid before this test is performed.

Occasionally one may find a lump in the pyloric region. Visible lump is more often a feature of congenital pyloric stenosis than adult acquired stenosis. In congenital pyloric stenosis palpation often reveals a thick pylorus. Otherwise, a palpable swelling of the stomach means either carcinoma or leaking perforation of a peptic ulcer. *In carcinoma*, the mass is irregular, hard with varying degrees of mobility. A leaking ulcer is firm, less mobile but more tender. But one thing should be borne in mind that *absence of a lump by no means excludes carcinoma of the stomach.*

B. **LIVER:** Liver is normally palpable in infancy up to the end of 3rd year. In adults the normal liver is impalpable. Only when the liver is pathologically enlarged it may become palpable under the right costal margin. To palpate for an enlarged liver one should place the hand on the right iliac fossa with the fingers pointing towards the left axilla (that means parallel to the right costal margin). If nothing abnormal is felt, the patient is asked to take deep breath in and out. Every time the patient expires, slide the hand a little towards the right costal margin. This is carried on till the edge of an enlarged liver strikes the lateral margin of the hand when the patient inspires. At this point the hand is kept static keeping a continuous pressure towards the abdomen. As the patient inspires the liver descends and the lateral margin of the index finger will be felt to ride over the free edge of the liver. At this time a few points should be noted as discussed below. If the students want to palpate the liver straight away by placing the fingers below the costal margin, they may miss gross enlargement of the liver. Attention is now directed to palpate the upper margin of the liver. Palpable liver may not be necessarily enlarged, as it may be dropped or pushed down by something from above. To demonstrate the upper limit of the liver it is necessary to percuss along the right midaxillary line commencing from the 4th interspace. When the resonance will be replaced by dullness the upper border of the liver is marked. It must be noted in the passing that hydatid cyst or amoebic abscess often causes an upward hepatic enlargement. When the liver becomes palpable note the following points: (i) *The extent of enlargement* below the costal margin in inches or finger-breadths; (ii) *The character of the edge*—sharp or rounded; (iii) The *surface*—smooth, irregular or nodular with or without umbilication in the nodules; (iv) The *consistency*—soft, firm or stony hard and (v) *Presence or absence of tenderness*. A stony hard and irregular liver is suggestive of metastatic carcinomatous deposits in the liver. A search should be made for the primary focus in the gastrointestinal tract (i.e., from the stomach down to the upper part of the rectum). The spread mainly occurs through blood via portal vein. Irregular firm liver with small nodules is characteristic of the liver cirrhosis. A soft and very tender liver is often come across in amoebic hepatitis.

C. **SPLEEN:** A normal spleen is not palpable. The spleen must be near two times larger than its normal size to be detected by clinical examination. When enlarged it extends from the left costal margin to the right iliac fossa. It moves freely with respiration. Splenic swelling has a sharp anterior border where one or two notches can be felt. This is very much characteristic of a splenic swelling.

The method of palpation of the spleen is very much similar to that of the liver except that this is tried on the left side **(Fig. 34.7)**. There are four methods of palpation: (1) The right hand of the clinician is placed parallel to the left costal margin at the level of the umbilicus and the patient is asked to breathe in and out. During expirations the hand is gradually slided towards the left costal margin till the splenic swelling touches the lateral border of the index finger during inspiration. (2) Some clinicians put their left hands on the left lower ribs and slide the skin downwards so that the right hand gets an extra bit of skin to insinuate beneath the left costal margin. By this method one can palpate a relatively smaller spleen which has not become big enough to reach below the level of the costal margin. Failure of palpation of an enlarged spleen is mostly due to palpating more medially than its actual position. An enlarged spleen appears just below the tip of the 10th rib. (3) Another method is that when the right hand reaches the costal margin at the tip of the 10th rib clinician's left hand is put round the lower left rib cage and it is pushed forward with each inspiration **(Fig. 34.7)**. This maneuver occasionally lifts a slightly enlarged spleen forwards enough to make it palpable. (4) From above spleen may be conveniently palpated with two hands arching below the left costal margin while the patient is asked to take deep breath in and out slowly. The hands are moved further downwards and laterally with each expiration waiting for the enlarged spleen to knock at the fingers during inspiration while the fingers are kept static.

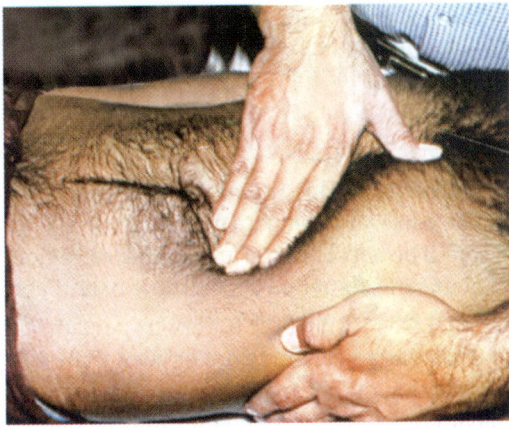

Fig. 34.7: Shows a maneuver to palpate the spleen. The right hand reaches the costal margin at the tip of the 10th rib and the clinician's left hand is put round the lower left rib cage and is pushed forward with each inspiration. A slightly enlarged spleen may be thus lifted forward enough to make it palpable by the right hand.

D. **GALLBLADDER:** When distended it can be felt as a tense globular swelling projecting downwards and forwards from below the liver just lateral to the outer border of the right rectus muscle (below the tip of the 9th rib). It moves freely with respiration and its upper limit is continuous with the liver. This can be moved slightly from side to side.

Gallbladder becomes palpable (a) in case of mucocele and empyema. Enlarged gallbladder (b) in a jaundiced patient is mainly due to carcinoma of the head of the pancreas or carcinoma of the common bile duct. Calculous jaundice is usually not associated with enlargement of the gallbladder owing to previous inflammatory fibrosis. This is called *Courvoisier's law* **(Figs. 34.8A and B)**. There are a few exceptions to this law, the notable of which are (i) double impaction of stones, i.e., one

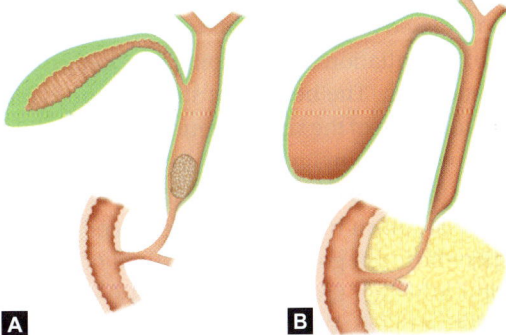

Figs. 34.8A and B: Diagrammatic representation of Courvoisier's law. In jaundice due to a calculus in the common bile duct the gallbladder is usually not distended owing to previous inflammatory fibrosis, whereas in obstruction of the common bile duct due to growth (e.g., carcinoma of the head of the pancreas) the gallbladder becomes distended in an attempt to reduce the pressure in the biliary system.

in the cystic duct and the other in the common bile duct; (ii) Oriental cholangiohepatitis; (iii) a pancreatic calculus obstructing the ampulla of Vater; (iv) Mucocele of gallbladder due to a stone in the cystic duct. (c) When the gallbladder swelling seems to be very hard—consider carcinoma of the gallbladder, a liver metastasis or very rarely a primary liver tumor.

E. **KIDNEY:** See Chapter 37— "Examination of a urinary case".

F. **PANCREAS:** This organ cannot be palpated normally unless a growth or cyst has developed in it. The best way to palpate the pancreas is to turn the patient to the right. The hips and knees are flexed. The left subcostal and epigastric regions are deeply palpated. This will evoke tenderness in acute and sometimes in chronic pancreatitis (*Mallet- Guy's sign*).

G. **COLON:** Inspection is very important in this case. A fullness of the right iliac fossa due to a distended cecum is better seen than felt. The cecum is distended in majority of cases of obstruction of the large intestine. When the cecum, the beginning of the ascending colon and pelvic colon are thickened they may be palpable. Look for tenderness. A lump in the line of the large intestine may be due to either a fecal mass or a neoplasm. To eliminate the first possibility one can re-examine the patient after a bowel wash, the fecal mass will disappear. Otherwise a fecal mass will yield to digital pressure showing indentation.

PERCUSSION: The limits of the solid organs can be mapped out by their dull note. The liver extends from the 6th rib to the costal margin on the right midaxillary line. The spleen extends from the 9th to the 11th rib on the left midaxillary line. When there is free fluid in the abdomen *shifting dullness* can be obtained. In case of distended cecum or pelvic colon tympanitic note may be obtained.

Differentiation between *ascites* and *ovarian cyst* can be made by percussion. In ascites there is a resonance anteriorly and dullness in the flanks whereas in an ovarian cyst there is dullness anteriorly and resonance on the flanks. Further, shifting dullness can be demonstrated in case of ascites but not in the case of ovarian cyst.

AUSCULTATION: It is not very helpful in the diagnosis of chronic abdominal conditions. In case of splenomegaly with portal hypertension, one may hear a venous hum louder on inspiration with a stethoscope placed just below the xiphoid process. This is due to engorgement of the splenic vein and the hum is due to the spleen being compressed during inspiration. This is known as *Kenawy's sign*. Auscultation with scraping may determine the size of the stomach. The bell of the stethoscope is placed below and to the left of the xiphisternum. Along the lines radiating downwards from this point the abdominal wall is scraped with a finger. So long as the finger remains within the limit of the stomach the sound so produced differs from that when the finger goes beyond the limit of the stomach. The point at which the sound changes is the boundary line of the stomach. When several such points are joined the greater curvature of the stomach can be delineated.

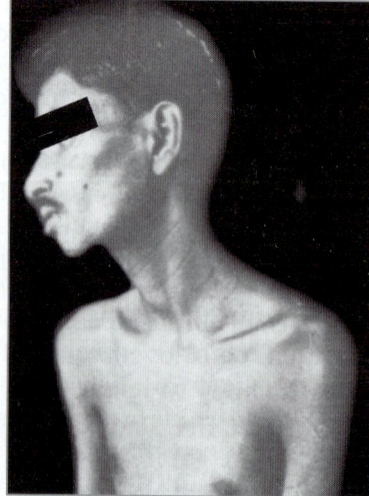

Fig. 34.9: Troisier's sign—i.e., enlargement of the left supraclavicular lymph node in a late case of a carcinoma of the stomach.

Examination of the left supraclavicular lymph nodes: This is highly important so far as the carcinoma of the stomach and other abdominal organs are concerned. But it is pity that only a small number of students can remember it. Enlargement of this group of lymph nodes in carcinoma of the stomach is known as *Troisier's sign* **(Fig. 34.9)**.

Rectal and vaginal examinations: Besides the rectal and colonic cases where these examinations are indispensable, in other chronic abdominal conditions the importance of rectal and vaginal examinations cannot be over-emphasized. In appendicitis, Crohn's disease, gastric carcinoma (where Krukenberg's tumor of the ovary may be revealed in vaginal examination), etc., these examinations may help in diagnosis.

GENERAL EXAMINATIONS

There are few conditions outside abdomen which may mimic chronic abdominal conditions. So, after examining the abdomen, if the clinician is not satisfied with the clinical findings to account for the pain of the abdomen, he should think of extra-abdominal causes. In these cases he should proceed as follows:
1. Examine the **chest** and **chest wall** for the presence of pleurisy, angina pectoris, coronary thrombosis, pericarditis, fibrosis of intercostal muscles or membranes (pleurodynia), herpes zoster, etc.
2. **The spine** for presence of Pott's disease and extradural abscess (very rare).
3. The **nervous system** for tabes dorsalis. Loss of ankle jerk and sluggish pupillary reaction to light with past history of syphilis and presence of lightning pain in the legs are diagnostic features of this condition.

SPECIAL INVESTIGATIONS

1. **GASTRIC FUNCTION TESTS:** These tests are performed as first things in the morning and are comprised of basal secretion and maximum secretion by stimulants such as insulin, histamine and pentagastrin.

    The patient should have had nothing to eat or drink from the previous night and should not have taken antacid or anticholinergic drugs for previous 24 hours. The patient should remove his shoes, jacket and tie and opens his collar. His weight and height are measured. The patient now lies comfortably on a couch and his nostril and throat are sprayed with a solution of 3% lignocaine in isotonic saline. A nasogastric tube, which was Ryle's tube previously and now it is a plastic, radio-opaque 125 cm long tube with holes close to the tip, is first well lubricated with liquid paraffin and is passed through the nose. The patient is asked to swallow repeatedly while the tube is being pushed steadily and rapidly down through the pharynx and esophagus into the stomach. A large 20–50 mL syringe is then fixed to the end of the tube and the stomach is emptied of juice and air by repeated aspirations. The patient is now taken to the fluoroscopy room and the position of the tube is adjusted so that its tip lies in the most dependent part of the stomach which is shown to be along the left border of the spinal column. The tube is now fixed to the face and the end of the tube is connected to a low continuous suction machine which works at a subatmospheric pressure of 3–5 cm Hg. Minor adjustment of tube position may be necessary to allow satisfactory aspiration. Normally the quantity of this aspiration is less than 70 mL. If it be more than this, it indicates presence of duodenal ulcer, pyloric obstruction, pylorospasm or hypersecretion. Now the time is recorded and one 60-minutes or four 15-minutes aspirates may be collected and labeled with the times. This is *basal secretion*.

    a. **Night fasting secretion (Dragstedt):** This is actually the night secretion of the stomach in its interdigestive and resting period. Gastric secretion is aspirated through continuous or intermittent low pressure suction for the period of 12 hours from 9 PM to 9 AM. Normally this secretion amounts to about 400 mL. Volumes above this level are suggestive of vagal hyperactivity. In Zollinger-Ellison syndrome this volume may be more than a liter. The juice is tested for HCl in mEq. In duodenal ulcer this figure is between 40 and 80, in gastric ulcer it is between 5 and 15, in Zollinger-Ellison syndrome it is between 100 and 300 (normal figure being between 10 and 20).

BASAL SECRETION: 12 hours over-night fasting secretion has little diagnostic advantage over the morning basal secretion. Moreover technically the former is unreliable. The mEq acid per hour of basal secretion in duodenal ulcer is about 5 mEq/hr, in gastric ulcer 1–2 mEq/hr (normal figure being 1 mEq/hr.). Basal secretion represents secretion of that portion of the patient's parietal cell mass which is being excited even under the resting condition.

MAXIMUM SECRETION: This can be found out with various stimulants. Whereas Kay's augmented histamine test is gradually losing popularity and Hollander's insulin test has got limited scope of application, pentagastrin is becoming a popular stimulant and is used more often than any other stimulant.

b. Pentagastrin test: The optimum dose of pentagastrin is 6 microgram per kg body weight. It is mostly injected IM. 15 minutes samples are collected during the next one hour. The term maximum acid output (MAO) is generally used to denote maximum acid output in the whole 60 minutes after injection of pentagastrin and is expressed as m mol/hr. This test not only has a diagnostic importance but also helps in assessing treatment of the patient, e.g., when the acid status is low operation like vagotomy and drainage procedure is enough whereas in case of high acid status individuals operation like vagotomy and antrectomy or partial gastrectomy should be called for. In gastric carcinoma MAO is very low.

c. Kay's augmented histamine test: This test determines the total mass of oxyntic cells in the stomach. At first the fasting stomach contents are collected. Mepyramine malleate is given intramuscularly at the dose of 100 mg to nullify the side effects of histamine except its stimulation of gastric acid. About 30 minutes later histamine acid phosphate at the dose of 0.04 mg per kg body weight is injected subcutaneously. The gastric acid secretion is collected during the next one hour. The average HCl response in mEq free acid per hour as follows: a gastric ulcer—15; duodenal ulcer—30–40; anastomotic ulcer—30–35.

d. Hollander's insulin test: This is based on the fact that hypoglycemia, caused by insulin, induces direct vagal stimulation on the parietal cell mass. Insulin given to a patient who has had a vagotomy performed should result in no increase in acid production. This test is of more value to assess the completeness of vagotomy in the postoperative period. After the fasting stomach contents are aspirated, soluble insulin in the dose of 0.2 unit per kg. of body weight is injected intravenously. 2 mL of venous blood is taken just before the introduction of insulin for estimation of sugar. Eight 15 minutes aspirates are collected and labelled. 2 mL of venous blood is taken at 30 and 45 minutes after introduction of insulin to estimate the level of blood sugar. It must be remembered that patient's comments and appearance should be noted. Dryness and slight impairment of the level of consciousness should immediately rouse the suspicion of imminent hypoglycemic coma. Dextrose (50%) in the dose of 50 mL should always be kept available during the test and injected immediately intravenously should the said condition arises. A fall in the blood sugar level below 45 mg per 100 mL will lead to hypersecretion of acid.

Maximum acid output is expected at that time. A rise in concentration of 20 m mol per liter above the basal level in the first hour suggests incomplete vagotomy. It must be remembered that a high acid concentration in basal secretion in the range of more than 20 m mol free acid per hour is indicative of Zollinger-Ellison syndrome.

2. **EXAMINATION OF BLOOD:** Hemoglobin level will be low in anemic patient with melena and hematemesis erythrocyte sedimentation rate (ESR) will be high in gastric carcinoma or carcinoma anywhere in the abdomen. During acute attack of appendicitis white blood count (WBC) count will be high. Estimation of circulating gastrin by radioimmunoassay is very much informative.

3. **EXAMINATION OF STOOL:** Melena, i.e., black and tarry stool indicates peptic ulcer with hemorrhage. Small hemorrhage may not be detectable by naked eye examination of the stool. In these cases *occult blood examinations* of the feces should be undertaken. In chronic pancreatitis there will be presence of neutral fat (steatorrhea) and striated muscle fibers (creatorrhea) in the stool. Blood and mucus in the stool is a feature of ulcerative colitis. So routine examination of the stool should be a must in chronic abdominal cases.

4. **RADIOLOGICAL INVESTIGATION: Barium meal X-ray** is very much informative so far as the diseases of the stomach, small intestine and appendix are concerned. Lesion of the cecum and proximal part of the colon can be diagnosed by barium follow-through examination. The students should follow the patient to the X-ray department and see how screening is done with barium meal or enema. The patient is given the barium sulphate meal, which is radio-opaque. Palpation of the organ which seems to be diseased under the screen is the most important part of the X-ray examination and is called fluoroscopy. A series of films are also taken 3, 6 and 24 hours after ingestion of the meal. Normally, the fundus of the stomach is seen to be filled with gas (if the film is taken in erect position). The first part of the duodenum appears as a cap, proximal to which a constriction appears caused by normal pyloric sphincter. A constriction also appears about 3–4 cm proximal to the pyloric sphincter. This signifies the junction of the body of the stomach and pyloric antrum.

Normally stomach empties within 4 hours. If any residue of barium meal is seen at the stomach at the level of the ulcer producing a notch or "incisura" on the greater curvature **(Fig. 34.10)**; (a) a constant deformity suggesting a chronic cicatricial process due to an ulcer; (b) "rugal convergence", i.e., the folds of scar tissue converge on the ulcer side; (c) coarseness and irregularity of the gastric mucosa and, (d) a tender spot on the lesser curvature under fluoroscopic examination.

It is difficult to determine the *development of malignancy in a gastric ulcer*. It may be stated that any ulcer on the lesser curvature more than 1 inch in diameter and all the ulcers on the greater curvature should be taken as malignant unless proved otherwise.

In a duodenal ulcer careful serial radiography may reveal an ulcer crater. But in majority of cases this is not so easily detected. It is important to recognize the shape of the normal duodenal cap in barium meal X-ray. Indirect

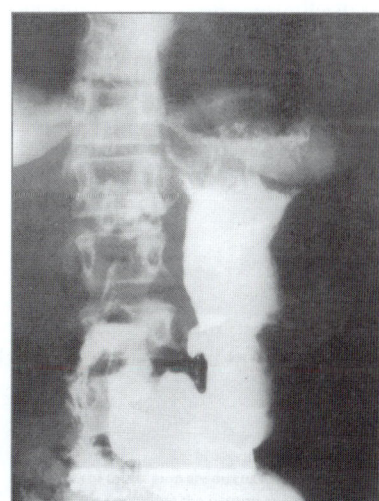

Fig. 34.10: Gastric ulcer showing the ulcer crater on the lesser curvature of the stomach and an incisura (indrawing) on the greater curvature just opposite to the crater. Note that the duodenal cap is normal.

signs are more common and they are persistent deformity of the dependent part of the stomach after 6 hours it may be due to hypotonia or pylorospasm. If however there is a residue after 24 hours a diagnosis of organic pyloric stenosis is almost certain.

A *gastric ulcer* is recognized by projecting bud of barium meal from normal smooth outline— which is known as *ulcer crater* or *niche*. This is usually seen in the lesser curvature of stomach. This is a direct sign of an ulcer. Since ulcers may lie on the posterior or anterior wall of the lesser curvature, it is obvious that the usual anteroposterior view will not show them. An oblique view may reveal some of them. In these cases, when the stomach has emptied or the barium has gone below the level of the ulcer, there may be left a fleck of barium in the crater with a clear zone around it and corona of mucosal rugae converging towards the crater. These, when seen, are also definite signs of ulcer. In addition to these direct signs one should look for the indirect signs of gastric ulcer. They are: (a) persistent spasm of duodenal cap, localized tenderness over the duodenum and rapid emptying of the stomach; (b) deformity of the duodenal cap may sometimes be caused by adhesions in gallbladder diseases.

Carcinoma of the stomach is diagnosed by persistent "filling-defect" which must be constant in all films **(Figs. 34.11 to 34.13)**. The presence of a long and segmental obliteration of mucosal pattern and segmental loss of peristalsis are considered as valuable additional signs of carcinoma.

In *carcinoma of the head of pancreas* the barium filled duodenum is widened—the "pad" sign **(Fig. 34.14)**. In case of ampulla of Vater carcinoma a filling defect is seen which may give the duodenum an appearance of a reversed 3 (ε).

In *pseudopancreatic cyst* the stomach is anteriorly displaced which is shown in lateral view **(Fig. 34.15)**.

In *appendicitis* the part played by X-ray examination is not very significant. The two cardinal signs are tenderness and fixity of the appendix *which has been visualized by barium meal*. A definite opinion cannot be given if the appendix is not properly visualized.

Barium meal follow-through examination: This is performed when a lesion at the distal end of the ileum, appendix, cecum or the proximal part of the ascending colon is suspected. After

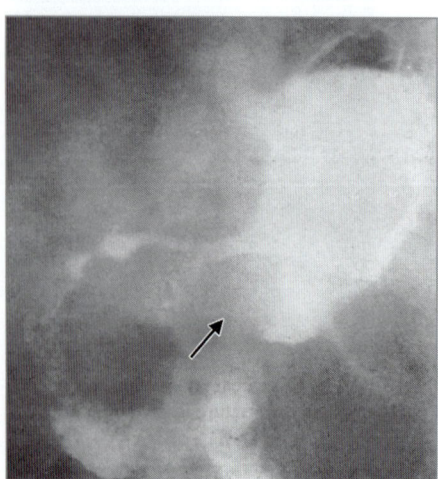

Fig. 34.11: Barium meal X-ray showing the typical filling defect (Shown by an arrow) of carcinoma of the pyloric region of the stomach.

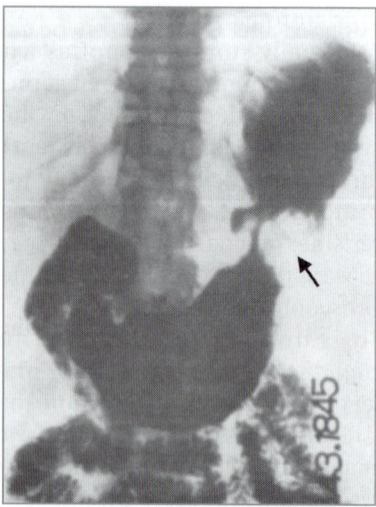

Fig. 34.12: Barium meal X-ray showing irregular filling defect of the pyloric region of the stomach due to carcinoma of the stomach.

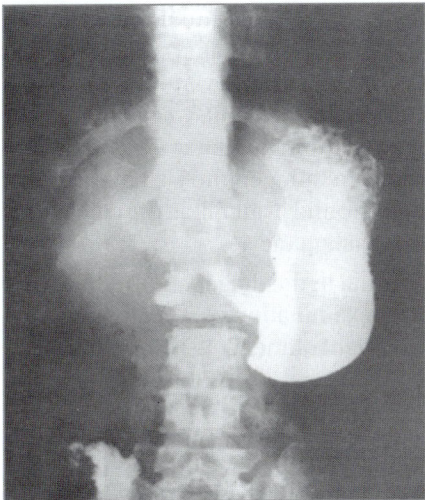

Fig. 34.13: Gastric carcinoma causing 'hour-glass' contracture (shown by an arrow).

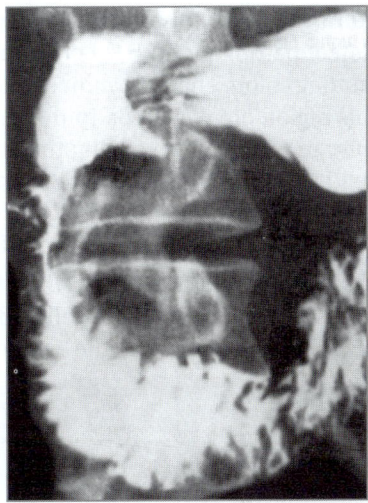

Fig. 34.14: Hypotonic duodenography showing filling defect due to carcinoma of the pancreas.

giving barium meal fluoroscopic examination of stomach and duodenum is performed. Then films are taken after 2, 3 and 4 hours. This is particularly helpful in diagnosis of (i) appendicitis (non- filling of appendix, fixity and tenderness on the appendix when it is filled with barium); (ii) Ileocecal tuberculosis (the cecum is displaced upwards and the distal part of the ileum becomes slightly narrowed and almost vertical); (iii) Crohn's disease (the terminal ileum becomes narrowed—'string sign of Kantor'); (iv) Carcinoma of cecum (irregular filling defect in cecum).

Hypotonic duodenography: Shows the pathology of the duodenum and the deformity of the duodenum due to the pathology of the pancreas in a much better way. Here the duodenum is made atonic by antrenyl injection, hypotonic barium is pushed through a gastroduodenal (Scott-Harden) tube and lastly the duodenum is distended with air to give a double-contrast effect. In chronic pancreatitis the earliest change is a definite flattening of the medial margin of the duodenal loop and later on inverted "3" sign is seen. In carcinoma of the pancreas small filling defects **(Fig. 34.15)**

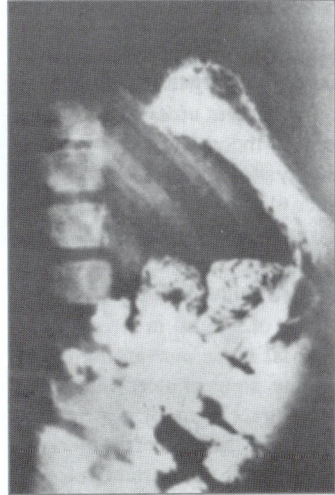

Fig. 34.15: Lateral view of barium meal X-ray showing anterior displacement of the stomach due to presence of pseudopancreatic cyst.

or areas of constriction are seen. Besides these, intrinsic lesions of the duodenum like diverticula, papilloma, carcinoma, etc., are better delineated than in conventional barium X-ray.

For the radiological investigation of the biliary tract: The patient should be prepared with an aperient, enema and pitressin in order to expel feces and gas which interfere with biliary shadows. At first straight X-ray is taken. In straight X-ray gallstones can be visualized in only 10% of cases. If visualized, they look like rings in which the centers remain radiotranslucent whereas the periphery shows calcification. This is typical of mixed stones. Cholesterol stones are not at all radio-opaque. Very rarely a calcified gallbladder or limy bile within the gallbladder may be seen.

Barium enema examination: Barium enema is introduced per anal canal and X-rays are taken to detect pathology in the rectum, sigmoid colon, descending colon, transverse colon and ascending colon. The deformities which are revealed by this examination in various pathologies of this region are discussed in the section of **'DIFFERENTIAL DIAGNOSIS'**. *Double contrast enema,* in which after keeping the enema for sometime the barium enema is evacuated and instead air is pumped through the anal canal. Thus the barium lining in the wall of the colon will be more clearly delineated against the contrast dark background of air filling the colon. This is ideal for small polyp, small ulcer of the mucosa and early malignancy.

Oral cholecystography (Figs. 34.16 to 34.21): This is essential in the diagnosis of gallbladder diseases. The function of the gallbladder is assessed by this examination. A straight X-ray will be taken in the morning. In the evening the patient is given a light dinner consisting of nonfatty

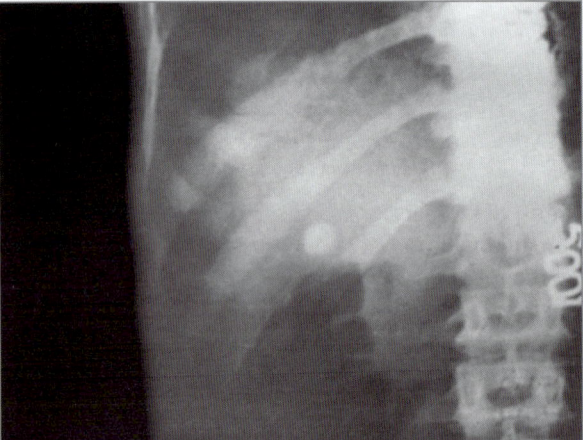

Fig. 34.16: Straight X-ray showing a typical radio-opaque gallstone. Note that the center of the stone is relatively radiotranslucent.

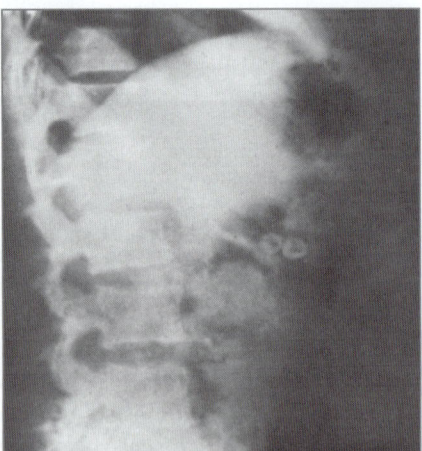

Fig. 34.17: In lateral view note that the gallstones (with relatively radiotranslucent center) are situated quite in front of the vertebral bodies (cf. renal stone).

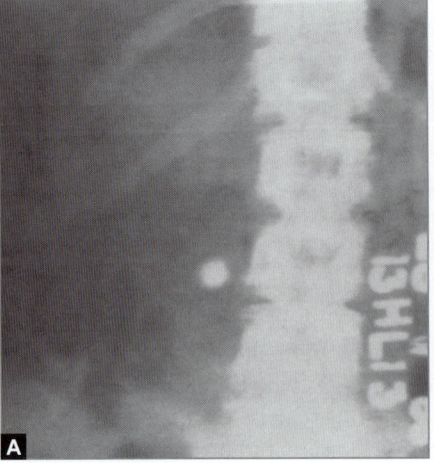

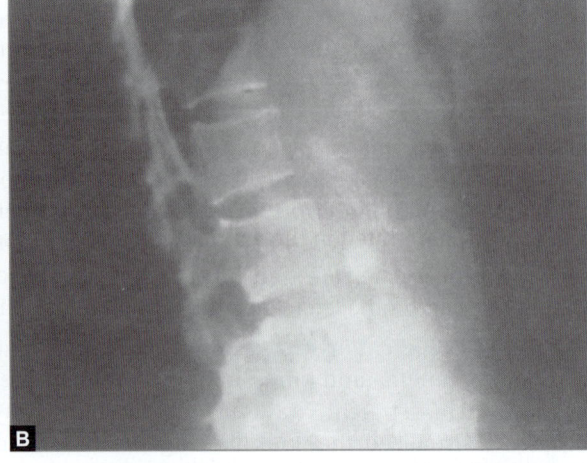

Figs. 34.18A and B: (A): Straight X-ray of the abdomen showing radio-opaque solitary stone in the gallbladder; (B) Note that the gallstone lies in front of the lumbar vertebra (cf. renal stone).

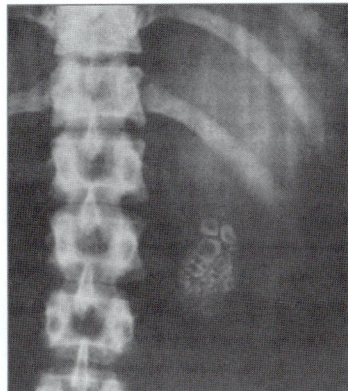

Fig. 34.19: Straight X-ray showing typical multiple mixed stones in the gallbladder.

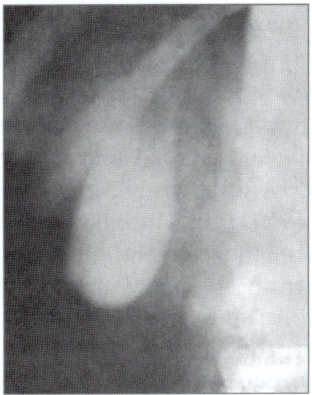

Fig. 34.20: Oral cholecystography showing a normal functioning gallbladder.

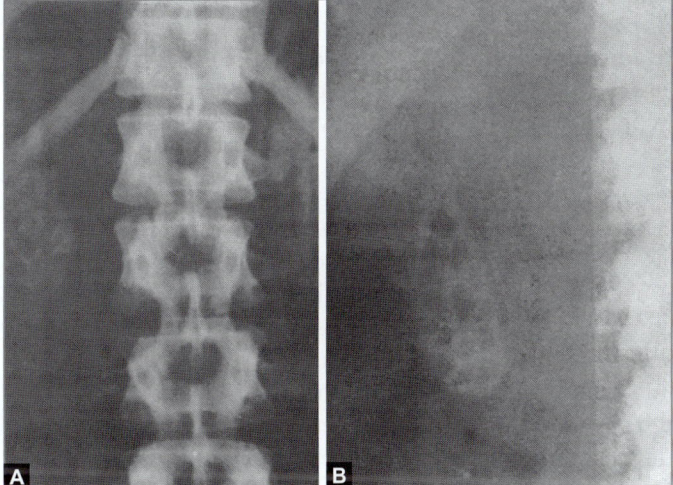

Figs. 34.21A and B: Oral cholecystogram showing negative shadows of gallstones. Obviously these gallstones are not radio-opaque and will not be revealed in straight X-ray.

food. After this the patient is given 6 tablets of 'Telepaque' to be ingested with water. The patient is not given anything to eat or drink till the radiological examination is made on the next morning after 14 hours of ingestion of the dye. The dye is absorbed from the intestine, excreted by the liver and concentrated in the gallbladder. If the dye is not eliminated by vomiting or excessive diarrhea a normal functioning gallbladder should be visualized in skiagraphy. Nonvisualization of the gallbladder means a nonfunctioning gallbladder. Of course, in a jaundiced patient with impaired liver function the dye may not be excreted and concentrated in the amount to make the gallbladder visible. After 2 or 3 films have been exposed the patient is given a drink containing sufficient amount of fat to cause contraction of the gallbladder. 10–20 minutes later films are taken in order to see that the gallbladder contracts normally. Biloptin in the evening and solu biloptin in the next morning followed 3 hours later by radiography may show the bile ducts as well as the gallbladder. Stones which were not in the control picture (straight X-ray) may now show as filling defects against uniformly opaque back ground—the 'negative shadows' of gallstones.

Intravenous cholangiography: Till today it has occupied a mediocre position so far as the disease of the biliary tree is concerned. "Biligrafin" is used for this purpose. 20 mL is injected very slowly into a vein. Skiagrams are taken 10–40 minutes after the injection. The biliary tract is frequently visualized due to higher concentration of the dye (about 50–100 times) within the bile. For the gallbladder this investigation is inferior to oral cholecystography.

By showing a good picture of the biliary tree, stone or other pathology can be easily detected. Though positive finding is of immense importance, yet a negative finding is of no value because the incidence of false negative is unacceptably high. *There are two places where this test surpasses oral cholecystography in diagnosing cholecystitis.* Firstly when the absorption of the dye is impaired as when the patient is vomiting or suffering from diarrhea and the secondly in case of acute cholecystitis.

Percutaneous transhepatic cholangiography (PTC) (Figs. 34.22 to 34.24): In the recent years by using a 23-guage thin walled needle the percentage of successful study has been increased and the incidence of complication has been decreased thus making this an important investigating method. This investigation shows intra- or extrahepatic biliary obstruction due to various causes. This should be done in the operation theatre keeping everything ready for operation, if be needed. The prothrombin level should be raised to normal by IM injection of vitamin K1. The needle ensheathed by a flexible polypropylene tube is pushed through the liver into dilated intrahepatic biliary canaliculi. The needle is withdrawn, the polypropylene tube is attached to a syringe and by trial and error aspiration of bile will be seen flowing into the syringe. At this time 20–40 mL of 45% hypaque is injected and X-ray exposures are made.

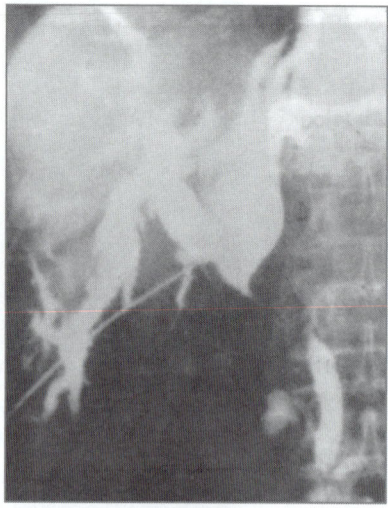

Fig. 34.22: Percutaneous transhepatic cholangiogram (PTC) showing obstruction of the common bile duct due to metastatic lymph nodes in the Porta-hepatis.

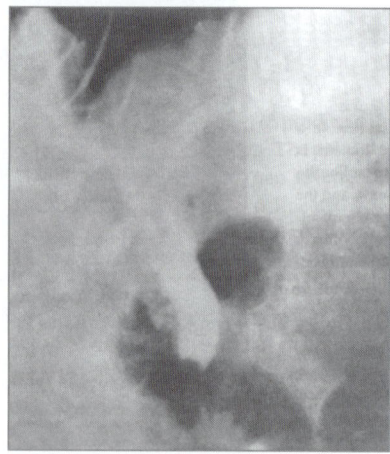

Fig. 34.23: PTC showing obstruction of the common bile duct due to a stone in its lower part shown by the concave margin of dye.

At least three attempts should be made before it is presumed that there is no dilatation of the intrahepatic bile duct. Hemorrhage, biliary leakage and sepsis are the three major complications of this investigation. It should be a routine practice to send some bile for culture and sensitivity test so that if sepsis ultimately develops one can use the most suitable antibiotic.

5. **FIBEROPTIC ENDOSCOPY**—is a great forward step so far as investigation of chronic abdominal conditions are concerned. Modern technique of fiberoptic gastroscopy gives more light and show the actual pathology distinctly. The patient is prepared in the following way: he should fast for 8–10 hours preceding endoscopy. In case of pyloric obstruction repeated aspirations are necessary. Antacids should not be given 10 hours prior to examination.

Barium meal X-ray, if required, should be done at least two days before endoscopy. The patient is sedated. The throat should be anesthetized locally and this remains for about an hour. Indications of gastroscopy are: (i) any gastric lesion shown or suspected in X-ray studies; (ii) upper gastrointestinal bleeding; (iii) persistent vomiting and; (iv) symptom complained by a postgastrectomy patient. It cannot be over emphasized that endoscopy occupies an important role in GI bleeding. Further one can detect a peptic ulcer which has not been shown by barium meal X-ray. It also can assess the improvement of the ulcer by medical treatment. A gastric ulcer—whether benign or malignant can also be diagnosed by endoscopy. Gastric camera will show still picture of the pathology in the stomach. Last but not the least is its 90 percent accuracy in finding out a stomach ulcer which is often missed by skiagraphy.

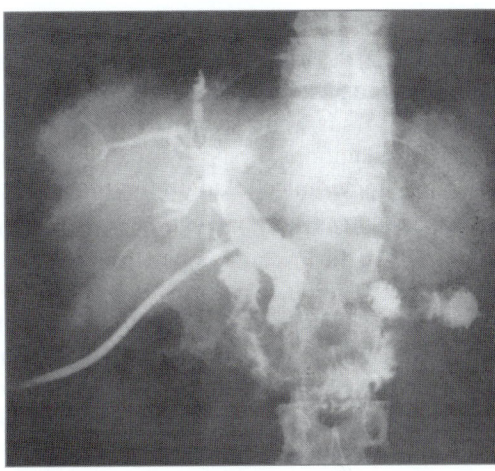

Fig. 34.24: T-tube cholangiography showing stone (negative shadow) at the distal end of the common bile duct. Note that the common bile duct and hepatic ducts are dilated.

The stomach has long been accessible to the endoscopist and gastritis, ulceration, hemorrhage, stomata and malignancy were diagnosed conveniently. But regular inspection of the duodenum was not possible till the advent of a slim endoscope which can be passed through the pylorus. The forward viewing Olympus GIFD and ACMI or side-viewing Olympus JFB can be used for duodenoscopy as a part of the esophagogastroduodenoscopy. Over all extreme flexibility and control of the instrument make it possible for every part of the stomach and duodenum to be inspected and a lesion may be biopsied. Thus radiology by barium meal which has traditionally been the primary method of gastric examination and is now regarded as complementary, may soon be less important than endoscopic studies. Besides the uses already described above, duodenoscopy is particularly indicated in the assessment of dyspepsia. There may be definite oedema, narrowing or permanent distortion of the round orifice of the pylorus. There may also be duodenitis in these cases. These are in fact examples of X-ray negative dyspepsia.

Endoscopic retrograde cholangiopancreatography (ERCP): Nowadays common bile duct and pancreatic ducts can be cannulated by side viewing fiber-optic duodenoscope through ampulla of Vater. Cannulation of the papilla of Vater is carried out with the instrument so positioned as to give an end-on view of the papilla from some 1 cm distance. A polythene cannula is made clear of air and flushed with 60% Urografin. The cannula is passed through the instrument taking care not to spill contrast medium into the duodenum since this stimulates peristalsis and makes cannulation difficult. Contrast medium is introduced slowly under fluoroscopic control. Both biliary and pancreatic ductal systems fill, but usually one duct fills first. If the pancreatic duct is filled first contrast medium more than 2–2.5 mL should not be injected. When the pancreatic ductules at the tail are filled injection must be stopped since overfilling will lead to extravasation and will cause pain. After pancreatography the tip of the cannula is readjusted to fill the biliary duct. Now 40 mL of contrast can be used and preferably 25% hypaque is used to prevent obscuring of the small stones. Its main indications are three:

(1) Jaundice: persistent and recurrent undiagnosed jaundice (cause of obstruction will be revealed); (2) Biliary tract problems: undiagnosed upper abdominal pain (suspected to be biliary in origin) and postoperative biliary symptoms. (3) Pancreatic diseases: undiagnosed abdominal or back pain (suspected to be pancreatic in origin), chronic and relapsing pancreatitis (stricture, irregular dilatations, cysts, etc., can be seen). The main complications of this procedure are infection (including cholangitis and serum hepatitis) and pancreatitis.

6. **ULTRASOUND:** The development of diagnostic ultrasound has definitely brought about a revolution in the investigations of chronic abdominal disorders. A sonar scan involves minimal patient preparation, takes an average of 15–20 minutes to perform and causes no discomfort to the patient. The barium has a deleterious effect on the scan so if possible ultrasonic examination should be carried out before barium studies. In a supine scan of the upper abdomen it is possible at various levels to outline the liver, spleen, aorta, vena cava and the kidneys. The gallbladder can frequently be identified and there is often a small echo-free area. Ultrasound is of particular value in the diagnosis of space- occupying lesions. The size, shape and consistency of the organs normally outlined can be assessed and relationships of the mass to these organs can be identified. Cysts present very well defined contour and are transonic. Their surfaces are usually echo-free although they may give rise to linear echoes due to presence of septa. Poor demarcation of the malignant tumor suggests infiltration of the surrounding tissues.

Carcinoma of stomach may even be diagnosed as the mass which remains deep to the left lobe of the liver. The patient is given 2–3 glasses of water to identify the gastric lumen. The palpable mass corresponds exactly to the area of fine echoes on the wall of the stomach.

In liver, not only anatomical abnormalities like Riedel's lobe can be diagnosed, but also cysts, abscesses, primary and secondary tumors can be diagnosed by ultrasound. The most frequently recognized appearance of metastatic tumor is either ring-shaped pattern or solid irregular mass with expansion of the adjacent liver outline.

So far as the gallbladder diseases are concerned, in the absence of jaundice ultrasonic B-mode scanning compares well with oral cholecystography, but in the presence of jaundice however ultrasonic scanning is considered to be the investigation of choice, as ultrasound can be used regardless of the state of the gallbladder and liver. Congenital anomalies like duplication of the gallbladder or Phrygian cap can be imaged with ultrasound, even gallbladder size is easily measured with this technique. Ultrasound can detect gallstones larger than a few mm in size. Biliary mud can also be appreciated **(Figs. 34.25 to 34.29)**. It may be confessed that ultrasound may even be preferred to oral cholecystography provided the necessary skills are available. The advantage of ultrasound is that additional information about the biliary tract, liver and pancreas can be obtained. Even a thick, edematous gallbladder without presence of gallstones as well as gangrenous

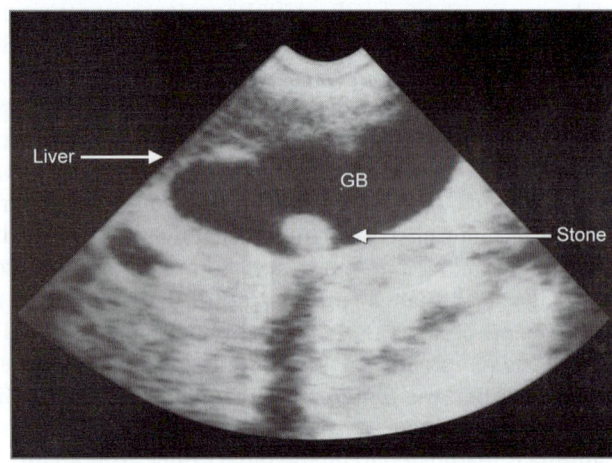

Fig. 34.25: Ultrasonography showing clearly a stone in a dilated gallbladder (GB).

Chapter 34: Examination of Chronic Abdominal Conditions

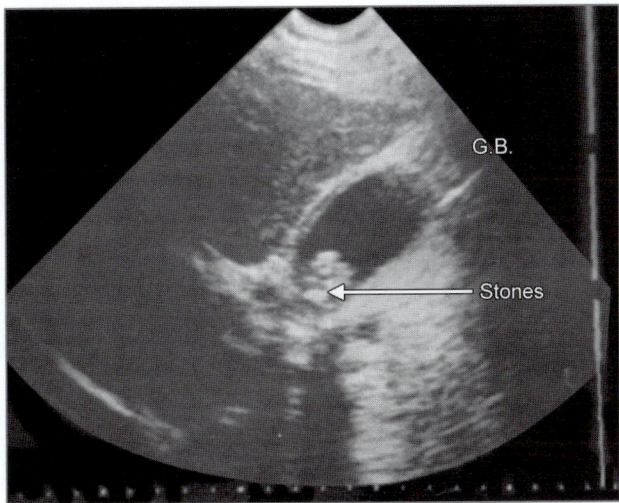

Fig. 34.26: Ultrasonography showing multiple stones inside a dilated gallbladder (GB).

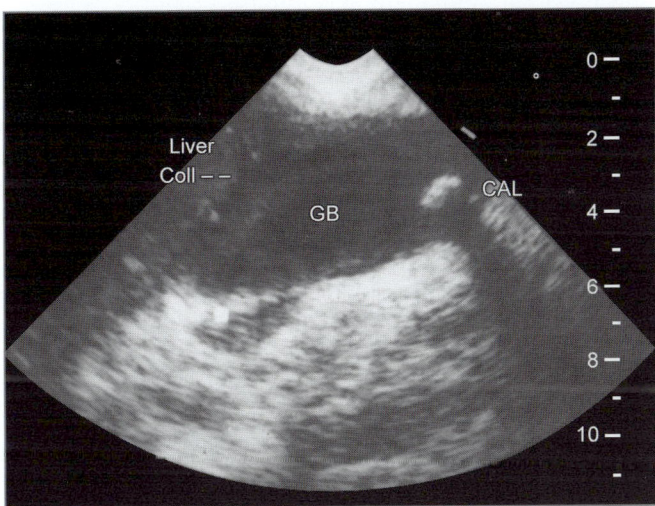

Fig. 34.27: Ultrasonography showing a calculus at the neck of the gallbladder, which is hugely dilated—a case of empyema gallbladder. One can also see fluid collection (Coll.) around the highly infected gallbladder (GB).

gallbladder may also be identified by ultrasound. It must be remembered that children may be rarely affected by gallbladder disease and ultrasound is an excellent imaging modality for these cases than oral cholecystography without the hazards of ionizing radiation.

Intrahepatic biliary tree and the common hepatic duct can be clearly identified by real-time ultrasound fluoroscopy. A diameter of more than 7 mm in case of common hepatic duct indicates dilatation of the intrahepatic biliary tree. Stone in the common bile duct can also be identified by this technique. It may even show an enlarged gallbladder with obstruction of the lower end of the common bile duct due to carcinoma of the pancreas when the gallbladder is not palpable clinically. *Here lies the importance of ultrasonic scanning over any method of*

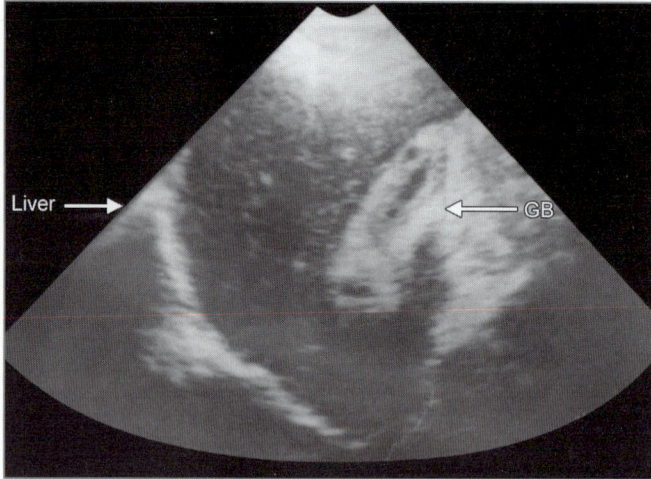

Fig. 34.28: Ultrasonography showing thick walled gallbladder (GB)—a case of acalculous acute cholecystitis.

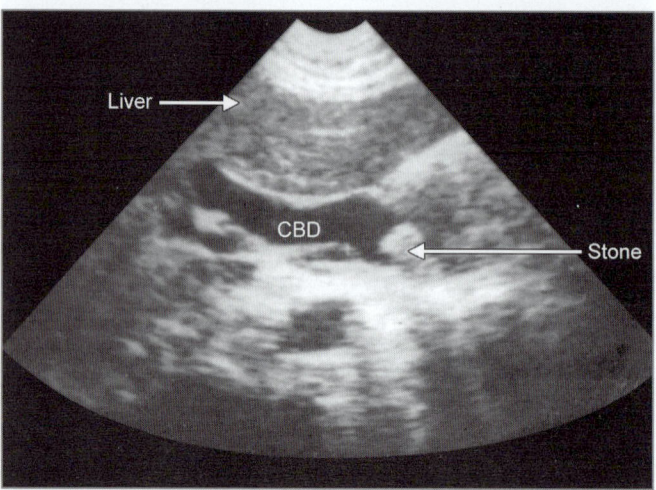

Fig. 34.29: Ultrasonography showing a big stone at the distal end of the common bile duct (CBD) which is dilated.

investigation. The pancreas is difficult to examine as it is effectively screened by the echo-reflecting bowel. Though a normal pancreas cannot be defined, yet an inflamed edematous pancreas can however be seen as a poorly defined mass in front of the aorta and the vertebral column. Cysts and pseudocysts can be readily outlined and tumors more than 3 cm in diameter can be identified with the ultrasonic equipment. An enlarged spleen can be recognized from its typical shape—the splenic notch. Cysts of the spleen whether congenital or traumatic are easily seen by ultrasound within the splenic substances. Splenomegaly associated with portal hypertension and cirrhosis of the liver is also not very difficult to detect. Lymph nodes can also be appreciated **(Fig. 34.30)**.

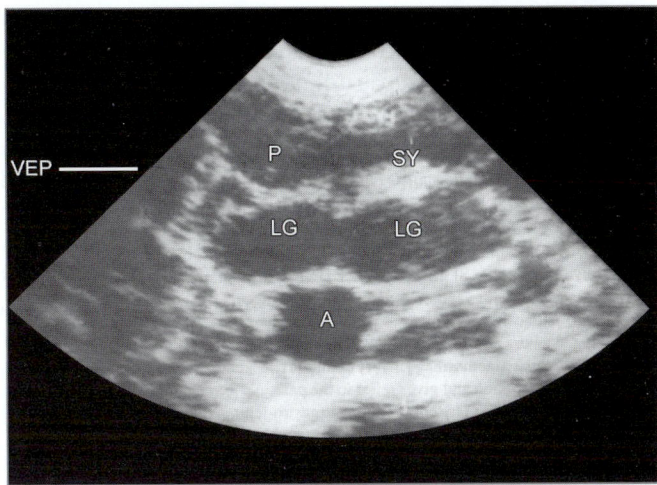

Fig. 34.30: Ultrasonography of the abdomen showing enlarged metastatic lymph nodes in front of the aorta (involving pre- and para-aortic groups of lymph nodes).

Ultrasonic guidance for biopsy and aspiration is an added advantage of this mode of investigation. Aspiration of the liver cyst has been performed guided by ultrasound. This technique is more popular in case of renal cyst.

7. **RADIO-ISOTOPE SCANNING:** Liver scans were found to be of value especially in the differential diagnosis of upper abdominal masses, of jaundice, of hepatomegaly and in the screening of patient with malignant disease. The method is as follows: The patient is given inorganic iodide orally for two days prior to scanning to block thyroid uptake of isotope. Scanning is performed with the patient in supine position 8–10 minutes after the administration of the isotope (this represents the time taken for the hepatic uptake). The isotopic agents normally used are ^{131}I-labelled human serum albumin and ^{99}technetium. In the cases of hepatomegaly of unknown etiology scanning may help in the differentiation between focal and diffuse diseases. Cirrhosis of liver gives rise to a characteristic pale, patchy scan owing to reduced and irregular hepatic uptake. Scanning may detect malignant nodes in the porta hepatic as a cause of jaundice. Scanning has at times been used to demonstrate right subphrenic abscess. The greatest application of liver scanning is in detection of intrahepatic lesion such as abscess, hydatid and other cysts, primary or secondary neoplasms. Reported figures of overall accuracy in detection of hepatic metastasis range from 77% to 93%.

Pancreatic scanning is performed by using ^{75}Se-labelled methionine in the dose of 3 μc per kg admitted intravenously. From a pancreatic scan information can be obtained whether the pancreas is functioning or not, its size, shape, various cysts and tumors within its substance.

8. **RADIOACTIVE ISOTOPES IN ALIMENTARY BLEEDING:** Following intravenous injection of erythrocytes labelled with ^{51}Cr the loss of blood into the lumen of the gut may be measured as ^{51}Cr is not reabsorbed. In clinical management of acute gastrointestinal bleeding, the site of hemorrhage is difficult to find by radiographic or endoscopic examination or even at laparotomy. If following injection of ^{51}Cr-labelled red cells fine polythene tube is passed slowly down the gut as far as the terminal ileum. Frequent samples of gut fluid are obtained and their blood contents are determined. As soon as bleeding is detected the position of the end of the tube is determined radiologically.

9. **SELECTIVE VISCERAL ANGIOGRAPHY:** Bleeding at the rate of 0.5–3 cc per minute can be diagnosed by this technique. Emergency angiography is indicated for acute hemorrhage when the site of hemorrhage is unknown. Angiography may not only accurately localize hemorrhage but also can control bleeding to some extent by selective infusion of vasoconstricting drugs. This significantly reduces blood loss and allows better preparation of an emergency patient. Percutaneous catheterization via the femoral or axillary approach by the Seldinger technique is followed by selective injection of iodinated water soluble contrast material into the celiac, superior mesenteric or inferior mesenteric artery. Thus the site of hemorrhage is identified. The vessels nearest to the site is selectively catheterized. Pitressin is infused at the rate of 0.2 unit per minute for 15 minutes. Later on this dose is adjusted according to the rate of hemorrhage. Immediate surgery is necessary when bleeding is not controlled by pitressin. Gelfoam mixed clot or a fogarty catheter can be used to occlude the bleeding vessel.

10. **LAPAROSCOPY**—in the investigation of patients with jaundice allows visualization of intra-abdominal pathology, target biopsy of intra-abdominal lesions and percutaneous intrahepatic cholangiography all carried out at one procedure is of great diagnostic value. Cholangiography is carried out into dilated intrahepatic ducts, but in cases with minimal dilatation, the gallbladder can be injected with contrast medium. To minimize biliary leakage from the gallbladder which may be under tension, the needle should be directed through the adjacent liver tissue across the gallbladder bed.

11. **EXPLORATORY LAPAROTOMY:** In places where there is not much scope of carrying out various investigations as stated above, exploratory laparotomy should be called for earlier and becomes the last court of appeal. It must be realized that even after the sophisticated investigations as discussed above have been utilized, a few cases will remain undiagnosed and in these circumstances exploratory laparotomy may be justified to arrive at a definite diagnosis.

DIFFERENTIAL DIAGNOSIS

CHRONIC GASTRIC ULCER

The majority of the patients are more than 40 years of age and men are more often affected than women. Occupationally the patients are mainly in the rank of executive and perhaps greater stress and strain of the responsibility of the job may predispose the ulcer formation. The patients are often thin due to restricted diet for fear of pain. The main symptom is epigastric discomfort or pain which may vary from vague and mild discomfort, dull aching or burning to very severe pain which compels the patient to lie down. The main feature of the pain is its "clock-like" regularity. The pain appears immediately after taking food, so the patient becomes afraid of it but appetite remains good (cf. duodenal ulcer). Thus the patient may lose a little weight. The pain may radiate to the back when the ulcer penetrates into the pancreas. Relief is obtained spontaneously as soon as the stomach is emptied, or by taking alkali or by vomiting which is often self-induced. Vomiting is sometime a notable symptom, but is not more than 15% of cases. Hematemesis and melena may associate chronic gastric ulcer in about 1/4 of the cases. On examination deep tenderness can be elicited with remarkable constancy in the midepigastric region. Investigation can be carried out as discussed above.

CHRONIC DUODENAL ULCER

Typically the patients are young (below 40 years of age), quite busy and swallows his meals hastily at an irregular intervals between cigarettes and telephone calls. Again men dominate. Pain is the main symptom, but it appears 2½–4 hours after meal when the stomach becomes empty, i.e., "hunger pain". The pain usually appears in the early morning or in the late afternoon. The heavier the meal, the longer is the interval but the worse is the pain. The pain is characteristically located 1½ inches to the right of the midline on the transpyloric plane (i.e. about a hand's breadth below the xiphisternal joint). Relief is obtained by taking food. The pain maintains a characteristic periodicity and the attacks come in the spring and autumn. It must be realized that it is precipitated by excessive work, worry and anxiety, cigarettes and alcohol. Eructation of water or acid and heartburn are also very common symptoms of this fail disease. It must be remembered that vomiting is an uncommon symptom of duodenal ulceration. Hematemesis and melena which are features of hemorrhage within the ulcer are more frequent than in case of gastric ulcer. Appetite is exceptionally good, moreover patients eat at frequent intervals to get rid of the pain, so the majority of the patients are well build. On examination, localized deep tenderness on the duodenal point is quite common. There is 2% chance of perforation and 5% chance of massive hemorrhage. Investigations should be carried out as mentioned earlier.

PYLORIC STENOSIS

This is due to cicatrization of a duodenal or a juxta-pyloric ulcer. Peculiarly this occurs more often in the female. The long history of duodenal ulcer, certain loss of its periodicity with enhancement of pain and fullness towards evening are the typical points in the history worth noting. Vomiting, which is large in amount also occurs characteristically in the evening. It is often foul and frothy and contains undigested food material eaten even 2–3 days earlier. On examination, visible peristalsis passing from left to right is pathognomonic. Succussion splash is often heard. Barium meal X-ray will clinch the diagnosis.

GASTROJEJUNAL ULCER

It may occur after Polya type of partial gastrectomy or after gastrojejunal anastomosis. The incidence becomes very high when gastrojejunostomy is not associated with vagotomy. Recurrent ulcer occurs in about 3% of cases after Polya gastrectomy and 5% of cases after vagotomy and gastrojejunostomy. Symptoms usually appear within 2 years or so after the operation. Pain is again an important symptom and usually boring in nature and appears within 1/2 hour after taking food. The pain characteristically radiates from above and left of the umbilicus to the left iliac fossa. Hemorrhage is very common and it may be manifested as hematemesis, melena or occult blood in the stool. Vomiting is also very common and gives relief to the pain. A gastrojejunal ulcer is more prone to perforation than a peptic ulcer. This ulcer may penetrate into the transverse colon leading to gastrojejunocolic fistula. With the appearance of this fistula symptoms of anastomotic ulcer disappear, but unfortunately severe diarrhea and eructation of foul gas take their places. Even the patients may vomit fragments of formed feces. The main pathology behind this dreadful condition is the fouling of the jejunum by colonic contents. This results in tremendous disturbance of the vital absorptive mechanism. X-ray examination with barium meal will show narrowing of the gastrojejunostomy stoma and spastic contraction of the stomach and jejunum. Actual ulcer crater is hardly seen. It must be remembered *that gastro jejunocolic fistula is better diagnosed by a barium enema* since in more than 1/2 the patients the barium meal fails to reveal the fistula.

CARCINOMA OF THE STOMACH

The clinical picture can be conveniently described under 4 headings: (1) insidious type, (the carcinoma occurring in the body of the stomach), (2) obstructive type (carcinoma occurring in the pylorus or at the cardiac end), (3) as a lump and (4) as a carcinoma superimposed on a gastric ulcer.

This is a disease of the elderly, but if suspected in the young, should not be turned down on the point of age only. This is again commoner in men.

(1) *The insidious type:* The history is usually short. The early symptoms are indigestion, vague discomfort, a sensation of fullness and heaviness after meals in the upper abdomen; loss of appetite; a feeling of weakness, etc. The pain in the true sense is usually conspicuous by its absence in the early stage. Pain may appear in the very late stage of the disease.

The late symptoms are vomiting which give no relief to the pain, loss of weight and constant epigastric pain which is neither caused by nor relieved by food. On examination, wasting and pallor are noticeable features. The patients may be jaundiced. The abdomen becomes scaphoid and the skin becomes wrinkled and inelastic. Paradoxically there may be ascites with abdominal distension. On palpation there may be slight epigastric tenderness.

Deep palpation with relaxed abdomen may reveal an epigastric mass which is hard, irregular, mildly tender and may or may not move with respiration. One should try to palpate the liver which when palpable indicates secondary involvement with hard nodules. Fluid thrill and shifting dullness may be present if there is free fluid in the peritoneal cavity. There may be hard subcutaneous metastatic nodules in the umbilical region. To seek secondary deposit elsewhere one should palpate the lymph node of the neck particularly the left supraclavicular lymph nodes (Virchow's). Rectal examination may reveal transcoelomic implantation of metastatic cells into the rectovesical pouch. Vaginal examination may reveal Krukenburg's ovarian tumor. Wandering thrombophlebitis (Trousseau's sign) should be looked for in late cases. Special investigations should be carried out as discussed above.

(2) *Obstructive type:* Gastric carcinoma at the cardiac end and at the pylorus may obstruct the passage of food. Growth at pylorus is much more common than the former variety. The clinical picture resembles pyloric stenosis. The characteristic features of carcinoma are:(a) The history is short—a few months. (b) There may not be any previous history of peptic ulcer. (c) Anorexia, nausea and vomiting are constant; the vomitus is offensive containing altered blood "coffee ground". (d) Loss of weight is marked. (e) Skiagraphy with barium meal will confirm the diagnosis.

(3) *Lump:* Sometimes the patients may present with epigastric lump and nothing else. The general appearance of the patient will be same as discussed above. The lump will be hard, irregular, mobile or fixed, may or may not move with respiration. One should look for secondary metastasis.

(4) *Peptic ulcer type:* The possibility of carcinoma supervening on a gastric ulcer is recognized but the percentage of such complication is questionable. Malignancy should be suspected when: (a) there is loss of periodicity of the attacks, remission being shorter or nil; (b) the sharp burning ulcer pain is replaced by a constant dull ache; (c) good appetite of the gastric ulcer is replaced by loss of appetite; (d) nausea is common but vomiting gives no relief as previously (vomiting may be coffee ground); (e) loss of weight is rapid.

HIATUS HERNIA

It is defined as prolapse of a part of stomach into the thoracic cavity through esophageal hiatus. It may be of (i) sliding type—85%, (ii) paraesophageal (rolling) type—10% or (iii) mixed type—5%. Middle-aged or elderly obese ladies are the usual victims. Patients may complain of heart-burn, which becomes aggravated in stooping or lying down position, belching or reflux of acidic gastric juice into the mouth. They may also present with the symptoms due to the presence of hernia in the chest, such as flatulent dyspepsia, fullness, shortness of breath, upper abdominal pain, tachycardia, etc. They may also come with the complications of esophagitis like dysphagia, slight hematemesis or anemia etc. Special investigations like barium meal X-ray **(Figs. 34.31A and B)**, esophagoscopy, etc., will diagnose the condition.

CHRONIC CHOLECYSTITIS AND CHOLELITHIASIS

Though the typical proverb is that the patients are usually **F**at, **F**ertile, **F**air, **F**emale of **F**orty, yet one should not give very much importance to this five 'F's as definite aid to diagnosis.

In many cases *the feeling of distension* is the first symptom and the patient may feel that she has eaten too much before she has finished the meal. Gradually the patients start complaining of pain over the upper part of the right rectus muscle often radiating to the inferior angle of the right scapula. The patients often notice that the pain becomes worse after taking fatty foods (qualitative dyspepsia). The patient may make attempts to get relief by inducing vomiting, but that is seldom achieved as in peptic ulcer case. Nausea is very common but vomiting is rare. *Postprandial belching,* often described as flatulent dyspepsia, is also a common symptom of this condition. Patient's appetite is maintained. Attacks of pain are irregular lasting for weeks or months or pain free intervals of varying length.

Jaundice is not a sign of cholecystitis although a slight icteric tinge may be present due to associated cholangitis. Inspection reveals a normally looking abdomen. On palpation the most important sign is that of Murphy (*see* page 567). In majority of cases the gallbladder is not palpable unless a mucocele or empyema develops. The various modes of X-ray are quite confirmatory and have already been discussed under the heading of "Special Investigations". Oral cholecystography and ultrasound are quite diagnostic.

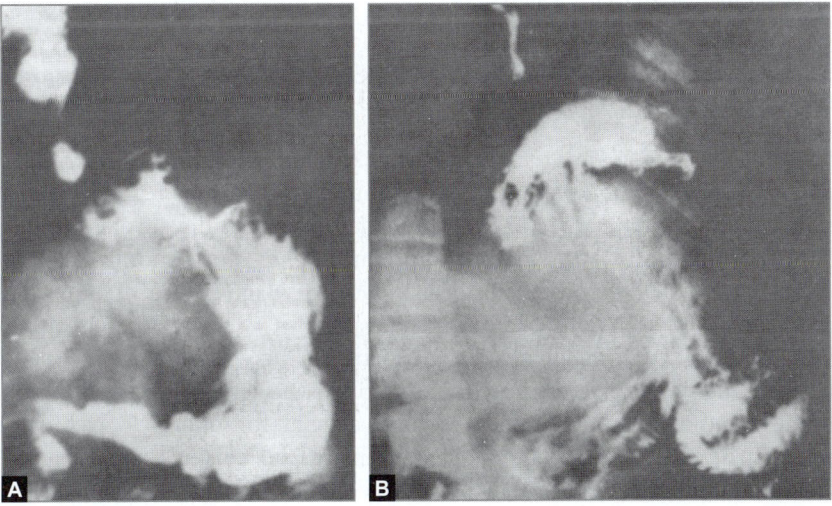

Figs. 34.31A and B: Barium meal X-ray showing sliding type and rolling type of hiatus hernia respectively.

STONE IN THE COMMON BILE DUCT

Typically the patients suffer from (a) biliary colic, (b) jaundice following each attack of colic and (c) intermittent fever (Charcot's)—the triad of choledocholithiasis. It should be differentiated from carcinoma of the head of pancreas.

Oriental cholangiohepatitis: This is a condition in which there are long standing stones in the common bile duct. This results from obstruction to the common bile duct due to infestation by the Chinese liver flukes (Clonorchis Sinensis). The patient presents with pain, jaundice and intermittent pyrexia (Charcot's triad). Urine contains bile and the stool becomes clay colored. This condition is common in Japan, China, Hong Kong, etc.

Choledochus cyst: In this condition weakness of a part or whole of the wall of the common bile duct leads to a cystic dilatation which ultimately gives pressure on the remaining bile duct and thus obstructs the flow of the bile to the duodenum. This condition is rare and females are affected more commonly than males. In Japan this condition is commoner than in any other countries. The patient never presents before six months of age and about half of the cases present only in adult life. Upper abdominal pain, obstructive jaundice and pyrexia from infection (Charcot's triad) are again the main presenting symptoms. Palpation may reveal the cyst, which may be confused with pancreatic cyst.

CHRONIC PANCREATITIS

It is a condition in which there is slow but progressive destruction of the acini with increasing fibrosis—the whole pathology leads to functional failure of the pancreas. Abdominal pain is the main presenting symptom which starts in the epigastrium and tends to pass through to the back. The pain varies from a boring pain to that of biliary colic. The pain is often quite intolerable which becomes slightly relieved when the patient sits up. The pain lasts for about 3-4 days. Vomiting is present in more than 50% of cases. Weakness is very common. Jaundice is present in less than 20% of cases but diabetes is more common (about 1/3 of cases). Steatorrhea is quite common. Best way to palpate the pancreas is to turn the patient to the right and hips and knees are flexed. The left subcostal region is deeply palpated. This will evoke tenderness in acute and chronic pancreatitis (Mallet-Guy's sign).

CARCINOMA OF THE PANCREAS

It usually affects the head, sometimes the body and rarely the tail of the organ. Men are usually the victims.

Carcinoma of the head of the pancreas **(Figs. 34.32A and B)**: Although it is often described as a painless condition, yet the patient may present with pain as his first symptom. Jaundice is very common and in majority of cases it precedes pain. Jaundice is classically said to be progressively deepening. Intermission may be seen in cases of carcinoma of the ampulla of Vater due to sloughing of the growth. Anorexia and loss of weight are very common as in other carcinomas. Diarrhea may be troublesome and foul smelling. The pale stools are quite common and steatorrhea from enzyme deficiency is also a feature of this condition. Occasionally patients may present with the symptoms very much similar to those of acute pancreatitis. So old patients when present with these symptoms one should investigate thoroughly to exclude carcinoma of the pancreas. The gallbladder is enlarged according to Courvoisier's law (see page 569). The tumor is seldom palpable. The liver may be enlarged. Ascites may be present only in the late cases.

Carcinoma of the body and tail of the pancreas: Pain in the epigastrium is the cardinal symptom. The peculiar feature of the pancreatic pain is that it passes through to the back. It is aggravated when the patient lies down and lessened when he sits up so the patient often spends the night sitting up with his arms folded across the chest. Thrombophlebitis migrans may be an indication of the presence of pancreatic carcinoma. Thrombophlebitis which appears spontaneously and resolves only to appear again elsewhere is the type one often comes across. This is known as *Trousseau's sign.*

CHRONIC APPENDICITIS

Young girls are the main victims of this condition. A vague pain in the abdomen which is more often complained at the right iliac fossa is probably the earliest symptom in the majority of cases. Definite localized pain may be absent instead a vague dyspepsia may be complained of Vomiting may be present but does not afford any relief to pain. This is commoner in pre- and postileal positions of the appendix. Constipation is a common accompaniment of this condition. Scalding pain on micturition or pain which mimics ureteric colic is often complained of. On examination the cardinal finding is a distinct tenderness over the appendix. Rectal examination often gives a clue to the diagnosis.

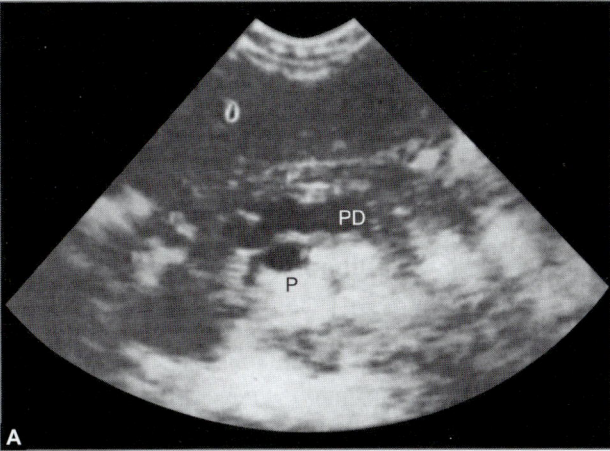
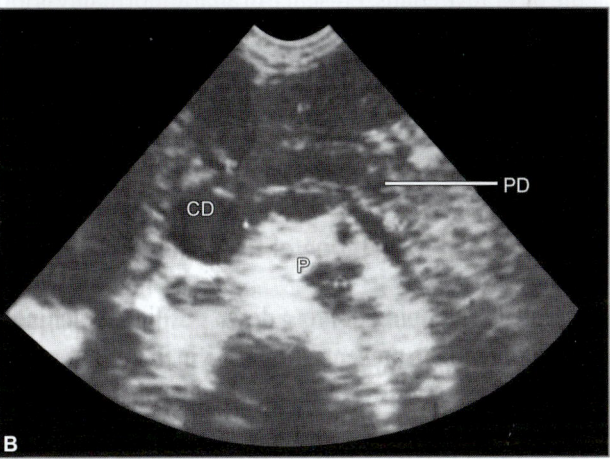

Figs. 34.32A and B: (A) Ultrasonography—one can see a mass in the head of the pancreas near ampulla of Vater with dilated pancreatic duct; (B) In the same case one can see the dilated pancreatic duct (PD) and also a very dilated common bile duct (CD) and the mass near the ampulla of Vater (P).

CROHN'S DISEASE

The patients often have diarrhea without obvious bleeding. Perianal lesions such as abscesses, fissure and fistulae are quite common in this condition. The clinical picture is best considered in 4 stages:(1) the inflammatory stage, when a mass is palpable in the right iliac region; (2) the colitis stage, when diarrhea, fever, anemia and loss of weight are present; (3) the stenotic stage, when the picture of small gut obstruction supervenes and (4) the fistula stage, either external or internal—communicating with the sigmoid colon, bladder, cecum, etc. Differentiation from an appendicular lump is made by the absence of origin of pain in the umbilical region, insidious onset and presence of occult blood in stool. Skiagraphy with a barium meal will reveal loss of peristalsis in the affected loop and the 'string sign' of Kantor when the lumen is narrowed to a fine cord (*see* **Fig. 35.12**).

If the condition has involved the colon, in barium enema a coarse cobblestone pattern may be present but it is often difficult to differentiate this from pseudopolyposis of ulcerative colitis. Segmental lesions strongly favor the diagnosis of Crohn's disease. An abrupt cut-off in the radiological abnormalities speaks in favor of Crohn's disease. The deep fissuring ulcers may give rise to spiky or rose-thorn appearance. Sigmoidoscopy may reveal Crohn's disease if the condition has involved the rectum.

Crohn's disease of the colon: The main three features of this condition are diarrhea, loss of weight and abdominal pain. Sometimes abdominal lump may be present due to pericolonic thickening or infection. Spontaneous fistula may develop either to the exterior or with the viscus. This type of fistula formation is never found in ulcerative colitis though occasionally seen in diverticulitis. In acute colonic Crohn's disease there will be toxic dilatation of the colon as seen in acute ulcerative colitis. Presence of anal abnormality is found in about 80% of colonic cases. Rectal bleeding is less frequent than that in ulcerative colitis and diverticulitis. In contradistinction to ulcerative colitis, rectum is involved in only half the cases, so in sigmoidoscopy normal rectal mucosa does not exclude this condition. The mucosa when affected shows edematous swelling, granularity and scattered small ulcers with normal mucosa in between (cf. ulcerative colitis, where there is uniform diffuse change without presence of intervening normal mucosa).

Systemic disorders like erythema nodosum, synovitis, iritis and minor septic skin conditions may be seen with this condition.

ABDOMINAL TUBERCULOSIS

Abdominal tuberculosis can be one of two types—(1) Intestinal tuberculosis and (2) Tuberculosis of mesenteric lymph nodes.

1. **Intestinal tuberculosis:** This is also of two varieties—(1) Ulcerative tuberculosis and (2) Hyperplastic ileocecal tuberculosis.
1. **ULCERATIVE TUBERCULOSIS:** This usually results from inhalation of tubercle bacilli (human type) in sputum in a case of pulmonary tuberculosis. This condition is characterized by multiple ulcers at the terminal ileum. The long axis of the ulcer lies transversely. The serous coat overlying the ulcer becomes thickened, so perforation is unusual. Healing of the ulcers leads to stricture formation. Loss of weight and diarrhea with fetid odor stools containing pus and occult blood are complained of. Often the patient is a known case of pulmonary tuberculosis. On examination nothing specific can be discovered except slight tenderness in the right iliac fossa. Barium meal follow-through may demonstrate nonfilling or inadequate filling of terminal ileum, cecum and proximal part of ascending colon due to narrowing and hypermotility of the ulcerated segment.
2. **HYPERPLASTIC TUBERCULOSIS** is described in the next chapter in the section of differential diagnosis of swellings in the right iliac region.
2. **Tuberculosis of mesenteric lymph nodes:** This is a rare entity and mainly seen in children. Tubercle bacilli (both human type and bovine types) enter the mesenteric lymph nodes through the Peyer's patches present in the terminal ileum. There are various types of presentation of this disease—(a) As a cause *of abdominal pain:* This central constant abdominal pain is more of a discomfort than severe pain. On examination slight tenderness can be elicited in the umbilical region. Enlarged lymph nodes may be palpable as firm, discrete, round nodules on the right

of the umbilicus. (b) As a cause *of general symptoms:* Patient only presents with loss of weight, loss of appetite, pale and evening rise of temperature. (c) As a cause *of intestinal obstruction:* A coil of small intestine may become adherent to a caseating node to become obstructed. (d) *Indistinguishable from appendicitis:* Sometimes this condition may present with abdominal pain, vomiting and slight tenderness in the right iliac fossa mimicking appendicitis. That the pain is persistent in the same place, negative Rovsing's sign, no high pulse rate and no high leukocytosis go against the diagnosis of appendicitis. Straight X-ray may reveal calcified lymph nodes. (e) As *pseudomesenteric cyst:* After caseation the cold abscess remains confined between the two leaves of the mesentery to form a cyst (mesenteric cyst).

DIVERTICULITIS

The diverticula are pulsion diverticula and infection occurs secondarily in them. Diverticula appear most commonly in the sigmoid colon. These diverticula are due to excessive intracolonic pressure from thickened circular fibers which interdigitate with each other. This leads to excessive segmentations and an increase in the intracolonic pressure. Inflammation usually starts at the wall of the diverticulum and spreads in the pericolic tissue and mesenteric fat. The only symptom in the *diverticulosis stage* is rectal bleeding. This bleeding may be profuse and occurs due to trauma round the neck of the diverticula when it steps in and out through the defect in the muscle under varying degree of intraluminal pressure. It must be remembered that profuse rectal bleeding in the elderly is more often due to diverticular disease than carcinoma.

Appearance of symptoms suggests that *diverticulosis has progressed to diverticulitis.* Intermittent abdominal pain especially in the left iliac fossa with flatulence and slight distension are the characteristic features of this condition. The pain may be due to over distension of an isolated section of the colon or due to a small localized abscess. Typically the bowel actions are small and leave a feeling of incompletion. The patient passes small, pebbly motion which may be accompanied by blood and/or mucus.

Pericolonic abscess may develop with surrounding fibrosis and adhesion. A pelvic mass may result which may be felt both per abdomen and per rectum. This may even lead to intestinal obstruction. Rarely necrosis involves the whole of the diverticulum leading to perforation. The result of perforation may be anything from small localized abscess (commoner) to general peritonitis. This localized abscess may be absorbed on its own by conservative treatment or may become adherent to the bladder or another loop of bowel forming a vesico-colic or enterocolic fistula.

Sigmoidoscopy is important largely for its negative value in excluding carcinoma. It is difficult or may be impossible to pass the sigmoidoscope beyond the rectosigmoid junction due to excessive spasm of the sigmoid colon.

Contrast radiography should be avoided in the acute stage. Barium meal follow through or barium enema may be helpful in diagnosing this condition. The latter is more useful in excluding carcinoma. In the first stage there may be small saw-tooth projections. Later large saw-tooth or accordion pleated outline will be obvious. In infective stage it shows a straight sigmoid colon without much convolutions and sacculations.

HIRSCHSPRUNG'S DISEASE OR PRIMARY MEGACOLON

This condition is due to failure of proper development of the myenteric plexus of the bowel to migrate leading to aganglionosis of the distal part of the bowel. The pathology starts in the distal rectum and spreads to a variable distance proximally and even may spread into the small intestine. This leads to inability of the bowel to adequately contract which leads to failure in peristalsis. Constipation or inability to pass meconium is the hallmark of this disease. It is the most common cause of intestinal obstruction in the new born babies. It shows a familial tendency and mostly occurs in the first year of life commonly within 3 days following birth. Occasionally if the defect is short enough, the condition may not be diagnosed until adult life; however, there will be a history of constipation from first few days of life. Inability to pass meconium which can only be helped by insertion of a little finger or a tube into the rectum, is very suggestive. Progressive abdominal distension with visible peristalsis is the pathognomonic feature of this condition. Rectal examination reveals that the rectum is empty and contracted and the anus is normal. After withdrawal of the finger a large gush of flatus and meconium are passed. As the time passes by the abdomen becomes increasingly distended with borborygmi and visible peristalsis.

Acquired or secondary megacolon: It occurs in older children and even adults. There is no aganglionic segment and hence colonic distension extends up to the anal canal. Rectal examination will reveal scybalous mass in the rectum and there may be anal fissure which indicates the cause of this condition.

ULCERATIVE COLITIS

This disease affects women more often than men and maximum incidence is between 20 and 30 years. Patients present with mucous, blood stained or purulent diarrhea. There may be abdominal discomfort or pain. The disease is characterized by remissions and relapses. It is rare in tropical countries like India. In chronic and recurrent type the patients gradually become wasted and anemic from diarrhea. In acute fulminating type patients run high temp. (103 –104°F) and incessant diarrhea containing blood and pus make the patients emaciated. The severity of the condition depends mainly on the extent of involvement of the disease, the depth of the mucosal ulceration and the age of the patient. When this condition is confined to the rectum and sigmoid colon it rarely causes severe illness. When the whole or a substantial portion of the colon is involved the attack is likely to be more severe with some systemic upset. Even though much of the colon is involved the illness can be mild if ulceration remains superficial. To the contrary, deep ulceration especially if the deep muscle is exposed over a moderately large area, severe illness will be the result. *Systemic manifestations* of this disease are erythema nodosum, pyoderma, arthritis, etc., and these have no relation with the extent of the ulceration but with the extent of the involvement of the disease. Depletion of the protein is always expected resulting in loss of muscle bulk and loss of body weight. Colitis in the elderly tends to be much more dangerous than in younger patients. Diagnosis is mainly confirmed by two investigations—(1) Barium enema and (2) Sigmoidoscopy, colonoscopy and biopsy.

Barium enema: It must be remembered that when the patient is extremely ill, preliminary straight X-ray is required. If they show colonic dilatation (megacolon), barium studies should be judged to be contraindicated. In the early stage barium enema will fail to show any ulceration in chronic disease. The mucosal surface will appear smooth. But the colon becomes shortened and looses its haustral pattern. Later on, pseudopolyps may be shown as multiple small filling defects. In acute disease mucosal ulceration may be shown. There will be ulceration and pseudopolyposis.

As the rectum is almost invariably involved in ulcerative colitis, the disease can be diagnosed with confidence by *sigmoidoscopy* and *biopsy*. In mild cases, hyperemia and granularity of mucosa can be seen. The mucosa becomes friable. In more severe conditions diffuse hemorrhagic inflammation becomes obvious. Ulcer exudate can be seen. Biopsy specimen may be taken either with bronchoscopy forceps or with a suction type of instrument.

Complications are stricture, pseudopolyposis, carcinoma, hemorrhage, ischiorectal abscess, fistula-in-ano, arthritis, cirrhosis of liver, ankylosing spondylitis.

ISCHEMIC COLITIS

Unlike mesenteric arterial obstruction, which is an acute condition, ischemic colitis is a chronic condition. The reason is that the vascular occlusion is always incomplete as the collateral supply comes from the marginal artery of Drummond to allow the ischemic bowel to recover.

The *signs* and *symptoms* are similar to other types of colitis. There is often left-sided abdominal pain and tenderness along the course of the descending colon, which is more often located in the region of the splenic flexure, as that is the watershed junction between the superior and inferior mesenteric arteries supply. Bloodstained diarrhea is a common complaint. Later on there may be stricture formation at the site of ischemic colitis leading to intestinal obstruction.

POLYPS

Polyps of the intestine are best classified as follows:

Solitary	Multiple
Neoplastic: Adenoma, papillary adenoma, villous papilloma	Polyposis coli
Hamartoma: Juvenile, Peutz-Zegher's	Juvenile, Peutz-Zeghers'
Inflammatory: Benign lymphoid polyp	Benign lymphoid polyposis, pseudopolyposis of ulcerative colitis

FAMILIAL POLYPOSIS COLI

It is a disease transmitted through genes. Multiple polyps are found mostly in rectum and sigmoid colon, but ultimately the whole colon will be involved. Patients present with diarrhea containing mucus and blood from early age. Rectal examination will reveal one or more polyps. Sigmoidoscopy and barium enema X-ray **(Fig. 34.33)** will diagnose the case. Adenocarcinoma is a fatal complication of this disease.

CARCINOMA OF THE COLON

The cauliflower or fungative type occurs in the right half of the colon and the annular or cirrhosis type is encountered in the left half. Clinical features depend on whether the growth is in the right or left half of the colon. In the right half of the colon, the intestinal contents being of the fluid nature, obstruction is not an early feature although the growth is of the hypertrophic type. The patient complains of certain vague symptoms, such as loss of appetite, loss of weight, weakness, flatulence, dyspepsia, etc. Anemia is often present. He may have diarrhea alone or alternating diarrhea and constipation. The most important diagnostic finding is the presence of a lump at the site of the cecum or ascending colon.

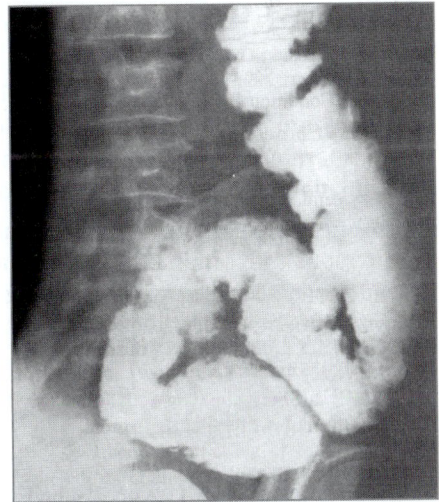

Fig. 34.33: Barium enema X-ray showing multiple polyposis coli.

In the left half of the colon, the contents being solid and the growth being of the annular type, the patient complains of increasing constipation requiring increasing dose of purgatives to move the bowel. No tumor is felt; what is felt is the loaded colon above the growth, as demonstrated by 'pitting on pressure' on the fecal matter. In either case, the diagnosis is confirmed by barium enema (or meal, in the case of the cecal growth) which reveals filling defect in the colon.

DISEASES OF THE UMBILICUS

A. **Umbilical fistulas:** (1) Fecal, due to patent vitello-intestinal duct. (2) Urinary, due to patent urachus. (3) Septic, due to infection, abscess formation and bursting. Sometimes umbilical calculus is formed inside the septic cavity. Any intra-abdominal abscess may leak through the umbilicus and form a sinus or fistula.

B. **Enteroteratoma** (syn. Umbilical Adenoma, Raspberry tumor). **(Fig. 34.34)**: It is due to prolapse of the mucosa of the unobliterated distal end of the vitellointestinal duct. (Persistence of the proximal part gives rise to Meckel's diverticulum*). It produces a red raspberry-like tumor with a tendency to bleed.

C. **Endometrioma:** Diagnosis of this condition is suggested when a history of bleeding at each menstruation is obtained in women of child bearing age. It is associated with similar growth of the uterus or ovary.

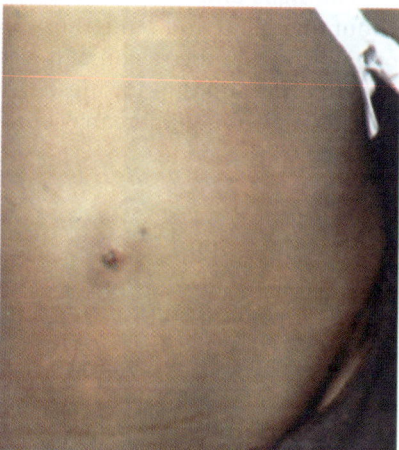

Fig. 34.34: Umbilical adenoma (raspberry tumor).

D. **Carcinoma:** (1) Primary growth may occur when the lymph nodes of both axillae and both groins are likely to be involved. (2) Secondary carcinoma may develop from primary in the stomach, colon, ovary or breast.

E. **Umbilical concretion (calculus):** This occurs in those who do not maintain hygiene of the umbilicus and mainly affects old individuals. Black concretions develop inside the umbilicus which is formed by desquamated epithelium and dirt. It remains symptomless for years, but inflammation may supervene to cause abscess formation with discharge.

F. **Umbilical abscess:** This is a simple abscess of the umbilicus due to its poor hygiene. It is not synonymous with omphalitis which is a condition of new born baby where adequate aseptic precaution is not taken while severing the umbilical cord. The stump of the umbilical cord becomes inflamed. Umbilical abscess however may or may not be associated with umbilical calculus and purulent discharge.

G. **Pilonidal sinus:** This sinus is very rarely seen in umbilicus when tuft of hair can be seen protruding through it. For characteristic features of this sinus see page 629.

---

* **Meckel's Diverticulum:** It occurs in about 2% of subjects, is about 2 inches long and is situated about 2 feet proximal to the Ileocecal junction at the antimesenteric border unlike jejunal diverticula which arise from the mesenteric border. It gives rise to following complications: (1) Meckel's diverticulitis resembling acute appendicitis; (2) Intestinal obstruction either by a band of fibrous tissue from the apex of the diverticulum, or by volvulus occurring around the band, or rarely by intussusception, the apex being formed by swollen heterotopic mucosa (the diverticulum itself may not be inverted); (3) Peptic ulcer resulting from the heterotopic gastric mucosa at the base of the diverticulum; this may lead to bleeding per annum or even perforation; (4) Littre's hernia—this term is applied when a Meckel's diverticulum lies within a hernial sac.

Chapter 34: Examination of Chronic Abdominal Conditions

Algorithmic Approach to Patient with Chronic Abdominal Conditions

Patient presents with chronic abdominal symptoms

↓

Is the pain localized or diffuse?
- Localized pain → Narrow down by **quadrant-based differentiation**
- Diffuse pain → Consider **IBS, functional dyspepsia, peritoneal disease**

↓

Is there unintentional weight loss?
- Yes → High suspicion for **malignancy, chronic infection, malabsorption**
- No → Consider **inflammatory or functional disorders**

↓

Are there associated symptoms?
- Jaundice → Hepatobiliary disease (cirrhosis, biliary obstruction, pancreatic cancer)
- Change in bowel habits → IBD, colorectal cancer, functional disorders
- Epigastric burning pain → GERD, peptic ulcer disease, gastroparesis
- RUQ pain postmeals → Chronic cholecystitis, biliary dyskinesia

↓

Perform diagnostic investigations
- CT scan with contrast → Preferred for **chronic pancreatitis, bowel cancer, mesenteric ischemia**
- Ultrasound abdomen → Identifies **gallstones, liver disease, ascites**
- Upper endoscopy (EGD) → Detects **peptic ulcer, gastritis, esophagitis**
- Colonoscopy → Essential for **colorectal cancer, IBD, diverticular disease**

↓

Confirm diagnosis and initiate appropriate management
- Surgical management → **Cancer, bowel obstruction, gallbladder disease**
- Medical therapy → **Peptic ulcer disease, IBD, GERD, functional disorders**
- Lifestyle and dietary modifications → For **GERD, IBS, chronic pancreatitis**

Examination of an Abdominal Lump

CHAPTER 35

HISTORY

See **Chapter 3 "Examination of a Lump or a Swelling"**, Chapter 34 "Examination of Chronic Abdominal Conditions" and Chapter 37 "Examination of a Urinary Case" to know various types of presentation.

History in abdominal lump

Aspect	Clinical significance	Patient-friendly questions
Onset and duration	Sudden → Inflammatory, hernia Gradual → Neoplasm, cyst	"When did you first notice the lump? Has it grown over time?"
Pain association	Painful lump → Abscess, inflamed hernia Painless lump → Malignancy, cyst	"Does the lump hurt when touched or all the time?"
Movement with respiration	Moves → Hepatic, gallbladder, splenic mass Fixed → Retroperitoneal tumor	"Do you feel the lump move when you take deep breaths?"
Associated symptoms	Jaundice → Liver, pancreas tumor Constipation → Colorectal cancer	"Have you noticed yellowing of your eyes or changes in your bowel habits?"
Previous medical history	Prior hernia repair → Recurrent hernia History of hepatitis → Liver tumor	"Have you had any previous surgeries or liver conditions?"

PHYSICAL EXAMINATION

The general appearance of the patient has been discussed in the chapter of "Examination of Chronic Abdominal Conditions".

EXAMINATION OF THE ABDOMEN

Causes of abdominal lump in different regions

Location	Possible causes
Epigastric	Gastric tumor, pancreatic cyst, aortic aneurysm
RUQ	Hepatomegaly, gallbladder tumor, liver abscess

Contd...

Contd...

Location	Possible causes
LUQ	Splenomegaly, gastric malignancy
Periumbilical	Mesenteric cyst, umbilical hernia, pancreatic pseudocyst
RLQ	Appendicular mass, cecal carcinoma, Crohn's disease
LLQ	Diverticular abscess, sigmoid carcinoma, ovarian cyst
Suprapubic	Bladder mass, uterine fibroid, ovarian tumor

A. INSPECTION

Besides the points which have already been discussed in the previous chapters, the followings should be particularly noted in a case of an abdominal lump:

1. **Condition of the skin over the swelling** whether it is tense, red, shining or pigmented? Are there engorged veins?
2. **Position, size and shape:** Of these the position is the most important and should be described in relation to the nine anatomical regions of the abdomen **(Fig. 35.1)**. Not much information can be elicited by inspection regarding size and shape.
3. **Movement with respiration:** Swellings arising from the liver, gallbladder, stomach and spleen move well with respiration. Swelling in connection with the kidney or suprarenal moves very little with respiration.
4. **Visible peristalsis:** One should spend sometime inspecting the abdomen to detect visible peristalsis if present. Carcinoma at the pylorus of the stomach may present with visible peristalsis. Similarly carcinoma of the transverse colon may produce visible peristalsis. In the former case the peristalsis will be from left to right, whereas in the latter it will be from right to left. Rare cases of obstruction in intestine from malignant growth or enlarged lymph nodes may demonstrate similar visible peristalsis.
5. **The hernial sites:** If the swelling is situated over one of the hernial sites, the patient is asked to cough to note the impulse on coughing. When the test is positive the case is one of a hernia. It must be remembered that a swelling over the hernial site may not necessarily be a hernia.
6. **The scrotum:** It should be made a routine to inspect the scrotum. Malignancy of the testis may lead to metastasis in the pre-and para-aortic lymph nodes. Swelling of these lymph nodes may be the first presenting symptom in these cases. If scrotum is not examined the entire diagnosis is missed **(Fig. 35.2)**.
7. **Left supraclavicular lymph node:** Before completing inspection, one should not forget to see the supraclavicular fossa particularly on the left

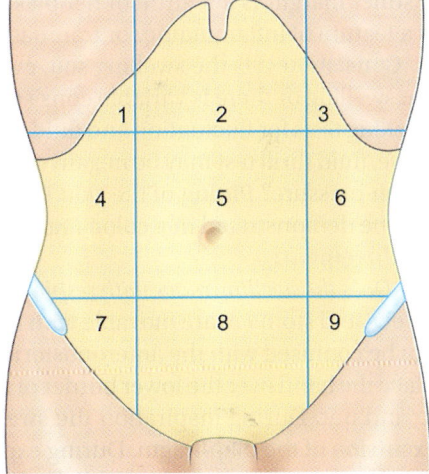

Fig. 35.1: The abdomen is divided into nine regions by two horizontal and two vertical lines. The upper horizontal or transpyloric line midway between the xiphisternum and the umbilicus, the lower horizontal or transtubercular line at the level of the two tubercles on the iliac crest about 2 inches behind the anterior superior iliac spines. The vertical lines are drawn on either side through the midpoint between the anterior superior iliac spine and symphysis pubis. The regions are: (1) Right hypochondrium, (2) Epigastrium, (3) Left hypochondrium, (4) Right lumbar, (5) Umbilical region, (6) Left lumbar, (7) Right iliac, (8) Hypogastrium, (9) Left iliac.

side to detect if there is any swelling. These nodes are often secondarily involved (Troisier's sign) in breast carcinoma, abdominal carcinoma (especially of the stomach, pancreas or of the colon) and in malignant tumor of the testis. Involvement of these nodes gives a hint towards inoperability of the tumor.

B. PALPATION

Deep palpation (*see* page 565) is required to know details about an abdominal swelling.

1. **Local temperature:** This is assessed as has been discussed in Chapter 3. Local rise of temperature indicates inflammatory swelling.

2. **Tenderness:** Pain on pressure is also a feature of an inflammatory swelling.

3. **Position, size, shape and surface:** These are important and give definite clue to the diagnosis. Position indicates the organ that has been involved. Size, shape and surface give indications as to the underlying pathology.

4. **Margin:** One must try to get all round the swelling. There may be difficulties when some part of the swelling disappears under the costal margin or the pelvis. Well-defined and distinct margin is a feature of neoplasm. Ill-defined margin is a feature of inflammatory or traumatic swelling.

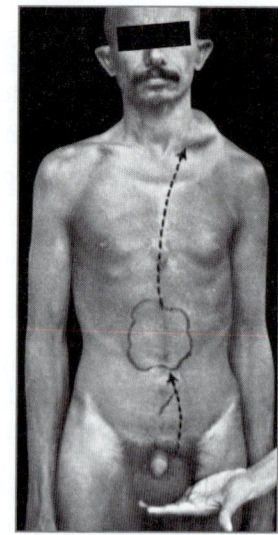

Fig. 35.2: The patient came with lumps in the abdomen and neck. Examination of the scrotum revealed a testicular growth. The lumps are obviously due to secondary deposit in the lymph nodes.

5. **Consistency:** Is the swelling soft, cystic, firm or hard? Is it of same consistency throughout the swelling or there is variable consistency at different parts of the swelling. In case of a cystic swelling tests for fluctuation and fluid thrill should be performed. Of course, if the cyst becomes tense, fluid thrill test may be negative and fluctuation will be difficult to elicit. Does the swelling pit on pressure? Pitting of the skin is the feature of a parietal abscess. Pitting on pressure can also be demonstrated in a colon loaded with feces.

6. **Movement:**

(a) *Does the swelling move with respiration or not?* Swelling associated with the liver, gallbladder, spleen and stomach are movable with respiration. This is an up and down movement and must not be confused with the anteroposterior movement of the abdominal wall during respiration. Place the hand over the lower border of the swelling and the patient is asked to take deep breath in and out. During inspiration the swelling will move downwards alongwith the downward excursion of the diaphragm. During expiration the swelling goes back to its normal position.

(b) *Is the swelling movable in all directions?* The swelling is held and tried to move in vertical and horizontal directions. Any restriction of movement is noted. A mesenteric cyst moves freely at right angle to the line of attachment of the mesentery but not so along the line (the line of attachment of the mesentery is an oblique line starting 1 inch to the left of the midline and 1 inch below the transpyloric plane and extending downwards and to the right for about 6 inches).

(c) *Is the swelling 'ballottable'?* One hand is placed behind the loin and the other hand in front of the abdomen and the swelling is moved anteroposteriorly between the two hands. A renal swelling is 'ballottable'.

7. **Parietal or intra-abdominal:** The abdominal muscles are made taut by asking the patient either (i) to raise his shoulders from the bed with the arms folded over the chest the 'rising-

test' **(Fig. 35.3)** or (ii) to raise both the extended legs from the bed the 'leg lifting test' (Carnett's test) **(Fig. 35.4)** or (iii) to try to blow out with his nose and mouth shut. If the swelling is parietal the swelling will be more prominent when the abdominal muscles are made taut and will be freely movable over the taut muscle. If the swelling is parietal but fixed to the abdominal muscle the swelling will not be movable when the muscles are made taut, e.g., recurrent fibroid of Paget and hematoma in the rectus muscle. If the swelling disappears or becomes smaller when the abdominal muscles are made taut, the swelling is an intra-abdominal one. Another differentiating point is that if the swelling moves vertically with respiration it is obviously an intra-abdominal swelling.

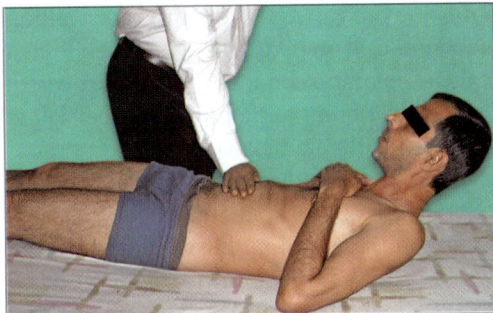

Fig. 35.3: The 'rising test' in which the patient raises his shoulder from the bed with the arms folded over the chest. This test is performed to know whether the swelling is parietal or intra-abdominal.

8. **Is the swelling pulsatile or not?** A swelling in front of the abdominal aorta is pulsatile. This pulsation is 'transmitted' one. An aneurysm of the abdominal aorta is also pulsatile. But this pulsation is 'expansile' one. To differentiate between 'transmitted' and 'expansile' pulsations one may put index finger of each hand over the swelling. With each pulsation the two fingers will be diverted in 'expansile' pulsation whereas fingers will not be diverted in case of 'transmitted' pulsation (*see* page 31). Another differentiating point is to place the patient in "knee elbow" position. A swelling in front of the abdominal aorta will be separated from the aorta and will become nonpulsatile, whereas an aneurysm will continue to pulsate.

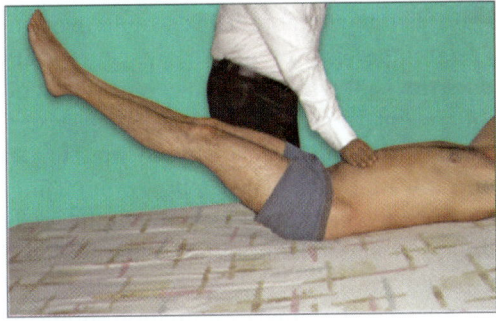

Fig. 35.4: The 'leg lifting test' (Carnett's test) to make the abdominal muscles taut to know whether the swelling is parietal or intra-abdominal.

9. A swelling at any of the **hernial sites** should be tested for expansile impulse on coughing and reducibility. These tests are positive in case of hernia.

10. Lastly, **palpate the liver, the spleen** and **kidney** to ascertain the relationship of the tumor to these organs. Try to insinuate fingers between the swelling and the costal margin. This is possible more readily in case of renal swelling but hardly in cases of hepatic and splenic swellings **(Fig. 35.5)**.

C. PERCUSSION

A swelling arising from a solid organ will be dull on percussion if the swelling is quite superficial. If the coils of intestine overlie the swelling the percussion note will be resonant even if the swelling is a solid one. That is why a swelling arising from a liver or a spleen is dull on percussion whereas a renal swelling is resonant. Only if the kidney is considerably enlarged that the coils of

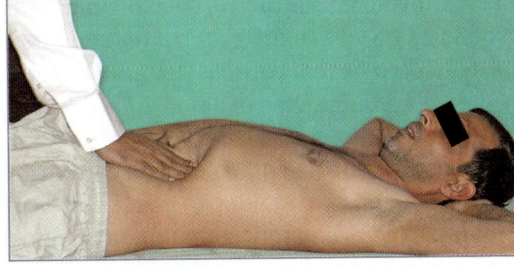

Fig. 35.5: Demonstrating that the hand can be insinuated between the swelling and the costal margin in case of a renal swelling but not in case of a splenic swelling.

intestine are moved aside and the swelling becomes dull on percussion, but even then a band of colonic resonance may be discovered. Another differentiating point between renal swelling and splenic swelling is to percuss the loin just outside the erector spinae. This area is normally resonant due to the presence of colon. In case of renal swelling this area will be dull as the colon is pushed out by the swelling but in case of a splenic swelling normal resonance is preserved **(Fig. 35.6)**.

Test for *shifting dullness* when free fluid is suspected in the peritoneal cavity. In ascites, dullness is present over the flanks and it shifts as the patient rolls over. In an ovarian cyst dullness is present over the center and does not shift with the change of position of the patient.

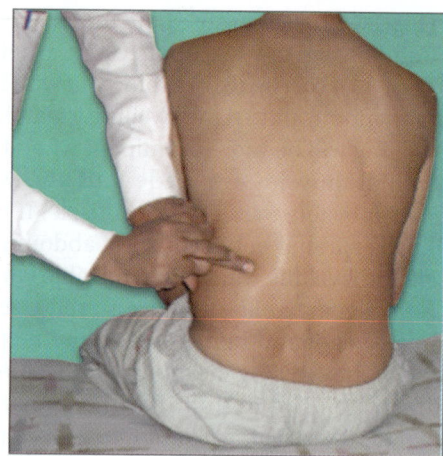

Fig. 35.6: Percussing the loin just outside the erector spinae. This area is normally resonant. With a renal tumor the resonance is replaced by dullness but with a splenic enlargement the normal resonance is preserved.

Hydatid thrill is elicited by placing 3 fingers over the swelling and percussing over the middle one and after thrill will be felt by other 2 fingers. This test is rarely demonstrable.

The area of liver and splenic dullness should be marked out. The upper limit of the liver dullness is raised in subphrenic abscess, liver abscess and hydatid cyst occurring at the superior aspect of the liver.

Rectal and vaginal examination should always be carried out.

SPECIAL INVESTIGATIONS

1. **Stomach and duodenum:** See the last chapter.
2. **Liver and gallbladder:** Examination of the stool for *Entamoeba histolytica,* liver function test, straight X-ray of abdomen, cholecystography, aspiration of the liver and subphrenic abscess should be carried out. In a hydatid cyst of the liver, a history of an attack of urticaria, the presence of eosinophilia in the blood, a positive complement fixation test and Casoni's intradermal reaction are of great help in arriving at a diagnosis. Should the cyst be situated at the upper surface of the liver, X-ray will confirm the diagnosis. Liver scan and selective angiography will help in the diagnosis of liver swelling particularly if the case is one of carcinoma (primary or secondary). Stone in the gallbladder and bile duct as well as empyema of the gallbladder can be diagnosed by noninvasive technique like ultrasound.
3. **Spleen:** Examination of blood and estimation of platelet count, reticulocyte count, bleeding time, etc. are imperative.
4. **Pancreas:** X-ray examination with barium meal will reveal, in a lateral view, that the swelling is behind the stomach pseudopancreatic cyst (*see* **Fig. 34.15**). Examination of stool for the presence of muscle fibers and for estimation of fat and fatty acids, and examination of the urine for its diastase index and for sugar should be carried out. Carcinoma of the head of the pancreas can be diagnosed by hypotonic duodenography (*see* under the chapter of "Examination of Chronic Abdominal Conditions").

Carcinoma near ampulla of Vater can be diagnosed by intravenous (IV) cholangiography and percutaneous transhepatic cholangiography. Retrograde fiberoptic endoscopy will also reveal this condition. Retrograde endoscopic pancreaticocholangiography will help in the diagnosis of ca-ampulla of Vater, stone near the ampulla and chronic pancreatitis. Carcinoma of the pancreas can also be diagnosed by selective angiography and pancreatic scan. Pancreatic cyst can be conveniently diagnosed by ultrasound.

5. **Colon:** In addition to occult blood test of the stool and sigmoidoscopy, radiological examination should be made with barium meal for the proximal colon and with barium enema for the distal region. The contrast enema, i.e., introduction of air into the colon after the barium enema is partly evacuated, is a valuable method of investigation. A thin film of barium lining the lumen of the colon demarcates its outlines and any filling-defect is readily demonstrated.

6. **Urinary Organs:** See Chapter 37 on 'Examination of a Urinary Case'.

DIFFERENTIAL DIAGNOSIS OF ABDOMINAL SWELLINGS

First ascertain the position of the swelling in respect to the nine anatomical regions of the abdomen and then whether the swelling is parietal or intra-abdominal. The causes and differential diagnosis of lumps in different regions of the abdomen are discussed below.

CAUSES AND DIFFERENTIAL DIAGNOSIS OF SWELLINGS IN THE RIGHT HYPOCHONDRIUM

A. **PARIETAL SWELLINGS:** Besides the swellings involving the skin and subcutaneous tissue, e.g., sebaceous cyst, lipoma, fibroma, neurofibroma, angioma, etc., as may occur in other situation, the special parietal swelling is a *cold abscess* arising from caries of the rib (commonly) or spine (rarely). It gives rise to a soft cystic and fluctuating swelling with no signs of inflammation. Irregularity in the affected rib or deformity of the spine, if present, clinches the diagnosis. An X-ray is helpful. A *hepatic, subphrenic* or *perigastric* abscess may burrow through the anterior abdominal wall to form a parietal abscess.

B. **INTRA-ABDOMINAL SWELLINGS:** They may occur in connection with: (1) liver, (2) gallbladder, (3) subphrenic space, (4) pylorus of the stomach and duodenum, (5) hepatic flexure of the colon, (6) right kidney and (7) right suprarenal gland.

1. **Liver:** Enlargement of the liver is determined by palpating its lower border and percussing its upper limit. Hepatic swellings are continuous with the liver dullness and move up and down with respiration. It is difficult to move the swellings sideways. Causes of enlargement of liver are many, but the important surgical conditions are considered here.

(a) *Congenital Riedel's* lobe is a tongue-shaped projection from the lower border of the right lobe of the liver. It is likely to be mistaken for an enlarged gallbladder but it is more wide and flat than the gallbladder and lacks the spherical outline of the distended gallbladder.

(b) *Amebic hepatitis and abscess:* The patient, who has suffered from amebic dysentery months or years ago and now complains of pain in the right hypochondrium often referred to the right shoulder with rise of temperature, is probably suffering from amebic hepatitis. When a swelling can be felt, an abscess has probably developed. The patient looks pale and slightly icteric. This will attract the attention of a keen observer. The liver is palpable and very tender. Even if the liver is not palpable, intercostal tenderness may be elicited. Upper limit of liver dullness is raised. When an abscess develops the swelling becomes softer with extreme tenderness. Subcutaneous

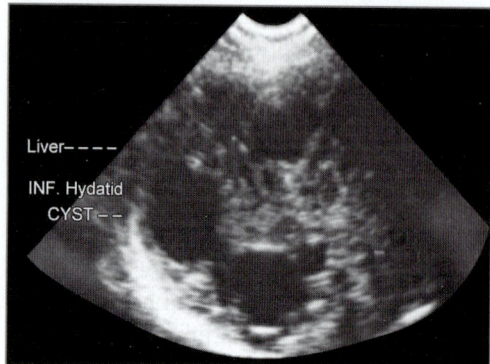

Fig. 35.7: Ultrasonography showing hydatid cyst in the liver.

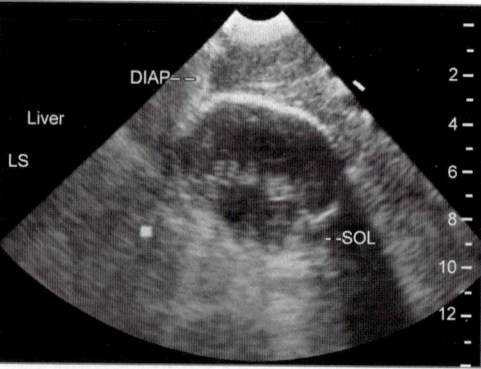

Fig. 35.8: Ultrasonography showing calcified hydatid cyst of the liver which is affecting the right lobe of the liver very near to diaphragm.

edema which pits on pressure is an additional finding and should always be looked for. In X-ray screening the diaphragm is abnormally *raised* and *relatively immobile.* Presence of *Entamoeba histolytica* in the stool is diagnostic. Aspiration of anchovy sauce (chocolate color) pus leaves no doubt about the diagnosis.

(c) *Suppurative pylephlebitis:* During the course of acute appendicitis or inflamed piles, if the patient suffers from a high rise of temperature with rigor one should suspect of this condition. The liver becomes palpable and tender.

(d) *Suppurative cholangitis:* Usually, a history of cholelithiasis is received. The stone becomes impacted in the common bile duct. There will

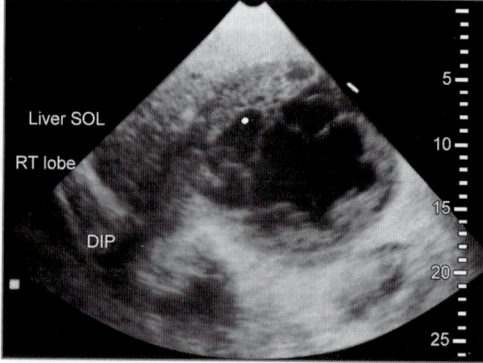

Fig. 35.9: Ultrasonography of the abdomen showing a typical hydatid cyst of the liver affecting upper part of the right lobe of the liver very close to the diaphragm (DIP).

be high rise of temperature and the liver becomes tender. Jaundice is usually associated with.

(e) *Gumma of the liver:* This condition is very rare nowadays. It resembles carcinoma having no symptom in the early stage. It is a manifestation of third stage of syphilis, Wassermann reaction (WR) and Kahn test will be positive. Presence of other syphilitic stigmas confirm the diagnosis.

(f) *Hydatid cyst* **(Figs. 35.7 to 35.9)***:* When it occurs near the lower margin of the liver it gives rise to a palpable spherical and smooth swelling, with hydatid thrill and fluctuations. Diagnosis is made by the history of attack of urticaria, eosinophilia, complement fixation test and Casoni's intradermal reaction. X-ray and ultrasound are helpful when the cyst occurs at the upper surface of the liver. If suppuration takes place the signs and symptoms of infection may dominate the picture.

(g) *Carcinoma of the liver:* Primary carcinoma is rare. It may be a hepatoma or cholangioma. Secondary carcinoma of the liver is much commoner and results from metastasis **(Figs. 35.10 and 35.11)** from carcinoma of the gastrointestinal tract via portal vein or from organs like breast through lymphatics. In this condition the liver is enlarged, irregular with nodules of varying size and shape and becomes hard. The nodules may show softening in the center and may become umbilicated. The patient may be jaundiced sooner or later and ascites may be associated with. Primary focus should be searched for and its recovery clinches the diagnosis.

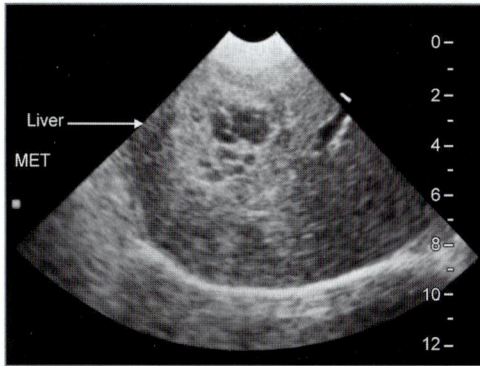

Fig. 35.10: Ultrasonography showing multiple liver metastasis.

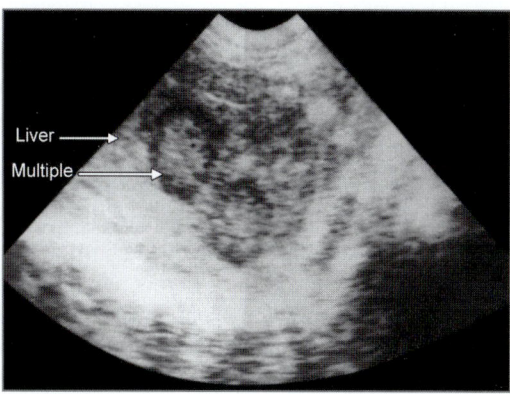

Fig. 35.11: Ultrasonography showing multiple metastases in the liver.

(h) *Melanotic carcinoma of the liver:* It occurs secondary to similar growth on the palm, foot or eye. An enlarged liver with malignant melanoma anywhere in the body should clinch the diagnosis.

(i) *Cirrhosis of the liver:* It must be remembered that in this condition the liver is not always enlarged; on the contrary it may be shrunk. In precirrhotic stage the liver may be firm, irregular with small nodules which are never umbilicated (cf. carcinoma). Portal hypertension will be present with enlargement of the spleen. Ascites may be associated with but jaundice is never present. These cases often come to the surgical clinic with hematemesis from rupture of esophageal varices.

2. **Gallbladder:** It feels as an oval smooth swelling which is tense and cystic. It comes out of the lower border of the liver and moves freely up and down with respiration along with liver. The swelling may be tender depending on the amount of inflammation present. It can be moved sideways a little. It is not ballottable as a kidney swelling. Diagnosis as to the cause of gallbladder swelling has been discussed in the previous chapter.

3. **Subphrenic abscess:** There are innumerable causes of accumulation of pus under the diaphragm. Majority follow intraperitoneal conditions, e.g., perforated peptic ulcer (most common), following abdominal trauma, following operations on biliary tract, following operation on the stomach or colon and acute appendicitis. Diagnosis mainly depends on suspicion. The patient looks very much anxious and drawn. They may complain of anorexia and nausea. A rise of temperature is always associated with. But its degree varies there may be high rise of temperature with rigor, sweating and rapid pulse, or there may be slight rise of temperature but the patient always looks abnormally ill. Rigor only occurs when there is concomitant pylephlebitis or a liver abscess. More important indicator is the pulse rate which always becomes abnormally fast irrespective of the temperature. Tachypnea is also often present. Pain is not a very prominent feature and should not be much relied on so far as the diagnosis is concerned. If present, it usually becomes localized to the site of lesion. Right hypochondrium or epigastrium is the usual site of pain. Very occasionally it may be complained of in the lower part of thorax, right lumbar region or even referred to the right shoulder. Jaundice is not a sign of this condition but if present indicates obstruction of the common bile duct with a stone or suppurative pylephlebitis.

Tenderness just below the costal margin or xiphoid process or more precisely tenderness over the 11th intercostal space though suggestive of this condition yet may be absurd. X-ray screening will show sluggish movement of the diaphragm. The diaphragm becomes raised and gas may be found beneath it. Aspiration of pus from the subdiaphragmatic space leaves no doubt about the diagnosis.

4. **Pylorus of the stomach and duodenum:**

(a) *Carcinoma* of this region usually gives rise to obstructive symptoms. The details of manifestations of carcinoma of the stomach have been discussed in earlier chapter. Barium meal X-ray will show 'filling-defect' which is very diagnostic.

(b) *Subacute perforation of peptic ulcer* forms a localized tender mass which is a rare condition. The patient gives history suggestive of peptic ulcer and sudden excruciating pain before formation of the mass. It may lead to a subphrenic abscess.

5. **Hepatic flexure of the colon:**

(a) *Intussusception* (*see* page 553).

(b) *Hypertrophic tuberculosis:* This usually starts in the ileocecal region and may move up into this region. See the right iliac fossa for more description.

(c) *Carcinoma of this part of the colon* may present with a lump only or with anemia, anorexia and occult blood in the stool. The lump is irregular and hard with slight or no movement. Barium enema X-ray reveals constant filling defect which is very diagnostic.

6. **Kidney:** The features of a kidney swelling are: (i) It is a reniform swelling; (ii) It moves very slightly with respiration as it comes down a little at the height of inspiration; (iii) It is ballottable; (iv) A sickening sensation is often felt during manipulation; (v) A hand can be easily insinuated between the upper pole of swelling and the costal margin; (vi) Percussion will reveal resonant note in front of a kidney swelling as coils of intestine and colon will always be in front of the kidney.

As regards the different causes of kidney swelling and differential diagnosis the reader is referred to the chapter on "Examination of a Urinary Case".

7. **Suprarenal tumors:** Suprarenal gland has got a cortex and a medulla. *In the adrenal cortex*, the causative lesion may be bilateral hyperplasia, a benign adenoma or a malignant carcinoma. *In the medulla* pheochromocytoma, which is usually a benign tumor, a benign ganglioneuroma or malignant neuroblastoma may appear. Hyperplasia of the medulla, though described, is exceedingly rare. The clinical syndromes vary with the hormones which are produced. Thus in the lesions of the cortex, excess of aldosterone causes aldosteronism, excess of cortisol causes Cushing's syndrome, excess of androgen causes andrenogenital syndrome and excess of estrogen causes feminisation in the male. In medullary tumors the clinical features depend on the relative amounts of adrenaline and noradrenaline which are produced.

CAUSES AND DIFFERENTIAL DIAGNOSIS OF THE SWELLINGS IN THE EPIGASTRIUM

A. **PARIETAL SWELLINGS:** In addition to the swellings discussed under the right hypochondrium, i.e., tumors of the skin and subcutaneous tissue, cold abscess, hepatic, subphrenic and perigastric abscesses, the swelling peculiar to this region is the epigastric hernia. *Epigastric hernia:* The usual sufferer is a strong muscular laborer. He presents with a small round swelling exactly in the midline anywhere between the xiphisternum and umbilicus. In the first stage, it is sacless herniation of the extraperitoneal fat through a weak spot in the linea alba. There is no symptom at this stage. In the second stage, a pouch of peritoneum is drawn after it. In the last stage, a small tag of omentum gets into the sac and becomes adherent to it. At this stage the patient complains of dragging pain, discomfort or pain after food, not unlike those in peptic ulcer.

B. **INTRA-ABDOMINAL SWELLINGS:** They occur in connection with the: (1) liver and subphrenic space, (2) stomach and duodenum, (3) transverse colon, (4) omentum, (5) pancreas, (6) abdominal aorta, (7) lymph nodes and (8) retroperitoneal structure.

1. **Liver** and **subphrenic abscess** have been discussed in the previous section.
2. **Stomach** and **duodenum.**
   (a) *Congenital pyloric stenosis:* Babies about 2–4 weeks old when present with projectile vomiting after meals, the diagnosis becomes obvious. On examination visible peristalsis of the stomach is always seen. Sometime a definite lump may be felt at the pylorus of the stomach.
   (b) *Subacute perforation of peptic ulcer:* See 'Swellings in the right hypochondrium'.
   (c) *Carcinoma of the stomach:* See 'Swellings in the right hypochondrium'.
3. **Transverse colon:** Intussusception, diverticulitis, hyperplastic tuberculosis and neoplasms are the causes of swellings which may originate from the transverse colon. In intussusception there will be emptiness at the right iliac fossa. The patient complains of colicky pain, a lump in the epigastrium and "red currant jelly" in the stool. In inflammatory conditions a tender and irregular mass may be felt. In carcinoma the swelling is the presenting symptom. The swelling is irregular, hard and may be mobile above downwards and very slightly in the sideways or may be fixed. Anemia, anorexia and occult blood in the stool are the features which help in the diagnosis. Barium enema X-ray reveals constant 'filling-defect' of the colon.
4. **Omentum:** In the tubercular peritonitis, the omentum is rolled up to form a transverse ridge in the epigastrium. Enlarged lymph nodes or adherent coils of intestine are also come across in this condition.
5. **Pancreas:** It hardly gives rise to a palpable swelling. The condition that forms lump in connection with this organ is the *pseudopancreatic cyst* **(Fig. 35.12)**. True cyst of the pancreas is extremely rare. The pseudocyst is a collection of fluid in the lesser sac of the peritoneal cavity resulting from acute pancreatitis or trauma. It forms a smooth rounded swelling with fluctuation test positive. X-ray with barium meal will show the exact position of the swelling which is situated behind the stomach and is best seen in the lateral X-ray.

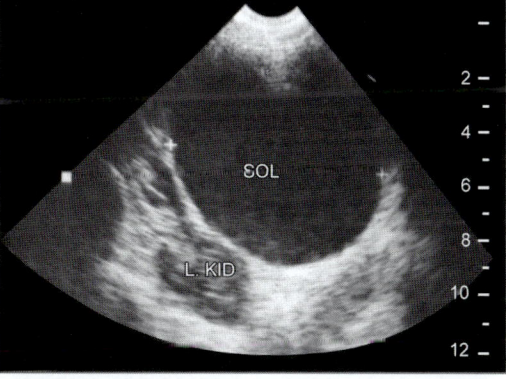

Fig. 35.12: Ultrasonography of the abdomen showing pseudocyst of the pancreas in the lesser sac of the peritoneum which has extended to in front of the left kidney.

6. **Abdominal aorta:** Aneurysm of this part of the aorta is not uncommon. It presents a swelling in the epigastrium with characteristic expansile pulsation. This pulsation should be differentiated from transmitted pulsation caused by a swelling, just in front of the aorta. Knee-elbow position is of great help in this respect. The swelling in front of the aorta will hang loose forward leaving contact with the aorta, hence losing its pulsatile property. Whereas an aneurysm of the aorta will be still pulsatile.

7. **Lymph nodes:** In addition to the usual causes of enlargement of lymph nodes, the followings are more important in this region: (i) tabes mesenterica, (ii) lymphosarcoma and (iii) secondary malignant growth from the neighboring organs and also from the testis.
8. **Retroperitoneal sarcoma** and **teratoma** are the two conditions commonly seen in the posterior abdominal wall arising from the retroperitoneal tissue.

CAUSES AND DIFFERENTIAL DIAGNOSIS OF SWELLINGS IN THE LEFT HYPOCHONDRIUM

A. **PARIETAL SWELLINGS:** As on the right side.
B. **INTRA-ABDOMINAL SWELLINGS:** These swellings occur in connection with the: (1) spleen, (2) stomach, (3) left lobe of liver, (4) splenic flexure of the colon, (5) tail of the pancreas, (6) left subphrenic space, (7) left kidney and (8) left suprarenal gland.
1. **Spleen:** An enlarged spleen is differentiated from a renal swelling by the following points: (i) The spleen enlarges towards the umbilicus, i.e., downwards, forwards and inwards, whereas the kidney enlarges forwards and directly downwards towards the iliac fossa. (ii) A splenic swelling is smooth and uniform, its anterior border is sharp with *one or more notches*, the characteristic feature of this organ. (iii) *On inspection,* a splenic swelling moves more freely with respiration than a renal swelling, (iv) *In palpation,* the spleen is palpated more easily from the anterior aspect and the kidney from the posterior aspect, as the spleen lies just under the anterior abdominal wall and the kidney on the posterior abdominal wall. (v) Further, for the same reason the hand can be insinuated between the swelling and the costal margin in case of the kidney but not in the case of the spleen. (vi) Always look for the notches while palpating a splenic swelling. (vii) *On percussion on anterior abdominal wall,* the splenic swelling is dull all throughout but in case of a renal swelling a band of colonic resonance is obtained. (viii) The loin just lateral to the erector spinae is resonant in splenic swelling but dull in renal swelling.

Causes of enlargement of the spleen are many. Malaria and kala-azar are common in this country but are of little surgical importance. Only the conditions of surgical importance are described below:
(a) **HEMOLYTIC ANEMIA:** There are two forms of this disorder: (i) congenital (hereditary spherocytosis) and (ii) acquired.
(i) **HEREDITARY SPHEROCYTOSIS:** The main pathology is congenital increase in permeability of the red cell membrane to sodium. As sodium leaks into the cell its osmotic pressure rises, the cell swells, becomes spherical and more fragile. In this condition the energy and oxygen requirement of the red cells increase. In the spleen there is deficiency of both glucose and oxygen in the pulp and therefore a large number of red cells are destroyed. Splenectomy reduces red cell destruction. Though it does not cure the congenital red cell membrane defect yet it makes the red cell survival time normal and thus lessens anemia. This defect is transmitted as a Mendelian autosomal dominant. The circulating excess bilirubin remains unconjugated with glycuronic acid and is attached to albumin. This is not excreted through urine. Hence it is called acholuric jaundice.

The patients present with anemia and jaundice. A family history may be elicited. Though it is a congenital condition yet it may not be manifested before puberty or even adult life. In adult cases there is often a history of biliary colic. In fact about 70% of untreated cases may show pigment stone in the gallbladder. Sometimes a severe crisis of red cell destruction is come across.

The RBC count may fall down to 2 millions during the attack. Such attacks are characterized by abdominal pain, nausea, vomiting and pyrexia besides usual extreme pallor and jaundice. These crises may be precipitated by acute infection and may be as dangerous as to cost lives.

On examination, the spleen is always large. The liver may be palpable and chronic ulcers of the legs are often seen in adult sufferers.

The fragility test will show increased fragility of the RBCs. Normal erythrocytes begin to hemolyze in 0.47% saline solution, whereas in this condition hemolysis occurs in 0.6% or even stronger solution.

The reticulocyte count will give an index as to the severity of this condition. After a crisis the count will be greatly increased. *Fecal urobilinogen* is increased as most of the urobilinogen is excreted by this route.

Measurement of fecal urobilinogen, if made possible, is the best guide to the extent of hemolysis in this condition. Finally use of radioactive chromium (^{51}Cr) by labeling the patient's own red cells and by daily scanning over the spleen will show the degree of red cell sequestration by the spleen. If the sequestration is high, splenectomy can be considered.

(ii) **ACQUIRED HEMOLYTIC ANEMIA:** In this condition autoantibodies are produced which attach themselves to the circulating erythrocytes and this results in their early dissolution. In this condition Coombs' test is usually, but not always positive. The patients are usually middle-aged or elderly subjects. Family history is usually absent. The spleen is palpable in 50% of cases. The liver may also be palpable and there is sometimes generalized enlargement of the lymph nodes.

(b) **IDIOPATHIC THROMBOCYTOPENIC PURPURA:** The disease manifests itself by hemorrhages of all grades of severity. It may occur in acute form which is mostly seen in children. Acute episode consists of cutaneous purpura, bleeding from the oral mucous membrane and epistaxis. This condition is also seen in chronic form which is the disease of the adult. The attacks tend to come in cyclic order and relapses are of increasing severity. Ecchymoses or purpuric patches in the skin and the mucous membrane are the main manifestations of this disease. These lesions are mainly seen in the dependent areas due to increased intravascular pressure. Sustained bleeding from the wounds which may even be trifle is also a noticeable feature. Bleeding from the mucous membrane either from the gums or in the form of epistaxis or in the form of menorrhagia is not uncommon. Urinary and gastrintestinal (GI) tract hemorrhages are rare, similarly rare is hemarthrosis. On examination there is hardly any abnormality detected except that the tourniquet test becomes positive. Enlargement of spleen is hardly noticed if so the spleen becomes just palpable and never hugely enlarged. So a huge spleen makes the diagnosis of thrombocytopenic purpura improbable.

In the *tourniquet test,* the cuff of a sphygmomanometer is applied to the upper arm and inflated to just below the systolic blood pressure for 10 minutes. This causes venous obstruction. Within 5 minutes petechial hemorrhages occur in the skin below the cuff. This test indicates excessive capillary fragility.

SECONDARY PURPURA is sometimes seen in conditions like acute septicemia; tuberculosis; brucellosis; Boeck's sarcoid; idiosyncrasy to certain drugs like alkylating agents, quinine and arsenical; associated with extensive burns; leukemia; carcinomatosis of bone; X-ray therapy, etc. Senile purpura and Henoch-Schoenlein purpura are also examples of this condition.

(c) **PORPHYRIA:** It is an inborn error of catabolism of hemoglobin. The main surgical importance is the association of abdominal crisis with this condition. The crisis is characterized by intestinal colic with constipation. The patient is anemic with neurological and mental symptoms. Splenic enlargement is a well marked feature and should always be looked for. This will save many unnecessary laparotomies from misdiagnosis. Slight jaundice following an abdominal pain is not unusual.

(d) **EGYPTIAN SPLENOMEGALY:** This condition is due to infestation by *Schistosoma mansoni* (in majority of cases) and *Schistosoma haematobium* (in ¼ of cases). Enlargement of the spleen with hypochromic anemia, eosinophilia, leukopenia and lymphocytosis are the usual features. The liver is moderately enlarged in ¾ of the cases. In late cases there will be enormous enlargement of the spleen and ascites due to liver atrophy.

(e) **FELTY'S SYNDROME:** Chronic rheumatoid arthritis, leukopenia and enlargement of the spleen constitute this syndrome. Associated pyogenic infections, infected ulcers around the ankles, anorexia, loss of weight and enlargement of lymph nodes help in the diagnosis.

(f) **LEUKEMIA** is characterized by a pronounced hyperplasia of the precursors of the white blood corpuscles throughout the entire reticuloendothelial system. Two types are known myeloid and lymphatic. The spleen is grossly enlarged in case of the former and not so in case of the latter. The blood count will reveal large number of white cells in both the types with more percentage of myelocytes in myeloid leukemia and very high percentage of lymphoblasts in lymphatic leukemia. Splenectomy is of doubtful value.

(g) **TUMORS AND CYSTS** are rare in spleen.

Swellings in connection with other organs are discussed under the right hypochondrium.

CAUSES AND DIFFERENTIAL DIAGNOSIS OF SWELLINGS IN THE LEFT AND RIGHT LUMBAR REGIONS

A. **PARIETAL SWELLINGS:** A *lumbar abscess* (cold) resulting from Pott's disease gives rise to a swelling which requires to be differentiated from a *lumbar hernia*. Both these conditions produce impulse on coughing. The hernia is reducible and tympanitic, whereas the abscess is partially reducible and dull on percussion. The features of caries spine deformity, tenderness, and rigidity will clinch the diagnosis. X-ray will show characteristic bony changes in Pott's disease.

B. **INTRA-ABDOMINAL SWELLINGS:** These swellings develop in connection with the ascending or descending colon, right or left kidney. In addition, swellings from the neighborhood may extend to this region, e.g., the liver, gallbladder on the right side and the spleen on the left side. These are discussed in appropriate sections.

CAUSES AND DIFFERENTIAL DIAGNOSIS OF SWELLINGS IN THE UMBILICAL REGION

A. **PARIETAL SWELLINGS:** Those occurring in connection with the umbilicus and rectus sheath are important.

1. **Umbilicus:** *Congenital polyp* or *adenoma* may occur in association with patent umbilical end of the vitelline duct. Sometimes a granulomatous mass resulting from deep seated infection, may look an adenoma.

Umbilical hernia: Three types are recognized: (a) congenital, (b) infantile and (c) para-umbilical hernia of the adult. The last type is described here. The classical patient is fat multiparous female above the age of 40. The hernia is usually seen just above the umbilicus where the two recti divaricate and this allows the hernia to come out. The two classical signs are always present, i.e., expansile impulse on coughing and reducibility. Irreducibility and incarceration (obstruction) are the two frequent complications. The clinician is warned against the diagnosis of incarceration, as the real event may be strangulation and valuable time may be lost by giving enema, waiting for the result and doing this or that. Incidence of strangulation is less in this hernia than in inguinal or femoral hernia.

Postoperative or incisional hernia. This hernia comes out through an incisional scar. The wall of this hernia consists of fibrous tissue and the contents may be adherent. These are readily diagnosed by the presence of scar with a history of previous operation, expansile impulse on coughing and reducibility.

2. **Rectus sheath:** *Hematoma* in the sheath resulting from trauma or following convulsion of tetanus and strychnine poisoning has been recorded. Tearing of the inferior epigastric artery will cause hematoma in the lower abdomen below the arcuate line. Following a severe bout of coughing or a sudden blow to the abdomen may cause an exquisitely tender lump in relation to the rectus abdominis. There will be bruising of the skin with discoloration suggesting a hematoma underneath.

Abscess within the rectus sheath though rare should be borne in mind.

Desmoid tumor is a type of fibroma which is not encapsulated and is hard. It arises from the deeper part of the rectus abdominis. Majority of the patients are women and have already borne children. This tumor also arises from the scar of the operational wound. Some form of trauma either stretching of the muscle fibers during pregnancy or operational wound will cause hematoma within the muscle fibers which may initiate the tumor formation. This tumor is notorious to recur after excision and is also called 'Recurrent fibroid of Paget'. So it requires wide excision. The recurrent growth is more malignant than the original one.

B. **INTRA-ABDOMINAL SWELLINGS:** These may develop in connection with the: (1) stomach and duodenum, (2) transverse colon, (3) omentum, (4) small intestine and mesentery, (5) lymph nodes, (6) pancreas, (7) aorta and (8) retroperitoneal connective tissue. Swellings from the neighborhood when much enlarged may invade this region, e.g., splenic, renal, uterine and ovarian swellings.

1. **Small intestine and mesentery:** In this group tuberculosis of the intestine together with tabes mesenterica, tumors of the small intestine, intussusception and cysts of the mesentery are included.

Matted coils of intestine with tuberculous mesenteric lymphadenitis is generally presented with a lump. The patient is usually a child. A pale looking child with loss of appetite, loss of weight and evening pyrexia is probably suffering from this condition. Sometimes the pain becomes the main symptom and on deep palpation infected mesenteric lymph nodes may be palpable. Each node is round or oval without regular outline and is not homogeneous. Radiologically calcified tuberculous lymph nodes may be seen. For calcification to occur in lymph nodes it takes about a year or more. So absence of calcified lymph node radiologically does not exclude this condition.

Tumors of the small intestine are rare compared to the large intestine. Even if they appear they hardly produce a palpable lump till late stage. Adenoma, submucous lipoma and leiomyoma are the benign tumors but they do not produce any palpable swelling. The tumors which may produce palpable lumps are lymphosarcoma and spindle-cell sarcoma. Carcinoma is very rare and only becomes palpable in late stage.

Cysts of the mesentery may be of various types of which chylolymphatic, enterogenous (derived from a diverticulum on the mesenteric border of the intestine) and dermoid (teratoma) cysts deserve mentioning. Besides these, tubercular abscess of the mesentery and hydatid cyst of the mesentery are rarely seen. These present as painless abdominal swellings, which are fluctuant and are situated near the umbilicus. The swellings move freely at right angle to the line of attachment of the mesentery but a little along the line of attachment. These cysts will be dull on percussion but will be surrounded by band of resonance. Recurrent attacks of abdominal pain may also be the presenting symptom. Temporary impaction of a food bolus in a segment of bowel narrowed by the cyst may produce features of intestinal obstruction. Torsion of the mesentery may produce acute abdomen which demands immediate relief. Rupture of the cyst and the hemorrhage of the cyst are the two complications of this condition which may give rise to acute abdominal catastrophe. Barium meal X-ray will show coils of intestine to be displaced around the cyst. A portion of the intestine may be shown to be narrowed.

2. **Retroperitoneal connective tissue:**

Retroperitoneal cyst: A cyst developing in the retroperitoneal tissue may attain very large dimensions. Pyelography may be required to differentiate cyst from a hydronephrosis. These cysts may be derived from remnants of the Wolffian ducts when the containing fluid will be clear or the cyst may be a teratoma when it is filled with sebaceous material.

Retroperitoneal lymphoma—mainly affects women and will also require pyelography for differential diagnosis.

Retroperitoneal sarcoma—presents with similar features as the previous one. An indefinite abdominal pain or subacute intestinal obstruction from pressure on the colon may be the presenting symptom. On examination, a fixed smooth swelling may be discovered which will require pyelography to rule out the possibility of a renal swelling.

CAUSES AND DIFFERENTIAL DIAGNOSIS OF SWELLINGS IN THE RIGHT ILIAC REGION

A. **PARIETAL SWELLINGS:** There is no special parietal swelling in this region. An *iliac abscess* (pyogenic) or an *appendicular abscess* may burrow through the anterior abdominal wall and may become parietal. Inguinal swellings are discussed elsewhere.

B. **INTRA-ABDOMINAL SWELLINGS:** These swellings may develop in connection with the structures which normally present in this region or may originate from organs lying in other regions and abnormally invade this region.

The structures which normally present in this region are: (1) the appendix, (2) cecum, (3) terminal part of the ileum, (4) lymph nodes, (5) iliac arteries, (6) retroperitoneal connective tissue, (7) iliopsoas sheath and (8) ilium (os ilii).

Swellings arising from organs lying in other regions which may invade right iliac region are: (1) renal swelling (unascended), (2) gallbladder swelling, (3) uterine swelling, (4) urinary vesical swelling, (5) undescended testis and (6) pelvic abscess.

1. **Appendix:** Appendicular lump is the most common swelling in the right iliac region. The lump may be either an appendicular mass or an appendicular abscess. The appendicular mass gradually develops on third day or earlier after commencement of an attack of acute appendicitis. The mass invariably coincides with the position of the appendix. There will be rigidity of the abdominal musculature, beneath which the tender mass may not be so easy to feel. The mass consists of inflamed appendix, greater omentum, edematous cecal wall surrounded by coils of small intestine matted together with lymph. This is an attempt by the nature to make a protective wall around the inflamed appendix to prevent general peritonitis even if the appendix perforates. With conservative treatment gradually the mass becomes smaller and disappears. This can be verified by outlining the mass with a skin pencil. The lump is irregular, firm, tender, and fixed.

It may be tympanitic on percussion, but it is so tender that the patient may not allow proper percussion to be performed. This appendicular mass should not be confused with appendicular abscess. Variable pyrexia and increase in the number of leukocytes with polymorphonuclear leukocytosis are features of appendicular abscess. Whereas appendicular mass does not contain any pus at all, the appendicular abscess contains pus. Appendicular abscess tends to approach towards the surface when inflammatory signs, i.e., redness and edema of the abdominal wall become evident.

2. **Ileocecal region:**
(a) *HYPERPLASTIC ILEOCECAL TUBERCULOSIS:* In this condition infection starts in the lymphoid follicles and then spreads to the submucous and subserous planes. The intestinal wall becomes thickened with narrowing of its lumen. There will be early involvement of regional lymph nodes which become matted along with the involved terminal part of ileum and cecum to produce the lump.

Recurrent attacks of abdominal pain with diarrhea and features of blind loop syndrome (i.e., anemia, loss of weight and steatorrhea) are the usual complaints. Along with these symptoms a lump in the right iliac fossa with ill health and evening rise of temperature should arouse the suspicion of this condition.

This condition should be differentially diagnosed from Crohn's disease, actinomycosis and carcinoma of the cecum. In Crohn's disease the cecum remains in its position and is not elevated as in this condition. Anal complications such as fissure and multiple fistulae are mainly seen in Crohn's disease. Fistulae may even be seen in the right iliac fossa in Crohn's disease. Carcinoma of the cecum is a disease of the elderly. Occult blood in the stool with anemia and rapid loss of weight are features of this condition. The lump, if felt, is hard, irregular and fixed (at a later stage). Moreover features of tuberculosis will always be present in hyperplastic ileocaecal tuberculosis. Barium meal X-ray and follow through can categorically differentiate these conditions. In hyperplastic ileocaecal tuberculosis a long narrow constricted terminal ileum and ascending colon with cecum in high up position can be noticed. In Crohn's disease a narrow and smooth terminal part of ileum (string sign of Kantor) can be seen. This part of ileum will be devoid of peristaltic waves and cecum will be normal in majority of cases (cf. Hyperplastic ileocecal tuberculosis). In carcinoma of the cecum there will be an irregular filling defect affecting the cecum with soft tissue shadow showing the extent of the tumors but terminal part of ileum is absolutely normal.

(b) *AMEBIC TYPHLITIS:* This condition hardly produces a lump. Diarrhea is the main manifestation of this disease. In tropical countries where amebiasis is endemic this is a constantly recurring problem. One must be very careful to exclude this condition before one does appendicectomy. Patient complains of pain mainly over two places over the cecum and the sigmoid colon. On examination, a thickened and tender colon may be palpable. Sigmoidoscope is of great help in diagnosis. Rectal hemorrhage, fibrous stricture, intestinal obstruction, paracolic abscess, ischiorectal abscess and fistula (from perforation by amebae of the intestinal wall followed by secondary infection) and even perforation are the complications of amebic typhlitis.

(c) *CROHN'S DISEASE OR REGIONAL ILEITIS:* The clinical feature can be best classified into four stages: (i) *Inflammatory stage,* when a tender mass is palpable in the right iliac fossa. The patient will run temperature and there will be moderate anemia. This condition is very much similar to acute appendicitis barring the fact that the patient will be having diarrhea instead of constipation. (ii) *The colitis stage,* when diarrhea, fever, anemia, loss of weight, etc., are present. Occult blood and mucus may be present in the stool. Majority of the patients will suffer from steatorrhea. High incidence of fissure-in-ano, perianal abscess and fistulae is significant diagnostic point at this stage. (iii) *The stenotic stage,* when the picture of small intestinal obstruction may supervene. (iv) *The fistulae,* either external or internal communicating with the sigmoid colon, the cecum, the urinary bladder, etc., are not infrequent in the late stage. Barium meal X-ray will reveal loss of peristalsis in the affected loop and the string sign of Kantor when the lumen is narrowed to a fine cord **(Fig. 35.13)**.

(d) **CARCINOMA OF THE CECUM:** Usually, the patient is above 40. The lump may be the first indication of this disease. There may not be any change in the bowel habit. If present, alternate constipation and diarrhea may be the complaint. Anemia, anorexia, and loss of weight are the associated signs and symptoms of this condition.

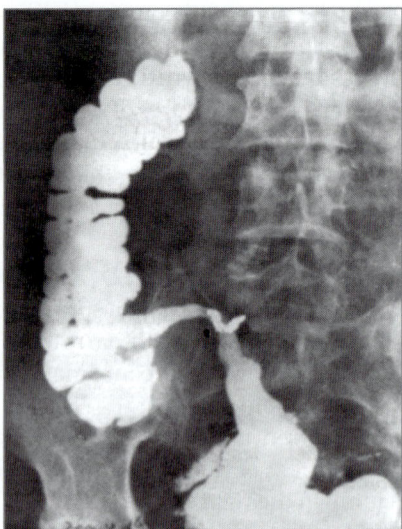

Fig. 35.13: Barium meal X-ray showing Crohn's disease affecting the terminal part of the ileum producing the typical 'string sign of Kantor'.

Occult blood in the stool is a diagnostic point in special investigation. Barium meal X-ray will show 'filling defect' in the cecum which is the main diagnostic feature of this condition. Soft tissue shadow of the tumor may be seen in case of a big lump.

(e) **ACTINOMYCOSIS** of the cecum and appendix may give rise to a hard and fixed mass in the right iliac fossa. Multiple sinuses are seen discharging sulfur granules. Discoloration of the affected skin is often noticed. This condition may follow after operation of the appendix.

(f) **IMPACTION OF ROUND WORMS** in the lower part of the ileum often produces a lump. History of passing worms with stool or vomiting is often obtained.

3. **Lymph nodes:** Enlargement of the iliac group of lymph nodes may produce lump in this region. The details of causes of enlargement of lymph nodes have been discussed in chapter 8 of 'Examination of the lymphatic system'. Filariasis, lymphosarcoma, secondary carcinoma and tuberculosis are the main causes of enlargement of lymph nodes in this region. Filarial nodes are suspected when the patient suffers from periodic attacks of fever with simultaneous tenderness and swelling of the nodes. Eosinophilia and demonstration of microfilaria in blood drawn at night will clinch the diagnosis. Lymphosarcoma gives rise to rapid enlargement of the nodes without other complaints in the young subject. Secondary carcinoma will be felt as a hard, nodular and fixed mass. Primary growth should be looked for and if found settles the diagnosis. Tuberculous nodes will be associated with other tuberculous features. These nodes may soon often produce cold abscess which shows a tendency to burrow through the tissues to come more superficially and gives rise to a cold abscess in the parietes.

4. **Iliac arteries:** Aneurysm of iliac artery is rare but easy to recognize by expansile pulsation.

5. **Retroperitoneal sarcoma:** See page 606.

6. **Iliopsoas sheath:** Two conditions iliac abscess of pyogenic origin and iliopsoas cold abscess from Pott's disease should be considered here.

ILIAC ABSCESS results from infection of a hematoma in the traumatized iliacus muscle. This condition mimics appendicular abscess and is differentiated by two points: (i) that there will be a history of trauma and the pain is only restricted to this region unlike appendicular abscess where pain started in the region of the umbilicus and then shifted to the right iliac fossa and (ii) that there will be a clear space between the abscess and the ilium in case of appendicular abscess but not in case of an iliac abscess.

ILIOPSOAS COLD ABSCESS gravitates from the affected thoracolumbar vertebrae down the psoas sheath deep to the inguinal ligament into the thigh. Therefore, cross fluctuation above and below the inguinal ligament can be easily demonstrated. Deformity of the spine (gibbus) and X-ray will confirm the diagnosis. Cold abscess arising from sacroiliac joint may fill up the right iliac fossa. Examination of this joint and X-ray should always be performed.

7. **Ilium:** The pathological conditions which may give rise to bony swellings from the ilium are same as those arising from any other bone. These have been discussed in Chapter 11 "Examination of Diseases of Bone".

The structures which abnormally present or those which invade this region from the neighborhood are:

8. **Kidney:**

(a) *Unascended kidney:* The first rudiment of the kidney makes its appearance in the pelvis. With the development of the fetus the kidney gradually ascends to take up its final position. Due to some unknown reason the kidney may fail to ascend and remain permanently either in the pelvis or in the iliac fossa as a lobulated mass. Intravenous pyelogram (IVP) alone can make the diagnosis with certainty.

(b) *Dropped kidney* or moveable kidney may come down to the right iliac fossa and create confusion in the diagnosis. But a kidney to drop to the iliac fossa is extremely rare.

9. **Gallbladder:** Very occasionally a hugely distended gallbladder (hydrops) with enlarged liver may descend as low as the right iliac fossa.

10. **Uterus and its appendages:** (a) *Tubo-ovarian mass,* (b) *pyosalpinx,* (c) *cyst and abscess of the broad ligament,* (d) *fibroid of the uterus* and (e) *ovarian cyst* may invade this region. History of their extension from the pelvis and findings of the vaginal examination should be taken into consideration in diagnosis.

11. **Urinary bladder:** If it be enlarged with retention of urine the swelling will be in the hypogastrium and not in this region. Only a huge diverticulum of the bladder may invade this region.

12. **Retained or undescended testis:** The testis develops in the lumbar region. As the fetus grows, the testis descends through the inguinal canal into the scrotum. The testis may abnormally fail to descend and become an abdominal organ or may remain within the inguinal canal. It hardly forms a swelling when it is an abdominal organ, though the chance of malignant transformation is higher in this region. When it is within the inguinal canal it forms a swelling which gives rise to the typical 'testicular feel'. It must be remembered that the most common position of an ectopic testis is the superficial inguinal pouch.

13. **Pelvic abscess,** as it enlarges, may overflow towards the iliac fossa. Besides other features, rectal and vaginal examinations are conclusive.

CAUSES AND DIFFERENTIAL DIAGNOSIS OF SWELLINGS IN THE HYPOGASTRIUM

The bladder must be emptied by a catheter before clinical examination is made.

A. **PARIETAL SWELLINGS:** In addition to those parietal swellings discussed under the umbilical region, a rare swelling urachal cyst may be considered here.

Urachal cyst: Normally, the urachus (the remnant of the allantois extending from the bladder to the umbilicus) becomes obliterated. If it remains patent, it forms a urinary fistula at the umbilicus in a newborn baby. Closure of the umbilical and vesical ends and persistence of the middle segment gives rise to the urachal cyst. This is a cystic swelling, which lies just deep to the abdominal musculature and is relatively fixed.

B. **INTRA-ABDOMINAL SWELLINGS:** These swellings may occur in connection with: (1) the urinary bladder, (2) small intestine, (3) sigmoid colon, (4) uterus and its appendages, (5) pelvis and (6) pelvic bone.

1. **Urinary bladder:** Distended urinary bladder forms a globular swelling that can be seen and palpated in the midline just above the pubis. It may reach up to the umbilicus in chronic retention of urine. It is dull on percussion which is a very significant point, as this area is normally resonant due to the presence of the terminal coils of the small intestine. Pressure on distended bladder will induce a desire for micturition. Differential diagnosis of causes of retention of urine is discussed in page 613.

2. **Uterus:** It is again emphasized that the urinary bladder should be catheterized before palpation for the uterus is made. Many a wrongly diagnosed uterine swelling melts away after catheterization. Two common swellings of the uterus are due to pregnancy and fibroid. Amenorrhea in a young woman with smooth uterine enlargement would suggest pregnancy to be confirmed by classical signs and symptoms of pregnancy. Menorrhagia of some standing in women above 30 years of age but before menopause with irregular enlargement of the uterus (except in the submucous type in which the swelling will be smooth) will lead one to think of fibroid.

3. **Fallopian tube and ovary:** Acute salpingitis rarely gives rise to a lump in early stage. The *TUBO-OVARIAN MASS* results from chronic salpingitis and oophoritis. The patient is a young woman and the mass is situated either in the midline or more often on one or the other side of the midline. This is usually preceded by an attack of pelvic peritonitis in the form of pain, rise of temperature, bladder disturbance, etc. Vaginal examination is confirmatory.

RUPTURED TUBAL GESTATION: No lump is normally felt in the early stage. When the leakage is slow, a mass can be felt a few days later, on one side of the uterus or behind it. History of missed period or periods is an important hint to the diagnosis.

OVARIAN TUMOR AND CYSTS: They spring up from one side of the pelvis but later on take up a central position. Their attachment to the uterine cornua as determined by the vaginal examination, is an important diagnostic feature. Menstruation will be normal or scanty depending on the amount of ovarian destruction. It should be differentiated from ascites by dullness over the front of the abdomen with resonant areas in the flanks, whereas in ascites there is dullness on the flanks with resonance over the front of the abdomen in supine position.

BROAD LIGAMENT CYST gives rise to a swelling that can be felt abdominally. It is not usually so big as the ovarian cyst. By vaginal examination this condition is more conveniently diagnosed.

4. **Pelvic abscess:** It may follow acute appendicitis, salpingo-oophoritis, perforated peptic ulcer, puerperal sepsis, etc. Besides constitutional disturbances it leads to copious discharge of mucus per anum and frequency of micturition. Patient will complain of pain in the lower abdomen and will run temperature. Rectal examination will reveal bulging of the anterior wall of the rectum.

5. **Pelvic bones:** Swellings in connection with the pelvic bones are rare. Their fixity to any of the pelvic walls, bony hard consistency and X-ray will make the diagnosis certain.

CAUSES AND DIFFERENTIAL DIAGNOSIS OF SWELLINGS IN THE LEFT ILIAC REGION

A. **PARIETAL SWELLINGS:** In this region iliac abscess (pyogenic) or cold abscess may form swelling. Appendicular abscess cannot be present here. Inguinal swellings have been discussed elsewhere.

B. **INTRA-ABDOMINAL SWELLINGS:** The same conditions that have been discussed under the right iliac region are applicable here, with the exception of the cecum and appendix, but in their stead the sigmoid (and descending) colon is substituted. Amongst the structures that may invade this region, the spleen should be considered instead of the gallbladder.

Sigmoid colon: There are two pathologies of the sigmoid colon which may give rise to a mass in the left iliac fossa. These are *diverticulitis* and *carcinoma*. The patient is above 40 years in both these conditions.

DIVERTICULITIS: Diverticulosis, which is the first stage of this condition often passes asymptomatic. But rectal hemorrhage and flatulent distension of the lower abdomen may be the presenting symptoms at this stage. When inflammation sets in diverticulitis develops. Fever, malaise, pain and tenderness on the left iliac fossa are the main features of this condition. All these sum up to mimic left sided appendicitis. This disease is rare in India. X-ray with barium enema will show multiple diverticula or 'saw tooth' appearance with narrowing of the colon. Sudden hemorrhage, perforation, local abscess, general peritonitis (very rare), fistulae (both internal and external) and even carcinoma are the complications of this disease.

CARCINOMA: In this region mainly annular type of carcinoma is seen. Increasing constipation requiring increasing doses of purgatives is the main presenting symptom. The carcinoma itself hardly produces a lump. What is felt is a loaded colon proximal to the stenosis as determined by pitting on pressure. X-ray with barium enema will show constant 'filling defect'.

Algorithmic Approach to Patient with Abdominal Lump

Patient presents with an abdominal lump

↓

Is the lump painful or painless?
- **Painful lump** → Consider **inflammation, abscess, hernia**
- **Painless lump** → Consider **malignancy, cystic lesion**

↓

Does the lump move with respiration?
- **Yes** → Likely **hepatic, gallbladder, splenic origin**
- **No** → Consider **retroperitoneal, fixed intra-abdominal mass**

↓

Is the lump fluctuant or solid?
- **Fluctuant** → **Cystic lesion, abscess**
- **Solid** → **Tumor, malignancy, organomegaly**

↓

Perform diagnostic investigations
- **Ultrasound** → Detects **cystic vs solid lesions, organ involvement**
- **CT scan/MRI** → Evaluates **malignancy, retroperitoneal lesions**
- **Blood work (LFT, tumor markers, infection markers)** → Helps in differential diagnosis

↓

Confirm diagnosis and initiate treatment
- **Surgical management** → Hernia, abscess drainage, tumor resection
- **Medical therapy** → Infectious causes, conservative management
- Follow-up for malignancy or chronic conditions

Examination of a Rectal Case

CHAPTER 36

HISTORY

The patient may present with bleeding, discharge of pus or mucus, pain, abnormality in bowel habit or prolapse.

1. **Bleeding:** Enquire about the ***AMOUNT OF BLEEDING***; the ***COLOR OF THE BLOOD*** lost—bright red (coming from the rectum or anal canal), dark red (coming from the ascending, transverse, descending or sigmoid colon) or black, i.e., melena (from the small intestine or higher); *Its relation with the feces*—unchanged blood may appear in four ways: (i) blood mixed with feces means that the blood has come from bowel higher than sigmoid colon where the softness of the stool remains giving chance to the blood to mix with the feces. (ii) Blood on the surface of the feces usually comes from the rectum or anal canal. (iii) Blood separate from the feces may occur when bleeding occurs at some other time defecation, e.g., bleeding carcinoma of the rectum when blood accumulates in the rectum and gives rise to desire to defecate and only blood and mucus come out. Such bleeding may also occur in diverticulosis, diverticulitis, ulcerative colitis, polyp, prolapsed piles, etc. (iv) Blood in the toilet paper is only seen in case of minor bleeding from the anal skin either due to fissure-in-ano or external hemorrhoids.

   When a child comes with bleeding per anum, a diagnosis of rectal polyp should be made until this is excluded by rectal examination.

2. **Discharge of pus or mucus:** Soiling of the clothes with purulent discharge coming from a sinus is the constant complaint of the patient with a fistula-in-ano. In ulcerative carcinoma of the rectum the patient often passes a considerable quantity of blood-stained, purulent and offensive discharge at the time of defecation. Excessive mucus is also discharged in colitis, Crohn's disease and colloid carcinoma of the rectum.

3. **Pain:** It is interesting to know that all pathological conditions below the Hilton's line are painful but above this line they are painless so long as they remain confined within the rectal wall. Inflammation or infiltration beyond the rectal wall is likely to be painful. Enquire about the *nature of pain*—whether throbbing (anorectal abscess) or sharp cutting (anal fissure) or intermittent in nature in case of fistula-in-ano (see below) and its *relation with defecation*. Pain is the main symptom of chronic fissure-in-ano. It starts with defecation and persists for sometime after the act. In a fistula-in-ano pain is intermittent. When the fistula becomes closed the pain appears and gradually increases as the discharge accumulates until the fistula is forced open, when the collection is voided and pain disappears. Uncomplicated piles are absolutely painless but when they are complicated by secondary infection or strangulation, they become painful. Carcinoma of the rectum is painless to start with. When pain appears it indicates a spread into the pelvic cellular tissue or sacral plexus (causing bilateral sciatica). An annular lesion high in the rectum may obstruct the lumen of the bowel and cause lower abdominal colic.

4. **Abnormality of the bowel habit:** In carcinoma of the rectum the bowel habit is altered and the *nature of alteration depends on the position of the growth*—whether occurring at the pelvirectal junction, in the ampulla or in the anal canal *and on the macroscopic feature of the growth*—either annular or ulcerative or proliferative. The growth at the pelvirectal junction or in the sigmoid colon is usually of the annular type. Increasing constipation is the earliest symptom in these cases. A proliferative growth in the ampulla causes a sensation of fullness in the rectum and the patient feels that his bowel has not been completely emptied after defecation. In ulcerative growth, mucus, pus, blood and feces accumulate overnight during the night and the patient on rising from the bed gets an urgent call to stool—this is called 'spurious morning diarrhea'. A growth in the lower part of the rectum and anal canal may alter the shape of the stool which becomes either pipestem or tape-like. *Tenesmus* is the painful straining to empty bowel without any result. Such tenesmus may be caused by a proliferative growth (space-occupying lesion) in the ampulla of rectum.

5. **Prolapse:** If the patient complains of something coming out of the anal canal during defecation, he is possibly suffering from prolapse, polypus or long standing internal piles. Enquire whether the prolapse that comes out with defecation is reduced automatically after the act or has to be replaced by pushing it in. Sometimes the patient comes with a prolapse remaining unreduced for two to three days. Enquire also about the length of the protruded mass. If the protrusion is slight, it is a partial prolapse (i.e., prolapse of the mucous membrane and submucosa only). If it is more than two inches in length, it is a complete prolapse or procidentia (i.e., prolapse of all coats of the rectum).

6. **Other complaints:** (a) *Pruritus ani* is a symptom often complained of by the patients. A list of the conditions which cause pruritus ani have been given at the end of this chapter.

Loss of weight and cachexia are often complained of by patients with malignant growth in this region. (c) Various types of indigestion may be complained of in case of carcinoma of rectum, ulcerative colitis, Crohn's disease and fissure-in-ano (particularly in old individuals when the rectum is full of feces as the patients try to avoid defecation which is so painful).

Past history: In a case of fistula-in-ano a previous history of anal abscess is often obtained. This abscess has either burst spontaneously or has been incised. Fistula-in-ano may be even found in cases of tuberculosis, Crohn's disease, ulcerative colitis, colloid carcinoma of the rectum etc. So relevant questions must be asked to find out if the patient is suffering or was suffering from any of these ailments. Habitual constipation is often associated with internal piles and fissures. In the case of prolapse a previous history of dysentery or severe diarrhea may be obtained. Wasting of the patient leads to weakening of the rectal support—this together with tenesmus as occurs in dysentery is responsible for the development of prolapse. Anal tag and perianal abscess are sometimes seen in Crohn's disease.

Family history: Polyposis is recognized to be a hereditary disease. A family history may be volunteered by the patients suffering from piles, fissures, prolapse and even carcinoma of the rectum.

History in rectal examination

Aspect	Clinical significance	Patient-friendly questions
Bleeding	Bright red → Anal canal/rectum Dark red → Colon, IBD	"Have you noticed blood in your stool? What color was it?"
Pain	Sharp → Anal fissure Throbbing → Abscess	"Do you feel pain before, during, or after passing stool?"

Contd...

Contd...

Aspect	Clinical significance	Patient-friendly questions
Bowel habits	Constipation → Tumor, stricture Urgency → Ulcerative colitis	"Have you had changes in your bowel habits recently?"
Prolapse	Partial (<2 cm) vs complete (>2 cm)	"Do you feel something coming out of your anus during defecation?"
Family history	Polyposis, colorectal cancer	"Does anyone in your family have a history of colon or rectal cancer?"

■ RECTAL EXAMINATION

Position of the patient: 1. *The left lateral position (Sims')*: This is the most popular position for anorectal examination. The patient lies on the left-side. The buttocks should project over the edge of the table. Both the hips and knees are well flexed so that the knees are taken near to the chest of the patient. This position is suitable for inspection of the perianal region and proctoscopy.
2. *Dorsal position*: The patient lies on his back with the hips flexed. The examiner passes his forearm beneath the right thigh and the index finger is pushed through the anal canal. This position is popular when the patient is too ill to alter the position. It is also convenient to do bimanual examination in this position. The right index finger remains in the rectum while the left hand on the abdomen to know the interior of the pelvis in a better way—the size and characteristics of a pelvic swelling and more information regarding recto-vesical or rectouterine pouch, but this position is not suitable for inspection around the anus.
3. *The knee-elbow position*: This position is particularly suitable for palpating the prostate and seminal vesicles.
4. *Right lateral position*—can be chosen in the case of carcinoma at the pelvirectal junction when it tends to fall downwards and towards the anus for better palpation by the examining finger.
5. *Lithotomy position*: The advantages of this position are that more informations regarding pelvic viscera can be obtained and bimanual examination can be conveniently performed. Moreover, a lesion high in the rectum is more likely to be felt.

The students should remember that about 10 cm from the anus can be explored by digital examination.

It cannot be emphasized too strongly *that the anal region must be inspected firstly, palpated secondly and digital examination lastly.*

A. INSPECTION

This part of examination should never be omitted. Anal tags (external piles), sentinel pile (a feature of chronic fissure), fistula-in-ano, pilonidal sinus, condyloma and carcinoma can be diagnosed by inspection alone. Swellings and ulcers may be seen in this region as in other regions of the body. Anal tag may be present anywhere around the anus but the position of the sentinel pile is more or less constant—on the midline posteriorly. The sentinel pile is associated with **fissure-in-ano**, which is a linear ulcer in the anal canal (mostly situated on the midline posteriorly). The lower end of the fissure can just be seen when the anal margins are separated—a procedure which causes extreme pain. When a **fistula-in-ano** is found note the distance of its orifice from the anus and its position—whether situated anteriorly or posteriorly to an imaginary line passing transversely through the middle of the anus. The position of the external opening of a fistula-in-ano gives an idea of the position of the internal opening. If the external orifice lies either behind the imaginary line referred to above or anterior to it but beyond 1½ inches from the anus, the internal opening will be found on the midline posteriorly between the two sphincters, the fistulous track being curved. When the external opening is situated in front of the line but within 1½ inches of the anus, the internal opening lies on the same radial line as the external opening, the track being straight (*Goodsall's rule*) **(Fig. 36.1)**. **Pilonidal sinus** is seen typically on the midline at the tip of the coccyx. A tuft of hair will be seen extruding through the sinus. **Condylomata** (*see* **Fig. 36.9**) at anal region are of two types: **CONDYLOMATA ACUMINATA** and **CONDYLOMATA LATA**. *Condylomata acuminata* are multiple, pedunculated papilliferous lesions that are easy to recognize. These are caused by a virus which is a variant of the papilloma virus responsible for skin warts. This type of warts may spread over a wider area to involve the perineum, labia majora and even back of the scrotum. *Condyloma lata* is a manifestation of secondary syphilis and is rare nowadays. These are flat, raised, white and hypertrophied epithelium at the mucocutaneous junction of the anus. **Anal carcinoma** is mostly seen as an extensive ulcer with everted margin **(Figs. 36.2 and 36.3)**.

Furthermore inspection will provide with informations regarding internal piles, prolapse, pruritus ani, etc. When there is a history of **prolapse** ask the patient to strain as he would do during defecation, if required, in the squatting position **(Figs. 36.4 and 36.5)**. Note the protruded mass. In case of prolapse if the protrusion is less than 1 inch it is a partial prolapse, whereas any protrusion more than 2 inches should be considered as complete. *Long-standing* **internal piles** may protrude through the anus, but this protruded mass is divided in segments whereas an incomplete prolapse is a single segment **(Fig. 36.6)**. It should be remembered that an external pile is covered with skin whereas an internal pile is covered with mucous membrane. Very rarely a **polypus** or an *intussusception* may come out of the anal orifice. **Melanoma** of the anus, though rare, may be seen as bluish-black soft mass which may be confused with a thrombotic pile.

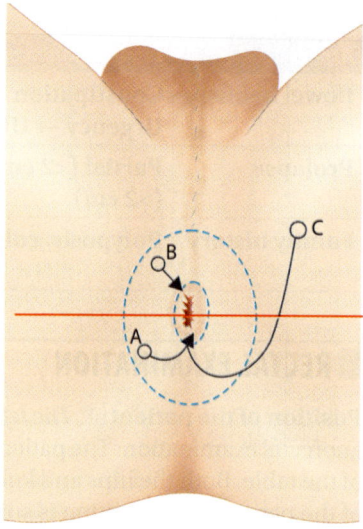

Fig. 36.1: Application of Goodsall's rule. When the external opening of a fistula-in-ano (A) lies behind the transverse line passing across the anus or (C) anterior to this line but beyond 1½ inches from the anus, the internal opening is found in the midline posteriorly between the sphincters, the fistula's track being curved. When the external opening (B) is situated in front of the transverse line, but within 1½ inches from the anus, the internal opening lies in the same radial line as the external orifice, the fistula track being straight.

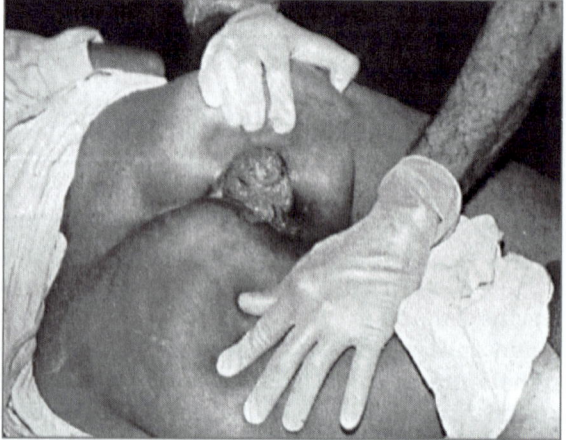

Fig. 36.2: Carcinoma of the rectum involving the anal canal.

B. PALPATION

Before digital examination palpation of the perianal region should be performed. A *swelling* or an *ulcer* may be present in this region

Chapter 36: Examination of a Rectal Case

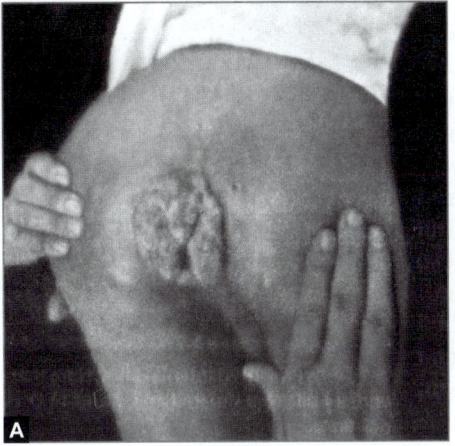
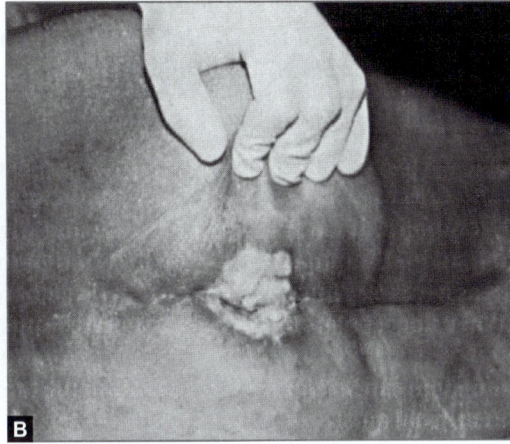

Figs. 36.3A and B: (A) Anal carcinoma; (B) Basal cell carcinoma of the anus.

and should be examined as has been described in the Chapters 3 and 4. An indurated tender swelling with brawny edema on one side of the anus is usually due to an *ischiorectal abscess*. One should not wait for fluctuation to develop. External opening of *fistula-in-ano* can be seen in this region. Careful palpation will indicate the track. An apex of long standing *intussusception* may be seen through the anus. This has to be differentiated from *prolapse* of the rectum. In the former a finger can be insinuated between intussusception and the anal margin, but in the latter this is not possible.

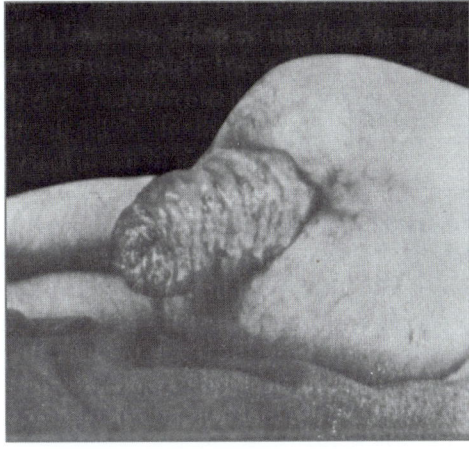

Fig. 36.4: Complete prolapse (procidentia) of the rectum.

C. DIGITAL EXAMINATION

Nowadays disposable gloves are being used. Then patient should be told what is about to be done. He is instructed to open his mouth and breathe in and out deeply. The gloved finger should be lubricated and the lubricant is wiped round the anus. The digital examination should be made gently and should not hurt the patient. The pulp of the index finger should be laid flat on the anal verge. Gentle pressure is exerted till the sphincter yields. More pressure will gradually push the finger into the anal canal with rotatory movement. The tip of the index finger should not be introduced straight into the anus. While the finger is

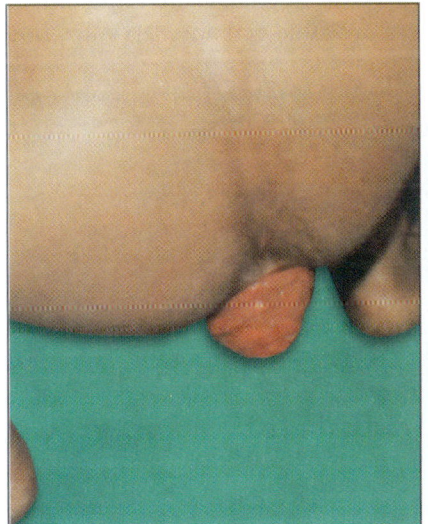

Fig. 36.5: A case of complete rectal prolapse.

within the anal canal and rectum a definite system should be established to get all the informations of rectal examination **(Figs. 36.7A and B)**.

When the finger is in the anal canal note the tone of the sphincter, any pain or tenderness and any thickening of the wall of the anal canal. Patients with fissures may have spasm of the sphincters and will complain of excruciating pain during digital examination. Examination may be deferred in these cases as necessary informations cannot be gathered.

When finger enters the rectum, it should be pushed as high as possible. Informations received in rectal examination can be divided into (a) within the lumen, (b) in the wall and (c) outside the wall.

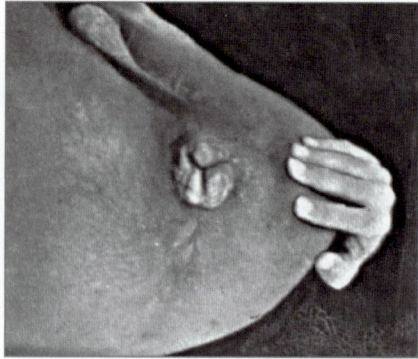

Fig. 36.6: Prolapsed internal piles. Note that the primary piles are situated at 3, 7 and 11 O'clock positions.

A. **Within the lumen:** Sometimes the rectum is found to be full of hard feces. At these instances a complete rectal examination is impossible. So it is a good practice to give enema before the rectal examination. The apex of an *intussusception* may occasionally be felt. Its freedom from the rectal wall can be easily assessed if the finger is passed between intussusception and the rectal wall. In *intestinal obstruction* there will be "ballooning" of the rectum. This is evident by the fact that rectal wall can only be felt by bending the examining finger in the rectum. However this sign is not much reliable. False positive results are sometimes seen after administration of enema or in obstruction of the urinary tract (presumably reflex in origin). If a *mass* can be felt ask the patient to strain down. This will bring the mass further down for proper palpation.

B. **In the wall:** Just inside the opening of the anus a circular groove can be felt. This lies between the external and internal sphincter muscles. This also marks the dividing line between the external and internal hemorrhoidal plexuses. Further up the anorectal ring can be felt. It is approximately 3 cm above the anal verge. This marks the junction between the anal canal and rectum. Posteriorly, the ring is felt best, then laterally due to presence of sling-like arrangement of the puborectalis component of the levator ani muscle. These landmarks are important in determining the location of different anorectal abscesses or fistula-in-ano. Above this ring

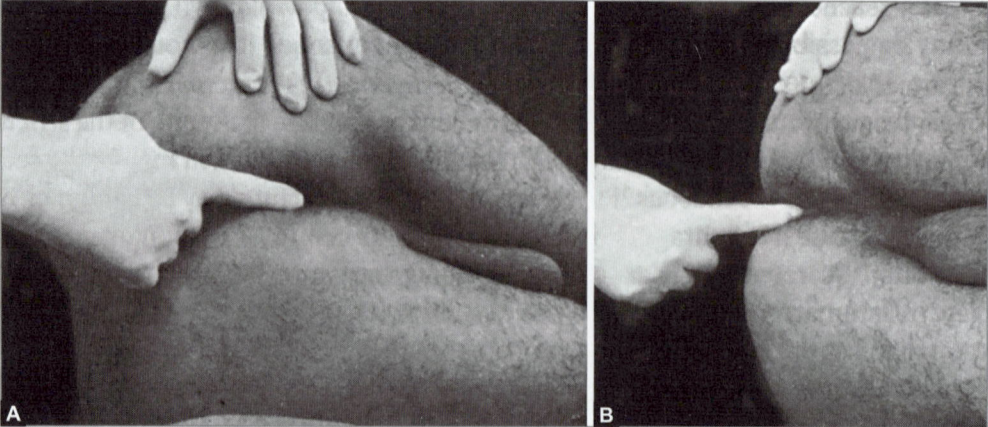

Figs. 36.7A and B: Showing the correct and the wrong methods of introducing the finger into the rectum.

the finger enters the spacious lower part of the rectum. The ascending finger may feel a soft fold of mucous membrane called valve of Houston. *It cannot be impressed too strongly that uncomplicated internal piles cannot be felt with the finger.* They are diagnosed by proctoscope. Only chronically inflamed and thrombosed piles can be felt by digital examination. The internal opening of the *fistula-in-ano* is usually felt as a small dimple in the center of an indurated area. Most frequently it is situated on the midline posteriorly between external and internal sphincters. A diagnosis of *ulcer* is made by absence of normal smoothness of the rectal mucous membrane. The edge of the ulcer should be carefully palpated for induration and eversion— the pathognomonic features of a malignant ulcer. Besides carcinoma, an ulcer may be due to tuberculosis, dysentery, gonorrhea, soft sore, syphilis, etc. History and isolation of the positive organism will establish the nature of the ulcer. A *polypus* of the rectum is felt as soft round growth about the size of a small grape slipping under the finger. It must be remembered that a soft lesion of the rectal wall is likely to be felt on the downward stroke of the finger than in its upward course. So, as soon as a soft lesion is felt the finger is pushed up clear of the lesion till it reaches its upper limit. The finger is now flexed and withdrawn partially to feel the lesion properly. It may be possible to pull a polypus out of the anus and examine it thoroughly.

When the lumen of the rectum is constricted a diagnosis of *stricture of the rectum* is made. Note the position and extent of such constriction and the character of the mucous membrane at the site of the stricture whether ulcerated or thickened. It must be remembered that narrowing of the rectal lumen may be caused by pressure from outside in which case the mucous lining is perfectly smooth. A stricture may be benign or malignant. A benign stricture feels like a diaphragm with a clean-cut hole in its center. A malignant stricture feels hard, irregular and is often ulcerated. There are various causes of benign stricture. Besides trauma and post-operative stricture, a few inflammatory conditions may give rise to such strictures. Lymphogranuloma inguinale is the most important in this group. In this case the stricture is rubbery and tubular in character. It is a form of venereal disease caused by ultramicroscopic virus. An enquiry should be made about previous history of genital sores and inguinal bubo. The diagnosis is established by Frei's intradermal test.

Carcinoma of the rectum is a condition in which rectal examination is of paramount importance. About 75% of carcinomata of the rectum occur in the lower part of the ampulla, where they tend to be papilliferous or ulcerative with everted edge. The remaining 25% occur in the upper part of the rectum and are annular in shape. About 90% of rectal cancer can be felt by digital examination and it is criminal not to perform rectal examination in patients with any rectal complaint. Determine how much of the circumference of the rectum is involved by the growth. The tumor may bleed readily during examination. Try to decide whether the tumor is fixed or mobile, how much is its local spread—whether the neighboring structures such as bladder and prostate (or uterus and vagina) anteriorly and the sacrum and the coccyx posteriorly are involved. It is useful to remember that the growth preserves its mobility so long as it remains within the fascia propria of the rectum.

C. **Outside the wall:** This is the most important part of rectal examination and probably more often used as a diagnostic procedure than the previous section. The structures around the rectum are explored systematically by palpating anteriorly, right lateral, left lateral and posteriorly.

ANTERIORLY: The anatomical structures on this aspect are the prostate, seminal vesicles, base of the bladder and rectovesical pouch of peritoneum in case of male; the uterus, the cervix, the vagina and rectouterine pouch (pouch of Douglas) in case of female. The examinations of the prostate, the seminal vesicles and base of the bladder are described under "Examination of a urinary case". To make summary of this examination it may be stated that the normal prostate is firm, rubbery, bilobed, its surface is smooth with a shallow central sulcus and the rectal mucosa can be moved freely over it. The seminal vesicles are palpable just above the upper lateral angles of the gland.

Uterus and cervix are easy to feel per rectum. The uterus is felt as a tumor whereas the cervix can be felt projecting through the anterior rectal wall which is popularly known as *pons asinorum*. It is a good practice to feel the cervix first and then follow to the uterus onwards. Bimanual palpation can define the shape and size of the uterus and any ovarian mass in a better way.

Now the attention is directed towards rectovesical or rectouterine pouch. The index finger when fully inserted reaches about one inch above the floor of pouch of Douglas in the female and about half that distance in the male. Presence of pus, blood, malignant deposit (e.g., from carcinoma of the stomach) or tumor of the sigmoid colon may be felt through the pouch.

LATERALLY: The structures which are felt laterally are the ischiorectal fossa, the lateral wall of the pelvis, lower end of the ureters and internal iliac arteries. The pelvic appendix can be felt on right side and the rectal examination is imperative in pelvic appendicitis as tenderness may not be so obvious per abdomen. In case of female fallopian tubes and ovaries may be palpable and rectal examination is of great help in diagnosing salpingitis, ovarian cysts and tumors. A mass may be palpable in a leaking ectopic gestation of some days standing.

Ischiorectal abscess is often felt per rectum as an extremely tender and tense swelling on the side of the rectum. Rarely, a stone in the lower end of the ureter and an aneurysm of the internal iliac artery may be felt per rectum. Inflammation and growth from the bony wall of pelvis, central dislocation of the hip joint, fracture of the pelvic girdle may be discovered by the finger in the rectum.

POSTERIORLY: The hollow of the sacrum and coccyx are easily felt through rectum. Any pathological condition affecting this region can be easily palpated through rectum. A suspected case of coccydynia can be detected by an index finger inside the rectum and a thumb over the coccyx to detect abnormal mobility and tenderness in this condition. Sacrococcygeal teratoma and postanal dermoid can also be felt and diagnosed per rectum.

Bimanual examination: The examination of the contents of the pelvis can be conveniently examined during rectal examination by placing another hand on the abdomen. This gives a better idea of the size, shape and nature of any pelvic mass. Its immense importance in staging of bladder carcinoma is discussed in Chapter 37.

At the end of the rectal examination always look at the examining finger for presence of feces, blood, pus or mucus.

Abdominal examination: In case of annular carcinoma at the upper part of the rectum an indistinct lump may be felt at the left side of the abdomen. This is nothing but the descending colon loaded with hard feces. This swelling pits on pressure and thus distinguishes it from any solid swelling at this region. Examine the liver for secondary metastasis. Note also if there is any jaundice, hard subcutaneous nodules and free fluid within the abdomen.

Lymph nodes: Carcinoma arising from the hind gut will metastasize to the iliac groups of lymph nodes. On deep palpation one may discover enlargement of these nodes particularly in thin patients. Carcinoma arising from or involving the lower part of the anal canal below the pectinate line commonly spreads to the inguinal group of lymph nodes and these are easily palpable.

SPECIAL INVESTIGATIONS

1. **Proctoscopy:** With the patient in the left lateral or 'knee-elbow' position the warm and lubricated proctoscope is gently inserted into the rectum (**Fig. 36.8**). The instrument is introduced at first in the direction of the axis of the anal canal, i.e., upwards and forwards towards the patient's umbilicus until the anal canal is passed. The instrument is then directed posteriorly to enter into the rectum properly. Now the obturator is withdrawn and the interior of the rectum and anal canal is seen with the help of a light. The internal piles, fissures, ulcer and growth can be seen if present. The piles will prolapse into the proctoscope as this instrument is being withdrawn. Note the position of the piles. They are generally positioned according to the main branches of the superior hemorrhoidal vein. The

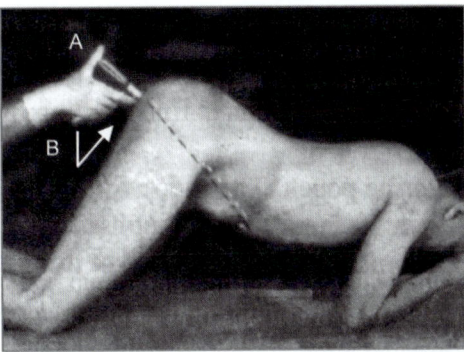

Fig. 36.8: Proctoscopy in the 'Knee-elbow' position. (A) The instrument is first pushed towards the patient's umbilicus as this is the direction of the anal canal. As soon as the anal canal is passed, the instrument is then depressed and pushed towards the sacrum along the rectum (B).

main three branches are situated in the left lateral, right anterior and right posterior positions. When the patient is in the lithotomy position these positions will correspond to the 3, 7 and 11 o'clock positions respectively, if a watch is imagined to be held against the anus. These are called *primary piles*. A few *secondary piles* (4–5) may frequently develop in between the primary ones. *Chronic fissure* is often situated on the midline posteriorly. By proctoscope one can also find inner opening of *fistula*. One can take biopsy from a *growth* or an *ulcer* through a proctoscope.

2. **Sigmoidoscopy:** The length of a sigmoidoscope is about 14 inches (35 cm). By this instrument whole of the rectum and a large part of the sigmoid colon can be examined. The conventional position for introduction of this instrument is the 'knee-elbow' position. But a few surgeons prefer left lateral position. The instrument is well lubricated and passed through the anus along the direction of the anal canal, i.e., upwards and forwards towards the umbilicus of the patient. As soon as its tip has entered the rectum all further introduction should be carried out under direct vision. The obturator is withdrawn, the glass eye-piece and the light-carrier are fitted and the bellow is attached. Now the instrument is pushed posteriorly (at right angle of the previous direction). While within the rectum, by circumduction movement the interior of the rectum is thoroughly inspected. The instrument is gradually pushed upwards following the sacral curve. Horizontal folds are come across and easily circumvented. As it comes nearer the pelvic-rectal junction the instrument will be directed more anteriorly on one side or the other (usually the left side). Introduction of the instrument into the pelvic colon is the most difficult part of the operation. By gentle inflation of the bowel under direct vision the lumen can be made to open out in advance of the instrument. By continuing in the same manner the sigmoidoscope can be passed up to its full extent so that the greater part of the pelvic colon can be examined.

This instrument is mainly used to detect presence of any growth, ulcer, diverticula, etc., in the rectum and lower part of the sigmoid colon. The growth can be biopsied and a smear may be taken from ulcer for bacteriological examination through this instrument. The proliferative type of carcinoma has an irregular nodular surface which is friable and bleeds easily. In case of ulcerative type of carcinoma the margin will be everted and raised. A benign growth is usually pedunculated. An adenoma may be smooth and lobulated. A sessile benign growth is often difficult to distinguish from carcinoma without biopsy.

A sigmoidoscopy should always be supported by contrast enema X-ray. There may be multiple tumors. Just by seeing a polyp through sigmoidoscopy one should not be content in removing it. If there be a carcinoma higher in the colon, this will implant cancer cells in the rectal wound.

3. **Colonoscopy:** Since barium enema was introduced there has been no practical diagnostic method in the colon after X-ray and before the surgeon's knife. With the advent of fibreoptic colonoscope, the whole of the colon up to the cecum can be viewed for practical purposes. This instrument is preferred to sigmoidoscope by majority of the patients.

The key to pleasant and successful colonoscopy lies in achieving a clean bowel before hand. Colonoscopy is never done under general anesthesia, but it may be done after satisfactory analgesia by injecting intravenously diazepam (Valium) 5–20 mg. and pethidine 25–75 mg. It is extremely important for the endoscopist to pay attention to any pain being experienced because of excessive stress on the bowel wall or on the attachments of the colon.

Colonoscopy and the contrast enema are complementary procedures. When the barium enema report is at hand, the *strong indications* of a diagnostic endoscopic examination following the contrast study are listed below: (i) X-ray study negative, but the symptoms persist including occult blood and anemia; (ii) X-ray study positive yet for confirmation; (iii) X-ray study positive for cancer, but for taking biopsy; (iv) X-ray study positive for cancer yet to exclude synchronous cancer or associated polyps; (v) X-ray study positive for polyp, but to exclude malignant change or for additional polyps; (vi) X-ray study positive for inflammatory disease, but to know the extent of disease and for biopsy.

Perforation is the most frequently reported complication. There are certain clinical conditions in which an attempt at endoscopic examination appears unwise. These are: (i) acute toxic dilatation of the colon, (ii) acute severe ulcerative colitis, (iii) acute diverticulitis, (iv) radiation necrosis, (v) recent bowel anastomosis and (vi) in uncooperative patients.

Endoscopic polypectomy has drastically reduced the need for the abdominal approach. Even in most instances malignant polyps can be controlled entirely by polypectomy via the colonoscope.

4. **X-ray:** 1. *Straight X-ray of the abdomen* may indicate evidence of intestinal obstruction due to annular growth at the rectosigmoid junction.
2. *Chest X-ray* is performed in an established case of carcinoma of the rectum to exclude pulmonary metastasis.

5. **Barium enema X-ray:** The importance of this examination in a case of bleeding per anum and in pathologies of the rectum and anal canal cannot be overemphasized. In any case of internal hemorrhoid barium enema X-ray must be performed to exclude any carcinoma above the rectum to be the cause of this condition. In case of rectal polyp, this polyp may be one of the multiple polyps in the colon which should be excluded by barium enema. Other pathologies like Crohn's disease, ulcerative colitis which often affect this region are mainly diseases of the GI tract above this region and better be revealed by barium enema X-ray.

DOUBLE CONTRAST BARIUM ENEMA examination is often used nowadays and it delineates the colonic and rectal walls more precisely to detect pathologies like polyps and carcinomas which may be missed in barium enema X-ray.

CT scan and **Ultrasonography** are only used in case of rectal carcinomas to detect intrapelvic or intra-abdominal lymph node enlargement and to detect the spread of such growth into neighboring viscera.

DIFFERENTIAL DIAGNOSIS

SACROCOCCYGEAL TERATOMA
It is the most common among the large tumors which are seen in a newborn baby. Teratoma may appear anywhere in the body, but frequent choice of this pre-coccygeal region is due to the fact that it is the site of the 'primitive node' which is composed of a group of totipotent cells. Females are more often affected than males. This tumor is firmly fixed to the coccyx and occasionally to the last piece of the sacrum. This tumor may assume a very huge size, but it may be small enough to pass unnoticed. This small variety may turn malignant.

POSTANAL DERMOID
A soft cystic swelling may sometimes be come across in the space behind the rectum and anal canal and in front of the lower part of the sacrum and coccyx. This is a postanal dermoid and is a form of teratoma. Though congenital such a cyst often remains symptomless till adult life, until and unless it becomes infected or becomes burst outside forming a sinus. The cyst however if exceptionally of big size may give rise to difficulty in defecation. The cyst is easily palpable by rectal examination and may be discovered accidentally by this examination.

HEMORRHOIDS (PILES)
Varicosities of the veins of the anal canal are known as hemorrhoids. It may be internal or external depending on the position of the varicosity. If it is above the Hilton's line it is called 'internal hemorrhoid' and if it is below the Hilton's line it is called 'external hemorrhoid'. So internal hemorrhoid is covered by mucous membrane whereas the external hemorrhoid is covered with skin.

Internal hemorrhoids are the varicosities of the internal hemorrhoidal plexuses. These could be divided into two main types: (a) *Vascular hemorrhoids* in which there is extensive dilatation of the terminal superior hemorrhoidal venous plexus—commonly found in younger individuals particularly men; (b) *Mucosal hemorrhoids* in which there is sliding down of the thickened mucous membrane which conceals the underlying veins. Piles may occur at all ages, but are uncommon below the age of 20 years barring piles secondary to vascular malformations which may occur in children. For practical purposes internal hemorrhoids can be divided into three degrees :—

First degree hemorrhoids are those in which hypertrophy of the internal hemorrhoidal plexus remains entirely within the anal canal as the mucosal suspensory ligaments remain intact. Patients in this stage usually present with rectal bleeding and discomfort or irritation. Bleeding is bright red and occurs during defecation as 'splash in the pan'. It may continue for months or years.

Second degree hemorrhoids occur when with further hypertrophy the mucosal suspensory ligaments become lax and piles will descend so that they prolapse during defecation but spontaneous reduction takes place afterwards. There may be small skin tag, some mucous discharge, soreness and irritation.

In *third degree* hemorrhoids, they remain prolapsed after defecation and require replacement. These often descend spontaneously or on exercise. The mucosa overlying such hemorrhoids undergoes squamous metaplasia. Mucous discharge and pruritus ani become troublesome and anemia becomes obvious. Secondary hemorrhoids occur between the three primary ones, the most common being the midposterior position. There may be a large skin tag.

General examination is intended to find out cause of this condition. Whether the patient is constipated or not? Causes of raised intra-abdominal pressure should be excluded. They are urethral stricture, an enlarged prostate, a big pelvic tumor pressing on the superior rectal veins. Pregnancy not only presses on the superior rectal veins but also excess progesterone during this period relaxes the smooth muscles on the walls of the said veins.

Rectal examination is usually not fruitful, as uncomplicated piles cannot be felt with finger unless they are thrombosed or fibrosed. Hemorrhoids are mainly diagnosed by *proctoscopy*. After the proctoscope has been fully introduced the obturator is taken out and with good light interior of the anal canal is seen. The proctoscope is slowly withdrawn. Red brown mucosa with the piles will bulge into the proctoscope. The three common primary piles are at 3, 7 and 11 o'clock positions (when the patient is in the lithotomy position). *Sigmoidoscopy* should always be performed to exclude any serious rectal pathology (such as carcinoma). If there is any doubt as to the origin of the blood passed per rectum or a history of altered bowel habit, a barium enema X-ray or colonoscopy must be performed.

FISSURE-IN-ANO

This is a longitudinal ulcer in the anal canal posteriorly situated in majority of cases. Fissures may be of two varieties: (a) Acute and (b) Chronic.

ACUTE FISSURE is a deep tear in the anal canal with surrounding edema and inflammatory induration. It is always associated with spasm of the anal sphincters. Bright streak of blood with the passage of stool and pain after defecation are the characteristic features. Acute fissures often heal spontaneously.

CHRONIC FISSURE: When acute fissure fails to heal, it will gradually develop into a deep undermined ulcer with continuing infection and edema. This ulcer stops above at the pectinate line. Below, there is hypertrophied papilla and skin tag known as 'sentinel pile'. As the fissure is mainly situated in the lower anal canal it is highly painful and associated with spasm of the sphincters. Rectal examination can feel the chronic ulcer. But due to extreme spasm of the Sphincter proctoscopy may be postponed till later stage.

Posterior angulation of the anal canal, relative fixation of the anal canal posteriorly, divergence of the fibers of the external sphincter muscle posteriorly and the elliptical shape of the anal canal are the theories of predominately posterior midline location of fissures.

The students should remember a few secondary causes of anal fissures, e.g., ulcerative colitis, Crohn's disease, syphilis, tuberculosis, etc.

ANORECTAL ABSCESSES

There are mainly three types of these abscesses—(i) Perianal, (ii) Ischiorectal and (iii) Pelvic-rectal abscesses. Two other types are also seen—(iv) Submucous and (v) Fissure abscess (associated with chronic fissure).

(i) **PERIANAL:** An acutely tender rounded cystic lump will be seen and felt by the side of the anal verge below Hilton's line. This can be conveniently palpated with an index finger inside the anal canal and a thumb superficial to the swelling. This abscess is less painful than the ischiorectal abscess as the skin can expand easily in this region.

(ii) **ISCHIORECTAL:** Patient will complain of excruciating throbbing pain by the side of the anal canal. Inspection will reveal brawny edematous swelling. It is very tender swelling with or without fluctuation. One should not wait for fluctuation to appear. By rectal examination one can feel the tender swelling on one side of the rectum. This abscess may travel to the opposite side posteriorly.

(iii) **PELVI-RECTAL ABSCESS:** Clinically, this abscess mimics the pelvic abscess in many respects. This abscess lies above the levator ani but below the pelvic peritoneum.

Submucous and *fissure abscesses* can be diagnosed by history and rectal examination. In any case of anorectal abscess, Crohn's disease must be eliminated.

FISTULA-IN-ANO

This is a track lined by granulation tissue which opens deeply in the anal canal or rectum and superficially on the skin around the anus. Sometimes the track does not open into the anal canal or rectum, when it should better be called a 'sinus'. Mostly these fistulae develop from anorectal abscess which burst spontaneously or was incised inadequately.

An anal fistula may occur with or without symptoms. A history of intermittent swelling with pain, discomfort and discharge in the perianal region can often be obtained. Inspection and palpation usually delineate the course and nature of the fistula. After discovery of an external opening it is possible to palpate the fibrous cord subcutaneously leading toward the anal canal. This is better palpated bidigitally—index finger inside the lumen of the anal canal and the thumb superficially around the anus. All sides should be palpated for presence of multiple fistulae or sinuses. The most important part in rectal examination is to feel the anorectal sling and to find out whether the internal opening is above or below that sling. When the internal opening is above the anorectal sling the fistula is said to be a '*high fistula*' and if the inner opening is below the anorectal sling the fistula is said to be a '*low fistula*'. While a low fistula can be laid open without fear of incontinence, treatment of a high fistula is very difficult and calls for expert hands in this speciality. Students are referred to page 620 for recapitulation of Goodsall's rule. Proctoscopy may indicate the inner opening. Sigmoidoscopy is mandatory to rule out 'proximal disease', be it inflammatory, neoplastic or otherwise. In every instance, a barium enema should be performed. Scrapings from fistula should be examined bacteriologically. In case of recurrent and multiple fistulae one should always try to eliminate tuberculosis, Crohn's disease, ulcerative colitis, lymphogranuloma inguinale and colloid carcinoma of the rectum. A high index of suspicion is necessary in this respect.

PILONIDAL SINUS

The word 'pilonidal' means nest of hairs. It is a sinus which *contains a free tuft of hairs.* These sinuses are commonly found in the skin covering the sacrum and coccyx, between the fingers (in hair dressers) and at the umbilicus. Hairs break off by friction and then find entry either through the open mouth of the sudoriferous gland or through the soften skin either by sweat or some form of dermatitis. This condition is mainly seen between 15 and 40 years. At this age the mouth of sudoriferous gland becomes wider. It is rare before puberty and after 40 years. It is common in men than women. It is typically common in dark-haired, hirsute white men.

The common symptoms are pain and discharge. Pain may be from dull ache to throbbing (particularly when the opening is closed and the discharge becomes purulent and stagnant inside). When the discharge comes out the pain is relieved. Discharge varies from a little serum to a sudden gush of pus. Pilonidal sinuses are always in the midline of the natal cleft over the lowest part of the sacrum and coccyx. This differentiates this condition from anal fistula. Palpation of the skin and subcutaneous tissues around the sinus reveals areas of subcutaneous induration. Inguinal lymph nodes do not enlarge because the infection is mostly mild and chronic. The skin around the sinus is usually normal. But when infected it becomes red and tender. There may be puckered scar of old infected sinus. Pilonidal sinus is also seen in interdigital cleft in barber's hand, axilla and umbilicus.

RECTAL PROLAPSE

This condition is seen at the extremes of life—in children between 1 and 3 years and in the elderly after 40 years of age. In children direct downward course of the rectum due to undeveloped sacral curve and reduced anal tone predispose. Women are more commonly affected than men. The main complaint is that something is coming out per rectum during defecation. It may come out spontaneously even on standing, walking or coughing. The prolapse may reduce spontaneously or require digital reduction. An enquiry should be made into the presence or absence of other symptoms, e.g., anorectal bleeding, mucous discharge, anal pain, the bowel habit, the control of defecation etc.

Inspection is probably the single most important part of examination. If the prolapse is not immediately visible, it is often possible to make it appear by asking the patient to perform a Valsalva maneuver. This examination is done in the left lateral position or squatting position. Hemorrhoids or polyps can be easily diagnosed. Main difficulty in diagnosis is between mucosal (partial) and complete rectal prolapse. However, this should not present a problem if it is remembered that a mucosal prolapse consists of only two layers of mucosa, whilst a complete prolapse consists of full thickness of rectal wall. Furthermore there may be a sulcus between the prolapse and the inside of the anal canal. If the length of the prolapse is less than 3.75 cm it is a partial prolapse and if it is more than this it is a complete prolapse. A finger in the anal canal can estimate the tone of the anal sphincter and levator ani. Proctoscopy will exclude other pathologies. Double contrast barium enema and colonoscopy will be required if no obvious cause of prolapse can be found out. There may be associated neoplastic lesion further up.

PERIANAL CROHN'S DISEASE

It must be remembered that 75% of patients with Crohn's disease develop perianal complication. This incidence of course depends on the site of gastrointestinal pathology—the more distal is the disease, higher is the rate of perianal complications. More interesting feature is that perianal complications of Crohn's disease may even appear before the Crohn's disease elsewhere in the GI tract even by a few years. The perianal complications can be classified into primary conditions and secondary conditions. *Primary conditions* are fissures, cavitating ulcers like intestinal disease and ulcerated piles. *Secondary conditions* are strictures, skin tags, fistulae and infective abscesses.

PERIANAL WARTS (CONDYLOMATA ACUMINATA) (FIG. 36.9)

These are warts caused by a virus which is a variant of the papilloma virus responsible

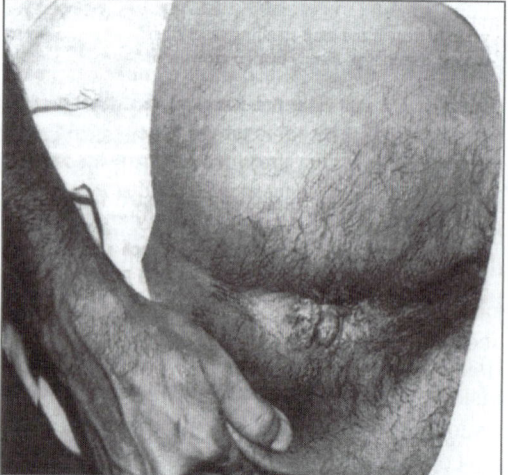

Fig. 36.9: Shows a case of condyloma acuminatum in the anal region.

for skin warts. These are often transmitted by sexual contact, hence these may be present or associated with sexually transmitted disease, e.g., gonorrhea, syphilis, AIDS and herpes genitalis. These are also noticed in patients whose immune response has been depressed with steroids or other forms of chemotherapy.

On inspection perianal warts are multiple, pedunculated, papilliferous lesions seen around the anus. Sometimes the whole perineum is affected, even including the labia majora or the back of the scrotum.

Main symptoms are irritation, discomfort and pain from rubbing against the clothings. These may ulcerate and become infected.

CONDYLOMA LATA

These are broad based, flat topped, raised and white papules. These are actually the manifestation of secondary syphilis. These are highly contagious.

PROCTALGIA FUGAX

Sometimes the patient presents to the doctor with severe rectal pain. The pain appears suddenly and cramp-like in nature, deep inside the anal canal and usually at night. Such pain usually passes off spontaneously after a few minutes or even hours. Nothing can be prescribed to relieve such pain.

Its cause is unknown, as general and rectal examinations are usually normal. It may be suggested that such pain is caused by spasm of the muscles of the pelvic floor.

CARCINOMA OF THE RECTUM

Unlike other carcinomas this condition may be seen even in young patients. So age is not criterion for diagnosis. If it occurs in the young it is very virulent. Bleeding is the most constant symptom. It may bleed during defecation or it may simply stain the underclothing. In case of proliferative growth in ampulla the patient feels the sense of incomplete defecation even after full opening of the bowel. The patient may endeavor to empty the rectum several times a day often with passage of blood and mucus ('spurious diarrhea'). The patient often gets up in the morning with an urgent urge for defecation. In case of annular carcinoma affecting the upper part of the rectum the patient complains of increasing constipation needing increasing dose of purgative and as a result diarrhea ensues. It is also due to the fact that hard feces irritate the colon leading to diarrhea. Pain is a late symptom, but pain of colicky character may be experienced by patients with annular growth of the rectosigmoid junction due to some degree of intestinal obstruction. When any growth has invaded beyond the rectal wall pain will be experienced. Weight loss and anemia are the usual features. Abdominal examination is usually negative. In annular growth of the rectosigmoid junction the colon loaded with feces may be felt. Pitting on pressure is diagnostic. Liver should always be palpated for metastasis. Peritoneum may be studded with secondary deposits. Ascites may be the result. About 90% of rectal cancers can be felt by finger for rectal examination. Induration of the base of growth is very significant be it an ulcerative or proliferative growth. After the finger has been withdrawn, it will be smeared with blood and mucus if the finger has touched the carcinoma. The mobility of the growth should be tested. At times enlarged iliac group of nodes can be felt through the rectum. One should always perform sigmoidoscopy, double-contrast barium enema X-ray, colonoscopy (if possible) and biopsy of the growth.

BLEEDING PER ANUM

Surgical causes will only be considered here. Causes can be best classified into A. Those which give rise to pain and B. Those which are painless.

A. In this group are: (i) Fissure-in-ano; (ii) Fistula-in-ano; (iii) Carcinoma of the anal canal; (iv) Ruptured perineal haematoma; (v) Ruptured-anorectal abscess; (vi) Endometriosis; (vii) Injury etc.

B. In this group are: (i) Blood alone—Polyp, villous adenoma and diverticular disease; (ii) Blood after defecation—hemorrhoids; (iii) Blood with mucus—ulcerative colitis, Crohn's disease, intussusception, ischemic colon, etc.; (iv) Blood mixed with stool—carcinoma of the colon; (v) Blood streaked on stool—carcinoma of the rectum.

Examination and investigation should be in the line discussed above.

ANAL CONDITIONS WITH PAIN

Pain alone: After defecation—anal fissure; spontaneously at night—proctalgia fugax.
Pain with bleeding: Anal fissure, thrombosed and strangulated anal piles, anal carcinoma, rupture of anorectal abscess.
Pain with lump: Perianal hematoma, anorectal abscess, carcinoma of the anal canal.
Pain with fistula: Fistula-in-ano.
Pain with something coming out with bleeding: Prolapse rectum, prolapsed hemorrhoid, prolapse rectal polyp, intussusception (rarely).

STRICTURE OF THE RECTUM AND ANAL CANAL

Causes and diagnosis

1. **Congenital** narrowing of the lumen occurs at the level of the anal membrane.
2. **Traumatic:** (i) Injury to the rectum (penetrating injury, impaction of the fetal head during parturition), (ii) Following operations like hemorrhoidectomy due to injudicious removal of the skin or mucous membrane. This may occur after operations for fistula, excision of villous growth or polypus. To prevent stricture formation following these operations frequent digital dilatation is advised during the healing process.
3. **Inflammatory:** In this group the most important is lymphogranuloma inguinale—a form of venereal disease. This disease is commoner in women and starts as a sore in the posterior vaginal wall. Frei's intradermal test is confirmatory. Stricture may also develop due to cicatricial contraction during healing process of the ulcers of the rectum caused by tuberculosis, syphilis, gonorrhea, soft sore, bilharziasis, dysentery, etc.
4. **Spasmodic:** Though spasmodic strictures are temporary, yet in untreated and long-standing cases fibrous stenosis may result.
5. **Neoplastic:** Commonly this is a malignant stricture, e.g., annular carcinoma. Rarely benign growths may lead to stenosis, e.g., villous adenoma.
6. **General:** In this group are endometriosis (frequent menstruation with pain in the first two days), senile anal stenosis due to chronic internal sphincter contraction, irradiation stricture, etc.

PERINEAL FISTULAE

Causes and diagnosis:
1. **Fistula-in-ano:** This is the most common cause of a fistula in the perineal region. Diagnosis is made by the previous history of an anal abscess which has incised or burst giving rise to a fistula. It may be incomplete or complete communicating with the rectum. Sometimes, the fistula track is extensive—the horse-shoe type—connecting the ischiorectal fossa of each side. Tuberculous proctitis, ulcerative colitis, Crohn's disease, colloid carcinoma of the rectum, lymphogranuloma, bilharziasis may be the cause of fistula-in-ano.
2. **Urethral fistula:** This is the result of a neglected periurethral abscess which develops proximal to the urethral stricture. When the abscess is incised or bursts urine leaks out through the wound during micturition. A hard fibrous tract is formed and can be traced up to the urethra. It may be single or multiple—when the term 'watering-can' perineum is used (*see* **Fig. 5.3**, page 87).
3. **Fistula or sinus in connection with bone:** Exceptionally, a sinus in the perineum may be due to osteomyelitis (pyogenic or tuberculous) of the tuber ischii, sacrum or coccyx.
4. **Pilonidal sinus**—so called because of the presence of a tuft of hair in its interior—is commonly situated in the internatal cleft near the tip of the coccyx.
5. **Infected postanal dermoid:** When a dermoid occurring in front of the coccyx becomes infected and opened, a sinus may develop in the perineum.

All fistulous tracks may be visualized by an X-ray film taken after injecting lipiodol.

PRURITUS ANI

Causes are best classified into: (a) causes in the rectum and anal canal, (b) in the vagina, (c) in the skin, (d) due to parasites and (e) general causes.
(a) *Pruritus from mucous discharge from the anus:* Hemorrhoids, fissures, fistula, polyps, carcinoma (particularly the colloid variety), skin tags, condyloma, etc.
(b) *Pruritus from the vaginal discharge*: Trichomonas vaginitis, Monilial vaginitis, gonorrhea, cervical erosions, etc.
(c) *Pruritus from skin diseases*: Tinea cruris, monilial infections, infections from diabetes (Monilial infections are also commoner in diabetes).
(d) *Pruritus from the parasites*—mainly thread worms.
(e) In the *general group* are poor hygiene, psychoneuroses and leakage of liquid paraffin from its excessive use.

Algorithmic Approach to Patient with Rectal Disorders

Patient presents with rectal symptoms (bleeding, pain, discharge, prolapse, altered bowel habits)

↓

Is there rectal bleeding?
- Yes → Determine **bright red (active/lower GI bleed)** vs **dark red blood (old/upper GI bleed)**
  - Bright red blood → **Hemorrhoids, anal fissure, rectal cancer, proctitis**
  - Dark red blood → **IBD, diverticulosis, ischemic colitis, rectal cancer**
- No → Proceed to next step

↓

Is there rectal pain?
- Yes → Determine **pain type**
  - Throbbing pain → Suggests **anorectal abscess, deep fistula**
  - Sharp, cutting pain → Suggests **anal fissure, acute thrombosed hemorrhoids**
  - Dull, persistent pain → Suggests **rectal cancer, advanced fistula**
- No → Proceed to next step

↓

Is there rectal prolapse or a palpable mass?
- Yes → Differentiate by **digital rectal examination (DRE)**
  - Soft, pedunculated mass → **Rectal polyp, mucosal prolapse**
  - Firm, Irregular Mass → **Rectal cancer, stricture**
- No → Proceed to next step

↓

Is there mucus or purulent discharge?
- Yes → Determine likely cause
  - Mucus discharge → Suggests **IBD (ulcerative colitis, crohn's), rectal prolapse**
  - Purulent discharge → Suggests **fistula-in-ano, perianal abscess, sti (Gonorrhea, chlamydia)**
- No → Proceed to next step

↓

Are there altered bowel habits (constipation, diarrhea)?
- Yes → Consider underlying conditions
  - Chronic constipation → Suggests **strictures, rectal cancer, IBS**
  - Recurrent diarrhea → Suggests **IBD, malabsorption, infectious colitis**
- No → Consider functional disorders

↓

Perform rectal examination (DRE, proctoscopy, sigmoidoscopy, imaging)
- Prolapsed mass → Determine **piles vs rectal prolapse**
- Digital rectal examination (DRE) → Evaluate **mass, strictures, ulcers, growths**
- Proctoscopy/Sigmoidoscopy → Identify **hemorrhoids, polyps, malignancy**
- Biopsy (If malignancy suspected) → Confirm diagnosis

↓

Confirm diagnosis and initiate treatment based on findings
- Medical therapy → **Hemorrhoids, fissure-in-Ano, IBD, mild proctitis**
- Surgical management → **Fistula-in-Ano, rectal cancer, strangulated hemorrhoids**
- Lifestyle modifications → **High-fiber diet, SITZ baths for mild cases**

Examination of a Urinary Case

CHAPTER 37

HISTORY

1. **Age:** Wilms' tumor (nephroblastoma) is a disease of childhood below 4 years of age. Adenocarcinoma or renal cell carcinoma (hypernephroma) of the kidney is mainly seen in middle-aged individuals above 40 years of age. Bilateral polycystic kidney is also seen in individuals above 40 years of age. Acute pyelonephritis may occur at puberty, just after marriage (honeymoon pyelitis) and during pregnancy. Majority of renal calculi are seen between the ages of 30 and 50 years. Both benign hypertrophy of prostate and carcinoma of prostate are diseases of old age above 50 years of age, mostly above 60 years.
2. **Sex:** Acute pyelonephritis and cystitis are more common in females due to their short and straight urethra through which organisms find easy access. Incidence of renal stone is seen equally in males and females. Adenocarcinoma or renal cell carcinoma occurs more commonly in men than women in the ratio of 2:1. Prostatic diseases are obviously seen in males only.
3. **Residence:** Vesical calculus is more common in Rajasthan and Punjab. Schistosomiasis is more common in greater part of Africa, Israel, Syria, Iran and Iraq.
4. **Social Status:** Both renal calculus and vesical calculus are more often seen in poorer class of people may be due to lack of regular adequate diet. Though such predilection cannot be given much importance.
5. **Occupation:** Bladder carcinoma is more seen among workers in aniline dye factories, of dyeing industry, rubber and cable industries, of printing industry and in gas workers. People working in leather industry, textile industry and hairdressers also have higher incidence of bladder cancer.

History taking in urinary case

Aspect	Clinical significance	Patient-friendly questions
Pain	Dull → Tumor, Colicky → Stone	"Where exactly do you feel the pain? Does it move anywhere?"
Hematuria	Initial → Urethra, Terminal → Bladder, Total → Kidney	"Have you noticed blood in your urine? Was it at the start, middle, or end?"
Urinary frequency	Daytime (UTI, diabetes), nighttime (BPH, bladder cancer)	"Do you need to urinate frequently? More during the day or night?"
Urinary retention	Acute → Painful, Chronic → Painless	"Do you feel you cannot empty your bladder completely?"
Family history	Bladder cancer, kidney stones, polycystic kidney	"Has anyone in your family had kidney or bladder issues?"

COMPLAINTS

1. **Pain:** Enquire about its *onset, duration, progress* and *nature*. One should also ask whether the pain has any radiation or not, whether it is referred or not and what is its *relation with micturition*. **RENAL PAIN** is usually felt as a *dull* and *constant ache* mainly at the angle between the outer border of the erector spinae muscle and the lower border of the 12th rib (renal angle). This pain may even be *severe*. This pain often spreads along the subcostal area towards the umbilicus. The patient typically describes renal pain by putting his hand on the waist with his fingers spreading backwards to cover the renal angle and his thumb forwards pointing towards the umbilicus

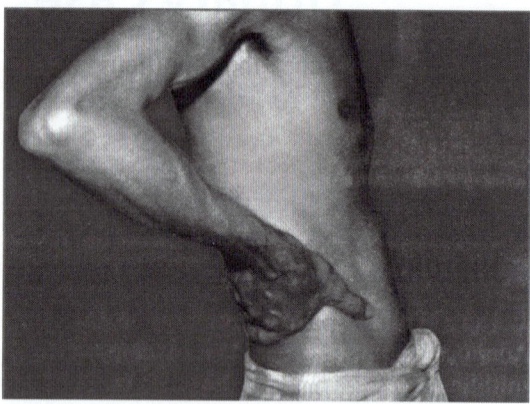

Fig. 37.1: When a patient experiences renal pain and he is asked to show with his hand the site of pain, this is the usual position of the hand of the patient as shown in the figure.

(Fig. 37.1). If there is significant enlargement of the kidney, the peritoneum is stretched and the pain is localized anteriorly at the upper and outer quadrant of the abdomen. Renal pain is mainly caused by distension of the renal capsule and the pelvis. Acute pyelonephritis, tuberculosis, renal stone may cause this typical pain. Sometimes the patient may feel pain in the opposite kidney which hypertrophies in order to compensate the impaired function of its fellow. It must be remembered that many renal diseases are painless because their progression is so slow that capsular distension does not occur. Such diseases include cancer, chronic pyelonephritis, staghorn calculus, tuberculosis, etc. The students are warned not to use the term "Renal Colic". Colicky pain only develops when a muscular conducting tube gets obstructed. In case of urinary organs such structure is the ureter and colic only develops from this structure. A severe renal pain which fluctuates in its severity is often called the 'renal colic' by mistake. This so called "colic" neither has the typical griping character nor disappears completely between the attacks.

URETERIC PAIN is mainly caused by acute obstruction either by passage of a stone or a blood clot. There is capsular distension along with severe *colicky pain* due to spasm of the renal pelvis and ureteric muscle. This characteristically starts from the renal angle and radiates downwards *along the course of the ureter,* around the waist obliquely across the abdomen to the groin, base of the penis and to the scrotum in case of males and to the labia majora in case of females and to the inner side of the upper part of the thigh (Fig. 37.2). The point where this ureteric pain begins usually corresponds to the level of the obstruction. This is a *referred pain* due to common innervation of the upper ureter and the testis (T11-12) and the lower ureter and the inner side of the upper part of the thigh (L1,

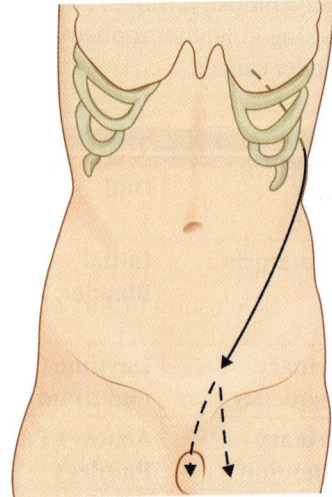

Fig. 37.2: Diagrammatic representation of radiation of pain in case of ureteric colic.

through genitofemoral nerve). The severity and colicky nature of this pain are caused by the hyperperistalsis and spasm of the smooth muscle of the ureter as it attempts to get rid of a foreign body. It is of griping nature and comes in waves with exacerbations and wanes. The pain passes off as suddenly as it came to give a pain-free interval between the attacks. The patient virtually tosses over the bed during the attacks trying in vain to get relief. This pain is often accompanied by nausea and vomiting.

The patient often gives history that his attacks of colic follow episodes of jolting or unusual movements. Such history suggests that he has a stone in the ureter, which moves by such jolting or unusual physical activity and thus causing the colic.

The clinician may be able to judge the position of the stone by the history of pain. If the stone is lodged in the upper ureter the pain radiates to the testicle (T11-12). When the stone is in the middle of the ureter the pain is referred to the McBurney's point on the right side resembling appendicitis and on the left side simulates diverticulitis (T12-L1). When the stone approaches the bladder, symptoms of vesical irritability appear and the pain may be referred to the penis, labia majora and inner side of the thigh.

VESICAL PAIN varies from mild discomfort to an intense strangury. Pain from bladder is usually dull, midline suprapubic pain which may become worse on micturition. *'Strangury' is a painful desire to micturate which starts in the bladder and radiates into the urethra, but it neither produces any urine nor relieves the pain.* The overdistended bladder in acute retention will cause agonizing pain in the suprapubic area. Interstitial cystitis and vesical ulceration caused by tuberculosis or bilharziasis may cause suprapubic discomfort when the bladder becomes full and is usually relieved by urination. In chronic retention of urine the patient experiences little or no suprapubic discomfort even though the bladder reaches the umbilicus. Cystitis, the most common cause of bladder pain, does not produce any pain over the suprapubic region but is referred to the distal urethra during micturition. Pain is often referred to the tip of the penis with or without hematuria towards the end of micturition and is diagnostic of vesical calculus. In children, vesical calculus is indicated by sudden screaming and pulling at the prepuce during micturition.

PROSTATIC PAIN is not common though occasionally come across when the prostate is inflamed. The patient may feel a vague discomfort or fullness in the perineal or rectal area (S2-4). It is often associated with difficulty in passing urine. Due to the location patient often thinks the pain is coming from the rectum. Throbbing pain in the perineum indicates prostatic abscess. Lumbosacral backache is occasionally experienced as referred pain from the prostate but is not a common symptom of prostatitis.

URETHRAL PAIN occurs during or at the end of micturition. Scalding pain during micturition is characteristic of acute urethritis.

2. **Swelling:** Enquire about its *mode of onset, duration, progress* and *unilateral* or *bilateral*. Patient may present with a swelling in the loin. When a middle-aged man comes with such a swelling with short history one must suspect a carcinoma in the kidney. This may or may not be associated with hematuria. It is generally a painless condition. Similar painless swelling may be the presenting feature in case of children under the age of 5 years. This is characteristic of nephroblastoma. Sometimes a swelling with long history may become diminished in size immediately after passing urine. This is a case of intermittent hydronephrosis. Bilateral renal swelling in a man of 40 years of age is typical of polycystic disease of the kidney. One kidney may be affected earlier or may be more swollen than the other kidney to cause confusion to the diagnosis (the case is then considered to be unilateral swelling of the kidney).

3. **Hematuria:** Bloody urine is a dangerous symptom which cannot be ignored. Enquiry must be made about its *quantity*, its *relation to micturition*—whether blood appears at the beginning of the act (urethral), towards the end of the act (vesical) or is intimately mixed throughout the process (prerenal, renal or vesical). Whether hematuria is *associated with pain* or not? Some individuals will pass red urine after eating beets or taking laxatives containing phenolphthalein, in which case the urine is translucent and does not contain red cells. Sometimes children may pass red urine after ingestion of cakes, cold drinks, fruit juice containing rhodamine B. Hemoglobinuria following hemolytic syndromes may also cause the urine to be red. Details of the causes of hematuria have been discussed later in this chapter.

4. **Frequency of micturition:** In a few diseases of the urinary system there will be increased frequency of micturition. Inflammation of the bladder and benign hypertrophy of the prostate are the most common conditions which cause increased frequency of micturition **(Figs. 37.3A and B)**. Retention of urine in the bladder following inadequate emptying may be one of the important causes of the frequency of micturition. This is often first noticed at night, so the patient must be asked whether the frequency of micturition is more at night (nocturnal micturition) or not. 24 hours frequency should be recorded as a day/night ratio. The various causes of increased frequency of micturition are discussed later in this chapter.

5. **Difficulty in urination (dysuria):** Progressive loss of force and caliber of the urinary stream is noted as a man grows older. In case of prostatic obstruction there is a delay in starting the act of micturition. The stream instead of being projectile tends to fall vertically. The patient should be asked whether straining improves the stream (e.g., urethral stricture) or retards the stream (e.g., enlarged prostate—the median lobe pressing on the internal urethral meatus). Sudden stoppage of the stream during micturition is suggestive of a vesical calculus or pedunculated papilloma of the bladder, the micturition may be started again by changing posture.

6. **Retention of urine:** When a patient fails to pass urine the condition is called retention of urine. There are two forms of retention—acute and chronic. Acute retention is painful whereas

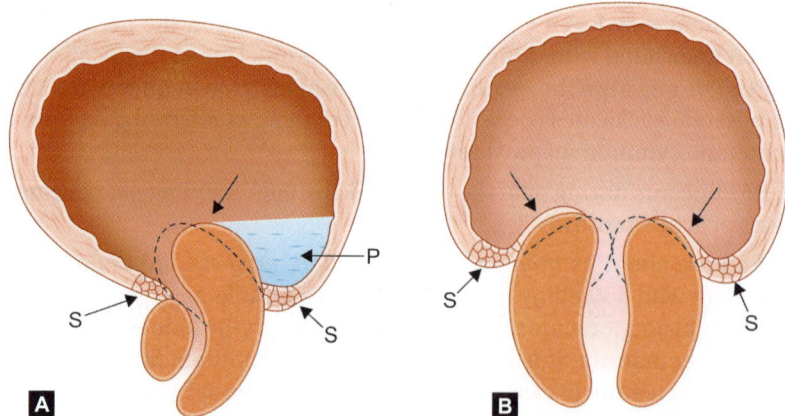

Figs. 37.3A and B: Diagrams showing how straining hinders the act of micturition when the prostate is enlarged. (A) The median lobe is enlarged and straining increases the intravesical pressure depressing the median lobe forward thus occluding the internal urethral meatus. (B) The lateral two lobes are enlarged and increased intravesical pressure will lead to approximation of the intravesical parts of the lateral lobes and thus occludes the internal urethral meatus. 'P'—post prostatic pouch holding the residual urine; 'S'—internal sphincter, note that the prostate enlarges through the sphincter and causes urgency.

chronic retention is painless. When infection supervenes chronic retention the condition becomes painful. In acute retention the patient cries in agony urgently begging to be relieved. In chronic retention the bladder may be distended up to the umbilicus, but the patient is absolutely ignorant of the condition and assumes a cheerful look.

7. **Anuria:** In this condition urine is not excreted by the kidneys therefore the bladder remains empty. In retention urine is formed but it cannot be voided due to obstruction in the urethra, so the bladder becomes full of urine and distended. The causes of anuria are: (a) prerenal, e.g., shock; (b) renal, e.g., pyelonephritis, glomerulonephritis, incompatible blood transfusion, crush syndrome and renal tuberculosis; (c) postrenal, e.g., calculus anuria, accidental ligature of both ureters during the operation of hysterectomy.

8. **Discharge from the urethra:** In acute gonococcal urethritis the discharge is profuse and purulent. In chronic urethritis or prostatitis a glairy fluid (gleet) is noticed to be discharged particularly in the morning just before micturition.

9. **Incontinence:** There are many reasons of incontinence. The history often gives a clue to the diagnosis. There are five types of incontinence:—(1) *True incontinence*—when the patient passes urine without warning. It must be remembered that the bladder remains empty in this condition. (2) *False (overflow) incontinence*—when urine overflows from the distended bladder. (3) *Automatic bladder*—when there is periodic contraction of the bladder without patient's knowledge. (4) *Urgency incontinence*—when the patient feels urgency to pass urine and if it is not possible a few drops may come out. This occurs in acute cystitis particularly in women and in benign hypertrophy of prostate in men. (5) *Stress incontinence*—when a few drops of urine come out during physical strain (e.g., coughing, laughing, rising from a chair, etc.), due to slight weakness of the sphincteric mechanism.

10. **Renal failure:** Symptoms of renal failure such as headache, drowsiness, insomnia, thirst, hiccough, vomiting, convulsion, etc., may be met with.

11. **Gastrointestinal syndromes:** Patients with acute pyelonephritis will not only suffer from localized backache, fever, chill, rigor, symptoms of irritability but also from generalized abdominal pain and distension. Patients with ureteric colic often suffer from severe nausea, vomiting and abdominal distension. Afferent stimuli from the renal capsule or musculature of the pelvis may cause pylorospasm (symptoms of peptic ulcer) by reflex action. Inflammations and swellings of the kidney may produce symptoms due to displacement and irritation of the intraperitoneal viscera lying in close relation with the kidney concerned (e.g., hepatic flexure of the colon, the duodenum, the head of the pancreas, the liver and the gallbladder in case of the right kidney; whereas splenic flexure of the colon, tail of the pancreas and stomach in case of left kidney). The symptoms arising from chronic renal diseases (e.g., chronic pyelonephritis, hydronephrosis, staghorn calculus, cancer, etc.), may in every way simulate those of other abdominal pathologies such as peptic ulcer, gallbladder, appendicitis, etc. So, if a thorough survey of the gastrointestinal (GI) tract does not reveal the cause of the symptoms, the clinician should keep every consideration to study the urinary tract.

Past history: This is very much important and should never be omitted. Whether the patient had suffered from any urinary trouble before? If he had suffered from gonorrhea, syphilis or tuberculosis? A patient, who had suffered from pulmonary tuberculosis or bone tuberculosis even in his childhood, if presents with vague symptoms this time (after about 20 years), may be suffering from tuberculous affection of the kidney. Enquiry must be made whether the patient was taking any medicine or not. Phenacetin, cyclophosphamide, saccharine and excessive caffeine intake have been incriminated to cause bladder cancer.

■ PHYSICAL EXAMINATION

A. **GENERAL SURVEY:** The tongue should be examined. Whether it is dry or moist (the protruded tongue is touched), clear or covered with white or brown fur. Whether the patient is drowsy or not. Dry and covered tongue with drowsiness and delirium are features of uremia. Cachexia is sometimes detected in cases of malignancy of kidney, urinary bladder and in renal tuberculosis. Pulse and temperature are always recorded. Cheyne-Stokes respiration may be noticed in uremia. Blood pressure is always examined, as hypertension is often present with various kidney diseases, e.g., renal ischemia, bilateral polycystic kidney, hydronephrosis, renal carcinoma etc. Skin is rough and dry and there is edema of face in renal failure.

B. **LOCAL EXAMINATION:**

1. **EXAMINATION OF THE KIDNEY:**

INSPECTION: In *recumbent position* a kidney swelling cannot be seen. However, a huge kidney swelling of hydronephrosis or nephroblastoma in case of children may be seen as the fullness of the corresponding lumbar region. The swelling moves slightly with respiration. In *sitting posture* from behind fullness of the area just below the last rib and lateral to the sacrospinalis muscle is more evident in case of renal swelling (particularly malignancy) and perinephric infection. Presence and persistence of indentations in the skin from lying on wrinkled sheets suggests edema of the skin secondary to the perinephric abscess.

PALPATION: The kidneys lie rather high under the lower ribs. The right kidney is slightly lower than the left. It is very difficult to palpate the kidney by traditional method of palpation of the abdomen. By this one can only feel the lower part of the right kidney though with extreme difficulty. The best method of palpation of the kidney is by bimanual palpation **(Fig. 37.4)**. The patient lies on his back. A pillow is placed beneath the knees. One hand is placed behind the loin at the renal angle which is used to lift the kidney. The other hand is placed in front of the abdomen just below the costal margin. The patient is now asked to breathe deeply. With each phase of expiration when the abdominal musculature becomes more relaxed the hand in front is gradually pressed posteriorly. The hand behind is used to push the kidney anteriorly. After third or fourth expiration the hand in front is sufficiently pushed deep to feel the kidney, if it is palpable. Once the kidney can be felt, an attempt must be made to feel the kidney during inspiration. At this time the kidney moves downwards and the hand in front can trap the kidney and thus palpate the size, shape and consistency of the organ as it slips back into its normal position.

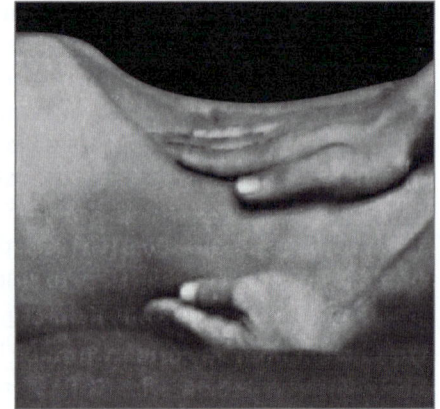

Fig. 37.4: Bimanual palpation of the kidney.

Another method of palpating the kidney is to ask the patient to lie on the sound side. The affected side is palpated by two hands in the similar way as has been discussed above (**Fig. 37.5**). This is quite a useful method of palpating a kidney. *In case of newborn babies* the hand is placed in such a way that the fingers will be on the renal angle and the thumb anteriorly. The two hands are used for two sides. The protagonists of this method have claimed it to be successful in 95% of cases.

In sitting posture one can feel the tenderness of the kidney and swelling quite effectively (**Fig. 37.6**). The patient sits up and folds his arms in front so that the back is stretched enough for better palpation. The clinician presses his thumb on the renal angle formed by the lower border of the 12th rib and outer border of erector spinae. This sign is of great value in determining tenderness of the kidney. This is known as 'the renal angle test' or 'Murphy's kidney punch' (**Fig. 37.7**).

A normal kidney is impalpable unless the patient is unusually thin. The *characteristics of a kidney swelling* are that: (i) it lies in the loin or can be moved into the loin, (ii) it is of reniform shape, (iii) it is a ballotable swelling, (iv) it moves slightly with respiration, (v) there is always a band of colonic resonance anteriorly, (vi) it is dull posteriorly, (vii) however, large may be in case of the renal swelling fingers can be insinuated between the costal margin and the swelling.

When palpable, note its size, shape, surface, consistency, etc. Whether the consistency is solid or cystic. A solid renal swelling suggests compensatory hypertrophy, a neoplasm, advanced tuberculosis, etc., whereas a cystic swelling is mainly due to hydronephrosis, pyonephrosis, a solitary cyst or polycystic kidney. Fluctuation can be elicited, though with difficulty, in a hydronephrosis or a large solitary cyst. In case of pyonephrosis this test cannot be positive due to inflammatory thickening of the surrounding tissues. Superficial edema as evidenced by pitting on pressure, is suggestive of perinephric abscess.

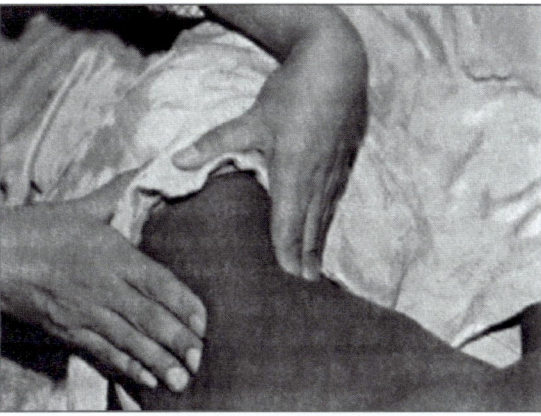

Fig. 37.5: The patient is turned laterally on his sound side. The diseased kidney is palpated bimanually as mentioned in the text. This is a useful method of palpating a kidney.

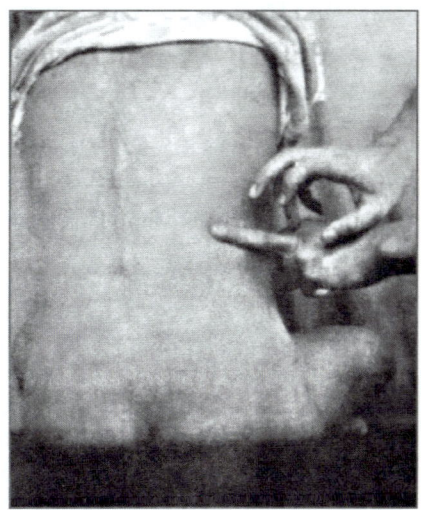

Fig. 37.6: A differentiating point between the renal swelling and splenic swelling is to percuss the loin just outside the erector spinae. This area is normally resonant due to the presence of colon. In case of renal swelling this area will be dull as the colon is pushed out by the swelling.

Ballottement: This is in fact a bimanual examination. With the patient supine one hand is insinuated behind the loin so that the pulps of the slightly flexed fingers are kept in contact with the area lateral to the erector spinae muscle and the other hand is laid flat on the abdomen so that the greater part of the flexor surfaces of the fingers overlie the kidney. Short, sharp, forward thrusts are made by the fingers of posteriorly placed hand (displacing). This will cause bouncing impact of the kidney swelling on the anteriorly placed hand (watching). So this is a ballotable swelling.

PERCUSSION: Anteriorly, there is always a band of resonance due to the presence of colon and small intestine, unless the tumor is large enough to push them aside. If there is difficulty in eliciting colonic resonance one can inflate the colon with air by means of a rubber catheter introduced through the anus (Baldwin's method). Posteriorly, a dull note will always be present lateral to the erector spinae muscle. At times a greatly enlarged kidney cannot be felt on palpation, particularly if it be soft (e.g., a large hydronephrosis). This swelling can be readily outlined by percussion both anteriorly and posteriorly. Percussion has got a special value in outlining an enlarging mass following renal trauma (progressive hemorrhage) where tenderness and muscle spasm prevent proper palpation.

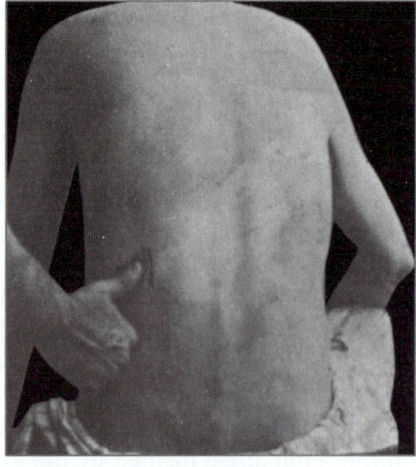

Fig. 37.7: Eliciting tenderness in the kidney by pressing at the renal angle (Murphy's kidney punch).

AUSCULTATION: Its importance particularly lies in cases of stenosis or aneurysm of the renal artery. A systolic bruit may be heard in these cases. Bruits may be heard over the femoral arteries in Leriche syndrome, which may be a cause of impotence.

2. **EXAMINATION OF THE URETER:** Ureter cannot be felt. But its terminal part may occasionally be felt, particularly when it is pathological, through the vagina or rectum.

3. **EXAMINATION OF THE BLADDER:** Bladder is a pelvic organ. It reaches abdomen when it is distended. At this time it can be palpated as an oval swelling just above the symphysis pubis. At least 150 mL of urine must be collected in the bladder to make it palpable above symphysis pubis. The swelling is elastic in feel and dull on percussion. Pressure induces a desire for micturition. In case of a swelling in the lower abdomen, one should always catheterize the bladder before examination is started. Many a swelling will be melted away by such catheterization. Sometimes in case of children a thickened hypertrophied bladder may be felt above symphysis pubis secondary to obstruction caused by posterior urethral valves. *Bimanual palpation* (abdominorectal or abdominovaginal) is the best way to determine the extent of vesical neoplasm. It must be done under general anesthesia. The finger in the rectum in case of male is pushed anteriorly above the prostate, whereas the other hand of the clinician is placed on suprapubic region and is gradually pressed posteriorly. Thus, the urinary bladder is felt bimanually (*see* **Fig. 37.8**).

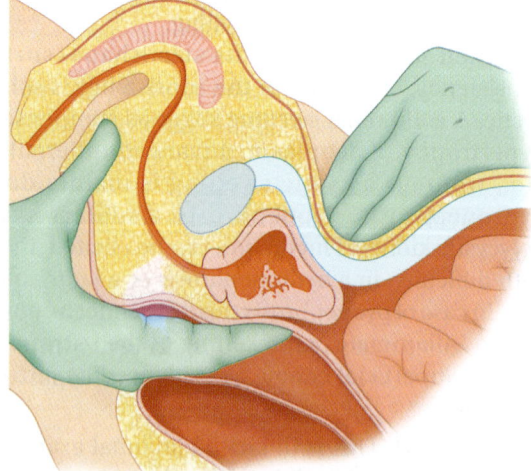

Fig. 37.8: Shows the method of bimanual palpation of the urinary bladder under general anesthesia. Note the position of the finger in the rectum and the hand on suprapubic region. The vesical neoplasm is indicated by dots. This is the best way clinically to determine the stage of the bladder cancer (see page 1282 of 'A Concise Textbook Of Surgery' by Dr. S. Das).

4. **EXAMINATION OF THE PROSTATE:** Prostate can only be palpated per rectum. The patient must empty his bladder first. If possible, watch the act of micturition—'how much is the loss of projectile force?' It is again emphasized that before doing rectal examination palpate the abdomen particularly the suprapubic region to know if the bladder is totally empty or not. Even after micturition if the bladder is not empty, this finding is important and predicts that the rectal examination will not be very reliable in providing necessary informations regarding the prostate. The findings of rectal examination are discussed below in the section of 'Rectal Examination'. Rectal examination for prostate is usually performed in Knee-elbow position or left lateral position. *Bimanual palpation* (abdominorectal or abdominovaginal) in lithotomy position is sometimes required. By this examination intravesical lobe of prostate can be felt. Fixity of this lobe in carcinoma can be ascertained. Residual urine in the postprostatic pouch can be felt as a soft swelling above the prostate. Seminal vesicles can be well palpated by this technique.

5. **EXAMINATION OF THE URETHRA**—for any discharge, fistula, tenderness, calculus or foreign body should be performed. In some instance, stricture may be felt as firm thickening.

6. **EXAMINATION OF THE EXTERNAL GENITALIA** is described in chapter 40.

7. **EXAMINATION OF THE PERINEUM** for swelling, redness and edema (periurethral abscess or perineal hematoma). Note if there are urethral fistulas.

8. **RECTAL EXAMINATION:** This examination is of tremendous importance in case of male patients. The prostate, the seminal vesicles and lower part of the base of the bladder can only be palpated through rectum. Rectal examination should be started by noting the tone of the external sphincter. Laxity of the sphincter suggests similar changes in the urinary sphincter. Before proceeding to palpate the seminal vesicles, it is customary to rule out pathologies in the lower part of the rectum and anal canal.

While palpating for the **prostate** the following points should be noted: (i) The *size*: Gradually the students will learn what is the normal size of prostate while palpating through the rectum. This is attained by practice. But it must be remembered that the clinical importance of prostatic hyperplasia is measured by the severity of symptoms and the amount of residual urine, and not by the size of the gland. (ii) *Consistency*: Normally the consistency of the prostate is like a rubber. It becomes mushy when congested, becomes indurated in chronic infection with or without calculi and becomes stony hard in carcinoma. (iii) *Surface*—whether smooth or irregular. (iv) Whether the *median groove* and the *lateral sulci* can be felt. It must be remembered that enlargement of median lobe may not be detected by rectal examination. But one can palpate this lobe per rectum with introduction of a urethral bougie. (v) *Mobility of the rectal mucosa* over the prostate is an important point to differentiate benign enlargement from malignant diseases of the prostate. (vi) *Prostatic massage* is important particularly in case of asymptomatic prostatitis. Diagnosis of such silent disease is important in preventing cystitis and epididymitis. Prostate should *not* be massaged in acute prostatitis, acute urethritis and obvious cancer of prostate.

Normally **seminal vesicles** are not palpable. They can only be palpated when they are diseased. These are best palpated in knee-elbow position. In case of acute inflammation (commonly gonococcal or *E. coli*) the vesicles feel cystic and tender. In case of chronic infection, particularly in tuberculous disease, they feel indurated and irregular.

The **base of the bladder** is also not felt normally per rectum. But a vesical calculus may be palpable per rectum. Malignant growth of the bladder can be well felt per rectum and bimanual palpation (abdominorectal in males and abdominovaginal in females) should always be performed under general anesthesia to detect the actual extent of the disease.

GENERAL EXAMINATION

Heart should be examined in case of suspected renal hypertension. **Lungs** should be examined in tuberculous affection of the kidneys as well as the seminal vesicles. Renal carcinoma mainly spreads by blood, and lungs are the most common site of metastasis. So, lungs should be examined as a routine in case of cancer of the kidney. One should examine for **Parathyroid** enlargement in recurrent renal calculi cases. One should also look for presence of other congenital abnormalities in cases of congenital anomalies of the kidney and ureter, e.g., double ureter, horseshoe kidney etc.

Radicular pain is often confused as kidney pain. Every patient who complains of flank pain should be examined for evidence of nerve root irritation. Arthritic changes in the costovertebral or costotransverse joints, hypertrophy of costovertebral ligaments pressing on a nerve, intervertebral disc disease and impingement of a rib spur on a subcostal nerve are the causes of such irritation. Radiculitis usually causes hyperesthesia of the area of skin supplied by the irritated peripheral nerve. Pressure exerted by the thumb over the costovertebral joints will reveal local tenderness at the point of emergence of the involved peripheral nerve.

SPECIAL INVESTIGATIONS

1. **BLOOD:** Erythrocytosis has been noted in association with renal carcinoma. The erythropoietin level in the plasma is also increased. Following radical surgery erythropoietin level and increased red cell count return to normal level. It is interesting to note that if metastases develop later erythrocytosis returns. Hypochromic anemia sometimes occurs in association with pyelonephritis, uremia and even carcinoma. Immunoassay examination of the blood for certain tumor markers is now possible. CEA (carcinoembryonic antigen) level becomes high in adenocarcinoma of the kidney. Alpha fetoprotein level also goes up in case of carcinoma of urinary bladder.

2. **URINE:** Proper collection of urine is of utmost importance. In both men and women the urethra harbors bacteria and few pus cells. Mid-stream urine should be collected for examination. In an infected case '2-glass' test affords valuable information. Urine is first voided in a test tube for about 10–15 mL and then the stream is directed to the 2nd test tube for the same amount of sample. Turbidity in the first glass suggests urethritis whereas turbidity in the 2nd glass suggests cystitis. First of all, general microscopic examination of the urine should be performed for the presence of RBC, crystals of oxalates, phosphates or cystine, bacteria, pus cells and malignant cells. *Cytological examination* of urinary sediment is sensitive and specific for poorly differentiated cancer cells anywhere in the urinary tract. Culture in ordinary or special culture media should be performed if bacteria and/or pus cells are detected in the urine. Sensitivity test to various antibiotics (antibiogram) should be performed when the culture becomes positive. Animal (guineapig) inoculation test is important if tuberculosis is suspected. When the urine is acid in reaction, contains pus cells and is sterile in ordinary culture, one should suspect renal tuberculosis. Acid-fast staining should be performed with the centrifuged sediments from 15 mL of urine. It will reveal tubercle bacilli in about 70–80% of cases. This may be confirmed by animal inoculation test or better by special culture. In the latter case the result is obtained in three weeks instead of six weeks as in animal inoculation. Urinary pH is important. It ranges normally from 4.5 to 7.5. A pH below 4.5 is typical of diabetic acidosis whereas a pH above 7.5 suggests presence of urea-splitting organisms. *Specific gravity* of the urine is also examined

particularly of the morning sample collected after 12 hours of overnight restriction of fluid. The specific gravity of this urine is normally about 1.020. If this specific gravity becomes less than 1.010 it is indicative of renal failure.

Dipsticks impregnated with chemicals which change color in presence of blood, sugar or protein are convenient way to screen urine for various abnormalities. These (Multistix or Labstix) are often used nowadays.

3. **RENAL FUNCTION TESTS:** (a) *Protein urea*: Amount of protein up to 100 mg per 24 hours is normal. Heavy protein urea is seen in nephrosis and at times glomerulonephritis. (b) *Specific gravity* of urine is a simple and significant test of renal function. Kidneys can concentrate up to 1.040 at the age below 40 and about 1.030 at the age of 50. Specific gravity of urine voided in the early morning is important and if it is less than 1.010 one may suspect poor function of the kidneys. (c) The *PSP* test: The patient is instructed to pass urine. Exactly 1 mL of phenol-sulfonphthalein is given intravenously. The patient is allowed to drink no more than 20 mL of water during each of the two subsequent half hour periods. Urine specimens are collected at half-hour intervals. The average amount of dye normally recovered in the first half-hour sample is 50–60%, the 2nd sample contains 10–15% (thus one hour excretion is about 60–75%). The PSP test is a test of renal blood flow and tubular function. (d) *Creatinine clearance:* The normal values vary between 72–140 mL/min. (e) *Blood nitrogen levels*: In the adult the upper limits of normal are—creatinine 1.4 mg/100 mL and blood urea nitrogen 20 mg/100 mL.

Levels of blood urea and serum creatinine are useful clinical guide to overall renal function. Creatinine clearance will give an approximate value for glomerular filtration rate. Estimation of clearance of chromium-51-labeled ethylenediaminetetraacetic acid is probably more accurate in this respect. It must be remembered that kidneys have large functional reserve and 70% of function of kidneys must be lost before renal failure becomes evident in various tests.

4. **CATHETERIZATION AND RESIDUAL URINE:** Introduction of a catheter may determine the type of obstruction in the urethra. With an enlarged prostate, obstruction is encountered after the catheter has gone beyond the apex of the prostate (i.e., above the perineal membrane) due to the kinking of the prostatic urethra. In case of urethral stricture, obstruction is obtained below the perineal membrane since the bulb of the urethra is the most common site of stricture formation. The position of the obstruction can be further determined by a finger in the rectum. The *residual urine*, i.e., the amount of urine collected by means of a catheter after the patient has voided urine is a good indication of the capacity of the rectoprostatic pouch particularly in case of prostatic enlargement.

5. **X-RAY EXAMINATION (STRAIGHT X-RAY):** *Preparation of the patient*: No food or fluids should be given to the patient for at least 6 hours before X-ray examination. A purgative is given the night before. Enema is sometimes prescribed but it is probably less effective. Plain film of the abdomen is taken of the kidney, ureter and bladder region (KUB region).

It gives a clue to the diagnosis if properly studied.

(a) KIDNEY—size can be assessed from this film. Congenital absence or unascended kidneys can be diagnosed. Similarly, an enlarged kidney from hydronephrosis, polycystic disease or renal cancer can be diagnosed. A normal kidney extends from the top of the 1st to the bottom of the 3rd or middle of the 4th lumbar vertebra. In 90% of cases the right kidney is lower than the left because of displacement by the liver. Localized swelling as may be caused by a carbuncle, a tubercular cyst, a simple cyst or a tumor can be diagnosed.

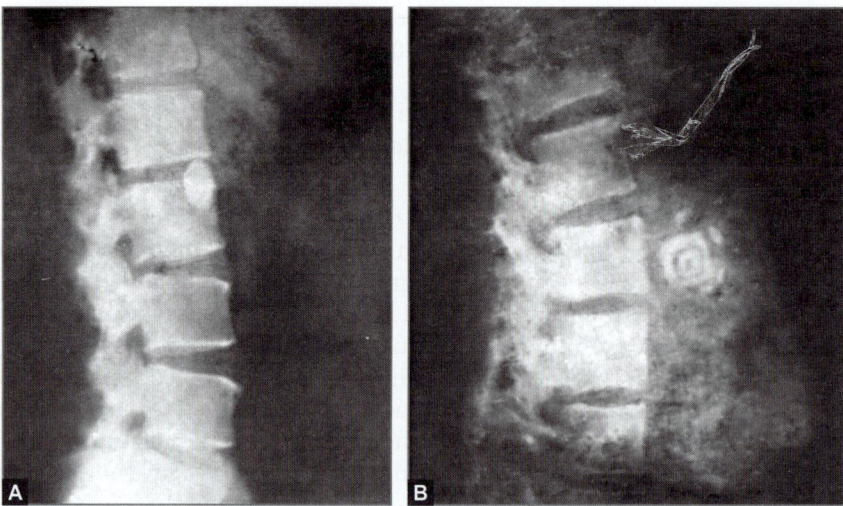

Figs. 37.9A and B: Lateral views showing a renal stone *in* (A) superimposed on the shadow of the vertebral column and gallstone; (B) Front of the vertebral column.

(b) STONES: Majority of the urinary calculi are radio-opaque except the pure uric acid stone *which* is not common. It is very difficult to assess the exact position of the radio-opaque stone in straight X-ray of the abdomen **(Figs. 37.9A and B)**. A lateral view or visualization of the urinary tract with radio-opaque dye is necessary. Numerous small calcific bodies in the parenchyma of the kidney may suggest tuberculosis or medullary sponge kidney or nephrocalcinosis caused by hyperparathyroidism. About 7% of malignant renal tumors contain some calcification.

A renal calculus has to be differentiated from (i) a gallstone, (ii) calcified lymph nodes, (iii) calcified costal cartilage, (iv) phlebolith, (v) calcified aneurysm of the abdominal aorta or renal artery and (vi) small calcific bodies in the substance of a kidney as discussed above. A stone in the appendix or a faecolith in the colon may be confused with a stone in the ureter. *It must be remembered that for the diagnosis of a stone either in the kidney, ureter or bladder, a straight film is all that is required, not a urogram.* Even dense round shadows in urogram may not be due to stone. They are often caused by the depths of the dye inside the end-on calyces (i.e., those directed anteriorly or posteriorly).

The *characteristics of a renal stone are*: (i) That a renal calculus moves with respiration which can be verified by taking two exposures, one at full inspiration and the other at full expiration. (ii) Density of a renal stone is uniform whereas gallstones are less dense in the center. (iii) Renal stones take the shape of the renal pelvis and calyces whereas a solitary gallstone may be round and multiple gallstones are squeezed into the gallbladder and become faceted. (iv) In lateral view the renal stone lies superimposed on the shadow of the vertebral column, whereas gallstones are seen in front of the vertebral bodies.

Ureteric stone **(Fig. 37.10)** is usually oval and lies in the line of the ureter. It is an imaginary line passing along the tips of the transverse processes of the lumbar vertebrae, over the sacro-iliac joint, down to the ischial spine from where this line deviates medially. *Vesical calculi* **(Fig. 37.11)** are seen just above the symphysis pubis. The *prostatic calculi* appear as small dots behind the symphysis pubis.

(c) **PSOAS SHADOWS** are normally seen quite distinctly. Obscure psoas shadows mean perinephric hematoma, abscess or cold abscess.

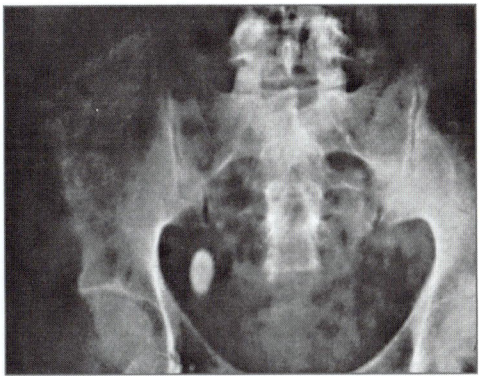

Fig. 37.10: Ureteric stone near the ischial spine.

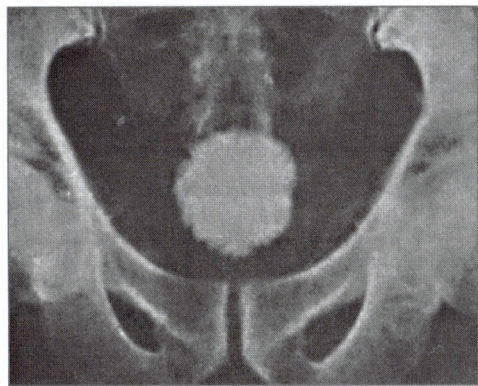

Fig. 37.11: Vesical calculus. Note its rough surface. This is typical of an oxalate stone.

(d) **BONES** should be carefully noticed to detect any arthritic change or presence of metastases (either osteolytic—commonly seen in a renal carcinoma or osteoblastic—commonly seen in prostatic carcinoma). Arthritic changes may well lead to radicular pain which may mimic a renal pain.

(e) **TOMOGRAPHY** will enhance the renal and psoas outlines thus clarifying renal size and shape. It may also reveal zones of calcification invisible in the plain film. A space-occupying lesion of the renal pelvis revealed in excretory urogram may show a faint opaque body compatible with stone but not tumor in the tomogram studies.

6. **EXCRETORY UROGRAMS (Fig. 37.12):** This is probably a better nomenclature than intravenous pyelography (IVP), since this does not only reveal the picture of the pelvis of the kidney, but also of the kidney, calyces, ureters and the urinary bladder. It is also called intravenous urography.

Preparation of the patient has been described in section 5. A straight X-ray of the abdomen (particularly the KUB region) is first taken. Then the radio-opaque fluid is injected intravenously. Generally, Hypaque (sodium diatrizoate) or Urografin is injected. Adult dose is about 20–25 mL injection is made slowly. Preliminary test of hypersensitivity is always performed. Subcutaneous injection of 0.1 mL of the contrast medium is made. If induration and erythema develop promptly the test is positive. If symptoms and signs of hypersensitivity appear during injection, it should be stopped immediately. Warning signs are respiratory difficulty, itching, urticaria, nausea, vomiting and fainting. Treatment consists of oxygen and intravenous dextrose for shock, intravenous injection of antihistaminic drug and intravenous injection of barbiturates for convulsion.

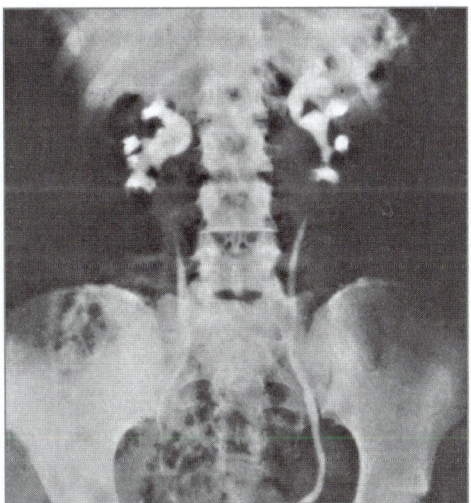

Fig. 37.12: Excretory urogram showing cavities suggesting cavernous tuberculosis.

Routine radiograms are taken at 10 seconds for nephrogram effect and at 5, 10 and 15 minutes with the patient in supine position. For hypertensive patients films should be taken 2–3 minutes after the beginning of the injection. Delayed concentration of dye in one kidney may suggest decreased renal blood flow and function. At 25 minutes a film is taken in erect posture to note the efficiency with which the renal pelvis and ureters drain, ureterograms and also the mobility of the kidneys. All films should include kidney, ureter and bladder areas, as fine changes in the ureters which imply the presence of vesicoureteral reflux may be detected. It is advisable to inject additional radio-opaque medium if there is impaired concentration in the initial films.

In infants and children the films should be taken at 3, 5, 8 and 12 minutes as their kidneys excrete the fluid more rapidly than do those of the adults.

X-ray of the bladder region after voiding should be routine in all urologic patients. At the conclusion of the urographic study, the patient is instructed to pass urine and a film of the bladder area is taken immediately. This will demonstrate the presence or absence of residual urine.

Excretory urogram is contraindicated in (i) allergic patients, (ii) multiple myeloma (the dye makes insoluble complex with Bence-Jones protein and precipitate in the renal tubules), (iii) congenital adrenal hyperplasia, (iv) diabetes and (v) primary hyperparathyroidism.

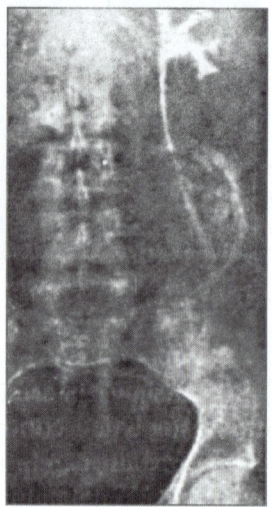

Fig. 37.13: Intravenous pyelogram showing double kidney. The normal upper kidney shows cupping of the minor calyces and the lower one shows inward direction of the calyces—a congenital abnormality.

Excretory urogram is a physiological and as well as an anatomical test since it not only determines the function of the kidney but also clearly demonstrates the contour of the renal pelvis and calyces.

INTRAVENOUS INFUSION UROGRAPHY (Fig. 37.13): This is indicated when there is a huge hydronephrosis or there is certain amount of renal failure (blood urea is in the range of 100 mg). About 2 mL per kg body weight of contrast medium in an equal volume of normal saline is infused in a subcutaneous vein slowly for over a period of 10 minutes. The films are taken at longer intervals.

SUBCUTANEOUS INFUSION UROGRAPHY: When a proper subcutaneous vein cannot be obtained for intravenous urography, this procedure is adopted. Diluted contrast medium is infused into the subcutaneous tissue along with hyaluronidase (hylase).

7. **RETROGRADE UROGRAMS (Fig. 37.14): INDICATIONS**: (i) *Inadequate excretory urograms* which have failed to demonstrate the renal pelvis, calyces and the ureters adequately, this investigation will be required. (ii) *Impaired renal function* which has failed to show the pelvis and calyces, this test is needed. (iii) *Sensitivity to intravenous contrast medium* is the

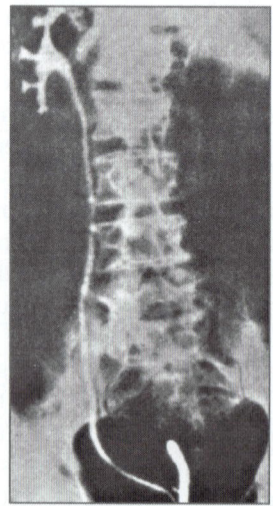

Fig. 37.14: Retrograde urogram showing normal cupping of the minor calyces. Note the end of the catheterizing cystoscope lying within the bladder.

definite indication for this test. (iv) If *pyuria is present* catheterization of the ureters may be needed to obtain separate specimens from each kidney for bacteriological study and then retrograde urograms may be performed. (v) Since in intravenous urogram the density of the dye may not be sufficient *for oblique and lateral radiograms*, retrograde urogram will be required.

PROCEDURE: (a) Preparation of the patient is similar to that of excretory urogram except for the fact that the patient may be allowed to take fluids unless general anesthesia is to be employed. (b) Cystoscopy and ureteral catheterization are performed. (c) Preliminary straight X-ray of the abdomen is taken to know the positions of the catheters besides the points already discussed earlier. (d) 25% sodium diatrizoate (Hypaque) is used as the contrast medium and 3 to 5 mL is first introduced to delineate normal size pelvis. For hydronephrosis more amount of medium is required. (e) Supine urogram is taken, developed and viewed. If filling is not complete, more dye is instilled before further X-rays are taken. (f) Oblique, lateral and upright radiograms are taken as indicated. (g) Pneumopyelography: To differentiate between a non-opaque stone and a papillary tumor of the renal pelvis, 4–6 mL of air is instilled into the catheters. A stone may show some opacification, but a tumor will not, but both these will cause a filling defect in the pelvis or calyx in excretory urogram.

8. **ANTEGRADE UROGRAM:** The clinical indication for this test is inadequate information from intravenous urogram with an unsuccessful or impossible retrograde examination. Under fluoroscopic or ultrasonic control an 18-gauge needle, 15 cm long should be passed into a dilated calyx or pelvis. Radio-opaque dye should then be instilled and appropriate films are taken. It is better to pass the needle into a dilated calyx rather than pelvis as there will be a better seal round the needle track and less danger of puncturing large hilar vessels. Temporary drainage can also be provided with by a small plastic catheter introduced through the needle, which will be subsequently removed. The tube now act as nephrostomy tube.

FINDINGS: All urograms, be it excretory, retrograde or antegrade are read in the following manner:

A. *Nephrogram*: From the soft tissue shadow of the kidney, various congenital deformities can be detected. Any tumor or cyst can be suspected. The position and sizecan be assessed.

B. *Calyces*: A normal calyx looks like a cup due to projection of the apices of the papillae into the calyces. The calyces are directed outwards. Inward directed calyces suggest congenital abnormality such as horseshoe shaped kidney.

C. *Pelvis*: The size, shape and position of the pelvis are noted. The lower border of the pelvis forms a uniform curve with the lower calyx. The right pelvi-ureteric junction is situated opposite the transverse process of the second lumbar vertebra whereas the left is slightly higher up. The most important is the shape of the pelvis and the students must learn the normal shape of the pelvis.

D. *The ureter*: Usually the upper portion of the ureter is visualized. If the whole of the ureter is seen there must be an obstruction further down. Note the shape—whether dilated or not. Dilated ureter indicates obstruction or vesico-ureteral reflux. Also look at the position of the ureter, whether it is kinking or not and whether there is any congenital deformity or not.

9. **CYSTOGRAMS:** (a) *Excretory cystograms* can be obtained as later films of excretory urograms. If these are not satisfied to delineate clearly the pathological conditions of the bladder, retrograde cystogram may be required.

(b) *Retrograde cystograms* are performed by instilling radio-opaque fluid into the bladder through a catheter. This will outline the bladder-wall including the diverticula. Besides these, this test has a diagnostic value in rupture of the bladder and recurrent infection (vesico-ureteral reflux is the most common cause of perpetuation of infection).

(c) *Voiding cystourethrograms* are essential as increased intravesical pressure generated at the time of voiding will show ureteral reflux when cystogram has failed to detect it. This will also reveal function of the bladder neck, presence of posterior urethral valves or urethral stricture.

10. **URETHROGRAPHY:** Water soluble viscous solution like umbradil viscous V is often used. This investigation is of special value to know the length of the stricture, presence of diverticulum, etc. Its importance also lies in revealing the dilated prostatic ducts in chronic or tuberculous prostatitis and bladder neck obstruction. The dye is pushed with some local anesthetic (lignocaine 20%) by a special Knutsson's apparatus which has a penile clamp.

11. **CYSTOSCOPY:** This is the most important urological investigation. It not only reveals all the pathological processes inside the bladder, e.g., cystitis, tuberculous affection, stone, growth, diverticulum, enlarged prostate, etc., but also detect some involving the kidney and ureter. The ureteric orifices are situated at 4 O'clock and 8 O'clock positions. By rotating the cystoscope the orifices should be noticed carefully. Note the efflux of urine. *Chromocystoscopy* can be employed to find out the ureteric orifices as also the function of the kidney. 5 mL of 0.4% sterile solution of Indigo carmine is injected intravenously. Normally a blue jet will be seen to emerge from the ureteric orifices within 3 to 5 minutes. Delay indicates partial obstruction. Feeble efflux or nonappearance means impaired renal function. *In case of hematuria*, cystoscopy should be performed *at the time of bleeding* to detect which kidney is bleeding. But when bleeding is coming from the bladder, cystoscopy should be repeated *when bleeding has ceased.*

12. **URETERIC CATHETERIZATION**—is another important method of investigation. This is performed through a catheterizing cystoscope. Its indications are : (i) to collect specimen of urine from individual kidney for 'split' renal function test; (ii) to perform retrograde urography; (iii) in anuria; (iv) to dislodge ureteric stone; (v) in case of stone in the lower 1/3 of the ureter Dormia basket may be passed through the ureteric orifice to extract the stone.

13. **URETHROSCOPY:** *Anterior urethroscopy* is conducted under air inflation. It is indicated in stricture, foreign body and chronic urethritis.

Posterior urethroscopy is conducted by irrigating urethroscope. Through this the membranous part and the prostatic part of the urethra can be inspected. Verumontanum is an eminence on the posterior aspect of the prostatic urethra at the apex of which is the sinus pocularis on each side of which the two ejaculatory ducts open. This will be reddened and dilated in chronic vesiculitis. Numerous prostatic ducts can be seen which will be enlarged and will be seen extruding pus.

14. **NEPHROSCOPY:** This procedure is now often used in different urologic units to detect various lesions of the kidney. It may be performed either percutaneously, i.e., percutaneous nephrostomy (PCN) or by retrograde route, i.e., ureterorenoscopy (URS).

15. **ANGIONEPHROTOMOGRAMS** (intravenous renal angiogram): In this investigation a bolus of radio-opaque medium (30–50 mL of 90% hypaque) is injected inside a vein (antecubital vein) rapidly, 4–6 tomograms are taken. This is an efficient method to differentiate a cyst from a tumor. Space occupied by a cyst or abscess fails to opacify, whereas a malignant tumor shows a normal or increased opacification. Renal angiography is, however, more efficient in this differential diagnosis.

16. **RENAL ANGIOGRAPHY:** Although renal angiogram can be performed by direct lumbar needle puncture of the aorta, yet this technique has been superseded by percutaneous femoral

angiography. A catheter is passed to the level of the renal arteries under fluoroscopic control. It is also possible to do the catheterization through the brachial or axillary artery. 12–24 mL of radio-opaque fluid suitable for intravenous urography is injected and 10 exposures are taken in 10 seconds time **(Fig. 37.15)**.

Selective renal angiography is accomplished by passing a femoral catheter into one of the renal arteries under fluoroscopic control. About 8 mL of the contrast medium is injected and 16 exposures are taken within a few seconds. This technique gives detailed demonstration of the arterial pattern in the kidney and thus differentiates efficiently between renal cyst and tumor. If this technique also fails to differentiate in case of small lesion or gets obscured by overlying arteries, epinephrine can first be injected into the catheter followed by instillation of radio-opaque medium. This technique causes spasm of normal vessels but has no effect on arteries in tumors.

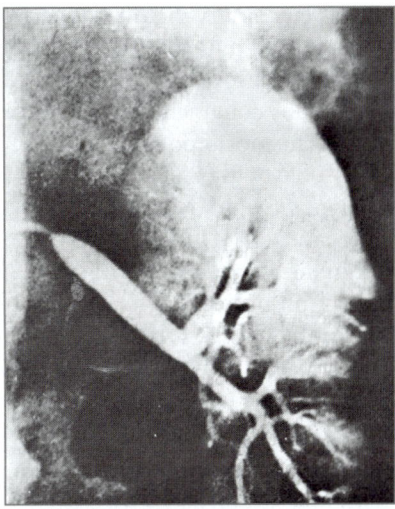

Fig. 37.15: Renal angiography showing the typical filling defect at the origin of the renal artery due to atheroma.

17. **VESICAL ANGIOGRAPHY:** A Seldinger catheter is passed to the bifurcation of the aorta and 30 mL of 90% contrast medium is injected. Alternatively each hypogastric artery is selectively catheterized and 10 mL of radio-opaque fluid is injected. Films are rapidly exposed in first 8 seconds. The series are repeated in oblique position to give tangential view of the tumor. This technique is occasionally required to judge the size and depth of penetration of the vesical neoplasms. Typical 'stain' of an invasive tumor can be revealed in X-ray.

18. **DIGITAL SUBTRACTION ARTERIOGRAPHY (DSA):** Satisfactory imaging of the renal vessels can be achieved by this technique after intravenous injection of contrast medium, though intra-arterial injection with a fine catheter inserted through the femoral artery using Seldinger technique offers more precise information. Nowadays flush venogram is more popular than arteriography in diagnosing renal carcinoma, where CT indicates tumor invasion of the renal vein. This is comparatively a newer technique and not available in many institutions in Indian subcontinent.

19. **LYMPHANGIOGRAPHY:** A lymphatic vessel in the foot is cannulated and oily contrast medium is injected. This leads to opacification of the inguinal, pelvic, aortic groups and supraclavicular lymph nodes. Metastatic infiltration can be demonstrated in regional lymph nodes by filling defect in malignant tumors of the testis, prostate, bladder and penis.

20. **COMPUTED TOMOGRAPHY (CT Scan):** In this examination the detector system is usually a scintillation phototube or gas-filled ionization chamber and not the X-ray film as in conventional radiography. The X-ray tube and the detector system are on opposite sides of the patient and during a scan they rotate around the patient recording informations about the internal structures of the thin transverse cross-section through which the X-ray beam is passing. Through a complex series of mathematical manipulations the computer 'reconstructs' and displays it as an integrated picture on a television monitor. In this examination, a renal mass is considered to be a simple benign cyst if it has a homogeneous density similar to that of water and has a very thin wall thickness that is virtually immeasurable. A renal cancer has density similar to or slightly higher than that of normal renal parenchyma but has a thick wall which is more significant.

It is customary that if urography demonstrates a solitary renal mass, it has to be evaluated by diagnostic ultrasound. If ultrasound demonstrates all the findings of a simple benign cyst, there is no reason to perform any other diagnostic imaging examination. Only if ultrasound fails to show any convincing result, CT offers an accurate and noninvasive method of evaluating the lesion. The most frequent causes of indeterminate results from ultrasound are (i) a mass in the upper pole of the kidney, (ii) a mass in the region of the renal pelvis, (iii) presence of multiple renal masses and (iv) markedly obese patient. CT is as accurate as angiography in determining the local extent of the cancer, presence of enlarged lymph nodes and presence of tumor thrombus within the renal vein and inferior vena cava.

Lymph nodes between renal hilum and the diaphragm are not adequately visualized by lymphography, but usually well delineated by CT. With the advance in technology in CT, lymphangiography should be reserved for suspected metastasis in normal-size lymph nodes. CT is accurate for staging of bladder cancer. Value of CT in the staging of prostatic cancer has not been adequately evaluated.

21. **ULTRASOUND:** With the static B scanner, the transducer is moved at a constant speed in a single sweep along the skin overlying the organ to be imaged. Conventional static B scan and real time instruments also visualize the bladder and prostate with the patient supine. Any change of renal outline and displacement or fragmentation of the collecting system of echoes is of pathological significance. With ultrasound, agenesis, hypoplasia, duplex or ectopic kidney can be diagnosed. Cysts can be differentiated from renal carcinomas. In case of hematuria, even if the intravenous urogram is normal, ultrasound can detect a peripheral lesion that does not deform the calyceal system or renal outline. Renal sonography should follow urography in evaluation of a renal mass. Renal sonography should be followed by percutaneous puncture (under sonographic visualization). If aspiration reveals clear fluid and the area is smooth-walled as demonstrated in X-ray following injection of a contrast medium, no further investigation is required. If sonogram fails to show the pattern of solid mass, arteriography is advised. Sonography is about 95% accurate in distinguishing between solid and cystic renal masses.

Large renal calculi can be diagnosed. Even exact position of a small calculus can be determined during operation by the application of a transducer direct to the kidney surface. A small needle can be passed through a slot guide of the probe to the stone.

B scanning of the bladder has been used to evaluate the intravesical extent of tumors. The *transrectal approach* is useful in detecting early asymptomatic tumors of the prostate and in accurately staging local disease of the prostate. This is now a routine investigation in carcinoma prostate.

22. **RADIOISOTOPE RENOGRAPHY:** 100 Ci of I^{131}-labeled hippuran is injected intravenous (IV) and radioactivity is measured over each kidney with a pair of scintillation detector. The tracing is in three segments—segment 1 (vascular phase) with a steep rise lasting 20–30 seconds due to the arrival of radioisotopes in the vascular bed; segment 2 (secretory phase) lasting for 2–5 mins. due to accumulation by the kidney and its subsequent secretion; segment 3 (excretory phase) indicates gradual tubular excretion. In renal hypertension the rise is too little (segment 1) and prolongation of third phase. In obstruction, the third phase is abnormally prolonged. It is the actual pattern of tracing which is more important. Function of kidney is very well assessed with this technique.

23. **RENAL SCINTISCAN:** This consists of measuring the rate of accumulation of ^{197}Hg-labeled neohydrin using an external detector up to 1 hour after injection. This test is not so efficient to

determine the function of kidney as the previous test, but in injury, it shows the portion of kidney affected and supersedes the previous test to determine the type of operation to be required.

24. **MAGNETIC RESONANCE IMAGING (MRI):** This is not superior to a good-quality CT. Still it may be used to know the local extent of bladder, prostate or kidney malignancies. Positron emission tomography may be better in staging urological malignancies.

25. **SERUM ACID AND ALKALINE PHOSPHATASE:** *Acid phosphatase* is present in small amount in normal blood serum (1–4 units). It is elevated in prostatic carcinoma with metastasis (10 units or more), but not so as long as the growth remains confined to the gland. It comes from the cancer cells but does not enter circulation as long as the capsule of the prostate is intact. *Alkaline phosphatase* is secreted by the liver. It enters the circulation from bone. When metastasis in bone occurs in prostatic carcinoma its level is elevated in the serum. It is well recognized fact that osseous metastasis in prostatic carcinoma is *osteosclerotic*, rather than osteolytic in character. *This is due to the elevation of alkaline phosphatase level.*

26. **CHEST X-RAY:** This is important to exclude blood-borne metastasis in the lungs. This is also used to exclude pulmonary tuberculosis in suspected cases of renal tuberculosis.

27. **BIOPSY:** In suspected prostatic carcinoma, a specimen of prostatic tissue may be obtained by transurethral resection or by aspiration with a needle through the perineum or through rectum and examined histologically. Very often bone marrow aspiration from the sternum or ilium reveals carcinoma cells even before the radiological evidence of metastasis.

28. **SMEARS** from the urethra or prostate (expressed by massage) should be examined microscopically for evidence of infection, when this is suspected. In carcinoma of the prostate, secretion obtained by prostatic massage may show cancer cells (exfoliate cytology).

29. **LAPAROSCOPY**—may be used to visualize intraperitoneal metastatic spread from a malignant lesion in the urinary system.

DIFFERENTIAL DIAGNOSIS OF DISEASES OF THE KIDNEY

Differential diagnosis of urinary case

Symptom	Possible causes
Flank pain (dull, aching)	Hydronephrosis, renal tumors, chronic pyelonephritis
Flank pain (colicky, radiating to groin)	Ureteric calculi, ureteric stricture, blood clots
Suprapubic pain	Cystitis, bladder outlet obstruction, interstitial cystitis
Hematuria (initial—beginning of urination)	Urethral trauma, urethritis, urethral stricture
Hematuria (terminal—end of urination)	Bladder tumors, prostatitis, bph
Hematuria (total—throughout urination)	Renal cell carcinoma, glomerulonephritis, trauma
Dysuria and urgency	Urinary tract infection (UTI), prostatitis, bladder stones

Contd...

Contd...

Symptom	Possible causes
Urinary retention (acute, painful)	Prostate enlargement, urethral stricture, bladder outlet obstruction
Urinary retention (chronic, painless)	Benign prostatic hyperplasia (BPH), neurogenic bladder
Increased urinary frequency and nocturia	Diabetes mellitus, bladder dysfunction, chronic kidney disease

HORSESHOE KIDNEY

Primary mesonephric buds which form the kidney on each side fuse when the embryo is only 30 to 40 days old. Usually the lower poles fuse. This kidney cannot ascend to its normal position. The bridge joining the lower poles lies in front of the fourth lumbar vertebra.

As the ureters are angulated as they pass over the fused isthmus, urinary stasis and stone formation are the usual complications. Tuberculosis and tumor formation are also noticed in this kidney. Horseshoe kidney is as such asymptomatic and only presents when the above complications appear.

Diagnosis is mainly confirmed by urography. Medially directed lowest calyx is confirmatory. Calyces of a normal kidney look outwards. Only occasionally, all the calyces of the horseshoe kidney may look inwards.

POLYCYSTIC KIDNEY

This disease is slightly more common in women. Infantile polycystic kidney disease is an hereditary autosomal recessive condition and is often fatal in the neonate.

Adult polycystic disease is an autosomal dominant condition and typically presents in mid-adult life (30–40 years). When an adult presents with bilateral renal swellings with dragging pain in the loin and hematuria in about 1/4th cases, the case is one of polycystic kidney. In case of unilateral renal swelling diagnosis becomes more difficult. This is seen when one kidney contains larger cysts than the other kidney. Patients with congenital cystic kidney pass abundant urine of low specific gravity (1.010 or less) with a trace of albumin but no casts and cells. Infection of the kidney in the form of pyelonephritis is a common complication. Renal hypertension is seen in more than half number of patients. Symptoms of uremia, e.g., anorexia, headache, drowsiness, vomiting, etc., with anemia may be present.

So polycystic kidney in adult is presented with one or more of the following features— (i) Abdominal swelling (enlarged kidney); (ii) Pain (due to enlargement of kidney); (iii) Hematuria (present in 25% of cases); (iv) Infection (presents with pyelonephritis); (v) Hypertension; (vi) Chronic renal failure.

Urography is confirmatory. If intravenous urography fails to delineate the pelvicalyceal system properly, retrograde urography should be advised. It must be remembered that one side should be performed and the other side is deferred for a week as edema may impair the renal function and if performed in both sides in one go there is every possibility of anuria. The calyces are stretched and elongated (spider-leg deformity) by the cysts **(Fig. 37.16)**. Similar deformity may be seen in renal cell carcinoma but in this case the spider legs are smooth and not irregular as seen in this carcinoma. Moreover in this condition the deformity is seen in both sides whereas in renal cell carcinoma the deformity is unilateral. In chromocystography there will be considerable delay in excretion of indigo carmine in the affected side.

Solitary renal cyst: This condition is rather asymptomatic. Renal swelling with or without dull ache in the loin is the usual presenting symptom. Occasionally hemorrhage inside the cyst may lead to acute renal pain or the cyst may press on the pelviureteric junction to cause urinary obstruction. Adenocarcinoma may appear in the walls of the cysts, which may be suspected on ultrasound or CT Scanning. These cases should be managed as renal cell carcinomas.

The condition is confirmed by urography. Filling defect of one or more calyces, which are actually stretched over the cyst, is the main abnormality detected. This, of course, is very much similar to what seen in renal neoplasm. Differentiation can be made by ultrasound, cyst puncture under sonographic control, CT and angiography.

Hydatid cyst of the kidney is very occasionally seen. That the patient passes 'grape skin' (ruptured daughter cysts) in the urine is confirmatory.

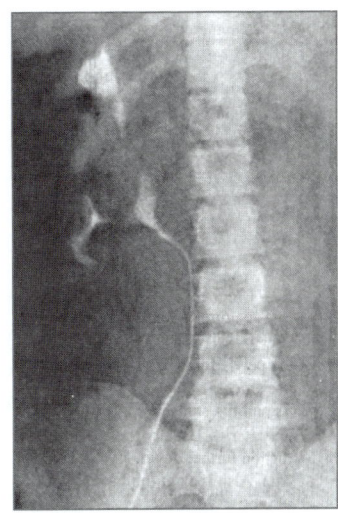

Fig. 37.16: Retrograde urogram showing polycystic kidney with 'spider-leg' elongation of the calyces.

HYDRONEPHROSIS

It is the distension of the calyces and pelvis of the kidney caused by an obstruction to the flow of urine.

The *causes* are:

Unilateral hydronephrosis	Bilateral hydronephrosis
A. *Pelviureteric obstruction:* 　(i) Idiopathic pelviureteric junction stenosis (common) 　(ii) Stone 　(iii) Tumor in the renal pelvis 　(iv) Pressure from aberrant artery	(i) Prostatic enlargement—benign or malignant (ii) Carcinoma of the bladder (iii) Schistosomiasis (iv) Urethral stricture or valve (v) Phimosis
B. Ureteric obstruction: 　(i) Stone 　(ii) Tumor of the ureter 　(iii) Tumor infiltrating from other organs, e.g., bladder, cervix, rectum or colon 　(iv) Ureterocele 　(v) Schistosomiasis 　(vi) Bladder tumor	

Females are more often affected than men and it occurs practically at all ages. Onset is insidious. Dull ache or a sense of weight may be felt in the loin. Sometimes the patients ignore it as mild backache. If the hydronephrosis develops quickly, the pain may be severe and colicky. It may be exacerbated by drinking excessive amount of water or alcohol or by taking diuretics. Sometimes the pain may be referred to the epigastrium, when it may be mistaken for duodenal ulcer. After a few hours, large quantity of urine may be passed and the swelling considerably reduces in size (Dietl's crisis). In bilateral cases the symptoms are mainly due to the causes.

On examination, a cystic large renal swelling is felt. It is ballotable and better palpable bimanually.

Urography is confirmatory. Conventional earlier films may fail to visualize the pelvis and calyces. Better delineation may be seen after 6 hours of injection. If pelvis and calyces are not seen properly retrograde urography should be called for. The earliest change is seen either in the renal pelvis or minor calyces according as the renal pelvis is extrarenal or intrarenal. In majority of cases the pelvis is extrarenal. Decreasing concavity and later on flattening of the minor calyces are the early changes in case of intrarenal pelvis. Gradually there will be dilatation of the major calyces and convexity (clubbing) of the minor calyces. The pelvis becomes so much distended (in late stages) that its convex lower margin forms an acute angle with the ureter. Sometimes the cause like stone may be found in X-ray.

Ultrasound scanning is also quite confirmatory, moreover it is the least invasive. It may be used to detect this case due to pelviureteric junction obstruction in utero.

Isotope renography may be used to detect dilatation of the renal collecting system due to obstruction.

Whitaker test is sometimes used in specialized unit to monitor intrapelvic pressure by percutaneous puncture of the kidney.

RENAL CALCULUS

Majority of the sufferers are between the ages of 30 and 50 years. Both sexes are equally affected, though males slightly dominate. Pain is the main symptom. Majority of the patients suffer from fixed dull ache in the angle between the lower border of the last rib and the lateral border of the sacrospinalis. Pain is also felt anteriorly in the corresponding hypochondriac region. This pain gets worse on movement like running, jolting and climbing up the stairs and gets better with rest. Ureteric colic is sometimes felt particularly when the stone obstructs the pelviureteric junction. Sudden griping pain is felt in the loin and tends to radiate towards the groin. The patient may toss over the bed in agony. Pain may be associated with profuse sweating and vomiting. Pain goes off as suddenly as it came. Hematuria may be complained of either during or after an attack. Pyuria is sometimes noticed but it must be remembered that increase in the number of white cells may be found in urine even in the absence of infection.

On examination, kidney cannot be palpated unless hydronephrosis has developed. Abdominal rigidity may be felt at the time of colicky pain. Tenderness can be elicited either in the renal angle or during bimanual palpation.

It must be remembered that quite a number of renal stones are asymptomatic. These are mainly phosphate stones. Patients may present with other gastrointestinal symptoms or may present quite late with supervening infection or uremia or during X-ray examination of the abdomen for some other complaints.

Straight X-ray of the KUB region **(Fig. 37.17)** will reveal 90% of the renal stones except the pure uric acid stones. When a stone is found, exposures are made during full inspiration and full expiration to see whether the stone moves slightly with the kidney during respiration. This is assessed by measuring the distance between the lower border of the kidney and the stone which will remain constant. A lateral film is also essential to exclude other conditions which will show similar type of shadow. A renal stone will be seen to be superimposed on the bodies of the lumbar vertebrae. The other conditions which mimic renal calculus in X-ray are—(i) gallstone, (ii) calcified lymph nodes, (iii) phleboliths, (iv) drugs or foreign bodies in the alimentary canal, (v) calcified tuberculous lesion of the kidney, (vi) calcified lesion of the suprarenal gland, (vii) fracture of the transverse process of the lumbar vertebra and (viii) calcified adrenal gland.

Excretory urography **(Fig. 37.18)** is essential to know (i) the position of the renal stone, (ii) if it has produced obstructive features or not, (iii) presence of nonopaque stone which can be visualized by filling defect and (iv) the functioning capacity of the affected as well as the sound kidney.

Ultrasound scanning is important to locate stones particularly for extracorporeal shock wave treatment.

ACUTE PYELONEPHRITIS

Females are more often affected due to their short urethra, which makes easy for the bacteria to enter the bladder. Acute pain is suddenly felt in both the loins. This may be preceded by the prodromal symptoms like headache, lassitude, aches in the joints, rise of temperature, nausea and vomiting. Pain may also be felt anteriorly to be confused with cholecystitis. Temperature rises sharply and may be accompanied by rigor. As cystitis gradually develops patient complains of frequency of micturition and burning pain along the length of the urethra during micturition and even after it. Patient may even complain of 'strangury', i.e., painful and fruitless desire to micturate. Urine may become cloudy and even blood-stained.

On examination, the patient looks ill and anemic. The tongue is dry and furred. Renal angle will be very tender. There may be rigidity anteriorly due to extreme tenderness.

Bacteriological examination of the urine is highly important. If culture detects the offending organism, sensitivity test must be performed to know which antibiotic will be effective most.

Excretory pyelography in an early case may show poor excretion of the dye and hence poor differentiation can be seen. Radio-isotope renogram will show diminished uptake in certain areas.

PERINEPHRIC ABSCESS

Diagnosis of this condition depends entirely on clinical examination. In case of pyrexia of unknown origin this condition should be borne in mind. Patient's back is inspected in sitting posture. Slight fullness may be detected just below the last rib and lateral to sacrospinalis muscle on comparing with the opposite side. There may be scoliosis of the lumbar spine with

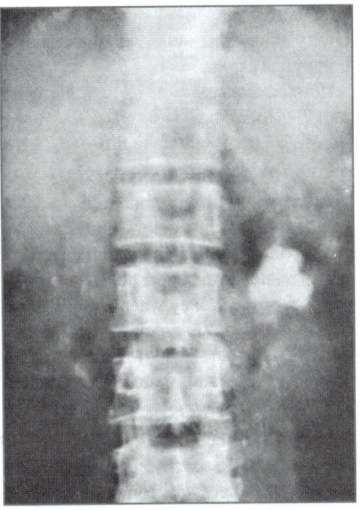

Fig. 37.17: Shows a typical stag horn calculus in straight X-ray.

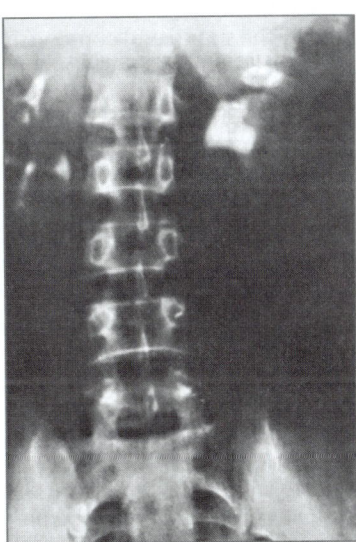

Fig. 37.18: IVP showing normal functioning kidney on right side and stag horn calculus with almost nonfunctioning kidney on left side.

concavity towards the affected side, which is a relatively early sign. The abscess is often related to the upper pole where no swelling can be detected. But less frequently such abscess may be related to the lower pole of the kidney when a swelling in the renal area can be seen. The patient is now instructed to lie prone on the examining table. While doing 'renal angle test' muscular rigidity is felt on the affected side.

In straight X-ray psoas shadow is obscured, there may be reactionary scoliosis with concavity towards the abscess. The diaphragm is raised and immobile on the affected side. Definite diagnosis is made by CT and ultrasonography.

RENAL TUBERCULOSIS

Men are more often affected than females and the majority of the victims are between 20 and 40 years of age, though no age is exempted. The earliest and the most common symptom is frequency of micturition both by day and night. Renal pain is absent (dull ache in the loin may be complained of) in majority of cases but if the bladder is involved patient will complain of suprapubic pain when the bladder is full and if the bladder is secondarily involved pain is felt at the tip of penis after micturition. If a tuberculous ulcer has affected a renal papilla painless hematuria will be the presenting symptom. Generalized symptoms like loss of weight, evening rise of temperature, cough, hemoptysis may or may not be associated with.

On examination, a tuberculous kidney is unlikely to be palpable. The palpable kidney is usually the sound and compensatory hypertrophied kidney (it may be tender). If this condition is suspected it is always worthwhile to examine the prostate, seminal vesicles and the epididymis.

Bacteriological examination is very important pathological test. The sediment of the morning urine should be stained and cultured for acid-fast bacilli. It must be remembered that presence of pus cells in acid urine without any organism in ordinary culture is probably a case of urinary tuberculosis and special culture and animal inoculation test should be called for. *Cystoscopy* will show pallor around the ureteric orifice in early case. Gradually the tubercles appear which coalesce to form a tuberculous ulcer. In late cases due to sclerosing periureteritis the ureter becomes shortened, so the ureteric orifice is pulled up giving rise to a 'golf-hole' ureteric orifice. The capacity of the bladder is gradually diminished and when secondarily infected the whole mucous membrane looks red and edematous. *Straight X-ray* may reveal calcification in healing foci or calcification around a caseous mass. In *urography* one may find irregular density in nephrogram. Irregular dilatation of the calyces or loss of one calyx due to edema and spasm of the calyceal neck may be the only finding. Cavity formation is also seen in ulcero-cavernous type. In late cases periureteric fibrosis makes the ureter wider and more straight losing its natural curves. Chest X-ray must be performed to exclude any active lung lesion.

TUMORS OF THE KIDNEY

Benign neoplasms are so rare in kidney that it is good to consider all neoplasms of the kidney as malignant. Three types are commonly seen—(A) Renal cell carcinoma or Carcinoma of kidney, (B) Nephroblastoma and (C) Papillary tumors of the renal pelvis.

1. **Renal cell carcinoma** (syn. **GRAWITZ TUMOR or HYPERNEPHROMA**): This tumor arises in the cortex from the cells of the uriniferous tubules. It is uncommon to see this tumor below the age of 50 years and it is twice as common in males than females. It can present in many ways but mainly three types of presentations are seen:—(1) *Painless intermittent hematuria;* (2) *A dragging pain* in the loin due to the presence of the kidney with the tumor and (3) *A palpable mass* due to enlarged kidney discovered by the patient accidentally. These main presentations

are always accompanied by general malaise, loss of weight, loss of energy, lassitude, anemia, etc., *Pain* in the kidney may be more disturbing when the tumor breaks through its capsule and invades neighboring structures. *Pyrexia of unknown origin* without any infection, tuberculosis, lymphoma, etc., may be the presenting symptom in odd cases. In about 1/4th of the cases the primary tumor remains silent and *secondary metastasis becomes the presenting features*, e.g., bone pain, fracture, persistent cough, hemoptysis, etc., (as blood borne metastasis is early in this tumor). *Polycythemia* with increased erythrocyte sedimentation rate (ESR) due to increased production of erythropoietin is the presenting feature in a few number of cases. This is evident by redness of the face and hands, heart failure and spontaneous venous and arterial thromboses. Occlusion of the left renal and testicular veins may lead to *varicocele* of recent onset and *edema of both legs* due to occlusion of the inferior vena cava. *Hypertension* due to increased production of renin is sometimes the presenting feature.

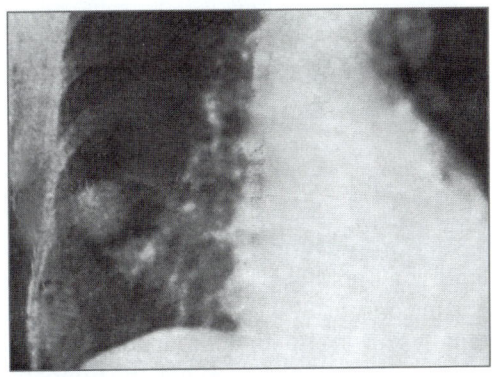

Fig. 37.19: Secondary deposit (cannon-ball appearance) at the right lower lung from renal cell carcinoma of the kidney.

On examination, an enlarged kidney may be palpable. If there is no palpable mass, cystoscopy should be done during hematuria to know from which kidney the blood is coming. Recent weight loss and anemia from hematuria are important general features. Large tumors are palpable and have all signs of an enlarged kidney described in page 604. A small tumor in the upper pole of the kidney may push the whole kidney downwards and make the lower pole easier to feel. Tenderness is conspicuous by its absence. Renal carcinoma often spreads along renal vein. The most common site for metastasis is the lung. The tumor cells reach the pulmonary vascular capillaries via the heart. The patient typically develops a number of isolated lesions within the lung field, known as cannon-ball metastases **(Fig. 37.19)**. Renal cell carcinoma is one of the tumors that commonly metastasis to bones. Areas of swelling and tenderness in the bones must be looked for carefully. Such metastases are often pulsatile with audible bruit.

Very rarely ectopic hormones may be produced which include parathyroid hormone or a parathyroid hormone-like substance which gives rise to hypercalcemia. There may be production of adrenocorticotropic hormone or human chronotropic hormone.

Clinical staging may be used for carcinoma of the kidney as devised by Robin—Stage I—tumor within the capsule;

Stage II—tumor invades the perinephric fat but within Gerota's fascia;

Stage III—tumor involvement of regional lymph nodes and/or renal vein;

Stage IV—tumor involvement of adjacent organs or distant metastasis.

Urography is extremely important. Renogram is important and may show the soft tissue shadow of the tumor. Otherwise excretory urography may be inconclusive due to lack of concentration of the contrast medium, yet it is important to know the function of the contralateral kidney. *Retrograde urography* may be necessary to know the exact changes of the calyceal system. Filling defect due to invasion of one or more minor and/or major calyces, elongation and stretching of the calyces over the tumor mass may show the 'spider-leg' deformity **(Fig. 37.20)**. The outline of this

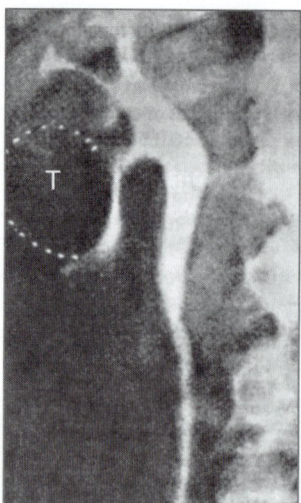

Fig. 37.20: Urogram showing the 'spider-leg' deformity due to adenocarcinoma (T) outlined by dots.

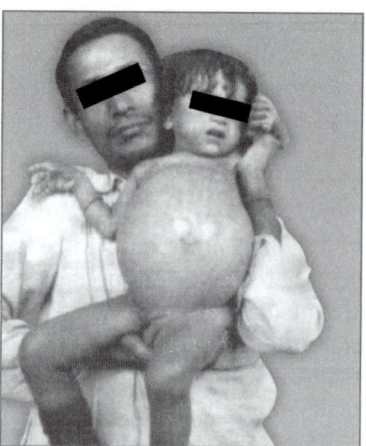

Fig. 37.21: Nephroblastoma (Wilms' tumor) of the left kidney.

spider-leg will be irregular in contradistinction to the same type of defect found in polycystic kidney where the outline will be smooth, the legs will be broadened and majority of the calyces will be affected besides the obvious fact that the defect is seen in both the kidneys. Filling defect may also be seen in the renal pelvis with various types of distortion. Ultrasound, CT, arteriography, Renal and bone scan, chest X-ray and tomography are the other investigations to be carried out to know more about the primary and secondaries of this fast growing tumors.

2. **Nephroblastoma** (Syn. **WILMS' Tumor**) (**Fig. 37.21**): It is a mixed tumor containing embryonic epithelial and connective tissue elements of the kidney. This is a tumor of children and majority of the victims are between 1–5 years of age. The main presenting feature is painless, rapidly growing tumor without hematuria. The tumor grows within its capsule pushing the rest of the kidney to one side. When the tumor bursts through the capsule into the pelvis hematuria results. So this is an ominous sign and indicates very bad prognosis. 50% of the patients suffer from rise in temperature which adds confusion to the diagnosis. On the right side this condition is confused with liver enlargement and on the left side with the splenic enlargement. Blood-borne metastasis is early and liver is mainly affected. Very rarely bones or brain may be involved.

Urography will show the soft tissue shadow of the tumor in nephrogram. Distortion and filling defects of the calyces are the main diagnostic points in urography.

3. **Papillary tumor** of the renal pelvis is discussed under the heading of 'Diseases of the ureter'.

DISEASES OF THE URETER

URETERIC CALCULUS

A stone in the ureter always originates from the kidney. Ureteric colic is the main symptom of this condition. Hematuria may be complained of. Ureteric colic starts as soon as the stone enters the pelvi-ureteric junction and recurs at longer or shorter intervals so long as the stone remains in the ureter. Ureteric colic ceases when the stone is ejected into the bladder or the stone is impacted in the ureter. When the stone is in the upper 1/3rd of the ureter, pain starts in the loin or near the renal angle and gradually radiates to the groin. Pain is griping in nature and starts suddenly. The patient almost tosses over the bed in agony often associated with profuse sweating and nausea. Pain suddenly goes off almost as suddenly as it appeared. At a lower level, pain commences rather anteriorly just above the iliac crest and is referred along the two branches of the genitofemoral nerve to the testis in the male and labium majus in the female and to the antero-medial aspect of the thigh in both sexes. The testis becomes retracted by the spasm of the cremaster. When the stone enters the intramural part of the ureter, pain is referred to the tip of the penis and the patient complains of strangury. When the stone becomes impacted, colic goes off, instead a dull ache arises according to the site of impaction. Such pain varies in intensity, increased by exercise and relieved by rest. On the right side this condition may be confused with appendicitis.

On examination, tenderness and rigidity may be felt along the course of the ureter.

A stone in the lower part of the ureter may be felt in rectal or vaginal examination.

Straight X-ray often reveals stone along the course of the ureter. *Urography* will reveal a nonopaque stone by filling defect. No excretion or delayed excretion is sometimes seen after an attack of ureteric colic. *Cystoscopy* will reveal a stone at the ureteric orifice. It will show delayed or no excretion after intravenous injection of Indigo carmine.

PAPILLARY TUMORS OF THE RENAL PELVIS

Transitional cell tumors can affect any part of the transitional cell epithelium, which lines the whole of the urinary tract. The frequency with which this tumor develops depends upon the length of time the urine, which contains the carcinogen, remains in contact with the epithelial surface. So, this tumor is mostly seen in the bladder (about 90%), then the renal pelvis (about 5%) and lastly in the ureter (about 1%). Painless hematuria is the main presenting symptom. There may be symptoms of ureteric obstruction when it occurs in the ureter. This tumor tends to be malignant. These tumors also spread by seeding into the ureter lower down and even bladder.

Urography is quite diagnostic which shows filling defect according to the position of the papillary tumor whether in the renal pelvis or ureter. Other radiological image and a combination of urinary cytology will confirm the diagnosis.

DISEASES OF THE BLADDER

ECTOPIA VESICAE OR EXSTROPHY OF THE BLADDER (FIGS. 37.22 AND 37.23)

This is a congenital anomaly in which there is defect in the formation or agenesis of the anterior wall of the allantois and lower abdominal wall. This is represented by a thin membrane, which after birth is separated with the umbilical cord. Thus, the posterior wall of the bladder is exposed. There is no umbilicus. Due to pressure of the viscera behind it, the deep red posterior surface extrudes. This surface may bleed. Urine constantly dribbles through the ureteric orifices. Penis is ill-developed and its dorsal surface is split open (epispadias) which is continuous above with the exstrophy of the bladder. There may be inguinal and umbilical hernia. There is always separation of the pubic bones without any symphysis pubis, instead a strong ligament holds the bones.

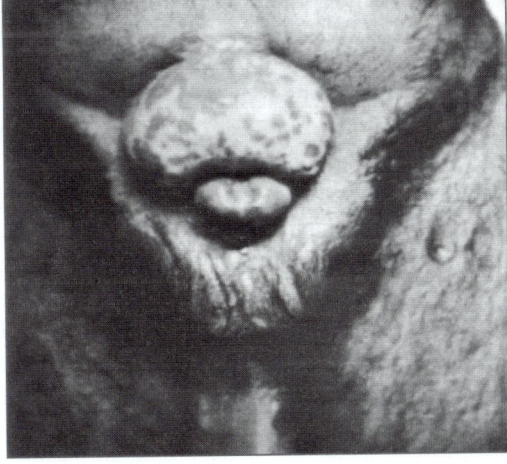

Fig. 37.22: Ectopia vesicae. Note the absence of umbilicus.

RUPTURE OF THE BLADDER: *See* page 613.

VESICAL CALCULUS (Fig. 37.24)

Stones may come to the bladder through the ureter and enlarge here. Otherwise stones may form in the bladder secondary to stasis and infection.

No age is exempt from this disease. Males are much more often affected than females. *Increased frequency of micturition* is the most common symptom. This is not experienced at night. The cause is that in standing posture the stone comes in contact with the trigone and initiates desire to micturate. During night the stone falls off the trigone and frequent desire to micturate goes off. Presence of stone in the bladder will give rise to *pain* in the suprapubic region *particularly after micturition*. This pain is often referred to the tip of the penis or to the labia majora and becomes aggravated by running and jolting. Children may scream and pull the Prepuce for pain after micturition. *Hematuria* at the end of micturition is also common symptom. This is caused by abrasion of the vascular trigone and gets worse on exercise. *Sudden interruption of the flow* due to blockage of the urethral meatus with the stone and subsequent continuation by change of posture is also not uncommon. *Symptoms of cystitis*, e.g., frequency of micturition, burning sensation, postpubic pain, etc., may overshadow those due to presence of stone.

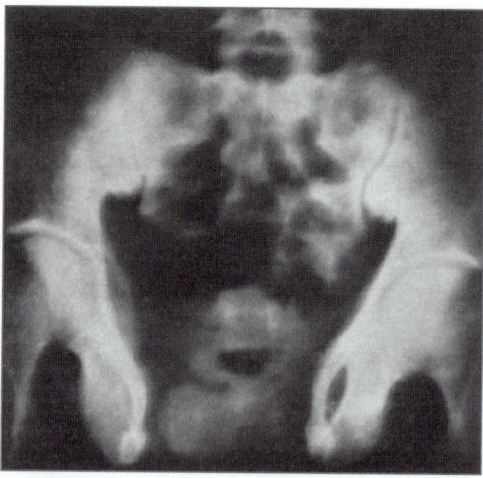

Fig. 37.23: The skiagram of a case of ectopia vesicae. It shows absence of the symphysis pubis resulting in a big gap between the two pubic bones.

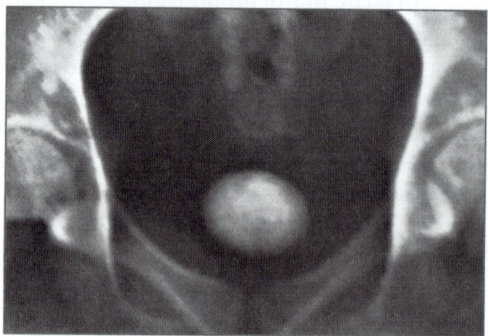

Fig. 37.24: Straight X-ray showing vesical calculus.

Sometimes stone may be situated in the postprostatic pouch or diverticulum without any typical symptom of stone and is only revealed in X-ray or cystoscopy for other complaints. These are known as 'latent stones'.

On examination, one may elicit suprapubic tenderness. A large stone can be felt per rectum (in male) or per vagina (in female). But bimanual palpation (one on the abdomen and the other in the rectum or vagina) may facilitate palpation.

Urine should be examined microscopically and bacteriologically. Straight X-ray will reveal about 95% of the vesical calculus. The whole KUB region should be exposed to exclude further stones in the ureter or kidney. Urography will show nonopaque stones by filling defect and demonstrate the functioning condition of the kidney. Cystoscopy and bladder sound will detect presence of stone as well.

DIVERTICULUM OF THE BLADDER

The usual victim is male over 50 years of age. There is no typical symptom of this condition. This condition usually develops from obstruction distal to the urinary bladder, e.g., bladder neck obstruction, senile enlargement of prostate, fibrous prostate, urethral stricture, posterior urethral valves, etc., So long it remains uninfected, it *remains dormant*. When it becomes infected *symptoms of cystitis* become evident. *Hematuria* may be complained of in a number of cases. *Double micturition* in rapid succession is very suggestive of this condition—first one is clear urine from the bladder and the second is the cloudy urine from the diverticulum.

Urography is confirmatory. Excretory urography will not only reveal this condition, but will also show its impact on the upper urinary tract. If excretory cystography fails to delineate the diverticulum, retrograde cystography will be necessary. Cystoscopy will actually show the diverticulum. For proper inspection the bladder should be fully distended.

CYSTITIS

Though this condition occurs at all times of life, yet young and middle aged subjects are the usual victims and women are more prone to suffer from this disease. Stasis, presence of foreign body (e.g., stone, catheter, neoplasm, etc.), avitaminosis and short urethra of females are the predisposing factors.

The most common symptom is *increased frequency of micturition* both during day and night. Desire to micturate occurs from every hour to every fifteen minutes. *Urgency* is usually associated with and if the bladder cannot be emptied forthwith incontinence results. *Pain* varies from mild discomfort to agonizing. When inflammation affects the dome of the bladder pain is complained of in the suprapubic region. When it affects the trigone pain is felt at the tip of penis or labia majora or even the perineum. Burning or scalding pain along the length of the urethra during micturition is a very typical symptom of this condition. *Hematuria* is quite common and in fact cystitis is the most common cause of hematuria. It is usually a few drops *at the end of micturition*, less often the whole specimen is blood-stained. *Cloudy urine* is also complained of in late cases.

On examination, one hardly finds a typical sign except suprapubic, per rectum or per vaginum tenderness of the urinary bladder. Urine should be examined for routine examinations and for culture and sensitivity tests. Cystoscopy confirms the diagnosis. This reveals hyperemia, mucosal hemorrhages, blistering, sloughing and ulceration of the mucosa.

TUBERCULOUS CYSTITIS

When tuberculosis affects the bladder there is invariably infection in the upper tract. The main complaint of the patient is increased frequency. There is often bladder pain and sometimes hematuria. Gradually the capacity of the bladder is decreased and frequency increases. General malaise, night fever and weight loss are the general features. It must be remembered that even when treated, subsequent scarring leads to a noncompliant bladder. The lower ends of the ureters may be involved to this process of fibrosis leading to obstruction. When the ureter is affected, sclerosing periureteritis may lead to shortening of the ureter, so that the ureteric orifice is pulled up giving rise to a 'golf-hole' ureteric orifice.

Cystoscopy reveals tuberculous ulceration. Early treatment may prevent cicatrization and bladder capacity may be maintained normal. So early treatment is of great importance.

INTERSTITIAL CYSTITIS

This condition is a chronic idiopathic cystitis involving the whole of the bladder. It usually occurs in women between 30 and 40 years of age. Mucosal ulceration with contact bleeding and marked muscular fibrosis are the main pathology which leads to a contracted bladder, the functional capacity of which is thus reduced. Intense frequency of micturition with hematuria and painful bladder are the presenting features.

TUMORS OF THE BLADDER

It can be broadly classified into two varieties clinically—(1) Papilloma and (2) Carcinoma.

Tumors of the bladder are commonly seen in males from middle age onwards. Certain chemicals when excreted in the urine may stimulate malignant change in the bladder. These are alpha- and beta-naphthylamine, benzidine, xylenamine, etc. The industries which use these chemicals are the rubber and cable industries, printers and dyers. Bilharziasis and the conditions which cause chronic irritation of the bladder mucosa may initiate tumor formation.

1. **PAPILLOMA:** Painless, profuse and paroxysmal hematuria is the main and only symptom for a long time. Hematuria may last for a few hours and days and then ceases to recur again after an interval of weeks or months. Sometimes clot retention or obstruction of the internal meatus may cause retention. Fragments of growth may be passed with urine which can be detected microscopically. Diagnosis is established by cystoscopy. A papilloma is pedunculated with villi which float in the fluid of the bladder. Malignant transformation is suspected when (i) the growth is sessile, (ii) the surrounding mucous membrane becomes edematous and more vascular, (iii) the villi are stunted and swollen like cauliflower, (iv) the surface of the growth ulcerates with areas of necrosis, (v) the tumor is accompanied by cystitis or (vi) submucosal lymphatic nodules appear around the growth.

2. **CARCINOMA:** Initial symptom is again profuse and intermittent hematuria. Later on symptoms of cystitis may appear, even strangury may be complained of. Loin pain may be a symptom from obstructed ureter. When the growth has invaded the tissues around the bladder, pain in the suprapubic region, buttock, perineum and even down the thigh may be complained of due to nerve involvement.

Cytology of urine may give a clue to the diagnosis. *Excretory urography* may show soft tissue shadow in case of large malignant growth. Obstruction of ureter may be evidenced in urography. Function of kidneys are generally not jeopardized. Mainly the filling defect of the growth is the diagnostic point in this investigation. *Cystoscopy* is the mainstay of diagnosis. A tumor which is sessile, lobulated, deep red and bleeds to touch is a carcinoma. The surface may become ulcerated in places. A carcinomatous ulcer may be seen. This is seen in the base of the bladder or on the trigone. Ulcer has everted margin and fixed indurated base. This is a fast growing carcinoma. *Bimanual palpation (recto-abdominally in the male and vagino-abdominally in the female) under general anesthesia* is very important to determine the stage of the cancer.

Unless a bladder tumor is large, it is not usually palpable. The majority of the bladder tumors (80%) are superficial, i.e., not involving the muscle of the bladder wall, at the time of first diagnosis. These are not detectable on clinical examination. The remaining 20% have already invaded the muscle of the bladder wall and farther; which can be palpable bimanually under general anesthesia. The size, position and mobility of the tumor must be assessed. The clinical staging of the disease should be performed in determining subsequent treatment. Staging is best achieved by a combination of bimanual examination under anesthesia followed by cystoscopic excision biopsy of the tumor.

DISEASES OF THE PROSTATE

BENIGN HYPERTROPHY OF THE PROSTATE

This is a disease of old age and almost never seen below fifty years of age. Hyperplasia and hypertrophy affect the inner glandular and fibrous tissue which compress the outer portion known as 'surgical capsule'. It is also called adenomatous enlargement of the prostate. The aetiology is not known, but the popular theory is that it is an involutional hypertrophy in response to a changing hormonal environment.

Though prostate starts enlarging at the age of 40 years, but patients usually present between 50 and 70 years.

Increased frequency of micturition particularly at night is the earliest symptom. Patient gets up in the middle of night twice or thrice to pass urine. This is due to inadequate emptying of the bladder and due to presence of sensitive prostatic mucous membrane of the intravesical enlargement of the prostate. Frequency gradually progresses and then presents both by day and night. Another symptom is *urgency* due to the fact that urine escapes through the stretched vesical sphincter into sensitive prostatic mucosa which causes reflex for intense desire to void. Gradually residual urine increases and frequency becomes more and more evident with advent of cystitis and polyuria due to renal insufficiency. *Difficulty in micturition* is quite common. The patient has to *wait* before the stream starts. The stream is weak and dribbles down instead of being projected. Straining hinders flow rather than increasing the flow. *Hematuria* is quite common. It is terminal in prostatic congestion but profuse due to rupture of 'vesical piles'. Some patients present with *retention of urine*—either acute or chronic. Others may present with *over-flow incontinence*. It may so happen that the patient may present with the *symptoms of uremia*—headache, drowsiness, vomiting and even hematemesis.

On examination, it is noted whether the patient is drowsy or not. The tongue should be noted—whether coated or not. The kidneys should be palpated. Tenderness there indicates pyelonephritis and enlargement may indicate hydronephrosis. Examine the penis, testis and epididymis.

Diagnosis is mainly made by *rectal examination*. The examination should be performed with the patient in the left lateral position or some prefer the knee-elbow position. The urinary bladder must be emptied before the examination. The index finger is usually used and should face the anterior surface of the rectum, so that the lobes of the prostate can be felt through the rectal wall. The prostate gland is enlarged. The finger may not even reach the upper limit of the prostate. The prostate may not be felt enlarged if only the median lobe is enlarged. It is not tender. The gland is firm, rubbery and lobulated. The two lateral lobes of the gland can be felt to bulge into the rectum divided by the central sulcus which is well defined. There may be some asymmetry of the enlargement, though both the lobes retain their smooth texture. Total prostatic volume is assessed by passing the examining finger from base to apex and also from side to side. It must be remembered that the size of the gland may not always correlate with the degree of obstruction by the gland or the symptoms of the patient. Consistency is homogeneous. The surface is smooth and bosselated. Persistence of median sulcus is a definite sign of this condition which is often obliterated in carcinoma. The rectal mucosa moves freely over the gland. It is advisable to empty the bladder first in retention for better palpation.

Clinically, the prostate is divided into 3 lobes, 2 lateral and 1 median. Histological process of benign prostatic hyperplasia usually affects all the lobes equally. Sometimes the median lobe may grow more than the lateral lobes. This lobe cannot be felt per rectum and the prostate may appear normal. However cystoscopically enlargement of this lobe can be detected. Enlargement of median lobe gives rise to mainly irritative symptoms, e.g., nocturia, frequency and urgency. Enlargement of lateral lobes mainly gives rise to obstructive symptoms, e.g., slow stream, terminal dribbling and hesitancy.

Blood is examined routinely for Hb%, total count (TC), differential count (DC), ESR, urea and sugar. *Urine* should be sent for routine examination, culture and sensitivity. Urography will indicate functional status of the kidneys and presence or absence of hydronephrosis. Cystography after voiding will indicate the amount of residual urine. Cystography may show filling defect due to projection of median lobe inside the bladder. *Cystoscopy* is essential to exclude presence of diverticulum, stone and growth. This is more important when the operation of prostatectomy is not performed transvesical.

Three recent advances have made diagnosis of this disease easier. These are estimation of prostate-specific antigen (PSA), transrectal ultrasound scanning and transrectal biopsy with ultrasound control. These are more elaborately discussed in the section of carcinoma of the prostate (see below).

ACUTE PROSTATITIS

Blood-borne infection seems to be the cause of this condition. High rise of temperature, rigor, pain all over the body particularly in the back are the prodromal symptoms which may mislead the clinician. Specific symptoms are perineal heaviness, pain during micturition and defecation. Increased frequency of micturition is only complained of when cystitis has supervened.

On examination, no abnormality can be detected except tenderness of the prostate on rectal examination. Initial specimen of urine which contains threads should be sent for culture and sensitivity.

CHRONIC PROSTATITIS

This generally occurs due to inadequate treatment of acute prostatitis. Aches all over with mild pyrexia and malaise are the usual symptoms. Premature ejaculation and impotence may be associated with. Dull ache in the perineum, low backache radiating downwards to the thigh and *gleety urine* are the only specific symptoms.

Diagnosis is based on rectal examination which may reveal a slightly tender prostate relatively firmer and irregular or softer than normal, examination of the fluid received by prostatic massage (which will contain pus cells and bacteria), microscopical examination, culture and sensitivity of the initial specimen of urine which contains the gleet and urethroscopy which reveals dilated prostatic ducts which may extrude pus.

CARCINOMA OF PROSTATE

This is the most common malignant condition in men over 60 years of age. Carcinoma of the prostate begins in the outer part of the gland, so it spreads easily into the floor of the pelvis. It often reaches an advanced stage before it causes symptoms. Symptoms are similar to those of benign hypertrophy of prostate—*frequency, urgency* and *difficulty of micturition* (collectively known as 'prostatism'). But the main difference is that the history is quite short and they get worse rapidly. About half the patients present with some form of *retention of urine*—acute or chronic. General debility, malaise, anemia and loss of weight are common. Sometimes urinary symptoms are absent or slight. *Pain in the back, sciatica* (from metastasis in the spine) and *pathological fractures* may be the symptoms first to appear.

On examination, the bladder may be felt suprapubically when there is retention. *Rectal examination* will reveal relatively hard nodular prostate, irregular and heterogenous in consistency. The median sulcus will be obliterated (very important sign) and the rectal mucosa is tethered to the gland (rectal mucosa cannot be moved over the prostate). The tissues lateral to the gland may be infiltrated giving rise to 'winging' of the prostate. Occasionally carcinoma may arise from an already adenomatous enlarged gland, so even in case of benign enlargement one should look for discrete induration. For clinical staging of the disease the students are referred to author's 'A CONCISE TEXTBOOK OF SURGERY', page 1323.

Digital rectal examination is an important screening examination for prostatic malignancy. Used in combination with measurement of serum level of the prostate-specific antigen and transrectal ultrasound and biopsy have led to a dramatic increase in the number of men diagnosed with prostatic carcinoma.

Special investigations are serum acid phosphatase (only raised when there is bony metastasis) and alkaline phosphatase, biopsy of the prostate, radiological examination (which shows osteoblastic lesion), bone scanning **(Fig. 37.25)**, lymphangiography, etc. Biopsy can be performed with a needle through the perineum, transurethral resection (which has the advantage of removing obstruction and providing large piece of tissue for examination and is mainly done during retention), but open perineal biopsy is still favored by a few urologists.

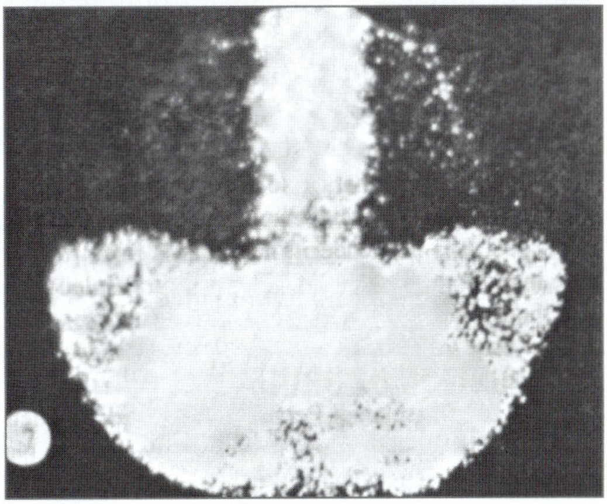

Fig. 37.25: Bone scan showing metastatic deposits in the iliac bones and lumbar vertebrae in a case of carcinoma of prostate.

Three recent advances are now used in specialized centers for precise diagnosis of this condition and also used as screening procedures to detect more patients with carcinoma of prostate. These are:

1. *Estimation of prostate-specific antigen:* prostate-specific antigen (PSA) is a glycoprotein, whose function is to facilitate liquefaction of semen. It is now being used as a marker for prostatic disease. It is measured by immunoassay technique and the normal upper limit is about 4 nmol/mL. It is more important in the diagnosis of carcinoma of prostate, in which case the level goes up to 15 nmol/mL in localized cancer to 30 nmol/mL in case of metastatic cancer. However in benign hyperplasia of prostate the level goes up to 4–10 nmol/mL.

2. *Transrectal ultrasound scanning*: This imaging technique offers accurate estimation of prostatic size. It is probably more effective in detection of associated early prostatic cancer. If such suspicion is not there, it is not required to use routinely. It is used when the level of PSA is high or the surface of prostate is hard and irregular. Though this investigation can be used in early detection of the tumor, however many such tumors are also missed with this technique. In fact only about 50% of cancers can be diagnosed with this technique.

3. Presently *transrectal biopsy* using an automated gun with appropriate antibiotic cover is used. Several cores are taken to make definite diagnosis.

URETHRAL STRICTURE

This is due to formation of fibrous tissue following damage to the urethral mucosa. The most common cause is gonococcal urethritis transmitted through sexual intercourse and obviously the sufferers are young adults.

Patient often gives a past history of exuding pus per urethra and later on glairy urethral discharge, particularly noticeable in the morning.

The most common symptom is *difficulty in micturition (dysuria)*. But the difference from benign hypertrophy of prostate is that the *flow increases on straining*. Normally the stream is thin and dribbles at the end. Gradually cystitis develops which increases frequency of micturition and causes urgency. *Acute retention* is quite common.

On examination, nothing abnormality could be detected except that the bladder may be palpable when it is distended. Examine the kidney region for back pressure and infection. Diagnosis is confirmed by passing bougie which will be obstructed at the bulb of the urethra (common site of stricture in gonococcal urethritis). Urethrography will demonstrate the site and length of the stricture. The *chief complications* are retention of urine and periurethral abscess which may burst to cause urethral fistula or extravasation of urine, according as it opens to the exterior or subcutaneous tissue respectively.

Other causes of urethral stricture are : (i) bad instrumentation (catheterization or bougienage); (ii) following prostatectomy; (iii) amputation of penis; (iv) direct injury (following treatment of rupture of urethra); (v) meatal ulcer; and (vi) urethral neoplasm.

▌RETENTION OF URINE

Retention of urine means accumulation of urine in the urinary bladder. Patient is unable to pass urine or passes small quantity of urine. It must be remembered that kidneys excrete urine normally. In anuria also patient does not pass urine but in this condition the kidneys fail to excrete urine and there is no urine in the bladder, hence collapsed. There are two forms of retention of urine—acute retention and chronic retention.

Acute retention is sudden inability to pass urine and it is a painful condition. *Chronic retention* is gradual accumulation of urine in the bladder due to inability of the patient to empty the bladder completely. The result is an enlarged painless bladder. If infection supervenes on chronic retention it becomes painful and it is often described as acute-on-chronic retention. It may be called 'infection-on-chronic retention'.

ACUTE RETENTION

It must be remembered that acute retention in a normal bladder is extremely rare and occurs only after anesthesia, an injury to the urethra or after a surgical operation. In majority of cases there has been a chronic retention before the acute attack. These cases may be called acute-on-chronic retention. The patient is likely to have some symptoms related to chronic retention previous to the acute episode. Sudden inability to pass urine with severe pain and with an exaggerated desire to micturate is the main presenting feature of this condition.

On examination, the urinary bladder is sufficiently enlarged to become palpable, tense and dull arising out of the pelvis. Pressure on this swelling increases the patient's desire to micturate.

Rectal examination will reveal that the prostate or uterus is pushed backwards and downwards by the bladder which can be easily felt as a cystic mass. It must be remembered that one cannot assess the size of the prostate gland when the bladder is full. One must try to feel the other organs of the pelvis as well. Sensory, motor and reflex functions of the nerves of the perineum and lower limbs should be assessed carefully.

CHRONIC RETENTION

Elderly individuals are mainly affected by this disease. Chronic retention is a painless condition and the patient is often unaware of his/her distended bladder. The symptoms may be in the form of increased frequency of micturition, difficulty of micturition or even overflow incontinence.

On examination the foreskin and urethral meatus should be examined for phimosis or meatal stenosis. The length of the urethra as far as the bulb should be palpated for a stricture, periurethral abscess or presence of a stone or a foreign body. Urethral discharge, if present, should be noted. The prostate must be examined, as this is the most common cause of retention of urine in the male. But the bladder should be deflated before proper assessment of the prostate. The bladder is always palpable. It may reach the umbilicus or somewhere in between the pubic symphysis and umbilicus. It is neither tense nor tender. Pressure on the bladder does not initiate the desire to micturate (cf. acute retention). The bladder is obviously dull to percussion and may elicit fluid thrill if the patient is thin. Examination of the nervous system is of immense importance. Bladder sensation/micturition reflex arc may be inhibited by a disease of CNS which is localized at the level of the mid sacral neural outflow. Absent ankle jerk and diminished or absent cutaneous sensation in the perineum and perianal regions are usually associated with such lesion.

In infants and *children* the urinary bladder is more of an abdominal organ and can be palpated without retention of urine. If there is difficulty or inability to pass urine the cause is most likely to be neurological in origin or due to obstruction from the presence of posterior urethral valves.

The **causes** of retention of urine are classified as follows:
A. **Mechanical:**
(a) *Urinary bladder*: Stone, tumor, blood clot and contracture of the bladder neck.
(b) *Prostate*: Prostatic abscess, benign and malignant enlargements.
(c) *Urethra*: Urethral stricture, rupture, congenital valves, foreign body, acute urethritis, stone, growth, pin-hole meatus, meatal ulcer.
(d) *Prepuce*: Phimosis.
From outside:
Pregnancy (retroverted gravid uterus), fibroid, ovarian cyst, carcinoma of the cervix uteri and rectum and any pelvic growth and paraphimosis.
B. **Neurogenic:**
(a) *Spinal cord diseases*, e.g., disseminated sclerosis, tabes dorsalis, transverse myelitis, etc.
(b) *Injuries and diseases of the spine*, e.g., fracture-dislocation, Pott's disease, etc.
(c) *Miscellaneous*, e.g., postoperative retention, hysteria, tetanus, drugs such as anticholinergics, smooth muscle relaxants, tranquillizers, etc.

HEMATURIA

Causes: These can be conveniently described under four headings—1. Lesions of the urinary tract; 2. Diseases of the adjacent viscera involving the urinary tract; 3. General disorders; 4. After ingestion of certain drugs.

1. **Lesion of the urinary tract:**
I. **KIDNEY:**
Congenital—polycystic kidney.
Traumatic—ruptured kidney.
Inflammatory—tuberculosis, acute nephritis (rare).
Neoplastic—angioma, carcinoma of the kidney, nephroblastoma of the kidney, papilloma or carcinoma of the renal pelvis.
Others—Stone, infarction, essential hematuria.
II. **URETER:** Stone, papilloma or carcinoma of urothelium.
III. **BLADDER:**
Traumatic—rupture.
Inflammatory—cystitis, Tuberculosis, Bilharziasis.
Neoplastic—papilloma and carcinoma.
Others—stone.
IV. **PROSTATE:** Benign and malignant enlargement. Sometimes prostatitis.
V. **URETHRA:**
Traumatic—Rupture.
Inflammatory—Acute urethritis.
Neoplastic—Transitional cell carcinoma.
Others—Stone.
2. **Diseases of the adjacent viscera:**
Acute appendicitis, salpingitis and *pelvic abscess.* The inflammatory process may spread to the ureter and bladder. *Carcinoma of the rectum* and *cervix uteri* may infiltrate the bladder to cause hematuria.
3. **General disorders:**
I. **BLOOD DISORDERS:** Purpura, sickle cell anemia, hemophilia, scurvy, malaria.
II. **INFARCTION:** Arterial emboli from myocardial infarct and subacute bacterial endocarditis.
III. **CONGESTION:** Right heart failure and renal vein thrombosis.
IV. **COLLAGEN DISEASES.**
D. **Drugs:** Anticoagulant drugs, hexamine, sulfonamides and salicylates—when given in large doses.

INCREASED FREQUENCY OF MICTURITION

In a normal person the act of micturition occurs 5–6 times during 24 hours. There will be increased frequency if the fluid intake is more than usual (physiological) or if the amount of urine formation is increased as in diabetes and chronic interstitial nephritis. If the total amount of urine remains normal, **causes** of increased frequency are:
1. *Renal*—any form of pyelitis, stone, tuberculosis and movable kidney.
2. *Ureteric*—stone (the lower the position of the stone the more is the frequency).
3. *Vesical*—any form of cystitis and stone; inflammatory condition of the pelvis, e.g., salpingitis, appendicitis; secondary infiltration from carcinoma of the uterus or rectum; mechanical obstruction to normal distension by a tumor, e.g., ovarian cyst, fibroid or retroverted uterus.
4. *Prostatic*—prostatitis, senile enlargement and malignant prostate.
5. *Urethral*—posterior urethritis (Gonococcal), stone, pin-hole meatus, phimosis and balanitis.

Investigation: History is taken as discussed above. Enquire whether frequency is more marked during the day or night, or there is no such distinction. Diurnal frequency is peculiar to vesical calculus and is due to irritation of the trigone in the erect position; nocturnal frequency, when complained of by an elderly man, is due to senile enlargement of the prostate; whereas in cystitis, frequency is equally marked by day and night. It must be remembered that frequency *in a young adult with sterile acid urine containing pus should be regarded as being due to renal tuberculosis* until this can be excluded. The other common cause in a young adult is gonococcal posterior urethritis in which the history is often helpful. In the middle-aged person one should think of diabetes in which the triad is polyuria (excessive discharge of urine), polydipsia (extreme thirst) and polyphagia (excessive eating). In the old, senile enlargement of the prostate is the most common cause.

Physical examination and *special investigations* are carried out as discussed above in order to arrive at a definite diagnosis.

Algorithmic Approach to Patient with Urinary Disorders

Patient presents with urinary symptoms (pain, hematuria, retention, frequency, discharge)

↓

Is there hematuria?
- Yes → Determine pattern
  - Initial hematuria (at the start of urination) → **Urethral origin** (infection, trauma)
  - Terminal hematuria (at the end of urination) → **Bladder origin** (bladder cancer, prostatitis)
  - Total hematuria (throughout urination) → **Renal origin** (glomerulonephritis, RCC, trauma)
- No → Proceed to next step

↓

Is there pain?
- Yes → Determine pain type and location
  - Dull flank pain → **Hydronephrosis, tumors, pyelonephritis**
  - Colicky pain (radiating to groin) → **Ureteric colic (renal calculi, blood clots)**
  - Suprapubic pain → **Cystitis, bladder outlet obstruction**
- No → Proceed to next step

↓

Is there urinary retention?
- Yes → Differentiate **acute vs chronic**
  - Acute retention (painful, sudden onset) → **Prostate obstruction, urethral stricture, neurogenic bladder**
  - Chronic retention (painless, progressive) → **BPH, detrusor dysfunction, diabetes**
- No → Evaluate **urinary frequency and nocturia**

↓

Is there increased urinary frequency?
- Yes → Differentiate **daytime vs nocturnal**
  - Daytime frequency → **UTI, diabetes mellitus, bladder stones**
  - Nocturia (frequent nighttime urination) → **BPH, bladder cancer, chronic kidney disease**
- No → Proceed to special investigations

↓

Perform physical examination (DRE, palpation, percussion, special tests)
- Digital rectal examination (DRE) → Assess for **prostatic enlargement, hard nodules (cancer), median lobe hypertrophy (BPH).**
- Palpate for bladder distension → Rule out **acute retention or chronic obstruction**
- Percussion of flank area → Renal enlargement in **hydronephrosis, tumors**
- Murphy's kidney punch test → Renal angle tenderness (pyelonephritis, renal abscess)

↓

Special investigations based on clinical suspicion
- Urinalysis and microscopy → Detect **hematuria, proteinuria, pyuria (infection), crystals (stones)**
- Renal function tests (creatinine, urea, electrolytes) → Evaluate **kidney function**
- Ultrasound (KUB region) → Identify **stones, tumors, hydronephrosis**
- CT scan (if required) → Detailed **renal pathology, mass lesions, obstruction sites**

↓

Confirm diagnosis and initiate treatment based on findings
- Medical management → UTI, pyelonephritis, BPH (alpha-blockers, 5-ARI inhibitors)
- Surgical interventions → Ureteroscopy for stones, TURP for BPH, cystectomy for bladder cancer
- Lifestyle modifications → Hydration, dietary changes for stone prevention

Examination of a Case of Hernia

CHAPTER 38

A *hernia* is defined as protrusion of whole or a part of a viscus through the wall that contains it. The term can be applied to protrusion of a muscle through its fascial covering or of brain through fracture of skull or through foramen magnum into the spinal canal. But by far the most common variety of hernia is protrusion of a viscus or a part of it through the abdominal wall and will be discussed here.

Of the abdominal herniae, the common varieties are inguinal, femoral, umbilical, incisional and epigastric, while the rare varieties are obturator, lumbar, gluteal and Spigelian.

Inguinal hernia comes out through the superficial inguinal ring. Indirect or oblique inguinal hernia **(Fig. 38.1)** comes out of the abdominal cavity through the deep inguinal ring, traverses all along the inguinal canal and ultimately becomes superficial through the superficial inguinal ring. Direct inguinal hernia enters the inguinal canal through the medial half

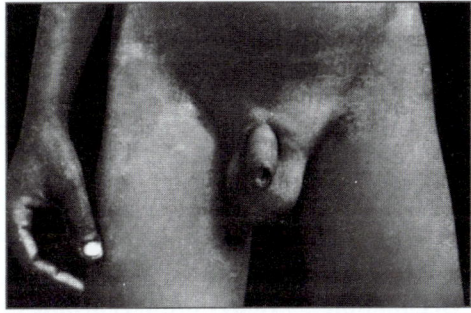

Fig. 38.1: A typical case of left oblique inguinal hernia.

of its weak posterior wall (through the Hesselbach's triangle) and becomes superficial through the same superficial inguinal ring. Inguinal hernia is said to be complete when the contents have reached the bottom of the scrotum. Otherwise the hernia is incomplete.

Femoral hernia comes out through the femoral canal and becomes superficial through the saphenous opening.

■ HISTORY

Comprehensive history-taking for hernia cases should include:
- **Age-based considerations:**
    - **Infants and children:** Congenital hernias (indirect inguinal, umbilical, diaphragmatic hernia).
    - **Young adults (20–40 years):** Inguinal hernia (most common), femoral hernia in women.
    - **Elderly (>50 years):** Incisional hernia (postsurgery), sliding hernia, richter's hernia.
- **Nature of swelling:**
    - **Reducible lump** → Likely uncomplicated hernia.
    - **Nonreducible lump (incarcerated)** → May indicate obstruction or strangulation.
    - **Sudden severe pain with redness (strangulated hernia)** → Emergency condition.

- **Location of swelling and its significance:**
  - **Groin region** → Inguinal or femoral hernia.
  - **Periumbilical swelling** → Umbilical hernia.
  - **Midline abdominal swelling** → Epigastric hernia.
  - **Postsurgical swelling** → Incisional hernia.
- **Associated symptoms:**
  - **Pain on straining (coughing, lifting weights)** → Common in uncomplicated hernias.
  - **Constipation, vomiting, abdominal distension** → Suggests obstruction (complicated hernia).
  - **Sudden onset of severe pain and redness over swelling** → Strangulation (emergency).
- **Occupation and lifestyle:**
  Heavy weightlifting, chronic cough, Constipation → Increased risk of hernia formation.

History in hernia cases

Aspect	Clinical significance	Patient-friendly questions
Onset and duration	Sudden → Strangulated hernia Gradual → Reducible hernia	"When did you first notice the swelling? Has it changed over time?"
Pain	Mild → Reducible hernia Severe, Persistent → Strangulated hernia	"Does the swelling hurt, especially when coughing or lifting?"
Reducibility	Yes → Uncomplicated hernia No → Incarcerated/strangulated hernia	"Can you push the swelling back in?"
Occupation and lifestyle	Heavy lifting, chronic cough → Increased hernia risk	"Do you frequently lift heavy objects or suffer from a chronic cough?"

■ COMPLAINTS

1. **Pain:** In the beginning when there is a 'tendency to hernia' the patient complains of a dragging and aching type of pain which gets worse as the day passes. Pain may appear long before the lump is noticed. It continues so long as the hernia is progressing but ceases when it is fully formed.

   When the hernia becomes very painful and tender, it is probably strangulated. At this time the patient may complain of pain all over the abdomen due to drag on the mesentery or omentum.

2. **Lump:** Many herniae may cause no pain and the patient presents because he noticed a swelling in the groin. But this is very rare and some sort of discomfort is almost always present. The followings are the set of questions to be asked in case of any inguinoscrotal swelling:

   (a) *How did it start?*—Whether on straining like coughing or lifting weight. This is usual in case of a hernia. (b) *Where did it first appear?* If it be in the groin and gradually extended into the scrotum—it is an inguinal hernia. If it had appeared below the groin crease and gradually ascends above it—the swelling is a femoral hernia. (c) *What was the size and extent when it was first seen?* If the hernia reaches the bottom of the scrotum at its first appearance, it is a congenital hernia developed into a preformed sac. It must be remembered that though it is a congenital hernia it may appear at any age. In the acquired type the swelling is small to start with and gradually increases in size. (d) *Does it disappear automatically on lying down?* Direct inguinal hernia disappears automatically as soon as the patient lies down. Indirect hernia has to be reduced.

3. **Systemic symptoms:** If the hernia is obstructing the lumen of the bowel (incarcerated hernia) cardinal symptoms of intestinal obstruction will appear. They are colicky abdominal pain, vomiting, abdominal distension and absolute constipation. If the patient is vomiting, note the character of the vomitus—whether bilious or fecal smelling. Fecal smelling vomitus heralds ominous sign.

4. **Other complaints:** The cause of the hernia must be enquired into. Persistent coughing of chronic bronchitis, constipation, frequency of micturition or urgency of benign enlargement of prostate may be the earlier complaints which the patients deliberately do not mention considering them to be irrelevant. Leading questions may be asked to find out these complaints.

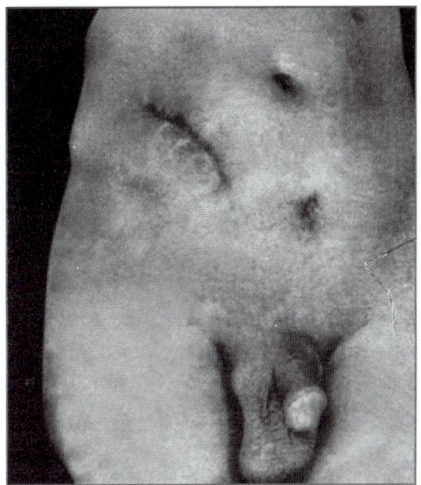

Fig. 38.2: A direct inguinal hernia may develop as a result of weakness of the abdominal wall caused by division of nerves during appendicectomy.

PAST HISTORY: Whether the patient had any operation or not? During appendicectomy division of nerve may lead to weakness of the abdominal muscles at the inguinal region and a subsequent direct inguinal hernia **(Fig. 38.2)**. Many a time the patient gives a previous history of hernia repair on the same side (recurrent hernia) or on the opposite side (right sided hernia generally precedes that of the left side).

LOCAL EXAMINATION

It must be realized that both the inguinal regions must be exposed from the level of the umbilicus to the midthigh level.

Position of the patient: Patient is first examined in the standing position and then in the supine position. Inguinal, femoral, epigastric, obturator, lumbar, gluteal and Spigelian herniae are best examined in the standing position and should not be omitted. The patient is asked to hold the clothes up during examination in the standing position. He must not bend forward while being examined.

A. INSPECTION

1. **Swelling:** If a swelling is already present, note (i) *Size and shape*: An indirect hernia is pyriform in shape, with a stalk at the external inguinal ring **(Fig. 38.3)**. It usually extends down into the scrotum. A direct hernia is spherical in shape and shows little tendency to enter into the scrotum. Femoral hernia, takes up a spherical shape starting from below and lateral to the pubic tubercle. (ii) *Position and extent:* Inguinal hernia extends from above the inner part of the inguinal ligament down to the scrotum. Note if the swelling goes right down to the bottom of the scrotum (congenital type) or stops just above the testis (funicular and acquired varieties). Femoral hernia extends from below the inguinal ligament and ascends over it **(Fig. 38.4)**. (iii) *Visible peristalsis:* If the covering is thin as in recurrent hernia peristalsis may be observed. Visible peristalsis is never seen in femoral hernia. In case of inguinal hernia the students should remember that the scrotal skin exhibits movements due to contraction of the dartos.

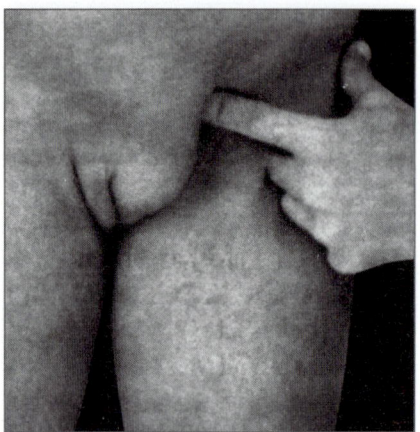

Fig. 38.3: In case of inguinal hernia, which is even commoner in case of females, the swelling lies medial to the pubic tubercle positioned by the tip of the index finger.

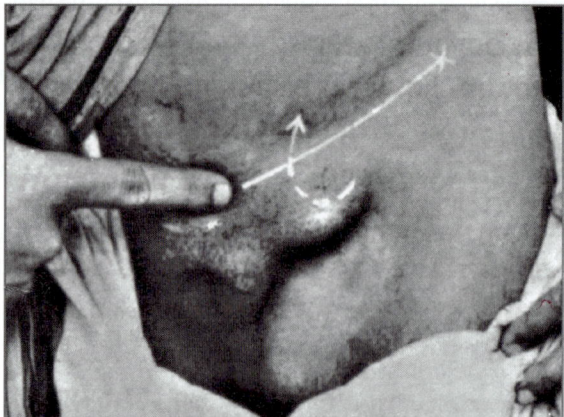

Fig. 38.4: The femoral hernia lies lateral to the pubic tubercle (positioned by the tip of the index finger) and below the inguinal ligament. When the hernia enlarges it travels upwards superficial to the inguinal ligament as shown by the arrow.

2. **Skin over the swelling:** In uncomplicated hernia the overlying skin should be normal. If the hernia is strangulated the skin may be reddened. If the patient is using truss for a long time, discoloration and streaks of brown pigmentation due to deposition of hemosiderin may be seen. The subcutaneous tissue may be atrophied, so the skin may be wrinkled. In case of recurrent hernia scar of previous operation will be evident. A wide, irregular and puckered scar indicates wound infection following previous operation. This is one of the common causes of recurrence.

3. **Impulse on coughing (Fig. 38.5):** The patient is asked to turn his face away from the clinician and to cough. This is done to avoid the salivary shower from the patient. Look carefully at the superficial inguinal ring. If a swelling already exists, it will expand during coughing as more abdominal contents will be driven out into the hernial sac due to increased abdominal tension (expansile cough impulse). If a swelling was not present a momentary bulge may be seen synchronously with the act of coughing. Presence of expansile cough impulse is almost diagnostic of a hernia, but absence of this sign does not exclude a diagnosis of hernia. If the neck of the sac is blocked by adhesions additional viscera will not get access into the sac during coughing.

4. **Position of the penis:** This is only important in case of inguinal hernia. A large hernia in the scrotum will push the penis to the other side.

B. PALPATION

If a swelling is present it is palpated systematically from in front, from the side and from behind noting all the points, e.g., temperature, tenderness, size and shape, etc., as discussed in Chapter 3

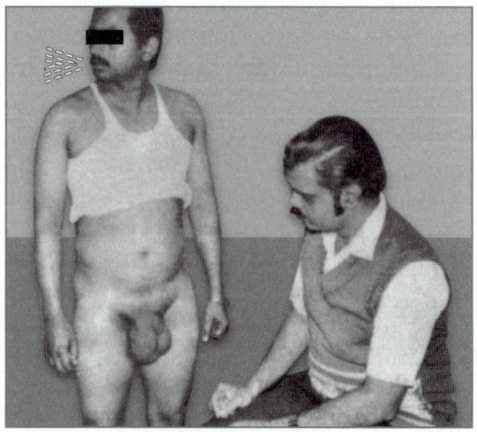

Fig. 38.5: Looking for an impulse on coughing while the patient coughs. Note the position of the patient (standing and that of the examiner—sitting).

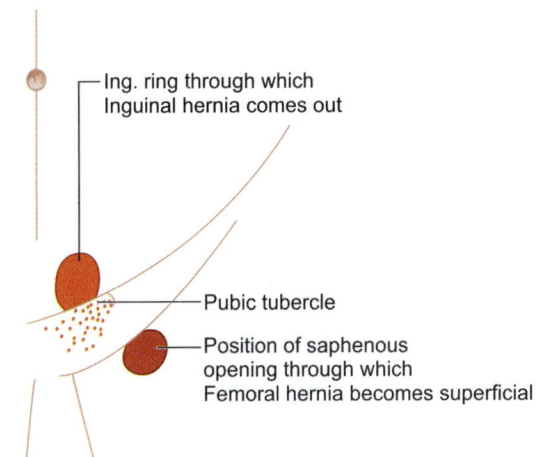

Fig. 38.6: Diagrammatic representation showing the relative positions of inguinal hernia and femoral hernia in respect to pubic tubercle. The superficial inguinal ring is placed above and medial to the pubic tubercle. The saphenous opening is situated 4 cm below and lateral to pubic tubercle.

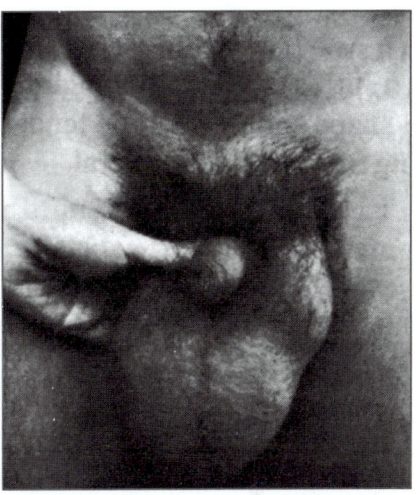

Fig. 38.7: Shows the method 'to get above the swelling'. In a case of inguinal hernia this is not possible. It is only possible in a pure scrotal swelling.

'Examination of a Swelling'. Only important points relevant to cases of hernia are discussed below:

1. **Position** and **extent**: If the swelling descends into the scrotum or labia majora, it is obviously an inguinal hernia. When it remains confined to the groin, it should be differentiated from a femoral hernia. Two anatomical structures are considered in this respect—(a) the pubic tubercle and (b) the inguinal ligament **(Fig. 38.6)**. An inguinal hernia is positioned above the inguinal ligament and medial to the pubic tubercle, whereas a femoral hernia lies below the inguinal ligament and lateral to the pubic tubercle. But it must be remembered that a large femoral hernia ascends superficial to the inguinal ligament though its base will still be below the inguinal ligament. In obese patients it is very difficult to feel the pubic tubercle. One may follow the tendon of adductor longus upwards to reach the pubic tubercle.

2. **To get above the swelling (Fig. 38.7)**: In case of a swelling this is important. This examination differentiates a scrotal swelling from an inguinoscrotal swelling. The root of the scrotum is held between the thumb in front and other fingers behind in an attempt to reach above the swelling. In case of inguinal hernia one cannot get above the swelling, whereas in case of the pure scrotal swelling one can feel nothing between the fingers except the structures within the spermatic cord. In case of femoral hernia this examination is of no use as femoral hernia does not give rise to a scrotal swelling.

3. **Consistency:** The swelling feels doughy and granular if the hernia contains omentum (omentocele or epiplocele). It is elastic if it contains intestine (enterocele). A strangulated hernia feels tense and tender. This is of great importance in diagnosing this condition.

4. **Relation of the swelling to the testis and spermatic cord:** Inguinal hernia remains in front and sides of the spermatic cord and testis which remain incorporated in the swelling. If the hernia is acquired or of funicular variety the hernia stops just above the testis. So the testis can be felt apart from the hernia.

TWO CLASSICAL SIGNS OF AN UNCOMPLICATED HERNIA ARE: (i) IMPULSE ON COUGHING AND (ii) REDUCIBILITY.

5. **Impulse on coughing** (Fig. 38.8): This examination should always be performed in standing position of the patient. When there is no swelling a finger is placed on the superficial inguinal ring and the patient is asked to cough. The root of the scrotum can also be held between the index finger and the thumb and felt for impulse on coughing. Contents of hernia will force out through the superficial inguinal ring and separate the thumb and the index finger. This is an expansile impulse. *Impulse on coughing will be absent in case of strangulated hernia, incarcerated hernia and when the neck of the sac becomes blocked by adhesions which prevent fresh entrance of the contents into the sac.* A distinguished method (Fig. 38.9) to find out whether the case is one of direct, indirect (oblique) or femoral hernia is to place the index finger over the deep inguinal ring (½ inch above the midinguinal point, which is the midpoint between anterior superior iliac spine and symphysis pubis), the middle finger over the superficial inguinal ring and the ring finger over the saphenous opening (4 cm below and lateral to the pubic tubercle). Remember this technique (*Zieman's technique*) can only be applied when there is no obvious swelling or after the hernia has been completely reduced. The patient is asked to hold the nose and blow (this is better according to Zieman) or to cough. When impulse is felt on the index finger the case is one of indirect hernia, when impulse is felt on the middle finger the case is one of direct hernia and when it is felt on the ring finger the case is one of femoral hernia.

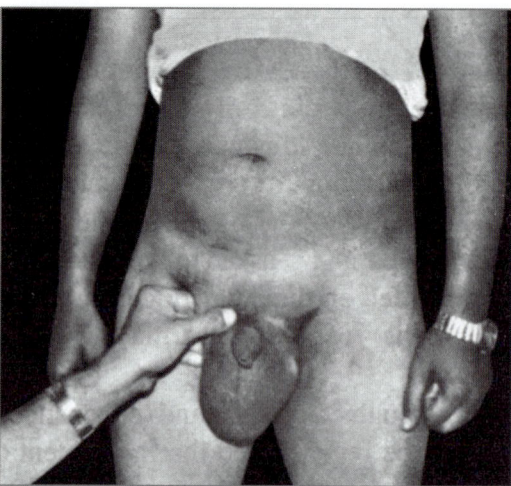

Fig. 38.8: Shows the method of palpation for impulse on coughing.

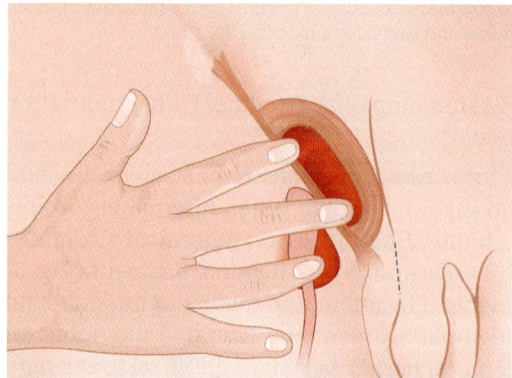

Fig. 38.9: Zieman's technique is shown in which the index finger is placed on the deep inguinal ring (to detect bulge of the indirect inguinal hernia when the patient coughs), the middle finger is placed on the superficial inguinal ring (to detect bulge of the direct inguinal hernia when the patient coughs) and the ring finger is placed on the saphenous opening (to detect bulge of the femoral hernia when the patient coughs). The patient is now asked to cough to diagnose the type of hernia the patient is suffering from.

In presence of swelling, coughing will expand (expansile impulse) the swelling and will increase tension within the swelling. It must be remembered that movement of the swelling is not a criterion. A localized swelling of the spermatic cord (encysted hydrocele of the cord) or an undescended testis will sometimes move down the inguinal canal and may come out through the external opening yet it is not a hernia. In case of a large femoral hernia many a time it is not so easy to elicit impulse on coughing. The whole mass is picked up between the thumb and the fingers to get at the root. Now the patient is asked to cough to palpate impulse on coughing.

6. **Is the swelling reducible?** The patient is first instructed to lie down on the bed. In many instances the hernia reduces itself when the patient lies down (direct hernia). You may ask the patient to reduce the hernia and in majority of cases the patients can reduce it aptly. In the remaining cases the patient is asked to flex the thigh of the affected side and to adduct and rotate it internally. This will not only relax the pillars of the superficial ring but also will relax the oblique muscles of the abdomen. The fundus of the sac is gently held with one hand and even pressure is applied to it to squeeze the contents towards and abdomen while the other hand will guide the contents through the superficial inguinal ring **(Fig. 38.10)**. *This is known as 'Taxis.'* Taxis must be carried out very gently. Rough handling will bring forth fatal complications. Note whether the contents reduce with gurgling. This occurs in an enterocele. In enterocele the first part is often difficult to reduce but the last part slips in easily. In an omentocele the first part goes in easily while the last part resents to be reduced.

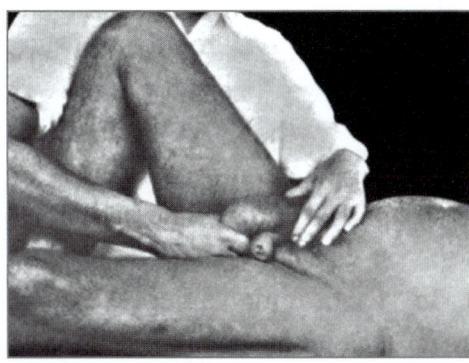

Fig. 38.10: Shows the method of reducing an inguinal hernia. Note that the thigh is flexed and internally rotated. With one hand the fundus of the sac is being squeezed while with the other hand the hernia is directed through the superficial inguinal ring.

In case of femoral hernia similar maneuver is employed to reduce except for the fact that the contents are reduced through the saphenous opening.

If a hernia cannot be reduced, it is an irreducible hernia or an obstructed hernia or a strangulated hernia.

7. **Invagination test (Figs. 38.11A and B):** *After reduction of the hernia,* this test may be performed to palpate the hernial orifice. It is better to perform this test in recumbent position of the patient. Little finger should be used to minimize hurting the patient. But if it becomes

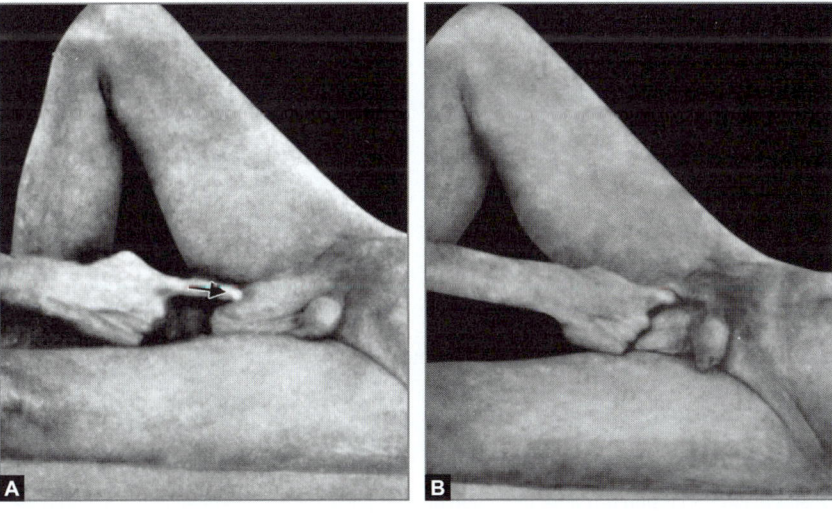

Figs. 38.11A and B: Invagination test. Commence invagination of the skin from the bottom of the scrotum so as to get free play of the finger for the second stage of examination.

inconvenient, one can use the index finger. Invaginate the skin from the bottom of the scrotum and the little finger is pushed up to palpate the pubic tubercle. Right hand should be used for the right side and left hand for the left side. The finger is then rotated and pushed further up into the superficial inguinal ring. The nail will be against the spermatic cord and the pulp will feel the ring. *Utmost gentleness is required for this examination.* Normal ring is a triangular slit which admits only the tip of a finger. If more than one finger can be easily introduced, the ring is abnormally large. But this will not always be associated with hernia. The patient is asked to cough. Normally, the examining finger will be squeezed by the approximation of the two pillars. A palpable impulse will confirm the diagnosis.

When the finger enters the ring—*does it go directly backwards* (direct hernia) or upwards, backwards and outwards (indirect hernia)? The finger is again rotated so that the pulp of the finger looks backwards. The patient is again asked to cough. If the *impulse is felt on the pulp of the finger the hernia is a direct one and if the impulse is felt on the tip it is an oblique hernia.*

8. **Ring occlusion test (Figs. 38.12A and B):** This test is performed in standing position and the hernia must be reduced first. This is a confirmatory test to differentiate an indirect inguinal hernia from a direct inguinal hernia. Since an indirect (oblique) hernia comes out through the deep inguinal ring and a direct hernia medial to the ring, pressure over the deep inguinal ring will occlude the indirect hernia but not the direct hernia. A thumb is pressed on the deep inguinal ring (½ inch above the midpoint between the anterior superior iliac spine and the symphysis pubis). The patient is asked to cough. A direct hernia will show a bulge medial to the occluding finger but an indirect hernia will not find access **(Figs. 38.12A and B)**.

In case of femoral hernia if pressure is exerted over the femoral canal the hernia will not be able to come out. This is a confirmatory test for femoral hernia.

9. **In case of child** a small inguinal hernia is often invisible due to presence of thick pad of fat over the inguinal region. To make visible such a hernia the child is asked to jolt or jump from the examining table or deliberately make it cry according to its age. Now palpate the spermatic cord as it emerges from the superficial inguinal ring. If there is a hernia the cord will be felt thicker than its fellow on the opposite side due to presence of hernial sac. Even when this test fails *Gornall's test* is performed. The child is held from back by both hands of the clinician on its

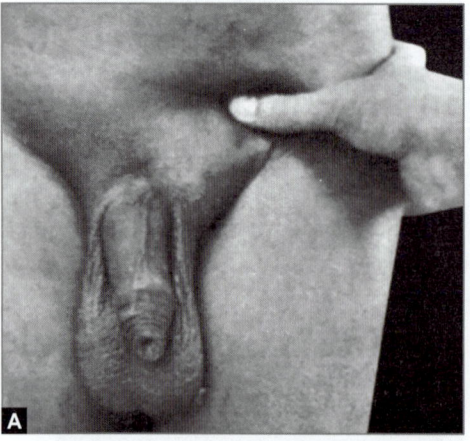 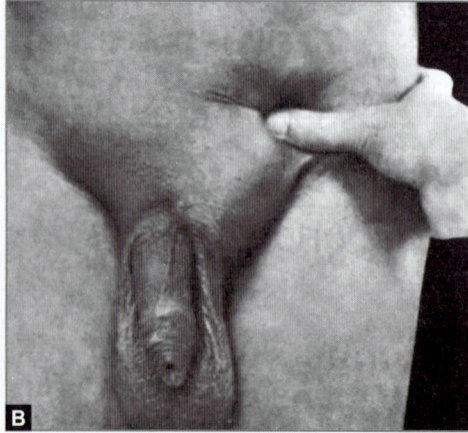

Figs. 38.12A and B: Ring occlusion test after reduction of an inguinal hernia. The deep inguinal ring is being occluded with the tip of the thumb. The patient is now asked to cough. In case of indirect hernia no bulging will be seen whereas in case of direct hernia (as shown in B) the hernia comes out.

abdomen. The abdomen is pressed and the child is lifted up. This will make the hernia apparent by increasing intra-abdominal pressure.

C. PERCUSSION

A resonant note over a hernia means it contains intestine (enterocele). Whereas if the note is dull it contains omentum or extraperitoneal fatty tissue. Percussion can differentiate acute epididymitis and acute filarial funiculitis from strangulated hernia. The note will be resonant in case of the latter whereas in case of former two cases the note will be dull **(Fig. 38.13)**.

D. AUSCULTATION

This does not give much diagnostic clue. Peristaltic sounds may be heard in an enterocele.

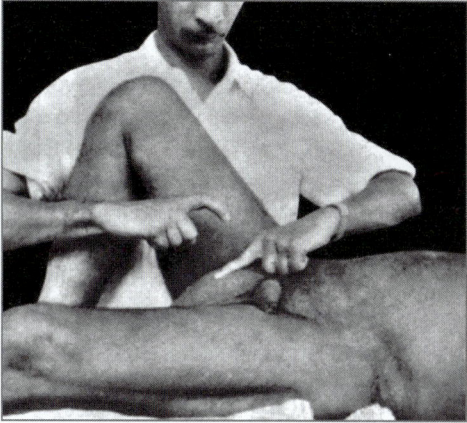

Fig. 38.13: Percussion on an inguinal hernia will give indication about its contents—an enterocele (resonant) or epiplocele (dull).

Examine the testis, epididymis and spermatic cord as discussed in Chapter 40. This part of examination is very important. In *traction test*, the testis is pulled downwards and with this the encysted hydrocele of the cord descends slightly and becomes fixed **(Fig. 38.14)**.

Examine the tone of the abdominal muscles to select the type of operation suitable for the particular case. The tone can be examined in the following ways: (a) To observe the patient in profile **(Fig. 38.15A)**. Undue protrusion of the lower abdomen denotes loss of tone. (b) In recumbent position the patient is asked to raise his shoulders against resistance. When oblique muscles are strong, retraction of the abdominal wall will be observed over the flanks. When the abdominal muscles are weak this test will demonstrate the '*Malgaigne's bulgings*' in the inguinal region or just above it **(Fig. 38.15B)**. These are oval-shaped longitudinal bilateral bulge produced on straining, above and parallel to the medial half of the inguinal ligament, i.e., along the inguinal canal. It indicates poor tone of the oblique muscles. (c) A finger is introduced into the superficial inguinal ring and the patient is asked to cough. The strength of the two pillars and the sphincteric action of the conjoined tendon can be assessed.

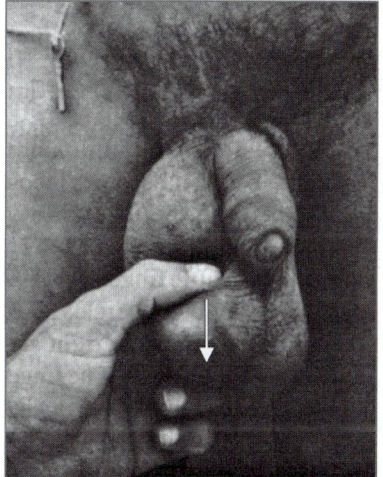

Fig. 38.14: An encysted hydrocele of the cord comes down and becomes fixed when the testis is pulled down.

■ GENERAL EXAMINATION

Thorough examination must be performed to exclude chronic bronchitis, enlarged prostate, stricture urethra, chronic constipation, etc., which will induce chronic strain as to cause hernia to develop.

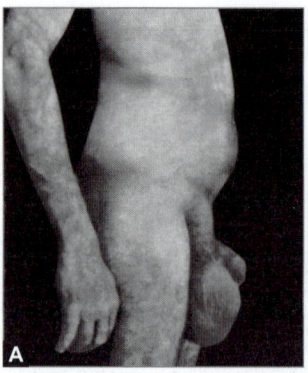 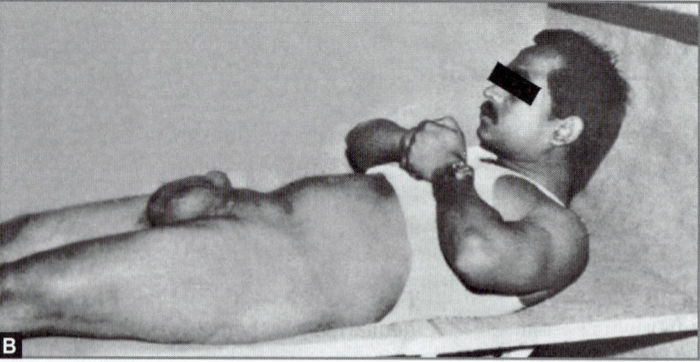

Figs. 38.15A and B: Methods of estimating the tone of the abdominal muscles: (A) by observing the patient in profile and (B) by 'rising test' to demonstrate Malgaigne's bulgings.

The **chest** must be thoroughly examined to exclude any cause of chronic cough. Rectal examination is obligatory to exclude chronic constipation and enlarged prostate. **Abdomen** should always be examined to exclude presence of intestinal obstruction.

DIFFERENTIAL DIAGNOSIS

Different locations of swellings and possible types of hernias

Location of swelling	Possible type of hernia
Groin (above inguinal ligament)	Indirect or direct inguinal hernia
Groin (below inguinal ligament)	Femoral hernia
Umbilical region	Umbilical hernia (congenital or acquired)
Midline abdomen	Epigastric hernia
Postsurgical site	Incisional hernia
Lower abdominal wall (obscure location)	Spigelian hernia
Obturator foramen	Obturator hernia (pain radiates to knee)

INGUINAL HERNIA

A. **ANATOMICAL TYPES:** Three types of classification can be made under this heading. **According to the extent** of the hernia it can be either: (a) a *bubonocele*—when the hernia does not come out of the superficial inguinal ring. (b) *an incomplete hernia* **(Fig. 38.16)**—when it comes out through the superficial inguinal ring but fails to reach the bottom of the scrotum, and (c) *a complete hernia*—when it reaches the bottom of the scrotum.

According to its site of exit it can be either: (a) *an oblique (indirect) hernia*—when the hernia comes through the deep inguinal ring, i.e., lateral to the inferior epigastric artery and (b) *a direct hernia*—when it comes out through the Hesselbach's triangle which is bounded medially by the lateral border of the rectus abdominis, laterally by the inferior epigastric artery and below by the inguinal ligament. That means the neck of the sac lies medial to the inferior epigastric artery.

According to the contents of the hernia, a hernia may be either: (a) *an enterocele*—when it contains the intestine (enteron); (b) *an epiplocele* or *omentocele*—when it contains omentum (epiploon); or (c) a *cystocele* when it contains the urinary bladder.

OBLIQUE (INDIRECT) HERNIA: It comprises more than 80% cases of inguinal hernia. Almost all the herniae in children **(Figs. 38.17A and B)** and women are of this type. It occurs earlier than a direct hernia. It is often complete, i.e., it reaches the bottom of the scrotum. The hernia descends obliquely downwards and inwards and it reduces obliquely in the opposite direction. This type of hernia does not reduce by itself and if reduced, does not come out at once, but requires a cough to bring it down. For reduction a little manipulation is required. If the internal ring is occluded the hernia cannot come out even if the patient coughs. Two forms of indirect inguinal hernia are found in practice: (i) congenital and (ii) acquired.

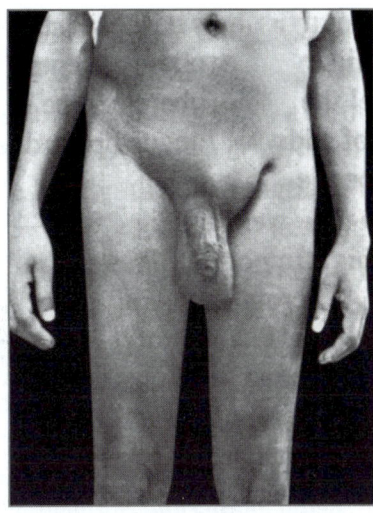

Fig. 38.16: An incomplete indirect left inguinal hernia.

Congenital hernia (Fig. 38.18): Normally, the funicular process of peritoneum becomes obliterated after the testis has reached the scrotum. The scrotal part of the process remains patent and acquires the name 'tunica vaginalis'. In case of congenital hernia the whole process remains patent. With increase in the abdominal pressure abdominal contents come out through the patent peritoneal process. Thus a congenital hernia reaches the bottom of the scrotum very quickly. It may so happen that the funicular process remains patent up to the top of the testis. So the hernia stops at the top of the testis and is known as a *congenital funicular hernia* **(Fig. 38.19)**. It must be remembered that congenital hernia, though so named, is usually seen in adults.

Acquired hernia (Fig. 38.20): As the name suggests it does not protrude into a preformed sac. Clinically, it can be differentiated from a congenital hernia by the fact that it does not become complete at once. Acquired hernia progresses gradually.

DIRECT HERNIA: This hernia is more common above the age of 40. It is frequently incomplete, but it may descend into the scrotum if remains untreated for years. The hernia comes out as soon as the patient stands and disappears immediately when he lies down. The swelling is more often spherical in shape. In case of invagination test the finger goes directly backwards instead

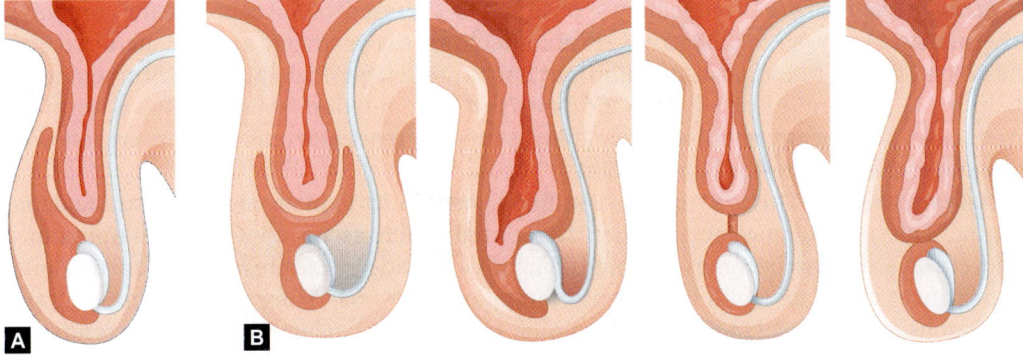

Figs. 38.17A and B: Two types of infantile hernia.

Fig. 38.18: Congenital vaginal hernia.

Fig. 38.19: Congenital funicular hernia.

Fig. 38.20: Acquired hernia.

of upwards, backwards and laterally (in case of indirect hernia). When the patient is asked to cough after occluding the deep inguinal ring the hernia comes out medial to the occluding finger. Direct hernia does not come out through the deep inguinal ring but a little medial to the ring. It becomes rarely strangulated as the neck of the sac is wide.

Enterocele is elastic in consistency, resonant on percussion and slips back into the abdomen with a distinct gurgle. Peristalsis may occasionally be seen if the coverings are thin. Peristaltic sound can be heard on auscultation. Reduction may be difficult in the beginning but easy towards the end.

Epiplocele feels doughy and granular. It is dull on percussion and reduces without gurgle. Reduction may be easy in the beginning but is difficult towards the end.

Cystocele only occurs in a direct hernia or in sliding hernia. It is suspected when the patient gives the history that the hernia gets enlarged just before micturition and smaller after micturition. Pressure on the hernia induces a desire for micturition particularly when it is distended.

B. **CLINICAL TYPES:** Clinically hernia may be of five types:

1. **Reducible hernia:** Normally an uncomplicated hernia is reducible. That means its contents can be returned into the abdominal cavity, but the sac remains in its position.

2. **Irreducible hernia**: In this hernia the contents cannot be returned to the abdomen, but it does not suggest any other complication whatsoever. Various causes of irreducibility are: (i) adhesion of its contents to each other, (ii) adhesion of its contents with the sac, (iii) adhesion of one part of the sac to the other part, (iv) sliding hernia and (v) very large scrotal hernia (scrotal abdomen). Irreducible hernia is often confused with strangulated hernia by the beginners. Clinically, a strangulated hernia is also irreducible, but it is extremely tender and tense and the overlying skin may be red. These signs are absent in a pure irreducible hernia.

3. **Obstructed** or **incarcerated hernia** (irreducibility+Intestinal obstruction): An obstructed hernia means the hernia is associated with intestinal obstruction due to occlusion of the lumen of the bowel. It must be remembered that there is no interference with the blood supply to the intestine in this hernia. One must be very careful to make this diagnosis, as strangulated hernia also possesses two of its features, i.e., irreducibility and intestinal obstruction. Of course the third and most important feature of a strangulated hernia is missing in this hernia, i.e., interference with the blood supply of the intestine. So it is a dangerous venture to diagnose obstructed hernia when strangulation may be the real state of affair and thus valuable time will be wasted until it becomes too late to save the patient's life.

4. **Strangulated hernia** (irreducibility + obstruction + arrest of blood supply to the contents): A hernia is said to be strangulated when the contents are so constricted as to be interfered with their blood supply. Intestinal obstruction may not be present particularly in case of omentocele, Richter's hernia and Littre's hernia. Diagnosis of strangulation is made when a hernia is irreducible, without any impulse on coughing, extremely tense and tender. These are followed by features of acute intestinal obstruction.

5. **Inflamed hernia:** This is a very rare condition and mimics in many respects a strangulated hernia. This hernia may occur when its content such as an appendix, a salpinx or a Meckel's diverticulum becomes inflamed. Diagnosis is made by the presence of constitutional disturbances associated with local signs of inflammation—overlying skin becomes red and edematous and the swelling becomes painful, tender and swollen. The only differentiating feature from a strangulated hernia is that this hernia is not tense and is not associated with intestinal obstruction.

Rare varieties of hernia are:
1. **Hernia-en-glissade or sliding hernia (Fig. 38.21):** In this type of hernia a piece of extraperitoneal bowel, usually the cecum on the right side or the pelvic colon on the left side or the urinary bladder on either side slides down outside the hernial sac forming a part of its wall being covered by the peritoneum on the hernial aspect only. There may be the usual contents in the sac. These herniae usually occur in older men. A large globular hernia when descends well into the scrotum this condition is suspected. It reappears slowly after reduction. This condition may be associated with strangulated small intestine within its sac or a strangulated large intestine outside the sac.
2. **Richter's hernia:** In this condition, only a portion of the circumference of the bowel becomes strangulated. This condition often complicates a femoral hernia and rarely an obturator hernia. This condition is particularly dangerous as operation is frequently delayed because the clinical features resemble gastroenteritis. Intestinal obstruction may not be present until and unless half of the circumference of the bowel is involved. The patient may or may not vomit, intestinal colic is present but the bowels are opened normally. There may be even diarrhea. Absolute constipation is delayed until paralytic ileus supervenes.
3. **Littre's hernia** is a hernia which contains Meckel's diverticulum.
4. **Maydl's hernia (Hernia-en-W)** *or retrograde strangulation (Fig. 38.22)*: In this condition two loops of bowels remain in the sac and the connecting loop remains within the abdomen and becomes strangulated. The loops of the hernia look like a 'W'. The loop within the abdomen becomes first strangulated and can only be suspected when tenderness is elicited above the inguinal ligament along with presence of intestinal obstruction.

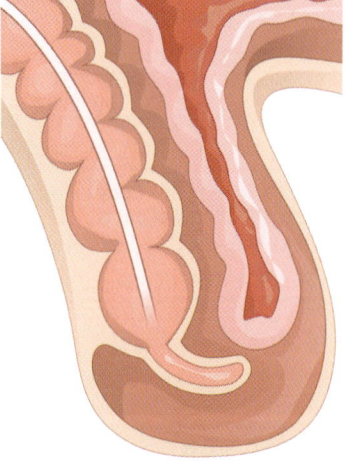

Fig. 38.21: Hernia-en-glissade or sliding hernia. The thick line represents the peritoneum, Note that the colon forms the wall of the sac.

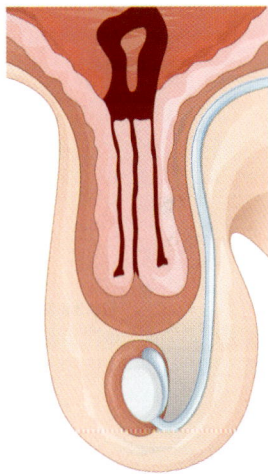

Fig. 38.22: Maydl's hernia. The loop in the abdomen is always found at a more advanced stage of strangulation than the loops in the sac.

FEMORAL HERNIA

A femoral hernia is a protrusion of extraperitoneal tissue, peritoneum and sometimes abdominal contents through the femoral canal. The femoral canal is bounded superoanteriorly by the inguinal ligament, inferoposteriorly by the pubic ramus and pectineus muscle, medially by the lacunar ligament (Gimbernat's ligament) and laterally by the femoral vein **(Fig. 38.23)**. The hernia actually comes out superficially through the saphenous opening situated 1½ inches below and lateral to the pubic tubercle. When the hernia is within the femoral canal it remains narrow, but once it escapes through the saphenous opening into the loose areolar tissues, it expands considerably. So a femoral hernia assumes the shape of a retort. Its bulbous extremity expands upwards even above the inguinal ligament. **Figure 38.24** shows anatomic representation of the position of the femoral ring and **Figure 38.25** shows the relative position of deep inguinal ring and femoral ring.

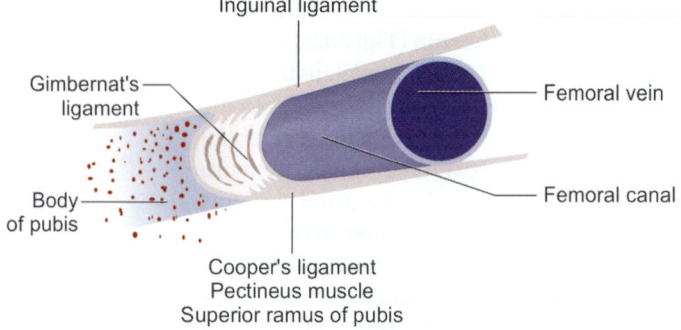

Fig. 38.23: Boundaries of the femoral canal.

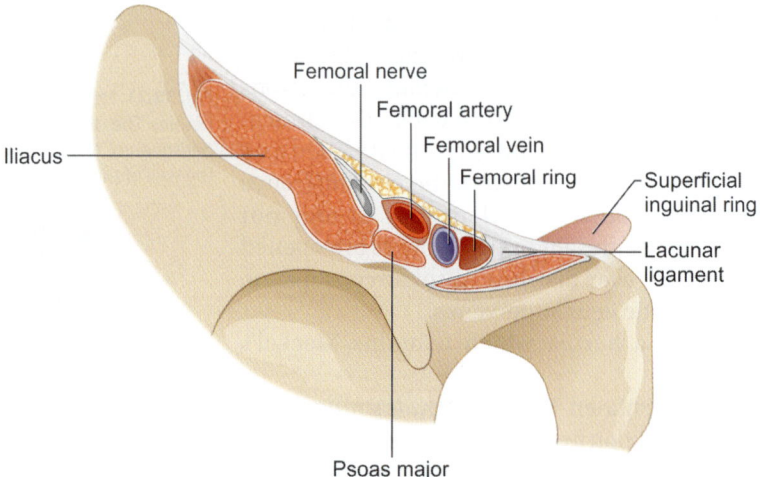

Fig. 38.24: Anatomic representation of the position of the femoral ring.

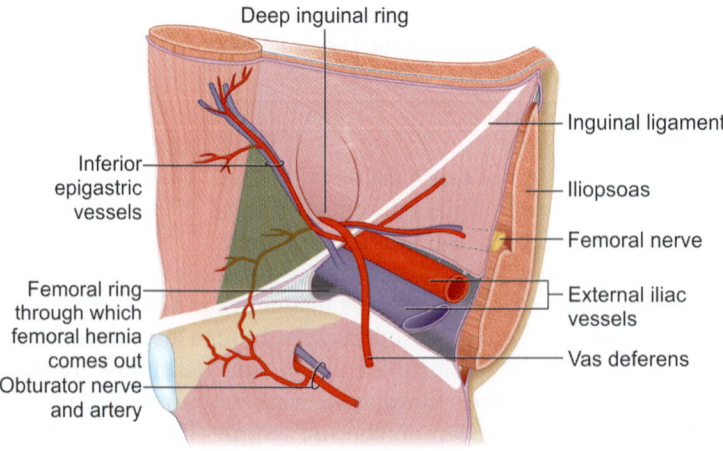

Fig. 38.25: Another anatomical representation of relative positions of deep inguinal ring and femoral ring which are shown from inside the abdomen through which inguinal hernia and femoral hernia come out respectively.

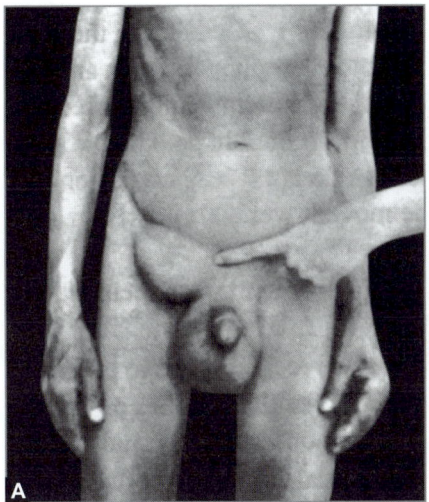 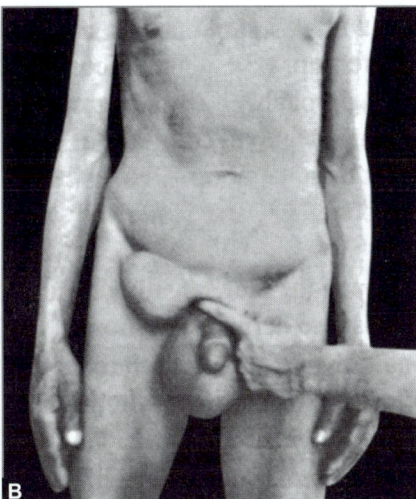

Figs. 38.26A and B: Femoral hernia in male, a rare occurrence. (A) The tip of the finger lies over the pubic tubercle. (B) 'invagination test' is being demonstrated. The inguinal canal is empty in a femoral hernia.

Femoral hernia is very rare before 20 years of age. The incidence gradually rises till the highest incidence is over 50 years. Femoral hernia is commoner in women (2:1). But the students must remember that even in women the most common hernia in the groin is the inguinal hernia. The right side is affected twice as common as the left side and in 20% of cases the condition is bilateral. The symptoms from femoral hernia are less pronounced than those of inguinal hernia. One thing must be borne in mind that the femoral canal being a rigid opening this hernia becomes *strangulated very often*. A very rare case of inguinal hernia is shown in **Figures 38.26A and B**.

The femoral hernia is *differentiated from an inguinal hernia* by the following points: (a) The femoral hernia lies lateral to the pubic tubercle and below the inguinal ligament but in late stage it may extend up above the inguinal ligament, whereas an inguinal hernia lies medial to the pubic tubercle and above the inguinal ligament. (b) In case of femoral hernia impulse on coughing can be seen and felt on the saphenous opening which is about 4 cm below and lateral to the pubic tubercle. (c) In case of femoral hernia the inguinal canal will be empty as determined by the 'invagination test'. (d) By occluding the deep inguinal ring an indirect hernia can be stopped coming out even if the patient coughs, but the direct hernia will bulge medial to the deep inguinal ring. Similarly, a femoral hernia can be prevented from coming out by pressure applied over the femoral canal or the saphenous opening.

PREVASCULAR FEMORAL HERNIA: This is a special variety of femoral hernia, which descends not through the femoral canal, but bulges down posterior to the inguinal ligament and in front of the femoral artery and vein. Obviously, it has a wide neck and a flattened wide sac. This hernia is not difficult to diagnose and can be reduced easily. Such hernia rarely gets strangulated and is very difficult to repair.

A femoral hernia should be differentiated from:
1. **Saphena varix:** It is a saccular enlargement of the termination of the long saphenous vein. This swelling usually disappears completely when the patient lies down. The so called impulse on coughing is present in this condition as well, but it is actually a fluid thrill and not

an expansile impulse to the examining fingers. Varicosity of the long saphenous vein is usually associated with.

Percussion on varicosities of the long saphenous vein will transmit an impulse upwards to the saphena varix felt by the fingers of the other hand—Schwartz's test. Sometimes a venous hum can be heard when the stethoscope is applied over the saphena varix.

2. **Enlarged lymph nodes:** A search for a possible focus of infection should be made in the drainage area which extends from the umbilicus down to the toes including the terminal portions of the anal canal, urethra and vagina (i.e., portions developed from the ectoderm). Causes of enlargement of lymph nodes are discussed in Chapter 8. The gland of Cloquet lying within the femoral canal may be enlarged and simulates exactly an irreducible femoral hernia. If any focus cannot be found out or any cause of enlargement of lymph nodes cannot be detected, the nature of the lump remains a matter of opinion which is best settled urgently in the operation theater.

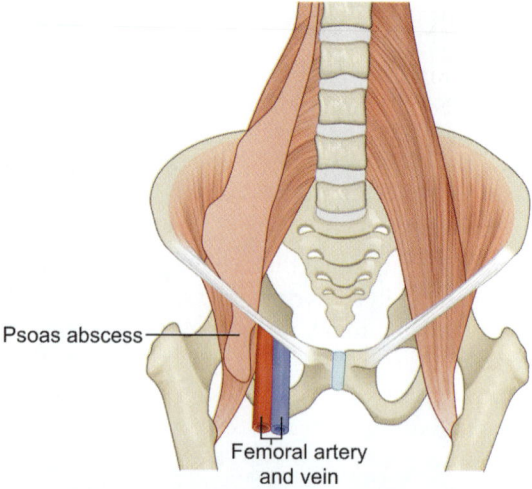

Fig. 38.27: Psoas abscess usually points in the groin lateral to the femoral vessels. The track of the psoas abscess from the caries spine is shown in the figure. It must be remembered that femoral hernia lies on the medial side of the femoral vessels.

3. **Psoas abscess** (Fig. 38.27): This is usually a cold abscess tracking down from Pott's disease. It is a reducible swelling and gives rise to impulse on coughing. It is a painless swelling and if the pulsation of the femoral artery can be palpated it will be appreciated that *the swelling is lateral to the artery*. Sometimes there is an iliac part of the abscess which is determined by cross-fluctuation. Examinations of the back and corresponding iliac fossa including X-rays clarify the diagnosis.

4. **An enlarged psoas bursa:** This bursa lies in front of the hip joint and under the psoas major muscle. It often communicates with the hip joint. In osteoarthritis of the hip joint this bursa becomes enlarged and produces a tense and cystic swelling below the inguinal ligament. *This swelling diminishes in size when the hip joint is flexed.* Presence of osteoarthritis in the hip joint, a cystic swelling, absence of impulse on coughing and that the swelling diminishes in size during flexion of the hip joint are the diagnostic points in favour of this condition.

5. **A femoral aneurysm:** Expansile pulsation is the pathognomonic feature of this condition.

6. **Lipoma:** The diagnostic points in favor of this condition are discussed in Chapter 3.

7. **Hydrocele of a femoral hernial sac (Fig. 38.28):** This is an extremely rare condition in which the neck of the sac becomes plugged with omentum or by adhesions. The hydrocele of the sac is thus produced by the secretion of the peritoneum.

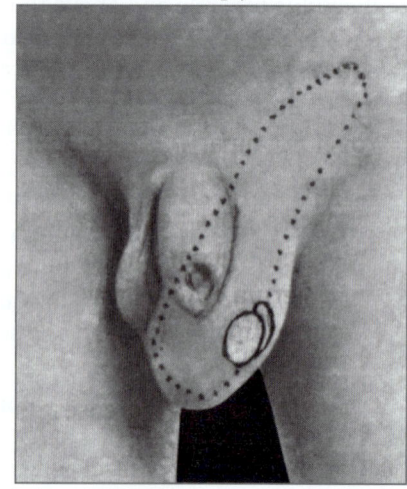

Fig.38.28: Inguinoscrotal swelling caused by an infantile hydrocele.

UMBILICAL HERNIA

Any hernia which appears to be closely related to the umbilicus can be called as "Umbilical hernia". Four definite varieties are seen:
1. **Exomphalos:** Abdominal contents are protruded *into the umbilical cord* being covered by a transparent membrane—a diaphanous membrane.
2. **Congenital umbilical hernia:** This hernia comes out through the center of a congenital weak umbilical scar. It is common in Negroes. It generally appears in the first few months after birth. Common symptom is the swelling rather than anything else. The neck of the hernia is generally wide and hardly gives rise to intestinal obstruction or strangulation. The main diagnostic features are: (i) Bulge through the center of the umbilical scar everting the whole umbilicus; (ii) Age of the patient; (iii) The swelling is easily reducible (spontaneously reduced when the child lies down) and there is definite impulse on crying; (iv) The size of the hernia varies—it may be a small defect admitting the tip of the little finger alone to quite a large opening admitting two or three fingers; (v) The content is usually small intestine, so resonant to percussion; (vi) About 90% of these herniae disappear spontaneously during the first 5 years of life as the umbilical scar thickens and contracts.
3. **Acquired umbilical hernia:** This hernia occurs in adult life and protrudes through the umbilical scar. It is very rare in comparison to the paraumbilical hernia which is described below. Almost invariably it is due to raised intra-abdominal pressure which has forced the hernia through the umbilical scar. One must try to find out the cause of raised intra-abdominal pressure in these cases. Common causes are—pregnancy, ascites, bowel distension, ovarian cyst and fibroid.
4. **Paraumbilical hernia:** It is the most common acquired umbilical hernia. It occurs *through a defect adjacent to the umbilicus*. The usual site is just above the umbilicus between the two recti, in fact lower half of the fundus of the sac is covered by the umbilicus. The diagnostic features are as follows: (i) Paraumbilical hernia develops in the middle and old age; (ii) Obese women are more commonly affected; (iii) Usual symptoms are pain and swelling. If the swelling is very small, it may not be noticed by the patient and the pain and discomfort become the main symptoms; (iv) The surface is smooth and the edge is distinct except when the patient is very fat; (v) It contains omentum or bowel. The lump is firm when it contains omentum. The lump is soft and resonant to percussion when the content is bowel; (vi) Many paraumbilical herniae are irreducible when the contents become adherent to the sac or the neck of the sac becomes narrow. If the hernia can be reduced, the firm fibrous edge of the defect in the linea alba can be felt; (vii) As the defect in the linea alba is firm and does not enlarge proportionately these herniae do give rise to intermittent abdominal pain, though strangulation is not common.

EPIGASTRIC HERNIA

An epigastric hernia is a protrusion of extraperitoneal fat and sometimes a small peritoneal sac through a defect in the linea alba. This defect is usually placed somewhere between the xiphisternum and the umbilicus. The main symptom is epigastric pain and swelling. Pain is usually located over hernia. It often begins after eating probably due to epigastric distension. If the patient could not see the lump, a self-diagnosis of peptic ulcer is often made. So whenever a patient will complain of epigastric discomfort or pain palpate the abdominal wall first to detect a small lump of epigastric hernia. It must be remembered that usually these herniae do not have impulse on coughing and cannot be reduced. Lipoma very much resembles this condition. That the swelling cannot be moved over the underlying structures favors the diagnosis of epigastric hernia.

INCISIONAL HERNIA is the hernial protrusion through the scar, usually due to previous surgical operation or accidental trauma. Infection of the wound and injury to the motor nerve predispose hernia formation.

DIVARICATION OF THE RECTI: In this condition, the linea alba stretches and allows the two recti muscles to part from each other. These two muscles are inserted to the pubis very close to the midline. By repeated contractions of the flat muscles of the abdomen the two recti show tendency to diverge particularly when the linea alba is weak. This condition is common in elderly multipara.

INTERSTITIAL HERNIA: This is also called an *Interparietal hernia*. In this condition the hernial sac passes between the layers of the anterior abdominal wall. This sac may be a continuation of an inguinal or femoral hernial sac.

SPIGELIAN HERNIA: This hernia occurs through the linea semilunaris at the level of the arcuate line, i.e., a few centimeters above the inguinal ligament. Usual victims are above 50 years of age.

LUMBAR HERNIA: This hernia comes out through the Petit's triangle being bounded below by the crest of the ilium, laterally by the external oblique and medially by the latissimus dorsi. There is another superior lumbar triangle being bounded by the 12th rib above, by the sacrospinalis medially and the posterior border of the internal oblique laterally. Through this triangle also the contents may come out of the abdomen. But the incidence is rarer than inferior lumbar hernia through Petit's triangle. Incisional lumbar hernia may follow an operation on kidney, the incisional wound being infected.

OBTURATOR HERNIA: This hernia comes out through the obturator foramen. As the hernia is covered by the pectineus muscle, it is often overlooked. This hernia causes more pain than any other type of hernia. Pain often radiates along the obturator nerve and may even be referred to the knee via its geniculate branch. The leg is usually kept in the semiflexed position and movement of the limb gives rise to pain. If the limb is flexed, abducted and rotated outwards the hernia becomes prominent. Patients are mostly over 60 years of age and women are more frequently affected than men. Incidence of Richter's hernia in this condition is only second to femoral hernia.

Algorithmic Approach to Patient with Hernia

Patient presents with swelling in groin, umbilical, or abdominal region

↓

Is the swelling reducible?
- Yes → Likely **uncomplicated hernia (routine surgical repair recommended)**
- No → Proceed to next step

↓

Is the swelling tender and nonreducible
- Yes → Consider **incarcerated or strangulated hernia (urgent surgical referral needed)**
- No → Proceed to next step

↓

Does the hernia show expansile cough impulse?
- Yes → Likely **hernia (requires further classification by location and characteristics).**
- No → Consider **differential diagnoses (lymphadenopathy, hematoma, tumor, abscess, lipoma, saphena varix)**

↓

Classify hernia based on location
- Above inguinal ligament → Direct or indirect inguinal hernia
- Below inguinal ligament → Femoral hernia (high risk of strangulation)
- Midline abdominal swelling → Umbilical or epigastric hernia
- Postsurgical swelling → Incisional hernia

↓

Perform special tests (deep ring occlusion, percussion, auscultation, reducibility tests)
- Deep ring occlusion test → Helps differentiate direct vs indirect inguinal hernia
- Percussion of hernia swelling → Resonant (intestinal content) vs dull (omental content)
- Auscultation over hernia site → Bowel sounds present → Suggests intestinal content in hernia
- Strangulation signs → Redness, severe pain, absent bowel sounds → Requires immediate surgery

↓

Confirm diagnosis and plan treatment
- Uncomplicated hernias → Elective surgical repair (herniorrhaphy, hernioplasty)
- Incarcerated hernias → Urgent reduction attempt + surgery
- Strangulated hernias → Emergency surgery to prevent bowel necrosis

Examination of a Swelling in the Inguinoscrotal Region or Groin
(Except Inguinal and Femoral Hernias)

CHAPTER 39

HISTORY

1. **Age:** Funiculitis (inflammation of the spermatic cord) is a disease of young age. Encysted hydrocele of the cord, lymph varix, varicocele, etc., may present at any age.
2. **Occupation:** Prolonged standing may be the cause of a varicocele.
3. **Residence:** Funiculitis and lymph varix are commoner in Odisha and adjoining districts of West Bengal.

COMPLAINTS

1. **Pain:** Funiculitis is always associated with pain and in fact pain is the presenting symptom in this disease. Tuberculous thickening of the cord, as an extension upwards from the epididymis, is also associated with pain. Malignant extension upward from the testis may be also associated with pain. Vague dragging pain is experienced on prolonged standing in case of a varicocele. Sudden agonizing pain over inguinoscrotal region and in the lower abdomen is complained of in torsion of the testis. On right side this condition often mimics appendicitis. So always examine the scrotum in case of sudden lower abdominal pain.

2. **Swelling:** Swelling is the main presenting feature in case of encysted hydrocele of the cord, diffuse lipoma of the cord, lymph varix, etc. Interrogations like "How did it appear?", "Where did it appear first?", "Does it disappear automatically on lying down?" will give a clue to the diagnosis. A varicocele appears spontaneously whereas a funiculitis starts with fever, ushered in with chill and rigor. An inguinal hernia appears from above whereas an infantile hydrocele, testicular growth and varicocele appear from below. An encysted hydrocele of the cord and diffuse lipoma of the cord appear first in the cord and then gradually enlarge. The most common place of ectopic testis is the superficial inguinal pouch. The patient will say that the swelling was in that position from the beginning. Undescended testis may give rise to the swelling in the inguinal region from the beginning. A varicocele disappears spontaneously when the patient lies down with the scrotum elevated. A lymph varix also reduces spontaneously on lying down although slower than a varicocele.

3. **Any other complaints:** The patient with tuberculous thickening of the cord may present other symptoms like evening rise of temperature, excessive coughing, hemoptysis, etc. Rapid onset of varicocele on the left side with hematuria indicates carcinoma of the kidney on that side. Sterility may be complained of in case of bilateral undescended testes (cryptorchism).

PAST HISTORY: Previous history of periodic attacks of fever accompanied by pain and swelling of the spermatic cord of scrotum is highly suggestive of filarial infection.

PERSONAL HISTORY: History of exposure may be obtained in gonococcal funiculitis.

History in cases with inguinoscrotal swelling

Aspect	Clinical significance	Patient-friendly questions
Onset and duration	**Sudden, acute painful swelling** → Torsion of testis, funiculitis, strangulated hernia **Gradual, painless swelling** → Hydrocele, varicocele, lipoma of cord **Intermittent swelling** → Suggests reducible hernia, lymph varix	"When did you first notice the swelling? Has it changed in size or characteristics over time?"
Pain	**Severe agonizing pain with radiation to lower abdomen** → Torsion of testis **Dull dragging pain, worse on standing** → Varicocele, hydrocele **pain with fever and redness over swelling** → Funiculitis, epididymo-orchitis	"Does the swelling hurt? Is the pain sudden and severe or dull and constant?"
Relation to posture	**Swelling disappears on lying down** → Varicocele, lymph varix **swelling persists in all positions** → Hydrocele, lipoma of cord	"Does the swelling reduce when you lie down or worsen when standing?"
Associated symptoms	**Hematuria with left-sided varicocele** → Consider renal cell carcinoma **Evening fever, cough, weight loss** → Suggestive of tuberculous epididymitis **Recurrent fever with scrotal Swelling** → Suggests filarial infection (lymph varix) **History of STDs or urethritis** → Risk of gonococcal funiculitis, epididymo-orchitis	"Have you noticed any blood in urine, fever, or weight loss?"
Past medical and surgical history	**History of previous groin Surgery** → Risk of incisional swelling, postsurgical hydrocele **Cryptorchidism in childhood** → Predisposes to testicular malignancy **Recurrent inguinal hernia repair** → May suggest lymphatic obstruction	"Have you had any previous surgeries in the groin or a history of testicular problems as a child?"

LOCAL EXAMINATION

Position of the patient: It is always convenient in these cases to examine the patient in the *standing position* first and later on in the *recumbent position*. The patient is asked to hold the clothes up to expose the parts completely. He must not be allowed to bend forwards while he is being examined.

INSPECTION

1. **Swelling:** *Position and extent* of the swelling are very important. A localized swelling in the spermatic cord is encysted hydrocele of the cord whereas a diffuse swelling of the cord may be a lipoma. A swelling in the superficial inguinal pouch (just above and slight lateral to the superficial inguinal ring) with absence of testis in the scrotum is probably an ectopic testis **(Fig. 39.1)**. Similarly a swelling in the inguinal region with absence of testis in the scrotum is an undescended testis.

2. **Skin over the swelling:** In funiculitis or in certain late cases of torsion of testis the skin over the swelling will be red and edematous. This must be differentiated from strangulated hernia which also shows signs of inflammation.

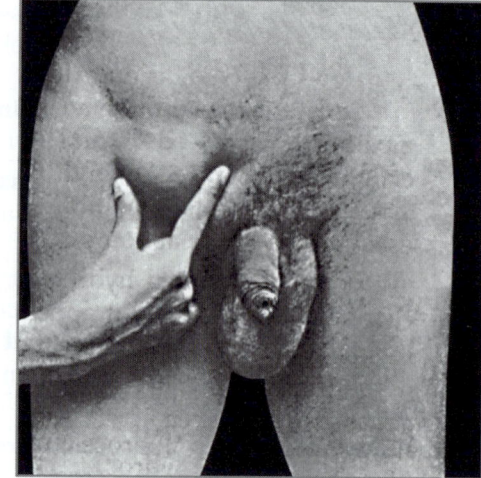

Fig. 39.1: Ectopic testis in the superficial inguinal pouch (the most common site). Note that the testis is absent from the right side of the scrotum.

3. **Impulse on coughing:** This differentiates a hernia from other conditions in this region. It must be remembered that lymph varix (lymphangiectasis) also gives an impulse (thrill-like) on coughing. Varicocele also gives an impulse on coughing like a fluid thrill. An undescended testis with associated hernia may also give impulse on coughing.

PALPATION

1. **Position and extent:** A cystic swelling in the middle of spermatic cord without any upward extension is an encysted hydrocele of the cord. A diffuse swelling of the cord may be a lipoma when it is noninflammatory and a funiculitis when it is inflammatory. The most common position of an ectopic testis is at the superficial inguinal pouch whereas an undescended testis may be felt in the inguinal canal.

2. **Consistency:** A localized cystic, fluctuant and translucent swelling is an *encysted hydrocele of the cord*. *A lymph varix* feels soft, cystic and doughy. A varicocele is diagnosed by its peculiar feel like a "bag of worms".

3. **Reducibility:** It is a classical sign of a hernia. But a lymph varix and a varicocele become spontaneously reduced when the patient lies down. This reduction occurs slowly and not abruptly as in the case of a hernia. After reduction the external abdominal ring is pressed with a finger and the patient is asked to stand up. A varicocele and a lymph varix will gradually fill from below. But a hernia is prevented from coming down.

4. **Impulse on coughing:** This is also a classical sign of a hernia. A *varicocele* and a *lymph varix* also give impulse on coughing, but the impulse is felt like a thrill and is not the typical expansile impulse as felt in the case of a hernia.

PERCUSSION and **AUSCULTATION** are not important in these cases. Percussion is helpful in differentiating a strangulated hernia from acute funiculitis, the former being resonant as it contains the intestine.

It is always advisable to **examine the testis**, **epididymis** and the **spermatic cord** in these cases.

GENERAL EXAMINATION

The **chest** should be examined particularly in the case of tuberculous epididymitis extending upwards. The **abdomen** should be examined thoroughly in case of malignant infiltration of the spermatic cord from the testis to exclude presence of palpable enlarged pre- and para-aortic groups of lymph nodes. In a case of rapidly growing varicocele in a middle-aged man one **should examine the kidney** as very often tumor of the kidney spreads along the lumen of renal vein (in case of left side) or inferior vena cava (in case of right side) to obstruct the testicular vein resulting in a varicocele.

CAUSES OF INGUINOSCROTAL AND GROIN SWELLINGS

A. **Inguinoscrotal swellings** (except inguinal hernia): (i) Encysted hydrocele of the cord; (ii) Varicocele; (iii) Lymph varix or lymphangiectasis; (iv) Funiculitis; (v) Diffuse lipoma of the cord; (vi) Inflammatory thickening of the cord extending upwards from the testis and epididymis; (vii) Malignant extension from the testis; (viii) Ectopic testis; (ix) Undescended testis; (x) Torsion of the testis; (xi) Retractile testis; (xii) Enlarged lymph nodes (external iliac and inguinal groups);(xiii) Abscess in the inguinal region; (xiv) Aneurysm of the external iliac artery.
B. **Femoral swellings** (except femoral hernia): (i) Enlarged lymph nodes (inguinal group); (ii) Saphena varix; (iii) Psoas abscess; (iv) An enlarged psoas bursa; (v) A femoral aneurysm; (vi) Lipoma; (vii) Hydrocele of a femoral hernial sac; (viii) Ectopic testis; (ix) Osteomyelitis and tumors of the upper end of the femur.

DIFFERENTIAL DIAGNOSIS

Differential diagnosis of inguniscrotal swelling and their key features

Condition	Key features
Encysted hydrocele of cord	Fluctuant, translucent, no cough impulse
Varicocele	Bag of worms feel, disappears on lying down, thrill on coughing
Funiculitis	Tender, indurated cord, fever, redness over swelling
Lymph varix	Soft, doughy swelling, slow reduction on lying down
Lipoma of cord	Soft, lobulated, irreducible, no cough impulse
Undescended testis	Empty scrotum, testis palpable in groin

Contd...

Contd...

Condition	Key features
Ectopic testis	Testis in superficial inguinal pouch, not moving down with chair test
Torsion of testis	Acute severe pain, absent cremasteric reflex, no cough impulse
Testicular malignancy extension	Hard, nodular cord, associated abdominal mass

A. INGUINOSCROTAL SWELLINGS

1. **Encysted hydrocele of the cord:** When a portion of the funicular process persists, remains patent and is shut off from the tunica vaginalis below and the peritoneal cavity above, it eventually becomes distended with fluid and presents a cystic swelling either in the inguinal or inguinoscrotal region or in the scrotum. Fluctuation test and translucency test will be positive. One can very well 'get above the swelling'. If the swelling is held at its upper limit and the patient is asked to cough there will be no impulse on coughing. This shows that it has got no connection with hernia nor with the peritoneal cavity. If the testis is pulled down the swelling will also come down and becomes immobile. This is the *traction test*. The testis can be felt apart from the swelling.

2. **Varicocele:** It is a condition in which the veins of the pampiniform plexus become dilated and tortuous. Usually the left side is affected, probably because: (i) the left spermatic vein is longer than the right, (ii) the left spermatic vein enters the left renal vein at a right angle, (iii) at times the left testicular artery arches over the left renal vein to compress it and (iv) the left colon when loaded may press on the left testicular vein. In the beginning the patient will experience aching or dragging pain particularly after prolonged standing. The swelling appears when the patient stands and disappears when he lies down with the scrotum elevated. The impulse on coughing is more like a thrill. On palpation it feels like a 'bag of worms'. After occluding the superficial inguinal ring with a thumb if the patient is asked to stand up the varicocele fills from below. It must be remembered that a rapid onset of varicocele suggests a carcinoma of the kidney. The renal vein is often involved earlier by permeation in these cases and thus compresses the left spermatic vein which drains into the left renal vein and on the right side the inferior vena cava is affected into which the right spermatic vein drains.

3. **Lymph varix or lymphangiectasis:** It is a condition in which the lymphatic vessels of the cord become dilated and tortuous caused by obstruction due to filariasis. Past history of periodic attacks of fever with simultaneous development of pain and swelling of the cord are the main symptoms of this condition. The swelling appears on standing and disappears spontaneously on lying down, although slower than in case of varicocele. The impulse on coughing is thrill like and not the typical expansile impulse found in a case of hernia. On palpation it feels soft, cystic and doughy. Presence of eosinophilia and living microfilariae in the blood drawn at night are very much diagnostic.

4. **Funiculitis:** Besides gonococcal infection funiculitis may be caused by filariasis particularly in this country. Aching in the groin with variable degree of fever are the presenting symptoms in majority of cases. Initial symptoms may be those of acute prostatitis. The inguinal and inguinoscrotal regions will be inflamed and the skin becomes red, edematous and shiny. It is

sometimes very difficult to differentiate it from a small strangulated hernia. While the former condition is mainly treated by conservative means, immediate operative intervention is the only life-saving measure for the latter condition. So differentiation is imperative. Palpation just above the deep inguinal ring is of great help in differentiating these two conditions. In a strangulated hernia the abdominal contents can be felt as they enter the deep inguinal ring whereas in funiculitis no such structures can be felt.

5. **Diffuse lipoma of the cord:** This is a very rare condition. The cord feels soft and lobulated. The swelling is irreducible having no impulse on coughing.

6. **Inflammatory thickening of the cord** (extending upwards from the testis and epididymis): Tuberculosis often gives rise to this condition. Slight ache in the testis with generalized symptoms of tuberculosis often ushers this condition. Indurated and slightly tender nodular thickening of the cord can be felt. Epididymis is obviously tender, enlarged and nodular. Rectal examination may reveal indurated seminal vesicle of the corresponding side and sometimes of the contralateral side. In late cases cold abscess develops in the lower and posterior aspect of the scrotum which may discharge itself resulting in formation of a sinus. In about two-thirds of the cases active tuberculosis of the renal tract may be evident.

7. **Malignant extension of the testis:** This can be easily diagnosed by presence of malignant growth in the testis. The cord feels hard and nodular. There may be secondary deposits in the pre- and para-aortic and even in left supraclavicular lymph nodes.

8. **Undescended and ectopic testis:** An *undescended testis* is one which is arrested at any point along its normal path of descent (Fig. 39.2). An *ectopic testis* is one which has deviated from its usual path of descent. In both these conditions the scrotum of the same side will be empty. If the swelling is within the inguinal canal it is probably an undescended testis. The testis is recognized by its shape, feel and 'testicular sensation'. Ascertain whether the testis is lying superficial or deep to the abdominal muscles by the 'rising test'. The most common site for an ectopic testis, is just above and lateral to the superficial inguinal ring and superficial to the external oblique aponeurosis (Fig. 39.3). It must be remembered that the undescended testis is always smaller and less developed than its fellow in the scrotum but an ectopic testis is usually well developed. Sometimes an undescended testis may be associated with an inguinal or an interstitial hernia.

Though the most common position of ectopic testis is at the superficial inguinal pouch, yet ectopic testis may be found (i) at the root of the penis (pubic type), (ii) at the perineum (perineal type) and (iii) rarely at the upper and medial part of the femoral triangle (femoral type).

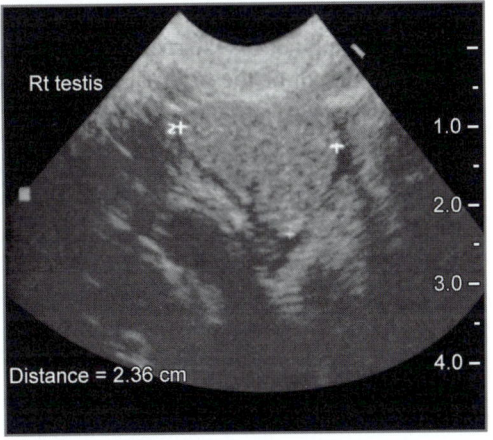

Fig. 39.2: Ultrasonography showing intra-abdominal right testis (undescended testis).

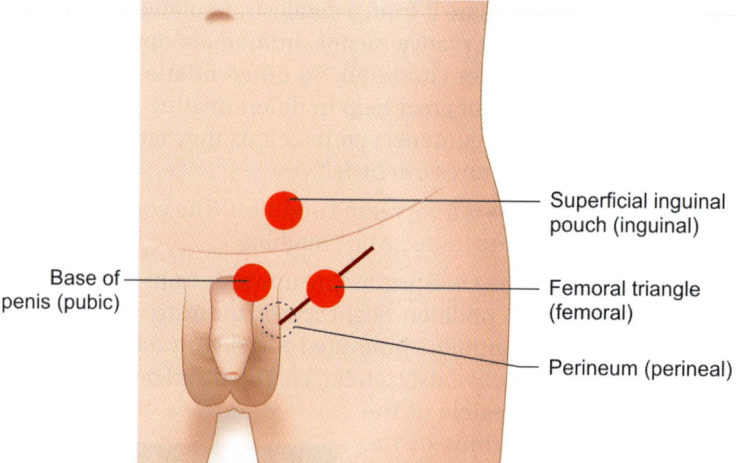

Fig. 39.3: Sites of ectopic testis. These sites are in accordance with the five tails of gubernaculum, of which the normal one is scrotal while the other four are inguinal, pubic, femoral and perineal.

The ectopic testis probably occurs due to rupture of the main scrotal tail of the gubernaculum testis. According to Lockwood, the gubernaculum testis has five tails (**Fig. 39.4**):
1. The scrotal tail—which is the main one.
2. Pubic tail—attached to the pubic tubercle.
3. Perineal tail—attached to the perineum.
4. Inguinal tail—attached to the front of the inguinal canal.
5. Femoral tail—attached to the saphenous opening.

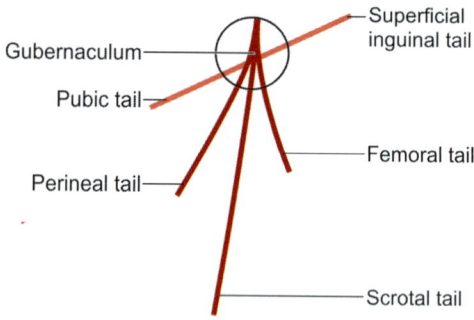

Fig. 39.4: Five tails of gubernaculum testis. See the text.

The scrotal tail is the strongest and the other tails normally disappear and that is why the testis normally descends to the scrotum. In case one of the four accessory tails becomes stronger, the testis is drawn towards the attachment of that tail and then the testis is called an '*ectopic testis*'.

9. **Torsion of the testis:** It is mainly a cause of the swelling of scrotum but an *undescended testis may frequently undergo torsion* which is a subject matter of this chapter. This condition mimics a strangulated hernia. It will give rise to a tense and a tender swelling without an impulse on coughing. Absence of testis in the scrotum should arouse suspicion of this condition. Slight fever, no constipation and dullness on percussion will go in favor of torsion.

10. **Retractile testis:** This condition is quite common in children and is often diagnosed as ectopic testis due to the fact that in majority of cases the testis lies in the superficial inguinal pouch. Strong contraction of the cremaster muscle may pull the testis up from the scrotum into the superficial inguinal pouch. The testis is usually well developed, the scrotum is also normally developed and the testis can be brought down to the bottom of the scrotum. In difficult cases

the child is asked to sit on a chair keeping both feet on its seat and the knees are flexed to the extreme and brought towards its chest. This puts pressure on the inguinal canal downwards and brings the retractile testis into the scrotum. This is known as '*Chair test*' **(Fig. 39.5)**. But probably the first maneuver to simply drag the testis into the scrotum is more successful.

B. **FEMORAL SWELLINGS:** These are discussed in the previous chapter under the heading of 'Femoral Hernia'.

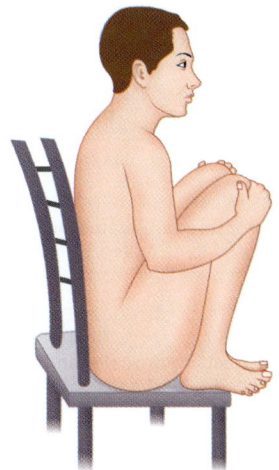

Fig. 39.5: Chair test (Orr). The young patient is asked to sit on a chair hugging his knees to his chest. By this maneuver the retractile testis is pushed down to the bottom of the scrotum. By this test retractile testis can be differentiated from ectopic testis.

Algorithmic Approach to Patient with Inguinoscrotal Swelling

Patient presents with swelling in groin or scrotum

↓

Is the swelling reducible?
- **Yes** → Likely **uncomplicated hernia** (check for cough impulse, further differentiation needed)
- **No** → Proceed to next step

↓

Is the swelling translucent on transillumination?
- **Yes** → Suggests **hydrocele** (encysted hydrocele of cord, tunica vaginalis hydrocele)
- **No** → Proceed to next step

↓

Does the swelling have a 'bag of worms' feel?
- **Yes** → Suggests **varicocele** (more common on left side, disappears on lying down)
- **No** → Proceed to next step

↓

Is the swelling tender, indurated, and associated with fever?
- **Yes** → Suggests **funiculitis or epididymo-orchitis** (infectious or inflammatory process)
- **No** → Proceed to next step

↓

Does the swelling disappear on lying down?
- **Yes** → Suggests **varicocele or lymph varix** (slow reduction, unlike hernia)
- **No** → Proceed to Next Step

↓

Is the testis palpable in the groin with an empty scrotum?
- **Yes** → Consider **undescended testis** (within inguinal canal) or **ectopic testis** (superficial inguinal pouch, perineum, femoral region)
- **No** → Proceed to next step

↓

Is the swelling hard, nodular, and associated with a testicular mass?
- **Yes** → Suggests **testicular malignancy extension** (check for para-aortic lymphadenopathy, metastatic symptoms)
- **No** → Consider other diagnoses **(lipoma of cord, aneurysm, abscess, chronic granulomatous disease)**

↓

Confirm diagnosis and plan treatment based on findings
- **Medical management** → Funiculitis, epididymo-orchitis, lymph varix (antibiotics, anti-inflammatory drugs, supportive care)
- **Surgical interventions** → Varicocele ligation, hydrocelectomy, hernia repair, orchidopexy (for undescended testis), orchidectomy (for malignancy)

Examination of Male External Genitalia

CHAPTER 40

THE SCROTUM

HISTORY

1. **Age:** Carcinoma of the skin of the scrotum is a disease of individuals above 50 years of age. But malignant condition of the testis is common in young individuals—teratoma between 20 and 30 years, whereas seminoma between 30 and 40 years. Torsion of the testis is commonly seen in teen-aged boys. Hydrocele is seen even in infants, but the primary hydrocele is most common over the age of 40 years. While the secondary hydrocele is commoner between 20 and 40 years of age. Tuberculous orchitis is the disease of the young. Majority of the epididymal cysts and spermatoceles occur in men above 40 years of age. Cysts of the epididymis, though congenital, appear in the middle-aged men.

2. **Occupation:** Except carcinoma of the scrotal skin, other conditions do not have a definite relation with occupation. The former condition is often caused by frequent contact with soot (chimney sweep's cancer), tar or oil (mule spinner's cancer). The skin is exposed to these irritants for many years before a cancer develops. Varicocele often develops in men who are involved in work which requires prolonged standing (Bus conductors, etc.).

3. **History of present illness:** *Malignant growth of the testis* often grows silently without the knowledge of the patient and in fact he may present a lump in the epigastric or umbilical region due to secondary deposits in the lymph nodes. A history of trauma followed immediately by a swelling is the usual history of a *hematocele*, which maintains this size for a long time. In *torsion of the testis* an exciting cause is almost always present like straining at stool, lifting a heavy weight or coitus. This is due to violent contraction of the spirally attached cremaster muscle, which favors rotation of the testis around a vertical axis. *Acute epididymo-orchitis* begins with an ache in the groin and slight rise of temperature. This is followed by severe pain, a considerable rise of temperature with redness and swelling of the scrotum. In *filariasis* periodic attacks of fever, pain and swelling of the spermatic cord and scrotum are the main features. In *tuberculous epididymitis*, a slight ache or a trivial injury call the patient's attention towards the testis. Injury to the bulb of the urethra or bursting of a periurethral abscess—a complication of gonococcal stricture is the usual history of *extravasation of urine*. In *gummatous orchitis*, a trivial injury calls the patient's attention towards the already diseased testis.

History in examination of male external genitalia

Aspect	Clinical significance	Patient-friendly questions
Onset and duration	Sudden painful swelling → Torsion of testis Gradual painless swelling → Hydrocele, epididymal cyst	"When did you first notice the swelling? Has it changed in size or characteristics over time?"

Contd...

Contd...

Aspect	Clinical significance	Patient-friendly questions
Pain	**Severe, acute pain with nausea** → Torsion **Mild dull ache** → Hydrocele, varicocele	"Does the swelling hurt? Is the pain sudden and severe or dull and constant?"
Associated symptoms	**Fever and redness** → Fournier's gangrene **Blood in urine** → Testicular malignancy	"Have you noticed fever, redness, or urinary symptoms?"

■ LOCAL EXAMINATION

A. INSPECTION

1. **Skin and subcutaneous tissue:** The skin of the scrotum is usually wrinkled and freely mobile over the testis. It becomes red and edematous in case of *acute epididymo-orchitis*.

In *hydrocele* the skin will be tense, so the normal rugosity of the skin will be lost and subcutaneous veins will be prominent. Normal rugosity of the skin will also be lost in presence of underlying pathology such as tuberculous epididymitis, gummatous orchitis, teratoma and seminoma of the testis, in an otherwise normal size scrotum.

Multiple sebaceous cysts are not uncommon in scrotal skin **(Figs. 40.1 and 40.2)**. Their features will be similar to sebaceous cyst anywhere in the body (*see* Page 63).

Carcinomatous ulcers may occur anywhere in the scrotum but the industrial cancers are common in the cleft between the scrotum and the thigh. These ulcers are small and circular with everted edge. The floor is covered with yellowish-gray infected necrotic tissue. Ulcers usually discharge offensive, purulent or serosanguineous fluid.

It must be remembered that *gummatous ulcer* of the scrotum resulting from extension of a gumma of the testis lies always on the *anterior aspect of the scrotum*. *Tuberculous ulcer* resulting from tuberculous epididymitis is always seen on the *posterior aspect of the scrotum*. These positions are reversed if the testis is anteverted. In severe infection the testis may protrude through the scrotum and appear as a granulating mass, which is known as *hernia testis*. Rarely the patient may present with *gangrene of the scrotum* for which no cause can be found out. This is known as *Fournier's gangrene (idiopathic gangrene)*. If there are multiple sinuses one should suspect *'Watering can' perineum*.

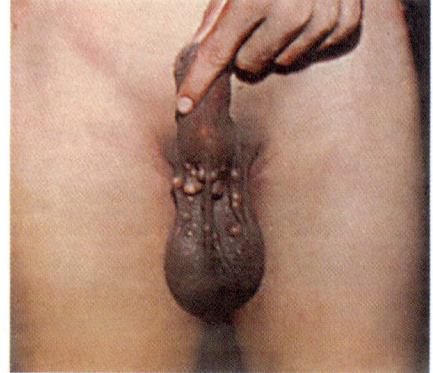

Fig. 40.1: Multiple sebaceous cysts of the scrotum.

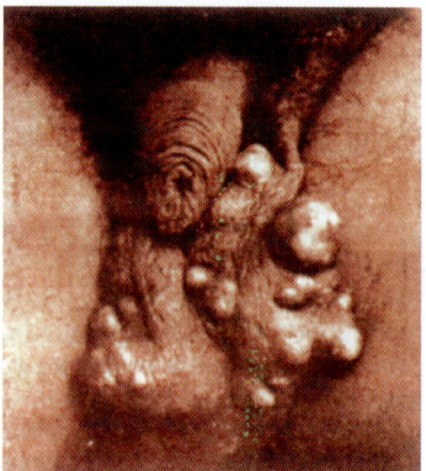

Fig. 40.2: Multiple sebaceous cysts of the scrotum.

One must remember that *edema* of the scrotum and penis may occur in medical conditions like nephritis, heart failure, etc. The surgical causes are cellulitis, filariasis, blocking of lymph vessels by cancer cells or following block dissection of inguinal lymph nodes and extravasation of urine. In case of **extravasation of urine** look at the perineum for evidence of injury or presence of periurethral abscess which bursts spontaneously to allow the urine to extravasate **(Fig. 40.3)**. A few cases of cellulitis of scrotum is misdiagnosed as suppurated hydrocele.

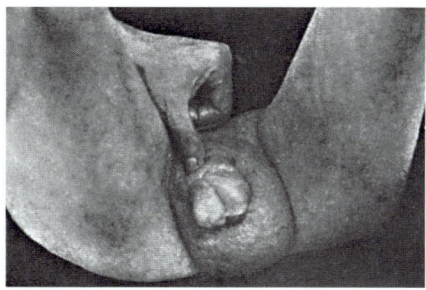

Fig. 40.3: Extravasation of urine.

Thickening of the skin and subcutaneous tissues of the scrotum may be so enormous that the scrotum assumes the size of a watermelon (*elephantiasis of the scrotum*), the penis becomes buried in the scrotal swelling **(Figs. 40.4 and 40.5)**. The skin and subcutaneous tissues of the penis may be similarly thickened to produce the typical *'Ram's Horn' penis* in filariasis **(Fig. 40.6)**. Another manifestation of filariasis is *lymph scrotum* in which the skin of the scrotum shows excessive rugosity with vesicles containing fluid (lymph) **(Fig. 40.7)**. Rupture of these vesicles from friction will lead to profuse exudation of lymph (lymphorrhagia).

2. **Swelling:** Slight swelling of the scrotum is evident by loss of normal rugosity of the scrotum. This is seen in any infection of testis and epididymis. Other conditions like cysts of the epididymis, spermatocele, etc., do not produce obvious swelling on inspection. Hydrocele may bring forth various degrees of swelling of the scrotum—small to very big so as to hang up to knee level. A peculiar constriction is often found around the swelling. If the hydrocele is tense it tends to stand out (forward projection).

Note the size, shape and extent of the swelling. Does it extend up along the spermatic cord to the groin?

3. **Impulse on coughing:** Many a time hydrocele is associated with hernia—a bubonocele or a complete inguinal hernia. Hernia shows impulse on coughing. So this part of examination cannot be dispensed with.

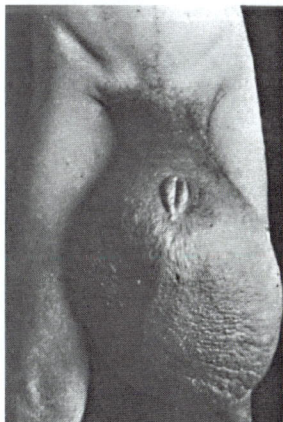 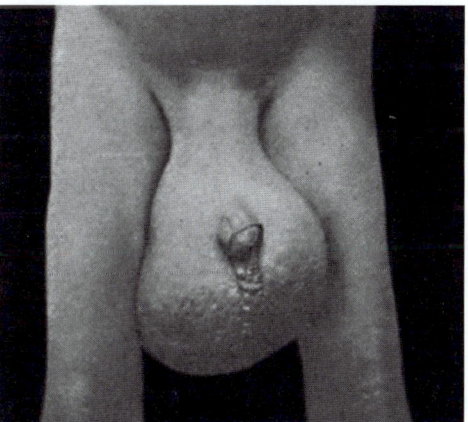 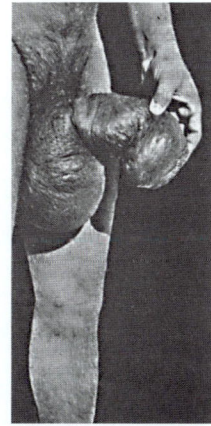

Fig. 40.4: Elephantiasis of the scrotum. Note that the penis is buried in the scrotal swelling.

Fig. 40.5: Another case of elephantiasis of scrotum.

Fig. 40.6: Elephantiasis of the scrotum with 'Ram's Horn' penis.

B. PALPATION

That the swelling is purely scrotal is confirmed by getting above the swelling.

1. **Skin:** If there is an ulcer, palpate it thoroughly as described in Chapter 4. *A carcinomatous ulcer* of the scrotum is diagnosed by yellowish-gray slough on the floor, hard base and everted margin. In the early stage the ulcer is freely mobile, but if the malignant ulcer becomes tethered to the underlying testis, it becomes fixed and moves with the testis. At this stage it is difficult to decide whether the lesion is a primary skin cancer or a testicular tumor ulcerating through the skin. An anteriorly placed ulcer which is fixed to the testis is probably a **gummatous ulcer**, whereas a

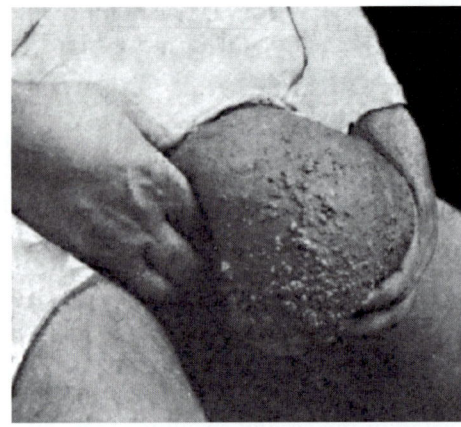

Fig. 40.7: Lymph scrotum with vesicles.

posteriorly placed ulcer which is fixed to the epididymis is a *tuberculous ulcer*. The testis cannot be separated from the protruded necrotic mass in case of *hernia testis*, but the testis can be easily separated in **hernia of a hydrocele**. Edema of the scrotum will 'pit on pressure'.

2. **Swelling:** This is first examined in the usual line as discussed in Chapter 3, noting *temperature, tenderness, extent, size, shape, surface, margin* and *consistency*. The most common cystic swelling is a vaginal hydrocele, i.e., a collection of serous fluid in the tunica vaginalis **(Fig. 40.8)**. The two cardinal signs of a hydrocele are: fluctuation and translucency.

FLUCTUATION (Fig. 40.9): This test cannot be performed in the traditional way, as the whole scrotum is very much mobile. So, this test is performed by holding the upper pole of the scrotal swelling between the thumb and the fingers of one hand to make the swelling tense and steady, while intermittent pressure is applied at the lower

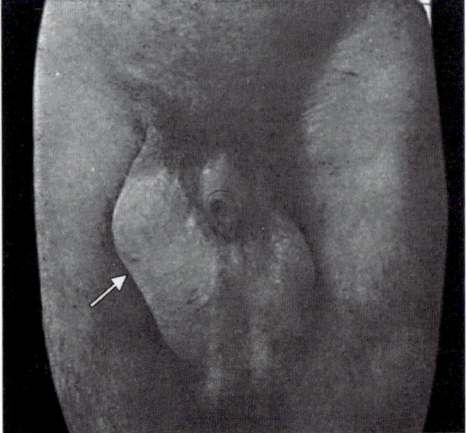

Fig. 40.8: A typical case of hydrocele of the tunica vaginalis. Note a faint constriction at the middle of the swelling shown by an arrow.

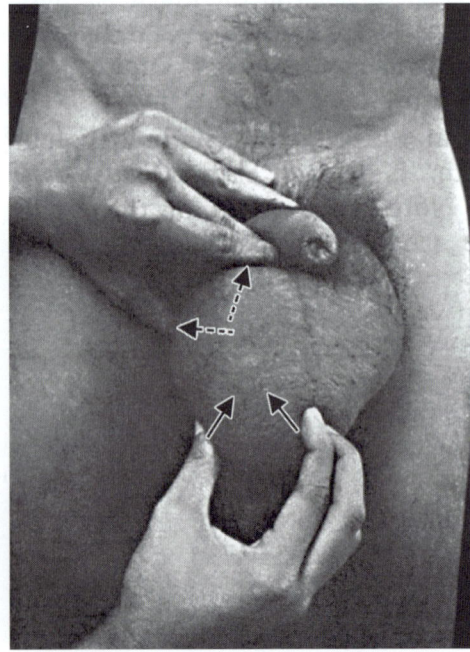

Fig. 40.9: The method of eliciting fluctuation in a case of hydrocele. See the text.

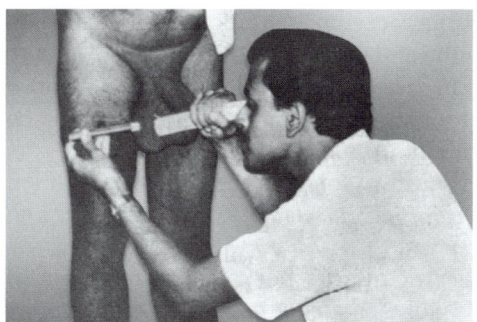

Fig. 40.10: The right method of performing the translucency test.

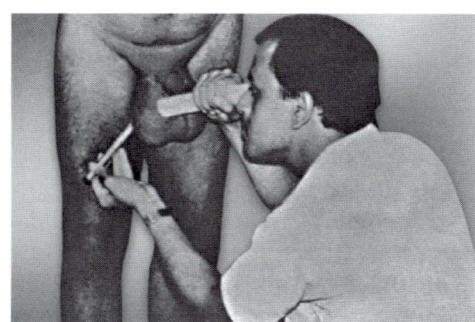

Fig. 40.11: The wrong method of performing the translucency test. The torch is placed behind the testis which will stand in the way of the light and will make the test negative even in presence of hydrocele.

pole with the thumb and the fingers of the other hand. This will push the fluid inside the tunica vaginalis upwards, the thumb and the fingers holding the upper pole of the swelling will be pushed apart from each other making this test positive.

TRANSLUCENCY (Figs. 40.10 and 40.11): This test is best performed in darkness. A pencil torch is placed *laterally* over the swollen scrotum. A red glow will be seen throughout the scrotum indicating presence of clear fluid inside the scrotum. This can be better visualized through a roll of paper placed on the other side of the scrotum even in daylight. The common mistake the students often make is to place the torch on the posterior aspect of the scrotum and the roll of paper anteriorly. The testis comes in the way of the light and this test becomes false negative. Uncomplicated hydrocele and the cyst of the epididymis are translucent but spermatocele is not translucent as the fluid it contains is not clear.

REDUCIBILITY: This is tested by raising the scrotum and compressing the swelling gently. Congenital hydrocele and a varicocele are reducible. In case of the former always examine the abdomen for ascites as congenital hydrocele is often associated with tuberculous peritonitis.

IMPULSE ON COUGHING: Many a time scrotal swelling may be associated with a hernia, varicocele or lymph varix. The root of the scrotum is held and the patient is asked to cough. An impulse either expansile in nature (hernia or congenital hydrocele) or thrill-like (varicocele or lymph varix) may be obtained. If this test is omitted, these conditions may be missed and treatment will be incomplete.

3. **Testis:** Examination of a scrotal swelling cannot be complete without palpation of the testis, epididymis and spermatic cord. Note its *position, size, shape, surface, consistency, weight, mobility* and *testicular sensation*. Note the *position* of the testis—whether normal, anteverted (the epididymis lies anteriorly and the body lies posteriorly), completely inverted, i.e., upside down (the globus major lies inferiorly) or incompletely inverted, i.e., the testis lies horizontally. These latter two positions predispose torsion of the testis. Whether the testis is normal in size, larger, or smaller than normal size? Smaller testis is an underdeveloped testis. Larger testis is often pathological—gummatous or with a tumor. Whether the *surface* is smooth or nodular? Whether the consistency is uniform or heterogenous? Note the *weight* of the organ in respect of its size. This is done by balancing the testis on the palm of the hand. The testis becomes relatively heavy in a case of neoplasm and old hematocele, but is comparatively light in a gumma of the testis.

Testicular sensation is very important. This is a peculiar sickening sensation felt by the patient when a mild pressure is applied on the testis. In gumma and malignant tumor of the testis, the testicular sensation quickly dwindles away (more so in case of gumma). In case of malignancy one should be very gentle and should not squeeze roughly lest the malignant cells should be dislodged and thrown into the venous and lymphatic channels.

It must be remembered that testis may be absent from the scrotum (in undescended testis, ectopic testis and retractile testis). *The testis is mainly affected in mumps, syphilis and neoplasm.*

4. **Epididymis:** This is normally felt as a firm nodular structure attached to the posterior aspect of the testis. Its large upper part is known as head (globus major), the middle part as body and the lower as tail (globus minor). Epididymis is mainly affected in tuberculosis, filariasis and acute (both gonococcal and nongonococcal) epididymo-orchitis. In **tuberculosis** the globus minor is first affected (the infection being mostly retrograde) and becomes enlarged, nodular and slightly tender. Only in blood-borne infection the globus major may be involved first. Gradually, the whole epididymis becomes enlarged, firm, craggy and slightly tender. Softening of the epididymis and formation of cold abscess in the posterior aspect of the scrotum is a great diagnostic point in favor of tuberculosis. In **filariasis** the epididymis also enlarges and becomes firm. **Acute epididymo-orchitis** is often gonococcal or *B. coli* infection (from retrograde passage of urine or 'reflux epididymitis' and postoperative epididymitis following prostatectomy) or from mumps.

Remember syphilis attacks the testis and tuberculosis affects the epididymis. Later on in both these conditions the disease spreads to the other organ. In filariasis, both the testis and epididymis are simultaneously involved.

5. **Spermatic cord:** This is best palpated at the root of the scrotum between the thumb and the index finger *simultaneously on both sides*. The vas deferens will be felt as hard whipcord slipping between the thumb and the index finger. Besides the vas, the fingers normally feel a number of strings, which are nothing but fibers of cremaster muscle. The spermatic cord is thickened and tender in any inflammatory condition of the epididymis—either acute or chronic. The vas is thickened and beaded in tuberculous epididymitis. The cord is not affected in syphilis but becomes thickened and slightly tender in filariasis. Lymph varix is also a feature of filariasis. A lymph varix feels soft and doughy whereas a varicocele feels like a 'bag of worms'. Both these conditions will yield a thrill-like impulse on coughing, but a varicocele more readily reduces than a lymph varix. In malignancy of the testis the growth may be extended upwards along the cord. In this case the cord will feel hard and nodular.

6. **Lymph nodes:** It is an extremely important part of examination. The skin of the scrotum drains into the inguinal group of lymph nodes whereas the testis and epididymis drain into the pre- and para-aortic lymph nodes at the level of the origin of the testicular artery from the aorta, i.e., at the transpyloric plane. These groups of lymph nodes must be palpated **(Fig. 40.12)**. The left supraclavicular group of lymph nodes may be

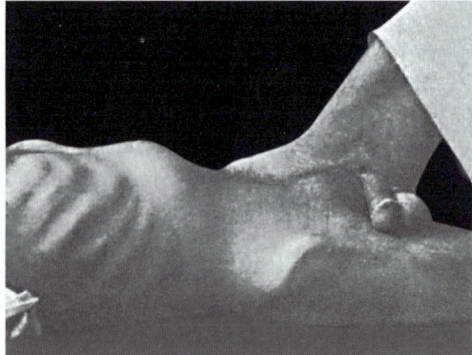

Fig. 40.12: A lump in the epigastric region of the abdomen from secondary deposits in the lymph nodes from malignant growth of the testis.

involved as in case of malignancies in other abdominal organs by lymphatic spread of malignant cells along the thoracic duct.

GENERAL EXAMINATION

Lungs should be examined particularly in case of tuberculous epididymo-orchitis to exclude tuberculous affection of the lung and malignancy of the testis to exclude secondary deposits in the lung.

One should look for other **syphilitic stigmas** (*see* page 75) in cases of gummatous orchitis.
Kidneys should be examined in cases of tuberculous epididymitis and varicocele of recent onset. In about 60% of cases there is either active tuberculosis in the renal tract or evidence of previous disease. Varicocele may be a sequel to adenocarcinoma of the kidney of the same side.
Rectal examination should always be performed in epididymo-orchitis either acute or chronic. Acute prostatitis often precedes epididymo-orchitis. The seminal vesicles are often enlarged and tender in cases of tuberculous epididymitis.

SPECIAL INVESTIGATIONS

Blood should be examined for eosinophilia and microfilaria in filariasis. Lymphocytosis and increased erythrocyte sedimentation rate (ESR) may be seen in cases of tuberculous epididymo-orchitis. Positive Wassermann reaction (WR) and Kahn tests favor the diagnosis of syphilitic orchitis.
Urine should be examined as a routine in cases of acute and chronic epididymo-orchitis. Acute epididymitis often results from retrograde passage of infected urine and presence of *E. coli, Streptococcus, Staphylococcus* or even proteus may be detected in urine. In tuberculous epididymitis many a time one will find tubercle bacilli in the urine.
Chest X-ray is an important investigation in tuberculous epididymo-orchitis to exclude presence of pulmonary tuberculosis. This is also important to exclude secondary deposits in the lungs in cases of testicular tumors particularly the teratomas.
Intravenous pyelography should also be performed in cases of testicular tumors to know the exact positions of the kidneys so that they may be properly shielded during radiotherapy and also to detect retroperitoneal lymphatic metastasis that might have displaced the ureters or brought about deformity of the renal pelvis.
Lymphangiography is an important part of investigation to determine secondary deposits in the para-aortic lymph nodes which have not shown clinical enlargement. Its value in assessing shrinkage of enlarged nodes by radiotherapy is also great.

Aschheim-Zondek test will be positive in cases of Sertoli cell tumor (interstitial cell tumor) and human chorionic gonadotrophin in 12 hour collection of urine will be higher than normal level (100 iu) in chorion carcinoma (malignant teratoma trophoblastic) of the testis.
Ultrasonography is extremely helpful not only to know the position of the testis, but also to know whether they are normal or not. This investigation is helpful in hydrocele, hematocele, secondary hydrocele, torsion of testis, etc.
Aspiration of a cystic swelling may clinch the diagnosis in a spermatocele or chylocele. The fluid is milky in spermatocele but in case of the cyst of the epididymis the fluid is clear. In hydrocele an amber color fluid may be obtained whose specific gravity remains in the range of 1.022–1.024; it

contains water, inorganic salts, cholesterol, fibrinogen and 6% of albumin. In case of secondary hydrocele from testicular tumor the fluid will be blood stained. To facilitate better palpation of testis and epididymis fluid should be aspirated out in case of secondary hydrocele.

Prostatic massage may demonstrate presence of gonococci in cases of acute gonococcal epididymo-orchitis and may demonstrate tubercle bacilli in cases of tuberculous epididymo-orchitis.

DIFFERENTIAL DIAGNOSIS

Differential diagnosis and their key features

Condition	Key features
Hydrocele	Soft, fluctuant, positive transillumination
Varicocele	Bag of worms feel, disappears on lying down
Funiculitis	Tender, indurated cord, fever, redness over scrotum
Lymph varix	Soft, doughy swelling, slow reduction on lying down
Lipoma of cord	Soft, lobulated, irreducible, no cough impulse
Testicular tumor	Hard, nodular, irregular mass, nontender
Torsion of testis	Acute severe pain, absent cremasteric reflex
Fournier's gangrene	Rapidly spreading gangrene, systemic toxicity

HYDROCELE

This can be classified into congenital and acquired varieties. *Acquired variety* can be further classified into *primary* (idiopathic) and *secondary* (from diseases of the testis and epididymis). In *congenital hydrocele* (Fig. 40.13), the processus vaginalis remains patent and it freely communicates with the peritoneal cavity. But usually the communicating orifice remains too small for hernia to develop. This condition is mainly diagnosed by the fact that the hydrocele gradually disappears when the patient lies down but it returns in the erect posture. The small opening prevents emptying of the hydrocele by digital pressure. In bilateral cases one should exclude ascites from tuberculous peritonitis.

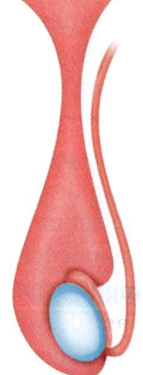

Fig. 40.13: Congenital hydrocele.

Primary hydrocele is mostly seen in middle-aged men but occasionally it is seen in early childhood. This may be unilateral or bilateral. The main and only complaint is the swelling of the scrotum and that is why the patient often presents with enormous swelling. One can 'get above the swelling' if it is a pure hydrocele, the only exception is the infantile hydrocele. The color and temperature of the overlying skin are normal. Primary hydrocele is not tender but secondary hydrocele may be tender. It is dull on percussion in contradistinction to the hernia, which is often resonant (due to presence of intestine inside the hernial sac). The fluid of the hydrocele surrounds the body of the testis making the testis impalpable.

If one can feel the testis separate from the scrotal swelling then the swelling is not a hydrocele but may be a cyst of the epididymis or spermatocele. In about 5% of cases inguinal hernia is associated with this condition. So one should not omit to look for impulse on coughing. The diagnosis of hydrocele is made by fluctuation and translucency tests.

Secondary hydrocele occurs secondary to acute and chronic epididymo-orchitis, syphilitic affection of the testis and occasionally in malignant tumor of the testis. A secondary hydrocele rarely attains a big size and in majority of cases it is lax in contradistinction to the primary hydrocele which is often tense. Generally, it does not interfere with the palpation of the testis and the epididymis but occasionally aspiration may be needed for better palpation.

Different other types of hydrocele:

a. *Infantile hydrocele (Fig. 40.14):* In this condition, the tunica and the processus vaginalis are distended upto the deep inguinal ring but do not communicate with the general peritoneal cavity. It does not necessarily appear in infants though its name suggests so.

b. *Funicular hydrocele (Fig. 40.15):* In this condition, the funicular process is closed just above the tunica vaginalis, so it does not produce a proper scrotal swelling but an inguinal swelling will be present. It is often confused with an inguinal hernia and it is a very rare condition.

c. *Hydrocele of the hernial sac (Fig. 40.16):* Sometimes the neck of a hernial sac becomes closed by adhesions or plugged with omentum. This results in retention of the serous fluid secreted by the peritoneum of the hernial sac resulting in a hydrocele.

d. *Encysted hydrocele of the cord (Fig. 40.17):* This has been discussed in the previous chapter. Bilocular hydrocele is shown in **Figure 40.18**.

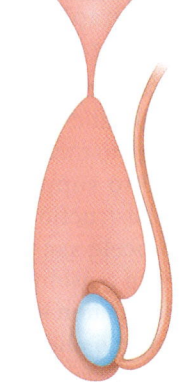

Fig. 40.14: Infantile hydrocele.

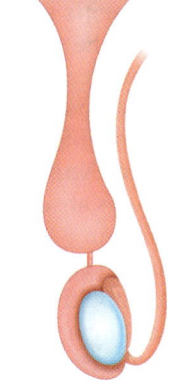

Fig. 40.15: Funicular hydrocele.

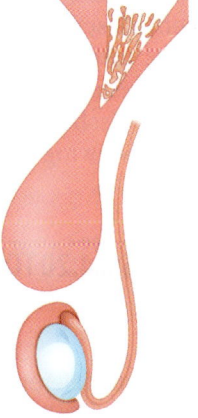

Fig. 40.16: Hydrocele of hernial sac.

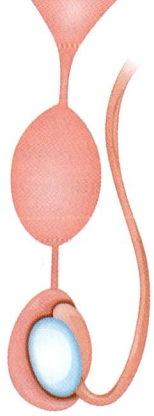

Fig. 40.17: Encysted hydrocele of the cord.

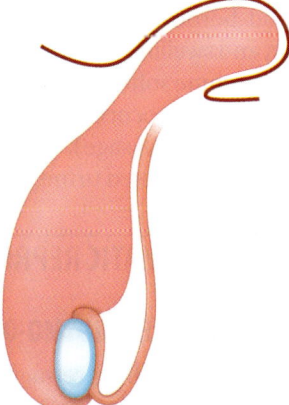

Fig. 40.18: Bilocular hydrocele 'enbissac'.

Ultrasonography can be used to detect the hydrocele **(Fig. 40.19)**.

Complications of a hydrocele are: (i) *Rupture*—either traumatic or spontaneous; (ii) Hematocele from injury to the hydrocele; (iii) Infection which may lead to suppurative hydrocele and even gradual destruction of the testis; (iv) Hernia of the hydrocele sac may result in long-standing cases when tension of the fluid within the tunica causes herniation through the dartos muscles; (v) Calcification of the sac wall and (vi) Atrophy of the testis in long-standing cases.

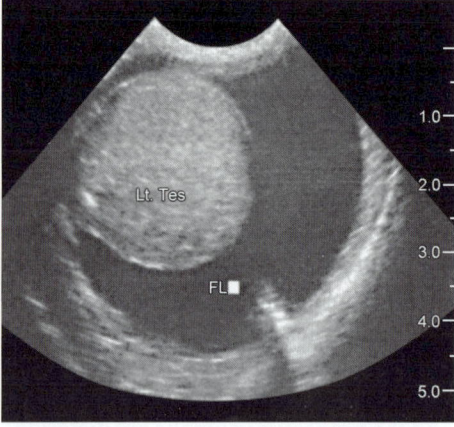

Fig. 40.19: Ultrasonography showing a typical case of hydrocele of left scrotum. FL indicates fluid and LT. TES indicates left testis.

Hematocele: Recent hematocele is usually the result of injury or during tapping of a hydrocele. Patient presents scrotal swelling with pain. On examination the swelling is quite tender, fluctuant but not translucent. *Old hematocele* may result from slow hemorrhage into the tunica vaginalis. This may be a painless condition which gives more confusion to the diagnosis. In majority of cases a history of trauma cannot be elicited. Thus this condition simulates testicular tumor in many respect. No history of gradual enlargement of the swelling, presence of testicular sensation (this is always absent in testicular tumors) and absence of metastasis favors the diagnosis of this condition.

Pyelocele (suppurated hydrocele): This is a sequel of infection in the hydrocele sac. This condition should be differentiated from cellulitis of the scrotal wall. Pressure on the hydrocele through a comparatively healthy area will elicit tenderness in the cases of suppurated hydrocele but not in the case of cellulitis.

ACUTE EPIDIDYMO-ORCHITIS

Infection usually starts in the epididymis and may gradually spread to the body of the testis giving the name epididymo-orchitis. It is actually a retrograde infection secondary to the infection of the urethra, prostate and seminal vesicles which spreads via the lumen of the vas deferens. Blood-borne infection, though rare, affects the globus major first. Patient presents with severe pain and swelling of the testis. The scrotal wall becomes red and edematous. Later on epididymis may become soften and adherent to the scrotal wall. Causative organism is usually gonococcus (following gonococcal urethritis and diagnosed by finding gonococci in the discharge collected by prostatic massage), *E. coli, Streptococcus, Staphylococcus* or *Proteus* (following retrograde passage of infected urine, following catheterization, prostatectomy or cystitis).

■ DIAGRAMMATIC REPRESENTATIONS OF SCROTAL SWELLINGS (FIGS. 4.20 TO 40.31)

TUBERCULOUS EPIDIDYMO-ORCHITIS

This also results from retrograde spread of infection from seminal vesicle via vas deferens. Blood-borne infection, though rare, will affect the globus major first. Slight aching is the only complaint of the patient and it does not attract attention of the patient till it is involved in a trivial injury. On examination, normal rugosity of the scrotal skin is lost and there is some restriction in the mobility

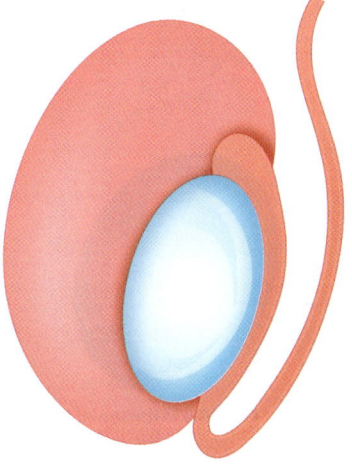
Fig. 40.20: Hydrocele or hematocele.

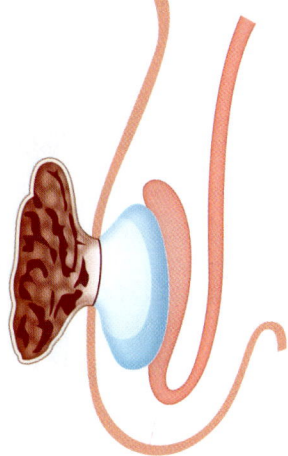
Fig. 40.21: Hernia testis.

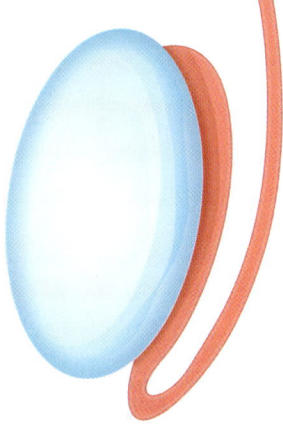
Fig. 40.22: Orchitis or gumma of the testis.

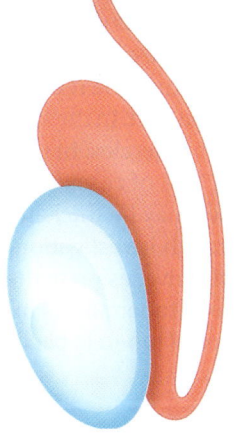
Fig. 40.23: Acute epididymo-orchitis.

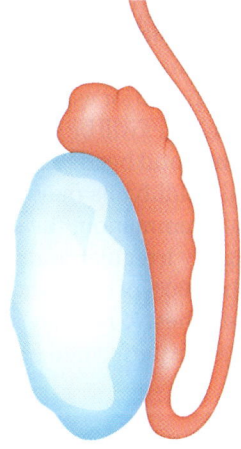
Fig. 40.24: Filaria epididymo-orchitis.

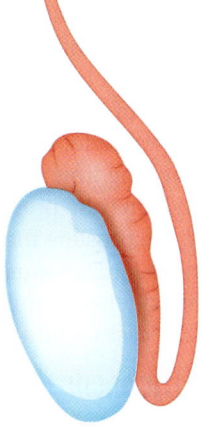
Fig. 40.25: Tuberculous epididymitis.

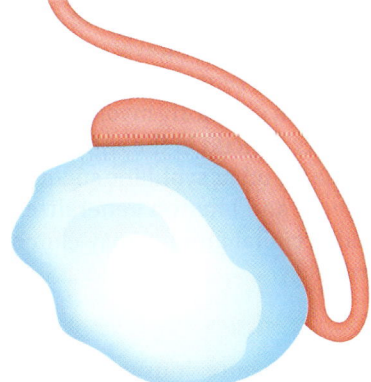
Fig. 40.26: Tumor of the testis.

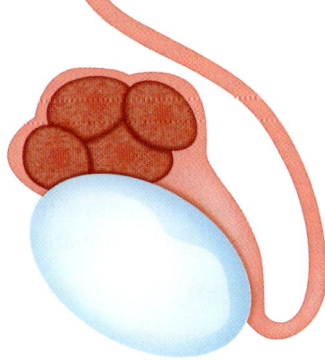
Fig. 40.27: Cysts of the epididymis.

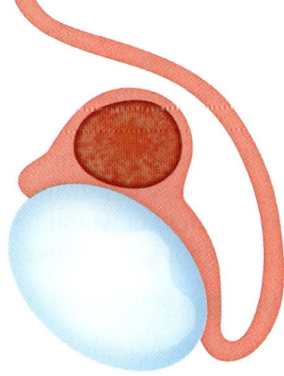
Fig. 40.28: Spermatocele

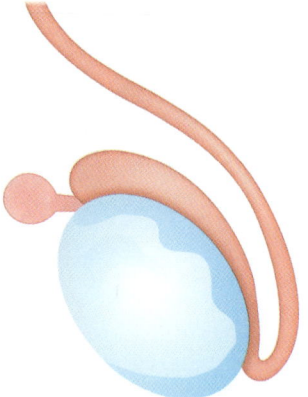
Fig. 40.29: Cyst of hydatid of Morgagni.

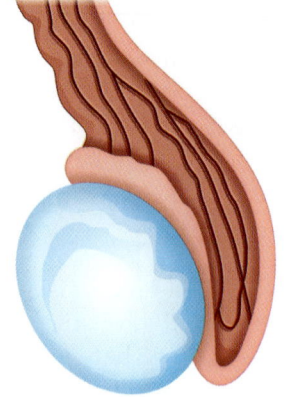
Fig. 40.30: Varicocele or lymph varix.

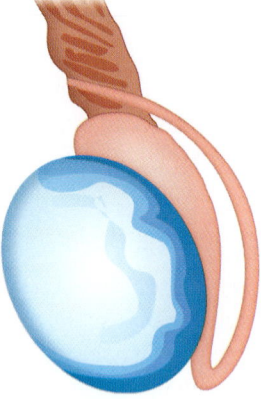
Fig. 40.31: Torsion of the spermatic cord.

of the testis. Slightly tender, indurated and nodular globus minor and later on the body of the epididymis can be detected. Gradually, the whole epididymis becomes thickened and it is felt as firm, craggy and tender nodules. The nodules gradually soften and cold abscess develops in the posterior aspect of the testis. This may adhere to the skin and burst out discharging thin pus, thus develops the tuberculous sinus on the posterior aspect of the scrotum. It must be remembered that in case of anteverted testis these changes will be seen on the anterior aspect. In the spermatic cord, the vas deferens may be thickened and beaded due to submucous tubercles. In untreated cases for long time the contralateral epididymis may be diseased. In 30% of cases secondary hydrocele may be present. On rectal examination, the seminal vesicles may be thickened and tender, the prostate may also be slightly irregular and tender. A thorough investigation of the urinary system is a must as no less than 60% of cases show presence of active lesion in the renal tract or evidence of previous disease. Chest X-ray may show evidence of tuberculosis in about 1/2 of the cases. Culture of semen may be performed to detect presence of tubercle bacilli.

SYPHILITIC ORCHITIS

Three types of late manifestations may be seen involving the testis in syphilis. These are: (i) *Bilateral orchitis*—mostly seen in congenital syphilis. (ii) *Interstitial fibrosis*—is a symptom less and bilateral affection in which there is gradual destruction of the seminiferous tubules. The testes are not enlarged but there will be loss of testicular sensation. (iii) *Gumma* —is the most common of these three varieties. It is always unilateral. The body of the testis slowly enlarges. It is a painless condition. The testis becomes hard with loss of testicular sensation. Secondary hydrocele is almost always present. Later on the testis becomes soften anteriorly involving the scrotal wall and ultimately a gummatous ulcer forms. It is often very difficult in the early stage to differentiate it from a testicular tumor. A search should be made for other syphilitic stigmas, but a history of previous exposure, development of hard chancre and later on generalized involvement of lymph nodes (particularly the epitrochlear and occipital groups) may clinch the diagnosis. Positive serological tests of the serum are confirmatory.

SUBACUTE EPIDIDYMO-ORCHITIS (FILARIAL)

In filariasis epididymo-orchitis is quite common and is of subacute nature. It usually affects the globus major of the epididymis. The epididymis feels swollen, firmer and slightly tender.

The digital fossa between the testis and the epididymis on the lateral aspect is obliterated with inflammatory adhesions. Gradually, the testis is involved. It becomes enlarged, firm, slightly tender and loses to certain extent testicular sensation. Secondary, hydrocele is not uncommon. Differentiation from tuberculous epididymitis is made by presence of a history of periodic fever, absence of 'craggy' epididymis leading to softening, formation of cold abscess and sinus; absence of involvement of the seminal vesicles on rectal examination, presence of eosinophilia and demonstration of microfilariae in the peripheral blood.

LYMPH VARIX

This is nothing but dilatation of the lymph vessels of the spermatic cord. This is a characteristic feature of filariasis. So it is often associated with filarial fever which has a periodicity. The onset is sudden and is ushered in with chill and rigor. The temperature may rise to 103°–104°. The features with which this condition may be differentiated from malarial fever is by simultaneous attack of tenderness and swelling of the spermatic cord. The spermatic cord gives rise to multilocular elongated cystic swelling, which can be designated as 'diffuse hydrocele of the cord'.

LYMPH SCROTUM

This term is applied to the condition of dilatation and tortuosity of the cutaneous lymphatics of the scrotum. Excessive rugosity and presence of vesicles are noticed in the skin of the scrotum. The vesicles may be of different sizes containing clear or slightly turbid fluid. Rupture of vesicles from friction may lead to exudation of lymph (lymphorrhagia). Secondary infection is the most important and frequent complication. In absence of infection the skin of the scrotum remains thickened but soft. Later on gradual fibrosis will give rise to elephantiasis.

CHYLOCELE

Presence of chylous fluid in the tunica vaginalis causes this condition. This condition may be suspected when a case of hydrocele presents with a periodic history of fever and a negative translucency test. The fluid may contain microfilaria.

ELEPHANTIASIS OF THE SCROTUM

It is a very common manifestation of filariasis. Lymphatic obstruction and later on fibrosis in the lymph-logged tissue will cause this condition. The disease comes through stages viz. filarial fever, lymphangitis, lymph stagnation and finally elephantiasis. So in the early stage the part becomes swollen and edematous, pitting on pressure, but later on when there is excessive growth of fibrous tissue it becomes nonyielding and firm. The lymph provides suitable nourishment for happy growth of the fibroblasts. The thickening commences at the most dependent part of the scrotum and gradually extends upwards. So the thickening is maximum at the bottom and minimum at the root. On section, the hypertrophied skin forms the outermost layer, under which is the dense fibrotic layer, deep to it is a layer of gelatinous lymphlogged blubbery tissue and deep to it is the hydrocele with the testis. This testis may be atrophied due to lack of nutrition and pressure.

EXTRAVASATION OF URINE (Fig. 40.32)

It may occur: (i) from ruptured urethra if the patient tries to pass urine after such injury or (ii) from bursting of periurethral abscess resulting from stricture of the urethra. This condition means urine has come out from its normal path. The knowledge of spread of extravasation of urine is essential in understanding the clinical picture of this condition. The bulbous urethra is the most common site of ruptured urethra, similarly it is the most common site of periurethral abscess following stricture of urethra. So extravasation of urine commonly occurs from this part of the urethra. The urine first collects in the superficial pouch of the perineum. This pouch is closed above by inferior fascia of the urogenital diaphragm (perineal membrane), closed below by fascia of Colles, laterally by ischiopubic rami and posteriorly by continuation of the perineal membrane with the fascia of Colles. So this pouch is open only anteriorly through which urine may come out and travel forwards in the subcutaneous tissue of the scrotum, penis and lower part of the anterior abdominal wall, lying deep to the fascia of Scarpa as it starts deep to the fascia of Colles. But students must remember that it cannot gravitate down the thigh as the fascia of Scarpa is attached to the fascia lata of the thigh a little distal to and parallel to the inguinal ligament.

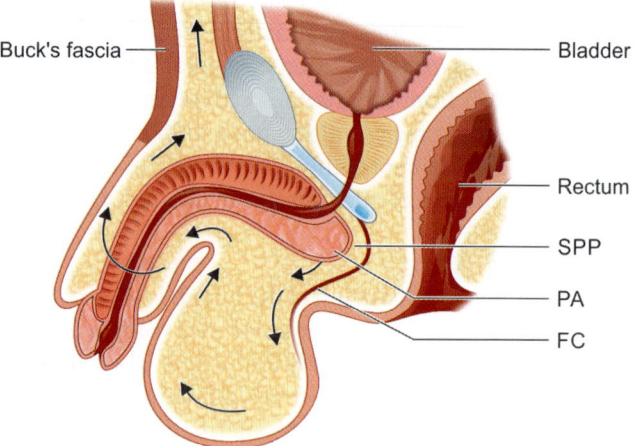

Fig. 40.32: The route of spread of extravasated urine. The urine at the time of micturition escapes through the periurethral abscess (PA) into the superficial pouch of the perineum (SPP) under the fascia of Colles (FC). It then spreads into the scrotum, penis and anterior abdominal wall under the fascia of Scarpa (FS) (for reasons see the text, page 523). A portion of the urinary bladder (BL) and that of the rectum are also shown.

The swelling due to this condition is of the nature of edema and the water-logged condition can be easily assessed by pinching the skin of the scrotum and penis. Rise of temperature with or without rigor is expected. In neglected cases sloughing may take place with formation of urinary fistulae. But the patient may not survive up to this stage. Diagnosis is made by previous history of urethral stricture with recent development of swelling and pain indicating periurethral abscess or an injury to the bulbous part of the urethra followed by swelling of the perineum, scrotum, penis and lower part of the anterior abdominal wall.

TORSION OF THE TESTIS

Some congenital abnormalities usually predispose to torsion of the testis and it must be remembered that the abnormality is usually bilateral so that the other side is always liable to undergo torsion. The **abnormalities are:** (i) Inversion of testis, (ii) Full coverage of the testis with tunica vaginalis so that the testis is suspended in the tunica and (iii) Presence of a long mesorchium which separates the testis from the epididymis. Torsion does occur in an undescended testis.

The most common incidence is between 10 and 15 years of age and it is extremely rare after 25 years of age. Sudden and agonizing pain in the groin and lower abdomen is the main symptom.

This condition is notoriously difficult to diagnose with confidence, but one must keep this condition in mind whenever a patient presents with acute testicular symptoms. Sudden and agonizing pain, which is quite severe occurring between the ages of 10 and 25 years, more commonly between 12 and 18 years is suspicious of a case of torsion. This condition is extremely rare after 25 years of age. The agonizing pain is often referred to the groin and lower abdomen instead of being restricted to the scrotum only. Nausea and vomiting are very common associated symptoms. Past history of similar attacks which subsided spontaneously may be obtained. Straining at stool, lifting heavy weight, coitus and blow on the scrotum as the boy jumps on his bicycle are the *exciting causes.*

On examination, the affected testis hangs higher in the scrotum. Generally, a fully developed testis does not undergo torsion as its anchorage prevents torsion. The scrotal skin remains normal in early hours, but after a lapse of 6 hours or so the skin becomes red, hot and edematous. The testis is exquisitely tender and the patient does not allow to touch. The testis is swollen and it is very difficult to differentiate the contour of the epididymis from the body of the testis.

Torsion of an undescended testis should be differentiated from a strangulated hernia. That the scrotum of that side is empty goes in favor of torsion. Greater problem is to *differentiate torsion of a testis inside the scrotum from an acute epididymo-orchitis.* One may feel the twisted spermatic cord to clinch the issue. In cases of acute epididymo-orchitis, the epididymis is initially the site of maximum swelling and tenderness and the testis remains normal; while in case of torsion, the testis occupies an elevated position and is itself tender on palpation. Moreover in case of the former the onset is less acute and may be associated with other urinary tract symptoms, e.g., frequency and dysuria. If the scrotum is elevated, pain is relieved to certain extent in case of acute epididymo-orchitis, but pain will be aggravated in case of torsion. Lastly if mumps can be excluded in case of a boy and urethritis can be excluded in case of a man, the diagnosis of the prevailing condition is torsion of the testis and not acute epididymo-orchitis.

Another condition that *mimics torsion of the testis* is *torsion of the testicular appendage or Morgagni's. hydatid* which is a mullerian duct remnant. The symptoms are very much similar, but less severe. The diagnosis is possible if the torted appendage can be felt. Often transillumination test may help.

If the diagnosis is still in doubt it is better to explore quickly, as torsion, if not relieved immediately, will lead to death of the testis, on the other hand exploration will not do any extra damage in case of acute epididymo-orchitis.

TUMORS OF THE TESTIS

Though these tumors only constitute 1% of all malignant tumors in man, yet these are one of the most common forms of malignant tumors in the young. Almost all (99%) testicular tumors are malignant. The two main varieties of testicular tumors are—(a) Seminoma (40%)—carcinoma of the seminiferous tubules and (b) Teratoma (35%)—malignancy in the rete testis from totipotent cells. 15% of the tumors are the mixed type containing both of the above two types. Of the remaining 10%–6% are lymphoma, 2% are interstitial cell tumors (arising from Leydig cells and cells of Sertoli) and the 2% other tumors. Clinically, it may not be possible to differentiate between seminoma from teratoma and final differentiation rests on histology.

Teratoma **(Fig. 40.33)** occurs between the ages of 20 and 30 years, whereas **seminoma** **(Fig. 40.34)** occurs between the ages of 30 and 50 years. The most common presentation is a painless swelling of the testis. Duration is about a few months. Trivial injury may draw the attention of the patient towards the swelling and he often incriminates trauma to be the cause of the swelling. Dull aching or dragging pain may be experienced in the scrotum if the swelling has grown very large. Acute pain and tenderness is very rare form of presentation which is indistinguishable from acute epididymo-orchitis. General malaise, wasting and loss of appetite are also complained of but in less number of cases. Rarely, this condition may present itself as abdominal pain and swelling of the legs due to secondary metastasis in the pre- and para-aortic groups of lymph nodes. It must be remembered that seminomas first metastasize by lymphatic spread and blood-borne metastasis is late; whereas in teratomas blood-borne metastasis is early.

Secondary hydrocele and infertility are very rare forms of presentation but should not be forgotten. Also remember that undescended testis is more vulnerable (about 50 times) to malignant transformation which is not reduced by late orchidopexy. Leydig cell tumors secrete male hormones and may lead to sexual precocity; whereas Sertoli cell tumors secrete female hormones and may lead to feminization and formation of gynecomastia.

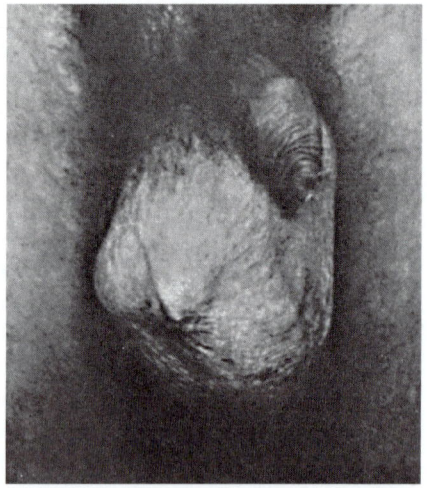

Fig. 40.33: Teratoma of the testis. Note the irregular surface of the testis.

On examination, the swelling is purely scrotal. The testis is enlarged, firm, smooth and heavy. This is more noticed in case of seminoma, but slight nodularity can be felt. In teratoma the surface is irregular or nodular. Consistency may be varying with soft bosses in between. Testicular sensation is always lost early, but one must be very gentle in finding out this sign. The spermatic cord remains normal for quite a long time. But eventually it may be thickened due to cremasteric hypertrophy and enlargement of testicular vessels, but the vas is never thickened. Rectal examination will reveal no abnormality of the prostate and seminal vesicles.

Now attention is directed towards examination for secondaries. Lymphatic metastasis will cause enlargement of the pre-and para-aortic groups of lymph nodes which are situated just above the level of the umbilicus. Liver should be palpated. Lungs should be examined including chest X-ray to exclude blood-borne metastasis there.

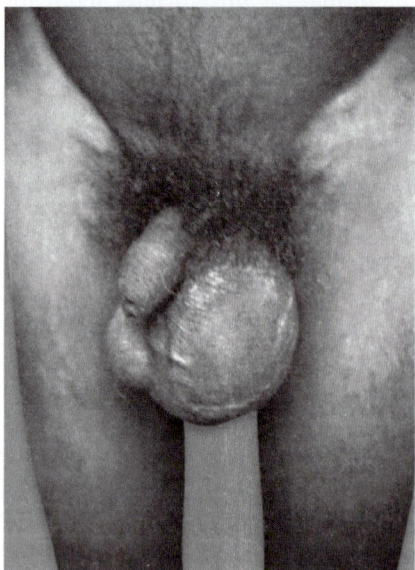

Fig. 40.34: A case of seminoma of the testis.

Investigations are done as discussed under the heading of 'Special Investigations'.

CYSTS

Barring the cyst of an appendage of the testis, these mainly arise in connection with the epididymis.

(i) **Cysts of the epididymis**: These are cystic transformation of the aberrant structures like paradidymis, hydatid of Morgagni (appendix of the epididymis), the vas aberrans of Haller, etc. Though congenital, yet the sufferers are usually middle-aged men. There are actually multiple cysts or multilocular cyst above and behind the body of the testis. In contradistinction to hydrocele these can be felt apart from the testis. The fluid it contains is crystal clear. These are tense, fluctuant and brilliantly translucent. But due to presence of multiple septa brilliant translucency is finely tesselated giving the appearance of a Chinese lantern. This condition may be bilateral. If the cyst grows bigger and encroaches downwards into the scrotum, it may mimic a hydrocele, but this cyst lies behind the testis, whereas hydrocele lies in front of the testis.

(ii) **Spermatocele:** This is unilocular cyst situated in the head of the epididymis. The fluid inside contains spermatozoa and resembles barley water. This is a lax swelling in comparison to the previous condition. This is less translucent than the previous condition.

(iii) **Cyst of an appendage of the testis:** This is a very rare condition and forms a globular swelling at the superior pole of the testis. It is usually unilateral and may undergo torsion if pedunculated.

FOURNIER'S GANGRENE (IDIOPATHIC GANGRENE OF THE SCROTUM) (FIG. 40.35)

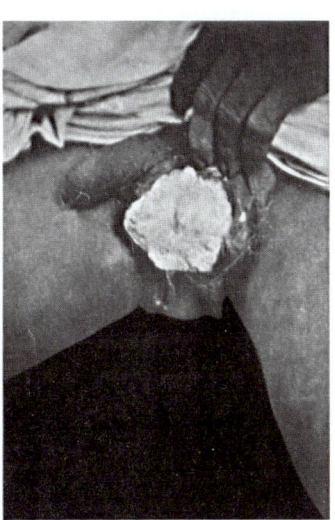

Fig. 40.35: A typical case of Fournier's gangrene of scrotum.

It is a rare condition in which: (i) there is sudden appearance of scrotal inflammation in an apparently healthy individual; (ii) There is rapid onset of gangrene and (iii) in majority of cases no cause can be found out. This condition is considered to be an infective gangrene in which fulminating inflammation causes obliterative arteritis of the subcutaneous tissue and hence the gangrene. Minor injuries in the perineum often start the disease, e.g., bruise and scratch in the perineum, injection of anal fissure or opening of a periurethral abscess. The causative organisms are hemolytic streptococci, staphylococci, *E. coli, Cl. welchii,* etc. Clinical features are sudden pain in the scrotum with pyrexia, prostration and pallor. If not treated properly the whole scrotum is sloughed off leaving the testes hanging exposed. Gradually gangrene spreads to the neighboring tissues as superficial extravasation of urine.

SEBACEOUS CYSTS OF THE SCROTUM (*SEE* FIGS. 40.1 AND FIG. 40.2)

Sebaceous cysts are commonly seen in the scrotum after puberty till middle-age. Multiple cysts are quite common of different sizes. Hardly any of these cysts attain very large size.

CARCINOMA OF SCROTUM

This disease has a distinct relation with occupation. Previously, this condition used to occur among chimney sweepers where soot was the carcinogen. Later on this condition occurred from soakage of the trousers of mule spinners with lubricating oil used in cotton industry. Now this lubricating oil has been made free from impurities and is no more causing this disease. Till today a few among tar and shale oil workers are affected, though majority are of unknown etiology. The growth starts as a painless nodule or ulcer. On examination hard feel of the nodule or base of the ulcer is of significance. Inguinal lymph nodes are almost always enlarged, discrete and hard.

THE PENIS

HISTORY

Age: Congenital lesions, e.g., phimosis, hypospadias, epispadias are commonly seen in children. Hunterian chancre, soft chancre, lymphogranuloma inguinale, granuloma inguinale are seen in adults. Carcinoma of penis is a disease of old age.

Race: Muslims and Jews are almost immune to carcinoma of penis due to their religious custom of early circumcision.

COMPLAINTS

Mother may complain that her son is not passing water satisfactorily. Either it is coming out in thin stream or falls by drops. It may be due to a pinhole meatus or more often phimosis. If the complaint is that the foreskin is ballooning during micturition, it is purely due to phimosis. **Phimosis** is a condition in which the prepucial opening is narrow and cannot be retracted over the glans penis. It must be remembered that the adults may present with such complaints. Long-standing chronic balanoposthitis may lead to cicartical contraction and hence develops phimosis. Similarly subprepucial carcinoma **(Fig. 40.36)** may lead to phimosis. Meatal ulcer may lead to acquired *pin-hole meatus.* Patient may complain with excruciating pain and swelling of the glans penis, with the foreskin fastened tight round the corona glandis. This is *paraphimosis*. Sometimes the patients present with **ulcers** in the penis. Enquire about any history of exposure. If the ulcer has developed after four days of exposure it is a soft sore (chancroid). If it has developed after four weeks of exposure it is a hard chancre (Hunterian chancre). There may be a fleeting, painless papule or ulcer often unnoticed by the patient in case of lymphogranuloma inguinale. In case of granuloma inguinale a painless vesicle or indurated papule develops in penis after 1-4 weeks of exposure. This erodes to form a slowly extending ulcer with red granulomatous floor. If there is no history of exposure one should keep in mind the possibility of cancer. If the patient complains of discharge, enquire particularly where is the **discharge** corning from—the urethra or the prepuci al sac. In balanoposthitis, carcinoma, etc. discharge may come from the prepucial sac. Even if the discharge is coming from the urethra, note particularly that it is not coming from the infected Morgagni's follicles which open by a pair of mouths just behind the lips of the external urethral meatus.

If the patient complains of **pain** in the penis, note its relation with micturition. *Pain during micturition* is complained of in acute urethritis, acute prostatitis, prostatic abscess and passage of a calculus. *Pain following micturition* is complained of in vesical calculus, cystitis and diverticulum of the bladder. *Pain independent of micturition* is come across in balanoposthitis, herpes, advanced carcinoma of penis, etc.

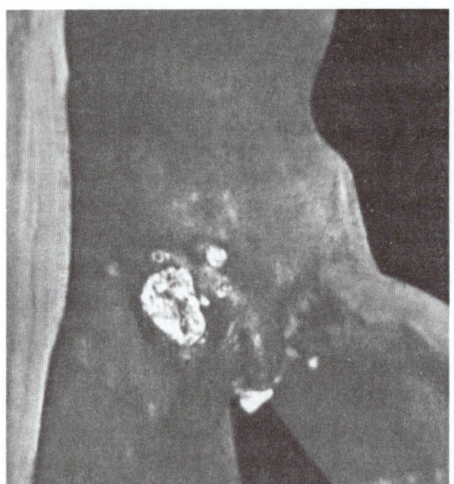

Fig. 40.36: Carcinoma of the penis with secondary involvement of the inguinal lymph nodes (fungating).

LOCAL EXAMINATION

Examine systematically, (a) the prepuce, (b) the external urethral meatus, (c) the glans penis and (d) the body of the penis.

Retract the prepuce over the glans up to the corona. Failure to do so is due to **phimosis**. When the prepuce becomes tight round the corona with swelling of the glans, the condition is known as **paraphimosis**.

Look for presence of *pinhole meatus*. This is mainly a congenital deformity but acquired type may be seen following a meatal ulcer. **An ulcer** may be due to either Hunterian chancre or chancroid or granulomatous inguinale or an epithelioma. A *Hunterian chancre* is painless with the well-defined edge and an indurated base. This feels like a button. *Chancroid* (soft sores) are multiple, painful ulcers with ill-defined and edematous margins discharging pus. *Epithelioma* may be anywhere on the skin of the prepuce or the glans penis. Two types are usually seen—a papilliferous tumor (cauliflower-like growth) and an ulcer with raised and everted edge and necrotic floor. A few **premalignant conditions** may be seen: (i) *Leukoplakia* (features are same as those more popularly known in the tongue). (ii) *Paget's disease*—as chronic red eczema on the glans or inside the prepuce. (iii) *Erythroplasia of Querat*-as dark red flat indurated patch on the glans or inner surface of the prepuce. This is also seen on vulva and in the mouth.

The **swellings** on the glans may be an epithelioma, erythroplasia of Querat and condylomata acuminata (venereal warts). Venereal warts are multiple papillomatous growths which are moist and discharge bad smelling serous fluid. They are mostly placed in the region of coronal sulcus. These are the most common benign neoplasm of the penis.

Balanitis is an infection of the glans penis and *posthitis* is infection of the inner surface of the prepuce. The patient complains of a bad smelling creamy discharge from beneath the prepuce.

Epispadias **(Fig. 40.37)** is a condition in which the urethral opening is on the dorsal surface of the penis. But more common *hypospadias* **(Figs. 40.38 to 40.40)** is a condition in which the urethra opens on the ventral surface of the penis. According to the position of the opening it is classified into a glandular type (opening is on the glans), a penile type (opening is on the body of the penis) **(Figs. 40.41 and 40.42)** or the perineal type (the opening is on the perineum with bifid scrotum).

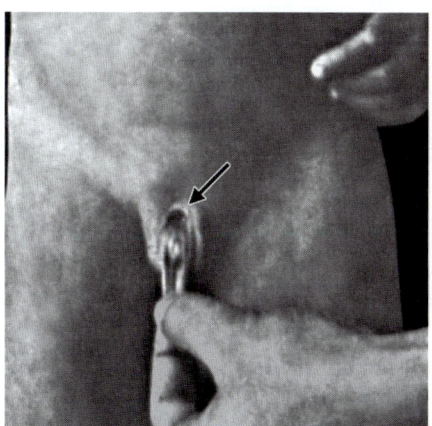

Fig. 40.37: Epispadias.

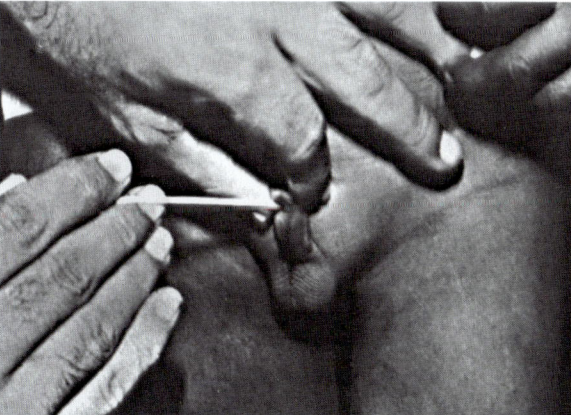

Fig. 40.38: Coronal hypospadias.

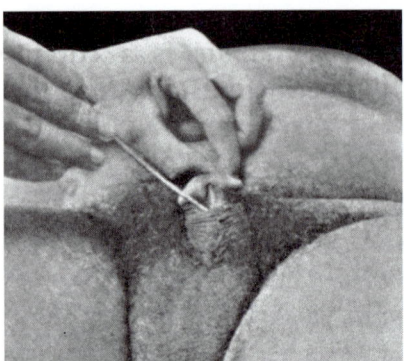

Fig. 40.39: A case of coronal hypospadias.

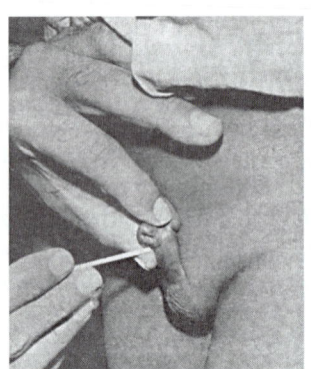

Fig. 40.40: A case of coronal hypospadias.

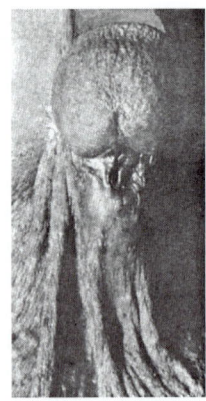

Fig. 40.41: Hypospadias—there is a distal penile opening.

Watch the patient passing urine: In case of phimosis the prepuce will balloon out or a very fine stream of urine can be seen. Both indicate phimosis which needs circumcision.

Body of the penis is palpated with index finger and thumb of both hands systematically. The deep part of the body is palpated through the scrotum and perineum.

If urethritis is suspected the penis can be milked with the thumb and the index finger to express some purulent discharge.

Examination of the draining lymph nodes: Carcinoma of the penis mainly drains into the inguinal group of lymph nodes. But it must be remembered that enlargement of these lymph nodes do not always signify the presence of metastasis. In fact, in about 50% of cases swelling of these lymph nodes is due to inflammation rather than lymphatic metastasis. Involvement of the urethra by inflammation or neoplasm will lead to enlargement of lymph nodes of the iliac group.

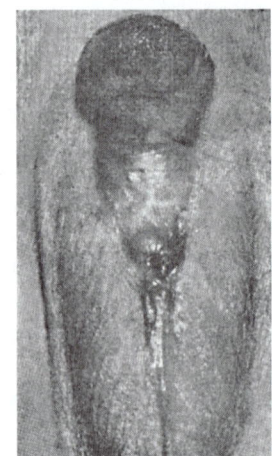

Fig. 40.42: Hypospadias—there is a proximal penile opening (penile type).

DIFFERENTIAL DIAGNOSIS

HYPOSPADIAS

This is the most common congenital malformation of the urethra. The external urinary meatus is not situated at the tip of the penis, but at some point on the undersurface of the penis or in the perineum. According to its location, hypospadias can be of the following types: (a) *Glandular* type in which the meatus is situated on the under-surface of the glans generally at a point where the frenum (which is absent) is normally attached. A blind depression marks the normal site of the meatus. This is the most common variety. (b) *Coronal* type, in which the meatus is at the corona. (c) *Penile* type, in which the meatus is situated at some point on the undersurface of the body of the penis between the glans and the penoscrotal junction. (d) *Penoscrotal* type, in which the meatus is at the penoscrotal junction. (e) *Perineal* type, in which the meatus is at the perineum about 3 cm in front of the anus. This is the least common. The scrotum is cleft. The testes are either undescended or if descended are very small. In all varieties the penis is curved downwards (chordee) (except the glandular type) due to presence of fibrous tissue from the meatus to the tip of the penis.

EPISPADIAS

This is quite rare and the external urinary meatus in this condition opens on the dorsal surface of the penis. Three varieties are usually seen: (a) *Glandular* type, where the meatus is situated on the dorsal aspect of the glans. (b) *Penile* type, in which the meatus is situated on the dorsal aspect of the body of the penis. The penis curves upward. (c) *Total* type, which is associated with ectopia vesicae and incontinence of urine.

PHIMOSIS

It is a condition in which the end of the prepuce is so narrow that it cannot be retracted over the glans up to the corona. It is a congenital abnormality. So, the children are the main sufferers. It may or may not be associated with pinhole meatus. It leads to difficulty in micturition and ballooning of the prepuce. Recurrent balanoposthitis causing pain and purulent discharge are the common complications. The smegma in the prepucial sac may become inspissated to form concretions. Urinary tract infection is not common.

Phimosis may develop in adults *(acquired type)* from long standing balanoposthitis or carcinoma occurring on the undersurface of the prepuce. So in case of phimosis in the adult it is better to make a dorsal slit for proper examination inside.

PARAPHIMOSIS (FIGS. 40.43 AND 40.44)

When a narrow prepuce is forcibly retracted behind the corona it may stick tight in this position. It impedes venous blood flow and causes edema and congestion of the glans which in turn makes reduction of the prepuce more difficult. The patient presents with swelling and pain of the glans penis. It needs immediate surgical intervention.

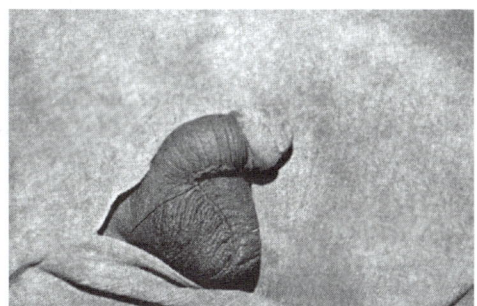

Fig. 40.43: Paraphimosis.

BALANOPOSTHITIS

This is infection of the glans penis and the prepucial sac. The patient complains of obnoxious smell and creamy discharge from beneath the prepuce. When the foreskin is retracted one will find red and edematous inner surface of the prepuce. If the retraction is not possible a dorsal slit or circumcision must be performed. Patient usually complains of itching, pain or discharge from the subprepucial space.

If the prepuce can be retracted, the glans and inside of the prepuce should be examined properly. The inguinal lymph nodes should be palpated. A thorough search for the cause of balanoposthitis should be made. The *main causes are:* (i) *Candida albicans* is common in sexually active persons and diabetes. Glans penis is itching with red patches. Prepuce becomes whitish with longitudinal fissuring particularly at the tip. (ii) Herpes genitalis—often involves glans, foreskin and even the shaft of penis. The initial itchy vesicles are soon replaced by shallow, painful erosions. There may be painful inguinal lymphadenopathy. (iii) Fixed drug eruptions are painless discoloration of the glans which develop from certain drug hypersensitivity.

(iv) Poor hygiene is a very common cause of this condition. (v) Diabetes which makes the patient more susceptible to infection, may cause this condition. (vi) Syphilitic chancre and carcinoma often associated with this condition and clinician must be careful about this. This condition should not be ignored as a subprepucial carcinoma may be the cause of this condition.

INFECTION OF MORGAGNI'S FOLLICLES

These are a pair of follicles that open laterally just behind the lips of the external urethral meatus. Openings are not usually seen except when the follicles become infected often as a complication of urethritis, when pus will be seen extruding through the prominent openings.

INFECTION OF TYSON'S GLANDS

These are a pair of sebaceous glands which secrete smegma. These glands are situated on either side of frenum and the ducts open in the prepucial sac and not in the urethra. These glands become infected as complication of gonococcal urethritis and give rise to firm, tender swellings on the undersurface of the glans just lateral to the frenum.

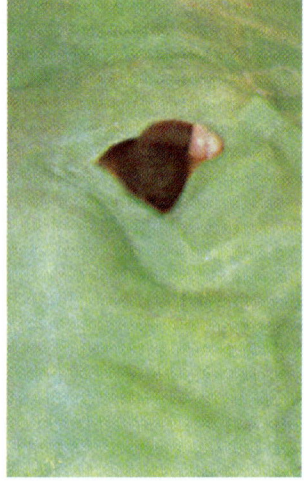

Fig. 40.44: A typical case of paraphimosis.

MEATAL ULCER

This occurs from abrasion to delicate unprotected mucosa by napkins following recent circumcision. It is characterized by alternating open ulceration which may slightly bleed to stain the undercloth and scabbing of the meatus leading to narrowing of the external meatus. In fact anteroposterior diameter of the external meatus is shortened. If untreated it may lead to pinhole meatus which causes retention of urine to varying extent.

SYPHILITIC CHANCRE (HUNTERIAN CHANCRE) (FIG. 40.45)

It is a sore or an ulcer on the prepuce or on the glans. It occurs in the primary stage of syphilis and the incubation period is 3–4 weeks from the exposure. It is a painless ulcer with well-defined margin raised above the surface with indurated base. It feels like a button. It must be remembered that chancre on genitalia is painless but on other sites such as fingers and lips they tend to be painful. *Spirochaeta pallida* can be demonstrated in the serous discharge on dark-ground illumination. The inguinal nodes are invariably enlarged. They feel rubbery, discrete, freely mobile and are not tender. The second stage of syphilis will begin 4–6 weeks after the appearance of the chancre.

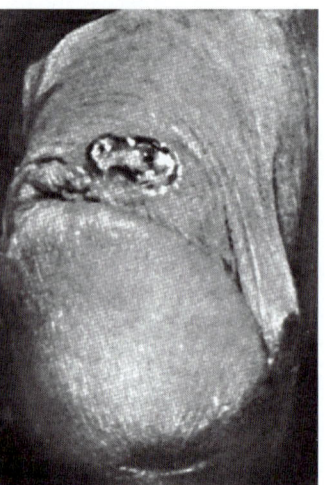

Fig. 40.45: A typical Hunterian chancre at the coronal sinus.

CHANCROID (SOFT SORES)

These are multiple painful sores affecting the glans and prepuce. They have ill-defined, inflammatory and edematous margins. Soft sores are caused by Ducrey's bacilli and the incubation period is about 3–5 days. The inguinal lymph nodes are invariably enlarged and they show tendency towards suppuration.

PREMALIGNANT CONDITIONS

(i) Leukoplakia, (ii) Paget's disease and (iii) Erythroplasia of Querat have been discussed under the heading of 'Local Examination'.

LYMPHOGRANULOMA INGUINALE

It is a venereal disease and transmitted by sexual intercourse, but accidental infection has occurred (e.g., handling the primary or the secondary lesion inadvertently). The infection is caused by a virus of the psittacosis lymphogranuloma inguinale group. The **primary lesion** is often ignored. These are sores in the anterior urethra (penis in case of male). The sores look like vesicles which are painless. These gradually disappear and the secondary lesion starts. The patients mainly present with the **secondary lesions**, the incubation period of which varies from three to six weeks after exposure. The lymph nodes in one or both the groins are enlarged. Pariadenitis occurs leading to matting of the lymph nodes. The overlying skin gradually becomes red. The matted lymph nodes tend to suppurate and gradually become superficial. Ultimately thick yellowish-white pus is discharged. The resulting sinus or sinuses persist for months or years. In case of females an additional complication arises if the primary lesion affects the posterior vaginal wall or cervix. In these cases pararectal lymph nodes enlarge and suppurate. Due to intense pararectal inflammation fibrosis of the rectal wall follows with the formation of a stricture of rectum. Due to lymphatic obstruction there may be occasional elephantiasis of the scrotum and penis as well as the vulva. Ischiorectal abscess, rectovaginal fistulae and perianal abscess may develop in females consequent upon intense pararectal inflammation. Complement fixation test and biopsy of the affected lymph nodes confirm the diagnosis. The Frei test is also confirmatory. 0.1 mL of sterile pus obtained from an unruptured bubo of a patient suffering from this disease is injected intradermally. If a red papule of at least 6 mm diameter appears in 48 hours the test is positive and the patient is suffering from this condition.

GRANULOMA INGUINALE

In contradistinction to the previous condition granuloma inguinale mainly manifests itself in the primary lesion. This is a vesicle surrounded by an area of erythema and induration. Gradually, the overlying epithelium disintegrates and ulcer develops. These ulcers may be seen in the genital, inguinal and perianal regions. Pain is conspicuous by its absence. *The lymph nodes are not involved.* This condition is caused by Donovan body, which is seen as a Gram-negative rod in the cytoplasm of mononuclear tissue cells.

ELEPHANTIASIS OF THE PENIS

Penis may be involved separately or alongwith the scrotum in filariasis. The subcutaneous tissue of the penis may be affected similar to the scrotum. Sometimes penis may be enormously thickened and distorted owing to unequal contraction of hypertrophied fibrous tissue and fascia around the penis. Such a distorted and swollen organ is called the 'Ram's horn penis'. At other times the penis may be completely buried under the enormously distended scrotum. Its orifice is then indicated by hypertrophied prepuce, from where a long channel goes upwards to meet the glans penis.

PEYRONIE'S DISEASE

This is due to indurated plaque formed at the dorsal aspect of one corpus cavernosum. The penis on erection becomes curved and painful. Probably trauma of unknown nature is the cause of this condition. Majority of the patients are over forty years of age.

PAPILLOMAS (VENEREAL WARTS)

This is the most common benign growth of the penis. It may occur in the uncircumcised as well as in the circumcised. These are actually condylomata acuminata. These appear on the glans, coronal sulcus, frenulum and also inside the urethral meatus. So these occur mainly in areas subject to trauma during intercourse. These are caused by human papilloma virus which are almost invariably sexually transmitted. These are moist, multiple papillomas without induration and discharges thin serous fluid. These warts may progress to intraepithelial neoplasia and later to invasive carcinoma.

CARCINOMA OF THE PENIS (FIGS. 40.46 AND 40.47)

A few pathological facts are to be remembered in this respect. *Firstly* circumcision, if correctly performed soon after birth, confers almost total immunity against this disease. But circumcision done in early infancy does not provide the same degree of immunity. *Secondly,* a few conditions ***predispose*** to the development of cancer. These are chronic balanoposthitis, leukoplakia, papillomas, Paget's disease and erythroplasia of Querat. *Thirdly,* majority of the carcinomas are of squamous variety, only rarely columnar variety may develop arising from Tyson's glands (situated on either side of the frenum). *Fourthly,* the earliest spread is to the lymph nodes (first to inguinal group and then to iliac group) and direct spread to the body of the penis is prevented by a fascial sheath for many months. *Lastly*, this is a slow growing tumor. Though majority of the patients are above 40 years of age yet 30% of the patients are under 40 years of age. The lesion may be anywhere on the skin of the prepuce or glans penis. It is a painless condition so in an uncircumcised individual mild irritation and purulent discharge from under the prepuce are often the first symptoms. Gradually, blood stained foul discharge may be noticed. At this stage the condition may be misdiagnosed as balanoposthitis. One must be clever enough to suspect this to be a case of carcinoma and a dorsal slit must be performed for proper inspection. Majority of the patients present with a lump or an ulcer. The lump is a sessile cauliflower growth with an indurated base whereas an ulcer has the same indurated base with rolled out and everted margin, the floor is formed by necrosed tissues.

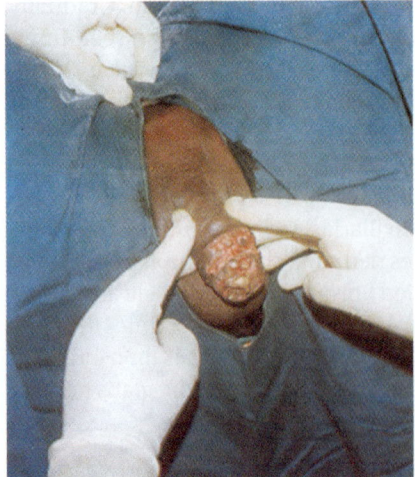

Fig. 40.46: A case of carcinoma of penis which is gradually affecting the body of the penis and has almost eroded the prepuce.

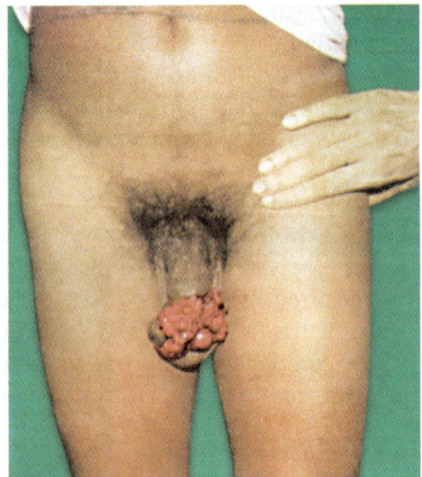

Fig. 40.47: A case of carcinoma of penis affecting glans penis. The inguinal lymph nodes are being palpated.

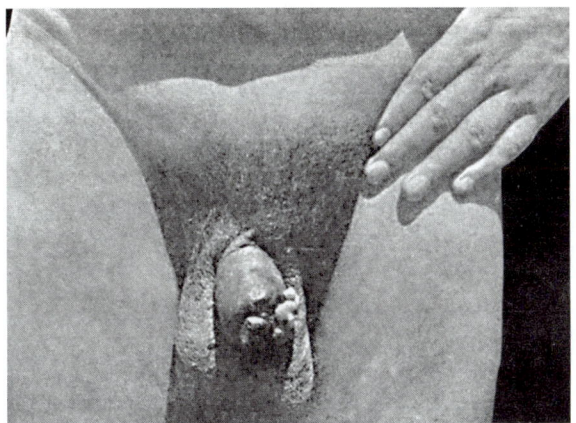 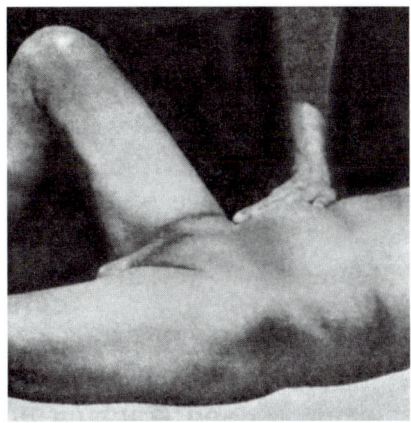

Fig. 40.48: Palpating the inguinal lymph nodes in a case of carcinoma of the penis.

Fig. 40.49: Palpating the external iliac lymph nodes. The thigh is flexed to relax the abdominal muscles.

The inguinal lymph nodes are often enlarged, but about half of these cases the enlargement is due to sepsis and the other half due to secondary deposits **(Fig. 40.48)**. One must palpate the iliac group of lymph nodes to exclude secondaries in these nodes **(Fig. 40.49)**. Death may occur due to bleeding from external iliac or femoral vessels from erosion by the metastatic lymph nodes.

PRIAPISM

This means persistent and painful erection of the penis. Most common cause is idiopathic thrombosis in the corpora cavernosa. But other causes are—sickle cell anemia, leukemia, secondary malignant deposit in corpora cavernosa, spinal cord injury and organic diseases of central nervous system.

Algorithmic Approach to Patient with Male External Genitalia Disorders

Patient presents with scrotal or penile swelling

↓

Is the swelling painful?
- Yes → Proceed to next step
- No → Consider **painless swellings (hydrocele, varicocele, tumor, lipoma of cord)**

↓

Is there sudden severe pain with nausea and vomiting?
- Yes → Suggests **torsion of testis (urological emergency, urgent surgery needed)**
- No → Proceed to next step

↓

Is there fever with redness over scrotum?
- Yes → Consider **epididymo-orchitis or fournier's gangrene (urgent IV antibiotics, surgical debridement if needed)**
- No → Proceed to next step

↓

Is the swelling translucent on transillumination?
- Yes → Suggests **hydrocele or epididymal cyst (benign, requires imaging for confirmation)**
- No → Proceed to next step

↓

Is the swelling hard, nodular, and irregular?
- Yes → Suggests **testicular tumor (requires scrotal ultrasound and tumor markers: AFP, β-HCG, LDH)**
- No → Consider other diagnoses **(lipoma, hernia, abscess, funiculitis, lymph varix)**

↓

Confirm diagnosis and plan treatment based on findings
- Medical management → Epididymo-orchitis (antibiotics), fournier's gangrene (IV antibiotics, Surgical debridement), Filariasis (antifilarial therapy).
- Surgical interventions → Varicocele ligation, hydrocelectomy, hernia repair, orchidopexy (for undescended testis), orchidectomy (for malignancy)

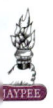 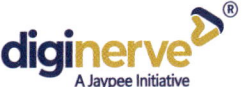

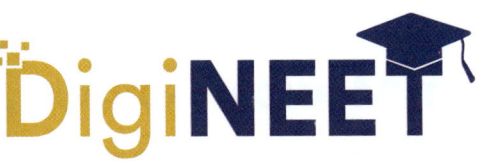

Simplify your undergraduate studies and NEET PG preparation with this comprehensive program covering all 19 subjects. Crafted by India's top faculty, it includes video lectures, printed notes, OSCEs, a QBank, test series, and the innovative Dr. Wise AI Chatbot.

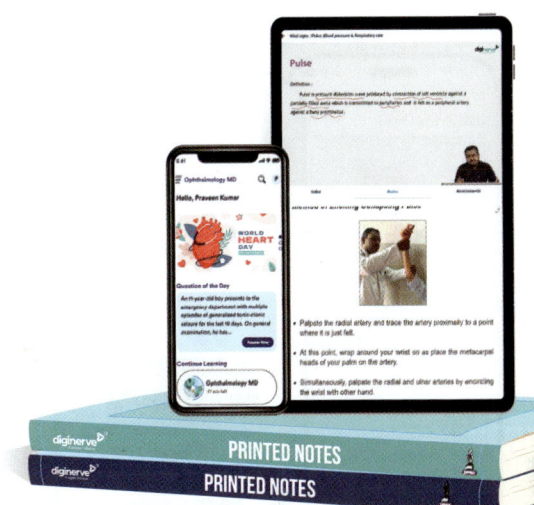

Course Features

1400+ hrs Video Lectures

1500+ Topics in Notes

15000+ Questions in QBank

1800+ GEMS

450+ OSCEs

Test Series

Dr. Wise AI Chatbot

Drug Chart

Regular Webinars by Esteemed Faculty

Access Anytime, Anywhere

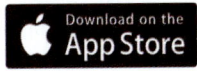 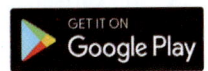 

+91-8800-418-418   marketing@diginerve.com

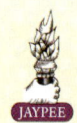
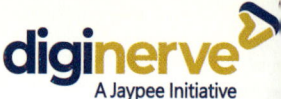

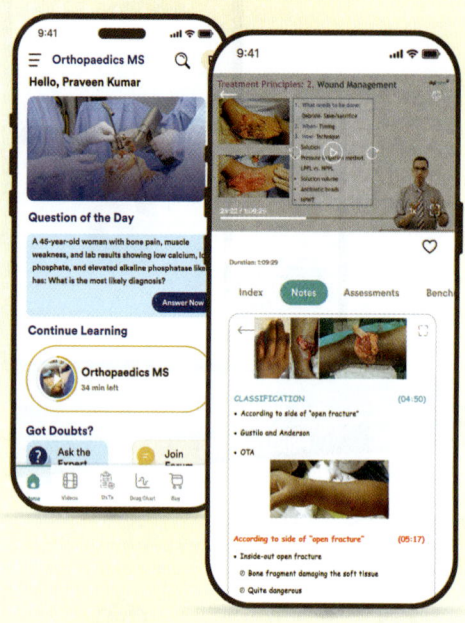

Premium Medical Content, Anytime, Anywhere

Trusted by 150K+ Users

20+ Courses | **3600+** Hrs of Video Content | **790+** Mentors

A host of features for **UnderGrads**, **PostGrads** and **Professionals**

Available on

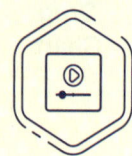 Video Lectures
 Notes
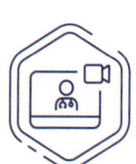 OSCEs
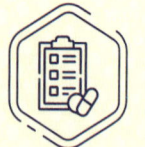 Drug Chart
 Question Bank
 Dr. Wise AI Chatbot

 +91-8800-418-418   marketing@diginerve.com

INDEX

Page numbers followed by *f* refer to figure.

A

Abdomen 11, 320, 506, 537f, 566f, 597f, 682, 685f, 695
   acute 527, 528, 529f, 532, 539f, 540f, 558
   auscultation of 518, 538f
   causes of 543
   contour of 533, 564
   CT scan of 547f
   epigastric region of 706f
   examination of 119, 527, 532, 596
   midline 682
   straight X-ray of 519, 576f
   ultrasonography of 583f, 605f
Abdominal disorders 357
Abdominal distension 516, 539, 674
Abdominal examination 564, 624
Abdominal flanks 567
Abdominal injuries 517, 520, 525
   examination of 516
Abdominal lump 596, 616
   causes of 596
   examination of 596
Abdominal muscles 566, 599f, 682f, 725f
   examine tone of 681
Abdominal organs, palpation of 568
Abdominal pain 540f
   cause of 590
   recurrent attacks of 611
Abdominal swelling 654
   differential diagnosis of 601
Abdominal wall 11, 81f, 536, 546f, 565, 606, 675f, 714
Abdominothoracic wall 516
Abducent nerve 317
   paralysis 317
Abduction 262f, 263f, 277, 284, 290
   injury 243, 244f
   movement of 262, 278f
   process of 265
   rotation 284
   tests 238
Abductor pollicis brevis 148, 148f, 160
   tendons of 271f
Abscess 52, 90, 601, 609
   alveolar 393, 396
   anorectal 628
   chronic 496, 499

   extradural 385, 571
   hepatic 601
   iliac 613
   intracutaneous 363
   intramammary 496
   ischiorectal 621
   pelvic 610, 613, 614
   pericolonic 591
   perigastric 601
   perinephric 640, 657
   popliteal 294, 295
   psoas 688, 688f, 695
   pyogenic 52
   recurrence of 480
   retromammary 496
   right subphrenic 583
   subcuticular 361
   subdiaphragmatic 549
   submucous 629
   subphrenic 549, 601, 603, 605
   terminal pulp-space 361
   umbilical 594
Accident, type of 299
Acetabular roof 282f
Acetabulum 283f
   floor of 229
Achalasia 504, 506, 509
Achilles
   tendinitis 164, 167
   tendon rupture 164, 168
Achondroplasia 181
Acid phosphatase 653
Acidophil adenoma 324
Acoustic neurofibroma 314, 324
Acoustic neuroma 56
Acrocyanosis 108
Acromioclavicular
   dislocation 211, 213
   joint 208, 263
Actinomycosis 135, 386, 397, 429, 612
   diagnosis of 87
Actinomycotic sinus 474
Active straight-leg raising test 344f
Acute appendicitis 528, 535f, 544-546
   pain 532
Adamantinoma 393, 394, 395f
Addison's disease 404, 457

Adduction 262f, 263f, 278, 280f, 290
   deformity 274f
   injury 243
   tests 238
Adductor pollicis 149, 150f, 367f
Adenocarcinoma 422, 635, 660f
Adenoid
   cystic carcinoma 422-424
   facies 388
Adenoma 593, 608
   papillary 593
   umbilical 594
Adhesion 205
Adrenal cortex 604
Adson's test 100, 100f
Adult polycystic disease 654
Ainhum 95f, 106
   affecting fourth toe 95f
Aird's test 358
Albright's disease 187
Albumin 176
Alcoholism 143
Alkaline phosphatase 653, 667
   level, elevation of 653
Alkaptonuria 254
Allen's test 96
Allergy, history of 5
Alpha-naphthylamine 664
Alveolar abscess 393, 396
   complications of 396
Amazia 495
Amebic hepatitis 568, 601
Amebic liver abscess 549
Amebic typhlitis 527, 611
Amelanotic melanoma 62
Ameloblastoma 394
Amnesia
   post-traumatic 299, 300
   retrograde traumatic 299
Amyloid disease 176
Anal canal 620f, 626f
   direction of 625f
   stricture of 632
Anal conditions 632
Anal fissure 617
Anatomical snuff box 227
Anemia 508, 532
Anesthesia, general 642f
Aneurysm 38f, 109, 110, 472
   acquired 110
   arteriovenous 111

complications of 111
congenital 110
false 109
popliteal 289, 294, 295
true 109
varicose 111
Aneurysmal dilatation 112
Aneurysmal varix 111
Angiography 45, 519
selective 102, 453
vertebral 322
Angionephrotomograms 650
Angiosarcoma 182
Angular cheilosis 409
Anhidrosis 446, 476
Ankle 241
absence of 540
adduction injury of 244f
clonus 319, 319f
examination of 295
extensors of 40f
flexors of 40f
jerk 249f, 319, 319f
joint 175f, 375
ligament of 375
passive movements of 296f
swelling of 378
tuberculosis of 296
mechanism of injury of 241
sprain of 242
unilateral edema of 296
Ankyloglossia 412
Ankylosing spondylitis 335, 351, 357
straight X-ray of 348f
Ankylosis 257, 393
false 257
true 257
Anterior compartment syndrome 108
Anterior horn tear 240f
Anterior superior iliac spine 231f, 278f, 280f, 597f
Anterior tibial artery 98
palpation of 99f
Antibiogram 644
Antibioma 496
Anticoagulant drugs 670
Anuria 639
Anus 633
basal cell carcinoma of 621f
Anvil test 340f
Aorta 609
abdominal 605, 646
aneurysm of 506
embolus obstructing bifurcation of 101f
Aortic aneurysm 556
leaking 556
ruptured 556

Aortic arch
development of 511
occlusive disease 108
Aortic embolism 109
Aortography 101f
Ape-like hand 160
Ape-thumb deformity 144
Apley's distraction test 238
Apley's grinding test 237
Appendicectomy 675f
scar 88f
Appendicitis 527, 533, 538, 548, 567, 574, 591
acute 528, 535f, 544-546
catarrhal 545
chronic 589
diagnosis of 539, 545
obstructive 545
Appendicular colic 542, 557
Appendicular tenderness 534
Appendix 610
non-filling of 575
Appetite 127, 128, 563
Apprehension test 292
Arch assessment 375
Areola 484
Argyll Robertson pupil 249f
Arm 484
length of 210
midposterior line of 215f
Arrhythmias, cardiac 439
Arterial embolus 108
Arterial occlusion, acute 108
Arterial puncture, direct 102
Arterial thrombosis, acute 109
Arteriography 101, 102f, 111, 180
pulmonary 477
Arteriovenous fistula 111, 119
congenital 50, 82
Artery 38f
brachial 99
iliac 610, 612
occlusion 104
popliteal 96f, 99
ulnar 99
Arthritis
acute 251, 267, 271, 285, 286
chronic 251, 267
gonococcal 252
pneumococcal 252
pyogenic 365
tuberculous 253, 259, 283f, 287f
Arthrogram 282
Arthrography 201, 250, 291
Arthropathy 200
hemophilic 260

Arthroscopy 200, 250, 291
Articular branch 159, 161
Articular cartilage 254
erosion of 252f
Aschheim-Zondek test 707
Asphyxia, traumatic 467
Aspiration 465, 472, 492
biopsy 181
pneumonia 476
pneumonitis 505
Astrocytoma 314, 321, 323
Ataxia 311
Atelectasis
massive 476
segmental 476
Atheroma 651f
Atherosclerosis 94
Atresia, esophageal 508
Attacks, periodicity of 560
Attitude 7, 196, 207, 214, 229, 234, 287, 337, 531
Auditory nerve 318
Auriculotemporal syndrome 420
Auscultation 9, 29, 41, 100, 119, 174, 249, 447, 464, 472, 552, 570
Autoimmune disorders 135
Autosomal dominant
disease 56
inheritant disorder 189
Avascular necrosis 204, 204f, 227
Avitaminosis 663
Avulsion fracture 228
Axilla 209f, 485, 488, 496f
lymph nodes of 489f
vertical circumference of 210
Axillary embolism 109
Axillary lymph nodes 129, 490f, 497, 500
Axillary nerve 146
Axillary tail 486
Axonotmesis 154

B

Babcock's triangle 283f
Bacillus fusiformis 409
Back, stiffness of 336
Backward hinge 332
Bacteria 666
Baker's cyst 294f
Balanitis 670, 719
Balanoposthitis 721, 724
Baldwin's method 642
Baldwing's test 535
Ballance's sign 521
Bamboo' spine 351
Barber's pilonidal sinus 371
Barium enema 541, 585, 592
examination 542, 576

Pincer-shaped ending of 541*f*
   X-ray 626
Barium meal 506, 574
   X-ray 573, 574*f*, 575*f*, 585, 587*f*, 612*f*
Barlow's test 279, 280*f*, 284
Basal cell
   carcinoma 60, 60*f*, 621*f*
   papilloma 66
Basal pneumonia 534
   pain 539*f*
Basal secretion 571, 572
Baseballer's elbow 268
Basophil adenoma 324
Bazin's disease 82
Beaten silver appearance 321*f*
Bed-shaking test 534
Bell nerve 157
Bence-Jones protein 648
Bennett's fracture 223, 225, 227
Benzidine 664
Beta-naphthylamine 664
Biceps brachii 39*f*
   long head of 168
Biceps jerk 320
Biceps tendon 41*f*
   rupture of 164, 266
Bicipitoradial bursitis 269
Bidigital palpation 418*f*
Bifid nose 384, 384*f*
Biliary system 569*f*
Biliary tract 529
   radiological investigation of 575
Biliary tree 542*f*
Bilocular hydrocele 709*f*
Bimanual palpation 209*f*, 391, 642, 643, 664
Biopsy 45, 75, 128, 133, 181, 322, 494, 592, 653
   incisional 46
   marrow 181
   open 45, 181
Black hairy tongue 21, 411
Bladder 517, 670
   base of 643
   cancer, stage of 642*f*
   carcinoma 635
   diseases of 661
   distended 329
   diverticulum of 662
   dysfunction 328
   examination of 642
   exstrophy of 661
   injury to 228
   rupture of 662
   tumors of 664
Blastomycosis 135
Bleeding 73
   alimentary 583

   amount of 617
   anorectal 630
   nasal 301
   per anum 632
Blood 132, 153, 519, 540, 644, 707
   borne infection 666
   cholesterol 103
   color of 617
   disorders 670
   examination of 573
   gases, estimation of 465
   lipids 103
      high level of 103
   pressure 304, 316, 469, 541
      elevation of 311
   routine examination of 74
   spread 413
   tests 128
   urea estimations of 540
   velocity, determination of 102
   vessels
      injury to 202, 307, 309
      palpation of 97
Blue nevus 60
Blumberg's sign 534
Boas's sign 533
Body
   carcinoma of 589
   height, vertebral 331
   parts of 131
   weight, loss of 28
Bolus obstruction 555
Bone 295, 473, 492, 647
   abnormalities 7
   around elbow 215
   crepitus 23
   cyst 177*f*, 179*f*
      aneurysmal 182, 190
   diseases 171*f*, 172
   disorder, differential diagnosis of 182
   examination of 171, 195
   iliac 667*f*
   injuries 206, 207
      examination of 198
   lengthening of 173
   scan 200, 348, 453, 473, 495, 495*f*, 667*f*
   secondary carcinoma of 182, 193
   shortening of 173
   solitary cyst of 171
   spotted 182
   X-ray of 75, 180
Bony
   irregularity 174, 197, 234
   points, relative position of 210, 217
   swellings, classification of 181

Boutonniere deformity 253, 371
Bowel
   anastomosis 626
   dysfunction 328
   gas-distended 552
   habit 530, 563
      abnormality of 618
Bowen's disease 66
Brachial group 489, 491*f*
Brachial plexus 142, 156
   lesion of 142, 156
Brachioradialis 40, 147
   muscle 147*f*
Bradycardia 316, 324, 441
Brain 473
   injury to 307, 309
   scan 306, 312, 322
   tumors 324
Branham's sign 97
Brawny edema 485
Breast 481*f*, 482, 486*f*, 488*f*, 490*f*, 499
   accessory 495, 496*f*
   cancer 492, 495*f*
      diagnosis of 494
      family history of 481
   carcinoma of 479, 485*f*, 486*f*, 489, 490*f*, 492*f*, 494, 494*f*, 502, 502*f*
   congenital absence of 495
   disease 480
      benign 497
   examination of 479
   lump 487*f*, 488*f*, 503
   lymph vessels 490*f*
   pendulous 496
   solitary cyst of 499
   substance 487
   tissue 486, 487
   tumors of 499
   ultrasonograms 494
   underdevelopment of 496
Breathing, difficulty of 441
Brittle bone 181, 185
Broad ligament
   abscess of 613
   cyst 614
Brodie's abscess 176, 177*f*, 181, 184
Brodie's serocystic disease 499
Brodie-Trendelenburg test 117
Bronchiectasis 475, 509
Bronchitis, chronic 476
Bronchoscopy 432, 473
Bronchus
   erosion of 511
   tear of 467
Brown tumor 459
Brown's vasomotor index 103
Brucellosis 357
Bryant's test 210

Bryant's triangle 229, 230, 230f
Bubonocele 682
Buccal mucosa 401
Bucket handle tear 240f
Buerger's disease 74, 92, 94, 103, 104
Burkitt's tumor 396
Burn
    contracture 370
    scar of 68f
Bursa superficial 378
Bursitis, crepitus of 23
Burst fracture 332, 332f
Butcher's wart 368

C

Cachexia 618
Calcanean spur 381
Calcaneum
    crush fracture of 244f
    fracture of 243
    tuberculous cavity of 380f
Calcaneus tuber-joint angle 242
Calcium, serum 540
Calculus 423
Calf tenderness 121f
Calyces 649, 655f
    minor 648f
Campbell de Morgan spot 50
Cancer 639
    cells 490f
    breast 492, 495f
Cancer-en-cuirase, part of 487
Cancrum oris 106, 386, 386f, 403, 409
Candida albicans 721
Candle bones 182
Cannon-ball
    appearance 659f
    metastasis 180f
Capener's sign 282
Capital epiphysis, displacement of 283f
Caput medusae 20
Carbon dioxide 466
Carbuncle 53, 106, 368, 385
Carcinoembryonic antigen 644
Carcinoid
    facies 388
    syndrome 388
Carcinoma 456, 475, 482f-485f, 500, 500f, 506, 594, 604, 615, 619, 664
    advanced 90, 483f
    anal 620, 621f
    anaplastic 438, 454
    annular 632
    branchiogenic 434
    breast 479, 485f, 486f, 489, 490f, 492f, 494, 494f, 502f
    bronchial 266
    bronchogenic 469
    cheek 404f
    early detection of secondary 179
    epidermoid 61, 80, 422
    esophageal 505
    follicular 438, 453, 456
    fungated 500f
    gastric 586
    impalpable 493
    inflammatory 501
    lip 386, 402, 404, 405f, 410
    medullary 454, 456, 457
    mucoepidermoid 422
    papillary 438, 447, 453, 456
    scirrhous 482, 484
    secondary 139, 180, 387, 612
Carcinomatous epulis 394
Card test 149, 149f
Cardiac failure, congestive 439
Cardioarterial embolization 108
Cardiospasm 504, 509, 509f
Cardiovascular disease 104
Cardiovascular system 450f
Caries
    sicca 264
    spine, skiagram of 347f
Carnett's test 599f
Carotid
    angiography 306, 322
    artery 99, 429f
    body tumor 428, 429f, 436
    occlusive disease 107
    pulsation 446f
    sheath 445
Carpal bones 224
Carpal tunnel syndrome 168, 272, 362
Carpometacarpal joint 363
Carpopedal spasm 460
Cartilaginous loose bodies 241
Casoni's test 43
Catheter 663
Cat-scratch disease 135, 137
Cauda equina syndrome 328
Causalgia 226
Cavity, tuberculous 380f
Cecum, carcinoma of 612
Cell types 135
Cellulitis 51, 363, 385, 434
Central dislocation 233
Cerebellar tumors 325
Cerebral
    compression 303, 304, 304f, 311
    concussion 303, 304, 309
    contusion 304, 309
    irritation 304, 309
    laceration 309
    puncture 322
Cerebration 324
Cerebrospinal fluid 314
    escape of 307
    Wassermann reaction of 321
Cervical lymph node 129f, 130, 391, 401, 406, 423
    enlargement 433f
    palpation of 447
    swelling 128f, 129f
Cervical rib 92, 105, 149f, 264, 266, 428
    symptoms of 106
    syndrome 361, 362
Cervical spine 332, 436
Cervical spondylosis 264
Cervical vertebra
    fracture dislocation of 44f
    tuberculosis of 266
Cervix 539, 624
Chair test 699, 699f
Chancre
    extragenital 386
    syphilitic 722
Chancroid 718, 719, 722
Charcot's joint 246, 249f, 255, 260, 268, 291
Chauffeur's fracture 225, 226
Cheek 404, 406
    carcinoma of 404f
    examination of 400
Chemical peritonitis 549
Chemosis 439, 448
    extensive 449f
Chest 462, 505, 539, 571, 682, 695
    barrel shaped 471
    contour of 470
    diseases 470, 478
    examination of 469
    flank 471
    injuries 462
        examination in 462
    trauma 468
    type of 10
    upper part of 430
    wall 488, 539, 571
        sinus of 474
    X-ray 75, 432, 495f, 506, 519, 653, 707
Chicken breast 470
Chiene's test 231
Cholangiogram, percutaneous transhepatic 578, 578f
Cholangiography, intravenous 542, 578

Index

Cholangiohepatitis, oriental 570, 588
Cholangitis 580, 587
   suppurative 602
Cholecystitis 529, 561, 578
   acute 533, 539, 541, 546
   chronic 587
   sign of 587
Choledochus cyst 588
Cholelithiasis
   chronic 587
   previous history of 553
Chondroblastoma 182
Chondroma 176, 178f, 182, 190
   multiple 181, 185
Chondromalacia patellae 291, 292
Chondromyxoid fibroma 182, 191
Chondrosarcoma 179, 182, 192
Chromocystoscopy 650
Chromophobe adenoma 324
Chronic abdominal lesions,
      diagnosis of 559
Chronic retention 668, 669
   infection on 668
Chvostek-Weiss sign 460
Chylocele 713
Chylous fluid 713
Cinephlebography, ascending
      functional 123
Cirrhosis 22
   hepatic 388
Cirsoid aneurysm 51f, 111
   extensive 41f
Clammy extremities 517
Claudication 94
Clavicle 186f, 208
   fracture of 211, 212, 212f
Claw
   foot 376f, 377
   hand 144, 144f, 361
   toe 377
Cleft
   lip 384f, 401
   palate 384, 384f, 403f
Cleidocranial dysostosis 182, 186, 186f
Clergyman's knee 293
Clinician's thumb 236f
Clinoid processes, posterior 321f
Cloudy urine 663
Club foot 376, 377
Clutton's joint 256, 288f
Coccidioidomycosis 135
Coccyx, injuries to 228
Cock's peculiar tumor 63, 387
Codman's method 260, 261f
Codman's triangle 179
Coffee-ground' appearance 18
Cold
   abscess 52, 264, 277, 341f, 341f,
      347, 380f, 471, 472, 474, 601

   iliac 341f, 613
   sinus 474
   effects of 93
   water test 96
Colic 16, 543, 556
   esophageal 509
   ureteric 528, 557
Colitis
   ischemic 593
   stage 612
   ulcerative 550, 592, 618, 628, 629
Collagen diseases 670
Collateral ligaments, injury to 239
Colles' fracture 200f, 223, 224, 225,
      225f, 371
   dinner-fork deformity of 223
   movement 224
   true reversed 226
Colloid
   carcinoma 501, 618
   goiter 438, 442, 442f, 444, 450f,
      453, 454, 454f
Colon 570, 601, 641f
   acute toxic dilatation of 626
   carcinoma of 593
   Crohn's disease of 590
   diverticular disease of 550
   hepatic flexure of 604, 639
   part of 604
Colonoscopy 626
Comedocarcinoma 501
Common bile duct 569f, 579f, 582f,
      588, 589f
   distal end of 579f
   gallbladder 569
   obstruction of 578f
Complete rectal prolapse 621f, 630
Compound palmar ganglion 271,
      372, 372f
Compression
   fracture 331f, 356
   test 464, 464f, 519
Computed tomography 43, 543
Concussion 304
Condyloma 63, 64f, 79, 386, 619, 620
   acuminata 79, 620, 630, 630f
   lata 79, 631
Congestion 670
Conjunctiva 439
Connective tissue tumors 422
Consciousness
   level of 6, 299, 302
   loss of 300
   stage of 311
Constipation 546, 674
   absolute 551
Constriction, congenital 378f
Constrictor muscle, inferior 508

Contrast radiography 75, 519
Contrecoup injury 307
Contusion 466
Cope's obturator test 536f
Cope's psoas test 535, 535f
Cord
   complete contusion of 333
   concussion 333
   diffuse
      hydrocele of 713
      lipoma of 697
   encysted hydrocele of 681f, 692,
      694-696, 709, 709f
   inflammatory thickening of 697
   injury to 333
   lipoma of 695, 708
   tumor 266
Coronal hypospadias 719f, 720f
Coronal sulcus 724
Costochondritis 473, 474
Costoclavicular compressive
      maneuver 97
Cough 469, 504, 676f
   impulse on 31, 36, 116, 676, 678,
      694, 703, 705
Courvoisier's law 569, 569f
Coxa vara 7, 275, 276f, 282, 283f,
      284
Cozen's test 268f
Craggy epididymis, absence of 713
Cranial fossa
   anterior 302f, 303f
   fracture of 308, 309
   middle 302
Cranial nerves 10, 305
   examination of 316
   injury to 308
Craniopharyngioma 321
C-reactive protein 540
Creatinine clearance 645
Cremasteric reflex 320
Crepitus 22, 97, 197, 392, 464
Crest, iliac 339f
Cretinism 388
   facies of 388
Cricoid cartilage 458
Crohn's disease 87, 507, 542, 575,
      589, 611, 612f, 617, 618,
      628-630
   diagnosis of 590
   perianal 630
Crossed leg test 96
Cruciate ligament
   anterior 238f
   injury to 240
   integrity of 238f
   posterior 238f

Crush fracture 243, 332f
Cubitus varus deformity 215f
Cullen's sign 546f
Curly toes 378
Cushing's syndrome 316, 388
Cutaneous naevi 320
Cyanosis 7, 532
    peripheral 7
Cylindroma 387, 423
Cyst 33f, 182, 293, 386, 580, 608,
        613, 716
    branchial 428f, 429f, 431, 434
    dentigerous 393, 394, 394f
    dermoid 30f, 42f, 48, 383, 385f,
        387, 428, 431
    mesenteric 591
    mucous 387, 404, 424
    ovarian 567, 570, 613, 614
    periapical 394
    pseudomesenteric 591
    pseudopancreatic 574, 575f, 605
    radicular 394
    retention 424
    retroperitoneal 610
    sebaceous 63, 63f, 387, 717
    solitary 182, 186
    suprasellar 321
Cystic hygroma 58, 58f, 427, 428,
        429f, 431, 431f, 435
    development of 58f
Cystic swelling 34f, 271, 295
    aspiration of 707
Cystitis 635, 663
    chronic idiopathic 663
    interstitial 663
    symptoms of 662, 663
    tuberculous 663
Cystocele 682
Cystograms 649
Cystosarcoma phyllodes 482, 499
Cystoscopy 650, 658, 661, 663, 664

D

Dactylitis 368
Dalrymple's sign 448
de Quervain's disease 164, 271f
de Quervain's thyroiditis 454
Decubitus 7
Deep fascia 38
Deep inguinal ring 678f, 686f
Deep vein thrombosis 22, 115, 121,
        123f
Deformity 153, 165, 166, 196, 207,
        215, 246, 254, 269, 297, 336,
        337, 361, 374, 380
    abnormal 196, 234
    angle of 274
    congenital 369

    nature of 274
    type of 338
Degeneration 354
Degenerative disc disease 357
Deglutition, movement on 32
Dehydration 551
    facies of 531
Deltoid muscle 265
Deltopectoral node 490f
Dental
    cyst 393, 394
    ulcer 411
Dequervain's disease 271
Dercum's disease 55
Dermoid, acquired 49
Diabetes mellitus 69, 143, 457
Diabetic gangrene 104, 107
Diaphragm 652
    injury to 467
    screening of 473
Diaphyseal aclasis 175f, 178f, 181,
        185
    multiple exostoses 176
Diarrhea 457, 588, 592
    ensues 631
    spurious 631
Diazepam 626
Dietl's crisis 656
Digital rectal examination 667
Digital subtraction arteriography
        651
Diphtheria 155, 504
Diplopia 439
Disc
    disease, history of 328
    prolapse 266
Discography 348
    normal 349f
Dislocation 201
    causes of pathological 275
    complications of 201, 202
    posterior 215f, 229f
Displaced articular cartilage 393
Dissecans 255
Disseminated lupus 457
Distal interphalangeal joint 365
Distal penile opening 720f
Distal tracheoesophageal fistula 508
Distension 16, 537, 551
    feeling of 587
Diverticula 591
    esophageal 509
Diverticulitis 542, 591, 615
    acute 542, 626
        colonic 547
    stage 591
Doppler ultrasonogram 123
Dorsal branch 160
Dorsal hand 362

Dorsal subaponeurotic space 367f
Dorsal subcutaneous space 367f
Dorsalis pedis pulse 98f, 100f
Dorsolumbar region, caries of 337f
Double contrast barium enema 576,
        626
Douglas pouch 623
Drawer sign 238, 238f
Drill biopsy 45, 494
Drowsiness, symptoms of 665
Dry gangrene 103
Duct 417
    carcinoma 502
    papilloma 493, 499
Dugas' test 211
Duodenal cap 573f
Duodenal point 566f
Duodenal ulcer, chronic 585
Duodenum 522, 600, 605, 609
    pylorus of 604
Dupuytren's contracture 164, 168,
        361, 369, 369f
Duramater, injury to 307
Dyspepsia
    flatulent 561
    qualitative 563
Dysphagia 412, 439, 441, 504, 505,
        508, 511, 512
    causes of 504, 507, 511
    examination of 504, 505
    lusoria 511
Dyspnea 439, 454, 469
Dysuria 638, 653, 668

E

Ear bleeding 301
Echoencephalography 306, 312, 322
Ectopia vesicae 661, 661f, 662f
Ectopic beats 439
Ectopic salivary
    glands 410, 424
    neoplasms 402
Ectopic testis 694f, 695-698, 699f
    site of 698f
Ectrodactylism 369
Eczema 120, 484
Edema 32f
    causes of 22
    legs 659
    periorbital 449f
    pitting 119
Elbow 161, 214
    anteroposterior broadening of 215
    dislocation of 109, 222
    joint 266, 267
        effusion of 267
    movements of 218
    posterior dislocation of 215f
    tunnel syndrome 269, 362

Index

Electroencephalography 306, 322
Electromagnetic flow meter 102
Elephantiasis 126*f*
    causes of 57
    neurofibromatosis 56
Elevated arms test 96
Embolic gangrene 105
Embolism, popliteal 109
Embolization, types of 108
Emphysema, surgical 463, 464, 466
Empty glenoid 213*f*
Empyema 469, 472*f*, 474, 549
    acute 469, 475
    chronic 475
    necessitatis 471*f*, 472*f*, 474
Encephalocele 383
Encephalography 322
Endocrinal disorder 182
Endocrine organ failure syndrome 457
Endometrioma 594
Endoscopic retrograde cholangiopancreatography 579
Endoscopy 519, 542
Enema 542
Enesmus 531
Enophthalmos 476
Entamoeba histolytica 600, 602
Enterocele 677, 681, 684
Enteroteratoma 594
Ependymoma 323
Epicondylitis
    lateral 164, 268
    medial 164, 268
Epididymis 681, 695, 706
    appendix of 716
    cysts of 711*f*, 716
Epididymitis 701
    acute 540*f*
    tuberculous 711*f*
Epididymo-orchitis 706
    acute 701, 702, 706, 710, 711, 715
    subacute 712
    tuberculous 710
Epidurography 348
Epigastric artery, tearing of inferior 557
Epigastrium 597*f*, 604
    direct blow to 516
Epileptic fits 300, 314
Epiphrenic diverticulum 510
Epiphysis 219*f*, 364*f*
    slipped 282, 284, 286
Epiplocele 684
Epispadias 661, 718, 719, 719*f*, 721
Epithelial debris 394
Epithelioma 61, 80, 719

Eponychium 364
Epulis 393
Equinus deformity 120
Erb's paralysis 145*f*
Erb-Duchenne paralysis 156
Erector spinae 600*f*, 641*f*
Erysipelas 51, 386
Erythema nodosum 590
Erythrocyte sedimentation rate 573
Erythroplasia 719, 724
Escherichia coli 707, 710
Esophageal spasm, diffuse 507, 509
Esophageal sphincter 507
Esophageal varix, barium meal X-ray of 510*f*
Esophagogastric junction 510
Esophagoscopy 432, 506
Esophagus 445, 507, 511, 511*f*
    achalasia of 506
    atresia of 507, 508
    benign stricture of 509*f*
    carcinoma of 504, 506, 510, 511*f*
    dilatation of 509*f*
    diverticula of 509
    lower end of 509*f*
    malignant growth of 511*f*
    rupture 467
Ewing's tumor 179, 179*f*, 182, 192
Excisional biopsy 46
Exfoliative cytology 43, 507
Exomphalos 689
Exophthalmos 448, 448*f*, 449, 449*f*
    malignant 449*f*
    progressive 449*f*
Exostosis 175*f*, 190, 190*f*
    multiple 178*f*, 181, 185
Extension injury 332
Extensor digitorum 147
Extensor pollicis
    brevis, tendons 271*f*
    longus
        attrition rupture of 371
        tendon, spontaneous rupture of 226
Extensor tendon 268*f*
    rupture 361
External rotation injury 243, 243*f*
Extradural hemorrhage 310, 310*f*, 311
    classical syndrome of 310
Extrahepatic biliary tree 542
Extraperitoneal rupture 523, 524*f*
Eye 10, 303, 448*f*
    malignant melanoma of 61*f*
    outer canthus of 30*f*
    signs 447
    symptoms 441
Eyelids, edema of 302*f*

F

Face
    blueness of 531
    cyanosis of 531
    development of 385*f*
    differential diagnosis of 388
    examination of 383
Facial bones, fractures of 385
Facial cleft 384, 401
Facial nerve 317, 318*f*, 418*f*
    examine 418
    paralysis of 418*f*
    position of 418*f*
Facial vein 157
Facial weakness 415
Facies 7, 441
    abdominal 531
    hippocratica 7, 531
Faetor 412
Fallopian tube 614
Fascia 257
    diseases 164
    disorders 170
        classification of 164
Fascial spaces 366*f*
    infections of 366
Fasciopathy 164
Fat
    infrapatellar pad of 234*f*
    necrosis, traumatic 496
Fatal spinal cord injury, cause of 342
Fecal urobilinogen 607
    measurement of 607
Fegan's method 119
Felty's syndrome 608
Femoral aneurysm 688, 695
Femoral artery 99, 277, 277*f*
Femoral canal, boundaries of 686*f*
Femoral condyles 291*f*, 293
Femoral head, destruction of 283*f*
Femoral hernia 673, 676*f*, 678*f*, 685, 686*f*-688*f*, 695
    sac, hydrocele of 688, 695
Femoral neck
    fracture of 229*f*
    inferior aspect of 283*f*
Femoral nerve stretch test 344
Femoral pulse 99*f*
Femoral ring 686*f*
Femoral vessels 688*f*
Femur 494
    fracture neck of 232, 233
    head of 230
    supracondylar fracture of 109
Fever 28, 86, 127, 469, 563
Fiberoptic endoscopy 578
Fibrinous loose bodies 241

Fibroadenoma 479, 482-484, 486, 494f, 499
Fibroadenosis 479, 480, 486, 497
   cystic hyperplasia of 499
Fibrocystic disease 186, 497
Fibroid, recurrent 599
Fibroma 53, 54, 182, 191
Fibrosarcoma 62f, 182, 192
Fibrosis 86, 511
   inflammatory 483, 569
   interstitial 712
Fibrositic nodule 167
Fibrositis 167, 357
Fibrous dysplasia 182, 186
Fibrous epulis 393, 394f
Fibrous septum 364f
Filarial elephantiasis 57
Filarial lymphadenitis 137f, 137f
Filariasis 540f, 612, 706
   epididymo-orchitis 711f, 712
   evidence of 539
Fine needle aspiration
   biopsy 43
   cytology 43, 453
Finger
   clawing of 361
   clubbing of 21
   congenital deformities of 378f
   drop 253
   extension 362
   extensor tendon of 169f
   Hunterian chancre of 368
   infection of 363
   palmar surface of 33, 486
   tip of 364
Fissure 484
   abscesses 629
   acute 628
   chronic 619, 625
Fissure-in-ano 619, 628
Fistula 85, 86, 89, 91, 418, 633, 629
   branchial 87, 88f, 403f, 427f, 429, 429f, 435
   causes of 85, 86
   chronic discharging 497
   classification of 90
   examination of 85, 87
   formation, type of 590
   track 620f
Fistula-in-ano 619, 620f, 621, 629, 633
Fixed adduction deformity 273, 274f
Fixed flexion deformity 274, 274f, 278f
   angle of 274, 274f
Fixed lateral deformity 274
Flail chest 463, 463f, 465

Flat foot 376, 376f, 377
   spasmodic 377
Flexion 262f, 277, 290, 342
   finger locking on 361
   injury 331f, 332
   range of 270
Flexor carpi
   radialis 160
   ulnaris 148, 161
Flexor digitorum superficialis 147, 159
Flexor pollicis longus 147, 148f, 160
   tendon of 367f
Flexor retinaculum 271, 372f
Flexor tendon 367f
   sheath 365
Fluctuation 34f, 487f
   test 288f, 341f, 431
Fluid
   levels 552
   thrill 36, 538, 567, 567f
Follicular cyst, rupture 531
Follicular odontome 394
Foot 241
   deformity of 242, 376, 376f
   diseases 374
   drop 143
   examination of 374
   fibroma of 54f
   forcible dorsiflexion of 121f
   infections of 379
   joints of 295
   malignant melanoma of 140f
   movements of 96f
   sensory supply of 152f
Forearm, branches in 159
Fossa, iliac 529f, 535f, 540f
Fournier's gangrene 702, 708, 717, 717f
Fracture 196, 201, 230f, 243, 464f
   capitulum 219, 221
   closed 201
   comminuted 201
   complications of 201, 202, 218
   dislocation 199f, 332f
   healing 495
   horse-shoe shaped 308, 654
   impacted 201
   incomplete 332
   line of 199
   metacarpal 223, 224, 227
   neck 232f
   oblique 201
   open 201
   pathological 180f, 199, 666
   presence of 174
   signs of 303f

   spiral 201
   split 243
   stable 331
   transverse 201
   T-shaped 219, 220
   types of 201
   unstable 331
   Y-shaped 219, 220
Fragility test 607
Freckles 59
Free flush arteriography 102
Free thyroxin index 451
Frei's intradermal test 623
Freiberg's disease 381
Frenulum 724
Frey's syndrome 420
Froment's sign 150f, 362
Frost bite 93
Frozen shoulder 265
Fungal origin 135
Fungation 482, 483f, 502f
Funicular hydrocele 709
Funiculitis 692, 695, 696, 708
Funnel chest 470
Furuncle 368
Fusion, besides lack of 356

G

Gait 7, 287, 338
   analysis 375
Galactocele 499
Galeazzi fracture 223, 225, 226f
Gallbladder 529f, 569, 576f, 577f, 581, 588, 600, 603, 608, 613
   dilated 580f
   disease 528, 559, 563, 580
      diagnosis of 576
   distended 601
   empyema of 600
   mucocele of 570
   normal functioning 577
   point 567
   region 557
   swelling 610
Gallstone 264, 509, 576f, 577f, 646f
   ileus 541, 542f, 554
   negative shadows of 578
Gammaglobulin 455
Ganglia 164
Ganglion 169, 169f, 269f, 271, 371, 378
Gangrene 92, 113, 717
   causes of 104
   idiopathic 702
   infective 104, 106
   moist 103
   neuropathic 107

Index

physical 104
signs of 103
syphilitic 107
traumatic 104
Gangrenous area 97
limb above 97
Gas gangrene 106
Gastrectomy, partial 585
Gastric content 551
reflux of 511
regurgitation of 511
Gastric function tests 571
Gastric ulcer 559, 566, 573, 573f, 574
chronic 584
pain 561
Gastroduodenal tube 575
Gastroesophageal reflux 507, 511
Gastrografin 519
Gastrointestinal syndromes 639
Gastrointestinal tract, perforation of 541
Gastrojejunal anastomosis 585
Gastrojejunal ulcer 585
Gastrojejunocolic fistula 585
Genital examination 519
Genitalia
disorders 726
examination 11, 701
Genitofemoral nerve 529, 637
distribution of 557
Genslen's test 345, 345f
Genu
recurvatum 287f
valgum 287f
Giant cell
granuloma 395
tumor 182, 191
Giant follicle lymphoma 135
Gigantism 316
Gillie's test 346, 346f
Gimbernat's ligament 685
Glandular fever 137
Glans penis 724f
Gleety urine 666
Glioblastoma 323
multiforme 314
Gliomas 323
Globular process 385f
Globus minor 706
Glomangioma 51
Glomus tumor 51, 371, 380
Glossitis 508
chronic superficial 410
Glossopharyngeal nerve 318
Gluteus
maximus 40f
medius 40f

Glycosuria 541
Goiters 442f, 450f, 453
diffuse parenchymatous 454
endemic simple 438
exophthalmic 447f, 455
hyperplastic 454
large solitary nodular 443f
multinodular 438, 444, 453, 454
nodular 442, 442f, 454
nontoxic 453
physiological 442
retrosternal 443, 455
simple 438
solitary nodular 438, 454, 455
toxic 453
types of 438
typical exophthalmic 449f
Goitrogens 440
Golfer's elbow 164, 167, 268
Golf-hole ureteric orifice 663
Goodsall's rule 629
application of 620f
Gordon's biological test 133
Gornall's test 680
Gout 254, 259
hysterical 255
Granulation tissue 74, 86f, 172f
Granuloma
inguinale 723
pyogenic 66
pyogenicum 66
Granulomatous epulis 393
Grave's sign 303
Graves' disease 452, 453, 455
Grawitz tumor 658
Gray-Turner's sign 546f, 547
Greater trochanter 229, 230f, 231f, 276, 281
elevation of 230f
palpation of 230f
Greater tuberosity 208f, 211, 214
fracture of 209, 214
Greenstick fracture 201
Grey Turner's sign 533
Groin swellings, causes of 695
Growth
benign 47
carcinomatous 429f
fungated 81f
nodular 81f
Gubernaculum testis 698f
Guineapig inoculation test 133
Gummatous orchitis 701
Gums 401, 403, 406
Gunshot wound 142
Gynecomastia 493f, 502, 716
Gynecomazia 492, 493f

H

Haemothorax 469
Hairs, free tuft of 629
Hairy mole 59
Hallux
rigidus 378
valgus 377, 377f
Hamartoma 593
Hamilton's ruler test 210, 210f
Hammer toe 377, 378
Hamstrings 40f
Hand 223
circumduction of 363
conditions 373
diseases 360
examination of 360, 383
infections of 363, 368
joints of 269
lesions of 369
swellings of 371
Hard palate 403f
gummatous perforation of 403f
Harrison's sulci 471
Hashimoto's disease 438, 442, 457
Hashimoto's thyroiditis 454
Head 10, 301
differential diagnosis of 388
injuries 300, 302, 303, 313, 385
classification of 306
complications of 312
examination of 299
local examination of 316
of pancreas, carcinoma of 569f, 574, 588
of radius
dislocation of 217
subluxation of 222
trauma 331
Headache 300, 315
post-traumatic 312
symptoms of 665
Hearing loss 315
Heart 464, 467, 644
apex beat of 464, 471
burn 561
failure, congestive 22
Heat, effects of 93
Heberden's nodes 371
Hemangioma 49, 182, 191, 386
capillary 49, 49f
cavernous 46f, 50
tongue 402f
Hematemesis 562
Hematocele 701, 710, 711f
Hematoma 499, 519, 609
subcapsular 521
Hematomyelia 327
Hematorrhachis 327

Hematuria 517, 635, 638, 650, 653, 662, 663, 665, 669
  painless 661
    intermittent 658
Hemiparalysis 130*f*
Hemivertebra 356
Hemolytic anemia 457, 606
  acquired 607
Hemopericardium 467
Hemophilic joint 251, 256
Hemopneumothorax 465*f*
Hemoptysis 466, 469
Hemorrhage 120, 543, 555, 584, 585
  extradural 310, 310*f*, 311
  fatal 129*f*
  infratentorial 311
  internal 462, 518
  intraperitoneal 556
  intraventricular 310
  middle meningeal 310*f*
  progressive 642
  retroperitoneal 518
  subconjunctival 303*f*
  subdural 310, 311
  supratentorial 310, 311
  traumatic intraspinal 333
Hemorrhagic fluid 546*f*
Hemorrhoids 627
  first degree 627
  internal 627
  mucosal 627
  second degree 627
  third degree 627
  vascular 627
Hemothorax, traumatic 466
Hepatic ducts 579*f*
Hepatitis 529
  serum 562, 580
Hernia 673, 674, 676*f*, 678*f*, 682, 684, 691
  abdominal 673
  acquired 683, 683*f*
  complete 682
  congenital 683
    funicular 683, 683*f*
    umbilical 689
    vaginal 683*f*
  diaphragmatic 467
  direct 680*f*, 682, 683
    inguinal 675*f*, 678*f*
  epigastric 604, 689
  examination of 673
  femoral 673, 676*f*, 678*f*, 685, 686*f*-688*f*, 695
  hiatus 507, 511, 586, 587*f*
  incarcerated 675, 684
  incisional 609, 690
  incomplete 682
  indirect inguinal 678*f*
  infantile 683*f*
  inflamed 684
  inguinal 673, 673*f*, 676*f*, 677*f*, 679*f*-681*f*, 682, 686*f*, 687, 695
  interparietal 690
  interstitial 690
  irreducible 684
  left inguinal 683*f*
  lumbar 341*f*, 690
  oblique 682, 683
  obstructed 684
  obturator 690
  paraumbilical 689
  postoperative 609
  presence of 587
  recurrent 675
  reduction of 679
  Richter's 673, 685
  sliding 673, 685, 685*f*
  spigelian 690
  strangulated 673, 678, 684
  tendency to 674
  testis 702, 704, 711*f*
  type of 682
  umbilical 608, 689
  varieties of 685
Hernia-en-glissade 685, 685*f*
Hernial orifice 533, 679
Hernial sac, hydrocele of 709, 709*f*
Hernial sites 597, 599
  palpation of 537
Herpes zoster 155
Hesselbach's triangle 673, 682
Hexamine 670
Hiatus hernia, paraesophageal 511
Hiccup 19
High arch foot 376
Hip 229
  acute arthritis of 292
  adduction of 278*f*
  central dislocation of 233*f*
  congenital dislocation of 275, 277*f*, 279*f*, 281, 282*f*, 284
  developmental dysplasia of 284
  dislocation of 232, 233
  fixed flexion deformity of 279*f*
  joint 272, 274*f*, 276*f*, 278*f*, 688
    effusion of 277
    palpation of 276
    rotation movement of 279*f*
    tuberculosis of 283
    tuberculous arthritis of 275
  pathological dislocation of 279*f*, 286
  rotation of 279*f*
  tuberculosis of 283*f*, 285, 285*f*, 286
Hippocratic facies 387, 388
Hirschsprung's disease 553, 591
Histiocytic lymphoma 138
Histoplasmosis 135
Hodgkin's disease 28, 129, 129*f*, 130, 131, 132*f*, 135, 138
  clinical staging of 139
Holdswath test 330
Hollander's insulin test 572
Homan's sign 121, 121*f*, 122
Honeymoon pyelitis 635
Horn
  calculus, typical stag 657*f*
  tear, posterior 240*f*
Horner's syndrome 266, 446, 476
Housemaid's knee 2, 293
Humeral epicondyle 217*f*
Humerus 494
  divides circular trochlea 219*f*
  lower third of 216
  neck of 211, 214
  subcoracoid dislocation of 208*f*
  supracondylar fracture of 109, 143*f*, 220*f*
  upper end of 209, 211, 211*f*
Hunter's disease 181
Hunterian chancre 70, 72, 73, 79*f*, 404, 718, 719, 722
  typical 722*f*
Hurler's disease 181
Hutchinson's freckle 60
Hutchinson's pupils 303
Hydatid cyst 182, 499, 602
Hydatid thrill 41, 600
Hydrocele 702, 704*f*, 705*f*, 708, 710*f*, 711*f*
  complications of 710
  congenital 708
  hernia of 704
  infantile 688*f*, 709
  primary 708
  secondary 709, 716
  types of 709
Hydrocephalus 383, 383*f*
Hydronephrosis 639, 640, 655
  bilateral 655
  unilateral 655
Hygroma, cystic 58, 58*f*, 427, 428, 429*f*, 431, 431*f*, 435
Hyoid arch 385*f*
Hyoid bone, greater cornu of 157
Hyperabduction maneuver 97
Hypercalcemia, symptoms of 459
Hyperesthesia 533
Hypergammaglobulinemia 425
Hypernephroma 635, 658

Index

Hyperparathyroidism 180, 182, 188, 459
   primary 459
   secondary 460
   tertiary 460
Hyperplasia 136
   cystic 497
   diffuse 496
Hyperplastic ileocecal tuberculosis 611
Hypertension 654, 659
Hypertrophic scar 64, 65f
Hypochondriac region, right 528
Hypochondrium 597f, 601, 606
Hypogastrium 529, 551, 613
Hypoglossal nerve 130f, 146, 157, 318
Hypospadias 718-720, 720f
   coronal type 720
   glandular type 720
   penile type 720
   penoscrotal type 720
   perineal type 721
Hypotension 517
Hypothalamic-pituitary axis, test of 451
Hypothenar eminence 366f
Hypothyroidism 388, 440
   congenital 388
Hypotonic duodenography 575, 575f

I

Idiopathic thrombocytopenic purpura 607
Ileitis, regional 542, 548, 611
Ileum
   terminal 575
   part of 610
Ileus, paralytic 553
Iliac fossa 528, 536
Iliac spine, superior 678
Iliopsoas sheath 612
Ilium 613
Immunization, history of 6
Implantation dermoid 34f, 49, 49f, 371
In vitro tests 451, 452
Incongruent joint surfaces 254
Incontinence 639
   false 639
Indigo carmine 661
Infarction 670
Infections 69, 203
   chronic 86
   deep space 363
   localized 363
   spreading 363
   subcutaneous 364

Inferior vena cava obstruction 564
Inflammation 543, 544
Infra-articular synovial membrane, layers of 265
Infrapatellar bursitis 293
Ingrowing toe-nail 379, 380
Inguinal ligament 341f, 675, 676f
Inguinal lymph nodes, secondary 718f
Inguinoscrotal swellings 688f, 693, 695, 696, 700
   causes of 695
   differential diagnosis of 695
Injury 212, 228f
   abdominal 517, 520, 525
   around elbow 219
   closed 520
   examination of 207, 214, 223, 228, 229, 233, 234, 241, 462
   extraperitoneal 522
   higher risk of 328
   multiple 523
   open 520
   renal 523
   types of 333
Insomnia 312
Intercostal nerve
   diseases of 544
   distribution 336
Internal jugular vein 431f
Interosseous nerve
   anterior 159
   posterior 158
Interstitial cell tumor 707
Intervertebral discs 345f
   disorders of 354
   prolapsed 335
Intervertebral space 347f
Intestinal colic 548, 551, 557
Intestinal obstruction 538f, 548, 527, 555, 591, 622
   acute 531, 541, 541f, 543, 550
   cause of 592
Intestine 592, 681
   large 522
   matted coils of 609
   small 522
Intra-abdominal lesions 584
Intra-articular adhesion 205
Intracranial abscess, diagnosis of 325
Intracranial non-malignant cystic lesions 323
Intracranial pressure 321f
   raised 314
Intracranial space-occupying lesions 326
   investigation of 314

Intracranial tumors
   classification of 323, 324
   diagnosis of 324
Intradermal mole 59f
Intraperitoneal rupture 522, 523
Intrathecal whitlow 365
Intrathoracic hernial sac 505
Intussusception
   acute 553
   pathognomonic feature of 541f
   screening 541
Invagination test 679, 679f, 687f
Iritis 590
Irritable hip 285
   causes of 286
Irritation, stage of 530
Ischemia 69
   renal 640
   severe 110
Ischial tuberosity, prominent part of 231f
Isolated pelvic ring fractures 228
Isotope technique 102
Itching 19
Ivory exostosis 190

J

Jaundice 8, 532, 557, 562, 580
   calculous 562
   causes of 562
   neoplastic 562
Jaw 399
   examination of 390
   movements of 418
   osteomyelitis of 397
   swellings 393
      classification of 393
Joffroy's sign 448
Joint 207, 212, 297
   abnormalities 7
   bony components of 250, 267
   complications 205
   costovertebral 342
   crepitus 23
   deformity of 247
   diseases of 251
   disorders, causes of 251
   examination 247
   injuries 202, 206, 212, 245
      examination of 195
   interphalangeal 147, 149f, 363
   malalignment of 254
   neuropathic 251
   palpation of 290
   pathologies 259
      causes of major 259
      examination of individual 259

position of 214, 247
sense 319
space 250
sternoclavicular 208, 263
tuberculous affection of 264
X-ray of 75
Jugular lymph sac 58f
Jugular vein 355
  engorgement of external 20
Junctional nevus 60
Juxta-pyloric ulcer 585

K

Kahn tests 79, 602
Kanavel's sign 366, 367f
Kangri cancer 3f, 81f
Kantor string sign 575, 611, 612f
Kaposi's sarcoma 379
Kay's augmented histamine test 572
Kehr's sign 521, 529f
Keloid 27f, 31f, 64, 65f
  fibrous tissue 64
Kenawy's sign 570
Keratoacanthoma 65
Keratosis, seborrheic 66
Kidney 523, 570, 599, 604, 613, 645, 670, 707
  bimanual palpation of 640f
  differential diagnosis of 653
  enlarged 654
  examination of 640
  hydatid cyst of 655
  lower part of 640
  polycystic disease of 637
  renal cell carcinoma of 659f
  swelling 641
  tumors of 658
Kienbock's disease 227
Kiss lesion 292, 387f, 405f
Klein's sign 548
Klumpke's paralysis 153, 156
Knee 238f
  elbow position 619, 625f
  flexion of 290f
  jerk 249f, 319, 320f, 540
  joint 234, 239, 278f, 280f, 286, 288f, 295f
    effusion of 288f
    examination of 290f
    extreme flexion of 256f
    flexion of 289f
    fluid in 288
    lateral aspect of 178f
    loose body of 241, 241f
    tuberculosis of 291, 291f
  local examination of 235
  osteoarthritis of 292
  tuberculosis of 292

Kocher's test 445
Koilonychia 21, 21f, 508
Krukenberg's tumor 490f, 492, 571
Kyphosis 338, 351, 355

L

Lacrimal glands 131, 425
  enlargement of 424
Lacunar ligament 685
Lahey's method 445f
Langer's lines 64
Laparoscopy 584, 653
Laparotomy 134
  exploratory 584
Large intestine 522
  rupture of 522
Laryngocele 435
Laryngoscopy 432, 473, 506
Lateral condylar epiphysis, fracture-separation of 221
Lateral flexion 343
  method of 343f
Latissimus dorsi 39f
Leg
  raising test, straight 343, 346
  swelling of 121
  symptoms 115
  ulcer of 81
Leiomyoma 507
Leprosy 143, 155, 362
  lepromatous 155
Lesions
  congenital 383, 718
  cystic 183, 324
  incomplete 156
  infective 324
  inflammatory 385
  ischemic 361
  malignant 493, 494
  primary 723
  secondary 723
  space-occupying 315, 618
  traumatic 385
  vascular 324
Lesser trochanter, avulsion fracture of 233
Leucine amino-peptidase 540
Leukemia 608
  lymphatic 135, 140
Leukocytosis 46, 176, 540
Leukoplakia 410, 719, 723
Lhermitte's sign 345, 345f
Lid retraction 448
Ligaments 257
Ligamentum patellae 236f, 293
Limb
  circumference of 198, 249

girth of 280
injury to 331
skin of 116
temperature of affected 145
Limp 272, 286
Lingual thyroid 402, 403f
Lip 401, 404
  benign neoplasms of 410
  carcinoma of 386, 402, 404, 405f, 410
  chancre of 402
  hemangioma of 386f
  Hunterian chancre of 409
  pigmentation of 401
  squamous cell carcinoma of 387f
  unilateral hare 384f
Lipiodol, injection of 472
Lipodermatosclerosis 119, 120
Lipoma 33f, 54, 55f, 182, 339f, 471f, 688, 695
  multiple 54, 55
  pedunculated 55f
  varieties of 54
Lipoproteins 103
Liposarcoma 182
Lithotomy position 619
Little finger, congenital contracture of 370
Littre's hernia 685
Liver 473, 492, 520, 528, 568, 600, 601, 605, 608
  carcinoma of 602
  cirrhosis of 603
  dullness 538f
    obliteration of 538
  gumma of 602
  melanotic carcinoma of 603
  palpate 599
  scan 495
Lobar pneumonia, acute 469
Lobular atelectasis 476
Loin, discoloration of 546f
London's sign 517, 522
Long thoracic nerve 146, 146f, 157
Loose bodies 251, 256
  classification of 241
Lordosis 275, 338, 351
Low back pain 356
  causes of 356
Lower jaw 391
  bimanual palpation of 392f
  tumors of 395
Lower limb 11, 94, 120, 329
  girth of 346
  length of 231, 343
  severe ischemia of 110
Lower lip, congenital fistulae of 385
Ludwig's angina 396, 434

Index

Lumbago 357
Lumbar cold abscess 341f
Lumbar disc
   prolapse 354, 355f
   protrusion 348f
Lumbar puncture 306, 320
Lumbosacral strain 356, 357
Lumbrical canals 366f
Lumen 622
Lump 26, 67, 88, 479, 488f, 498, 537, 586, 706f
   abdominal 596, 616
   breast 487f, 488f, 503
   carcinomatous 483f
   consistency of 34
   examination of 26, 29
   painless 499
Lunate bone, dislocation of 223, 225, 227
Lung 180, 464, 490f, 492, 644, 707
   abscess 469, 475, 509
   actinomycosis of 472
   atelectasis of 476
   carcinoma of 475
   collapse of 476
   deformity 223f
   function test 473
   hernia of 474
   laceration of 466
   radio-isotope scanning of 477
Lupus vulgaris 71f, 79, 386
Lutein cyst, rupture 531, 556
Lymph cyst 499
Lymph node 126, 129f, 131, 281, 291, 418, 431, 492, 582, 583f, 598f, 606, 609, 612, 624, 652, 706, 706f
   axillary group of 489
   biopsy of 250
   carcinomatous 433
   enlarged 427, 432f, 688, 695
   enlargement 132f, 135, 431f, 432
   causes of generalized 136
   epitrochlear 267
   examination of 9, 73, 88, 100, 175, 249, 472, 488, 720
   external iliac 725f
   groups of 431, 489
   iliac 131
   inguinal 79f, 129f, 132f, 724f, 725, 725f
   metastatic 578f
   pectoral group of 489f
   popliteal 295
   regional 41, 119, 405
   secondary carcinoma of 429f
   supraclavicular group of 490f
   swellings 433
   tuberculous 433
Lymph scrotum 703, 704f, 713
Lymph varix 692, 695, 696, 708, 712f, 713
Lymph vessels 140f, 407f
Lymphadenitis
   acute 135, 136
      nonspecific mesenteric 548
   chronic 135
      nonspecific 136
   granulomatous 135
   pyogenic 136
   syphilitic 137
   tuberculous 86f, 136
   mesenteric 609
Lymphangiectasis 694-696
Lymphangiography 128, 134, 134f, 651, 707
Lymphangioma 57, 402f
   capillary 57
   cavernous 57
   circumscriptum 57
Lymphangitis 363
   acute 132
   chronic 132
Lymphatic
   disease of 132, 141
   disorders 127, 128
   drainage 490f
   system 126
      examination of 126
Lymphedema 126f, 132
Lymphlogged blubbery tissue 713
Lymphogranuloma
   inguinale 129, 137, 629, 723
   venereum 135
Lymphography 349
Lymphoid polyposis, benign 593
Lymphoma 434
   lymphocytic 138
   malignant 456, 457
   mixed 138
   primary malignant 135
   retroperitoneal 610
   undifferentiated 138
Lymphorrhagia 713
Lymphosarcoma 135, 612

M

Macrocheilia 384, 402
Macrodactylism 369
Macroglossia 20, 402, 411
Macrostoma 384, 384f
Macules 8
Madelung's deformity 223, 226, 369, 369f
Madura foot 379
Magnuson's test 358
Malformation syndromes 182
Malgaigne's bulgings 681, 682f
Malignancy 69, 128, 323
   development of 573
Malignant lymphoma 456, 457
   histiocytic type 135
   Hodgkin's type 135
   lymphocytic type 135
Malignant tumor 386, 387, 456, 500
   proliferates 26
Malingerer's low back pain 357
Mallet finger 223, 225, 227, 361, 370
Malunion 204, 205
   site of 204
Mammary abscess 480
Mammary duct
   ectasia 497
   fistula 497
Mammary dysplasia 479, 480
   benign 497
Mammary fistula 484, 497
Mammography 493, 494f
   contrast 493
Mandible
   evidence of fracture of 391
   osteomyelitis of 429
Mandibular arch 385f
Mandibular cleft 384, 385f
Mandibular fracture assessment 391
Mandibular prognathism 398
Manometric examination 507
Manometry, esophageal 509
Mantoux test 133, 250
Manus valgus 223f
March fracture 381
Marfan's syndrome 189
Marjolin's ulcer 68f, 72f, 79, 81
Martorell's ulcer 82
Mass, palpable 658
Mastectomy 500f
   radical 126, 126f
Mastitis
   acute 496, 496f
   carcinomatosa 501
   chronic 497
   subareolar 496
   suppurative 480
Mastopathy, cystic 497
Maxilla, nasal surfaces of 390f
Maydl's hernia 685, 685f
McMurray's test 237, 237f
Meckel's diverticulitis 527, 548, 594
Meconium 24
   ileus 554
Medial collateral ligament
   deep fibers of 234f

rupture of 238f, 293
sprain of 234f
Medial epicondyle, fracture-
separation of 221
Medial meniscus 240f
anterior horn of 236f
cyst of 293
Medial nasal process 385f
Medial rotation deformity 274
Medial semilunar cartilage 234f
Median nerve 147, 159, 362
branches of 159
Mediastinal emphysema 464, 466
Mediastinal nodes 128
Mediastinoscopy 432, 473
Mediastinum 463f
Medulla 604
Medulloblastoma 314, 323
Megacolon
acquired 592
primary 591
secondary 592
Melaena 24
Melanocytes conglomerate 59f
Melanoma 620
benign 59
malignant 61, 139, 379, 380
Melena 562
Meleney's ulcer 80, 82
Meningiomas 323
Meningocele 342f, 349, 383, 383f
occipital 342f
Meningoencephalocele 383
Meningomyelocele 350
Meniscus, lateral 293
Menstrual history 531
Mental sinus, median 397
Mental state 7, 316, 441
Mental symptoms 314
Mesenteric arteries
inferior 593
superior 593
Mesenteric lymph nodes 131
tuberculosis of 590
Mesentery 522
cysts of 609
lymphadenitis, nonspecific 527
vascular obstruction 555
Mesonephric buds, primary 654
Metabolic disorder 155, 182, 254
Metacarpals, dislocations of 227
Metacarpophalangeal joints 362, 363
Metaphyseal aclasis 175f
Metastasis 495f, 501
disseminated 140f
multiple 603f
secondary 131, 659

Metastatic lymph nodes, enlarged 583f
Metatarsal bone, fracture of 244
Metatarsalgia 381
Methaemalbumin, serum 540
Microfilaria 713
Micrognathism 397
Micturition 531, 638f
difficulty of 665, 666, 668
end of 663
frequency of 638, 663
increased frequency of 662, 665, 670
pain independent of 718
Midcarpal joints 363
Middle palmar space 366f, 367f
infection of 367
Midesophageal diverticulum 510
Mid-gut, volvulus of 554
Mikulicz's disease 419, 419f, 424
Mikulicz's syndrome 415, 424
Mill's maneuver 268f
Miosis 476
Mobile scoliosis 350
Moebius' sign 448
Mole
juvenile 60
non-hairy 59
smooth 59
Molluscum sebaceum 65
Monilial stomatitis 408
Mononucleosis, infectious 137
Monostotic fibrous dysplasia 186
Monteggia fracture 222, 222f
Montgomery's glands 484, 496
Montgomery's tubercles 484
Moon face 7, 388
Morgagni
follicles, infection of 722
hydatid 712f
Morquio-Brailford disease 181
Morrant-Baker's cyst 294, 294f
Morris' bitrochanteric test 231
Morrissey's test 119
Morton's metatarsalgia 381
Morvan's disease 92
Moses' sign 121, 121f, 122
Motion, range of 392
Motor car collision 229
Motor function 317, 376
investigation of 318
Motor supply 362
Mouth
examination of 400, 505
floor of 404, 406
Movements, limitation of 248
Moynihan's method 567, 567f

Mucopolysaccharide disorders 181, 185
Mucous membrane, prolapse of 618
Mucous patches 79, 386
Mucous retention 404
cyst 400, 405f, 407
Multilocular cystic
disease 394
hygroma 58f
Multiple endocrine neoplasia
syndrome 459
Multiple myeloma 176, 180, 182, 193
Multiple nerves involvement, causes of 155
Mumps 421, 421f, 706
Murphy's kidney punch 641, 642f
Murphy's sign 567, 567f
Murphy's syndrome 532, 545
Muscle 257
abdominal 566, 599f, 682f, 725f
complications 203
diseases of 7, 164
disorders 170
classification of 164
dystrophy 7
fatigue 440
guard 518, 536, 536f
and rigidity 518
absence of involuntary 536
interosseous 149f
power 145, 148f, 329
gradation of 146
sternocleidomastoid 88f
underlying 38
wasting of 144
weakness 143
Muscular branches 159, 160
Muscular disorders 165
examination of 166
Muscular rigidity 536, 536f
Muscular violence 195
Muscular wasting 173, 235, 248, 266, 275
Musculocutaneous nerve 152f
Musculoskeletal disorders 479
Myasthenia gravis 457
Mycobacterium leprae 155
Myelocele 350
Myelography 348
Myelomatous epulis 393, 394
Myenteric plexus, development of 591
Mylohyoid 157
Myositis 357
ossificans 205
traumatica 205, 218, 218f
Myxedema 388
symptoms of 440
Myxomatous degeneration 55

Index

N

Naffziger's test 345, 355
Nails 21, 21*f*
    examination of 21
    lesions around 380
Nasal process, lateral 385*f*
Nausea 315, 561
Neck 10
    arm junction 266
    examination of 40, 427, 430*f*, 505
    fasciae of 430*f*, 431*f*
    hydrocele of 58
    lymph nodes of 392
    midline swellings of 433
    posterior triangle of 431*f*
    rigidity of 304
    swellings of 429*f*, 430, 432
    veins 471
        engorgement of 447
Needles
    biopsy 45
    sensation 16
Neighboring joints 173
    examination of 175, 250
Nelaton's line 231, 231*f*
Neoplasm 26, 663, 706
    benign 53, 658
    malignant 396
Nephroblastoma 635, 660, 660*f*
Nephrogram 649
Nephroscopy 650
Nephrotic syndrome 22
Nerve 152, 295
    accessory 146, 146*f*, 156, 318
    conduction study 153
    injury 71*f*, 202
    lesion 156
        examination for 74
    tumors 294
Nervous diseases 104
Nervous system 450*f*, 539, 571
    examination of 316
Neuralgia, brachial 265
Neurilemmoma 55, 57
Neurofibroma 55, 182
    local 55
Neurofibromatosis
    generalized 55
    multiple 351
        swellings of 28*f*
Neurolipomatosis 55
Neurological deficits 315
    presence of 304
Neurological disease 7
Neurological signs 346
Neuropraxia 153
Niche 574
Nicholson's maneuver 565
Nicoladonis sign 97
Night cramps 115
Night fasting secretion 571
Nipple 483, 484*f*, 486
    changes 481
    discharge 480, 481
    extreme retraction of 500*f*
    palpation of 488
    retraction of 480, 482*f*-485*f*
Nodular leprosy, elephantiasis graecorum of 57
Noisy abdomen 538
Non-Hodgkin's lymphomas 138
Nonostotic fibrous dysplasia 187*f*
Nonunion, causes of 204
Nuclear magnetic resonance 44, 323
Numbness 301
Nutrition, build and state of 7, 441
Nutritional disorder 182
Nystagmus 311

O

Obliterate compensatory lordosis 274*f*
Obstruction
    cause of 553
    nature of 552
    ureteric 655
Obturator foramen 281*f*
Obturator internus 536*f*
Obturator test 535
Occupational exposure 143
Ochsner's clasping test 147, 148*f*, 160
Ocular torticollis 436
Oculomotor nerve 303, 317
    paralysis 317
Odontomes 394
Olecranon 219*f*
    position of 214
    process 215*f*, 217
        fracture of 221
Olfactory nerve 316
Olfactory pit 385*f*
Oligodendroglioma 323
Ollier's disease 181, 185
Omentocele 682
Onychogryphosis 380
Onychomycosis 380
Ophthalmoplegia 439, 448
Opponens pollicis 148, 148*f*, 160
Optic nerve 316
Oral cavity
    disorders 414
    examination of 401
    steps 401
Oral cholecystography 576, 577*f*
Orange peel' appearance 482
Orchitis 711*f*
    syphilitic 712
Ortolani's test 279, 280*f*, 284
Oscillometry 103
Osteitis
    deformans 189
    fibrosa 180
        cyst with generalized 182
        cystica 459
    syphilitic 181
Osteoarthritis 205, 253, 259, 264, 286, 292, 335, 347, 357, 392, 495
Osteoblastic lesion 667
Osteoblastoma 182
Osteocartilaginous loose bodies 241
Osteochondritis 251, 255
    crushing 255
    dissecans 241*f*, 256*f*, 267, 268*f*, 293
    juvenilis 284
    splitting 255
Osteochondroma 178*f*, 182
    huge 178*f*
Osteoclastoma 177*f*, 179*f*, 182, 191, 393
    X-ray of 176
Osteogenesis imperfecta 181, 185
Osteoid osteoma 176, 182, 190
Osteolytic lesion 178*f*, 193*f*
Osteoma 175*f*, 176, 178*f*, 182, 190, 386
    compact 190
Osteomalacia 182, 188
Osteomyelitic sinus 86*f*, 90
Osteomyelitis 87, 176, 365, 393, 397, 429
    acute 181, 183, 354, 397
    chronic 172*f*, 177*f*, 181, 183, 397
        pyogenic 173
    pneumococcal 181, 184
    pyogenic 356
    subacute 397
    syphilitic 184
    tuberculous 181, 184
Osteoporosis 182, 188, 328
    widespread 351
Osteosarcoma 173*f*, 179, 179*f*, 180*f*, 182, 191
    malignant growth 171
Otitis media 314
Ovarian cyst 567, 570, 613, 614
    twisted 556
Ovary 614
Oxyphil adenoma 423

P

Pachydermatocele 57, 57f
Paget's disease 180, 189, 200, 347, 351, 387, 484, 495, 502, 719, 723, 724
Paget's recurrent fibroid 54
Paget's sarcoma 181
Pain 14, 25, 27, 86, 127, 143, 150, 151, 195, 246, 297, 400, 401, 469, 479, 504, 535f, 545, 548, 560, 617, 632, 635
  abdominal 540f
  acute 540f
  back 666
  bilateral 529f
  brachial embolism 109
  breast 481
  burning 15, 529
  character of 529
  colicky 529, 636
  constricting 16
  deep 14, 15
  dragging 658
  duration of 16
  effect of pressure on 530
  epigastric 689
  flank 653
  foot 381
  forearm 106
  forefoot 381
  heel 381
  midfoot 381
  migration of 17
  movements of 16
  nature of 15, 27, 335, 617
  neck 441
  night 272
  onset of 336
  original site of 15
  pancreatic 589
  pattern 115
  periodicity of 17
  precordial 455
  progression of 16
  prostatic 637
  psychogenic 14, 15
  radiation of 16, 374, 528, 636f
  radicular 644
  referred 16, 17, 529, 636
  relief of 562
  renal 636
  rest 93, 94
  scalding 15, 589
  sciatica 666
  segmental 14
  shifting of 528
  shooting 16
  site of 216f, 528
  spread, types of 17
  stabbing 16
  sudden onset of 188
  superficial 14
  suprapubic 653
  twisting 16
  types of 14
  urethral 637
  vesical 637
Painful arc syndrome 263f, 264
Pallor 7
Palm, cross section of 367f
Palmar cutaneous branch 159, 160
Palmar fascia thickening 361
Palmar interosseous 149
Palmar space, superficial 367f
Palmar surface 33, 33f, 486, 486f
Palpate spleen 569f
Palpate trachea 446f
Palpation 9, 29, 119, 121, 130, 173, 208, 234, 266, 404, 405f, 444, 463, 471, 485, 518, 533, 565, 620, 694, 704
  deep 586
  method of 417f
  wrong method of 406f, 534f
Pancoast's syndrome 266, 476
Pancoast's tumor 476
Pancreas 570, 600, 605, 609
  carcinoma of 575f, 588
  pseudocyst of 605f
  tail of 589
Pancreatic diseases 580
Pancreatic duct 589f
Pancreatitis 509, 580
  acute 496, 537, 540, 541, 547, 547f
  hemorrhagic 531, 546f
  chronic 559, 563, 588
Papillary cystadenoma lymphomatosum 422
Papilloma 31f, 53, 664, 724
Papules 8
Parabronchial diverticulum 510
Paracolic gutter, right 528
Paradoxical respiration 463, 463f
Parafollicular cells 457
Paralysis 312, 418f
  bulbar 507
  partial 154
Paraphimosis 718, 719, 721, 721f, 722f
Paraplegia 339
Parasites 633
Parathyroid 644
  tetany 460
Paresthesia 93
  types of 93
Parkinsonism, mask face in 7
Parona's space, infection of 368
Paronychia 361, 364
  chronic 364
Parotid duct, terminal part of 417f
Parotid gland 131, 415, 418f, 420, 429f
  benign tumor of 418
  carcinoma of 422
  deep lobe of 417f
Parotid tumor, mixed 416f
Parotitis
  acute 421, 421f
  chronic 421
  subacute 421
Pars interarticularis 352f
Patella
  fracture of 239
  recurrent dislocation of 292
Patellar clonus 319
Patellar tap 288, 288f
Paterson-Kelly syndrome 504, 508, 510
Pathological joints 258
  examination of 246
Pauwel's angle 232f
Pearly-white beaded edge 71
Peau d' orange 482, 483f, 485f, 500
Pectoral fascia 488f
Pectoralis major 39f, 488f
Pectoralis muscle 488f
Pectus
  carinatum 470
  excavatum 470
Pedicle, torsion of 543
Pellegrini Stieda's disease 293, 370
Pelvic
  appendicitis 536f, 545
  bones 614
  disorders 357
  ring disruption 228
Pelvi-rectal abscess 629
Pelvis 228, 228f, 233f, 344f, 649
  fracture of 228
  injury to 331
  movement of 278f
Pelviureteric junction 655, 660
Pelviureteric obstruction 655
Pemberton's sign 447
Pen test 148, 148f
Pencil-shaped bird-beak 509
Penile opening, proximal 720f
Penis 718
  body of 720
  carcinoma of 129f, 718f, 724, 724f, 725f
  elephantiasis of 723
  position of 676

Pentagastrin test 572
Peptic perforation 527, 549
Peptic ulcer 528f, 536-538, 559, 603
   disease 509
   pain, perforation of 529f
   perforation of 531
   subacute perforation of 604, 605
   symptoms of 639
   type 586
   vomiting, perforation of 530
Percussion 9, 29, 41, 119, 341, 447, 464, 472, 537
Perianal warts 630
Periductal mastitis 479
Perilunate dislocation 225, 227
Perineal fistulae 633
Perineal membrane 645, 714
Perineum, examination of 643
Periosteal fibroma 182
Periostitis 120
Peripheral nerve 142
   diseases 143
   lesion 163
      causes of 155
      examination of 40, 142
      paralysis 153
   types of injury of 153
Peripheral vascular disease 94, 113
   examination of 92
Peristalsis 31, 592, 597, 675
Peristaltic movements 533
Peristaltic sound 538f
   absence of 538
Peritoneal aspiration 521
Peritoneal fluid, diagnostic aspiration of 519
Peritoneal lavage 520
Peritoneocentesis 519
Peritoneum 685f
   lesser sac of 605f
   parietal 545
Peritonism 549
Peritonitis 388, 538f
   abdomen 538f
   perforation of 555
   pneumococcal 527
   stage of diffuse 550
Peritonsillar abscess 507
Perkin's lines 281, 281f
Permanent tooth, unerupted 394
Peroneal nerve 150, 162
Peroneal tendon sheath 296
Perthes' disease 7, 273, 281f, 282, 282f, 284, 286, 381
Perthes' test 118, 118f, 124
Pes cavus 376, 377
Pes planus 376, 377
Petit's triangle 339, 341f, 353

Peutz-Jegher's syndrome 404
Peyronie's disease 723
Phalanges 224
   dislocations of 227
   fractures of 227
Phalanx, proximal 148f
Phalen's sign 272
Pharyngeal pouch 435, 506, 508, 510
   barium meal X-ray of 506f
Pharyngo-esophageal diverticulum 510
Pharynx 507
   examination of 505
Phenol-sulfonphthalein 645
Pheochromocytoma 457, 459
Phimosis 670, 718, 719, 721
Phlebitis 120
   superficial 93
Phlebography 123
   ascending functional 123f
Phlebothrombosis 121
Phlegmasia
   alba dolens 121, 122
   cerulea dolens 121, 122
Pigeon chest 470
Pigmented naevus 59
Piles 627
   external 619
   internal 620
      prolapsed 622f
      uncomplicated 623
   primary 622f, 625
Pilonidal sinus 87, 594, 619, 620, 629, 633
Pin-hole meatus 670, 718, 719
Pins sensation 16
Pipestem stool 24
Pituitary adenoma 321, 324
Pizzillo's method 442, 442f
Pizzillo's technique 442f
Plantar fasciitis 164, 167
Plantar flexion 375
Plantar reflex 319
Plantar wart 378
Plasma
   cell mastitis 497
   fibrinogen 540
Plasmacytoma 182, 193
Platysma 429f
Pleomorphic adenoma 415, 422
Plethysmography 103
Pleural cavity 549
Pleural empyema 472f
Pleurisy 469
   diaphragmatic 534
Plexiform hemangioma 50
Plexiform neurofibromatosis 56, 56f, 57f

Plummer-Vinson syndrome 21, 504, 508
Plunging ranula 404f, 413, 428, 428f
Pneumonia 509
Pneumothorax 464, 466, 469, 470
   closed 466
   open 466
   traumatic 466
Pointing index 144, 147, 160
Pointing sign 517
Pointing test 522, 533
Policeman receiving tip 144
Policeman taking tip 153
Poliomyelitis 7, 286
Polycystic kidney 640, 654, 655f
Polycythemia 659
Polydactylism 369, 369f
Polymazia 495
Polyostotic fibrous dysplasia 186
Polyp 507, 593
   congenital 608
Polyposis coli 593
   familial 593
   multiple 593f
Polypus 620, 623
Polythene catheter 101
Pons asinorum 624
Popliteal fossa 290f, 294
   examination of 290f
   palpation of 289
Popliteal nerve
   lateral 150, 151f, 175f, 239
   medial 162
Popliteal pulse 99f
Porphyria 607
Port-wine stain 49, 50f
Positive telescopic test 279
Postauricular dermoid 30f
Posthitis 719
Postvagotomy 507
Pott's disease 331, 341f, 347f, 353, 436, 506, 540f, 571
   abscess 339
   examine spine for 539
Pott's paraplegia 354
Pott's puffy tumor 385
Pratt's test 118
Pregnancy 116, 546
Prepatellar bursitis 293
Pressure effect 111, 127, 173, 175
   examination for 42
Pressure symptoms 128
Priapism 725
   incontinence of 329
Primitive node 627
Proctalgia fugax 631
Proctoscopy 625, 625f

Profuse salivation 412
Prolapse 618
    history of 620
Prostate 643, 670
    benign hypertrophy of 665
    biopsy of 667
    carcinoma of 493f, 666, 667f
    diseases of 665
    examination of 643
    specific antigen 667
        estimation of 667
Prostatic calculi 646
Prostatic diseases 635
Prostatic massage 643, 708, 710
Prostatitis
    acute 666
    chronic 666
Protein
    content 321
    urea 645
Proteus 710
Protrusion 441
Proximal volar spaces, infection of 365
Pruritus 633
    ani 618, 633
Pseudocoxalgia 284
Pseudogout 255, 259
Pseudolipoma 55
Pseudoptosis 446
Pseudovomiting 510
Psoas bursa, enlarged 688, 695
Psoas test 545
Psychiatric diseases 7
Ptosis 476
Pubic bones 662f
Pubic tubercle 676f, 687f
Puboprostatic ligaments 524f
Pulled elbow 222
Pulmonary embolism 469, 476, 477
    diagnosis of 476
Pulp space 364f
    infection 364, 364f
Pulsatile 565
    mass 110
    swelling 111, 112, 295
Pulsation 31
Pulse 8, 304, 316, 531
    rate 441
Pump-handle test 346, 346f
Punch biopsy 45
Purpura 457
Purulent stools 24
Pus
    bacteriological examination of 181
    cells 666
    discharge of 617

Pustules 8
Pyelocele 710
Pyelogram, intravenous 648f
Pyelography
    excretory 657
    intravenous 707
Pyelonephritis
    acute 635, 657
    chronic 639
Pyemic abscess 52
Pylephlebitis, suppurative 602
Pyloric stenosis 585
    congenital 605
Pyogenic arthritis, acute 252f, 292
Pyorrhea alveolaris, sign of 403
Pyosalpinx 613
Pyrexia of unknown origin 659
Pyuria 649

Q

Quadriceps femoris 40f
Querat erythroplasia 723
Quinine, intramuscular injection of 145f

R

Rachitic chest 471
Radial arteries 99
Radial bursa 366f-368f
    infection of 366
Radial epiphysis 233f
Radial groove 158
Radial head, dense epiphysis of 268f
Radial nerve 142, 147, 147f, 157, 158, 362
    injury, recovery of 154
    paralysis 147f, 362
Radial styloid process 224f
Radiation 17, 336
    necrosis 626
Radioactive
    chromium 607
    fibrinogen test 76, 122
    isotopes 583
    scanning 180
Radioiodine therapy 449f
Radio-isotope
    renogram 652, 657
    scanning 477, 543, 583
Radio-opaque
    dye 348f
    gallstone 576f
Radius
    fracture neck of 219, 221
    lower third of 223
    palpate head of 216f
    upper end of 216

Ram's horn
    nail 380
    penis 703, 723
Ranula 407f, 413
    deep 428f
    typical 404f
Rat-tail deformity 511f
Raynaud's disease 92, 103, 105, 361
Raynaud's phenomenon 93
Rectal disorders 634
Rectal examination 232, 320, 346, 492, 524f, 538, 552, 571, 618, 619, 628, 643, 665, 668, 707
Rectal mucosa, mobility of 643
Rectal prolapse 630
Rectum
    ballooning of 622
    carcinoma of 617, 620f, 631
    colloid carcinoma of 617
    complete prolapse of 621f
    procidentia of 621f
    stricture of 623, 632
Rectus
    abdominis muscle, rupture of 557
    divarication of 690
    sheath 609
Recurrent laryngeal nerve 445
Red eczema, chronic 719
Red-currant jelly 538, 605
Reflex 152, 317, 329
    abdominal 320
    testing 376
Reflux esophagitis 504, 505, 506
Reiter's disease 252
Renal angiogram, intravenous 650
Renal angiography 650, 651, 651f
Renal artery 651f
Renal calculus 656
Renal cell carcinoma 635, 658, 659f
Renal colic 542, 636
Renal failure 639
Renal function test 645, 650
Renal hilum 652
Renal pelvis, papillary tumors of 661
Renal stone 576f, 646, 656
Renal tubule ricket 187
Respiration 9, 304, 463, 532
    irregular 311
    movement with 31, 597
    nature of 329
Respiratory movement 471, 517, 533
Retention, chronic 668, 669
Reticulocyte count 607
Reticulum cell sarcoma 135, 182
Retrocecal appendicitis 535f, 545
Retrograde cystograms 649

Retrograde percutaneous
      catheterization 101
Retrograde permeation 490f
Retroperitoneal conditions 544
Retroperitoneal connective tissue
      610
Retroperitoneal ruptures 522
Retroperitoneal tissue 606
Retrosternal prolongation 444f
Rheumatism, nonarticular 164
Rheumatoid arthritis 246, 253, 264,
      356, 371, 457
   juvenile 136
Rhomboid glossitis, median 411
Ribs
   chest for fracture of 305
   fracture of 23, 465
   palpation of 463
   tumors 473
Richter's hernia 673, 685
   incidence of 690
Rickets 180, 182, 187
   infantile 187
   renal 187
   types of 187
Riedel's lobe, congenital 601
Riedel's thyroiditis 454, 458
Ring occlusion test 680
Rising test 599f
Risser's sign 350
Risus sardonicus 7
Robertson pupil 540
Romberg's sign 249
Root transection 333
Round worms, impaction of 612
Rovsing's sign 534, 535, 535f, 545,
      591
Rupture ectopic gestation 527, 533,
      537, 539, 555
Ryle's tube 541

S

Sacral sympathetic supply 529
Sacrococcygeal teratoma 26f, 31f,
      624, 627
   congenital 339
Sacroiliac arthritis 358
Sacroiliac joint 345
   tuberculosis of 358
Sacroiliac lesion 344f
Sacroiliac strain 358
Sacrospinalis muscle 656, 657
Sacrum, injuries to 228
Saegesser's splenic point 521
Salicylates 670

Salivary gland 419f, 425
   disorders 426
   examination of 415
   sublingual 424
   tumors of minor 424
Salmon patch 49
Salpingitis, acute 529f, 548
Saphena varix 687, 695
Saphenofemoral valve 117
Saphenous nerve 152f
Sarcoidosis 137
Sarcoma 32f, 62, 502
   retroperitoneal 606, 610, 612
Sarcomatous epulis 393
Sartorius, tendons of 293
Saturday night palsy 153
Scabbard' trachea 446
Scalene node biopsy 473
Scalenus anticus syndrome 92, 106,
      361
Scalp
   cock's peculiar tumor of 63f
   hematoma of 385
   injury to 306
Scaphoid bone 204f
Scaphoid fracture 204f, 225, 226
Scapula 263f
   fracture 211, 213
   neck of 208
   neck of 208f
   palpation of 209
   winging of 143, 144f, 157f
Scar 68f, 145
Schatzki's ring 504, 510
Scheuermann's disease 347, 351
Schistosoma haematobium 608
Schoemaker's line 231
Schwann cells, sprouts of 154
Schwannoma 55, 57
Schwartz test 118, 119, 124
Sciatic nerve 150, 161
Sciatica 355
   bilateral 617
   mimicking 336
Sciatic-scoliosis 350
Scintillation-encephalography 322
Scleroderma 509
   diagnosis of 507
Sclerosis 200
   presence of 204
Scoliosis 338, 338f, 350
   compensatory 350
   paralytic 350
   postural 350
Scott-Harden tube 575
Scrotum 539, 540f, 597, 694f, 699f,
      701

anterior aspect of 702
carcinoma of 717
   skin of 701
edema of 703
elephantiasis of 703, 713
examination of 598f
Fournier's gangrene of 717f
idiopathic gangrene of 717
posterior aspect of 702
sebaceous cysts of 717
Scurvy 182
Seat-belt injury 327, 516
Sebaceous cysts, multiple 702
Sebaceous horn 64f
   over knee 64f
Seizures 300, 301, 315
Seldinger technique 101, 584
Semilunar cartilage 234f
   cyst of 234f
   injury to 240
Semimembranosus bursa 289f, 295f
   typical positions of 294f
Seminal vesicles 643
Seminiferous tubules 712
Seminoma 715
Senile
   gangrene 104
   keratosis 66
   kyphosis 351
   osteoporosis 347, 357
Senile wart 66
Sensation 329, 362
   loss of 143, 154
   testing 376
Sensory function 317
Sensory loss 151f, 154
Sentinel pile 619
Septic arthritis 259
Serratus anterior 40, 146
Serum
   acid 653
   amylase estimation 540
   bilirubin 540
   deoxyribo-nuclease 540
   glutamic oxaloacetic
      transaminase 477
   protein bound iodine 451
   thyroid stimulating hormone 451
Shenton's line 281, 281f
Sherren's triangle 533, 535f
Shifting dullness 537, 567, 600
   test 518
Shock 333, 462, 523
   evidence of 198
   severe 523
   signs of 517
Short saphenous system 118
Shoulder 207

bony arch of 208
contour of 208
dislocation of 109, 208, 208f
    anterior 213f
girdle 259
recurrent dislocation of 213
roundness of 208f
X-ray of 213f
Shoulder joint 211, 259, 261, 261f, 263f
  arthritis of 264
  diseases of 259
  dislocation of 208f, 211, 213
  movement of 210, 262f
  palpation of 261f
Shoveller's fracture 332
Sialectasis, congenital 420
Sialography 418
Sideropenic dysphagia 504
Sigmoid colon 615
  volvulus of 554
Sigmoidoscopy 591, 592, 625, 628
Sign-de-dance 537
Single nerve involvement, causes of 155
Sinus 85, 86, 89, 91, 172, 174, 269, 429, 471, 472, 633
  causes of 85, 86
  classification of 89
  examination of 85, 87
  formation 173, 470
  opening of 88
  preauricular 87, 89, 384
  wall of 88
Sjogren's syndrome 424
Skiagraphy 281, 284, 321, 473, 590
Skin 257, 429, 442, 463, 473, 533, 564, 702, 704
  abdominal 517
  changes 115, 375
  color of 7
  diseases 19, 633
  eruption 8
  fixity to 487
    overlying 37
  infiltration of 429f
  involvement of 431
  lymphatic drainage of 131f
  moist 449
  neuromas of 457
  pale 517
  palpation of 629
  redness of 86
  surrounding 73
  swelling arising from 295
  temperature 96
  test 43, 75
  thickening of 703

Skin over
  abdomen 517
  breast 482
  joint 248
  parotid gland 417
  swelling 32, 676, 694
    condition of 597
Skull
  erosion of 42f
  injury to
    base of 307, 308
    vault of 307, 308
  metastasis 495f
  X-ray of 312
Sleeping pulse rate 441
Sleepless nights 438
Slip sign 34f, 54
Slow pulse rate 315
Small artery occlusion 104
Small intestine 522, 609
  rupture of 522
  tumors of 609
Smith's fracture 225, 226
Smooth muscle 448
Snail track ulcer 409
Sodium diatrizoate 101
Soft chancre 70, 80
Soft cystic swelling 627
Soft palate 562
Soft sores 719, 722
Soft tissue shadow, abnormal 250
Solar keratosis 66
Solid lesions 494
Solitary bone cyst 395
Solitary renal cyst 655
Sore 80
Spastic paralysis 286
Spermatic cord 539, 540f, 677, 681, 695, 706, 716
  inflammation of 692
  torsion of 712f
Spermatocele 711f, 717
Spherocytosis, hereditary 606
Sphincter 620f
  proctoscopy 628
Spider leg deformity 655f, 659, 660f
Spider nevus 49, 50f
Spina bifida 335, 339, 356, 376f
  occulta 335, 339f, 349
Spinal abnormalities 336, 359
  examination of 335
Spinal column
  examination of 330
  pathologies of 340f
  tumors of 356
Spinal cord
  diseases of 544, 669

injuries, examination of 327, 328
  tumor of 45f
Spinal dura, irritation of 345f
Spinal injury 327, 334
  type of 327
Spinal nerve 151f
  root 355f
Spinal screening 376
Spine 338f, 340f, 506, 540f, 571
  acute osteomyelitis of 354
  deformities of 350
  diseases of 544, 669
  dislocation of 332
  extension of 343f
  fractures of 331, 332f
  lateral flexion of 343f
  movements of dorsal and lumbar 342
  rigidity of 342
  rotation of 338f, 344f
  tuberculosis of 353
Spinoumbilical line 567
Spinous process 338f, 340f
Spirochaeta pallida 722
Spleen 520, 568, 599, 600, 606
  causes of enlargement of 606
  cysts of 582
  method of palpation of 569
Splenic enlargement 600f
Splenic pain 529f
Splenic rupture 264
Spondylolisthesis 338, 339f, 352, 352f, 356
  congenital 348f
  moderate 352f
  skiagram of 348f
Spondylosis 357
  lumbar 355
Spongioblastoma 323
  polare 314
Sprain 201
Springing fibula 236, 236f, 242
Springing radius 216f, 223
Sputum 463
Squamous cell 80
  carcinoma 61, 72, 79, 81, 379, 379f, 422
  cauliflower surface of 31f
Squamous metaplasia 627
Staghorn calculus 639, 657f
Staphylococcus 707, 710
Steatorrhea 24
Stellwag's sign 448
Stereognostic sense, absence of 319
Sternoclavicular dislocation 211, 212
Sternomastoid muscle 40, 429f, 430, 430f

Sternum, palpation of 464
Stewart's sign 541
Stiffness 271, 286
Stilbestrol, ingestion of 493f
Still's disease 136
Stomach 563, 568, 600, 605
  anterior displacement of 575f
  carcinoma of 559, 568, 570f, 574, 574f, 580, 586, 605
  lesser curvature of 573f
  part of 586
  pyloric region of 574f
  pylorus of 604
Stomatitis 407
  angular 409
  aphthous 408
  catarrhal 408
  gangrenous 409
  ulcerative 409
  varieties of 408
Stone 588, 646, 663, 670
Stool
  abnormal 24
  blood in 24
  examination of 573
  types of 24
Stove-in-chest 465
Straight-leg raising test, passive 344f, 346
Strawberry
  angioma 50
  hemangioma 49f
  nevus 50f
  tongue 21
Streptococcal peritonitis 527
Streptococcus 707, 710
Stress
  fracture 381
  incontinence 639
Stricture 511
Stridor 439
Student's elbow 268
Styloid processes, relative position of 224
Subacromial bursitis 265
Subaponeurotic space, infection of 367
Subareolar plexus 490f
Subclavian artery 99
Subclavian steal syndrome 107
Subcoracoid dislocation 208
Subcutaneous emphysema, crepitus of 23
Subcutaneous infusion urography 648
Subcutaneous tissue 38, 257, 295, 472f, 473, 564, 702

Subcutaneous veins, dilated 173f
Subdeltoid bursitis 265
Subdiaphragmatic organs, injury to 467
Subhyoid bursal cyst 431
Sublingual dermoid 404, 413
Submandibular duct 157
  inspection of orifices of 419
Submandibular gland 418f
  carcinoma of 424
Submandibular lymph nodes 392, 405f
  palpation of 405f
Submandibular salivary
  duct 424, 424f
  gland 157, 418, 420, 423, 424, 424f, 428, 429f
    bimanual palpation of 420f
    swelling of 419f
    tumors of 424
Submandibular triangle 404f, 428f, 430f
Submucosa 618
Subperitoneal lymph plexus 490f
Subungual exostosis 379, 380
Succussion splash 568
Sudeck's osteodystrophy 205, 226
Sulfonamides 670
Sunray appearance, typical 179f
Superficial fascial space, infection of 380
Superficial inguinal
  pouch 694f
  ring 676f, 678f, 679f
Superficial vein
  abnormal 20
  rombosis 122
Superior vena cava superior 20
Supraclavicular fossa 485
Supraclavicular group 491f, 492
Supraclavicular lymph node, left 570, 570f, 597
Supraclavicular nerves 529
Supraclavicular nodes 432
Supracondylar fracture 142, 215f, 216f, 219, 220
  complications of 220
Suprahyoid position 459f
Supraspinatus tendinitis 164, 166
  chronic 264
Supraspinatus tendon 264f
  degeneration of 265
  rupture of 164, 167, 209, 265
Supratrochlear lymph node, examination of 267
Sural nerve 152f
Surpasses oral cholecystography 578
Swan-neck deformity 253, 371

Sweating 441
  excessive 439
Swelling 26, 33f, 34f, 41f, 67, 115, 116, 128, 165, 166, 172, 173, 197, 207, 215, 229, 237, 247, 248, 261, 266, 267, 269, 270, 276, 287, 288, 339, 340, 378, 403f, 416, 428, 430f, 438, 463, 464, 471, 472f, 485f, 518, 533, 565, 599f, 637, 677, 677f, 703, 704
  abdominal 654
  abnormal 196, 234
  acute 433
    inflammatory 46
  beneath artery 111
  cases of 29
  causes of 601, 604, 606, 608, 610, 613, 615
  chronic 433
    inflammatory 46
  congenital 46, 49
  cystic 34f, 271, 295
  diagnosis of 46
  different locations of 682
  differential diagnosis of 432, 601, 604, 606, 608, 610, 613, 615
  edge of 30
  examination of 26, 29, 692
  fast-growing 439
  femoral 695, 699
  fluctuates 34
  inflammatory 46, 427
  inguinoscrotal 688f, 693, 695, 696, 700
  intra-abdominal 599, 601, 605, 606, 608-610, 614, 615
  lies 676f
  location of 682
  malignant 42
  meal-related 415
  middle of 704f
  mucoperiosteal 393
  nature of 673
  neck 437
  neoplastic 47
  over arteries 111
  parietal 601, 604, 606, 608, 610, 614, 615
  progress of 28
  pulsatile 599
  quickly-grown 427
  recurrence of 28
  reducible 679
  relation of 430f
  renal 599f, 641f
  scrotal 677f, 710
  solid 295

splenic 599f, 641f
spontaneous development of 171
temperature of 32
traumatic 46
Swollen ankle 296
Swollen thenar eminence 368f
Symphysis pubis 597f, 662f, 678
Syndactylism 369, 369f
Synovial membrane of joints 371
Synovial sarcoma 62, 192
Synovitis 590
   chronic 286
   transient 286
Syphilis 69, 130, 628, 706
   mucous patch of 409
Syphilitic stigmas 131, 707
   common sites of 75f
Syphilitic synovitis, bilateral serous 288f
Syringomyelocele 350

T

Tabes dorsalis, exclude 539
Tachycardia 448f, 449, 517
Tactile sensitivity 150, 151
Tailor's bursa 296
Takayasu's arteritis 108
Talipes 376
   calcaneovalgus 376, 377
   calcaneus 376
   equinovarus 376, 376f, 377
   equinus 376
   valgus 376
   varus 376
Talocrural joint 375
Tamponade, cardiac 467
Tanyol's sign 564
Tardy ulnar palsy 142
Tear, types of 240f
Telescopic test 279, 279f, 284
Temporal artery, superficial 99
Temporal lobe tumors 325
Temporomandibular joint 392
   dislocation of 393
   disorders 399
   examination of 390
Tender spot 566
Tenderness 32, 72, 88, 166, 173, 197, 230, 248, 260, 276, 339, 340f, 518, 533
   absence of 568
   exact point of 235
   generalized 518
   method of 340f
   over hypogastrium 529f
   points of 234f

Tendinitis 203
   acute supraspinatus 264, 264f
Tendinopathy 164
Tendon 41, 257
   complications 203
   diseases of 164
   disorders 170
      classification of 164
   late rupture of 203
   ruptures 164
   sheath
      anatomical disposition of 366f
      infections 363
Tenesmus 618
Tennis elbow 164, 167, 268
Tenosynovitis 164
   chronic stenosing 296
   crepitus of 23
   stenosing 168
   stenosing 271, 271f
   suppurative 365
Tension pneumothorax 466
Teratoma 715
   retroperitoneal 606
Teratomatous dermoid 49
Terminal phalanx 364f
   epiphyseal line of 364f
   osteomyelitis of 365
Terry's nail 21
Testicular growth 598f
Testicular malignancy extension 696
Testicular sensation 697, 706
Testis 529f, 540f, 613, 681f, 705, 706, 712
   anteverted 712
   cyst of appendage of 717
   ectopic 694f, 695-698, 699f
   examine 681, 695
   gumma of 702, 711f
   hernia 702, 704, 711f
   inversion of 714
   malignant
      extension of 697
      growth of 701, 706f
   position of 705
   retractile 698, 699f
   torsion of 540f, 696, 698, 701, 708, 714
   tumor of 715, 711f
   undescended 610, 613, 695, 697, 697f, 714
Tetanus 7
Thenar space 366f, 367f
   infection 367, 368f
Thermography 494
Thickened synovial membrane 288
Thomas' test 274f

Thoracic aorta
   dissecting aneurysm of 110f
   rupture of 467
Thoracic cage 464f
Thoracic compression 539
Thoracic conditions 543
Thoracic disease 534, 537
Thoracic duct, rupture of 467
Thoracic injury 331
Thoracic kyphoscoliosis 471
Thoracic kyphosis 188
Thoracic outlet syndrome 105, 361, 362
Thoracic tuberculosis 336
Thoracic wall
   cystic swellings of 474
   solid swellings of 473
Thoracotomy, exploratory 473
Thorax 10, 484
Throbbing pain 15, 415, 529
Thromboangiitis obliterans 104
Thrombocytopenic purpura, diagnosis of 607
Thrombophlebitis 122
   migrans 589
Thrombosis 111
Thumb
   numbness in 362
   terminal phalanx of 148f
Thyroglossal cyst 429f, 431, 443, 443f, 454, 458, 458f
   inflamed 440
   typical position of 443f
Thyroglossal fistula 443, 459, 459f
Thyroid 447f, 458, 459
   auscultation of 447f
   bruit 449
   carcinomas 438
   cartilage 458
   disease, family history of 441
   disorders 438, 440
   enlargement 446f
   function tests 450
   gland 427, 442, 444, 445, 445f, 446f, 450, 455
      examination of 438
      palpation of 444f
   lower margin of 444f
   malignancies 453
   malignant 446f
   nodule, single non-functioning 452
   papillary carcinoma of 447
   pulse 446f
   scan 452
   solitary nodule of 443f

Index

swelling 442, 444*f*, 448*f*, 461
    differential diagnosis of 453
    examination of 442
    moves 442
  tissue 444*f*
Thyroiditis 454
  acute suppurative 457
  autoimmune 457
  chronic 457
  granulomatous 458
  struma 458
Thyrotoxicosis 438, 449*f*, 453
  primary 439, 444, 450*f*
  secondary 439, 449, 450*f*
Thyroxin, serum 451
Tibia, lateral condyle of 178*f*
Tibial artery, posterior 98, 98*f*
Tibial collateral ligament 236*f*
Tibial nerve 150
  posterior 152*f*
Tibial pulse, posterior 98*f*
Tibial spine, fracture of 241
Tinel's and Phalen's test 362
Toe
  bilateral gangrene of 97*f*
  deformities of 375, 376
Tongue 20, 21, 130*f*, 130*f*, 405, 458, 532
  carcinoma of 403*f*, 406*f*, 412, 412*f*
  color of 20
  congenital fissuring of 411
  examination of 400
    papillae of 20
  lymph drainage of 407*f*
  massive 402
  mobility of 402
  muscles of 146
  pale 21
  palpation of 406*f*
  protruded 20, 455*f*
  protrusion of 32, 143*f*
  syphilis in 411
  syphilitic furrowing of 411
  tremor of 20
  ulcer of 411
  volume of 402
Tongue-tie 410
Tonsillar node 432
Tonsils 432*f*
Toothpaste stool 24
Torn tendon 203
Torsion 555
Torticollis 436, 436*f*
Totipotent cells 26*f*
Tourniquet test 117, 124, 607
Toxic goiter 449*f*, 450*f*, 453, 455, 455*f*
  cardinal signs of primary 448*f*
  primary 438, 449*f*, 450*f*, 455, 455*f*

Toxic manifestation 447
Toxic megacolon 542
Toxic multinodular goiter 453
Toxoplasmosis 135
Trachea, position of 471
Traction diverticula 508
Traction osteochondritis 255
Traction test 696
Transcoelomic implantation 490*f*
Transformation, malignant 48, 422
Transillumination test 289, 431, 487
Transitional cell tumors 661
Translucency test 289*f*, 705*f*
Transmitted movements, absence of 197
Transpyloric plane 706
Transrectal biopsy 667
Transrectal ultrasound scanning 667
Transverse colon 605, 609
Trapezius 39*f*, 146
  actions of 40
  muscle 55*f*, 146*f*
Trauma
  abdominal 331
  arterial 109
  blunt 516
  urethral 517
Tremor 448*f*, 449
Trendelenburg's gait 7, 272
Trendelenburg's sign 284
Trendelenburg's test 117*f*, 124, 273*f*
Treponema pallidum 79
Triceps 39*f*
  jerk 320
Trigeminal nerve 391
  ophthalmic division of 56*f*
Trigger finger 164, 361, 370
Triglycerides 103
Tri-iodothyronine, serum 451
Trismus 393
Trochlear nerve 317
  paralysis 317
Troisier's sign 432, 570, 570*f*, 598
Trophic ulcer 71*f*, 78, 83, 378*f*
  presence of 329
Trousseau's sign 460, 589
T-tube cholangiography 579*f*
Tubercle bacilli 590
Tuberculin test 43
Tuberculoma 324
Tuberculosis 69, 128, 128*f*, 131, 271, 286, 356, 379, 433*f*, 628, 706
  abdominal 590
  cavernous 647*f*
  cervical 336
  cutaneous 71*f*
  first stage of 276*f*

  hyperplastic 590
  hypertrophic 604
  intestinal 590
  lumbar 336
  renal 658
  second stage of 276*f*
  ulcerative 590
Tuberculous sinus 86*f*, 87, 90, 429
Tuberculous ulcer 70, 70*f*, 73, 78, 412, 702, 704
  closer view of 70*f*
Tuber-joint angle 244*f*
Tubo-ovarian mass 613, 614
Tumor 26, 38*f*, 111, 182, 190, 379, 386, 424, 456, 608
  benign 26, 47, 182, 386, 456, 499
  desmoid 54, 609
  extracerebral 323
  frontal lobe 324
  histopathological examination of 181
  intracerebral 323
  malignant 386, 387, 456, 500
  metastatic 324, 422
  mixed 424
  mucoepidermoid 423
  odontogenic 393
  osseous 393
  ovarian 614
  parathyroid 457
  parietal lobe 325
  parotid 421, 421*f*
  raspberry 594
  root 266
  smooth outline of 494*f*
  sternomastoid 427, 428, 435, 436
  subcutaneous 294
  suprarenal 604
  testicular 708
  types of 474, 476
  universal 54
Tunica vaginalis 683
  hydrocele of 704*f*
Turban tumor 387
Two enema' test 542
Typhoid 184
  arthritis 252
  osteomyelitis 181
  ulcer 537
    perforation of 550
Typical multiple mixed stones 577*f*
Tyson's glands, infection of 722

U

Ulcer 68, 73*f*, 82, 84, 115, 120, 174, 379, 379*f*, 386, 429, 482, 484, 625, 718

acutely inflamed 73
aphthous 411
arterial 77, 82
base of 717
carcinomatous 70, 412, 702, 704
chronic 68f, 72f, 76
   nonspecific 412
classification of 76
clinical features of 76
crater 574
dental 411
diabetic 78
diagnosis of 623
differential diagnosis of 77
duodenal 566, 573, 584
dyspeptic 411
edge of 72f
   types of 71
epitheliomatous 68f
erythrocyanoid 82
examination of 68, 74, 642
gastric 559, 566, 573, 573f, 574
gradual-onset 69
gummatous 73, 79, 80f, 82, 429, 702, 704
healing 76
hypertensive 82
infective 82
ischemic 77
malignant 73, 77
meatal 668, 719, 722
nonspecific 76
painful 69
pathological features of 76
peptic 528f, 536-538, 559, 603
postpertussis 412
rodent 60, 60f, 70, 70f, 73, 386
specific 77
spreading 71, 76
sudden-onset 69
syphilitic 79, 412
traumatic 77
tuberculous 70, 70f, 73, 78, 412, 702, 704
types of 77
   edge of 72
varicose 70
venous 70f, 78, 81
with various diseases 83
Ulcerative colitis 550, 592, 618, 628, 629
   acute 542, 548
      severe 626
   perforation of 550
   pseudopolyposis of 593
Ulna
   lower end of 179f
   upper part of 217

Ulnar bursa 271, 366f, 367f
   infection of 366, 366f
Ulnar drift 253, 371
Ulnar nerve 144f, 148, 150f, 158, 160, 161, 362
   lesion 226
   palsy 361, 362
Ulnar styloid process 224f
Ultrasonography 43, 306, 424f, 580f, 582f, 589f, 697f, 710f
Umbilical region 589, 682
Umbilicus 604
   absence of 661f
   diseases of 594
Unconsciousness
   depth of 302
   duration of 299
   onset of 299
Upper brachial plexus lesion 156
Upper deep cervical lymph nodes, secondary carcinoma of 130f
Upper eyelid 446
   drooping of 317
   hemangioma of 37f
   lid retraction of 448f
Upper femoral epiphysis, congenital dislocation of 281f
Upper jaw 390
   mucoperiosteum of 394f
   tumors of 395
Upper limbs 10, 94, 328
Upper lip, congenital short frenum of 384
Urachal cyst 614
Uremia, symptoms of 665
Ureter 649, 670
   diseases of 660
Ureteric calculus 660
Ureteric catheterization 650
Ureteric stone 646
Urethra 670
   discharge 639
      Gonococci in 250
   examination of 643
   fistula 633
   injury to 228
   meatus, internal 638f
   membranous part of 524f
   neoplasm 668
   part of 523
   short 663
   stricture 638, 668
      causes of 668
   treatment of rupture of 668
Urethritis
   gonococcal 722
   posterior 670

Urethrography 650
Urethroscopy 650
   posterior 650
Uric acid, serum 254
Urinary bladder 523, 613, 614
   bimanual palpation of 642f
Urinary cytology 661
Urinary diastase, estimation of 541
Urinary disorders 672
Urinary frequency 635
Urinary organs 601
Urinary retention 328, 635, 654
Urinary sediment, cytological examination of 644
Urinary tract, lesion of 670
Urinary vesical swelling 610
Urine 43, 153, 176, 200, 519, 541, 644, 707
   bacteriological examination of 657
   causes of retention of 669
   cytology of 664
   deep extravasation of 524f
   examination of 74, 101
   excessive discharge of 671
   extravasation of 701, 703, 713
   incontinence of 329
   mid-stream 644
   retention of 638, 665, 666, 668
   specific gravity of 644
Urogenital diaphragm 714
Urogram 660f
   excretory 647, 647f, 648
   retrograde 648, 648f, 655f, 659
Urography 654, 658, 659
   excretory 657, 664
   intravenous infusion 648
Uterine
   pathology 546
   swelling 610
Uterus 613, 614, 624
   fibroid of 613

V

Vaginal discharge 633
Vaginal examinations 346, 492, 571
Vague
   aching pain 15
   dyspepsia 589
Vagus nerve 318
Valsalva maneuver 123
Varicocele 659, 692, 695, 696, 708, 712f
Varicose veins 73, 115, 116, 119, 125
   causes of 120
   complications of 120
   examination of 114, 124
   presence of 72

Index

Vascular diseases 69
Vascular disorders 357
Vasospasm, investigation for 103
Vater
　ampulla 579, 589f, 601
　papilla 579
Vein 20
　calcification of 120
　engorged 482
　varicosities of 627
Venereal disease research laboratory 250
Venous thrombosis 121
　types of 121
Ventriculography 306, 321
Vermooten's sign 523
Verruca necrogenica 368
Vertebra
　collapsed fracture of 44f
　pathology of 340f
　tuberculosis of 356
Vertebral column 285, 330f
Vertebral process fracture 356
Vesical angiography 651
Vesical calculus 646, 662, 662f
Vesicle 8, 704f
Villous adenoma 632
Villous papilloma 593
Vin rose patch 49
Vincent's angina 409
Vincent's stomatitis 403
Violence, nature of 195
Virchow's nodes 432
Virus hepatitis 562
Viscera, injury to 203
Visceral angiography, selective 584
Visceroptosis 565

Vision
　changes 301
　deamness of 315
　dimness of 324
　double 439, 441
　problems 315
Vocal cords, edema of 440
Vocal fremitus 464
　feel for 471
Voiding cystourethrograms 650
Volar spaces, infection of middle 365
Volkmann's ischemic contracture 202, 204, 218, 361, 370, 370f
Voluntary muscular rigidity 518, 536
Volvulus neonatorum 554
Vomiting 18, 300, 315, 516, 530, 545, 551, 561, 674
　postprandial 511
　symptoms of 665
Vomitus 18, 504, 530
　types of 19
von Graefe's sign 448
von Recklinghausen's disease 28f, 55, 56f, 180, 182, 188

W

Waddling gait 7, 272
Wallerian degeneration 154
Wandering acetabulum 283
Warm water test 96
Warmth, application of 92
Warthin's tumor 422, 423
Warts 63
　seborrheic 66
　venereal 724
Watering-can perineum 87f, 702
Water-sipping' test 507

Weakness 297, 301
Web-space
　abscess 361
　infection 365
Weight loss 127, 128, 470, 480, 505, 563
Wet gangrene 103
Wharton's duct 419, 419f
Whitaker test 656
Wilms' tumor 635, 660f
Worms, bag of 696
Worsen spinal cord damage 330
Wound 145, 198
Wrist 161, 223, 269, 362
　dorsal aspect of 169f, 269f
　drop 143, 143f, 362
　extensors of 39f
　flexion 361
　　test 272
　flexors of 39f
　ganglion 164
　joint 363
　　extensor muscles of 147
　　flexion of 270f
　loss of 362
Wuchereria bancrofti 135

X

Xiphisternal joint 585
Xiphisternum 597f, 604
Xylenamine 664

Y

Yaws 83

Z

Zenker's diverticulum 508
Zieman's technique 678, 678f